# PETERSON'S NURSING PROGRAMS 2015

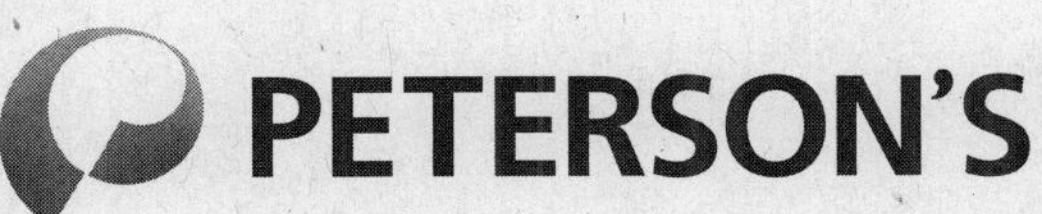

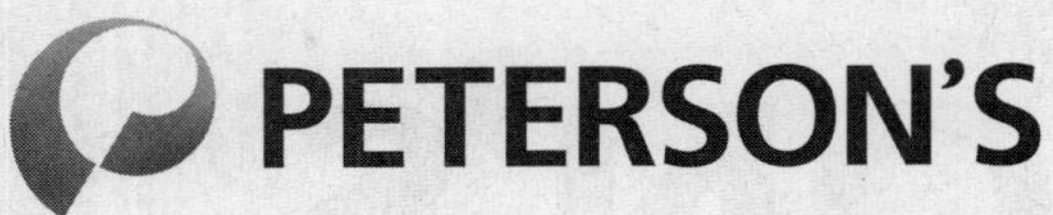



**About Peterson's**

Peterson's provides the accurate, dependable, high-quality education content and guidance you need to succeed. No matter where you are on your academic or professional path, you can rely on Peterson's print and digital publications for the most up-to-date education exploration data, expert test-prep tools, and top-notch career success resources—everything you need to achieve your goals.

For more information, contact Peterson's, 3 Columbia Circle, Suite 205, Albany, NY 12203-5158; 800-338-3282 Ext. 54229; or find us on the World Wide Web at www.petersonsbooks.com.



Peterson's makes every reasonable effort to obtain accurate, complete, and timely data from reliable source Nevertheless, Peterson's and the third-party data suppliers make no representation or warranty, either expressed or implied, as to the accuracy, timeliness, or completeness of the data or the results to be obtaine from using the data, including, but not limited to, its quality, performance, merchantability, or fitness for a particular purpose, non-infringement or otherwise.

NOTICE: Certain portions of or information contained in this book have been submitted and paid for by t educational institution identified, and such institutions take full responsibility for the accuracy, timeliness completeness and functionality of such contents. Such portions or information include (i) each display ad the "Profiles of Nursing Programs" section from pages 79 through 466 that comprises a one-half page of information covering a single educational institution, and (ii) each two-page in-depth description in the "-Page Descriptions" section from pages 468 through 493.



ISSN 1552-7743
ISBN: 978-0-7689-3864-7

Printed in the United States of America

10 9 8 7 6 5 4 3 2 1 16 15 14

Twentieth Edition

By producing this book on recycled paper (10% post-consumer waste) 51 trees were saved.

# CONTENTS

# FOREWORD

The American Association of Colleges of Nursing (AACN) is proud to collaborate on *Peterson's Nursing Programs 2015*.

According to the U.S. Bureau of Labor Statistics' (BLS) Employment Projections 2010–2020 released in February 2012, the registered nursing workforce is the top occupation in terms of job growth through 2020. It is expected that the number of employed nurses will grow from 2.74 million in 2010 to 3.45 million in 2020, an increase of 712,000 or 26 percent. The projections further explain the need for 495,500 replacements in the nursing workforce, bringing the total number of job openings for nurses due to growth and replacements to 1.2 million by 2020. In March 2012, the BLS reported that job growth in the health-care sector was outpacing the growth realized in 2011, accounting for 1 out of every 5 new jobs created in that year. Hospitals, long-term care facilities, and other ambulatory-care settings added 49,000 new jobs in February 2012, up from 43,300 new jobs created in January. As the largest segment of the health-care workforce, RNs likely will be recruited to fill many of these new positions.

As registered nurses find employment beyond hospitals in such areas as home care, community health, and long-term care, newly licensed RNs must have the proper education and training to work in these settings. It is vital that those seeking to enter or advance in a nursing career find the appropriate nursing program. This guide allows readers to find the program that best fits their needs, whether beginning a new career in nursing or attempting to advance one.

According to AACN's most recent annual institutional survey, enrollment in entry-level B.S.N. programs continues to climb. Gains were reported in all parts of the country in 2013, with an overall 2.6 percent increase in enrollments nationwide.

Although the health-care environment is complex and dynamic, there continues to be a significant demand for professional-level nurses. The primary route into professional-level nursing is the four-year baccalaureate degree. The professional nurse with a baccalaureate degree is the only basic nursing graduate prepared to practice in all health-care settings, including critical care, public health, primary care, and mental health. In addition, advanced practice nurses (APNs) deliver essential services as nurse practitioners, certified nurse-midwives, clinical nurse specialists, and nurse anesthetists. APNs typically are prepared in master's degree programs, and the demand for their services is expected to increase substantially.

Higher education in nursing expands the gateway to a variety of career opportunities in the health-care field. In addition to providing primary care to patients, graduates can work as case managers for the growing numbers of managed-care companies or can assume administrative or managerial roles in hospitals, clinics, insurance companies, and other diverse settings.

**The Nursing School Adviser** section of this guide is instructive and invaluable. Whether you are a high school student looking for a four-year program, an RN returning to school, or a professional in another field contemplating a career change, this section will address your concerns. This information presents various nursing perspectives to benefit students from diverse backgrounds.

Peterson's effort in making this guide well organized and convenient to read cannot be overstated. Peterson's has worked with AACN in producing a publication that is comprehensive and user-friendly. Like the previous editions, this edition is a genuine collaborative work, as AACN provided input from start to finish.

AACN's dedication and achievements in advancing the quality of baccalaureate and graduate nursing education are appreciated by Peterson's. We at AACN are fortunate to work with an organization that prides itself on being the leading publisher of education search and selection.

Furthermore, this publication would not be possible without the cooperation of the institutions included in this guide. We acknowledge the time and effort of those who undertook the task of completing and returning the surveys regarding their programs. We certainly appreciate their contribution.

*Peterson's Nursing Programs 2015* is the only comprehensive and concise guide to baccalaureate and graduate nursing education programs in the United States and Canada. We hope its contents will serve as the impetus for those looking for a rewarding and satisfying career in health care. AACN is proud to present this publication to the nursing profession and to those who seek to enter it.

—Eileen Breslin, Ph.D., RN, FAAN
President, AACN

—Geraldine D. Bednash, Ph.D., RN, FAAN
Chief Executive Officer and Executive Director, AACN

# A Note from the Peterson's Editors

For more than forty years, Peterson's has given students and parents the most comprehensive, up-to-date information on undergraduate and graduate institutions in the United States, Canada, and abroad.

*Peterson's Nursing Programs 2015* provides prospective nursing students with the most comprehensive information on baccalaureate and graduate nursing education in the United States and Canada. Our goal is to help students find the best nursing program for them.

To this end, Peterson's has joined forces with the American Association of Colleges of Nursing (AACN), the national voice for America's baccalaureate-and higher-degree nursing education programs. AACN's educational, research, governmental advocacy, data collection, publications, and other programs work to establish high-quality standards for bachelor's- and graduate-degree nursing education, assist deans and directors to implement those standards, influence the nursing profession to improve health care, and promote public support of baccalaureate and graduate education, research, and practice in nursing—the nation's largest health-care profession.

For those seeking to enter the nursing profession or to further their nursing careers, *Peterson's Nursing Programs 2015* includes information needed to make important nursing program decisions and to approach the admissions process with knowledge and confidence.

**The Nursing School Adviser** section contains useful articles to help guide nursing education choices, with information on nursing careers today, selecting a nursing program, financing nursing education, returning to school, and more. It also includes listings that provide valuable contact information for financial aid resources and specialty nursing organizations. And if you are one of the many people interested in accelerated nursing programs, there is an article that offers an in-depth look at this increasingly popular approach to nursing education. It is a must-read for those wishing to enter an accelerated baccalaureate or generic master's degree program.

At the end of **The Nursing School Adviser** is the "How to Use This Guide" article, which explains some of the key factors to consider when choosing a nursing program. In addition, it explains how the book is organized and shows you how to maximize your use of *Peterson's Nursing Programs 2015* to its full potential.

If you already have specifics in mind, such as a particular program or location, turn to the **Quick-Reference Chart.** Here you can search through "Nursing Programs At-a-Glance" for particular degree options offered by schools, listed alphabetically by state.

In the **Profiles of Nursing Programs** section you'll find expanded and updated nursing program descriptions, arranged alphabetically by state. Each profile provides all of the need-to-know information about accredited nursing programs in the United States and Canada. Display ads, which appear near some of the institutions' profiles, have been provided and paid for by those colleges or universities that wished to supplement their profile data with additional information about their institution.

If you are looking for additional information, you can turn to the **Two-Page Descriptions** section. Here you will find in-depth narrative descriptions, with photos, of those nursing programs that chose to pay for and provide additional information.

When you turn to the back of the book, you'll find eight **Indexes** listing institutions offering *baccalaureate, master's degree, concentrations within master's degree, doctoral, post-doctoral, online,* and *continuing education* programs. The last index lists every college and university contained in the guide along with its corresponding page reference.

Peterson's publishes a full line of resources to help guide you and your family through the admission process. Peterson's publications can be found at high school guidance offices, college and university libraries and career centers, your local bookstore or library, and at petersonsbooks.com. Peterson's guides are also available as eBooks.

We welcome any comments or suggestions you may have about this publication.

Publishing Department
Peterson's, a Nelnet company
3 Columbia Circle, Suite 205
Albany, NY 12203-5158

Your feedback will help us make your educational dreams possible. The editors at Peterson's wish you great success in your nursing program search.

# THE NURSING SCHOOL ADVISER

# NURSING FACT SHEET

Misconceptions about nursing have contributed to misinformation about the profession in the media. Here are the real facts:

- **Nursing is the nation's largest health-care profession, with more than 3.1 million registered nurses nationwide.** Of all licensed RNs, 2.6 million or 84.8 percent are employed in nursing.[1]
- **Registered Nurses compose one of the largest segments of the U.S. workforce as a whole and are among the highest paying large occupations.** Nearly 58 percent of RNs worked in general medical and surgical hospitals, where RN salaries averaged $66,700 per year. RNs composed the largest segment of professionals working in the health-care industry.[2]
- **Nurses compose the largest single component of hospital staff, are the primary providers of hospital patient care, and deliver most of the nation's long-term care.**
- **Most health-care services involve some form of care by nurses.** In 1980, 66 percent of all employed RNs worked in hospitals. By 2008, that number had declined slightly to 62.2 percent as more health care moved to sites beyond the hospital, and nurses increased their ranks in a wide range of other settings, including private practices, health maintenance organizations, public health agencies, primary care clinics, home health care, nursing homes, outpatient surgicenters, nursing-school-operated nursing centers, insurance and managed care companies, schools, mental health agencies, hospices, the military, industry, nursing education, and health-care research.[3]
- **Though often working collaboratively, nursing does not "assist" medicine or other fields.** Nursing operates independent of, not auxiliary to, medicine and other disciplines. Nurses' roles range from direct patient care and case management to establishing nursing practice standards, developing quality assurance procedures, and directing complex nursing care systems.
- **With more than four times as many RNs in the United States as physicians, nursing delivers an extended array of health-care services, including primary and preventive care by advanced nurse practitioners in such areas as pediatrics, family health, women's health, and gerontological care.** Nursing's scope also includes services by certified nurse-midwives and nurse anesthetists, as well as care in cardiac, oncology, neonatal, neurological, and obstetric/gynecological nursing and other advanced clinical specialties.
- **The primary pathway to professional nursing, as compared to technical-level practice, is the four-year Bachelor of Science in Nursing (B.S.N.) degree.** Registered nurses are prepared either through a B.S.N. program; a three-year associate degree in nursing; or a three-year hospital training program, receiving a hospital diploma. All take the same state licensing exam. (The number of diploma programs has declined steadily—to less than 10 percent of all basic RN education programs—as nursing education has shifted from hospital-operated instruction into the college and university system.)
- **To meet the more complex demands of today's health-care environment, the National Advisory Council on Nurse Education and Practice has recommended that at least two-thirds of the basic nurse workforce hold baccalaureate or higher degrees in nursing.**[4] Aware of the need, RNs are seeking the B.S.N. degree in increasing numbers. In 1980, almost 55 percent of employed registered nurses held a hospital diploma as their highest educational credential, 22 percent held the bachelor's degree, and 18 percent an associate degree. By 2008, a diploma was the highest educational credential for only 13.9 percent of RNs, while the number with bachelor's degrees as their highest education had climbed to 36.8 percent, with 36.1 percent holding an associate degree as their top academic preparation.[5] In 2010, 22,531 RNs with diplomas or associate degrees graduated from B.S.N. programs.[6]
- **In 2008, 13.2 percent of the nation's registered nurses held either a master's or doctoral degree as their highest educational preparation.**[7] The current demand for master's- and doctorally prepared nurses for advanced practice, clinical specialties, teaching, and research roles far outstrips the supply.
- **According to the U.S. Bureau of Labor Statistics, Registered Nursing is the top occupation in terms of the largest job growth from 2008–2018.**[8] Government analysts project that more than 581,500 new RN jobs will be created through 2018. Other projections indicate that by 2025, the U.S. nursing shortage will grow to more than 260,000 registered nurses.[9] Even as health care continues to shift beyond the hospital to more community-based primary care and other outpatient sites, federal projections say the rising complexity of acute care will see demand for RNs in hospitals climb by 36 percent by 2020.[10]

## REFERENCES


1. Health Resources and Services Administration. (September 2010). *The Registered Nurse Population: Findings From the 2008 National Sample Survey of Registered Nurses.* Washington, DC: U.S. Department of Health and Human Services.

2. U.S. Bureau of Labor Statistics, (2010, May). *Occupational Employment and Wages for 2009.* Access online at http://www.bls.gov/oes

3. See Note 1.

4. National Advisory Council on Nurse Education and Practice. (October 1996). *Report to the Secretary of the Department of Health and Human Services on the Basic Registered Nurse Workforce.* Washington, DC: U.S. Department of Health and Human Services, Division of Nursing.

5. See Note 1.

6. American Association of Colleges of Nursing (2011). *2010–2011 Enrollment and graduations in baccalaureate and graduate programs in nursing.* Washington, DC: Author.

7. See Note 1.

8. Lacey, T. A. and B. Wright. (2010). *Occupational Employment Projections to 2018.* Washington, DC: U.S. Department of Labor, Bureau of Labor Statistics.

9. Buerhaus, P. I., D. I. Auerbach, and D. O. Staiger. (2009, July–August). The recent surge in nurse employment: causes and implications. *Health Affairs,* 28(4), w657–w668.

10. See Note 4.

# Creating a More Highly Qualified Nursing Workforce

High-quality patient care hinges on having a well-educated nursing workforce. Research has shown that lower mortality rates, fewer medication errors, and positive outcomes are all linked to nurses prepared at the baccalaureate and graduate degree levels. The American Association of Colleges of Nursing (AACN) is committed to working collaboratively to create a more highly qualified nursing workforce since education enhances both clinical competency and care delivery.

## Snapshot of Today's Nursing Workforce

According to the National Center for Health Workforce Analysis within the Health Resources and Services Administration (HRSA), approximately 2.8 million registered nurses (RNs) are currently working in nursing (HRSA, 2013). This count reflects an increase from the last National Sample Survey of Registered Nurses conducted by HRSA in 2008 which found that 2.6 million RNs were employed in nursing (out of a population of more than 3 million licensed RNs).

HRSA's 2013 report, "The U.S. Nursing Workforce: Trends in Supply and Education," also found that 55 percent of the RN workforce held a baccalaureate or higher degree. In a separate study conducted by the National Council of State Boards of Nursing and The Forum of State Nursing Workforce Centers in 2013, the percentage of nurses in the United States with a baccalaureate or higher degree was 61 percent.

Graduates of entry-level nursing programs (baccalaureate degree, associate degree, and diploma) sit for the NCLEX-RN® licensing examination. The fact that new nurses pass the licensing exam at the same rate does not mean that all entry-level nurses are equally prepared for practice. The NCLEX tests for minimum technical competency for safe entry into basic nursing practice. Passing rates should be high across all programs preparing new nurses. This exam does not test for differences between graduates of different programs, measure performance over time, or test for all of the knowledge and skills developed through a baccalaureate program.

In October 2010, the Institute of Medicine released its landmark report on The Future of Nursing, initiated by the Robert Wood Johnson Foundation, which called for increasing the number of baccalaureate-prepared nurses in the workforce to 80 percent and doubling the population of nurses with doctorates. The expert committee charged with preparing the evidence-based recommendations contained in this report state that to respond "to the demands of an evolving health-care system and meet the changing needs of patients, nurses must achieve higher levels of education."

In March 2005, the American Organization of Nurse Executives (AONE) released a statement calling for all for registered nurses to be educated in baccalaureate programs in an effort to adequately prepare clinicians for their challenging and complex roles. AONE's statement, titled Practice and Education Partnership for the Future, represents the view of nursing's practice leaders and a desire to create a more highly educated nursing workforce in the interest of improving patient safety and providing enhanced nursing care.

## Research Linking Nursing Education to Patient Outcomes

AACN and other authorities believe that education has a strong impact on a nurse's ability to practice, and that patients deserve the best educated nursing workforce possible. A growing body of research reinforces this belief and shows a connection between baccalaureate education and lower mortality rates.

In an article published in the March 2013 issue of *Health Affairs,* nurse researcher Ann Kutney Lee and colleagues found that a 10-point increase in the percentage of nurses holding a B.S.N. within a hospital was associated with an average reduction of 2.12 deaths for every 1,000 patients—and for a subset of patients with complications, an average reduction of 7.47 deaths per 1,000 patients.

In the February 2013 issue of the *Journal of Nursing Administration,* Mary Blegen and colleagues published findings from a cross-sectional study of 21 University Health-System Consortium hospitals, which found that hospitals with a higher percentage of RNs with baccalaureate or higher degrees had lower congestive heart failure mortality, decubitus ulcers, failure to rescue, and postoperative deep vein thrombosis or pulmonary embolism as well as shorter length of stay.

In the October 2012 issue of *Medical Care,* researchers from the University of Pennsylvania found that surgical patients in Magnet hospitals had 14 percent lower odds of inpatient death within 30 days and 12 percent lower odds of failure-to-rescue compared with patients cared for in non-Magnet hospitals. The study authors conclude that these better outcomes were attributed in large part to investments in highly qualified and educated nurses, including a higher proportion of baccalaureate-prepared nurses.

In an article published in *Health Services Research* in August 2008 that examined the effect of nursing practice environments on outcomes of hospitalized cancer patients undergoing surgery, Dr. Christopher Friese and colleagues found that nursing education level was significantly associated with patient outcomes. Nurses prepared at the baccalaureate level were linked with lower mortality and failure-to-rescue rates. The authors conclude that "moving to a nurse workforce in which a higher proportion of staff nurses have at least a baccalaureate-level education would result in substantially fewer adverse outcomes for patients."

In a study released in the May 2008 issue of the *Journal of Nursing Administration,* Dr. Linda Aiken and her colleagues confirmed the findings from their landmark 2003 study (see details later in this article), which show a strong link between RN education level and patient outcomes. The noted nurse researchers found that every 10 percent increase in the proportion of B.S.N. nurses on the hospital staff was associated with a 4 percent decrease in the risk of death.

In the January 2007 *Journal of Advanced Nursing,* a study of 46,993 patients conducted by researchers at the University of Toronto found that hospitals with higher proportions of baccalaureate-prepared nurses tended to have lower 30-day mortality rates. The findings indicated that a 10 percent increase in the proportion of baccalaureate prepared nurses was associated with 9 fewer deaths for every 1,000 discharged patients.

In a study published in the March/April 2005 issue of *Nursing Research,* Dr. Carole Estabrooks and her colleagues at the University of Alberta found that baccalaureate-prepared nurses have a positive impact on mortality rates following an examination of more than 18,000 patient outcomes at 49 Canadian hospitals. This study, "The Impact of Hospital Nursing Characteristics on 30-Day Mortality," confirmed the findings from Dr. Aiken's landmark study from 2003.

In a study published in the September 24, 2003 *Journal of the American Medical Association,* Dr. Linda Aiken and her colleagues at the University of Pennsylvania identified a clear link between higher levels of nursing education and better patient outcomes. This extensive study found that surgical patients have a "substantial survival advantage" if treated in hospitals with higher proportions of nurses educated at the baccalaureate or higher degree level. A 10 percent increase in the proportion of nurses holding B.S.N. degrees decreased the risk of patient death and failure to rescue by 5 percent.

For more information on the link between nursing education and patient outcomes, see www.aacn.nche.edu/media-relations/fact-sheets/impact-of-education.

## Moving Towards a More Highly Educated Nursing Workforce

In September 2012, the Joint Statement on Academic Progression for Nursing Students and Graduates was endorsed by the American Association of Colleges of Nursing, American Association of Community Colleges, Association of Community Colleges Trustees, National League for Nursing, and the National Organization for Associate Degree Nursing. This historic agreement represents the first time leaders from the major national organizations representing community college presidents, boards, and program administrators have joined with representatives from nursing education associations to promote academic progression in nursing. With the common goal of preparing a well-educated, diverse nursing workforce, this statement represents the shared view that nursing students and practicing nurses should be supported in their efforts to pursue higher levels of education. Read the statement at www.aacn.nche.edu/aacn-publications/position/joint-statement-academic-progression.

In March 2012, the Robert Wood Johnson Foundation funded the Academic Progression in Nursing (APIN) Program to advance state and regional strategies to create a more highly educated nursing workforce. A total of $4.3 million in funding was awarded to the Tri-Council for Nursing to steer this initiative. Tri-Council members include the American Association of Colleges of Nursing, National League for Nursing, American Nurses Association, and the American Organization of Nurse Executives. For additional information, visit: www.aone.org/membership/about/press_releases/2012/032312.shtml

The nation's Magnet hospitals, which are recognized for nursing excellence and superior patient outcomes, have moved to require all nurse managers and nurse leaders to hold a baccalaureate or graduate degree in nursing by 2013. Settings applying for Magnet designation must also show what plans are in place to achieve the IOM recommendation of having an 80 percent baccalaureate-prepared RN workforce by 2020. Visit www.nursecredentialing.org for more information.

In its October 2010 report, "The Future of Nursing," the Institute of Medicine states, "an increase in the percentage of nurses with a BSN is imperative as the scope of what the public needs from nurses grows, expectations surrounding quality heighten, and the settings where nurses are needed proliferate and become more complex."

In May 2010, the Tri-Council for Nursing, a coalition of four steering organizations for the nursing profession (AACN, ANA, AONE, and NLN), issued a consensus statement calling for all RNs to advance their education in the interest of enhancing quality and safety across health-care settings. In the statement titled Education Advancement of Registered Nurses, the Tri-Council organizations present a united view that a more highly educated nursing workforce is critical to meeting the nation's nursing needs and delivering safe, effective patient care. In the policy statement, the Tri-Council finds that "without a more educated nursing workforce, the nation's health will be further at risk." See www.aacn.nche.edu/education-resources/TricouncilEdStatement.pdf.

In December 2009, Dr. Patricia Benner and her team at the Carnegie Foundation for the Advancement of Teaching released a new study titled, "Educating Nurses: A Call for Radical Transformation," which recommended preparing all entry-level registered nurses at the baccalaureate level and requiring all RNs to earn a master's degree within ten years of initial licensure. The authors found that many of today's new nurses are "undereducated" to meet practice demands across settings. Their strong support for high-quality baccalaureate degree programs as the appropriate pathway for RNs entering the profession is consistent with the views of many leading nursing organizations, including AACN.

In the July/August 2009 issue of *Health Affairs,* Dr. Linda Aiken and colleagues call for adapting federal funding mechanisms (i.e. Title VIII and Medicare) to focus on preparing more nurses at the baccalaureate and higher degree levels. This policy emphasis is needed to adequately address the growing need for faculty and nurses to serve in primary care and other advanced practice roles. The researchers reported that new nurses prepared in B.S.N. programs are significantly more likely to complete the graduate-level education needed to fill nursing positions where job growth is expected to be the greatest.

More than 690 RN-to-Baccalaureate programs are available nationwide, including more than 390 programs that are offered at least partially online. These programs build on the education provided in diploma and associate degree programs and prepare graduates for a broader scope of practice. In addition, 400 RN-to-Master's degree programs are available, which cover the baccalaureate content missing in the other entry-level programs as well as graduate-level course work.

Articulation agreements support education mobility and facilitate the seamless transfer of academic credit between associate degree and baccalaureate nursing programs. In addition to hundreds of individual agreements between community colleges and four-year schools, statewide articulation agreements exist in many areas including Florida, Connecticut, Arkansas, Texas, Iowa, Maryland, South Carolina, Idaho, Alabama, and Nevada to facilitate educational advancement. See media-relations/fact-sheets/articulation-agreements.

## References


Aiken, L.H., Cheung, R.B. & Olds, D.M. (2009, June 12). Education policy initiatives to address the nurse shortage in the United States. Health Affairs Web Exclusive. Accessed June 22, 2009 at http://content.healthaffairs.org/cgi/content/abstract/hlthaff.28.4.w646.

Aiken, L.H., Clarke, S.P., Sloane, D.M., Lake, E.T. & Cheney, T. (2008, May). Effects of hospital care environment on patient mortality and nurse outcomes. *Journal of Nursing Administration,* 38(5), 223–229.

Aiken, L.H., Clarke, S.P., Cheung, R.B., Sloane, D.M., & Silber, J.H. (2003, September 24). Educational levels of hospital nurses and surgical patient mortality, *Journal of the American Medical Association,* 290, 1617–1623.

American Association of Colleges of Nursing (2013). 2012-2013 Enrollment and graduations in baccalaureate and graduate programs in nursing. Washington, DC: Author.

American Organization of Nurse Executives. (2005). Practice and education partnership for the future. Washington, DC: American Organization of Nurse Executives.

Benner, P., Sutphen, M., Leonard, V. & Day, L. (2009). Educating Nurses: A Call for Radical Transformation. Carnegie Foundation for the Advancement of Teach. San Francisco: Jossey-Bass.

Blegen, M.A., Goode, C.J., Park, S.H., Vaughn, T. & Spetz, J. (2013, February). Baccalaureate education in nursing and patient outcomes. *Journal of Nursing Administration,* 43(2), 89–94.

Budden, J.S., Zhong, E.H., Moulton, P., & Cimiotti. J.P. (2013, July 13). The National Council of State Boards of Nursing and The Forum of State Nursing Workforce Centers 2013 National Workforce Survey of Registered Nurses. *Journal of Nursing Regulation,* 4(2), S1-S72.

Estabrooks, C.A., Midodzi, W.K., Cummings, G.C., Ricker, K.L. & Giovanetti, P. (2005, March/April). The impact of hospital nursing characteristics on 30-day mortality. *Nursing Research,* 54(2), 72–84.

Friese, C.R, Lake, E.T., Aiken, L.H., Silber, J.H. & Sochalski, J. (2008, August). Hospital nurse practice environments and outcomes for surgical oncology patients. *Health Services Research,* 43(4), 1145–1163.

Health Resources and Services Administration, National Center for Health Workforce Analysis. (2013, April). The U.S. nursing workforce: Trends in supply and education. Accessible online at http://bhpr.hrsa.gov/healthworkforce/reports/nursingworkforce/index.html.

Institute of Medicine. (2010). The Future of Nursing: Leading Change, Advancing Health. Washington, DC: National Academies Press.

Kutney-Lee, A., Sloane, D.M. & Aiken, L. (2003, March). An increase in the number of nurses with baccalaureate degrees is linked to lower rates of postsurgery mortality. *Health Affairs,* 32(3), 579–586.

McHugh, M.D., Kelly, L.A., Smith, H.L., Wu, E.S., Vanak, J.M. & Aiken, L.H. (2012, October). Lower Mortality in Magnet Hospitals. *Medical Care,* Publication forthcoming (published ahead of print).

National Council of State Boards of Nursing (See Budden, et al. reference above)

Tourangeau, A.E, Doran, D.M., McGillis Hall, L., O'Brien Pallas, L., Pringle, D., Tu, J.V. & Cranley, L.A. (2007, January). Impact of hospital nursing care on 30-day mortality for acute medical patients. *Journal of Advanced Nursing,* 57(1), 32–41.

Tri-Council for Nursing. (2010, May). Educational advancement of registered nurses: A consensus position. Available online at http://www.aacn.nche.edu/education-resources/TricouncilEdStatement.pdf.

Van den Heede, K., Lesaffre, E., Diya, L., Vleugels, A., Clarke, S.P., Aiken, L.H. & Sermeus, W. (2009). The relationship between inpatient cardiac surgery mortality and nurse numbers and educational level: Analysis of administrative data. *International Journal of Nursing Studies,* 46(6), 796–803.

# Counselors of Care in the Modern Health-Care System

**Geraldine D. Bednash, Ph.D., RN, FAAN**
*Chief Executive Officer and Executive Director*
*American Association of Colleges of Nursing*

## A Different Era

The nursing profession is alive and reshaping itself. The role of nurses as those who minister exclusively to a patient's basic-care needs has changed. Much of the effectiveness and productivity of the future health-care industry will derive from the training of and services provided by nurses.

Modern nurses take a proactive role in health care by addressing health issues before they develop into problems. They oversee the continued care of patients who have left the health-care facility. Nurses are expected to make complex decisions in areas ranging from patient screening to diagnosis and education. They explore and document the effects of alternative therapies (e.g., guided imagery) and address public health problems, such as teen pregnancy. They explore and understand new technology and how it relates both to patient care and to their own job performance. They work in a variety of settings and are held accountable for their decisions. In today's health-care environment, health-care administrators must recruit nurses with a broad, well-rounded education.

Health-care providers must change the way they administer care. Instead of focusing on the treatment of illness, they must promote wellness. Nurses will oversee patient treatment and medication and must understand the repercussions of these health-care processes for the patient and his or her family.

Cost is the driving force behind this industry-wide transformation. Insurance companies have, for the most part, instigated changes in the way health-care benefits are paid. The old fee-for-service system is no longer the only option. The trend toward managed care, in which a fixed amount of money is allocated for the care of each patient, is changing the way care is provided. It seems that employers of the future will recruit nurses who understand the overall structure of the health-care industry, who possess highly developed critical-thinking skills, and who bring to their positions a well-rounded understanding of the risks and benefits of every health-care decision.

## Counselors of Care

Job prospects for graduates of nursing programs are positive. Although many graduates receive associate degrees as registered nurses (RNs), hospital administrators and other employers want applicants with at least a Bachelor of Science in Nursing degree.

To practice in a fast-changing health system, entry-level RNs must understand community-based primary care and emphasize health promotion and cost-effective coordinated care—all hallmarks of baccalaureate education. In addition to its broad scientific curriculum and focus on leadership and clinical decision-making skills, a Bachelor of Science in Nursing degree education provides specific preparation in community-based care not typically included in associate degree or hospital diploma programs. Moreover, the nurse with a baccalaureate degree is the only basic nursing graduate prepared for all health-care settings—critical care, outpatient care, public health, and mental health—and so has the flexibility to practice in outpatient centers, private homes, and neighborhood clinics where demand is fast expanding as health care moves beyond the hospital to more primary and preventive care throughout the community.

Health-care administrators realize that patients are becoming more sophisticated about the care they receive, requiring an explanation and understanding of their health needs. Nurses will have to be knowledgeable care providers, working with physicians, pharmacists, and public health officials in interdisciplinary settings to satisfy these requirements.

Broader training enables graduates of baccalaureate programs to provide improved and varying types of care, and ensures stability and security in an industry now noted for its instability.

## Promising Opportunities

One of the rewards of a baccalaureate education can be a competitive salary. Graduates of four-year degree programs can expect salaries starting around $37,000 per year, a figure that might fluctuate depending on geographic area and, more specifically, by the demand in that area. Obviously, the greater the need for nurses, the higher their salaries.

The baccalaureate degree also serves as a foundation for the pursuit of a master's degree in nursing, which prepares students for the role of advanced practice nurse (APN). Students can earn degrees as clinical nurse specialists in neonatology, oncology, cardiology, and other specialties or as nurse practitioners, nurse-midwives, or nurse anesthetists. Master's-prepared nurses can also enjoy rewarding careers in nursing administration and education.

These programs generally span one to two years. Graduates can expect starting salaries of approximately $50,000 annually in advanced practice nursing settings, and demand for these graduates is expected to be high over the next fifteen years. In some localities, for example, the nurse practitioner may be the sole provider of health care to a family.

## Overall Transformation

The nursing field must be transformed to be compatible with the overall changes in the health-care industry. According to 2008 statistics, the average age of nurses was 46, with only 16.6 percent of nurses under the age of 35. It is projected that over the next ten years much of the nursing population will retire. Employment is projected to increase 23 percent by 2020.

The traditional career path of nurses is expected to change. More nurses will enter master's programs directly from baccalaureate programs, and more master's degree graduates will pursue doctoral degrees at a younger age. Since nurses will play a critical role in providing health care, a four-year baccalaureate degree is a crucial first step in preparing nurses to assume increased patient responsibilities within the health-care system.

# RNs Returning to School: Choosing a Nursing Program

**Marilyn Oermann, Ph.D., RN, FAAN, ANEF**
*Professor and Adult/Geriatric Health Chair*
*College of Nursing*
*The University of North Carolina at Chapel Hill*

If you are thinking about returning to school to complete your baccalaureate degree or to pursue a graduate degree in nursing, you are not alone. Registered nurses (RNs) are returning to school in record numbers, many seeking advancement or transition to new roles in nursing. Over the last two decades, the number of RNs prepared initially in diploma and associate degree in nursing programs who have graduated from baccalaureate nursing degree programs has more than doubled, according to the AACN. There are expanded opportunities for nurses with baccalaureate degrees in nursing. Although the decision to return to school means considerable investment of time, financial resources, and effort, the benefits can be overwhelmingly positive.

Higher education in nursing opens doors to many opportunities for career growth not otherwise available. By continuing your education, you can do the following:

- Update your knowledge and skills, critical today in light of rapid advances in health care
- Move more easily into a new role within your organization or in other health-care settings
- Pursue a different career path within nursing

Moreover, returning to school brings personal fulfillment and satisfaction gained through learning more about nursing and the changing health-care system and using that knowledge in the delivery and management of patient care.

## More Skills and Flexibility Needed

If you are contemplating returning to school, here are some facts to consider. The health-care system continues to undergo dramatic changes. These changes include hospitalized patients who are more acutely ill; an aging population; technological advances that require highly skilled nursing care; a greater role for nurses in primary care, health promotion, and health education; and the need for nurses to care for patients and families in multiple settings, such as schools, workplaces, homes, clinics, and outpatient facilities, as well as hospitals. With the nursing shortage, nurses are in great demand in hospitals. Moreover, as hospitals continue to become centers for acute and critical care, the nurse's role in both patient care and management of other health-care providers in the hospital has become more complex, requiring advanced knowledge and skills.

Because of the complexity of today's health-care environment, AACN and other leading nursing organizations have called for the baccalaureate degree in nursing as the minimum educational requirement for professional nursing practice. In fact, nurse executives in hospitals have indicated their desire for the majority of nurses on staff to be prepared at least at the baccalaureate level to handle the increasingly complex demands of patient care and management of health-care delivery. The baccalaureate nursing degree is essential for nurses to function in different management roles, move across employment settings, have the flexibility to change positions within nursing, and advance in their career. Baccalaureate nursing degree programs prepare the nurse for a broad role within the health-care system and for practice in hospitals, community settings, home health care, neighborhood clinics, and other outpatient settings where opportunities are expanding. Continuing education provides the means for nurses to prepare themselves for a future role in nursing.

The demand for nurses with baccalaureate and more advanced degrees will continue to grow. There is an excess of nurses prepared at the associate degree level, a mounting shortage of baccalaureate-prepared nurses, and only half as many nurses prepared at master's and doctoral levels as needed. Nurses with baccalaureate nursing degrees are needed in all areas of health care, and the demand for nurses with master's and doctoral preparation for advanced practice, management, teaching, and research will continue.

## Identifying Strategies

The decision to return to school marks the beginning of a new phase in your career development. It is essential for you to plan this future carefully. Why are you thinking about returning to school, and what do you want to accomplish by doing so? Understanding why you want to go back to school will help you select the best program for you. Knowing what you want to accomplish will help you to focus on your goals and overcome the obstacles that could prevent you from achieving your full potential.

Even if you decide that additional education will help you reach your professional goals, you may also have a list of reasons why you think you cannot return to school—no time, limited financial resources, fear of failure, and concerns about meeting family responsibilities, among others. If you are concerned about the demands of school combined with existing responsibilities, begin by identifying strategies for incorporating classes and study time into your present schedule or consider taking an online course. Remember, you can start your program with one course and reevaluate your time at the end of the term.

Research and anecdotal evidence from adults returning to college indicate that, despite their need to balance school work with a career and often with family responsibilities, these adult learners experience less stress and manage their lives better than they had thought possible. Many of these adult learners report that the satisfaction gained from their education more than compensates for any added stress. Furthermore, studies of nurses who have returned to school suggest that while their education may create stress for them, most nurses cope effectively with the demands of advanced education.

If costs are of concern, it is best to investigate tuition-reimbursement opportunities where you are employed, scholarships from the nursing program and other nursing organizations, and loans. The financial aid officer at the program you are considering is probably the best available resource to answer your financial assistance questions.

If you are unsure of what to expect when returning to school, remember that such feelings are natural for anyone facing a new situation. If you are motivated and committed to pursuing your degree, you will succeed. Most nursing programs offer resources, such as test-taking skills, study skills, and time-management workshops, as well as assistance with academic problems. You can combine school, work, family, and other responsibilities. Even with these greater demands, the benefits of education outweigh the difficulties.

## Clarifying Career Goals

Nursing, unlike many other professions, has a variety of educational paths for those who return for advanced education. You should decide if baccalaureate- or graduate-level work is congruent with your career goals. The next step in this process is to reexamine your specific career goals, both immediate and long-term, to determine the level and type of nursing education you will need to meet them. Ask yourself what you want to be doing in the next five to ten years. Discuss your ideas with a counselor in a nursing education program, nurses who are practicing in roles you are considering, and others who are enrolled in a nursing program or who have recently completed a nursing degree.

Baccalaureate degree nursing programs prepare nurses as generalists for practice in all health-care settings. Graduate nursing education occurs at two levels— master's and doctoral. Master's programs vary in length, typically between one and two years. Preparation for roles in advanced practice as nurse practitioners, certified nurse midwives, clinical nurse specialists, certified registered nurse anesthetists, nursing administrators, and nursing educators requires a master's degree in nursing. Many programs meet the needs of RNs by offering options such as accelerated course work, advanced placement, evening and weekend classes, and distance learning courses.

A trend in education for RNs is accelerated programs that combine baccalaureate and master's nursing programs. These combined programs are designed for RNs without degrees whose career goals involve advanced nursing practice and other roles requiring a master's degree. Nurses who complete these combined programs may be awarded both a baccalaureate and a master's degree in nursing or a master's degree only.

At the doctoral level, nurses are prepared for a variety of roles, including research and teaching. Doctoral programs generally consist of three years of full-time study beyond the master's degree, although some programs admit baccalaureate graduates and include the master's-level requirements and degree within the doctoral program.

## Matching a Program to Your Needs

Once you have defined your career goals and the level of nursing education they will require, the next step is matching your needs with the offerings and characteristics of specific nursing programs. Some of the criteria you may want to consider in evaluating potential schools of nursing include the types of programs offered, the length of the program and its specific requirements, the availability of full-and part-time study and number of credits required for part-time study, the flexibility of the program, whether distance education courses are available, and the days, times, and sites at which classes and clinical experiences are offered as they relate to your work schedule. Take into consideration the program's accreditation status; faculty qualifications in terms of research, teaching, and practice; and the resources of the school of nursing and of the college/university, such as library holdings, computer services, and statistical consultants. You should also consider the clinical settings used in the curriculum and their relationship to your career goals, as well as the availability of financial aid for nursing students.

Carefully review the admission criteria, including minimum grade point average requirements; scores required on any admission tests, such as the Graduate Record Examinations (GRE) for master's and doctoral programs; and any requirements in terms of work experience. For students returning for a baccalaureate degree, prior nursing knowledge may be validated through testing, transfer of courses, and other mechanisms. Review these options prior to applying to a program.

While the intrinsic quality and characteristics of the program are important, your own personal goals and needs have to be included in your decision. Consider commuting distance, whether courses are offered online, costs in relation to your financial resources, program design, and flexibility of the curriculum in relation to your work, family, and personal responsibilities. While the majority of nursing programs offer part-time study, many programs also schedule classes to accommodate work situations.

Many schools offer nursing courses online, and in some places, the entire baccalaureate and master's programs are available through distance learning. The largest enrollment in nursing distance learning is in baccalaureate programs for

RNs. Distance learning allows RNs to further their education no matter where they live. Many nurses prefer online courses because they can learn at times convenient for them, especially considering competing demands associated with their jobs, families, and other commitments.

## Ensure Your Success

Once you have made the decision to return to school and have chosen the program that best meets your needs, take an additional step to ensure your success. Identify the support you will need, both academic and personal, to be successful in the nursing program. Academic support is provided by the institution and may include tutoring services, learning resource centers, computer facilities, and other resources to support your learning. You should take advantage of available support services and seek out resources for areas in which you are weak or need review. Academic support services, however, need to be complemented by personal support through family, friends, and peers. With a firm commitment to pursuing advanced education, a clear choice of a nursing program to meet your goals, and support from others, you are certain to find success in returning to school.

# BACCALAUREATE PROGRAMS

**Linda K. Amos, Ed.D., RN, FAAN**
***Former Associate Vice President for Health Sciences***
***Dean Emerita***
***University of Utah***

The health-care industry has continued to change dramatically over the past few years, transforming the roles of nurses and escalating their opportunities. The current shortage of nurses is caused by an increasing number of hospitalized patients who are older and more acutely ill, a growing elderly population with multiple chronic health problems, and expanded opportunities in HMOs, home care, occupational health, surgical centers, and other primary-care settings. Expanding technological advances that prolong life also require more highly skilled personnel.

The increasing scope of nursing opportunities will grow immensely as nurses become the frontline providers of health care. They are assuming important roles in the provision of managed care, and they will be responsible for coordinating and continuing the care outside traditional health-care facilities. Nurses will play a major role in educating the public and addressing the social and economic factors that impact quality of care.

## Worldwide Standards

Nursing students of the future will receive a wealth of information. Understanding the technology used to manage that information will be essential to their ability to track and assess care. In this area, nurses will be able to provide care over great distances. In some areas, care is being managed by the nurse via tele-home health over the Internet. Use of the Internet and other computer-oriented systems is now an integral tool used by nurses. Nurses of the future, therefore, will have to become aware of worldwide standards of care. Nevertheless, the primary job of a nurse will be making sure that the right person is providing the right care at the right cost.

This goal will be accomplished as the industry turns away from the hospital as the center of operation. Nurses will work in a broad array of locations, including clinics, outpatient facilities, community centers, schools, and even places of business.

Much of the emphasis in health care will shift to preventive care and the promotion of health. In this system, nurses will take on a broader and more diverse role than they have in the past.

## Unlimited Opportunities, Expanded Responsibilities

The four-year baccalaureate programs in today's nursing colleges provide the educational and experiential base not only for entry-level professional practice, but also as the platform on which to build a career through graduate-level study for advanced practice nursing, including careers as nurse practitioners, nurse-midwives, clinical specialists, and nurse administrators and educators. Nurses at this level can be expected to specialize in oncology, pediatrics, neonatology, obstetrics and gynecology, critical care, infection control, psychiatry, women's health, community health, and neuroscience. The potential and responsibilities at this level are great. Increasingly, many families use the nurse practitioner for all health-care needs. In almost all U.S. states, the nurse practitioner can prescribe medications and provide health care for the management of chronic non-acute illnesses and preventive care.

The health-care system demands a lot from nurses. The education of a nurse must transcend the traditional areas of study, such as chemistry and anatomy, to include health promotion, disease prevention, screening, genetic counseling, and immunization. Nurses should understand how health problems may have a social cause, such as poverty and environmental contamination, and they must develop insight into human psychology, behavior, and cultural mores and values.

The transformation of the health-care system offers unlimited opportunities for nurses at the baccalaureate and graduate levels as care in urban and rural settings becomes more accessible. According to the U.S. Bureau of Labor Statistics, employment of RNs will grow more quickly than the average employment for all occupations through 2018, due largely to growing demand in settings such as health maintenance organizations, community health centers, home care, and long-term care. The increased complexity of health problems and increased management of health problems outside of hospitals require highly educated and well-prepared nurses at the baccalaureate and graduate levels. It is an exciting era in nursing that holds exceptional promise for nurses with a baccalaureate nursing degree.

The compensation for new nurses is once again becoming competitive with that of other industries. Entry-level nurses with baccalaureate degrees in nursing can expect a salary range of about $31,000 to $46,000 per year, depending on geographic location and experience. Five years into their careers, the national average for nurses with four-year degrees is more than $50,000 per year, with many earning more than $65,000. The current shortage has prompted some employers to offer sign-on bonuses and other incentives to attract and retain staff.

## Applying to College

Meeting your chosen school's general entrance requirements is the first step toward a university or college degree in nursing. Admission requirements may vary, but a high school diploma or equivalent is necessary. Most accredited colleges consider SAT scores along with high school grade point average. A strong preparatory class load in science and mathematics is generally preferred among nursing schools. Students may obtain specific admission information by writing to a school's nursing department.

To apply to a nursing school, contact the admission offices of the colleges or universities you are interested in and request the appropriate application forms. With limited spaces in nursing schools, programs are competitive, and early submission of an application is recommended.

## Accreditation

Accreditation of the nursing program is very important, and it should be considered on two levels—the accreditation of the university or college and the accreditation of the nursing program itself. Accreditation is a voluntary process in which the school or the program asks for an external review of its programs, facilities, and faculty. For nursing programs, the review is performed by peers in nursing education to ensure program quality and integrity.

Baccalaureate nursing programs in the United States undergo two types of regular systematic reviews. First, the school must be approved by the state board of nursing. This approval is necessary to ensure that the graduates of the program may sit for the licensing examinations offered through the National Council of State Boards of Nursing, Inc. The second is accreditation administered by a nursing accreditation agency that is recognized by the U.S. Department of Education.

Although accreditation is a voluntary process, access to federal loans and scholarships requires it, and most graduate schools accept only students who have earned degrees from accredited schools. Further, accreditation ensures an ongoing process of quality improvement based on national standards. Canadian nursing school programs are accredited by the Canadian Association of University Schools of Nursing, and the Canadian programs listed in this book must hold this accreditation. There are two recognized accreditation agencies for baccalaureate nursing programs in the United States: the Commission on Collegiate Nursing Education (CCNE) and the National League for Nursing Accrediting Commission (NLNAC).

## Focusing Your Education

Academic performance is not the sole basis of acceptance into the upper level of the nursing program. Admission officers also weigh such factors as student activities, employment, and references. Moreover, many require an interview and/or essay in which the nursing candidate offers a goal statement. This part of the admission process can be completed prior to a student's entrance into the college or university or prior to the student's entrance into the school of nursing itself, depending on the program.

In the interview or essay, students may list career preferences and reasons for their choices. This allows admission officers to assess the goals of students and gain insights into their values, integrity, and honesty. One would expect that a goal statement from a student who is just entering college would be more general than that of a student who has had two years of preprofessional nursing studies. The more experienced student would be likely to have a more focused idea of what is to be gained by an education in nursing; there would be more evidence of the student's values and the ways in which she or he relates them to the knowledge gained from preprofessional nursing classes.

## Baccalaureate Curriculum

A standard basic or generic baccalaureate program in nursing is a four-year college or university education that incorporates a variety of liberal arts courses with professional education and training. It is designed for high school graduates with no previous nursing experience.

Currently, there are more than 700 baccalaureate programs in the United States. Of the 683 programs that responded to a 2009 survey conducted by the American Association of Colleges of Nursing, total enrollment in all nursing programs leading to a baccalaureate degree was 214,533.

The baccalaureate curriculum is designed to prepare students for work in the growing and changing health-care environment. As nurses take a more active role in all facets of health care, they are expected to develop critical thinking and communication skills in addition to receiving standard nurse training in clinics and hospitals. In a university or college setting, the first two years include classes in the humanities, social sciences, basic sciences, business, psychology, technology, sociology, ethics, and nutrition.

In some programs, nursing classes begin in the sophomore year; others begin in the junior year. Many schools require satisfactory grade point averages before students advance into professional nursing classes. On a 4.0 scale, admission into the last two years of the nursing program may require a minimum GPA of 2.5 to 3.0 in preprofessional nursing classes. The national average is about 2.8, but the cutoff level varies with each program.

In the junior and senior years, the curriculum focuses on the nursing sciences, and emphasis moves from the classroom to health facilities. This is where students are exposed to clinical skills, nursing theory, and the varied roles nurses play in the health-care system. Courses include nurse leadership, health promotion, family planning, mental health, environmental and occupational health, adult and pediatric care, medical and surgical care, psychiatric care, community health, management, and home health care.

This level of education comes in a variety of settings: community hospitals, clinics, social service agencies, schools, and health-maintenance organizations. Training in diverse settings is the best preparation for becoming a vital player in the growing health-care field.

## Reentry Programs

Practicing nurses who return to school to earn a baccalaureate degree will have to meet requirements that may include possession of a valid RN license and an associate degree or hospital diploma from an accredited institution. Again, it is best to check with the school's admissions department to determine specifics.

Nurses returning to school will have to consider the rapid rate of change in health care and science. A nurse who passed an undergraduate-level chemistry class ten years ago would probably not receive credit for that class today because of the growth of knowledge in that and all other scientific fields. The need to reeducate applies not only to practicing nurses returning to school, but also to all nurses throughout their careers.

In the same vein, nurses with diplomas from hospital programs who want to work toward a baccalaureate degree must meet the common requirements for more clinical practice, and must develop a deeper understanding of community-based nursing practices such as health prevention and promotion.

Colleges and universities available to the RN in search of a baccalaureate give credit for previous nurse training. These programs are designed to accommodate the needs and career goals of the practicing nurse by providing flexible course schedules and credit for previous experience and education. Some programs lead to a master's-level degree, a process that can take up to three years. Licensed practical nurses (LPNs) can also continue their education through baccalaureate programs.

Nurses considering reentering school may also consider other specialized programs. For example, some programs are aimed at enabling nurses with A.D.N. degrees or LPN/LVN licenses to earn B.S.N.'s. Also, accelerated B.S.N. programs are available for students with degrees in other fields.

## RN-to-Baccalaureate Programs Fact Sheet

More than 692 RN-to-baccalaureate programs are available nationwide, including programs offered in a more intense, accelerated format. Program length varies from one to two years depending upon the school's requirements, program type, and the student's previous academic achievement.

Concerns about the limited availability of RN-to-baccalaureate programs are unfounded. In fact, there are more RN-to-baccalaureate programs available than there are four-year nursing programs or accelerated bachelor's degree programs for non-nursing college graduates. Access to RN-to-baccalaureate programs is further enhanced when programs are offered completely online or on-site at various health-care facilities.

Enrollment in RN-to-baccalaureate programs is increasing in response to calls for a more highly educated nursing workforce. From 2011 to 2012, enrollments increased by 15.5 percent, marking the tenth year of increases in RN-to-baccalaureate programs.

Hundreds of articulation agreements between A.D.N. and diploma programs and four-year institutions exist nationwide (including some statewide agreements), to help students who are seeking baccalaureate-level nursing education. Before enrolling in diploma and A.D.N. programs, students are encouraged to check with school administrators to see what articulation agreements exist with baccalaureate degree–granting schools and to determine which course work will be transferable.

## Choosing a Program

With more than 700 baccalaureate programs in the United States, the prospective student must do research to determine which programs match his or her needs and career objectives.

If you have no health-care experience, it might be best to gain some insight into the field by volunteering or working part-time in a care facility such as a hospital or an outpatient clinic. Talking to nurse professionals about their work will also help you determine how your attributes may apply to the nursing field.

When considering a nursing education, consider your personal needs. Is it best for you to work in a heavily structured environment or one that offers more flexibility in terms of, say, integrating a part-time work schedule into studies? Do you need to stay close to home? Do you prefer to work in a large health-care system such as a health maintenance organization or a medical center, or do you prefer smaller, community-based operations?

As for nursing programs, ask the following questions: How involved is the faculty in developing students for today's health-care industry? How strong is the school's affiliation with clinics and hospitals? Is there assurance that a student will gain an up-to-date educational experience for the current job market? Are a variety of care settings available? How much time in clinics is required for graduation? What are the program's resources in terms of computer and science laboratories? Does the school work with hospitals and community-based centers to provide health care? How available is the faculty to oversee a student's curriculum? What kind of student support is available in terms of study groups and audiovisual aids? Moreover, what kind of counseling from faculty members and administrators is available to help students develop well-rounded, effective progress through the program?

Visiting a school and talking to the program's guidance counselors will give you a better understanding of how a particular program or school will fit your needs. You can get a closer look at the faculty, its members' credentials, and the focus of the program. It's also not too early to consider what each program can offer in terms of job placement.

# MASTER'S PROGRAMS

**Tommie L. Norris, DNS, RN**
*Professor and Associate Dean, Chair*
*BSN and MSN Programs*
*College of Nursing*
*The University of Tennessee Health Science Center*
*Memphis, Tennessee*

The complexities of the health-care environment accompanied by The Affordable Care Act and the Institute of Medicine's (IOM) report *To Err is Human* have challenged health-care providers, educators, and consumers to redesign healthcare. The IOM report informed health-care providers and consumers that healthcare is fragmented, unsafe, and exists in a crisis situation. The IOM's *Future of Nursing Report* apprised the nation that nurses must practice to the full extent of their scope of practice, training, and education while also pursing higher levels of education. The Affordable Care Act will provide funds to train 600 new nurse practitioners and nurse midwives in just the next year. With improved access to healthcare, consumers will look toward advance practice nurses to manage their health-care needs. As the most trusted profession and largest sector of the health-care workforce, nurses are ready to meet the challenge to be a full partner in redesigning healthcare.

The American Association of Colleges of Nursing's (AACN) *The Essentials of Master's Education in Nursing* describes master's education as a "critical component of the nursing education trajectory to prepare nurses who can address the gaps resulting from growing healthcare needs" and to improve health outcomes. They further define how master's education prepares the nursing graduate to:

- Be the forerunner to improve quality outcomes.
- Exude excellence as a result of lifelong learning.
- Develop and direct interdisciplinary care teams.
- Serve as integrators of patient care across health-care systems.
- Manage innovative nursing practices.
- Incorporate evidenced-based practice.

Consumers of healthcare no longer are content to be passive but are active partners in their healthcare. Consumers can already see the changes in place and those being planned to transform healthcare:

- A Clinical Nurse Leader conducts patient rounds with an interdisciplinary health-care team to brainstorm processes aimed to streamline medication administration, ensuring medications are delivered and administered in a timely, safe, and accurate manner.
- A patient with a pacemaker places the phone's receiver over the implant allowing an advanced practice nurse to evaluate pacemaker function and manage care after oxygen saturation, BMI, and vital signs are transmitted.
- The Certified Nursing Administrator of a home health agency collaborates with the Chief Financial Officer to formulate the agency's budget, then later meets with the Director of the Human Resources Department to review policies related to current hiring practices.
- A Clinical Nurse Specialist consults with other nurses caring for diabetic patients to design cost-effective, patient-centered, high-quality care to reduce recidivism and chronic complications. Clinical Nurse Specialists manage the treatment of specific populations.
- The parents of a child preparing for an appendectomy are visited by a certified registered nurse anesthetist (CRNA) to obtain a preoperative history and answer any questions related to the anesthesia that the CRNA will administer.

## Master's Education in Nursing

Master's prepared nurses may assume the role as Advanced Practice Registered Nurses (APRNs), as well as, advanced roles such as Clinical Nurse Leaders (CNLs), nurse administrators, public health nurses, and nurse educators. The demand for master's prepared nurses is expected to remain high. There are more than 536 master's degree programs accredited by the Commission on Collegiate Nursing Education (CCNE) or by the National League for Nursing Accrediting Commission (NLNAC).

The Advanced Practice Registered Nurse (APRN) Consensus Model defines advance practice nurses as being educated at the Master's or Doctoral level and certified to prescribe, treat, and manage all aspects of patient care. AACN recognizes Clinical Nurse Specialists (CNS), Certified Nurse Practitioners (CNP), Certified Registered Nurse Anesthetists (CRNA), and Certified Nurse Midwives (CNM) as APRNs with advanced clinical skills and knowledge. With the Affordable Care Act improving access to healthcare for many Americans who were previously uninsurable or without affordable healthcare, it is clear more APRNs are needed.

APRNs practice in a wide range of practice arenas to provide primary and specialty care.

**Nurse Practitioners (NP)** manage care for patients across the lifespan with acute and chronic conditions and are key to providing access to care in underserved areas. NPs manage care across the wellness-illness continuum to include health screening and examinations/assessments, diagnosing, treating, health education, and disease prevention/promotion. Family/individual, pediatrics, adult-gerontology, neonatal, psychiatric/mental health, and women's health/gender-related are the six population foci.

**Nurse-Midwives** provide primary care that includes care of gynecologic and obstetric patients, newborns, and childbirth. Preventative and primary care are managed across diverse settings and could include screening for sexually transmitted diseases and risk factors that increase birth defects or infertility.

**Registered Nurse Anesthetists** deliver anesthesia across the lifespan in both acute and outpatient settings for general surgery, specialties such as trauma, pain management, and childbirth and outpatient procedures.

**Clinical Nurse Specialists (CNS)** focus nursing practice by populations, disease, and or practice venue. A CNS is responsible for the management of disease, health promotion/prevention, and assessment of risk behaviors in areas such as adult health, critical care, community health, psychiatric nursing, or neonatal nursing.

Master's-prepared nurses who are not APRNs also have many opportunities. Roles and practice settings are diverse and ever evolving with the dynamic healthcare environment. Such roles may include, but are not limited to, direct care foci such as the Clinical Nurse Leaders and nurse educators. Other roles include nurse administrators, public health nurses, nurse informaticists, and public policy.

In 2003, the American Association of Colleges of Nursing (AACN) in partnership with other national leaders and professionals developed the new Clinical Nurse Leader (CNL) role aimed to improve health-care outcomes by reducing fragmentation of care, decreasing the number of errors, and improving quality outcomes of care. The CNL is a master's-prepared generalist who works across health-care settings as a lateral care integrator. However, it is important to point out that the CNL role is not one of manager or administration—rather, the CNL is responsible for patient care outcomes whether by providing the care directly in complex situations or managing care in a microsystem. Their advanced skills and knowledge allow them to facilitate care in complex and dynamic systems.

**Nurse educators** advance the knowledge and skills of nurses entering the field, novice nurses, and experienced nurses. With an emphasis on lifelong learning and advancing education, there is a growing demand for nurse educators. Educators may choose to teach theory courses or supervise nursing students in a clinical setting, advance the knowledge of practicing nurses by offering classes on new technologies or evidence-based practice, or they may even serve as consultants to health-care agencies seeking better patient outcomes. The preparation for the nurse educator varies; however, those seeking faculty positions are advised to specialize in a clinical area such as adult health, women's health, pediatrics, psychiatric mental health, or community health. In addition, those seeking faculty roles will need formal course work in curriculum development, pedagogy, and student/program evaluation.

**Nurse administrators** practice in managerial and leadership roles to ensure high-quality patient care is delivered in a cost-effective manner. Entry-level nurse administrators may manage a microsystem; whereas, experienced nurse administrators may lead an entire organization. Certification programs are available for graduates of accredited nursing administration programs from the American Nurses Credentialing Center and the American Organization of Nurse Executives.

**Public health nurses** are specialists with an emphasis on the health and well- being of the public. Their diverse roles are applicable to many settings and may include epidemiology, managing a clinic that provides immunizations and health screenings, investigating and managing communicable disease, providing programs to address environmental risks, and working with government and community leaders to improve and or eliminate health risks.

**Nurse informaticists** apply the nursing process to computer and information science to support patients and healthcare providers in clinical decisions. The need to share healthcare information across care venues to provide patient-centered care along with the need to ensure privacy provides the perfect environment to promote the role of the nurse informaticist.

**Public policy nurses** interested in this role use nursing knowledge to educate the public and legislators concerning health-care issues to shape policy. Nurses with advanced education in public policy are poised to serve as consultants to local, state, and national policy-making bodies and associations that influence healthcare.

## Overview of the Master's Curriculum

Those looking to earn a master's degree in nursing have many options for entry:

- **Entry-level or Generic degree**—allows individuals who are non-nurses to meet the baccalaureate-level requirements gaining eligibility to sit for the initial RN licensure and earn a master's degree. The new Clinical Nurse Leader role is one popular choice that utilizes this option.
- **RN to Master's Degree**—allows registered nurses (RN) who have an earned an associate degree in nursing to complete the missing baccalaureate content and progress through the master's-level curriculum. The online delivery format is gaining popularity to accommodate the working RN's schedule. The time for completion varies depending whether the part-time or full-time program of study is selected.
- **Baccalaureate to Master's Degree**—thought of as the traditional postbaccalaureate master's degree, this option remains the most popular. Since the undergraduate content has been mastered, students focus solely on graduate-level course work, with most degrees awarded in 18 to 24 months. The Master of Science in Nursing (M.S.N.), Master of Nursing (M.N.), or Master of Science (M.S.) may be offered, all of which prepare students to meet the master's degree competencies.
- **Dual Master's Degree Programs**—provide an extensive concentration in a related field of study that is combined with nursing courses. More than 120 dual master's degrees are available that combine nursing coursework with business (MSN/MBA); public administration (MSN/MPA), and health administration (MSN/MSA).
- **Post Master's Certificate Programs**—allow nurses who have a master's degree in nursing to gain advanced skills

and knowledge in an additional area of nursing. Nursing education, administration, informatics, and clinical nurse leader are such options. A current trend is for nurses certified as Family Nurse Practitioners to return to earn certification as an Acute Care Nurse Practitioner to deliver care in such areas as the emergency department or intensive care.

The master's nursing curriculum builds on the skills and competencies gained in the baccalaureate nursing program. Content related to health-care economics/policy, genetics, organizational sciences, information sciences, complexity science, bioethics, and quality improvement science might be included. The master's curriculum includes three components:

1. Foundational core content for all individuals pursing a master's degree regardless of functional focus
2. Essential content aimed at advanced direct patient care
3. The functional area focus (clinical and didactic) experiences required by certification bodies and professional nursing organization as essential for specific roles.

Graduates of any one of the four APRN roles (CNP, CNS, CNM, or CRNA) must complete three separate graduate-level courses in physiology/pathophysiology, health assessment, and pharmacology (known as the direct care core or 3 Ps). Graduates pursing non-APRN roles but who have a direct care focus (CNL and nurse educator) must have content/course work in the 3 Ps, although three separate graduate-level courses are not required. Master's degrees preparing students for a practice profession must provide planned clinical experiences to ensure competence to enter nursing practice.

## Admission Requirements

The admissions requirements for master's programs in nursing vary depending on entry point and even by specialty. Schools may elect to use standardized admission exams such as the Graduate Record Examinations (GRE) or Miller Analogies Test (MAT). Others may choose to base admission on grade point average, letters of reference, college transcripts, and personal statements/essays. Schools may choose to give more importance to certain requirements—for example a school may weigh grade point average more heavily than the standardized exam score. Carefully select individuals to write letters of reference; faculty and employers may be seen as having more value than those written by personal friends or coworkers. When beginning the application process or just considering which master's programs is right, take the time to research any specific requirements. Some CRNA programs require a year of experience in critical care, and some neonatal nurse practitioner programs require a year in the neonatal ICU or related area for admission eligibility.

### RN-to-Master's Degree Programs Fact Sheet

Currently, there are 159 programs available nationwide to transition RNs with diplomas and associate degrees to the master's-degree level (M.S.N., M.S., or Master of Science in Nursing degree). These programs prepare nurses to assume positions requiring graduate preparation, including roles in administration, teaching, research, and as Clinical Nurse Leaders. Master's degree-prepared nurses are in high demand as expert clinicians, nurse executives, clinical educators, health-policy consultants, and research assistants.

RN-to-M.S.N. programs generally take about three years to complete, with specific requirements varying by institution and the student's previous course work. Though the majority of these programs are offered in traditional classroom settings, some RN-to-M.S.N. programs are offered largely online or in a blended classroom/online format.

The baccalaureate-level content missing from diploma and ADN programs is built into the front-end of the RN-to-M.S.N. program. Mastery of this upper-level basic nursing content is necessary for students to move on to graduate study. Upon completion, many programs award both the baccalaureate and master's degree.

The number of RN-to-M.S.N. programs has more than doubled in the past 15 years, from 70 programs in 1994 to 159 programs today. According to AACN's 2012 survey of nursing schools, 29 new RN-to-M.S.N. programs are in the planning stages.

When considering a master's program, consider the program length, delivery format such as face-to-face or online, accreditation status, financial aid availability, and employment rates. If considering transitioning into a doctoral program, determine if an articulation plan is in place. Career fairs, webinars, and college websites provide valuable information related to admission requirements.

## Benefits of a Master's Degree in Nursing

The perceived benefits of a master's degree in nursing vary from person to person. However, there is evidence that earning a master's degree boosts your nursing career and earning potential. A master's degree in nursing provides greater knowledge and fulfills the requirement for lifelong learning needed to keep pace with the complex dynamic healthcare system. A master's degree provides entry into leadership and managerial roles while broadening the scope of practice. With the aging of our nation and improved access to healthcare, advanced practice nurses will be pivotal to transform the health-care system. Faculty shortages at nursing schools are limiting the number of nurses when a shortage of nurses exists. A master's degree in nursing is the entry point into a nursing faculty position. The master's degree also provides the foundation for doctoral education whether it is advanced practice or research focused.

For the most part, nurses prepared at the master's-level garner higher wages than those with a bachelor's degree. Salaries differ by geographic regions and specializations. When comparing the salary of the four APN roles, the CRNA has the highest average salary, with an average yearly income of $156,000. Comparably, the average salary of a nurse practitioner is $94,050, with the median salary of a nurse midwife at $92,806. Clinical nurse specialists have an average yearly salary of $94,487. Master's-prepared nurses with a direct care focus but who are not APRNs, such as nursing faculty, are receiving $80,690. Chief nursing officers command $194,477 on average, with nurse informaticist earning $80,500.

# The Clinical Nurse Leader

The Clinical Nurse Leader or CNL® is a rapidly emerging nursing role developed by the American Association of Colleges of Nursing (AACN) in collaboration with leaders from the nursing education and practice arenas. The national movement to advance the CNL is fueled by the critical need to improve the quality of patient care and better prepare nurses to thrive across the health-care system. The CNL role was developed following research and discussion with stakeholder groups as a way to engage highly skilled clinicians as leaders in outcome-based practices.

CNL provide lateral integration at the point of care and combine evidence-based practice with the following:

- Microsystems-level advocacy
- Centralized care coordination
- Outcomes measurement
- Risk assessment
- Quality improvement
- Interprofessional communication

In practice, the CNL oversees the care coordination of a distinct group of patients and actively provides direct patient care in complex situations. CNLs have master's degrees and are advanced generalists, evaluating patient outcomes, assessing risks, and using their authority to change care plans when necessary. CNLs are leaders in the health-care delivery system; the implementation of their roles will vary across settings.

## Connecting Nursing Practice and Education

To support the creation of this new nursing role, AACN launched a national initiative involving more than 100 education-practice partnerships across the nation. Partners from schools of nursing and nursing practice sites are working together to transform care delivery by educating new CNLs and integrating them into the health delivery system.

More than seventy schools of nursing are now preparing CNLs for advanced generalist programs offered at the graduate level. Students may choose from traditional post-baccalaureate master's programs, degree completion programs for registered nurses (RNs), and accelerated programs for those seeking to make the transition into nursing. Most CNL programs are directly connected with practice sites interested in employing graduates to enhance care delivery, patient safety, and quality outcomes.

The Veterans Health Administration, the nation's largest employer of RNs, has embraced the CNL role and is planning to introduce it into all Veterans Affairs hospitals nationwide. Support for the clinical role is gaining momentum as many practice sites are reporting on the pioneering outcomes of the CNL staff.

## The Key to Positive Patient Outcomes

CNLs provide efficient and cost-effective patient care services, as well as the leadership needed to repair fragmented health-care delivery systems. CNLs are having a measurable impact on the quality of nursing services with practice sites reporting that CNLs are

- quickly making significant progress on raising patient, nurse, and physician satisfaction; improving care outcomes; and realizing sizable cost-savings.
- elevating the level of practice for all nurses on the unit by promoting critical thinking and innovation in nursing care.
- constructively managing change and promoting a team-based approach to care.
- understanding the bigger picture, including outcomes and patient satisfaction, when considering next steps, needed changes, and improvements to the practice setting.

## The CNL Mark of Excellence

The CNL Mark of Excellence certification is a unique credential that recognizes graduates of master's and post-master's CNL programs who have demonstrated accepted standards of practice. The CNL Mark of Excellence promotes safe, quality practice through its ongoing requirements for personal and professional growth. In 2007, AACN established a new certification commission—the Commission on Nurse Certification (CNC)—to oversee all aspects of the CNL certification program.

## Becoming a CNL

Those interested in becoming a CNL are encouraged to visit the AACN website, www.aacn.nche.edu/CNL, to find out more about this nursing career option. Detailed information is available online, including frequently asked questions, the white paper on the CNL role, and a directory of Web links for related programs.

# Accelerated Baccalaureate and Master's Degrees in Nursing

With the Bureau of Labor Statistics projecting the need for more than one million new and replacement registered nurses by the year 2020, nursing schools around the country are exploring creative ways to increase student capacity and reach out to new student populations. One innovative approach to nursing education that is gaining momentum is the accelerated degree program for non-nursing graduates. Offered at the baccalaureate and master's degree levels, these programs build on previous learning experiences and provide a way for individuals with undergraduate degrees in other disciplines to transition into nursing.

## Program Basics

- Accelerated baccalaureate programs offer the quickest route to licensure as a registered nurse (RN) for adults who have already completed a bachelor's or graduate degree in a non-nursing discipline.
- Fast-track baccalaureate programs take between 11 and 18 months to complete, including prerequisites. Fast-track master's degree programs generally take about 3 years to complete.
- Accelerated nursing programs are available in 46 states plus the District of Columbia and Puerto Rico. In 2012, there were 255 accelerated baccalaureate programs and 71 accelerated master's programs available at nursing schools nationwide. In addition, 25 new accelerated baccalaureate programs are in the planning stages, and 7 new accelerated master's programs are also taking shape. See www.aacn.nche.edu/education-resources/nursing-education-programs for a list of accelerated nursing programs.

## Fast-Track Nursing Education

- Accelerated baccalaureate programs accomplish programmatic objectives in a short time by building on previous learning experiences. Instruction is intense with courses offered full-time with no breaks between sessions. Students receive the same number of clinical hours as their counterparts in traditional entry-level nursing programs.
- Admission standards for accelerated programs are high, with programs typically requiring a minimum of a 3.0 GPA and a thorough prescreening process. Identifying students who will flourish in this environment is a priority for administrators. Students enrolled in accelerated programs are encouraged NOT to work given the rigor associated with completing degree requirements.
- Accelerated baccalaureate and master's programs in nursing are appropriately geared to individuals who have already proven their ability to succeed at a senior college or university. Having already completed a bachelor's degree, many second-degree students are attracted to the fast-track master's program as the natural next step in their higher education.

## Accelerated Program Graduates

- The typical second-degree nursing student is motivated, older, and has higher academic expectations than traditional entry-level nursing students. Accelerated students excel in class and are eager to gain clinical experiences. Faculty members find the accelerated students to be excellent learners who are not afraid to challenge their instructors.
- Graduates of accelerated programs are prized by nurse employers who value the many layers of skill and education they bring to the workplace. Employers report that these graduates are more mature, possess strong clinical skills, and are quick studies on the job.
- Given their experience and level of educational achievement, many graduates of accelerated master's programs are being encouraged to pursue roles as nurse educators to help stem the growing shortage of nurse faculty.

## Supporting Accelerated Programs

- Financial aid for students enrolled in accelerated baccalaureate and master's programs in nursing is limited. Many practice settings are partnering with schools and offering tuition repayment to graduates as a mechanism to recruit highly qualified nurses.
- Hospitals, health-care systems, and other practice settings are encouraged to form partnerships with schools offering accelerated programs to remove the student's financial burden in exchange for a steady stream of new nurse recruits. Nurse employers including Tenet Healthcare, Carondelet Health Network, University of Missouri Health Care, North Carolina Baptist Hospital, Duke University Health System, and many others are actively supporting the

development and growth of accelerated baccalaureate programs in nursing.

- Legislators on the state and federal levels are encouraged to increase scholarship and grant funding for these programs that produce entry-level nurses faster than any other basic nursing education program. These programs are ideal career transition vehicles for those segments of the labor force impacted by fluctuations in the economy.

## Research on Accelerated Nursing Programs

Bentley, R. Comparison of traditional and accelerated baccalaureate nursing graduates. *Nurse Educator*, 31(2), 79–83, May/June 2006.

Brewer, C. S., C. T. Kovner, S. Poornima, S. Fairchild, H. Kim, and M. Djukic. A comparison of second-degree baccalaureate and traditional-baccalaureate new graduate RNs: Implications for the workforce. *Journal of Professional Nursing,* 25 (1), 5–14, January-February 2009.

Kearns, L. E., J. R. Shoaf, and M. B. Summey. Performance and satisfaction of second-degree BSN students in Web-based and traditional course delivery environments. *Journal of Nursing Education*, 43(6), 280–284, June 2004.

Meyer, G. A., K. G. Hoover, and S. Maposa. A profile of accelerated BSN graduates, 2004. *Journal of Nursing Education*, 45(8), 324–327, August 2006.

Oermann, M.H., K. Poole-Dawkins, M. T. Alvarez, B. B. Foster, and R. O'Sullivan. Managers' perspectives of new graduates of accelerated nursing programs: How do they compare with other graduates? *Journal of Continuing Education in Nursing*, 41(9), 394–399, October 2010.

Ouellet, L. L., J. MacIntosh, C. H. Gibson, and S. Jefferson. Evaluation of selected outcomes of an accelerated nursing degree program. *Nursing Education Today*, 28(2), 194–201, February 2008.

Raines, D. A. and A. Spies. One year later: Reflections and work activities of accelerated second-degree Bachelor of Science in Nursing graduates. *Journal of Professional Nursing*, 23(6), 329–334, November/December 2007.

Roberts, K., J. Mason, and P. Wood. A comparison of a traditional and an accelerated basic nursing education program. *Contemporary Nurse*, 11(2/3), 283–287, December 2001.

Rouse, S. M. and L. A. Rooda. Factors for attrition in an accelerated baccalaureate nursing program. *Journal of Nursing Education*, 49(6), 359–362, June 1, 2010.

Seldomridge, L. A. and M. C. DiBartolo. The changing face of accelerated second bachelor's degree students. *Nurse Educator*, 32(6), 240–245, November/December 2007.

Seldomridge, L. A. and M. C. DiBartolo. A profile of accelerated second bachelor's degree nursing students. *Nurse Educator*, 30(2), 65–68, March-April 2005.

White, K., W. Wax, and A. Berrey. Accelerated second degree advanced practice nurses: how do they fare in the job market? *Nursing Outlook*, 48(5), 218–222, September-October 2000.

Ziehm, S. R., I. C. Uibel, D. K. Fontaine, and T. Scherzer. Success indicators for an accelerated masters entry nursing program: Staff RN performance. *Journal of Nursing Education*, 49(7), 395–403, July 2011.

# The Doctor of Nursing Practice (DNP)

On October 25, 2004, the member schools affiliated with the American Association of Colleges of Nursing (AACN) voted to endorse the *Position Statement on the Practice Doctorate in Nursing***.** This decision called for moving the current level of preparation necessary for advanced nursing practice from the master's degree to the doctorate-level by the year 2015. This endorsement was preceded by almost three years of research and consensus-building by an AACN task force charged with examining the need for the practice doctorate with a variety of stakeholder groups.

## Introducing the Doctor of Nursing Practice (DNP)

- In many institutions, advanced practice registered nurses (APRNs), including Nurse Practitioners, Clinical Nurse Specialists, Certified Nurse Mid-Wives, and Certified Nurse Anesthetists, are prepared in master's-degree programs that often carry a credit load equivalent to doctoral degrees in the other health professions. AACN's position statement calls for educating APRNs and nurses seeking top systems/organizational roles in DNP programs.
- DNP curricula build on traditional master's programs by providing education in evidence-based practice, quality improvement, and systems leadership, among other key areas.
- The DNP is designed for nurses seeking a terminal degree in nursing practice and offers an alternative to research-focused doctoral programs. DNP-prepared nurses are well-equipped to fully implement the science developed by nurse researchers prepared in PhD, DNSc, and other research-focused nursing doctorates.

## Why Move to the DNP?

- The changing demands of this nation's complex health-care environment require the highest level of scientific knowledge and practice expertise to assure high-quality patient outcomes. The Institute of Medicine, Joint Commission, Robert Wood Johnson Foundation, and other authorities have called for re-conceptualizing educational programs that prepare today's health professionals.
- Some of the many factors building momentum for change in nursing education at the graduate level include: the rapid expansion of knowledge underlying practice; increased complexity of patient care; national concerns about the quality of care and patient safety; shortages of nursing personnel, which demands a higher level of preparation for leaders who can design and assess care; shortages of doctorally prepared nursing faculty; and increasing educational expectations for the preparation of other members of the health-care team.
- In a 2005 report titled *Advancing the Nation's Health Needs: NIH Research Training Programs*, the National Academy of Sciences called for nursing to develop a non-research clinical doctorate to prepare expert practitioners who can also serve as clinical faculty. AACN's work to advance the DNP is consistent with this call to action.
- Nursing is moving in the direction of other health professions in the transition to the DNP. Medicine (MD), Dentistry (DDS), Pharmacy (PharmD), Psychology (PsyD), Physical Therapy (DPT), and Audiology (AudD) all offer practice doctorates.

## Sustaining Momentum for the DNP

- After a two-year consensus-building process, AACN member institutions voted to endorse the *Essentials of Doctoral Education for Advanced Nursing Practice* on October 30, 2006. Schools developing a DNP are encouraged to use this document, which defines the curricular elements and competencies that must be present in a practice doctorate in nursing.
- In July 2006, the AACN Board of Directors endorsed the final report of the *Task Force on the Roadmap to the DNP,* which was developed to assist schools navigating the DNP program approval process. This report includes recommendations for securing institutional approval to transition an MSN into a DNP program; preparing faculty to teach in DNP programs; addressing regulatory, licensure, accreditation, and certification issues; and collecting evaluation data. The Roadmap report and accompanying tool kit are posted at http://www.aacn.nche.edu/dnp.
- Schools nationwide that have initiated the DNP are reporting sizable and competitive student enrollment. Employers are quickly recognizing the unique contribution these expert nurses are making in the practice arena, and the demand for DNP-prepared nurses continues to grow. According to the 2009 salary survey conducted by *ADVANCE for Nurse Practitioners* magazine, DNP-prepared NPs earned $7,688 more than master's-prepared NPs.
- The Commission on Collegiate Nursing Education (CCNE), the leading accrediting agency for baccalaureate-

and graduate-degree nursing programs in the United States, began accrediting DNP programs in fall of 2008. To date, 116 DNP programs have been accredited by CCNE.

## Current DNP Program Statistics

- 184 DNP programs are currently enrolling students at schools of nursing nationwide, and an additional 101 DNP programs are in the planning stages.
- DNP programs are now available in 40 states plus the District of Columbia. States with the most programs (more than 5) include Florida, Massachusetts, Minnesota, New York, Pennsylvania, and Texas.
- From 2010 to 2011, the number of students enrolled in DNP programs increased from 7,034 to 9,094. During that same period, the number of DNP graduates increased from 1,282 to 1,595.

# THE NURSE PH.D.: A VITAL PROFESSION NEEDS LEADERS

**Carole Anderson**
*Former Dean of the College of Dentistry*
*The Ohio State University*
*Past President, American Association of Colleges of Nursing*

There is no doubt that education is the path for a nurse to achieve greater clinical expertise. At the same time, however, the nursing profession needs more nurses educated at the doctoral level to replenish the supply of faculty and researchers. The national shortage of faculty will soon reach critical proportions, making a significant impact on educational programs and their capacity to educate future generations of nursing students.

Although the number of doctorate programs has continued to increase, the total enrollment of students in these programs has remained fairly constant, resulting in a shortage of newly trained Ph.D.'s to renew faculty ranks. As a result, approximately 50 percent of nursing faculty possess the doctorate as a terminal degree. Furthermore, with many advances being made in the treatment of chronic illnesses, there is a continuing need for research that assists patients in living with their illness. This research requires individual investigators who are prepared on the doctoral level.

One reason there is a lack of nurses prepared at the doctoral level is that, compared to other professions, nurses have more interruptions in their careers. Many in the profession are women who work as nurses while fulfilling responsibilities as wives and mothers. As a result, many pursue their education on a part-time basis. Also, the nursing profession traditionally has viewed clinical experience as being a prerequisite to graduate education. This career path results in fewer individuals completing the doctorate at an earlier stage in their career, thereby truncating their productivity as academics, researchers, and administrators. To reverse this trend, many nursing schools have developed programs that admit students into graduate (doctoral and master's) programs directly from their undergraduate or master's programs.

## Nursing Research

When nurses do research for their doctorates, many people tend to think that it focuses primarily on nurses and nursing care. In reality, nurses carry out clinical research in a variety of areas, such as diabetes care, cancer care, and eating disorders.

In the last twenty years advances in medicine have involved, for the most part, advancing treatment, not cures. In other words, no cure for the illness has been discovered, but treatment for that illness has improved. However, sometimes the treatment itself causes problems for patients, such as the unwelcome side effects of chemotherapy. Nurses have opportunities to devise solutions to problems like these through research, such as studies on how to manage the illness and its treatment, thereby allowing individuals to lead happy and productive lives.

## The Curricula

Doctoral programs in nursing are aimed at preparing students for careers in health administration, education, clinical research, and advanced clinical practice. Basically, doctoral programs prepare nurses to be experts within the profession, prepared to assume leadership roles in a variety of academic and clinical settings, course work, and research. Students are trained as researchers and scholars to tackle complex health-care questions. Program emphasis may vary from a focus on health education to a concentration on policy research. The majority of doctoral programs confer the Doctor of Philosophy (Ph.D.) degree, but some award the Doctor of Nursing Science (D.N.S. or D.N.Sc.), the Doctor of Science in Nursing (D.S.N.), the Nursing Doctorate (N.D.), and the Doctor of Education (Ed.D.).

Doctoral nursing programs traditionally offer courses on the history and philosophy of nursing and the development and testing of nursing and other health-care techniques, as well as the social, economic, political, and ethical issues important to the field. Data management and research methodology are also areas of instruction. Students are expected to work individually on research projects and complete a dissertation.

Doctoral programs allow study on a full-or part-time basis. For graduate students who are employed and therefore seek flexibility in their schedules, many programs offer courses on weekends and in the evenings.

## Admission Requirements

Admission requirements for doctoral programs vary. Generally, a master's degree is necessary, but in some schools a master's degree is completed in conjunction with fulfillment of the doctoral degree requirements. Standard requirements include an RN license, Graduate Record Examinations (GRE) scores, college transcripts, letters of recommendation, and an essay. Students applying for doctoral-level study should have a solid foundation in nursing and an interest in research. Programs are usually the equivalent of three to five years of full-time study.

## Selecting a Doctoral Program

Selecting a doctoral program comes down to personal choice. Students work closely with professors, and thus the support and mentoring you receive while pursuing your degree is as vital as the quality of the facilities. The most important question is whether there is a "match" between your research interest and faculty research. Many of the same questions you would ask about baccalaureate and master's degree programs apply to doctoral programs. However, in a doctoral program, the contact with professors, the use of research equipment and facilities, and the program's flexibility in allowing you to choose your course of study are critical.

Other questions to consider include: Does the university consider research a priority? Does the university have adequate funding for student research? Many nurses with doctoral degrees make the natural transition into an academic career, but there are many other career options available for nurses prepared at this level. For example, nurses prepared at the doctoral level are often hired by large consulting firms to work with others in designing solutions to health-care delivery problems.

Others are hired by large hospital chains to manage various divisions, and some nurses with doctoral degrees are hired to manage complex health-care systems at the executive level. On another front, they conduct research and formulate national and international health-care policy. In short, because of the high level of education and a shortage of nurses prepared at this level, there are a number of options.

Needless to say, a doctoral education does provide individuals with a wide range of opportunities, with salaries commensurate with the type and level of responsibilities. Are there opportunities to present research findings at professional meetings? Is scholarship of faculty, alumni, and students presented at regional and national nursing meetings and subsequently published? Has the body of research done at a university enhanced the knowledge of nursing and health care?

Salaries are related to the various positions. Faculty salaries vary by the type of institution and by faculty rank, typically ranging from approximately $50,000 at the assistant professor level to above $100,000 at the professor level. Salaries of nurse executives also vary, with the lowest salaries being in small rural hospitals and the highest being in complex university medical centers. In the latter, average salaries are well above $100,000 and often reach close to $200,000 annually. Consultant salaries are wide-ranging but often consist of a base plus some percentage of work contracted. Clinical and research positions vary considerably by the type of institution and the nature of the work.

# AACN Indicators of Quality in Research-Focused Doctoral Programs in Nursing

Schools of nursing must consider the indicators of quality in evaluating their ability to mount research-focused doctoral programs. High-quality programs require a large number of increasingly scarce resources and a critical mass of faculty members and students. The "AACN Indicators of Quality in Research-Focused Doctoral Programs in Nursing" represent those indicators that should be present in a research-focused program.

There is considerable consensus within the discipline that while there are differences in the purpose and curricula of Ph.D. and Doctor of Nursing/Doctor of Nursing Science programs; most programs emphasize preparation for research. Therefore, AACN recommends continuing with a single set of quality indicators for research-focused doctoral programs in nursing, whether the program leads to a Ph.D. or to a Doctor of Nursing or Doctor of Nursing Science degree.

The following indicators apply to the Doctor of Philosophy (Ph.D.) in nursing, Doctor of Nursing Science (D.N.S. or D.N.Sc.), and Doctor of Nursing (N.D.) degrees.

## Faculty

I. Represent and value a diversity of backgrounds and intellectual perspectives.

II. Meet the requirements of the parent institution for graduate research and doctoral education; a substantial proportion of faculty hold earned doctorates in nursing.

III. Conceptualize and implement productive programs of research and scholarship that are developed over time and build upon previous work, are at the cutting edge of the field of inquiry, are congruent with research priorities within nursing and its constituent communities, include a substantial proportion of extramural funding, and attract and engage students.

IV. Create an environment in which mentoring, socialization of students, and the existence of a community of scholars is evident.

V. Assist students in understanding the value of programs of research and scholarship that continue over time and build upon previous work.

VI. Identify, generate, and utilize resources within the university and the broader community to support program goals.

VII. Devote a significant proportion of time to dissertation advisement. Generally, each faculty member should serve as the major adviser/chair for no more than 3 to 5 students during the dissertation phase.

## Programs of Study

The emphasis of the program of study is consistent with the mission of the parent institution, the discipline of nursing, and the degree awarded. The faculty's areas of expertise and scholarship determine specific foci in the program of study. Requirements and their sequence for progression in the program are clear and available to students in writing. Common elements of the program of study are outlined below.

I. Core and related course content—the distribution between nursing and supporting content is consistent with the mission and goals of the program, and the student's area of focus and course work are included in the following:

   A. Historical and philosophical foundations to the development of nursing knowledge

   B. Existing and evolving substantive nursing knowledge

   C. Methods and processes of theory/knowledge development

   D. Research methods and scholarship appropriate to inquiry

   E. Development related to roles in academic, research, practice, or policy environments

II. Elements for formal and informal teaching and learning focus on the following:

   A. Analytical and leadership strategies for dealing with social, ethical, cultural, economic, and political issues related to nursing, health care, and research

   B. Progressive and guided student scholarship

research experiences, including exposure to faculty's interdisciplinary research programs

C. Immersion experiences that foster the student's development as a nursing leader, scholarly practitioner, educator, and/or nurse scientist

D. Socialization opportunities for scholarly development in roles that complement students' career goals

III. Outcome indicators for the programs of study include the following:

A. Advancement to candidacy requires faculty's satisfactory evaluation (e.g., comprehensive exam) of the student's basic knowledge of elements I-A through I-E identified above

B. Dissertations represent original contributions to the scholarship of the field

C. Systematic evaluation of graduate outcomes is conducted at regular intervals

D. Within three to five years of completion, graduates have designed and secured funding for a research study, or, within two years of completion, graduates have utilized the research process to address an issue of importance to the discipline of nursing or health care within their employment setting

E. Employers report satisfaction with graduates' leadership and scholarship at regular intervals

F. Graduates' scholarship and leadership are recognized through awards, honors, or external funding within three to five years of completion

## Resources

I. Sufficient human, financial, and institutional resources are available to accomplish the goals of the unit for doctoral education and faculty research.

A. The parent institution exhibits the following characteristics:

1) Research is an explicit component of the mission of the parent institution

2) An office of research administration

3) A record of peer-reviewed external funding

4) Postdoctoral programs

5) Internal research funds

6) Mechanisms that value, support, and reward faculty and student scholarship and role preparation

7) A university environment that fosters interdisciplinary research and collaboration

B. The nursing doctoral program exhibits the following characteristics:

1) Research-active faculty as well as other faculty experts to mentor students in other role preparations

2) Provide technical support for the following:

(a) Peer review of proposals and manuscripts in their development phases

(b) Research design expertise

(c) Data management and analysis support

(d) Hardware and software availability

(e) Expertise in grant proposal development and management

3) Procure space sufficient for the following:

(a) Faculty research needs

(b) Doctoral student study, meeting, and socializing

(c) Seminars

(d) Small-group work

C. Schools of exceptional quality also have the following:

1) Centers of research excellence

2) Endowed professorships

3) Mechanisms for financial support to allow full-time study

4) Master teachers capable of preparing graduates for faculty roles

II. State-of-the-art technical and support services are available and accessible to faculty, students, and staff for state-of-the-science information acquisition, communication, and management.

III. Library and database resources are sufficient to support the scholarly endeavors of faculty and students.

## Students

I. Students are selected from a pool of highly qualified and motivated applicants who represent diverse populations.

II. Students' research goals and objectives are congruent with faculty research expertise and scholarship and institutional resources.

III. Students are successful in obtaining financial support through competitive intramural and extramural academic and research awards.

IV. Students commit a significant portion of their time to the program and complete the program in a timely fashion.

V. Students establish a pattern of productive scholarship, collaborating with researchers in nursing and other disciplines in scientific endeavors that result in the presentation and publication of scholarly work that continues after graduation.

## Evaluation

The evaluation plan includes the following:

I. Is systematic, ongoing, comprehensive, and focuses on the university's and program's specific mission and goals.

II. Includes both process and outcome data related to these indicators of quality in research-focused doctoral programs.

III. Adheres to established ethical and process standards for formal program evaluation, e.g., confidentiality and rigorous quantitative and qualitative analyses.

IV. Involves students and graduates in evaluation activities.

V. Includes data from a variety of internal and external constituencies.

VI. Provides for comparison of program processes and outcomes to the standards of its parent graduate school/ university and selected peer groups within nursing.

VII. Includes ongoing feedback to program faculty, administrators, and external constituents to promote program improvement.

VIII. Provides comprehensive data in order to determine patterns and trends and recommend future directions at regular intervals.

IX. Is supported with adequate human, financial, and institutional resources.

---

Approved by AACN Membership, November 2001.

# What You Need to Know About Online Learning

**Sally Kennedy Ph.D., APRN, FNP-C, CNE**
*Assistant Professor*
*College of Nursing*
*Medical University of South Carolina*

Today's college students are more diverse than at any time in recent history. Potentially three generations, all with varied life experiences that shaped them, can be found in the classroom. The youngest baby boomers will turn 50 in 2014, and their motivation for returning to school can range from seeking a second career or returning for a graduate degree to finally having the time and money to enter college after having put their own children through school. Realizing the dangers of overgeneralizing, this group may not be particularly tech savvy and may prefer to learn via lecture and taking notes. They are highly motivated and independent thinkers. The GenXers—now between 33 and 50 years of age—may want to be taught only what is necessary to learn a new career, and they consider leisure time as important as school. For them, school is often a means to a career that will support their lifestyles. Millennials, on the other hand, grew up with technology, the Internet, and immediate access to information. They prefer to multi-task. Raised by doting or "helicopter" parents as they are commonly referred to, this generation expects immediate feedback and prefers to work within groups, most likely the result of close family ties.

Because the learning needs of these generations are quite diverse, the classroom experience is much different than in previous generations. The baby boomers may have difficulty with younger students reviewing their Facebook pages, sending e-mails, or chatting during class instead of attending to the instructor or the material. The younger generations may be bored with lectures, want to cut to the chase, and prefer in-class group activities to help them learn the content. The generational differences and many other variables should be considered when deciding whether the classroom experience or an online program is the best choice. Let's explore online education in more depth.

## Understanding the Basics

First consider what is meant by **online learning** versus **distance education** as colleges and universities may define them differently. "Distance education" may mean meeting in a classroom with other students to watch a live video feed of a professor lecturing from a remote location. Or, "distance education" may be synonymous with online education. Online education, or e-learning, refers to an online virtual classroom accessed from the Internet that uses a learning management system (LMS), such as Moodle, Blackboard, or Desire2Learn as the platform.

Online education can be delivered synchronously or asynchronously in a fully online or hybrid format—four different variables. **Synchronous delivery** means that students must be online at a specific time to meet with the instructor and classmates. Similar to a classroom-based course, this format removes the flexibility online education typically provides. **Asynchronous course delivery** means "not occurring at the same time." Even if the program is marketed as asynchronous, synchronous meetings could still be required, which will limit flexibility and thus negating a major benefit of online education.

Some programs marketed as online may really be **hybrid**. This means that some of the learning occurs online, but face-to-face meetings are also required. A course delivered **fully online** requires no synchronous meetings, or if they are held, attendance may be optional. Understanding how a school defines "online education" is essential.

## The Online Learning Experience

So what is an online class like? Content is typically delivered through reading assignments, posted PowerPoint slides, podcasts (audio recordings), or YouTube videos. Some faculty members will record their lectures on video. However, the actual learning usually takes place in **small group discussions** within the learning management system. Students post their responses to a discussion question posed by the instructor that will help explore the content of the lesson. The assumption is that students will be self-directed and review the materials independently before responding. This approach provides opportunities to learn from both classmates and faculty.

Expectations for the **frequency of participation** in weekly discussions will vary. Some schools prescribe the number of days students must post each week. It is important to understand the expectations of being online and involved in class discussions. Dedicating a few hours, three to five days each week to being online reviewing classmates' posts and then researching and writing a response may be more time on the computer than anticipated.

While **assignments** can vary in online courses, a group project may be required—sometimes in every class. Group projects entail frequent communication, often synchronously, and may entail face-to-face meetings. This removes some of the flexibility of taking classes online. Depending on the group members' comfort with technology, various real-time options are available, such as chat rooms or Skype. Text-based, real-time applications (e.g., GoogleDocs or Wikis) allow students to collaborate on a document and see each other's contribution immediately.

Students who prefer to work independently may find this requirement challenging, especially if **group grades** are given. This means that each student in the group will earn the same grade regardless of how the workload was divided. The flip side of group work is that team-building skills are learned, which will be valuable in the job market. Inquiring about requirements of group work will avoid surprises.

Expectations of **faculty feedback** should be considered. While every student in an online course is required to participate in online discussions, frequent feedback from faculty may not be forthcoming. Faculty may reply to a few posts in each discussion, but not all. Students, on the other hand, will be required to respond to classmates. Students bring a wealth of life experiences to online discussions. Being open to learning from peers may seem foreign, but it can be an enriching experience.

## Making the Decision

Before making the decision, students should consider their educational goals as well as personal preferences, such as preferred learning style, learner characteristics, family support, comfort with technology, and a reliable Internet connection.

Understanding **educational goals** and deciding what is important is a first step. If the full college campus experience including attending football games, meeting new people in the student union, and having direct contact with faculty in a classroom setting is desired, online education may not be the best choice. However, if the flexibility of studying "anytime and anywhere" there is an Internet connection is appealing, then earning a degree online can be a viable option. Many adults have other considerations such as family obligations, a full-time job, or the distance to travel to find the right program of study. These variables can make on-campus classroom attendance at the same time each week problematic.

People also have a preferred **learning style,** and it can be visual, auditory, hands-on, or interpersonal. While students can learn from other methods, they typically prefer one over the others. Visual learners prefer pictures and diagrams. Auditory learners prefer to listen to lectures or recordings. Others are hands-on and like to be actively involved doing a task, while others prefer to learn in groups.

Many learning style inventories are available online to determine one's preferred learning style. Googling "learning style inventory" will bring up multiple options. Keep in mind that online education is primarily text-based, so consideration should be given to spending hours reading on the computer. However, more and more faculty members are using technology in their online courses, creating YouTube videos or audio recordings, called podcasts, which can be listened to online or downloaded into an MP3 player. Instructors realize the importance of providing a variety of methods to engage students with various learning style preferences.

Think about the **ideal individual characteristics of online learners.** Students must be motivated to reach their educational goals and be self-directed, organized, and able to meet deadlines. Being committed to completing a degree and having the motivation to do so are key factors in pursuing higher education, regardless of the setting. However, these attributes are essential for taking classes online. Having **support** from family or loved ones is also ideal. Because schoolwork is often done from home, having a dedicated room or space and an atmosphere conducive to studying is essential.

Intimidated by **technology**? Being somewhat familiar with how to use the computer is necessary. How much? When pursuing a college degree, it is important that you are able to focus on your studies and not spend a great deal of time learning technology. Being able to send an e-mail with an attachment and use a word processing program, such as Microsoft Word, is essential. Inquiring about the necessity of using other types of software, such PowerPoint or Excel, is a good idea. Often schools provide support to help students learn program-specific software. Knowing up front what type of software is required and if learning support is available may provide peace of mind.

On the flip side, many students who grew up with technology may have a different set of questions. Knowing whether the learning management system is accessible on an iPad or a smartphone may be a concern. Having an alternate means of accessing the learning management system from work during a lunch break, for example, where the company's firewall may block certain Internet sites may be desired to maximize study time.

A fast and reliable **Internet connection** is a necessity. Dial-up connections (linked to a telephone line) may have download capabilities too slow for today's online courses. With slower connections, the video is often downloaded in pieces resulting in an interrupted feed when listening to a podcast or watching a YouTube Video. Although widespread Internet access exists in most metropolitan areas linked directly via cable, this may not the case in more rural communities.

In addition, many popular gathering places, such as coffee shops and some fast-food restaurant chains provide "hotspots" or free wireless (Wi-Fi) connection. This leads to another consideration for taking classes online, that of having a "Plan B" in place in case problems with the home Internet connection occur.

Finally, consider the cost of online education. Inquire about how tuition is charged—by the course or by the program. Some schools charge an extra fee to take a course online. Ask if financial aide covers this additional fee. Also, having up-to-date hardware including a computer and printer is important. Older computers may not have the processing speed or most current software to access the learning management system or complete assignments effectively and efficiently. Will this be an added cost? Additional technology requirements may be added by the particular program of study, such as a video camera, webcam, headset, or software such as the entire Microsoft Office Suite. Unexpected costs such as these can add up.

In summary, online education offers many advantages. It is flexible, accessible, creates opportunities for great student interaction, helps build team-based skills, provides immediate access to materials, fosters the development of needed technology skills for life, and decreases time and access barriers to achieving educational goals. The disadvantages are best viewed from an individual standpoint. Hopefully, what has been discussed here will assist students in making an informed decision about seeking a higher education online.

# THE INTERNATIONAL NURSING STUDENT

For many international students completing baccalaureate, master's, or doctoral nursing programs, their choice of learning institutions is obvious. U.S. and Canadian colleges and universities are thought to offer the finest programs of nursing education available anywhere in the world. U.S. and Canadian nursing programs are renowned for their breadth and flexibility, for the excellence of their basic curriculum structure, and for their commitment to extensive on-site clinical training. Nursing study in the United States and Canada also affords students the opportunity for hands-on learning and practice in the world's most technologically advanced health-care systems. For many international nursing students, and especially for students from countries that are medically underserved, these features make U.S. and Canadian nursing programs unsurpassed.

## Applying to Nursing School

The application process for international students often involves the completion of two separate written applications. Many colleges screen international candidates with a brief preliminary application requesting basic biographical and educational information. This document helps the admission officer determine whether the student has the minimum credentials for admission before requiring him or her to begin the lengthy process of completing and submitting final application forms.

Final applications to U.S. and Canadian colleges and universities vary widely in length and complexity, just as specific admission requirements vary from institution to institution. However, international nursing students must typically have a satisfactory scholastic record and demonstrated proficiency in English. To be admitted to any postsecondary institution in the United States or Canada, you must have satisfactorily completed a minimum of twelve years of elementary and secondary education. The customary cycle for this education includes a six-year elementary program, a three-year intermediate program, and a three-year postsecondary program, generally referred to as high school in the United States. In addition, nursing school programs generally require successful completion of several years of high school-level mathematics and science.

The documentation of satisfactory completion of secondary schooling (and university education, in the case of graduate-level applicants) is achieved through submission of school reports, transcripts, and teacher recommendations. Because academic records and systems of evaluation differ widely from one educational system to the next, request that your school include a guide to grading standards. If you have received your secondary education at a school in which English is not the language of instruction, be certain to include official translations of all documents.

International students who have completed some university-level course work in their native country may be eligible to receive credit for equivalent courses at the U.S. or Canadian institution in which they enroll. Under special circumstances, practical nursing experience may also qualify for university credit. Policies regarding the transfer of or qualification for credits based on education or nursing experience outside the United States (or Canada for Canadian schools) vary widely, so be certain to inquire about these policies at the universities or colleges that interest you.

Language skills are a key to scholastic success. "The ability to speak, write, and understand English is an important determinant of success," says Joann Weiss, former Director of the Nursing and Latin American Studies dual-degree programs at the University of New Mexico in Albuquerque. Her advice for potential international applicants is simple: "Develop a true command of written and spoken English." English proficiency for students who have not received formal education in English-speaking schools is usually demonstrated via the Test of English as a Foreign Language (TOEFL); minimum test scores of 550 to 580 are commonly required. This policy, as well as the level of proficiency required, varies from school to school, so be sure to investigate each college's policies.

In addition, most universities offer some form of English language instruction for international students, often under the rubric ESL (English as a second language). Students who require additional language study to meet admission requirements or students who wish to deepen their skills in written or verbal English should inquire about ESL program availability.

Many colleges and universities also require that all undergraduate applicants take a standardized test—either the SAT and three SAT Subject Tests or the ACT. Like their U.S. and Canadian counterparts, international applicants to graduate-level nursing programs are required by most institutions to take the standardized Graduate Record Examinations (GRE).

Applicants should also be aware that financial assistance for international students is usually quite limited. To spare international students economic hardship during their schooling in the United States or Canada, many colleges and universities require them to demonstrate the availability of sufficient financial resources for tuition and minimum living expenses and supplies. As with so many admission requirements, policies regarding financial aid vary considerably; find out early what the policies are at the colleges that interest you.

## Attending School in the United States or Canada

Once you are accepted by the college or university of your choice, take full advantage of the academic and personal advising systems offered to international students. Most institutions of higher education in the United States and Canada maintain an international student advisory office staffed with trained counselors. In addition to general academic counseling and planning, an international adviser can assist in a broad range of matters ranging from immigration and visa concerns to employment opportunities and health-care issues.

With few exceptions, all university students also obtain specialized academic counseling from an assigned faculty adviser. Faculty advisers monitor academic performance and progress and try to ensure that students meet the institutional requirements for their degree. Faculty advisers are excellent sources of information regarding course selection, and some advisers offer tutorials or special language or educational support to international students.

Although all university students face academic challenges, international students often find life outside the classroom equally demanding. Suddenly introduced into a new culture where the way of life may be dramatically different from that of their native country, international students often face a variety of social, domestic, medical, religious, or emotional concerns. Questions about social conventions, meal preparation, or other personal concerns can often be addressed by your international or faculty adviser.

Lorraine Rudowski, Assistant Professor and Coordinator of the International Health Program at the College of Health and Human Services at George Mason University in Fairfax, Virginia, emphasizes the benefits of a strong relationship with your advisers: "My job as an adviser is to provide comprehensive support to my students—from academic counseling and opportunities for language development to emotional support and guidance to attending parties or other informal social events to ease the sense of social and personal isolation often experienced by foreign students."

Dr. Rudowski says that international students would do well to find a sponsor or confidant within the university who understands the conventions of the student's native country. "A culturally sensitive sponsor is better equipped to understand the unique needs of each international student and is much more likely to help students obtain the assistance they need, whether we're talking about religious issues, help with study methods or social skills, or simply knowing how to deal with such everyday chores as cooking and cleaning. All of these matters can be sources of deep concern to international students."

Yet for all the academic, social, and personal challenges facing international nursing students, there is good news. Deans of nursing, professors, and advisers typically praise the motivation and determination of their international students, and international nursing students often boast matriculation rates that match or exceed those of their U.S. and Canadian counterparts.

For more information about the rules and regulations governing international students' entrance to U.S. schools, log on to educationUSA, part of the U.S. Department of State's website, at http:// educationusa.state.gov.

# Specialty Nursing Organizations

**Academy of Medical-Surgical Nurses**
East Holly Avenue
Box 56
Pitman, NJ 08071-0056
866-877-AMSN (2676) (toll-free)
E-mail: amsn@ajj.com
www.amsn.org

**Air & Surface Transport Nurses Association**
7995 East Prentice Avenue
Suite 100
Greenwood Village, CO 80111
800-897-NFNA (6362) (toll-free)
Fax: 303-770-1614
www.astna.org

**American Academy of Ambulatory Care Nursing**
East Holly Avenue
Box 56
Pitman, NJ 08071-0056
800-262-6877 (toll-free)
E-mail: aaacn@ajj.com
www.aaacn.org

**American Association of Critical-Care Nurses**
101 Columbia
Aliso Viejo, CA 92656-4109
949-362-2000
800-899-AACN (2226) (toll-free)
E-mail: info@aacn.org
www.aacn.org

**American Association of Diabetes Educators**
200 West Madison Street
Suite 800
Chicago, IL 60606
800-338-3633 (toll-free)
Fax: 312-424-2427
E-mail: education@aadenet.org
www.aadenet.org

**American Association of Legal Nurse Consultants**
330 N. Wabash Avenue
Chicago, IL 60611
877-402-2562 (toll-free)
Fax: 312-673-6655
E-mail: info@aalnc.org
www.aalnc.org

**American Association of Neuroscience Nurses**
8735 W. Higgins Road
Suite 300
Chicago, IL 60631
847-557-2266
888-557-2266 (toll-free in the U.S. only)
Fax: 847-375-6430
E-mail: info@aann.org
www.aann.org

**American Association of Nurse Anesthetists**
222 South Prospect Avenue
Park Ridge, IL 60068-4001
855-526-2262 (toll-free)
Fax: 847-692-6968
E-mail: info@aana.com
www.aana.com

**The American Association of Nurse Attorneys**
3416 Primm Lane
Birmingham, AL 35216
205-824-7615
877-538-2262 (toll-free)
Fax: 205-823-2760
E-mail: taana@primemanagement.net
www.taana.org

**American Association of Nurse Practitioners (AANP)**
AANP National Administrative Office
PO Box 12846
Austin, TX 78711
512-442-4262
Fax: 512-442-6469
E-mail: admin@aanp.org
www.aanp.org/about-aanp

**American Association of Occupational Health Nurses**
7794 Grow Drive
Pensacola, FL 32514
850-474-6963
800-241-8014 (toll-free)
Fax: 850-484-8762
E-mail: aaohn@dancyamc.com
www.aaohn.org

**American College of Nurse-Midwives**
8403 Colesville Road
Suite 1550
Silver Spring, MD 20910
240-485-1800
Fax: 240-485-1818
www.midwife.org

**American Holistic Nurses Association**
100 SE 9th Street
Suite 3A
Topeka, KS 66612-1213
785-234-1712
800-278-2462 (toll-free)
Fax: 785-234-1713
E-mail: info@ahna.org
www.ahna.org

**American Nephrology Nurses' Association**
East Holly Avenue
Box 56
Pitman, NJ 08071-0056
856-256-2320
888-600-2662 (toll-free)
Fax: 856-589-7463

E-mail: anna@ajj.com
www.annanurse.org

**American Psychiatric Nurses Association**
3141 Fairview Park Drive
Suite 625
Falls Church, VA 22042
855-863-APNA (2762; toll-free)
Fax: 855-883-APNA (2762)
www.apna.org

**American Public Health Association**
800 I Street, NW
Washington, DC 20001-3710
202-777-APHA
Fax: 202-777-2534
E-mail: comments@apha.org
www.apha.org

**American Society for Pain Management Nursing**
P.O. Box 15473
Lenexa, KS 66285-5473
888-34ASPMN (toll-free)
913-895-4606
Fax: 913-895-4652
E-mail: aspmn@goamp.com
www.aspmn.org

**American Society of Ophthalmic Registered Nurses**
P.O. Box 193030
San Francisco, CA 94119-3030
415-561-8513
Fax: 415-561-8531
E-mail: asorn@aao.org
www.asorn.org

**American Society of PeriAnesthesia Nurses**
90 Frontage Road
Cherry Hill, NJ 08034-1424
877-737-9696 (toll-free)
Fax: 856-616-9601
E-mail: aspan@aspan.org
www.aspan.org

**American Society of Plastic Surgical Nurses**
500 Cummings Center
Suite 4550
Beverly, MA 01915
877-337-9315 (toll-free)
Fax: 978-524-8890
www.aspsn.org

**Association for Death Education and Counseling**
111 Deer Lake Road
Suite 100
Deerfield, IL 60015
847-509-0403
Fax: 847-480-9282
www.adec.org

**Association for Professionals in Infection Control and Epidemiology**
1275 K Street, NW
Suite 1000
Washington, DC 20005-4006
202-789-1890
800-650-9570 (toll-free)
Fax: 202-789-1899
E-mail: info@apic.org
www.apic.org

**Association for Radiologic & Imaging Nursing (ARIN)**
390 Amwell Road
Suite 402
Hillsborough, NJ 08844
908-359-5308
866-486-2762 (toll-free)
Fax: 908-450-1398
E-mail: info@arinursing.org
www.arinursing.org

**Association of Nurses in AIDS Care**
3538 Ridgewood Road
Akron, OH 44333-3122
800-260-6780 (toll-free)
330-670-0101
Fax: 330-670-0109
E-mail: anac@anacnet.org
www.anacnet.org

**Association of Pediatric Hematology/Oncology Nurses**
8735 W. Higgins Road
Suite 300
Chicago, IL 60631
855-202-9760 (toll-free in the U.S. only)
Fax: 847-375-6478
E-mail: info@aphon.org
www.aphon.org

**Association of Perioperative Registered Nurses**
2170 South Parker Road
Suite 400
Denver, CO 80231
800-755-2676 (toll-free)
303-755-6300
Fax: 800-847-0045 (toll-free)
E-mail: custsvc@aorn.org
www.aorn.org

**Association of Rehabilitation Nurses**
8735 W. Higgins Road
Suite 300
Chicago, IL 60631-2738
800-229-7530 (toll-free)
E-mail: info@rehabnurse.org
www.rehabnurse.org

**Association of Women's Health, Obstetric and Neonatal Nurses**
2000 L Street, NW
Suite 740
Washington, DC 20036
202-261-2400
800-673-8499 (toll-free in the U.S.)
800-245-0231 (toll-free in Canada)
Fax: 202-728-0575
E-mail: customerservice@awhonn.org
www.awhonn.org

**Dermatology Nurses' Association**
15000 Commerce Parkway
Suite C
Mount Laurel, NJ 08054
800-454-4362 (toll-free)
Fax: 856-439-0525
E-mail: dna@dnanurse.org
www.dnanurse.org

**Developmental Disabilities Nurses Association**
P.O. Box 536489
Orlando, FL 32853-6489
800-888-6733 (toll-free)
407-835-0642
Fax: 407-426-7440
www.ddna.org

**Emergency Nurses Association**
915 Lee Street
Des Plaines, IL 60016-6569
800-900-9659 (toll-free)
E-mail: www.ena.org/Pages/ContactUs.aspx
www.ena.org

**Hospice and Palliative Nurses Association**
One Penn Center West
Suite 229
Pittsburgh, PA 15276-0100
412-787-9301
Fax: 412-787-9305
E-mail: hpna@hpna.org
www.hpna.org

**Infusion Nurses Society**
315 Norwood Park South
Norwood, MA 02062
781-440-9408
Fax: 781-440-9409
E-mail: ins@ins1.org
www.ins1.org

**International Nurses Society on Addictions**
P.O. Box 14846
Lenexa, KS 66285-4846
877-6-INTNSA (646-8672) (toll-free)
Fax: 913-895-4652
E-mail: intnsa@intnsa.org
www.intnsa.org

**National Association for Home Care & Hospice**
228 Seventh Street, SE
Washington, DC 20003
202-547-7424
Fax: 202-547-3540
E-mail: exec@nahc.org
www.nahc.org

**National Association of Clinical Nurse Specialists**
100 North 20th Street
4th Floor
Philadelphia, PA 19103
215-320-3881
Fax: 215-564-2175
E-mail: info@nacns.org
www.nacns.org

**National Association of Directors of Nursing Administration/Long Term Care**
11353 Reed Hartman Highway
Suite 210
Cincinnati, OH 45241
800-222-0539 (toll-free)
513-791-3679
Fax: 513-791-3699
www.nadona.org

**National Association of Neonatal Nurses**
8735 W. Higgins Road
Suite 300
Chicago, IL 60631
847-375-3660
800-451-3795 (toll-free)
Fax: 866-927-5321
E-mail: info@nann.org
www.nann.org

**National Association of Nurse Practitioners in Women's Health**
505 C Street, NE
Washington, DC 20002
202-543-9693, Ext. 1
E-mail: info@npwh.org
www.npwh.org

**National Association of Orthopaedic Nurses**
330 N. Wabash Avenue
Suite 2000
Chicago, IL 60611
800-289-NAON (6266) (toll-free)
Fax: 312-673-6941
E-mail: naon@orthonurse.org
www.orthonurse.org

**National Association of Pediatric Nurse Practitioners**
5 Hanover Square
Suite 1401
New York, NY 10004
917-746-8300
Fax: 212-785-1713
E-mail: info@napnap.org
www.napnap.org

**National Association of School Nurses**
1100 Wayne Avenue #925
Silver Spring, MD 20910
240-821-1130
E-mail: nasn@nasn.org
www.nasn.org

**National Gerontological Nursing Association**
3493 Lansdowne Drive
Suite 2
Lexington, KY 40517
800-723-0560 (toll-free)
859-977-7453
Fax: 859-271-0607
E-mail: info@ngna.org
www.ngna.org

**National Organization of Nurse Practitioner Faculties**
1615 M Street, NW
Suite 270
Washington, DC 20006
202-289-8044
Fax: 202-289-8046
E-mail: nonpf@nonpf.org
www.nonpf.com

**Oncology Nursing Society**
125 Enterprise Drive
Pittsburgh, PA 15275
866-257-4ONS (4667) (toll-free)
412-859-6100
Fax: 877-369-5497 (toll-free)
E-mail: customer.service@ons.org
www.ons.org

**Preventive Cardiovascular Nurses Association**
613 Williamson Street
Suite 200
Madison, WI 53703
608-250-2440
E-mail: info@pcna.net
www.pcna.net

**Respiratory Nursing Society**
Donna C. Bond
3816 Hawthorne Avenue
Richmond, VA 23222
E-mail: dcbond@carilionclinc.org
www.respiratorynursingsociety.org

**Society for Vascular Nursing**
100 Cummings Center
Suite 124A
Beverly, MA 01915
888-536-4SVN (4786) (toll-free)
978-927-7800
Fax: 978-927-7872
www.svnnet.org

**Society of Gastroenterology Nurses and Associates, Inc.**
330 N. Wabash Avenue
Suite 2000
Chicago, IL 60611-7621
800-245-7462 (toll-free)
312-321-5165 (in Illinois)
Fax: 312-673-6694
E-mail: sgna@smithbucklin.com
www.sgna.org

**Society of Otorhinolaryngology and Head-Neck Nurses**
207 Downing Street
New Smyrna Beach, FL 32168
386-428-1695
Fax: 386-423-7566
E-mail: info@sohnnurse.com
www.sohnnurse.com

**Society of Urologic Nurses and Associates**
East Holly Avenue
Box 56
Pitman, NJ 08071-0056
888-827-7862 (toll-free)
E-mail: suna@ajj.com
www.suna.org

**Wound, Ostomy and Continence Nurses Society**
15000 Commerce Parkway
Suite C
Mt. Laurel, NJ 08054
888-224-WOCN (9626) (toll-free)
Fax: 856-439-0525
E-mail: wocn_info@wocn.org
www.wocn.org

# PAYING FOR YOUR NURSING EDUCATION

Whether you are considering a baccalaureate degree in nursing or have completed your undergraduate education and are planning to attend graduate school, finding a way to pay for that education is essential.

The cost to attend college is considerable and is increasing each year at a rate faster than most other products and services. In fact, the cost of a nursing education at a public four-year college can be more than $14,000 per year, including tuition, fees, books, room and board, transportation, and miscellaneous expenses. The cost at a private college or university, at either the graduate or undergraduate level, can be more than $30,000 per year.

This is where financial aid comes in. Financial aid is money made available by the government and other sources to help students who otherwise would be unable to attend college. In 2012-13, $238.5 billion in financial aid was distributed to undergraduate and graduate students in the form of grants, Federal Work-Study, federal loans, and federal tax credits and deductions. In addition, students borrowed about $8.8 billion from private, state, and institutional sources. (College Board, *Trends in Student Aid 2013*). Most college students in this country receive some form of aid, and all prospective students should investigate what may be available. Most of this aid is given to students because neither they nor their families have sufficient personal resources to pay for college. This type of aid is referred to as need-based aid. Recipients of need-based aid include traditional students just out of high school or college and older, nontraditional students who are returning to college or graduate school.

There is also merit-based aid, which is awarded to students who display a particular ability. Merit scholarships are based primarily on academic merit, but may include other special talents. Many colleges and graduate schools offer merit-based aid in addition to need-based aid to their students.

## Types and Sources of Financial Aid

There are four types of aid:

1. Scholarships
2. Grants
3. Loans
4. Student employment (including fellowships and assistantships)

Scholarships and grants are outright gifts and do not have to be repaid. Loans are borrowed money that must be repaid with interest, usually after graduation. Student employment provides jobs during the academic year for which students are paid. For graduate students, student employment may include fellowships and assistantships in which students work, receive free or reduced tuition, and may be paid a stipend for living expenses.

Most of the aid available to students is need-based and comes from the federal government through nine financial aid programs. Four of these programs are grant-based and are only available to undergraduate students:

1. Federal Pell Grants
2. Academic Competitive Grants
3. SMART Grants
4. Federal Supplemental Educational Opportunity Grants

Four are loan programs:

1. Federal Perkins Loan
2. Direct Stafford Loans (subsidized and unsubsidized)
3. Federal Direct Graduate PLUS loans
4. Federal Direct PLUS Loans

The final program is a student employment program called the Federal Work-Study Program, which is also awarded to undergraduate and graduate students based on financial need.

The federal government also offers a number of programs especially for nursing students. For example, the U.S. Department of Health and Human Services offers Nursing Student Scholarships, Nursing Student Loans, the Nursing Education Loan Repayment Program, and the Scholarship for Disadvantaged Students (SDS) program. Some of these programs require that the student work in a designated nursing shortage area for a period of time. These programs are administered by the nursing school's financial aid office. For more information, log on to http://bhpr.hrsa.gov/dsa.

The second-largest source of aid is from the colleges and universities themselves. Almost all colleges have aid programs from institutional resources, most of which are grants, scholarships, and fellowships. These can be either need-or merit-based.

A third source of aid is from state governments. Nearly every state provides aid for students attending college in their home state, although most only have programs for undergraduates. Most state aid programs are scholarships and grants, but many states now have low-interest loan and work-study programs. Most state grants and scholarships are not "portable," meaning that they cannot be used outside of your home state of residence.

A fourth source of aid is from private sources such as corporations, hospitals, civic associations, unions, fraternal organizations, foundations, and religious groups that give scholarships, grants, and fellowships to students. Most of

### *Federal Financial Aid Programs*

| Program | Who Benefits? | Maximum/Year |
|---|---|---|
| Federal Pell Grants | Undergraduate students | $5550 |
| Federal Supplemental Educational Opportunity Grants (FSEOG) | Undergraduate students | $4000 |
| Academic Competitivess Grants | Undergraduate students who are eligible for Federal Pell Grants | $750 (first-year students)<br>$1300 (second-year students) |
| SMART Grants | Undergraduate students who are eligible for Federal Pell Grants | $4000 (third- and fourth-year students) |
| Federal Perkins Loans | Undergraduate students | $5500 |
| | Graduate students | $8000 |
| Federal Direct Loans (subsidized) | Undergraduate students | $3500 (first-year students)<br>$4500 (second-year students)<br>$5500 (third-year students and above) |
| | Graduate students* | $8500 |
| Federal Direct Loans (unsubsidized) | Dependent undergraduate students | $2000 |
| | Independent undergraduate students | $6000 (first- and second-year students)<br>$7000 (third-year students and above) |
| | Graduate students | $12,000 |
| Federal Direct PLUS Loans | Dependent undergraduate students | Up to cost of attendance (less other financial aid received) |
| Federal Direct Graduate PLUS loans | Graduate and professional students | Up to cost of attendance (less other financial aid received) |

**Only eligible if period(s) of enrollment began prior to 7/1/2012.*

***The unsubsidized Federal Direct Loan amounts provided are in addition to the subsidized Federal Direct Loan amounts.***

these are not based on need, although the amount of the scholarship may vary depending upon financial need. The competition for these scholarships can be formidable, but the rewards are well worth the process. Many companies also offer tuition reimbursement to employees and their dependents. Check with the personnel or human resources department at your or your parents' place of employment for benefit and eligibility information.

## Eligibility for Financial Aid

Since most of the financial aid that college students receive is need-based, colleges employ a process called "need analysis" to determine student awards. For most applicants, the student and parents (if the student is a dependent) fill out one form on which family income, assets, and household information are reported. This form is the Free Application for Federal Student Aid (FAFSA). The end result of this need analysis is the student's "Expected Family Contribution," or EFC, representing the amount a family should be able to contribute toward education expenses.

### Dependent or Independent

The basic principle of financial aid is that the primary responsibility for paying college expenses resides with the family. In determining your EFC, you will first need to know who makes up your "family." That will tell you whose income is counted when the need analysis is done.

***Graduate Students:*** By definition, all graduate nursing students are considered independent for federal aid purposes. Therefore, only your income and assets (and your spouse's if you are married) count in determining your expected family contribution. (Due to the recent Supreme Court ruling, the use of "marriage" and "spouse" now includes same-sex marriages.)

***Undergraduate Students:*** If you are financially dependent upon your parents, their income and assets, as well as yours, are counted toward the family contribution. If you are financially independent of your parents, only your income (and your spouse's if you are married) counts in the calculation.

According to the U.S. Department of Education, in order to be considered independent for financial aid for 2014–15, you must meet any ONE of the following:

- You were born before January 1, 1987.
- You are or will be enrolled in a master's or doctoral program (beyond a bachelor's degree) during the 2014–15 school year.
- You are married on the day you apply (even if you are separated but not divorced).
- You have children who receive more than half their support from you.
- You have dependents (other than your children or spouse) who live with you and who receive more than half of their support from you and will continue to receive more than half their support from you through June 30, 2014.
- Both your parents are deceased, or you are an orphan or ward of the court (or were a ward of the court until age 18).
- You are engaged in active duty in the U.S. Armed Forces or are a National Guard or Reserves enlistee and are called to active duty for purposes other than training.
- You are a veteran of the U.S. Armed Forces. ("Veteran" includes students who attended a U.S. service academy and who were released under a condition other than dishonorable. Contact your financial aid office for more information.)
- You were verified on or after the start of the award year for which the FAFSA is filed, as either an unaccompanied youth who is homeless or at risk of being homeless and self-supporting.

If you meet any one of these conditions, you are considered independent and only your income and assets (and your spouse's if you are married) count toward your family contribution. Remember, if you are attending school as a graduate student, you are automatically independent for federal aid consideration.

If there are extraordinary circumstances, the financial aid administrator at the college you will be attending has the authority to make a change to your dependency status. You will need to provide extensive documentation of your family situation.

## Determining Cost and Need

Now that you know approximately how much you and your family will be expected to contribute toward your college expenses, you can subtract the EFC from the total cost of attending a college or graduate school to determine the amount of need-based financial aid for which you will be eligible. The average cost listed assumes that you will be attending nursing school full-time. If you will be attending part-time, you should adjust costs accordingly. For a more accurate estimate of the cost of attendance at a particular college, check the financial aid information usually available on the college's website or in its publications.

## Applying for Financial Aid

After you have subtracted your EFC from the cost of your education and determined your financial need, you will have a better understanding of how much assistance you will need. Even if you do not demonstrate financial need, you are still encouraged to file the FAFSA, as you may be eligible for assistance that is not based on need. The process for applying for aid can be confusing if you are not familiar with completing these types of applications. If you need assistance, you should contact the financial aid office for help.

Undergraduate and graduate students applying for aid must fill out the FAFSA. This application is available in high school guidance offices, college financial aid offices, state education department offices, and many local libraries. You are strongly encouraged to file the FAFSA online at www.fafsa.ed.gov. If you file online, you will need to have a Personal Identification Number (PIN). The PIN can easily be obtained at www.pin.ed.gov. Dependent students will need a PIN for themselves and one parent. When you file online, your application is processed more rapidly, and you are far less likely to make major errors. The FAFSA, whether you file a paper application or online, becomes available in November or December, almost a year before the fall term in which you will enroll, but you cannot complete it until after January 1.

If you file a paper application, you and your parents (if appropriate) must sign your completed FAFSA and mail it to a processing center in the envelope provided. Do not send any additional materials, but do make copies of everything you filled out.

The processing center enters the data into a computer that runs the federal methodology of need analysis to calculate your EFC. This center then distributes the information to the schools and agencies you listed on the FAFSA. The actual determination of need and the awarding of aid are handled by each college financial aid office.

It is generally recommended that you complete the FAFSA as soon as possible after January 1. You should check with each college to which you are applying to determine its filing deadline. It is important to meet all college deadlines for financial aid, since there is a limited amount of funds available. However, students who procrastinate can still file for federal aid any time during the year.

## What Happens After You Submit the FAFSA?

Two to four weeks after you send in your completed FAFSA, you will receive a Student Aid Report (SAR) that shows the information you reported and your official EFC. This is an opportunity for you to make corrections or to have the information sent to any new school you are considering that you did not list on the original FAFSA. The SAR contains instructions on how to make corrections or to designate additional schools. If you provided an e-mail address on the FAFSA, this information will be sent to this address rather than through conventional mail.

At the same time that you receive the SAR, the college(s) you specified also receive the information. The financial aid office at the school may request additional information from you or may ask you to provide documentation verifying the information you reported on the FAFSA. For example, they may ask you for a copy of your (and your parents') income tax return or official forms verifying any untaxed income you or your parents received (e.g., Social Security, disability, or welfare benefits).

Once the financial aid office is satisfied that the information is correct, you will receive a financial aid offer. Many colleges like to make this offer in the spring prior to the fall enrollment so that students have ample opportunity to make their plans. However, some colleges will wait until summer to notify you.

## Other Applications

The FAFSA is the required form for applying for federal and most state financial aid programs. Most schools also use the FASFA to determine eligibility for institutional aid; however, some colleges and graduate schools require additional information to determine eligibility for institutional aid. Nearly 500 colleges and universities, plus more than 200 private scholarship programs, employ a form called the Financial Aid PROFILE® from the College Scholarship Service (CSS). While the form is similar to the FAFSA, several additional questions must be answered for colleges that award their own funds. You begin the process in October or November by completing a PROFILE Registration form on which you designate the schools to which you are applying. A few weeks later, you will receive a customized, individualized application that you complete and send back to CSS, which, in turn, forwards your application information to the schools you selected. There is a fee charged for each school listed on the application.

## Financial Aid Offer

If you qualify for need-based aid, a college will typically offer a combination of different types of assistance— scholarship, grant, loan, and work-study—to meet this need. An offer of aid usually is made after you have been admitted to the college or program. You may accept all or part of the financial aid package. If you will be enrolling part-time (fewer than 12 credits per term), be sure to contact the financial aid office in advance since this may have impact on your overall aid eligibility.

If you are awarded Federal Work-Study Program aid, the amount you are awarded represents your earnings limit for the academic year under the program. In general, schools assume you will earn this money on an hourly basis, so it cannot be used to pay your term bill charges. On most campuses there are many jobs available for students. Not all of these are limited to students in the Federal Work-Study Program. Check with your placement office or financial aid office for more information.

Keep in mind that the student budget used to establish eligibility for financial aid is based on averages. It may not reflect your actual expenses. Student budgets usually reflect most expenses for categories of students (for example, single students living in their parents' home, campus-provided housing, or living in an apartment or house near campus, etc.). But if you have unusual expenses that are not included, you should consult with your school's financial aid office regarding a budget adjustment.

## If Your Family or Job Situation Changes

Because a family contribution is based on the previous year's income, many nursing students find they do not qualify for need-based aid (or not enough to pay their full expenses). This is particularly true of older students who were working full-time last year but are no longer doing so or who will not work during the academic year. If this is your situation, you should speak to a counselor in the financial aid office about making an adjustment in your family contribution need analysis. Financial aid administrators may make changes to any of the elements that go into the need analysis if there are conditions that merit a change. Contact the financial aid office for more information.

## Don't Qualify for Need-Based Aid?

If you don't qualify for need-based aid but feel you do not have the resources necessary to pay for college or graduate school, you still have several options available.

First, there is a student loan program for which need is not a consideration. This is the Federal Direct Loan (unsubsidized) program. There is also a non-need-based loan program for parents of dependent students or for graduate or professional students called the Direct PLUS Loan program. If you or your parents are interested in borrowing through one of these programs, you should check with the financial aid office for more information. There are also numerous private or alternative loan sources available. For many students, borrowing to pay for a nursing education can be an excellent investment in one's future. At the same time, be sure that you do not overburden yourself when it comes to paying back the loans. Before you accept a federal student loan, the financial aid office will schedule a counseling session to make certain that you know the terms of the loan and that you understand the ramifications of borrowing. If you can do without, it is often suggested that you postpone student loans until they are absolutely necessary.

For graduate nursing students, Federal Direct PLUS Loans are available to graduate and professional students. Students who are looking into alternative loan programs should be sure to compare any terms and conditions with this federal program. Students can borrow Federal Direct Graduate PLUS loans and alternative loan funds up to the cost of attendance less any other financial aid received.

A second option if you do not qualify for need-based aid is to search for scholarships. Be wary of scholarship search companies that promise to find you scholarships but require you to pay a fee. There are many resources that provide lists of scholarships, including the annually published *Peterson's Scholarships, Grants & Prizes* and *How to Get Money for College,* which are available in libraries, counselors' offices, and bookstores. Non-need scholarships require application forms and are extremely competitive; only a handful of students from thousands of applicants receive awards.

Another option is to work more hours at an existing job or to find a paying position if you do not already have one. The student employment or placement office at your college should be able to help you find a job, either on or off campus. Many colleges have vacancies remaining after they have placed Federal Work-Study Program eligible students in their jobs.

You should always contact the financial aid office at the school you plan to attend for advice concerning sources of college-based and private aid.

## Employer-Paid Financial Aid

Robert Atwater is a certified personnel consultant and certified medical staff recruiter and founder of Atwater Consulting in Lilburn, Georgia, a consulting firm for the employment and recruitment of physician assistants, nurse practitioners, certified nurse midwives, nurses, and nursing managers.

Health-care administrators, Atwater says, have coined a phrase to characterize their efforts to meet the growing demand for nurses with better skills and training: "Grow your own."

"Constant training through the course of a nursing career is the only way to keep pace with the technological and medical advances, but it can be a financial burden on the nurse," Atwater says.

That is why many employers now give qualified employees a benefits package that includes a continuing education allowance.

For the employer, this type of benefits package can help to recruit candidates willing to further their careers through education. Administrators feel it is the best way to build a staff of nurses with up-to-date certifications in all areas.

In a constantly expanding field, nurses should be required to continue and update their education. The nurses get a paid education, can keep their job, and work flexible hours while they are going to school. Inquiries about these allowances should be made during an interview with the company's human resources department. Additional information can be obtained from the nursing school, local hospitals in the area, or from other health-care professionals. There are many attractive options available because of the nationwide shortage of qualified nurses. Check with a number of potential employers before agreeing to any long-term contract.

# Sources of Financial Aid for Nursing Students

The largest proportion of financial aid for college expenses comes from the federal government and is given on the basis of financial need. Beyond this federal need-based aid—which should always be the primary source of financial aid that a prospective student investigates and which is given regardless of one's field of study—a sizable amount of scholarship assistance specifically meant to help students in nursing programs is also available from government agencies, associations, civic or fraternal organizations, and corporations. These sources of aid can be particularly attractive for students who may not be eligible for need-based aid. The following list presents some of the major sources of financial aid specifically for nursing students. Not listed are scholarships that are specific to individual colleges and universities or are limited to residents of a particular place or to individuals who have relatively unusual qualifications. Students seeking financial aid should investigate all appropriate possibilities, including sources not listed here. You can find this information in libraries, bookstores, and guidance offices guides, including two of Peterson's annually updated publications: *Peterson's How to Get Money for College: Financing Your Future Beyond Federal Aid,* for information about undergraduate awards given by the federal government, state governments, and specific colleges, and *Peterson's Scholarships, Grants & Prizes,* for information about awards from private sources.

**Air Force Institute of Technology**

*Award Name:* Air Force Active Duty Health Professions Loan Repayment Program

*Program Description:* Program provides up to $40,000 (2009) to repay qualified educational loans in exchange for active duty service in the U.S. armed forces.

*Application Contact:*
Air Force Institute of Technology
AFIT/ENEM
Attn: Ms. Patricia Faustman
2950 Hobson Way
Wright Patterson AFB, OH 45433-7765
800-543-3490, Ext. 3015 (toll-free)
E-mail: enem.adhplrp@afit.edu
www.afit.edu/adhplrp

**Alaska Native Tribal Health Consortium**

*Award Name:* ANTHC Scholarship Program

*Program Description:* Provides undergraduate and graduate scholarships for Alaska Native/American Indian students pursuing an education in the health-care field. Must be enrolled in at least 6 credits, be a permanent Alaska resident, and be enrolled in or descended from a federally recognized tribe.

*Application Contact:*
Juliann Pico, Director of Education
Education, Development & Training
Alaska Native Tribal Health Consortium
3900 Ambassador Drive
Suite 101
Anchorage, Alaska 99508
907-729-1301
E-mail: learning@anthc.org
http://anthctoday.org/business/int.html

**American Association of Colleges of Nursing (AACN)**

*Award Name:* AfterCollege/AACN Scholarship Fund

*Program Description:* The AfterCollege-AACN Scholarship Fund supports students who are seeking a baccalaureate, master's, or doctoral degree in nursing. Special consideration is given to students in a graduate program with the goal of becoming a nurse educator; students completing an RN-to-B.S.N. or RN-to-M.S.N. program; and those enrolled in an accelerated program.

*Application Contact:*
American Association of Colleges of Nursing
One Dupont Circle, NW
Suite 530
Washington, DC 20036
202-463-6930
Fax: 202-785-8320
E-mail: scholarship@aacn.nche.edu
http://bit.ly/aftercollege_AACN

**American Association of Critical-Care Nurses**

*Award Name:* AACN Educational Advancement Scholarships

*Program Description:* Nonrenewable scholarships for AACN members who are RNs currently enrolled in undergraduate or graduate NLNAC-accredited programs. The undergraduate award is for use in the junior or senior year. Minimum 3.0 GPA.

*Application Contact:*
American Association of Critical-Care Nurses
Scholarships
101 Columbia
Aliso Viejo, CA 92656-4109
800-899-2226 (toll-free)
E-mail: scholarships@aftercollege.com
www.aacn.org/scholarships

**American Cancer Society**

*Award Name:* Scholarships in Cancer Nursing

*Program Description:* Renewable awards for graduate students in nursing pursuing advanced preparation in cancer nursing: research, education, administration, or clinical practice. Must be U.S. citizen.

*Application Contact:*
American Cancer Society
Extramural Grants Program
250 Williams Street, NW
Atlanta, GA 30303-1002
800-ACS-2345 (toll-free)
Fax: 404-417-5974
E-mail: grants@cancer.org
www.cancer.org

**American Holistic Nurses' Association (AHNA)**
*Award Name:* Charlotte McGuire Scholarship Program
*Program Description:* Open to any licensed nurse or nursing student pursuing holistic education. Experience in holistic health care or alternative health practices is preferred. Must be an AHNA member with a minimum 3.0 GPA.
*Application Contact:*
Charlotte McGuire Scholarships
American Holistic Nurses' Association
100 SE 9th Street
Suite 3A
Topeka, KS 66612
800-278-2462 Ext. 10 (toll-free)
E-mail: info@ahna.org
www.ahna.org/About-Us/Donate-Sponsor/Charlotte-McGuire-Scholarships

**American Indian Graduate Center (AIGC)**
*Award Name:* AIGC Fellowships
*Program Description:* Graduate fellowships available for American Indian and Alaska Native students from federally recognized U.S. tribes. Applicants must be pursuing a postbaccalaureate graduate or professional degree as a full-time student at an accredited institution in the U.S., demonstrate financial need, and be enrolled in a federally recognized American Indian tribe or Alaska Native group or provide documentation of Indian descent.
*Application Contact:*
American Indian Graduate Center Fellowships
American Indian Graduate Center
3701 San Mateo, NE
Suite 200
Albuquerque, NM 87110
800-628-1920 (toll-free)
505-881-4584
E-mail: web@aigcs.org
www.aigc.com

**Association of Perioperative Registered Nurses (AORN)**
*Award Name:* AORN Foundation Scholarships
*Program Description:* Applicant must be an active RN and a member of AORN for twelve consecutive months prior to application. Reapplication for each period is required. For baccalaureate, master's of nursing, or doctoral degree at an accredited institution. Minimum 3.0 GPA required.
*Application Contact:*
AORN Foundation Scholarship Program
2170 South Parker Road
Suite 400
Denver, CO 80231-5711
800-755-2676 (toll-free)
E-mail: foundation@aorn.org
www.aorn.org/

**Bethesda Lutheran Communities**
*Award Name:* Nursing Scholastic Achievement Scholarship
*Program Description:* Award for college nursing students with a minimum 3.0 GPA who are Lutheran and have completed their sophomore year of a four-year nursing program or one year of a two-year program. Must be interested in working with people with developmental disabilities.
*Application Contact:*
Chris Dovnik, Program Coordinator
Bethesda Lutheran Communities
Executive Assistant for Mission Advancement
600 Hoffmann Drive
Watertown, WI 53094
800-383-8743, Ext. 4428 (toll-free)
E-mail: chris.dovnik@mailblc.org
http://bethesdalutherancommunities.org/scholarships

**Foundation of the National Student Nurses' Association, Inc.**
*Award Names:* Scholarship Program
*Program Description:* One-time awards available to nursing students in various educational situations: enrolled in programs leading to an RN license, RNs enrolled in programs leading to a bachelor's or master's degree in nursing, enrolled in a state approved school in a specialty area of nursing, and minority students enrolled in nursing or prenursing programs. High school students are not eligible. Funds for graduate study are available only for a first degree in nursing. Based on financial need, academic ability, and health-related nursing and community activities. Application fee of $10. Send self-addressed stamped envelope with two stamps along with application request.
*Application Contact:*
Scholarship Chairperson
Foundation of the National Student Nurses' Association, Inc.
45 Main Street
Suite 606
Brooklyn, NY 11201
718-210-0705
E-mail: nsna@nsna.org
www.nsna.org/FoundationScholarships.aspx

**Heart and Stroke Foundation of Canada**
*Award Name:* Nursing Research Fellowships
*Program Description:* In-training awards for study in an area of cardiovascular or cerebrovascular nursing. Award is directed toward preparing nurses who have completed their doctoral degree and who intend to undertake independent research pro-

grams. For master's degree candidates, the programs must include a thesis or project requirement.
*Application Contact:*
Heart and Stroke Foundation of Canada
222 Queen Street, Suite 1402
Ottawa, Ontario K1P-5V9
Canada
613-569-4361, Ext. 275
E-mail: research@hsf.ca
www.heartandstroke.com

**International Order of the King's Daughters and Sons, Inc.**
*Award Name:* International Order of King's Daughters and Sons Health Careers Scholarships
*Program Description:* For study in the health fields. B.A./B.S. students are eligible in junior year. Application must be for at least third year of college. RN students must have completed first year of schooling. Send #10 self-addressed stamped envelope for application and information.
*Application Contact:* Director
Health Careers Scholarship Department
P.O. Box 1040
Chautauqua, NY 14722
716-357-4951
E-mail: healthcareersdirector.kds@gmail.com
www.iokds.org/scholarship.html

**March of Dimes**
*Award Name:* Graduate Scholarships
*Program Description:* Scholarships for registered nurses enrolled in graduate programs in maternal-child nursing. Must be a member of the Association of Women's Health, Obstetric and Neonatal Nurses; the American College of Nurse-Midwives; or the National Association of Neonatal Nurses (NANN).
*Application Contact:* Education Services
March of Dimes
1275 Mamaroneck Avenue
White Plains, NY 10605
914-997-4609
E-mail: mlavan@marchofdimes.com
www.marchofdimes.com/professionals/grants.html

**National Association of Hispanic Nurses (NAHN)**
*Award Name:* National Scholarship Awards
*Program Description:* One-time award to an outstanding Hispanic nursing student. Must have at least a 3.0 GPA and be a member of NAHN. Based on academic merit, potential contribution to nursing, and financial need.
*Application Contact:*
National Association of Hispanic Nurses
Awards/Scholarship Committee
1455 Pennsylvania Avenue
Suite 400
Washington, DC 20004
202-387-2477
E-mail: info@thehispanicnurses.org
www.thehispanicnurses.org

**National Black Nurses Association, Inc. (NBNA)**
*Award Names:* NBNA Scholarships
*Program Description:* Scholarships available to nursing students who are members of NBNA and are enrolled in an accredited school of nursing. Must demonstrate involvement in African-American community and present letter of recommendation from local chapter of NBNA.
*Application Contact:*
National Black Nurses Association, Inc.
Scholarship Committee
8630 Fenton Street, Suite 330
Silver Spring, MD 20910
301-589-3200
E-mail: info@nbna.org
www.nbna.org/

**National Student Nurses' Association (NSNA)**
*Award Name:* Educational Advancement Scholarships
*Program Description:* Scholarships are awarded based on academic achievement and demonstrated commitment to nursing through involvement in student organizations and school and community activities related to health care.
*Application Contact:*
National Student Nurses' Association Foundation
45 Main Street
Suite 606
Brooklyn, NY 11201
718-210-0705
E-mail: nsna@nsna.org
www.nsna.org

**Nurses' Educational Funds, Inc.**
*Award Name:* Nurses' Educational Fund Scholarships
*Program Description:* Awards for full-time students at master's level, full-time or part-time at doctoral level, or RNs who are U.S. citizens and members of a national professional nursing association. Application fee: $10.
*Application Contact:*
Nurses' Educational Funds, Inc.
304 Park Avenue South
11th Floor
New York, NY 10010
212-590-2443
E-mail: info@n-e-f.org
www.n-e-f.org

**Oncology Nursing Society**
*Award Name:* Scholarships
*Program Description:* ONF offers nearly a dozen one-time scholarships and awards at all levels of study, with various requirements and purposes, to nursing students who are interested in pursuing oncology nursing. Contact the foundation for details about appropriate awards. Application fee: $5.
*Application Contact:*
Oncology Nursing Society
Development Coordinator
125 Enterprise Drive
Pittsburgh, PA 15275-1214
866-257-4667 (toll-free)

E-mail: awards@ons.org
www.ons.org/awards

**United States Air Force Reserve Officer Training Corps**
*Award Name:* Air Force ROTC Nursing Scholarships
*Program Description:* One- to four-year programs available to students of nursing and high school seniors. Nursing graduates agree to accept a commission in the Air Force Nurse Corps and serve four years on active duty after successfully completing their licensing examination. Must have at least a 2.5 GPA for one- and four-year scholarships or at least a 2.65 GPA for two- and three-year scholarships. Two exam failures result in a four-year assignment as an Air Force line officer.
*Application Contact:*
Air Force ROTC
551 East Maxwell Boulevard
Maxwell AFB, AL 36112
866-423-7682 (toll-free)
www.afrotc.com/scholarships

**United States Army Reserve Officers' Training Corps**
*Award Name:* Army ROTC Nursing Scholarships
*Program Description:* Two- to four-year programs available to students of nursing and high school seniors. Nursing graduates agree to accept a commission in the Army Nurse Corps and serve in the military for a period of eight years. This may be fulfilled by serving on active duty for two to four years, followed by service in the Army National Guard or the United States Army Reserve or in the Inactive Ready Reserve for the remainder of the eight-year obligation.
*Application Contact:*
Army ROTC Cadet Command
Army ROTC Scholarship
Fort Monroe, VA 23651-1052
800-USA-ROTC (toll-free)
www.goarmy.com/rotc/scholarships.html

**United States Department of Health and Human Services, Health Resources and Services Administration**
*Award Names:* NURSE Corps Scholarship Program
*Program Description:* Awards for U.S. citizens enrolled or accepted for enrollment as a full- or part-time student in an accredited school of nursing in a professional registered nurse program (baccalaureate, graduate, associate degree, or diploma)
*Application Contact:*
Division of Nursing
U.S. Dept. of Health and Human Services
5600 Fishers Lane, Room 8-37
Parklawn Building
Rockville, MD 20857
800-221-9393 (toll-free)
GetHelp@hrsa.gov
www.hrsa.gov/loanscholarships/scholarships/Nursing

# How to Use This Guide

The following includes an overview of the various components of *Peterson's Nursing Programs 2015,* along with background information on the criteria used for including institutions and nursing programs in the guide, and explanatory material to help users interpret details presented within the guide.

## Profiles of Nursing Programs

The **Profiles of Nursing Programs** section contains detailed profiles of schools that responded to our online survey and the nursing programs they offer. This section is organized geographically; U.S. schools are listed alphabetically by state or territory, followed by Canadian schools listed alphabetically by province.

The profiles contain basic information about the colleges and universities, along with details specific to the nursing school or department, the nursing student body, and the nursing programs offered.

Schools that are members of a consortium appear with an abbreviated profile. The abbreviated profile lists only the school heading and the specific college or university information, followed by a reference line that refers readers to the consortium profile, which contains detailed program information.

An outline of the profile follows. The items of information found under each section heading are defined and displayed. Any item discussed below that is omitted from an individual profile either does not apply to that particular college or university or is one for which no information was supplied. Each profile begins with a heading with the name of the institution (the college or university), the nursing college or unit, the location of the nursing facilities, the school's Web address, and the institution's founding date, specifically the year in which it was chartered or the year when instruction actually began, whichever date is earlier. In most cases, the location is identical to the main campus of the institution. However, in a few instances, the nursing facilities are not located in the same city or state as the main campus of the college or university.

Basic information about the college follows:

***Nursing Program Faculty:*** The total number of full-time and part-time faculty members, followed by, if provided, the percentage of faculty members holding doctoral degrees.

***Baccalaureate Enrollment:*** The total number of matriculated full-time and part-time baccalaureate program students as of fall 2013 is given. This snapshot of the nursing student body indicates the total number of matriculated students, both full-time and part-time, in the baccalaureate-level nursing program; the school's estimate of the percentage of nursing students in each of the following categories is provided, if applicable: Women, Men, Minority, International, and Part-time.

***Graduate Enrollment:*** The total number of matriculated full-time and part-time students in graduate programs in fall 2013 and the percentages of **Women, Men, Minority, International,** and **Part-time** students are given.

***Distance Learning Courses:*** This section appears if distance learning courses are available.

***Nursing Student Activities:*** This section lists organizations open only to nursing students, including nursing clubs, Sigma Theta Tau (the international honor society for nursing), recruiter clubs, and Student Nurses' Association.

***Nursing Student Resources:*** This section lists special learning resources available for nursing students within the nursing school's (or unit's) facilities.

***Library Facilities:*** Figures are provided for the total number of bound volumes held by the college or university, the number of those volumes in health-related subjects, and the number in nursing and the number of periodical subscriptions held and the number of those in health-related subjects.

### BACCALAUREATE PROGRAMS

***Degree:*** Baccalaureate degree or degrees awarded are specified.

***Available Programs:*** If, in addition to a generic baccalaureate program in nursing, a school has other baccalaureate nursing programs (e.g., accelerated programs or programs for RNs, LPNs, or college graduates with non-nursing degrees) they are specified here.

***Site Options:*** Locations other than the nursing program's main campus at which baccalaureate programs may be taken are listed. Off-campus classes generally are held in health-care facilities or other educational facilities that are part of or affiliated with the college or nursing school.

***Study Options:*** Lists full-time and part-time options.

***Online Degree Options:*** This section appears if online baccalaureate degrees are available. It also specifies if the distance learning options are only available online.

***Program Entrance Requirements:*** Lists special requirements typically required to enter a program of nursing leading to a baccalaureate degree, including completion of a specific program of prerequisite courses, sometimes called prenursing courses. These are specific course credits that must be earned by students who wish to enter the generic baccalaureate program. Students entering into other tracks may be required to prove that they have completed analogous courses. Often the minimum GPA requirement for prerequisite courses differs from that expected for general college courses. Other requirements are generally self-explanatory. This paragraph also indicates if transfer students are accepted into the program. Special tracks will require appropriate proof of experience, diplomas, or other credentials. Finally, application deadlines and fees are given.

***Advanced Placement:*** This entry indicates that program credits may be granted on the basis of examinations or evaluations of earned credits at other facilities by the program's faculty and administrators.

***Expenses:*** In this section, figures are provided for tuition, mandatory and other fees, and room and board, as well as an estimate of costs for books and supplies, based on the 2013–14 academic year. If a school did not return a survey, expenses for the 2011–12 or 2012–13 academic year are listed. Unless otherwise indicated, tuition is for one full academic year. If applicable, distinct tuition figures are given for state residents and nonresidents. Part-time tuition is expressed in terms of the per-unit rate (per credit, per semester hour, etc.) specified by the institution. The tuition structure at some institutions is very complex, with different rates for freshmen and sophomores than for juniors and seniors or with part-time tuition prorated on a sliding scale according to the number of credit hours taken. Mandatory fees include such items as activity fees, health insurance, and malpractice insurance.

***Financial Aid:*** This section combines data from our online nursing survey with data received on available financial aid programs. It provides information on college-administered aid for baccalaureate-level students, including the percentage of undergraduate nursing students receiving financial aid, all types of aid offered, and application deadlines. Financial aid programs are organized into these categories: gift aid (need-based), awards based on a student's formally designated inability to pay some or all of the cost of education; gift aid (non-need-based), scholarships given on the basis of a student's special achievements, abilities, or personal characteristics; loans, subsidized low-interest student loans that can be need-based or not; and work-study, a need-based program of part-time work offered to help pay educational expenditures. The application deadline is the deadline by which application forms and need calculations, such as the FAFSA, must be submitted to the institution in order to qualify for need-based and institutional aid.

***Contact:*** This section lists the name, title, mailing address, telephone number, and, if available, fax number and e-mail address of the person to contact for admission information about the baccalaureate program.

## GRADUATE PROGRAMS

The first three paragraphs provide information that is common to the college's graduate programs in nursing.

***Expenses:*** In this section, figures are provided for tuition, room and board, and required fees based on the 2013–14 academic year. If a school did not return a survey, expenses for the 2011–12 or 2012–13 academic year are listed. Unless otherwise indicated, tuition is for one full academic year. If applicable, distinct tuition figures are given for state residents and nonresidents. Part-time tuition is expressed in terms of the per-unit rate (per credit, per semester hour, etc.) specified by the institution.

***Financial Aid:*** This section combines data from our online nursing survey with data received on available financial aid programs. It provides information on college-administered aid including the percentage of graduate nursing students receiving financial aid, all types of aid offered, and application deadlines. The major kinds of aid available are listed, including traineeships, low-interest student loans, fellowships, research assistantships, teaching assistantships, and full and partial tuition waivers. If aid is available to part-time students, this is indicated. The application deadline is the deadline by which application forms must be submitted to the college's financial aid office.

***Contact:*** Lists the name, title, mailing address, telephone number, and, if available, fax number and e-mail address of the person to contact for admission information about graduate programs.

## MASTER'S DEGREE PROGRAM

***Degree(s):*** Master's degree or degrees awarded are specified. Joint degrees specify which two degrees are given, e.g., M.S.N./Ed. D., M.S.N./M.B.A., M.S./M.H.A., M.S.N./M.P.H., in programs that combine a master's degree (or doctorate) in nursing with a master's degree in another discipline, such as business administration, hospital administration, or public health.

***Available Programs:*** If a college has special tracks that give credit, accelerated programs, or advanced courses designed for students with previous nursing experience or higher education credentials that enable students to complete programs in less time than regularly required, these are specified here in three categories:

1. For RNs—programs that admit registered nurses with associate degrees or diplomas in nursing and award a master's degree. These include RN-to-master's programs that combine the baccalaureate and master's degrees into one program for nurses who are graduates of associate or hospital diploma programs and programs that admit registered nurses with non-nursing baccalaureate degrees.
2. For LPNs—programs that admit licensed practical nurses and award a master's degree.
3. For College Graduates with Non-Nursing Degrees—programs that admit students with baccalaureate or master's degrees in areas other than nursing and award a master's degree in nursing.

***Concentrations Available:*** Specific areas of study and concentrations offered by the school are listed. Areas of specialization in case management, health-care administration, legal nurse consultant, nurse anesthesia, nurse-midwifery, nursing administration, nursing education, and nursing informatics are noted. Clinical nurse specialist and nurse practitioner programs and areas of specialization within them are noted.

***Site Options:*** Locations other than the nursing program's main campus at which the master's degree programs are offered are listed. Off-campus classes generally are held in health-care facilities or other educational facilities that are part of or affiliated with the nursing school.

***Study Options:*** Lists full-time and part-time options.

***Online Degree Options:*** This section appears if online master's degrees are available. It also specifies if the distance learning options are only available online.

***Program Entrance Requirements:*** Lists generally self-explanatory requirements.

***Advanced Placement:*** Indicates that program credits may be granted on the basis of examinations or evaluations of earned credits at other facilities by the program's faculty and administrators.

***Degree Requirements:*** Indicates the number of master's program credit hours required to earn the master's degree and the need for a thesis or qualifying score on a comprehensive examination.

### POST-MASTER'S PROGRAM

***Areas of Study:*** Listed here are the specific areas of clinical nurse specialist programs, nurse practitioner programs, and other specializations offered as postmaster's programs.

### DOCTORAL DEGREE PROGRAM

***Degree:*** Doctoral degree awarded is specified.

***Areas of Study:*** Lists specific areas of study and concentration offered by the school.

***Program Entrance Requirements:*** Lists generally self-explanatory requirements.

***Degree Requirements:*** Indicates the number of program credit hours required to earn the doctorate and the need for a dissertation, oral examination, written examination, or residency.

### POSTDOCTORAL PROGRAM

***Areas of Study:*** Lists areas of study currently reported. These may change, dependent upon the individuals in the program.

***Postdoctoral Program Contact:*** Lists the name, title, mailing address, telephone number, and, if available, fax number and e-mail address of the person to contact for information about postdoctoral programs.

### CONTINUING EDUCATION PROGRAM

***Contact:*** The appearance of this heading indicates that the nursing school has a program of continuing education. If provided, the name, title, mailing address, telephone number, fax number, and e-mail address of the person to contact regarding the program are given.

## Display Ads

**Display ads,** which appear near some of the institutions' profiles, have been provided by those colleges or universities that wished to pay for and supplement the profile data with information about their institutions or nursing programs.

## Two-Page Descriptions

The **Two-Page Descriptions** section is an open forum for nursing schools to communicate their particular message to prospective students. The absence of any college or university from this section does not constitute an editorial decision on the part of Peterson's Publishing. Those who have submitted and paid for these inclusions are responsible for the accuracy of the content. Statements regarding a school's objectives and accomplishments represent its own beliefs and are not the opinions of the editors. The **Two-Page Descriptions** are arranged alphabetically by the official institution name.

## Indexes

**Indexes** at the back of the book provide references to profiles by baccalaureate, master's, doctoral, postdoctoral, online, and continuing education programs offered; for master's-level programs, by area of study or concentration; and by institution name.

## Abbreviations Used in This Guide

| | |
|---|---|
| AACN | American Association of Colleges of Nursing |
| AACSB | AACSB International—The Association to Advance Collegiate Schools of Business |
| AAHC | Association of Academic Health Centers |
| AAS | Associate in Applied Science |
| ABSN | Accelerated Bachelor of Science in Nursing |
| ACT | American College Testing, Inc. |
| ACT ASSET | American College Testing Assessment of Skills for Successful Entry and Transfer |
| ACT COMP | American College Testing College Outcomes Measures Program |
| ACT PEP | American College Testing Proficiency Examination Program |
| AD | Associate Degree |
| ADN | Associate Degree in Nursing |
| AHNP | Adult Health Nurse Practitioner |
| ALE | American Language Exam |
| AMEDD | Army Medical Department |
| ANA | American Nurses Association |
| ANP | Adult Nurse Practitioner |
| APN | Advanced Practice Nurse |
| ARNP | Advanced Registered Nurse Practitioner |
| AS | Associate of Science |
| ASN | Associate of Science in Nursing |
| BA | Bachelor of Arts |
| BAA | Bachelor of Applied Arts |
| BN | Bachelor of Nursing |
| BNSc | Bachelor of Nursing Science |

| | |
|---|---|
| BRN | Baccalaureate for the Registered Nurse |
| BS | Bachelor of Science |
| BScMH | Bachelor of Science in Mental Health |
| BScN | Bachelor of Science in Nursing |
| BSEd | Bachelor of Science in Education |
| BSN | Bachelor of Science in Nursing |
| CAI | computer-assisted instruction |
| CAUSN | Canadian Association of University Schools of Nursing |
| CCNE | Commission on Collegiate Nursing Education |
| CCRN | Critical-Care Registered Nurse |
| CFNP | Certified Family Nurse Practitioner |
| CGFNS | Commission on Graduates of Foreign Nursing Schools |
| CINAHL | Cumulative Index to Nursing and Allied Health Literature |
| CLAST | College-Level Academic Skills Test |
| CLEP | College-Level Examination Program |
| CNA | Certified Nurse Assistant, Certified Nursing Assistant, Certified Nurses' Aide |
| CNAT | Canadian Nurses Association Testing |
| CNL | Clinical Nurse Leader |
| CNM | Certified Nurse-Midwife |
| CNS | Clinical Nurse Specialist |
| CODEC | coder/decoder |
| CPR | cardiopulmonary resuscitation |
| CRNA | Certified Registered Nurse Anesthetist |
| CS | Certified Specialist |
| CSS | College Scholarship Service |
| DAP | Doctor of Anesthesia Practice |
| DNP | Doctor of Nursing Practice |
| DNS | Doctor of Nursing Science |
| DNSc | Doctor of Nursing Science |
| DOE | U.S. Department of Education |
| DrPH | Doctor of Public Health |
| DSN | Doctor of Science in Nursing |
| EdD | Doctor of Education |
| EFC | expected family contribution |
| ERIC | Educational Resources Information Center |
| ESL | English as a second language |
| ETN | Enterostomal Nurse |
| FAAN | Fellow in the American Academy of Nursing |
| FAF | Financial Aid Form |
| FAFSA | Free Application for Federal Student Aid |
| FC | family contribution |
| FNP | Family Nurse Practitioner |
| FSEOG | Federal Supplemental Educational Opportunity Grants |
| GED | General Educational Development test |
| GMAT | Graduate Management Admission Test |
| GPA | grade point average |
| GPO | Government Printing Office |
| GRE | Graduate Record Examinations |
| Gyn | gynecology |
| HIV | human immunodeficiency virus |
| HMO | health maintenance organization |
| ICEOP | Illinois Consortium for Educational Opportunities Program |
| ICU | intensive care unit |
| ISP | Internet service provider |
| ITV | interactive television |
| LD | Licensed Dietician |
| LPN | Licensed Practical Nurse |
| LVN | Licensed Vocational Nurse |
| MA | Master of Arts |
| MAEd | Master of Arts in Education |
| MAT | Miller Analogies Test |
| MBA | Master of Business Administration |
| MCSc | Master of Clinical Science |
| MDiv | Master of Divinity |
| MEd | Master of Education |
| MEDLINE | MEDLARS On-Line |
| MELAB | Michigan English Language Assessment Battery |
| MHA | Master of Hospital Administration<br>Master of Health Administration |
| MHD | Master of Human Development |
| MHSA | Master of Health Services Administration |
| MN | Master of Nursing |
| MNSc | Master of Nursing Science |
| MOM | Master of Organizational Management |
| MPA | Master of Public Affairs |
| MPH | Master of Public Health |
| MPS | Master of Public Service |
| MS | Master of Science |
| MSBA | Master of Science in Business Administration |
| M Sc | Master of Science |
| MSc(A) | Master of Science (Applied) |
| MScN | Master of Science in Nursing |
| MTS | Master of Theological Studies |
| MSEd | Master of Science in Education |
| MSN | Master of Science in Nursing |
| MSOB | Master of Science in Organizational Behavior |
| NCAA | National Collegiate Athletic Association |
| NCLEX-RN | National Council Licensure Examination for Registered Nurses |
| ND | Doctor of Nursing |
| NLN | National League for Nursing |
| NNP | Neonatal Nurse Practitioner |
| NP | Nurse Practitioner |
| NSNA | National Student Nurses' Association |
| OB | Organizational Behavior |
| OB/GYN | obstetrics/gynecology |
| OCLC | Online Computer Library Center |
| OM | Organizational Management |
| PEP | Proficiency Examination Program |
| PhD | Doctor of Philosophy |
| PHEAA | Pennsylvania Higher Education Assistance Agency |
| PHS | Public Health Service |
| PLUS | Parents' Loan for Undergraduate Students |
| PNNP | Perinatal Nurse Practitioner |

| | |
|---|---|
| PNP | Pediatric Nurse Practitioner |
| PSAT | Preliminary SAT |
| RD | Registered Dietician |
| RN | Registered Nurse |
| RN, C | Registered Nurse, Certified |
| RN, CAN | Registered Nurse, Certified in Nursing Administration |
| RN, CNAA | Registered Nurse, Certified in Nursing Administration, Advanced |
| RN, CS | Registered Nurse, Certified Specialist |
| ROTC | Reserve Officers' Training Corps |
| RPN | Registered Psychiatric Nurse |
| SAR | Student Aid Report |
| SAT | SAT and SAT Subject Tests |
| SLS | Supplemental Loans to Students |
| SNA | Student Nurses' Association |
| SNAP | Student Nurses Acting for Progress |
| SNO | Student Nurses Organization |
| SUNY | State University of New York |
| TAP | Tuition Assistance Program |
| TB | tuberculosis |
| TOEFL | Test of English as a Foreign Language |
| TSE | Test of Spoken English |
| TWE | Test of Written English |
| USIS | United States Information Service |
| WHNP | Women's Health Nurse Practitioner |

## Data Collection Procedures

The data contained in the preponderant number of nursing college profiles, as well as in the indexes to them, were collected through *Peterson's Survey of Nursing Programs* during winter 2013–14. Questionnaires were posted online for more than 800 colleges and universities with baccalaureate and graduate programs in nursing. With minor exceptions, data for those colleges or schools of nursing that responded to the questionnaires were submitted by officials at the schools themselves. All usable information received in time for publication has been included. The omission of a particular item from a profile means that it is either not applicable to that institution or was not available or usable. In the handful of instances in which no information regarding an eligible nursing program was submitted and research of reliable secondary sources was unable to elicit the desired information, the name, location, and some general information regarding the nursing program appear in the profile section to indicate the existence of the program. Because of the extensive system of checks performed on the data collected by Peterson's, we believe that the information presented in this guide is accurate. Nonetheless, errors and omissions are possible in a data collection and processing endeavor of this scope. Also, facts and figures, such as tuition and fees, can suddenly change. Therefore, students should check with a specific college or university at the time of application to verify all pertinent information.

## Criteria for Inclusion in This Book

*Peterson's Nursing Programs 2015* covers accredited institutions in the United States, U.S. territories, and Canada that grant baccalaureate and graduate degrees. The institutions that sponsor the nursing programs must be accredited by accrediting agencies approved by the U.S. Department of Education (USDE) or the Council for Higher Education Accreditation (CHEA) or be candidates for accreditation with an agency recognized by the USDE for its preaccreditation category. Canadian schools may be provincially chartered instead of accredited.

Baccalaureate-level and master's-level nursing programs represented by a profile within the guide are accredited by the National League for Nursing Accrediting Commission (NLNAC) or the Commission on Collegiate Nursing Education (CCNE). Canadian nursing schools are members of the Canadian Association of University Schools of Nursing (CAUSN).

Doctoral, postdoctoral, continuing education, and other nursing programs included in the profiles are offered by nursing schools or departments affiliated with colleges or universities that meet the criteria outlined above.

NOTICE: Certain portions of or information contained in this book have been submitted and paid for by the educational institution identified, and such institutions take full responsibility for the accuracy, timeliness, completeness and functionality of such contents. Such portions or information include (i) each display ad in the "Profiles of Nursing Programs" section from pages 79 through 466 that comprises a one-half page of information covering a single educational institution, and (ii) each two-page in-depth description in the "Two-Page Descriptions" section from Pages 468 through 493.

# QUICK REFERENCE CHART

# NURSING PROGRAMS AT-A-GLANCE

| | Baccalaureate | Masters | Accelerated | Joint Degree | Post-Masters | Doctoral | Postdoctoral | Continuing Education |
|---|---|---|---|---|---|---|---|---|
| **UNITED STATES** | | | | | | | | |
| **Alabama** | | | | | | | | |
| Auburn University | • | • | | | | | | • |
| Auburn University at Montgomery | • | • | | | | | | |
| Jacksonville State University | • | • | | | | | | • |
| Oakwood University | • | | | | | | | |
| Samford University | • | • | B | | • | • | | • |
| Spring Hill College | • | • | M | | | | | |
| Stillman College | • | | | | | | | |
| Troy University | • | • | | | • | • | | |
| Tuskegee University | • | | | | | | | |
| The University of Alabama | • | • | | | • | • | | |
| The University of Alabama at Birmingham | • | • | M | • | • | • | • | • |
| The University of Alabama in Huntsville | • | • | | | • | • | | • |
| University of Mobile | • | • | | | | | | • |
| University of North Alabama | • | • | | | | | | • |
| University of South Alabama | • | • | B,M | | • | | | |
| **Alaska** | | | | | | | | |
| University of Alaska Anchorage | • | • | | | | | | |
| **Arizona** | | | | | | | | |
| Arizona State University at the Downtown Phoenix Campus | • | • | B | • | • | • | | • |
| Brookline College | • | | B | | | | | |
| Chamberlain College of Nursing | • | • | B | | | | | |
| Grand Canyon University | • | • | | • | • | | | • |
| Northern Arizona University | • | • | B | | • | • | | |
| The University of Arizona | • | • | M | | • | • | | |
| University of Phoenix–Online Campus | • | • | B | • | • | • | | • |
| University of Phoenix–Phoenix Campus | • | • | B | • | • | | | • |
| University of Phoenix–Southern Arizona Campus | • | • | B | | • | | | • |
| **Arkansas** | | | | | | | | |
| Arkansas State University | • | • | B | | • | • | | |
| Arkansas Tech University | • | • | | | | | | |
| Harding University | • | | | | | | | • |
| Henderson State University | • | | | | | | | |
| Southern Arkansas University–Magnolia | • | | | | | | | |
| University of Arkansas | • | • | | | | | | • |
| University of Arkansas at Little Rock | • | | | | | | | |
| University of Arkansas at Monticello | • | | | | | | | |
| University of Arkansas at Pine Bluff | • | | | | | | | |
| University of Arkansas for Medical Sciences | • | • | B | | | • | • | • |
| University of Arkansas–Fort Smith | • | | | | | | | |
| University of Central Arkansas | • | • | | | • | | | |

***B = Baccalaureate; M = Masters***

| | Baccalaureate | Masters | Accelerated | Joint Degree | Post-Masters | Doctoral | Postdoctoral | Continuing Education |
|---|---|---|---|---|---|---|---|---|
| **California** | | | | | | | | |
| American University of Health Sciences | • | | B | | | | | |
| Azusa Pacific University | • | • | B,M | | • | • | | • |
| Biola University | • | | | | | | | |
| Brandman University | • | • | | | | • | | • |
| California Baptist University | • | • | M | | | | | |
| California State University, Bakersfield | • | | | | | | | • |
| California State University Channel Islands | • | | | | | | | |
| California State University, Chico | • | • | | | | | | • |
| California State University, Dominguez Hills | • | • | | | • | | | |
| California State University, East Bay | • | | | | | | | |
| California State University, Fresno | • | • | M | | • | • | | • |
| California State University, Fullerton | • | • | | | | • | | |
| California State University, Long Beach | • | • | B,M | | • | | | |
| California State University, Los Angeles | • | • | M | | • | | | |
| California State University, Northridge | • | | B | | | | | |
| California State University, Sacramento | • | • | | | | | | |
| California State University, San Bernardino | • | • | | | | | | |
| California State University, San Marcos | • | | B | | | | | |
| California State University, Stanislaus | • | | | | | | | |
| Charles Drew University of Medicine and Science | | • | M | | | | | |
| Concordia University | • | | B | | | | | |
| Dominican University of California | • | • | | | | | | • |
| Fresno Pacific University | • | | | | | | | |
| Holy Names University | • | • | | • | • | | | |
| Loma Linda University | • | • | B | | • | • | | |
| Mount St. Mary's College | • | • | B | | | | | |
| National University | • | • | | | | | | |
| Pacific Union College | • | | | | | | | • |
| Point Loma Nazarene University | • | • | | | • | | | • |
| Samuel Merritt University | • | • | B | | • | • | | |
| San Diego State University | • | • | | | • | | | • |
| San Francisco State University | • | • | B,M | | • | | | • |
| San Jose State University | • | • | | | • | | | |
| Sonoma State University | • | | | | | | | |
| University of California, Davis | | • | | | | • | • | • |
| University of California, Irvine | • | • | | | • | • | | • |
| University of California, Los Angeles | • | • | | • | • | • | • | • |
| University of California, San Francisco | | • | | | • | • | • | |
| University of Phoenix–Bay Area Campus | • | • | B | • | | | | |
| University of Phoenix–Central Valley Campus | • | | | | | | | |
| University of Phoenix–Sacramento Valley Campus | • | • | B,M | | • | | | • |
| University of Phoenix–San Diego Campus | • | • | B | | | | | |
| University of Phoenix–Southern California Campus | • | • | B | • | • | | | • |
| University of San Diego | | • | M | | | • | | |

***B = Baccalaureate; M = Masters***

| | Baccalaureate | Masters | Accelerated | Joint Degree | Post-Masters | Doctoral | Postdoctoral | Continuing Education |
|---|---|---|---|---|---|---|---|---|
| University of San Francisco | • | • | M | | • | • | | |
| Vanguard University of Southern California | • | | | | | | | |
| West Coast University | • | | B | | | | | |
| Western University of Health Sciences | | • | M | | • | • | | |
| **Colorado** | | | | | | | | |
| Adams State University | • | | | | | | | |
| American Sentinel University | • | • | | | | | | |
| Aspen University | | • | | | | | | |
| Colorado Christian University | • | | | | | | | |
| Colorado Mesa University | • | | | | | | | |
| Colorado State University–Pueblo | • | • | B | | • | | | |
| Denver School of Nursing | • | | B | | | | | |
| Metropolitan State University of Denver | • | | B | | | | | |
| Platt College | • | | B | | | | | |
| Regis University | • | • | B | | | | | |
| University of Colorado Colorado Springs | • | • | B | | • | • | | • |
| University of Colorado Denver | • | • | B | | • | • | • | • |
| University of Northern Colorado | • | • | B | | • | • | | |
| **Connecticut** | | | | | | | | |
| Central Connecticut State University | • | | | | | | | |
| Fairfield University | • | • | B | | | • | | • |
| Quinnipiac University | • | • | B | | • | • | | |
| Sacred Heart University | • | • | | | • | • | | |
| St. Vincent's College | • | | B | | | | | |
| Southern Connecticut State University | • | • | B | | • | • | | |
| University of Connecticut | • | • | B | | • | • | • | • |
| University of Hartford | • | • | | | • | | | • |
| University of Saint Joseph | • | • | | | • | | | |
| Western Connecticut State University | • | • | | | • | | | |
| Yale University | | • | | • | • | • | • | |
| **Delaware** | | | | | | | | |
| Delaware State University | • | • | | | | | | |
| University of Delaware | • | • | B | | • | | | • |
| Wesley College | • | • | M | | • | | | • |
| Wilmington University | • | • | B,M | • | • | | | |
| **District of Columbia** | | | | | | | | |
| The Catholic University of America | • | • | B | • | • | • | | |
| Georgetown University | • | • | B | | | • | | |
| The George Washington University | • | • | B | | • | • | | |
| Howard University | • | • | | | • | | | |
| Trinity Washington University | • | | | | | | | |
| University of the District of Columbia | • | | | | | | | |

*B = Baccalaureate; M = Masters*

| | Baccalaureate | Masters | Accelerated | Joint Degree | Post-Masters | Doctoral | Postdoctoral | Continuing Education |
|---|---|---|---|---|---|---|---|---|
| **Florida** | | | | | | | | |
| Adventist University of Health Sciences | • | | | | | | | |
| Barry University | • | • | B | • | • | • | | |
| Bethune-Cookman University | • | | | | | | | |
| Broward College | • | | | | | | | |
| Edison State College | • | | | | | | | |
| Florida Agricultural and Mechanical University | • | • | | | • | • | | • |
| Florida Atlantic University | • | • | B | | • | • | | |
| Florida Gulf Coast University | • | • | | | • | | | • |
| Florida International University | • | • | B,M | | • | • | | |
| Florida Southern College | • | • | B | • | • | | | |
| Florida State College at Jacksonville | • | | | | | | | |
| Florida State University | • | • | B | | • | • | | |
| Indian River State College | • | | | | | | | |
| Jacksonville University | • | • | B | • | • | • | | |
| Kaplan University Online | • | • | | | | | | |
| Keiser University (Fort Lauderdale) | • | • | | | | | | |
| Keiser University (Fort Myers) | • | • | | | | | | |
| Keiser University (Jacksonville) | • | • | | | | | | |
| Keiser University (Lakeland) | • | • | | | | | | |
| Keiser University (Melbourne) | • | • | | | | | | |
| Keiser University (Miami) | • | • | | | | | | |
| Keiser University (Orlando) | • | • | | | | | | |
| Keiser University (Port St. Lucie) | • | • | | | | | | |
| Keiser University (Sarasota) | • | • | | | | | | |
| Keiser University (Tallahassee) | • | • | | | | | | |
| Keiser University (Tampa) | • | • | | | | | | |
| Miami Dade College | • | | | | | | | |
| Northwest Florida State College | • | | B | | | | | |
| Nova Southeastern University | • | • | | | | | | |
| Palm Beach Atlantic University | • | | | | | | | |
| Polk State College | • | | | | | | | |
| Remington College of Nursing | • | | B | | | | | |
| St. Petersburg College | • | | | | | | | • |
| State College of Florida Manatee-Sarasota | • | | | | | | | |
| University of Central Florida | • | • | B | | • | • | | |
| University of Florida | • | • | B | • | • | • | | |
| University of Miami | • | • | B | | • | • | | • |
| University of North Florida | • | • | B | | • | | | |
| University of Phoenix–North Florida Campus | • | • | B | | | | | |
| University of Phoenix–South Florida Campus | • | • | | • | | | | |
| University of Phoenix–West Florida Campus | • | | B | | | | | |
| University of South Florida | • | • | B | • | | • | | • |
| The University of Tampa | • | • | | | • | | | • |
| University of West Florida | • | • | | | | | | |

***B = Baccalaureate; M = Masters***

| | Baccalaureate | Masters | Accelerated | Joint Degree | Post-Masters | Doctoral | Postdoctoral | Continuing Education |
|---|---|---|---|---|---|---|---|---|
| **Georgia** | | | | | | | | |
| Albany State University | • | • | B | | • | | | |
| Armstrong Atlantic State University | • | • | B | | • | | | |
| Brenau University | • | • | M | | • | • | | |
| Clayton State University | • | • | | | | | | |
| College of Coastal Georgia | • | | | | | | | |
| Columbus State University | • | | | | | | | |
| Emory University | • | • | B | • | • | • | | |
| Georgia College & State University | • | • | | | • | • | | |
| Georgia Regents University | • | • | M | | • | • | | |
| Georgia Southern University | • | • | | | • | • | | |
| Georgia Southwestern State University | • | • | | | | | | |
| Georgia State University | • | • | B | | • | • | | |
| Gordon State College | • | | | | | | | |
| Kennesaw State University | • | • | B | | | | | • |
| LaGrange College | • | | | | | | | |
| Middle Georgia State College | • | | | | | | | |
| Piedmont College | • | | | | | | | |
| Shorter University | • | | | | | | | |
| Thomas University | • | • | B,M | • | • | | | |
| University of North Georgia | • | • | | | • | | | |
| University of Phoenix–Atlanta Campus | | | | | | | | |
| University of West Georgia | • | • | B | | • | • | | |
| Valdosta State University | • | • | | | | | | • |
| **Guam** | | | | | | | | |
| University of Guam | • | | | | | | | |
| **Hawaii** | | | | | | | | |
| Chaminade University of Honolulu | • | | | | | | | |
| Hawai`i Pacific University | • | • | | • | • | | | |
| University of Hawaii at Hilo | • | | | | | | | |
| University of Hawaii at Manoa | • | • | M | • | • | • | | |
| University of Phoenix–Hawaii Campus | • | • | B | | | | | |
| **Idaho** | | | | | | | | |
| Boise State University | • | • | B | | | | | |
| Brigham Young University–Idaho | • | | | | | | | |
| Idaho State University | • | • | B | | • | • | | |
| Lewis-Clark State College | • | | | | | | | |
| Northwest Nazarene University | • | • | | | | | | |
| **Illinois** | | | | | | | | |
| Aurora University | • | • | | | | | | |
| Benedictine University | • | • | B,M | | | | | |
| Blessing–Rieman College of Nursing | • | • | B | | | | | |
| Bradley University | • | • | B | | | | | |

*B = Baccalaureate; M = Masters*

| | Baccalaureate | Masters | Accelerated | Joint Degree | Post-Masters | Doctoral | Postdoctoral | Continuing Education |
|---|---|---|---|---|---|---|---|---|
| Chicago State University | • | | | | | | | |
| DePaul University | | • | | | • | • | | |
| Eastern Illinois University | • | | | | | | | |
| Elmhurst College | • | • | | • | | | | |
| Governors State University | • | • | | | • | | | |
| Illinois State University | • | • | B | | • | • | | |
| Illinois Wesleyan University | • | | | | | | | |
| Lakeview College of Nursing | • | | B | | | | | |
| Lewis University | • | • | B,M | • | • | • | | • |
| Loyola University Chicago | • | • | B | • | • | • | | |
| MacMurray College | • | | | | | | | |
| McKendree University | • | • | | • | • | | | |
| Methodist College | • | | B | | | | | |
| Millikin University | • | • | M | | | • | | |
| Northern Illinois University | • | • | | • | • | | | |
| North Park University | • | • | | • | • | | | |
| Olivet Nazarene University | • | • | B | | | | | • |
| Resurrection University | • | • | B,M | | • | | | |
| Rockford University | • | | | | | | | |
| Rush University | | • | | | • | • | | • |
| Saint Anthony College of Nursing | • | • | | | • | | | |
| Saint Francis Medical Center College of Nursing | • | • | M | | • | • | | |
| St. John's College | • | | | | | | | |
| Saint Xavier University | • | • | B | • | • | | | • |
| Southern Illinois University Edwardsville | • | • | B | | • | • | | • |
| Trinity Christian College | • | | | | | | | |
| Trinity College of Nursing and Health Sciences | • | | B | | | | | |
| University of Illinois at Chicago | • | • | | • | • | • | • | • |
| University of St. Francis | • | • | B | | • | • | | |
| Western Illinois University | • | | | | | | | |
| **Indiana** | | | | | | | | |
| Anderson University | • | • | | • | • | | | |
| Ball State University | • | • | B | | • | • | | |
| Bethel College | • | • | | | • | | | |
| Goshen College | • | • | | | | | | |
| Huntington University | • | | | | | | | |
| Indiana State University | • | • | B | | • | • | | • |
| Indiana University Bloomington | • | | | | | | | |
| Indiana University East | • | | | | | | | |
| Indiana University Kokomo | • | | B | | | | | • |
| Indiana University Northwest | • | | B | | | | | |
| Indiana University–Purdue University Fort Wayne | • | • | | | | | | |
| Indiana University–Purdue University Indianapolis | • | • | B | | • | • | • | • |
| Indiana University South Bend | • | • | B | | | | | |
| Indiana University Southeast | • | | | | | | | |

***B = Baccalaureate; M = Masters***

| | Baccalaureate | Masters | Accelerated | Joint Degree | Post-Masters | Doctoral | Postdoctoral | Continuing Education |
|---|---|---|---|---|---|---|---|---|
| Indiana Wesleyan University | • | • | B | | • | | | |
| Marian University | • | | B | | | | | • |
| Purdue University | • | • | B | | • | • | | • |
| Purdue University Calumet | • | • | B | | • | | | |
| Purdue University North Central | • | | B | | | | | |
| Saint Joseph's College | • | | B | | | | | |
| Saint Mary's College | • | | | | | | | |
| University of Evansville | • | | | | | | | |
| University of Indianapolis | • | • | B,M | | • | • | | |
| University of Saint Francis | • | • | | | • | | | |
| University of Southern Indiana | • | • | | | • | • | | • |
| Valparaiso University | • | • | B | • | • | | | • |
| Vincennes University | • | | | | | | | |
| **Iowa** | | | | | | | | |
| Allen College | • | • | B | | • | • | | • |
| Briar Cliff University | • | • | | | | • | | • |
| Clarke University | • | • | | | • | | | • |
| Coe College | • | | | | | | | |
| Dordt College | • | | | | | | | |
| Grand View University | • | • | | | | | | • |
| Iowa Wesleyan College | • | | | | | | | |
| Luther College | • | | | | | | | • |
| Mercy College of Health Sciences | • | | | | | | | |
| Morningside College | • | | | | | | | |
| Mount Mercy University | • | • | B | | | | | • |
| Northwestern College | • | | | | | | | |
| St. Ambrose University | • | • | | | | | | • |
| University of Dubuque | • | | | | | | | |
| The University of Iowa | • | • | M | • | • | • | • | • |
| Upper Iowa University | • | | | | | | | |
| **Kansas** | | | | | | | | |
| Baker University | • | | | | | | | |
| Benedictine College | • | | | | | | | |
| Bethel College | • | | | | | | | |
| Emporia State University | • | | | | | | | |
| Fort Hays State University | • | • | | | • | | | |
| Kansas Wesleyan University | • | | | | | | | |
| MidAmerica Nazarene University | • | • | B | | | | | |
| Newman University | • | • | | | | | | |
| Pittsburg State University | • | • | | | • | | | • |
| Tabor College | • | | B | | | | | |
| The University of Kansas | • | • | | • | • | • | • | • |
| University of Saint Mary | • | | | | | | | |
| Washburn University | • | • | | | • | | | • |
| Wichita State University | • | | B | | | • | | |

*B = Baccalaureate; M = Masters*

| | Baccalaureate | Masters | Accelerated | Joint Degree | Post-Masters | Doctoral | Postdoctoral | Continuing Education |
|---|---|---|---|---|---|---|---|---|
| **Kentucky** | | | | | | | | |
| Bellarmine University | • | • | B | • | • | • | | • |
| Berea College | • | | | | | | | |
| Eastern Kentucky University | • | • | B | | | | | |
| Frontier Nursing University | | • | M | | | • | | |
| Kentucky Christian University | • | | | | | | | • |
| Kentucky State University | • | | | | | | | |
| Midway College | • | | B | | | | | • |
| Morehead State University | • | | | | | | | |
| Murray State University | • | • | | | • | | | • |
| Northern Kentucky University | • | • | B | | • | • | | • |
| Spalding University | • | • | B,M | | • | | | • |
| Thomas More College | • | | | | | | | |
| Union College | • | | | | | | | |
| University of Kentucky | • | • | | | • | • | | • |
| University of Louisville | • | • | B | | • | • | | • |
| University of Pikeville | • | | | | | | | |
| Western Kentucky University | • | • | M | | | • | | • |
| **Louisiana** | | | | | | | | |
| Dillard University | • | | | | | | | • |
| Grambling State University | • | • | | | • | | | |
| Louisiana College | • | | | | | | | |
| Louisiana State University at Alexandria | • | | | | | | | |
| Louisiana State University Health Sciences Center | • | • | B | | | • | | • |
| Loyola University New Orleans | • | • | | | • | • | | |
| McNeese State University | • | • | | | • | | | • |
| Nicholls State University | • | | | | | | | • |
| Northwestern State University of Louisiana | • | • | | | • | | | • |
| Our Lady of Holy Cross College | • | | | | | | | |
| Our Lady of the Lake College | • | • | B | | | | | • |
| Southeastern Louisiana University | • | • | B | | • | • | | |
| Southern University and Agricultural and Mechanical College | • | • | | | • | • | | |
| University of Louisiana at Lafayette | • | • | B | | • | | | • |
| University of Louisiana at Monroe | • | | | | | | | • |
| University of Phoenix–Louisiana Campus | • | | B | | | | | |
| **Maine** | | | | | | | | |
| Husson University | • | • | | | • | | | |
| Saint Joseph's College of Maine | • | • | | | | | | • |
| University of Maine | • | • | | | | | | |
| University of Maine at Fort Kent | • | | B | | | | | |
| University of New England | • | | B | | | | | • |
| University of Southern Maine | • | • | B | • | • | • | | • |

*B = Baccalaureate; M = Masters*

| | Baccalaureate | Masters | Accelerated | Joint Degree | Post-Masters | Doctoral | Postdoctoral | Continuing Education |
|---|---|---|---|---|---|---|---|---|
| **Maryland** | | | | | | | | |
| Bowie State University | • | • | B | | | | | |
| Coppin State University | • | • | B | | • | | | |
| Frostburg State University | • | | | | | | | |
| The Johns Hopkins University | • | • | B | • | • | • | • | • |
| Notre Dame of Maryland University | • | | B | | | | | |
| Salisbury University | • | • | B | | • | • | | |
| Stevenson University | • | • | B,M | | | | | |
| Towson University | • | • | | | • | | | |
| University of Maryland, Baltimore | • | • | M | • | • | • | | • |
| Washington Adventist University | • | | B | | | | | |
| **Massachusetts** | | | | | | | | |
| American International College | • | • | | | | | | |
| Anna Maria College | • | | | | | | | • |
| Becker College | • | | | | | | | |
| Boston College | • | • | M | • | • | • | | • |
| Curry College | • | • | B | | | | | |
| Elms College | • | • | | | | | | |
| Emmanuel College | • | • | | | | | | |
| Endicott College | • | • | | | | | | • |
| Fitchburg State University | • | • | B | | • | | | |
| Framingham State University | • | • | | | | | | • |
| Labouré College | • | | | | | | | |
| MCPHS University | • | | B | | | | | • |
| MGH Institute of Health Professions | • | • | B | | • | • | | |
| Northeastern University | • | • | | | | • | | • |
| Regis College | • | • | B,M | | • | • | | • |
| Salem State University | • | • | B,M | • | | | | • |
| Simmons College | • | • | B,M | | | • | | |
| University of Massachusetts Amherst | • | • | B | | | • | | • |
| University of Massachusetts Boston | • | • | B | | • | • | • | • |
| University of Massachusetts Dartmouth | • | • | | | • | • | | • |
| University of Massachusetts Lowell | • | • | M | | • | • | | • |
| University of Massachusetts Worcester | | • | M | | • | • | | • |
| Worcester State University | • | • | | | • | | | • |
| **Michigan** | | | | | | | | |
| Andrews University | • | • | | | • | | | |
| Calvin College | • | | | | | | | |
| Davenport University | • | | | | | | | |
| Davenport University | • | | | | | | | |
| Eastern Michigan University | • | • | | | | • | | |
| Ferris State University | • | • | B,M | • | | | | |
| Finlandia University | • | | | | | | | |
| Grand Valley State University | • | • | B | | | • | | • |

*B = Baccalaureate; M = Masters*

| | Baccalaureate | Masters | Accelerated | Joint Degree | Post-Masters | Doctoral | Postdoctoral | Continuing Education |
|---|---|---|---|---|---|---|---|---|
| Hope College | • | | | | | | | |
| Lake Superior State University | • | | | | | | | |
| Madonna University | • | • | | • | • | • | | • |
| Michigan State University | • | • | B | | • | • | | • |
| Northern Michigan University | • | • | B | | • | | | • |
| Oakland University | • | • | | | • | | | • |
| The Robert B. Miller College | • | | | | | | | |
| Rochester College | • | | | | | | | |
| Saginaw Valley State University | • | • | B,M | | • | • | | • |
| Siena Heights University | • | | | | | | | |
| Spring Arbor University | • | • | | • | | | | |
| University of Detroit Mercy | • | • | B,M | | • | | | |
| University of Michigan | • | • | B,M | • | • | • | • | |
| University of Michigan–Flint | • | • | B,M | | | • | | |
| Wayne State University | • | • | B | | • | • | | |
| Western Michigan University | • | • | | | | | | • |
| **Minnesota** | | | | | | | | |
| Augsburg College | • | • | | | | | | |
| Bemidji State University | • | | | | | | | • |
| Bethel University | • | • | | | | | | |
| Capella University | • | • | M | | | • | | |
| College of Saint Benedict | • | | | | | | | |
| The College of St. Scholastica | • | • | B | | • | • | | |
| Concordia College | • | • | B | | | | | |
| Crown College | • | | | | | | | |
| Globe University–Woodbury | • | | | | | | | |
| Gustavus Adolphus College | • | | | | | | | |
| Herzing University | • | | | | | | | |
| Metropolitan State University | • | • | | | • | • | | |
| Minnesota Intercollegiate Nursing Consortium | • | | | | | | | |
| Minnesota State University Mankato | • | • | B,M | | • | • | | • |
| Minnesota State University Moorhead | • | • | | | | | | |
| St. Catherine University | • | • | | | • | • | | |
| St. Cloud State University | • | | | | | | | |
| Saint Mary's University of Minnesota | • | | | | | | | |
| St. Olaf College | • | | | | | | | |
| University of Minnesota, Twin Cities Campus | • | | | | | • | | • |
| Walden University | • | • | | | • | • | | |
| Winona State University | • | • | | | • | • | | |
| **Mississippi** | | | | | | | | |
| Alcorn State University | • | • | | | • | | | |
| Delta State University | • | • | | | • | • | | |
| Mississippi College | • | | | | | | | |
| Mississippi University for Women | • | • | | | • | • | | |

***B = Baccalaureate; M = Masters***

| | Baccalaureate | Masters | Accelerated | Joint Degree | Post-Masters | Doctoral | Postdoctoral | Continuing Education |
|---|---|---|---|---|---|---|---|---|
| University of Mississippi Medical Center | • | • | B | | • | • | | • |
| University of Southern Mississippi | • | • | | | • | • | | |
| William Carey University | • | • | | | | • | | |
| **Missouri** | | | | | | | | |
| Avila University | • | | | | | | | |
| Central Methodist University | • | • | B | | | | | |
| Chamberlain College of Nursing | • | | B | | | | | |
| College of the Ozarks | • | | | | | | | |
| Cox College | • | • | B | | | | | • |
| Goldfarb School of Nursing at Barnes-Jewish College | • | • | B | | • | • | | |
| Graceland University | • | • | B | | • | • | | |
| Lincoln University | • | | | | | | | |
| Maryville University of Saint Louis | • | • | B,M | | | • | | |
| Missouri Southern State University | • | • | | | | | | |
| Missouri State University | • | • | B,M | | • | • | | • |
| Missouri Western State University | • | • | | | | | | • |
| Research College of Nursing | • | • | B | | • | | | |
| Saint Louis University | • | • | B,M | | • | • | | • |
| Saint Luke's College of Health Sciences | • | | | | | | | |
| Southeast Missouri State University | • | • | | | • | | | |
| Southwest Baptist University | • | • | | | | | | |
| Truman State University | • | | | | | | | |
| University of Central Missouri | • | • | | | | | | |
| University of Missouri | • | • | B | • | • | • | | • |
| University of Missouri–Kansas City | • | • | B | | • | • | | • |
| University of Missouri–St. Louis | • | • | B | | • | • | | • |
| Webster University | • | • | | | | | | |
| William Jewell College | • | | B | | | | | |
| **Montana** | | | | | | | | |
| Carroll College | • | | | | | | | |
| Montana State University | • | • | B | | • | • | | |
| Montana State University–Northern | • | | | | | | | |
| Salish Kootenai College | • | | | | | | | |
| University of Great Falls | • | | | | | | | |
| **Nebraska** | | | | | | | | |
| Bryan College of Health Sciences | • | • | | | | | | |
| Clarkson College | • | • | B | | • | | | • |
| College of Saint Mary | • | • | | | | | | |
| Creighton University | • | • | B | | • | • | | |
| Midland University | • | | | | | | | |
| Nebraska Methodist College | • | • | B | | • | | | • |
| Nebraska Wesleyan University | • | • | B,M | | • | | | |
| Union College | • | | | | | | | |
| University of Nebraska Medical Center | • | • | B | | • | • | • | • |

*B = Baccalaureate; M = Masters*

| | Baccalaureate | Masters | Accelerated | Joint Degree | Post-Masters | Doctoral | Postdoctoral | Continuing Education |
|---|---|---|---|---|---|---|---|---|
| **Nevada** | | | | | | | | |
| Great Basin College | • | | | | | | | |
| Nevada State College at Henderson | • | | B | | | | | |
| Roseman University of Health Sciences | • | | B | | | | | |
| Touro University | • | • | | | | • | | |
| University of Nevada, Las Vegas | • | • | B | | • | • | | • |
| University of Nevada, Reno | • | • | B | • | • | • | | |
| **New Hampshire** | | | | | | | | |
| Colby-Sawyer College | • | | | | | | | |
| Franklin Pierce University | • | • | | | | | | |
| Rivier University | • | • | | | • | | | |
| Saint Anselm College | • | | | | | | | • |
| University of New Hampshire | • | • | | | • | | | |
| **New Jersey** | | | | | | | | |
| Bloomfield College | • | | | | | | | |
| Caldwell College | • | | B | | | | | |
| The College of New Jersey | • | • | | | • | | | |
| College of Saint Elizabeth | • | | B | | | | | • |
| Fairleigh Dickinson University, Metropolitan Campus | • | • | B,M | | • | • | | • |
| Felician College | • | • | B,M | • | • | | | |
| Georgian Court University | • | | | | | | | |
| Kean University | • | • | M | • | | | | |
| Monmouth University | • | • | | | • | | | • |
| New Jersey City University | • | | B | | | | | |
| Ramapo College of New Jersey | • | • | | | • | | | • |
| The Richard Stockton College of New Jersey | • | • | | | | | | |
| Rowan University | • | | | | | | | |
| Rutgers, The State University of New Jersey, Camden | • | | B | | | | | |
| Rutgers, The State University of New Jersey, Newark | • | • | B | • | • | • | | • |
| Saint Peter's University | • | • | | | • | | | |
| Seton Hall University | • | • | B,M | • | • | • | | |
| Thomas Edison State College | • | • | | | | | | |
| William Paterson University of New Jersey | • | • | B | | • | • | | |
| **New Mexico** | | | | | | | | |
| Eastern New Mexico University | • | | | | | | | |
| New Mexico Highlands University | • | | | | | | | |
| New Mexico State University | • | • | | | | • | | • |
| Northern New Mexico College | • | | | | | | | |
| University of New Mexico | • | • | | | • | • | | |
| University of Phoenix–New Mexico Campus | • | • | B | | | | | |
| Western New Mexico University | • | | | | | | | |
| **New York** | | | | | | | | |
| Adelphi University | • | • | B | • | • | • | | • |

*B = Baccalaureate; M = Masters*

| | Baccalaureate | Masters | Accelerated | Joint Degree | Post-Masters | Doctoral | Postdoctoral | Continuing Education |
|---|---|---|---|---|---|---|---|---|
| Binghamton University, State University of New York | • | • | B | | • | • | | • |
| The College at Brockport, State University of New York | • | | | | | | | |
| College of Mount Saint Vincent | • | • | | | | | | |
| The College of New Rochelle | • | • | B | | • | | | |
| College of Staten Island of the City University of New York | • | • | | | • | | | |
| Columbia University | • | • | B,M | • | • | • | • | • |
| Concordia College–New York | • | | B | | | | | |
| Daemen College | • | • | B,M | | • | • | | |
| Dominican College | • | • | B | | | | | |
| D'Youville College | • | • | | | • | | | |
| Elmira College | • | | | | | | | • |
| Excelsior College | • | • | | | • | | | |
| Farmingdale State College | • | | | | | | | |
| Hartwick College | • | | B | | | | | |
| Hunter College of the City University of New York | • | • | B | • | • | • | | • |
| Keuka College | • | | B | | | | | |
| Lehman College of the City University of New York | • | • | B | | • | • | | • |
| Le Moyne College | • | • | B | | • | | | |
| Long Island University–LIU Brooklyn | • | • | B | | • | | | |
| Long Island University–LIU Post | • | • | | | • | | | |
| Maria College | • | | | | | | | |
| Medgar Evers College of the City University of New York | • | | B | | | | | |
| Mercy College | • | • | B,M | | • | | | |
| Molloy College | • | • | B | • | • | • | | • |
| Mount Saint Mary College | • | • | B | | • | | | |
| Nazareth College of Rochester | • | | | | | | | |
| New York City College of Technology of the City University of New York | • | | | | | | | |
| New York Institute of Technology | • | | | | | | | |
| New York University | • | • | B | • | • | • | | • |
| Niagara University | • | | B | | | | | |
| Pace University | • | • | B | | • | | | |
| Roberts Wesleyan College | • | • | | | • | | | |
| The Sage Colleges | • | • | B,M | • | • | • | | • |
| St. Francis College | • | | | | | | | |
| St. John Fisher College | • | • | B | | • | • | | |
| St. Joseph's College, New York | • | • | | | | | | |
| State University of New York at Plattsburgh | • | | | | | | | |
| State University of New York College of Technology at Alfred | • | | | | | | | |
| State University of New York College of Technology at Delhi | • | | | | | | | |
| State University of New York Downstate Medical Center | • | • | B | • | • | | | • |
| State University of New York Empire State College | • | | | | | | | |
| State University of New York Institute of Technology | • | • | B,M | | • | | | • |
| State University of New York Upstate Medical University | • | • | M | | • | | | • |
| Stony Brook University, State University of New York | • | • | B | | • | • | | • |
| Trocaire College | • | | | | | | | |

***B = Baccalaureate; M = Masters***

| | Baccalaureate | Masters | Accelerated | Joint Degree | Post-Masters | Doctoral | Postdoctoral | Continuing Education |
|---|---|---|---|---|---|---|---|---|
| University at Buffalo, the State University of New York | • | • | B | | | • | | |
| University of Rochester | • | • | B,M | • | • | • | | • |
| Utica College | • | | B | | | | | |
| Wagner College | • | • | | | • | | | |
| York College of the City University of New York | • | | | | | | | |
| **North Carolina** | | | | | | | | |
| Appalachian State University | • | | | | | | | |
| Barton College | • | | | | | | | |
| Cabarrus College of Health Sciences | • | | | | | | | |
| Duke University | • | • | B | • | • | • | | |
| East Carolina University | • | • | M | | • | • | | |
| Fayetteville State University | • | | | | | | | |
| Gardner-Webb University | • | • | | • | | • | | |
| Lees-McRae College | • | | | | | | | |
| Lenoir-Rhyne University | • | • | | | | | | |
| North Carolina Agricultural and Technical State University | • | | B | | | | | |
| North Carolina Central University | • | | | | | | | |
| Queens University of Charlotte | • | • | B | • | | | | • |
| The University of North Carolina at Chapel Hill | • | • | B | | • | • | • | • |
| The University of North Carolina at Charlotte | • | • | | | • | | | |
| The University of North Carolina at Greensboro | • | • | | • | • | • | | |
| The University of North Carolina at Pembroke | • | | | | | | | |
| The University of North Carolina Wilmington | • | • | | | • | | | |
| Western Carolina University | • | • | B | | • | | | |
| Winston-Salem State University | • | • | B | | | | | • |
| **North Dakota** | | | | | | | | |
| Dickinson State University | • | | | | | | | |
| Minot State University | • | | | | | | | |
| North Dakota State University | • | • | | | | • | | |
| Sanford College of Nursing | • | | | | | | | |
| University of Jamestown | • | | | | | | | |
| University of Mary | • | • | | | | | | |
| University of North Dakota | • | • | B | | • | • | | |
| **Ohio** | | | | | | | | |
| Ashland University | • | | B | | | | | |
| Capital University | • | • | B | • | • | | | |
| Case Western Reserve University | • | • | M | • | • | • | • | • |
| Cedarville University | • | • | | | | | | |
| Chamberlain College of Nursing | • | • | B | | | | | |
| Cleveland State University | • | • | B | • | • | • | | • |
| College of Mount St. Joseph | • | • | B,M | | | | | |
| Defiance College | • | | B | | | | | |
| Franciscan University of Steubenville | • | • | | | | | | |
| Franklin University | • | | B | | | | | |

*B = Baccalaureate; M = Masters*

| | Baccalaureate | Masters | Accelerated | Joint Degree | Post-Masters | Doctoral | Postdoctoral | Continuing Education |
|---|---|---|---|---|---|---|---|---|
| Hiram College | • | | | | | | | |
| Hondros College | • | | | | | | | |
| Kent State University | • | • | B,M | • | • | • | | • |
| Kettering College | • | | | | | | | |
| Lourdes University | • | • | | | | | | |
| Malone University | • | • | | | | | | |
| Mercy College of Ohio | • | | | | | | | |
| Miami University | • | | | | | | | |
| Miami University Hamilton | • | | | | | | | |
| Mount Carmel College of Nursing | • | • | B | | • | | | |
| Mount Vernon Nazarene University | • | | | | | | | |
| Muskingum University | • | | | | | | | |
| Notre Dame College | • | | | | | | | |
| Ohio Northern University | • | | B | | | | | |
| The Ohio State University | • | • | | • | • | • | | • |
| Ohio University | • | • | | | | | | |
| Otterbein University | • | • | B | | • | | | • |
| Shawnee State University | • | | | | | | | • |
| The University of Akron | • | • | B | | • | • | | • |
| University of Cincinnati | • | • | B,M | • | • | • | | • |
| University of Phoenix–Cleveland Campus | • | • | B | | | | | |
| University of Rio Grande | • | | | | | | | |
| The University of Toledo | • | • | | | • | • | | • |
| Urbana University | • | • | | | | | | • |
| Ursuline College | • | • | B,M | • | • | • | | |
| Walsh University | • | • | B,M | | | • | | |
| Wright State University | • | • | B | • | • | • | | • |
| Xavier University | • | • | M | • | | | | |
| Youngstown State University | • | • | | | | | | |
| **Oklahoma** | | | | | | | | |
| Bacone College | • | | B | | | | | |
| East Central University | • | | | | | | | |
| Langston University | • | | | | | | | |
| Northeastern State University | • | • | B | | | | | |
| Northwestern Oklahoma State University | • | | B | | | | | |
| Oklahoma Baptist University | • | • | B | | | | | |
| Oklahoma Christian University | • | | | | | | | |
| Oklahoma City University | • | • | B,M | • | | • | | • |
| Oklahoma Panhandle State University | • | | | | | | | |
| Oklahoma Wesleyan University | • | | B | | | | | |
| Oral Roberts University | • | | | | | | | |
| Rogers State University | • | | | | | | | |
| Southern Nazarene University | • | • | M | | | | | |
| Southwestern Oklahoma State University | • | | | | | | | |
| University of Central Oklahoma | • | • | | | | | | |

***B = Baccalaureate; M = Masters***

| | Baccalaureate | Masters | Accelerated | Joint Degree | Post-Masters | Doctoral | Postdoctoral | Continuing Education |
|---|---|---|---|---|---|---|---|---|
| University of Oklahoma Health Sciences Center | • | • | B | | • | • | | • |
| University of Phoenix–Oklahoma City Campus | | | | | | | | |
| University of Phoenix–Tulsa Campus | | | | | | | | |
| University of Tulsa | • | | | | | | | |
| **Oregon** | | | | | | | | |
| George Fox University | • | | | | | | | |
| Linfield College | • | | B | | | | | • |
| Oregon Health & Science University | • | • | B,M | • | • | • | • | • |
| University of Portland | • | • | | | | • | | |
| **Pennsylvania** | | | | | | | | |
| Alvernia University | • | • | | | | | | • |
| Bloomsburg University of Pennsylvania | • | • | | • | | | | |
| California University of Pennsylvania | • | | | | | | | |
| Carlow University | • | • | B,M | | • | | | • |
| Cedar Crest College | • | • | | | | | | |
| Chatham University | • | • | | | | • | | |
| Clarion University of Pennsylvania | • | • | | | • | | | |
| DeSales University | • | • | B,M | • | • | | | • |
| Drexel University | • | • | B | | • | • | | • |
| Duquesne University | • | • | B | | • | • | | • |
| Eastern University | • | | B | | | | | |
| East Stroudsburg University of Pennsylvania | • | | | | | | | |
| Edinboro University of Pennsylvania | • | | B | | | | | |
| Gannon University | • | • | M | | • | • | | |
| Gwynedd Mercy University | • | • | B | | • | | | |
| Holy Family University | • | • | B | | • | | | • |
| Immaculata University | • | • | B | | | | | |
| Indiana University of Pennsylvania | • | • | | | | • | | |
| La Roche College | • | • | B | | | | | • |
| La Salle University | • | • | | • | • | | | • |
| Lock Haven University of Pennsylvania | • | | B | | | | | |
| Mansfield University of Pennsylvania | • | • | | | | | | |
| Marywood University | • | • | | • | | | | • |
| Messiah College | • | • | | | | | | |
| Millersville University of Pennsylvania | • | • | | | • | | | |
| Misericordia University | • | • | B | | • | | | |
| Moravian College | • | • | B | | | | | • |
| Mount Aloysius College | • | | B | | | | | • |
| Neumann University | • | • | B | | • | | | |
| Penn State University Park | • | • | | • | • | • | • | • |
| Pennsylvania College of Health Sciences | • | | | | | | | |
| Pennsylvania College of Technology | • | | | | | | | |
| Robert Morris University | • | • | | | | • | | |
| Saint Francis University | • | | | | | | | |

*B = Baccalaureate; M = Masters*

| | Baccalaureate | Masters | Accelerated | Joint Degree | Post-Masters | Doctoral | Postdoctoral | Continuing Education |
|---|---|---|---|---|---|---|---|---|
| Slippery Rock University of Pennsylvania | • | | | | | | | |
| Temple University | • | • | | | • | • | | • |
| Thomas Jefferson University | • | • | B,M | | • | • | | • |
| University of Pennsylvania | • | • | B,M | • | • | • | • | • |
| University of Pittsburgh | • | • | B | | • | • | • | • |
| University of Pittsburgh at Bradford | • | | | | | | | |
| The University of Scranton | • | • | M | | • | | | |
| Villanova University | • | • | B | | • | • | | • |
| Waynesburg University | • | • | B,M | • | | • | | |
| West Chester University of Pennsylvania | • | • | B | | | | | |
| Widener University | • | • | | • | • | • | | • |
| Wilkes University | • | • | B,M | | • | | | • |
| York College of Pennsylvania | • | • | | | • | • | | |
| **Puerto Rico** | | | | | | | | |
| Inter American University of Puerto Rico, Aguadilla Campus | • | | | | | | | |
| Inter American University of Puerto Rico, Arecibo Campus | • | | | | | | | |
| Inter American University of Puerto Rico, Metropolitan Campus | • | | B | | | | | |
| Pontifical Catholic University of Puerto Rico | • | | | | | | | |
| Universidad Adventista de las Antillas | • | | | | | | | • |
| Universidad del Turabo | • | | | | | | | |
| Universidad Metropolitana | • | | | | | | | |
| University of Puerto Rico in Arecibo | • | | | | | | | |
| University of Puerto Rico in Humacao | • | | | | | | | |
| University of Puerto Rico, Mayagüez Campus | • | | | | | | | • |
| University of Puerto Rico, Medical Sciences Campus | • | • | | | | | | • |
| University of the Sacred Heart | • | • | | | | | | |
| **Rhode Island** | | | | | | | | |
| Rhode Island College | • | • | | | | | | |
| Salve Regina University | • | | | | | | | • |
| University of Rhode Island | • | • | | | • | • | | |
| **South Carolina** | | | | | | | | |
| Charleston Southern University | • | • | | | | | | |
| Clemson University | • | • | B | | • | | | |
| Coastal Carolina University | • | | | | | | | |
| Francis Marion University | • | | | | | | | |
| Lander University | • | | B | | | | | |
| Medical University of South Carolina | • | • | B | | | • | • | |
| Newberry College | • | | | | | | | |
| South Carolina State University | • | | | | | | | |
| University of South Carolina | • | • | | | • | • | • | • |
| University of South Carolina Aiken | • | | | | | | | |
| University of South Carolina Beaufort | • | | | | | | | |
| University of South Carolina Upstate | • | | | | | | | |

*B = Baccalaureate; M = Masters*

| | Baccalaureate | Masters | Accelerated | Joint Degree | Post-Masters | Doctoral | Postdoctoral | Continuing Education |
|---|---|---|---|---|---|---|---|---|
| **South Dakota** | | | | | | | | |
| Augustana College | • | | | | | | | |
| Mount Marty College | • | | B | | | | | |
| National American University | • | | | | | | | |
| Presentation College | • | | | | | | | |
| South Dakota State University | • | • | B | | • | • | | • |
| University of Sioux Falls | • | | B | | | | | |
| The University of South Dakota | • | | | | | | | |
| **Tennessee** | | | | | | | | |
| Aquinas College | • | • | B | | • | | | |
| Austin Peay State University | • | • | | | • | | | |
| Baptist College of Health Sciences | • | | | | | | | |
| Belmont University | • | • | B | | • | | | |
| Bethel University | • | | | | | | | |
| Carson-Newman University | • | • | B,M | | • | | | |
| Christian Brothers University | • | | | | | | | |
| Cumberland University | • | | B | | | | | |
| East Tennessee State University | • | • | B | | • | • | | • |
| King College | • | • | B,M | • | | | | |
| Lincoln Memorial University | • | • | B | | • | | | |
| Lipscomb University | • | | | | | | | |
| Martin Methodist College | • | | | | | | | |
| Middle Tennessee State University | • | • | M | | • | | | |
| Milligan College | • | | | | | | | |
| South College | • | | | | | | | |
| Southern Adventist University | • | • | M | • | • | • | | • |
| Tennessee State University | • | • | | | • | | | • |
| Tennessee Technological University | • | • | | | | | | |
| Tennessee Wesleyan College | • | | | | | | | |
| Union University | • | • | B | | • | | | • |
| University of Memphis | • | • | B,M | | • | | | |
| The University of Tennessee | • | • | B | • | • | • | | • |
| The University of Tennessee at Chattanooga | • | • | | | • | • | | |
| The University of Tennessee at Martin | • | | | | | | | |
| The University of Tennessee Health Science Center | • | • | B | | | • | | |
| Vanderbilt University | | • | | • | • | • | • | |
| **Texas** | | | | | | | | |
| Angelo State University | • | • | | | | | | |
| Baylor University | • | • | B | | | • | | |
| Concordia University Texas | • | | | | | | | |
| East Texas Baptist University | • | | | | | | | |
| Houston Baptist University | • | | | | | | | |
| Lamar University | • | • | | • | • | | | • |
| Lubbock Christian University | • | | | | | | | |

***B = Baccalaureate; M = Masters***

| | Baccalaureate | Masters | Accelerated | Joint Degree | Post-Masters | Doctoral | Postdoctoral | Continuing Education |
|---|---|---|---|---|---|---|---|---|
| Midwestern State University | • | • | | | • | | | • |
| Patty Hanks Shelton School of Nursing | • | • | | | • | | | • |
| Prairie View A&M University | • | • | | | • | | | |
| Sam Houston State University | • | | | | | | | |
| Southwestern Adventist University | • | | | | | | | |
| Stephen F. Austin State University | • | | | | | | | |
| Tarleton State University | • | | | | | | | • |
| Texas A&M Health Science Center | • | | B | | | | | |
| Texas A&M International University | • | • | | | | | | |
| Texas A&M University–Corpus Christi | • | • | B | | • | | | • |
| Texas A&M University–Texarkana | • | • | | | | | | |
| Texas Christian University | • | • | B | | • | • | | • |
| Texas State University–San Marcos | • | • | | | | | | |
| Texas Tech University Health Sciences Center | • | • | B | | • | • | | |
| Texas Tech University Health Sciences Center-El Paso | • | | B | | | | | |
| Texas Woman's University | • | • | | • | • | • | | |
| University of Houston–Victoria | • | • | B | | | | | |
| University of Mary Hardin-Baylor | • | • | | | • | | | |
| The University of Texas at Arlington | • | • | B | • | • | • | | • |
| The University of Texas at Austin | • | • | | • | • | • | | |
| The University of Texas at Brownsville | • | • | | | | | | • |
| The University of Texas at El Paso | • | • | B | | • | | | |
| The University of Texas at Tyler | • | • | B,M | • | • | • | | |
| The University of Texas Health Science Center at Houston | • | • | B | • | • | • | | • |
| The University of Texas Health Science Center at San Antonio | • | • | B | | • | • | | • |
| The University of Texas Medical Branch | • | • | B | | • | • | | |
| The University of Texas–Pan American | • | • | | | • | | | |
| University of the Incarnate Word | • | • | M | | • | • | | |
| Wayland Baptist University | • | | | | | | | |
| West Texas A&M University | • | • | | | • | | | |
| **Utah** | | | | | | | | |
| Brigham Young University | • | • | | | • | | | |
| Dixie State University | • | | | | | | | |
| Southern Utah University | • | | | | | | | |
| University of Phoenix–Utah Campus | | | | | | | | |
| University of Utah | • | • | B | | • | • | • | |
| Utah Valley University | • | | | | | | | |
| Weber State University | • | • | | | | | | |
| Western Governors University | • | • | B,M | | | | | |
| Westminster College | • | • | | | • | | | |
| **Vermont** | | | | | | | | |
| Norwich University | • | | | | | | | |
| Southern Vermont College | • | | | | | | | |
| University of Vermont | • | • | | | • | | | |

*B = Baccalaureate; M = Masters*

| | Baccalaureate | Masters | Accelerated | Joint Degree | Post-Masters | Doctoral | Postdoctoral | Continuing Education |
|---|---|---|---|---|---|---|---|---|
| **Virgin Islands** | | | | | | | | |
| University of the Virgin Islands | • | | | | | | | |
| **Virginia** | | | | | | | | |
| Bon Secours Memorial College of Nursing | • | | | | | | | |
| Eastern Mennonite University | • | • | | | | | | |
| ECPI University | • | | | | | | | |
| George Mason University | • | • | B | | • | • | | • |
| Hampton University | • | • | B | | | • | | |
| James Madison University | • | • | | | | • | | |
| Jefferson College of Health Sciences | • | • | | | | | | • |
| Liberty University | • | • | | | | | | |
| Longwood University | • | | | | | | | |
| Lynchburg College | • | • | B | | | | | |
| Marymount University | • | • | B | | • | • | | |
| Norfolk State University | • | | B | | | | | |
| Old Dominion University | • | • | B | | • | • | | • |
| Radford University | • | • | | | • | • | | |
| Sentara College of Health Sciences | • | | | | | | | |
| Shenandoah University | • | • | B | • | • | • | | • |
| Stratford University | • | | | | | | | |
| University of Virginia | • | • | | • | • | • | • | |
| The University of Virginia's College at Wise | • | | | | | | | |
| Virginia Commonwealth University | • | • | B | | • | • | | |
| **Washington** | | | | | | | | |
| Gonzaga University | • | • | M | | • | | | |
| Northwest University | • | | | | | | | |
| Olympic College | • | | | | | | | |
| Pacific Lutheran University | • | • | M | • | | | | • |
| Seattle Pacific University | • | • | | | • | | | |
| Seattle University | • | • | M | | • | • | | |
| University of Washington | • | • | B | • | • | • | • | • |
| Walla Walla University | • | | | | | | | |
| Washington State University College of Nursing | • | • | M | | • | • | | • |
| **West Virginia** | | | | | | | | |
| Alderson Broaddus University | • | | | | | | | |
| American Public University System | • | | | | | | | |
| Bluefield State College | • | | | | | | | |
| Fairmont State University | • | | B | | | | | • |
| Marshall University | • | • | B | | • | | | |
| Shepherd University | • | | | | | | | • |
| University of Charleston | • | | | | | | | |
| West Liberty University | • | | B | | | | | |
| West Virginia University | • | • | B,M | | • | • | | • |

***B = Baccalaureate; M = Masters***

| | Baccalaureate | Masters | Accelerated | Joint Degree | Post-Masters | Doctoral | Postdoctoral | Continuing Education |
|---|---|---|---|---|---|---|---|---|
| West Virginia Wesleyan College | • | • | | | | | | |
| Wheeling Jesuit University | • | • | B | | • | | | |
| **Wisconsin** | | | | | | | | |
| Alverno College | • | • | | | | | | • |
| Bellin College | • | • | B | | | | | |
| Cardinal Stritch University | • | • | M | | | | | |
| Carroll University | • | | | | | | | |
| Columbia College of Nursing/Mount Mary College Nursing Program | • | | | | | | | |
| Concordia University Wisconsin | • | • | | | • | | | |
| Edgewood College | • | • | B | • | | | | |
| Herzing University Online | • | • | | | | | | |
| Maranatha Baptist Bible College | • | | | | | | | |
| Marian University | • | • | | | • | | | |
| Marquette University | • | • | M | • | • | • | | |
| Milwaukee School of Engineering | • | | B | | | | | • |
| Silver Lake College of the Holy Family | • | | | | | | | |
| University of Phoenix–Milwaukee Campus | • | • | | | | • | | |
| University of Wisconsin–Eau Claire | • | • | B | | • | • | | • |
| University of Wisconsin–Green Bay | • | • | | | | | | |
| University of Wisconsin–Madison | • | | | | | • | • | • |
| University of Wisconsin–Milwaukee | • | • | | | | • | | |
| University of Wisconsin–Oshkosh | • | • | B | | • | • | | • |
| Viterbo University | • | • | | | | • | | • |
| Wisconsin Lutheran College | • | | | | | | | • |
| **Wyoming** | | | | | | | | |
| University of Wyoming | • | • | B | | • | • | | |
| **CANADA** | | | | | | | | |
| **Alberta** | | | | | | | | |
| Athabasca University | • | • | | | • | | | |
| University of Alberta | • | • | B | | • | • | | |
| University of Calgary | • | • | B | | • | • | | |
| University of Lethbridge | • | • | B | | | | | |
| **British Columbia** | | | | | | | | |
| British Columbia Institute of Technology | • | | | | | | | • |
| Kwantlen Polytechnic University | • | | B | | | | | |
| Thompson Rivers University | • | | | | | | | • |
| Trinity Western University | • | • | | | | | | |
| The University of British Columbia | • | • | B | • | | • | • | |
| University of Northern British Columbia | • | • | | | | | • | |
| University of Victoria | • | • | | | | • | | |
| Vancouver Island University | • | | | | | | | • |

***B = Baccalaureate; M = Masters***

| | Baccalaureate | Masters | Accelerated | Joint Degree | Post-Masters | Doctoral | Postdoctoral | Continuing Education |
|---|---|---|---|---|---|---|---|---|
| **Manitoba** | | | | | | | | |
| Brandon University | • | | | | | | | |
| University of Manitoba | • | • | | | | • | | • |
| **New Brunswick** | | | | | | | | |
| Université de Moncton | • | • | | | | | | • |
| University of New Brunswick Fredericton | • | • | B | | | | | • |
| **Newfoundland and Labrador** | | | | | | | | |
| Memorial University of Newfoundland | • | • | B | | • | | | |
| **Nova Scotia** | | | | | | | | |
| St. Francis Xavier University | • | | B | | | | | • |
| **Ontario** | | | | | | | | |
| Brock University | • | | | | | | | |
| Lakehead University | • | | B | | | | | |
| Laurentian University | • | • | | | | | | • |
| McMaster University | • | • | | • | | • | | |
| Nipissing University | • | | | | | | | |
| Queen's University at Kingston | • | • | B | | | • | | |
| Ryerson University | • | • | | | | | | • |
| Trent University | • | | B | | | | | |
| University of Ottawa | • | • | B | | | • | • | |
| University of Toronto | • | • | B | | • | • | • | • |
| The University of Western Ontario | • | • | B | | | • | • | |
| University of Windsor | • | • | | | | | | • |
| York University | • | | | | | | | • |
| **Prince Edward Island** | | | | | | | | |
| University of Prince Edward Island | • | | | | | | | |
| **Quebec** | | | | | | | | |
| McGill University | • | • | B | | | • | • | |
| Université de Montréal | • | • | | | • | • | • | • |
| Université de Sherbrooke | • | • | | | | • | • | |
| Université du Québec à Chicoutimi | • | • | B,M | • | • | | | |
| Université du Québec à Rimouski | • | • | | | | | | • |
| Université du Québec à Trois-Rivières | • | • | | | | | | |
| Université du Québec en Abitibi-Témiscamingue | • | | | | | | | |
| Université du Québec en Outaouais | • | • | | | | | | • |
| Université Laval | • | • | B,M | | • | • | • | • |
| **Saskatchewan** | | | | | | | | |
| University of Saskatchewan | • | • | B | | • | • | | • |

***B = Baccalaureate; M = Masters***

# PROFILES OF NURSING PROGRAMS

# U.S. AND U.S. TERRITORIES

## ALABAMA

### Auburn University

**School of Nursing**
**Auburn University, Alabama**

*http://www.auburn.edu/academic/nursing/*
Founded in 1856

**DEGREES • BSN • MSN**

**Nursing Program Faculty** 15 (90% with doctorates).

**Baccalaureate Enrollment** 289 **Women** 90% **Men** 10% **Minority** 3%

**Graduate Enrollment** 93 **Women** 96% **Men** 4% **Minority** 7% **Part-time** 20%

**Nursing Student Activities** Nursing Honor Society, Sigma Theta Tau, Student Nurses' Association, nursing club.

**Nursing Student Resources** Academic advising; academic or career counseling; assistance for students with disabilities; bookstore; campus computer network; career placement assistance; computer lab; computer-assisted instruction; e-mail services; employment services for current students; interactive nursing skills videos; Internet; library services; nursing audiovisuals; placement services for program completers; remedial services; resume preparation assistance; skills, simulation, or other laboratory; tutoring.

**Library Facilities** 4.3 million volumes; 256,354 periodical subscriptions.

#### BACCALAUREATE PROGRAMS

**Degree** BSN

**Available Programs** Generic Baccalaureate.

**Study Options** Full-time.

**Program Entrance Requirements** Minimum overall college GPA of 2.5, transcript of college record, CPR certification, health exam, health insurance, immunizations, interview, minimum GPA in nursing prerequisites of 2.5, professional liability insurance/malpractice insurance, prerequisite course work. Transfer students are accepted. *Application deadline:* 2/1 (fall), 5/1 (spring).

**Expenses (2013–14)** *Tuition, state resident:* full-time $28,098. *Tuition, nonresident:* full-time $44,610. *Required fees:* full-time $2000.

**Financial Aid** 85% of baccalaureate students in nursing programs received some form of financial aid in 2012–13.

**Contact** Pam Hennessey, Academic Advisor, School of Nursing, Auburn University, 118 Miller Hall, Auburn University, AL 36849. *Telephone:* 334-844-5665. *Fax:* 334-844-4177. *E-mail:* hennepp@auburn.edu.

#### GRADUATE PROGRAMS

**Expenses (2013–14)** *Tuition, state resident:* full-time $28,104. *Tuition, nonresident:* full-time $44,628.

**Financial Aid** 80% of graduate students in nursing programs received some form of financial aid in 2012–13.

**Contact** Dr. Barbara Wilder, Director, MSN Program, School of Nursing, Auburn University, 118 Miller Hall, Auburn University, AL 36849. *Telephone:* 334-844-5665. *E-mail:* wildebf@auburn.edu.

**MASTER'S DEGREE PROGRAM**

**Degree** MSN

**Available Programs** Master's.

**Concentrations Available** Nursing education. *Clinical nurse specialist programs in:* adult health, gerontology, pediatric.

**Study Options** Full-time and part-time.

**Program Entrance Requirements** Minimum overall college GPA of 3.0, transcript of college record, nursing research course, statistics course. *Application deadline:* 7/1 (fall), 10/1 (spring), 3/1 (summer).

**Degree Requirements** 51 total credit hours, thesis or project.

#### CONTINUING EDUCATION PROGRAM

**Contact** Dr. Stuart Pope, Outreach Coordinator, School of Nursing, Auburn University, Miller Hall, Auburn University, AL 36849-5505. *Telephone:* 334-844-5665. *Fax:* 334-844-4177.

### Auburn University at Montgomery

**School of Nursing**
**Montgomery, Alabama**

*http://www.aum.edu/nursing*
Founded in 1967

**DEGREES • BSN • MSN**

**Nursing Program Faculty** 20 (70% with doctorates).

**Baccalaureate Enrollment** 650 **Women** 80% **Men** 20% **Minority** 33% **International** 1% **Part-time** 20%

**Graduate Enrollment** 30

**Nursing Student Activities** Nursing Honor Society, Sigma Theta Tau, Student Nurses' Association.

**Nursing Student Resources** Academic advising; academic or career counseling; assistance for students with disabilities; bookstore; campus computer network; career placement assistance; computer lab; computer-assisted instruction; daycare for children of students; e-mail services; housing assistance; interactive nursing skills videos; Internet; learning resource lab; library services; nursing audiovisuals; remedial services; resume preparation assistance; skills, simulation, or other laboratory; tutoring.

**Library Facilities** 9,568 volumes in nursing; 273 periodical subscriptions health-care related.

#### BACCALAUREATE PROGRAMS

**Degree** BSN

**Available Programs** Generic Baccalaureate; RN Baccalaureate.

**Study Options** Full-time.

**Program Entrance Requirements** Transcript of college record, CPR certification, health exam, high school transcript, immunizations, interview, minimum GPA in nursing prerequisites of 2.5, professional liability insurance/malpractice insurance, prerequisite course work. Transfer students are accepted. *Application deadline:* 2/1 (fall), 5/1 (spring).

**Contact** *Telephone:* 334-244-3431. *Fax:* 334-244-3243.

#### GRADUATE PROGRAMS

**Contact** *Telephone:* 334-844-5613. *Fax:* 334-844-4177.

**MASTER'S DEGREE PROGRAM**

**Degree** MSN

**Available Programs** Master's.

**Concentrations Available** Nursing education. *Clinical nurse specialist programs in:* adult health, gerontology, pediatric. *Nurse practitioner programs in:* primary care.

**Study Options** Full-time and part-time.

**Program Entrance Requirements** Clinical experience, minimum overall college GPA of 3.0, written essay, 3 letters of recommendation, resume, statistics course.

**Advanced Placement** Credit given for nursing courses completed elsewhere dependent upon specific evaluations.

**Degree Requirements** 42 total credit hours, thesis or project, comprehensive exam.

# Jacksonville State University
## College of Nursing and Health Sciences
## Jacksonville, Alabama

***http://www.jsu.edu/nursing/***
Founded in 1883

**DEGREES • BSN • MSN**
**Nursing Program Faculty** 37 (35% with doctorates).
**Baccalaureate Enrollment** 541 **Women** 85% **Men** 15% **Minority** 23% **International** 2% **Part-time** 20%
**Graduate Enrollment** 49 **Women** 94% **Men** 6% **Minority** 45% **International** 2% **Part-time** 94%
**Distance Learning Courses** Available.
**Nursing Student Activities** Sigma Theta Tau, Student Nurses' Association.
**Nursing Student Resources** Academic advising; academic or career counseling; assistance for students with disabilities; campus computer network; computer lab; computer-assisted instruction; e-mail services; employment services for current students; externships; interactive nursing skills videos; Internet; learning resource lab; nursing audiovisuals; remedial services; resume preparation assistance; skills, simulation, or other laboratory; tutoring.
**Library Facilities** 685,991 volumes (23,363 in health, 1,679 in nursing); 14,376 periodical subscriptions (7,511 health-care related).

### BACCALAUREATE PROGRAMS

**Degree** BSN
**Available Programs** Generic Baccalaureate; RN Baccalaureate.
**Study Options** Full-time and part-time.
**Online Degree Options** Yes.
**Program Entrance Requirements** Transcript of college record, CPR certification, health exam, health insurance, high school transcript, immunizations, minimum GPA in nursing prerequisites, professional liability insurance/malpractice insurance, prerequisite course work. Transfer students are accepted. *Application deadline:* 6/1 (fall), 10/1 (spring).
**Expenses (2013–14)** *Tuition, area resident:* full-time $6792; part-time $283 per credit hour. *Tuition, state resident:* full-time $8280; part-time $345 per credit hour. *Tuition, nonresident:* full-time $13,584; part-time $566 per credit hour. *International tuition:* $13,584 full-time. *Room and board:* $6562; room only: $3812 per academic year. *Required fees:* full-time $300; part-time $150 per term.
**Financial Aid** 70% of baccalaureate students in nursing programs received some form of financial aid in 2012–13.
**Contact** Mr. David Hofland, Student Services Coordinator, College of Nursing and Health Sciences, Jacksonville State University, 700 Pelham Road North, Jacksonville, AL 36265-1602. *Telephone:* 256-782-5276. *Fax:* 256-782-5406. *E-mail:* hofland@jsu.edu.

### GRADUATE PROGRAMS

**Expenses (2013–14)** *Tuition, state resident:* full-time $7902; part-time $439 per credit hour. *Tuition, nonresident:* full-time $7902; part-time $439 per credit hour. *International tuition:* $7902 full-time. *Room and board:* $6562; room only: $3812 per academic year. *Required fees:* full-time $300; part-time $150 per term.
**Financial Aid** 60% of graduate students in nursing programs received some form of financial aid in 2012–13.
**Contact** Dr. Rebecca D. Peinhardt, Director, Graduate Studies, College of Nursing and Health Sciences, Jacksonville State University, 700 Pelham Road North, Jacksonville, AL 36265-1602. *Telephone:* 256-782-5960. *Fax:* 256-782-5406. *E-mail:* rpeinhardt@jsu.edu.

### MASTER'S DEGREE PROGRAM

**Degree** MSN
**Available Programs** Master's.
**Concentrations Available** *Clinical nurse specialist programs in:* community health.
**Study Options** Full-time and part-time.
**Online Degree Options** Yes (online only).
**Program Entrance Requirements** Minimum overall college GPA of 3.0, transcript of college record, written essay, interview, 3 letters of recommendation, nursing research course, physical assessment course, statistics course. *Application deadline:* Applications may be processed on a rolling basis for some programs.
**Advanced Placement** Credit given for nursing courses completed elsewhere dependent upon specific evaluations.
**Degree Requirements** 36 total credit hours, thesis or project, comprehensive exam.

### CONTINUING EDUCATION PROGRAM

**Contact** Mr. David Hofland, Student Services Coordinator, College of Nursing and Health Sciences, Jacksonville State University, 700 Pelham Road North, Jacksonville, AL 36265-1602. *Telephone:* 256-782-5276. *Fax:* 256-782-5406. *E-mail:* hofland@jsu.edu.

# Oakwood University
## Department of Nursing
## Huntsville, Alabama

***http://www.oakwood.edu/academics/academic-departments/nursing***
Founded in 1896

**DEGREE • BS**
**Nursing Program Faculty** 10 (33% with doctorates).
**Baccalaureate Enrollment** 85 **Women** 90% **Men** 10% **Minority** 99% **International** 5%
**Nursing Student Activities** Nursing club.
**Nursing Student Resources** Academic advising; academic or career counseling; assistance for students with disabilities; bookstore; campus computer network; computer lab; computer-assisted instruction; e-mail services; interactive nursing skills videos; Internet; learning resource lab; library services; nursing audiovisuals; remedial services; skills, simulation, or other laboratory; tutoring; unpaid internships.
**Library Facilities** 133,106 volumes (5,147 in health, 3,474 in nursing); 726 periodical subscriptions (47 health-care related).

### BACCALAUREATE PROGRAMS

**Degree** BS
**Available Programs** Generic Baccalaureate; RN Baccalaureate.
**Study Options** Full-time and part-time.
**Program Entrance Requirements** Minimum overall college GPA of 3.0, transcript of college record, CPR certification, written essay, health exam, health insurance, high school transcript, immunizations, interview, 3 letters of recommendation, minimum high school GPA of 3.0, minimum GPA in nursing prerequisites of 3.0, prerequisite course work. Transfer students are accepted. *Application deadline:* 1/16 (fall), 1/15 (winter).
**Expenses (2013–14)** *Tuition:* full-time $12,773; part-time $658 per hour. *International tuition:* $12,773 full-time. *Room and board:* $12,773; room only: $7354 per academic year. *Required fees:* full-time $965; part-time $625 per term.
**Financial Aid** 95% of baccalaureate students in nursing programs received some form of financial aid in 2012–13.
**Contact** Mrs. Denise Finley, Secretary, Department of Nursing, Oakwood University, 7000 Adventist Boulevard, Huntsville, AL 35896. *Telephone:* 256-726-7287. *Fax:* 256-726-8338. *E-mail:* dfinley@oakwood.edu.

# Samford University
## Ida V. Moffett School of Nursing
## Birmingham, Alabama

***http://www.samford.edu/nursing/***
Founded in 1841

**DEGREES • BSN • DNP • MSN**
**Nursing Program Faculty** 39 (59% with doctorates).
**Baccalaureate Enrollment** 434 **Women** 94% **Men** 6% **Minority** 15% **International** 1% **Part-time** 6%
**Graduate Enrollment** 275 **Women** 76% **Men** 24% **Minority** 17% **Part-time** 9%
**Distance Learning Courses** Available.
**Nursing Student Activities** Nursing Honor Society, Sigma Theta Tau, Student Nurses' Association, nursing club.
**Nursing Student Resources** Academic advising; academic or career counseling; assistance for students with disabilities; bookstore; campus computer network; career placement assistance; computer lab; computer-assisted instruction; e-mail services; employment services for current students; externships; housing assistance; interactive nursing skills videos; Internet; learning resource lab; library services; nursing audiovisuals; paid internships; resume preparation assistance; skills, simulation, or other laboratory; tutoring; unpaid internships.

**Library Facilities** 688,371 volumes (7,242 in health, 836 in nursing); 85,762 periodical subscriptions (2,597 health-care related).

## BACCALAUREATE PROGRAMS

**Degree** BSN
**Available Programs** Accelerated Baccalaureate for Second Degree; Baccalaureate for Second Degree; Generic Baccalaureate.
**Site Options** Birmingham, AL.
**Study Options** Full-time and part-time.
**Program Entrance Requirements** Minimum overall college GPA of 2.7, transcript of college record, CPR certification, written essay, health exam, health insurance, high school biology, high school chemistry, 2 years high school math, 2 years high school science, high school transcript, immunizations, minimum high school GPA of 3.0, minimum GPA in nursing prerequisites of 2.0, professional liability insurance/malpractice insurance, prerequisite course work. Transfer students are accepted. *Application deadline:* 5/1 (fall). Applications may be processed on a rolling basis for some programs. *Application fee:* $35.
**Advanced Placement** Credit given for nursing courses completed elsewhere dependent upon specific evaluations.
**Expenses (2013–14)** *Tuition:* full-time $25,528; part-time $853 per credit. *International tuition:* $25,528 full-time. *Room and board:* $9372; room only: $5172 per academic year. *Required fees:* full-time $800.
**Financial Aid** 87% of baccalaureate students in nursing programs received some form of financial aid in 2012–13.
**Contact** Mrs. Janice G. Paine, Director, Undergraduate Student Services, Ida V. Moffett School of Nursing, Samford University, 800 Lakeshore Drive, Birmingham, AL 35229. *Telephone:* 205-726-2872 Ext. 2746. *Fax:* 205-726-4269. *E-mail:* jgpaine@samford.edu.

## GRADUATE PROGRAMS

**Expenses (2013–14)** *Tuition:* full-time $18,500; part-time $740 per credit. *International tuition:* $18,500 full-time. *Room and board:* $9500 per academic year. *Required fees:* full-time $840.
**Financial Aid** 76% of graduate students in nursing programs received some form of financial aid in 2012–13. Institutionally sponsored loans, scholarships, and traineeships available. *Financial aid application deadline:* 3/1.
**Contact** Mrs. Allyson Maddox, Director, Graduate Student Services, Ida V. Moffett School of Nursing, Samford University, 800 Lakeshore Drive, Birmingham, AL 35229. *Telephone:* 205-726-2047. *Fax:* 205-726-4235. *E-mail:* amaddox@samford.edu.

### MASTER'S DEGREE PROGRAM

**Degree** MSN
**Available Programs** Master's; RN to Master's.
**Concentrations Available** Nurse anesthesia; nursing administration; nursing education. *Nurse practitioner programs in:* family health.
**Site Options** Birmingham, AL.
**Study Options** Full-time and part-time.
**Online Degree Options** Yes.
**Program Entrance Requirements** Clinical experience, computer literacy, minimum overall college GPA of 3.0, transcript of college record, CPR certification, immunizations, interview, 3 letters of recommendation, nursing research course, physical assessment course, professional liability insurance/malpractice insurance, prerequisite course work, MAT; GRE (for nurse anesthesia). *Application deadline:* 6/1 (fall), 9/1 (spring). *Application fee:* $65.
**Degree Requirements** 38 total credit hours, thesis or project.

### POST-MASTER'S PROGRAM

**Areas of Study** Nurse anesthesia. *Nurse practitioner programs in:* family health.

### DOCTORAL DEGREE PROGRAM

**Degree** DNP
**Available Programs** Doctorate.
**Areas of Study** Advanced practice nursing, nursing administration.
**Site Options** Birmingham, AL.
**Online Degree Options** Yes (online only).
**Program Entrance Requirements** Clinical experience, minimum overall college GPA of 3.5, interview by faculty committee, interview, 3 letters of recommendation, MSN or equivalent, vita, writing sample. *Application deadline:* 9/1 (spring), 2/1 (summer). *Application fee:* $65.
**Degree Requirements** 38 total credit hours, oral exam.

## CONTINUING EDUCATION PROGRAM

**Contact** Mrs. Suzanne Scharf, Continuing Education Coordinator, Ida V. Moffett School of Nursing, Samford University, 800 Lakeshore Drive, Birmingham, AL 35229. *Telephone:* 205-726-2045. *Fax:* 205-726-2219. *E-mail:* shscharf@samford.edu.

# Spring Hill College
## Division of Nursing
## Mobile, Alabama

***http://www.shc.edu/***
Founded in 1830

**DEGREES • BSN • MSN**
**Nursing Program Faculty** 8 (84% with doctorates).
**Baccalaureate Enrollment** 124 **Women** 86% **Men** 14% **Minority** 12%
**Graduate Enrollment** 62 **Women** 95% **Men** 5% **Minority** 45% **Part-time** 40%
**Distance Learning Courses** Available.
**Nursing Student Activities** Nursing Honor Society, Sigma Theta Tau, Student Nurses' Association.
**Nursing Student Resources** Academic advising; academic or career counseling; assistance for students with disabilities; bookstore; campus computer network; career placement assistance; computer lab; computer-assisted instruction; e-mail services; employment services for current students; externships; interactive nursing skills videos; Internet; learning resource lab; library services; nursing audiovisuals; placement services for program completers; resume preparation assistance; skills, simulation, or other laboratory; tutoring; unpaid internships.
**Library Facilities** 330 volumes in health, 300 volumes in nursing; 58 periodical subscriptions health-care related.

## BACCALAUREATE PROGRAMS

**Degree** BSN
**Available Programs** Baccalaureate for Second Degree; Generic Baccalaureate.
**Study Options** Full-time.
**Program Entrance Requirements** Minimum overall college GPA of 2.75, transcript of college record, CPR certification, written essay, health exam, health insurance, high school transcript, immunizations, 1 letter of recommendation, minimum GPA in nursing prerequisites of 2.75, prerequisite course work. Transfer students are accepted. *Application deadline:* 3/1 (spring).
**Advanced Placement** Credit by examination available.
**Contact** *Telephone:* 334-380-4492. *Fax:* 334-380-4495.

## GRADUATE PROGRAMS

**Contact** *Telephone:* 251-380-3067. *Fax:* 251-460-2190.

### MASTER'S DEGREE PROGRAM

**Degree** MSN
**Available Programs** Accelerated AD/RN to Master's; Master's; RN to Master's.
**Concentrations Available** Clinical nurse leader.
**Study Options** Full-time and part-time.
**Online Degree Options** Yes (online only).
**Program Entrance Requirements** Clinical experience, minimum overall college GPA of 3.0, transcript of college record, immunizations, professional liability insurance/malpractice insurance, prerequisite course work, resume, statistics course. *Application deadline:* Applications may be processed on a rolling basis for some programs.
**Advanced Placement** Credit by examination available. Credit given for nursing courses completed elsewhere dependent upon specific evaluations.
**Degree Requirements** 36 total credit hours, thesis or project.

# Stillman College
## Nursing Major
## Tuscaloosa, Alabama

***http://www.stillman.edu/***
Founded in 1876

**DEGREE • BSN**
**Library Facilities** 116,945 volumes; 31,867 periodical subscriptions.

## BACCALAUREATE PROGRAMS

**Degree** BSN

**Available Programs** RN Baccalaureate.
**Contact** *Telephone:* 205-349-4240. *Fax:* 205-366-8996.

# Troy University
## School of Nursing
## Troy, Alabama

*http://www.troy.edu/*
Founded in 1887

**DEGREES • BSN • DNP • MSN**
**Nursing Program Faculty** 39 (49% with doctorates).
**Baccalaureate Enrollment** 800 **Women** 88% **Men** 12% **Minority** 35% **International** 4% **Part-time** 10%
**Graduate Enrollment** 200 **Women** 97% **Men** 3% **Minority** 23% **Part-time** 29%
**Distance Learning Courses** Available.
**Nursing Student Activities** Sigma Theta Tau, Student Nurses' Association.
**Nursing Student Resources** Academic advising; academic or career counseling; assistance for students with disabilities; bookstore; campus computer network; career placement assistance; computer lab; computer-assisted instruction; e-mail services; employment services for current students; externships; housing assistance; interactive nursing skills videos; Internet; learning resource lab; library services; nursing audiovisuals; placement services for program completers; resume preparation assistance; skills, simulation, or other laboratory; tutoring; unpaid internships.
**Library Facilities** 612,668 volumes (45,006 in health, 3,843 in nursing); 30,072 periodical subscriptions (703 health-care related).

### BACCALAUREATE PROGRAMS

**Degree** BSN
**Available Programs** Generic Baccalaureate; RN Baccalaureate.
**Site Options** Montgomery, AL; Phenix City, AL; Dothan, AL.
**Study Options** Full-time.
**Program Entrance Requirements** Minimum overall college GPA of 2.5, transcript of college record, CPR certification, health exam, health insurance, immunizations, professional liability insurance/malpractice insurance, prerequisite course work. Transfer students are accepted. *Application deadline:* 3/15 (fall), 9/15 (spring). *Application fee:* $20.
**Advanced Placement** Credit by examination available. Credit given for nursing courses completed elsewhere dependent upon specific evaluations.
**Contact** *Telephone:* 334-670-3428. *Fax:* 334-670-3744.

### GRADUATE PROGRAMS

**Contact** *Telephone:* 334-834-2320. *Fax:* 334-241-8627.

#### MASTER'S DEGREE PROGRAM

**Degree** MSN
**Available Programs** Master's.
**Concentrations Available** Nursing administration; nursing education; nursing informatics. *Clinical nurse specialist programs in:* adult health, maternity-newborn. *Nurse practitioner programs in:* family health.
**Site Options** Montgomery, AL; Phenix City, AL.
**Study Options** Full-time and part-time.
**Online Degree Options** Yes.
**Program Entrance Requirements** Minimum overall college GPA of 3.0, transcript of college record, CPR certification, immunizations, 3 letters of recommendation, physical assessment course, professional liability insurance/malpractice insurance. *Application deadline:* Applications may be processed on a rolling basis for some programs. *Application fee:* $20.
**Advanced Placement** Credit given for nursing courses completed elsewhere dependent upon specific evaluations.
**Degree Requirements** 39 total credit hours, thesis or project, comprehensive exam.

#### POST-MASTER'S PROGRAM

**Areas of Study** *Nurse practitioner programs in:* family health.

#### DOCTORAL DEGREE PROGRAM

**Degree** DNP
**Available Programs** Doctorate; Post-Baccalaureate Doctorate.
**Areas of Study** Advanced practice nursing.
**Site Options** Montgomery, AL; Phenix City, AL.
**Online Degree Options** Yes (online only).
**Program Entrance Requirements** Clinical experience, minimum overall college GPA of 3.0, interview by faculty committee, 2 letters of recommendation, MSN or equivalent, vita, writing sample. *Application deadline:* 2/1 (fall). *Application fee:* $75.
**Degree Requirements** 74 total credit hours, oral exam, residency.

# Tuskegee University
## Program in Nursing
## Tuskegee, Alabama

*http://www.tuskegee.edu/home.aspx*
Founded in 1881

**DEGREE • BSN**
**Nursing Program Faculty** 7 (43% with doctorates).
**Baccalaureate Enrollment** 145 **Women** 99% **Men** 1% **Minority** 100%
**Nursing Student Activities** Nursing Honor Society, Student Nurses' Association, nursing club.
**Nursing Student Resources** Academic advising; academic or career counseling; assistance for students with disabilities; bookstore; campus computer network; career placement assistance; computer lab; computer-assisted instruction; e-mail services; interactive nursing skills videos; Internet; learning resource lab; library services; nursing audiovisuals; placement services for program completers; remedial services; resume preparation assistance; skills, simulation, or other laboratory; tutoring; unpaid internships.
**Library Facilities** 623,824 volumes (4,500 in health, 600 in nursing); 81,157 periodical subscriptions (250 health-care related).

### BACCALAUREATE PROGRAMS

**Degree** BSN
**Available Programs** ADN to Baccalaureate; Generic Baccalaureate; RN Baccalaureate.
**Study Options** Full-time and part-time.
**Program Entrance Requirements** Minimum overall college GPA of 3.0, transcript of college record, CPR certification, written essay, health exam, health insurance, high school biology, high school chemistry, 2 years high school math, 1 year of high school science, high school transcript, immunizations, interview, minimum high school GPA of 3.0, minimum GPA in nursing prerequisites of 3.0, professional liability insurance/malpractice insurance, prerequisite course work. Transfer students are accepted. *Application deadline:* 5/30 (fall), 11/30 (spring), 4/30 (summer). Applications may be processed on a rolling basis for some programs. *Application fee:* $35.
**Advanced Placement** Credit given for nursing courses completed elsewhere dependent upon specific evaluations.
**Contact** *Telephone:* 334-727-8382. *Fax:* 334-727-5461.

# The University of Alabama
## Capstone College of Nursing
## Tuscaloosa, Alabama

*http://nursing.ua.edu/*
Founded in 1831

**DEGREES • BSN • DNP • MSN • MSN/ED D**
**Nursing Program Faculty** 62 (65% with doctorates).
**Baccalaureate Enrollment** 1,603 **Women** 90% **Men** 10% **Minority** 19% **Part-time** 14%
**Graduate Enrollment** 360 **Women** 87% **Men** 13% **Minority** 38% **Part-time** 62%
**Distance Learning Courses** Available.
**Nursing Student Activities** Sigma Theta Tau, Student Nurses' Association.
**Nursing Student Resources** Academic advising; academic or career counseling; assistance for students with disabilities; bookstore; campus computer network; career placement assistance; computer lab; computer-assisted instruction; e-mail services; interactive nursing skills videos; Internet; learning resource lab; library services; paid internships; placement services for program completers; skills, simulation, or other laboratory; tutoring; unpaid internships.
**Library Facilities** 4 million volumes (21,000 in health, 350 in nursing); 118,753 periodical subscriptions (1,500 health-care related).

## BACCALAUREATE PROGRAMS

**Degree** BSN
**Available Programs** Baccalaureate for Second Degree; Generic Baccalaureate; RN Baccalaureate.
**Study Options** Full-time.
**Program Entrance Requirements** Minimum overall college GPA of 3.0, transcript of college record, CPR certification, health exam, health insurance, 4 years high school math, 4 years high school science, high school transcript, immunizations, minimum high school GPA of 2.5, minimum GPA in nursing prerequisites of 3.0, professional liability insurance/malpractice insurance, prerequisite course work. Transfer students are accepted. *Application deadline:* 6/1 (fall), 3/1 (summer). *Application fee:* $25.
**Expenses (2013–14)** *Tuition, state resident:* full-time $4725; part-time $1505 per course. *Tuition, nonresident:* full-time $11,975; part-time $3340 per course. *International tuition:* $11,975 full-time. *Room and board:* $11,800; room only: $8800 per academic year. *Required fees:* full-time $800; part-time $33 per credit.
**Financial Aid** 75% of baccalaureate students in nursing programs received some form of financial aid in 2012–13.
**Contact** Ms. Rebekah Welch, Director of Nursing Student Services, Capstone College of Nursing, The University of Alabama, Box 870358, Tuscaloosa, AL 35487-0358. *Telephone:* 205-348-6639. *Fax:* 205-348-6589. *E-mail:* rebekah.welch@ua.edu.

## GRADUATE PROGRAMS

**Expenses (2013–14)** *Tuition, state resident:* part-time $340 per contact hour. *Tuition, nonresident:* part-time $340 per contact hour.
**Financial Aid** 49% of graduate students in nursing programs received some form of financial aid in 2012–13.
**Contact** Dr. Joe Burrage, Assistant Dean, Graduate Program, Capstone College of Nursing, The University of Alabama, Box 870358, Tuscaloosa, AL 35487-0358. *Telephone:* 205-348-1020. *Fax:* 205-348-6674. *E-mail:* jwburrage@ua.edu.

### MASTER'S DEGREE PROGRAM

**Degrees** MSN; MSN/Ed D
**Available Programs** Master's; RN to Master's.
**Concentrations Available** Clinical nurse leader; nurse case management; nursing administration; nursing education. *Nurse practitioner programs in:* family health, psychiatric/mental health.
**Study Options** Full-time and part-time.
**Online Degree Options** Yes (online only).
**Program Entrance Requirements** Computer literacy, minimum overall college GPA of 3.0, transcript of college record, CPR certification, written essay, immunizations, 2 letters of recommendation, professional liability insurance/malpractice insurance, resume. *Application deadline:* 6/1 (fall). Applications may be processed on a rolling basis for some programs. *Application fee:* $50.
**Degree Requirements** 38 total credit hours.

### POST-MASTER'S PROGRAM

**Areas of Study** Clinical nurse leader; nurse case management.

### DOCTORAL DEGREE PROGRAM

**Degree** DNP
**Available Programs** Doctorate.
**Areas of Study** Advanced practice nursing, nursing administration.
**Online Degree Options** Yes (online only).
**Program Entrance Requirements** Minimum overall college GPA of 3.0, interview by faculty committee, interview, 3 letters of recommendation, MSN or equivalent, vita, writing sample. *Application deadline:* 4/1 (fall). Applications may be processed on a rolling basis for some programs. *Application fee:* $50.
**Degree Requirements** 34 total credit hours.

# The University of Alabama at Birmingham

**School of Nursing**
**Birmingham, Alabama**

***http://www.uab.edu/***
Founded in 1969
**DEGREES • BSN • DNP • MSN • MSN/MPH • PHD**
**Nursing Program Faculty** 116 (70% with doctorates).
**Baccalaureate Enrollment** 518 **Women** 82% **Men** 18% **Minority** 31% **International** 2% **Part-time** 44%
**Graduate Enrollment** 1,796 **Women** 81% **Men** 19% **Minority** 22% **International** 1% **Part-time** 88%
**Distance Learning Courses** Available.
**Nursing Student Activities** Sigma Theta Tau, Student Nurses' Association, nursing club.
**Nursing Student Resources** Academic advising; academic or career counseling; assistance for students with disabilities; bookstore; campus computer network; career placement assistance; computer lab; computer-assisted instruction; e-mail services; housing assistance; interactive nursing skills videos; Internet; learning resource lab; library services; nursing audiovisuals; paid internships; placement services for program completers; resume preparation assistance; skills, simulation, or other laboratory; tutoring.
**Library Facilities** 1.1 million volumes (131,721 in health, 7,003 in nursing); 36,371 periodical subscriptions (9,184 health-care related).

## BACCALAUREATE PROGRAMS

**Degree** BSN
**Available Programs** Baccalaureate for Second Degree; Generic Baccalaureate; RN Baccalaureate.
**Study Options** Full-time.
**Program Entrance Requirements** Minimum overall college GPA of 2.75, transcript of college record, CPR certification, written essay, health exam, health insurance, high school transcript, immunizations, minimum high school GPA of 2.0, minimum GPA in nursing prerequisites of 2.75, prerequisite course work. Transfer students are accepted. *Application deadline:* 4/11 (fall), 9/13 (spring).
**Expenses (2013–14)** *Tuition, state resident:* full-time $9850; part-time $337 per credit hour. *Tuition, nonresident:* full-time $13,210; part-time $457 per credit hour. *International tuition:* $13,210 full-time. *Room and board:* $8395; room only: $5955 per academic year. *Required fees:* full-time $1650; part-time $825 per term.
**Financial Aid** 65% of baccalaureate students in nursing programs received some form of financial aid in 2012–13.
**Contact** Mr. Peter Tofani, Assistant Dean for Student Affairs, School of Nursing, The University of Alabama at Birmingham, NB 1003, 1720 2nd Avenue South, Birmingham, AL 35294-1210. *Telephone:* 205-975-7529. *Fax:* 205-934-5490. *E-mail:* tofanip@uab.edu.

## GRADUATE PROGRAMS

**Expenses (2013–14)** *Tuition, state resident:* full-time $8847; part-time $457 per credit hour. *Tuition, nonresident:* full-time $19,953; part-time $1074 per credit hour. *International tuition:* $19,953 full-time. *Room and board:* $7495; room only: $5955 per academic year. *Required fees:* full-time $2100; part-time $700 per term.
**Financial Aid** 51% of graduate students in nursing programs received some form of financial aid in 2012–13. Fellowships, research assistantships, teaching assistantships, Federal Work-Study available. Aid available to part-time students.
**Contact** Mr. Peter Tofani, Assistant Dean for Student Affairs, School of Nursing, The University of Alabama at Birmingham, NB 1003, 1720 2nd Avenue South, Birmingham, AL 35294-1210. *Telephone:* 205-975-7529. *Fax:* 205-934-5490. *E-mail:* tofanip@uab.edu.

### MASTER'S DEGREE PROGRAM

**Degrees** MSN; MSN/MPH
**Available Programs** Accelerated AD/RN to Master's; Accelerated Master's for Non-Nursing College Graduates; Master's.
**Concentrations Available** Clinical nurse leader; health-care administration; nurse anesthesia; nursing administration; nursing education; nursing informatics. *Nurse practitioner programs in:* acute care, adult health, family health, neonatal health, occupational health, pediatric, psychiatric/mental health,women's health.
**Study Options** Full-time and part-time.
**Program Entrance Requirements** Clinical experience, computer literacy, minimum overall college GPA of 3.0, transcript of college record, CPR certification, written essay, immunizations, 3 letters of recommendation, prerequisite course work, resume, statistics course, GRE, GMAT, or MAT. *Application deadline:* 3/16 (fall), 10/28 (summer). *Application fee:* $45.
**Advanced Placement** Credit given for nursing courses completed elsewhere dependent upon specific evaluations.
**Degree Requirements** 44 total credit hours, comprehensive exam.

### POST-MASTER'S PROGRAM

**Areas of Study** *Nurse practitioner programs in:* acute care, adult health, family health, neonatal health, pediatric, psychiatric/mental health.

### DOCTORAL DEGREE PROGRAM

**Degree** DNP
**Available Programs** Doctorate.
**Areas of Study** Advanced practice nursing, health-care systems, nursing administration.
**Program Entrance Requirements** Minimum overall college GPA of 3.0, clinical experience, 3 letters of recommendation, statistics course, vita, writing sample. *Application deadline:* 1/18 (fall). *Application fee:* $45.
**Degree Requirements** 66 total credit hours, dissertation, residency, written exam.

**Degree** PhD
**Available Programs** Doctorate; Post-Baccalaureate Doctorate.
**Areas of Study** Nursing research, nursing science.
**Program Entrance Requirements** Clinical experience, minimum overall college GPA of 3.0, interview by faculty committee, interview, 3 letters of recommendation, scholarly papers, statistics course, vita, writing sample, GRE General Test. *Application deadline:* 1/18 (fall). *Application fee:* $45.
**Degree Requirements** 66 total credit hours, dissertation, oral exam, written exam, residency.

### POSTDOCTORAL PROGRAM

**Areas of Study** Nursing research, outcomes, vulnerable population.
**Postdoctoral Program Contact** Dr. Patricia Patrician, Donna Brown Banton Endowed Professorship and Associate Professor, School of Nursing, The University of Alabama at Birmingham, 1720 2nd Avenue South, Birmingham, AL 35294-1210. *Telephone:* 205-996-5211. *Fax:* 205-934-5490. *E-mail:* ppatrici@uab.edu.

## CONTINUING EDUCATION PROGRAM

**Contact** Dr. Cynthia S. Selleck, Associate Dean of Clinic Affairs and Partnerships, School of Nursing, The University of Alabama at Birmingham, School of Nursing, NB 443A, 1720 2nd Avenue South, Birmingham, AL 35294. *Telephone:* 205-934-6569. *Fax:* 205-996-6585. *E-mail:* cselleck@uab.edu.

# The University of Alabama in Huntsville

**College of Nursing**
**Huntsville, Alabama**

***http://www.uah.edu/nursing/***
Founded in 1950

**DEGREES • BSN • DNP • MSN**

**Nursing Program Faculty** 46 (30% with doctorates).
**Baccalaureate Enrollment** 662 **Women** 90% **Men** 10% **Minority** 14% **International** 1% **Part-time** 22%
**Graduate Enrollment** 106 **Women** 92% **Men** 8% **Minority** 15% **International** 1% **Part-time** 65%
**Distance Learning Courses** Available.
**Nursing Student Activities** Sigma Theta Tau, Student Nurses' Association.
**Nursing Student Resources** Academic advising; academic or career counseling; assistance for students with disabilities; bookstore; campus computer network; career placement assistance; computer lab; computer-assisted instruction; e-mail services; employment services for current students; housing assistance; interactive nursing skills videos; Internet; learning resource lab; library services; nursing audiovisuals; placement services for program completers; remedial services; resume preparation assistance; skills, simulation, or other laboratory; tutoring.
**Library Facilities** 302,503 volumes (13,004 in health, 3,480 in nursing); 628 periodical subscriptions (3,200 health-care related).

## BACCALAUREATE PROGRAMS

**Degree** BSN
**Available Programs** Baccalaureate for Second Degree; Generic Baccalaureate; RN Baccalaureate.
**Study Options** Full-time and part-time.
**Program Entrance Requirements** Minimum overall college GPA of 2.0, transcript of college record, CPR certification, health exam, health insurance, immunizations, minimum GPA in nursing prerequisites of 2.0, professional liability insurance/malpractice insurance, prerequisite course work. Transfer students are accepted. *Application deadline:* 3/1 (fall), 9/1 (spring).
**Advanced Placement** Credit by examination available. Credit given for nursing courses completed elsewhere dependent upon specific evaluations.
**Contact** *Telephone:* 256-824-6742. *Fax:* 256-824-2850.

## GRADUATE PROGRAMS

**Contact** *Telephone:* 256-824-6742. *Fax:* 256-824-6026.

### MASTER'S DEGREE PROGRAM

**Degree** MSN
**Available Programs** Master's; RN to Master's.
**Concentrations Available** Clinical nurse leader; health-care administration. *Clinical nurse specialist programs in:* adult health. *Nurse practitioner programs in:* acute care, family health.
**Study Options** Full-time and part-time.
**Online Degree Options** Yes.
**Program Entrance Requirements** Minimum overall college GPA of 3.0, transcript of college record, CPR certification, immunizations, 3 letters of recommendation, professional liability insurance/malpractice insurance, statistics course, MAT or GRE. *Application deadline:* 4/15 (fall).
**Advanced Placement** Credit given for nursing courses completed elsewhere dependent upon specific evaluations.
**Degree Requirements** 42 total credit hours, thesis or project, comprehensive exam.

### POST-MASTER'S PROGRAM

**Areas of Study** Nursing education. *Nurse practitioner programs in:* family health.

### DOCTORAL DEGREE PROGRAM

**Degree** DNP
**Available Programs** Doctorate.
**Areas of Study** Advanced practice nursing, nursing administration.
**Online Degree Options** Yes (online only).
**Program Entrance Requirements** Interview by faculty committee, letters of recommendation, MSN or equivalent, vita, writing sample. *Application deadline:* 4/15 (fall). *Application fee:* $40.
**Degree Requirements** 34 total credit hours, oral exam, written exam.

## CONTINUING EDUCATION PROGRAM

**Contact** *Telephone:* 256-824-2456. *Fax:* 256-824-6026.

# University of Mobile

**School of Nursing**
**Mobile, Alabama**

***http://www.umobile.edu/***
Founded in 1961

**DEGREES • BSN • MSN**

**Nursing Program Faculty** 14 (22% with doctorates).
**Baccalaureate Enrollment** 105 **Women** 93% **Men** 7% **Minority** 34%
**Graduate Enrollment** 19 **Women** 90% **Men** 10% **Minority** 54% **Part-time** 21%
**Nursing Student Activities** Sigma Theta Tau, Student Nurses' Association.
**Nursing Student Resources** Academic advising; academic or career counseling; assistance for students with disabilities; bookstore; campus computer network; career placement assistance; computer lab; computer-assisted instruction; e-mail services; employment services for current students; interactive nursing skills videos; Internet; learning resource lab; library services; nursing audiovisuals; remedial services; resume preparation assistance; skills, simulation, or other laboratory; tutoring; unpaid internships.
**Library Facilities** 221,828 volumes (10,000 in health, 6,500 in nursing); 190 periodical subscriptions (4,373 health-care related).

## BACCALAUREATE PROGRAMS

**Degree** BSN
**Available Programs** ADN to Baccalaureate; Generic Baccalaureate; RN Baccalaureate.
**Study Options** Full-time.
**Program Entrance Requirements** Minimum overall college GPA of 2.75, transcript of college record, CPR certification, health exam, health

insurance, high school transcript, immunizations, minimum GPA in nursing prerequisites of 2.75, prerequisite course work. Transfer students are accepted. *Application deadline:* 3/1 (fall).
**Advanced Placement** Credit given for nursing courses completed elsewhere dependent upon specific evaluations.
**Expenses (2012–13)** *Tuition:* full-time $17,110; part-time $609 per credit hour. *International tuition:* $17,110 full-time. *Room and board:* $8650; room only: $5100 per academic year. *Required fees:* full-time $570; part-time $346 per term.
**Financial Aid** 96% of baccalaureate students in nursing programs received some form of financial aid in 2011–12.
**Contact** Mrs. Mattie Easter, Assistant Professor, School of Nursing, University of Mobile, 5735 College Parkway, Mobile, AL 36613-2842. *Telephone:* 251-442-2337. *Fax:* 251-442-2520. *E-mail:* measter@mail.umobile.edu.

## GRADUATE PROGRAMS

**Expenses (2012–13)** *Tuition:* full-time $8604; part-time $478 per credit hour. *International tuition:* $8604 full-time. *Required fees:* full-time $146; part-time $73 per term.
**Financial Aid** 50% of graduate students in nursing programs received some form of financial aid in 2011–12.
**Contact** Dr. Janith C. Wood, Department Chair, School of Nursing, University of Mobile, 5735 College Parkway, Mobile, AL 36613-2842. *Telephone:* 251-442-2446. *Fax:* 251-442-2520. *E-mail:* jwood@mail.umobile.edu.

### MASTER'S DEGREE PROGRAM

**Degree** MSN
**Available Programs** Master's.
**Concentrations Available** Nursing administration; nursing education.
**Study Options** Full-time and part-time.
**Program Entrance Requirements** Minimum overall college GPA of 3.0, transcript of college record, CPR certification, immunizations, 3 letters of recommendation, statistics course. *Application deadline:* Applications may be processed on a rolling basis for some programs. *Application fee:* $40.
**Advanced Placement** Credit given for nursing courses completed elsewhere dependent upon specific evaluations.
**Degree Requirements** 39 total credit hours, thesis or project, comprehensive exam.

## CONTINUING EDUCATION PROGRAM

**Contact** Dr. Janith C. Wood, Dean, School of Nursing, School of Nursing, University of Mobile, 5735 College Parkway, Mobile, AL 36613. *Telephone:* 251-442-2446. *Fax:* 251-442-2520. *E-mail:* Jwood@mail.umobile.edu.

# University of North Alabama

**College of Nursing and Allied Health**
**Florence, Alabama**

***http://www.una.edu/nursing/***
Founded in 1830

**DEGREES • BSN • MSN**
**Nursing Program Faculty** 37 (22% with doctorates).
**Baccalaureate Enrollment** 390 **Women** 87% **Men** 13% **Minority** 20.5% **International** 1% **Part-time** 31%
**Graduate Enrollment** 36 **Women** 97% **Men** 3% **Minority** 17% **Part-time** 25%
**Distance Learning Courses** Available.
**Nursing Student Activities** Sigma Theta Tau, Student Nurses' Association.
**Nursing Student Resources** Academic advising; academic or career counseling; assistance for students with disabilities; bookstore; campus computer network; career placement assistance; computer lab; e-mail services; employment services for current students; housing assistance; interactive nursing skills videos; Internet; learning resource lab; library services; nursing audiovisuals; remedial services; resume preparation assistance; skills, simulation, or other laboratory; tutoring.
**Library Facilities** 670,168 volumes; 24,421 periodical subscriptions.

## BACCALAUREATE PROGRAMS

**Degree** BSN
**Available Programs** Generic Baccalaureate; RN Baccalaureate.
**Study Options** Full-time and part-time.
**Online Degree Options** Yes (online only).
**Program Entrance Requirements** Transcript of college record, CPR certification, health exam, health insurance, high school transcript, immunizations, minimum GPA in nursing prerequisites of 2.5, professional liability insurance/malpractice insurance, prerequisite course work. Transfer students are accepted.
**Contact** *Telephone:* 256-765-4984. *Fax:* 256-765-4935.

## GRADUATE PROGRAMS

**Contact** *Telephone:* 256-765-4931. *Fax:* 256-765-4701.

### MASTER'S DEGREE PROGRAM

**Degree** MSN
**Available Programs** Master's.
**Concentrations Available** Nursing administration; nursing education.
**Study Options** Full-time and part-time.
**Online Degree Options** Yes (online only).
**Program Entrance Requirements** Clinical experience, minimum overall college GPA of 3.0, transcript of college record, written essay, 3 letters of recommendation, professional liability insurance/malpractice insurance.
**Degree Requirements** 42 total credit hours, thesis or project.

## CONTINUING EDUCATION PROGRAM

**Contact** *Telephone:* 256-765-4787. *Fax:* 256-765-4872.

# University of South Alabama

**College of Nursing**
**Mobile, Alabama**

***http://www.southalabama.edu/nursing/***
Founded in 1963

**DEGREES • BSN • MSN**
**Nursing Program Faculty** 57 (30% with doctorates).
**Baccalaureate Enrollment** 316 **Women** 82% **Men** 18% **Minority** 24% **International** 3% **Part-time** 11%
**Graduate Enrollment** 368 **Women** 86% **Men** 14% **Minority** 19% **Part-time** 22%
**Nursing Student Activities** Sigma Theta Tau, Student Nurses' Association.
**Nursing Student Resources** Academic advising; academic or career counseling; assistance for students with disabilities; bookstore; campus computer network; career placement assistance; computer lab; learning resource lab; library services; nursing audiovisuals; resume preparation assistance.
**Library Facilities** 794,249 volumes (2,406 in health, 2,300 in nursing); 980 periodical subscriptions (299 health-care related).

## BACCALAUREATE PROGRAMS

**Degree** BSN
**Available Programs** ADN to Baccalaureate; Accelerated Baccalaureate; Generic Baccalaureate; RN Baccalaureate.
**Site Options** Fairhope, AL.
**Study Options** Full-time and part-time.
**Program Entrance Requirements** Minimum overall college GPA of 2.5, transcript of college record, CPR certification, health exam, health insurance, immunizations, minimum GPA in nursing prerequisites of 2.5, professional liability insurance/malpractice insurance, prerequisite course work. Transfer students are accepted.
**Advanced Placement** Credit given for nursing courses completed elsewhere dependent upon specific evaluations.
**Contact** *Telephone:* 251-434-3410. *Fax:* 251-434-3413.

## GRADUATE PROGRAMS

**Contact** *Telephone:* 251-434-3410. *Fax:* 251-434-3413.

### MASTER'S DEGREE PROGRAM

**Degree** MSN
**Available Programs** Accelerated Master's; Master's; Master's for Nurses with Non-Nursing Degrees.
**Concentrations Available** Nursing administration; nursing education. *Clinical nurse specialist programs in:* acute care, community health, family health, gerontology, maternity-newborn, pediatric, psychiatric/mental health,women's health. *Nurse practitioner programs in:*

acute care, family health, gerontology, neonatal health, pediatric, psychiatric/mental health,women's health.
**Study Options** Full-time and part-time.
**Program Entrance Requirements** Computer literacy, minimum overall college GPA of 3.0, transcript of college record, immunizations, nursing research course, physical assessment course, resume.
**Advanced Placement** Credit given for nursing courses completed elsewhere dependent upon specific evaluations.
**Degree Requirements** 30 total credit hours, thesis or project.

**POST-MASTER'S PROGRAM**
**Areas of Study** Nursing administration; nursing education. *Clinical nurse specialist programs in:* acute care, community health, family health, gerontology, maternity-newborn, pediatric, psychiatric/mental health,women's health. *Nurse practitioner programs in:* acute care, family health, gerontology, neonatal health, pediatric, psychiatric/mental health,women's health.

# ALASKA

## University of Alaska Anchorage
### School of Nursing
### Anchorage, Alaska

***http://www.uaa.alaska.edu/schoolofnursing/***
Founded in 1954

**DEGREES • BS • MS**
**Nursing Program Faculty** 26 (42% with doctorates).
**Baccalaureate Enrollment** 224 **Women** 80% **Men** 20% **Minority** 31% **International** 3% **Part-time** 18%
**Graduate Enrollment** 60 **Women** 94% **Men** 6% **Minority** 9% **Part-time** 12%
**Nursing Student Activities** Sigma Theta Tau, Student Nurses' Association.
**Nursing Student Resources** Academic advising; academic or career counseling; assistance for students with disabilities; bookstore; campus computer network; career placement assistance; computer lab; computer-assisted instruction; daycare for children of students; e-mail services; interactive nursing skills videos; Internet; learning resource lab; library services; nursing audiovisuals; placement services for program completers; remedial services; resume preparation assistance; skills, simulation, or other laboratory; tutoring.
**Library Facilities** 23,000 volumes in health, 150 volumes in nursing; 780 periodical subscriptions health-care related.

### BACCALAUREATE PROGRAMS
**Degree** BS
**Available Programs** Generic Baccalaureate; RN Baccalaureate.
**Study Options** Full-time and part-time.
**Program Entrance Requirements** Minimum overall college GPA of 2.7, transcript of college record, CPR certification, written essay, immunizations, 3 letters of recommendation, minimum GPA in nursing prerequisites of 2.7, professional liability insurance/malpractice insurance, prerequisite course work. Transfer students are accepted.
**Advanced Placement** Credit given for nursing courses completed elsewhere dependent upon specific evaluations.
**Contact** *Telephone:* 907-786-4550. *Fax:* 907-786-4558.

### GRADUATE PROGRAMS
**Contact** *Telephone:* 907-786-4570. *Fax:* 907-786-4559.

**MASTER'S DEGREE PROGRAM**
**Degree** MS
**Available Programs** Master's.
**Concentrations Available** Health-care administration; nursing education. *Clinical nurse specialist programs in:* community health, psychiatric/mental health. *Nurse practitioner programs in:* family health, psychiatric/mental health.
**Study Options** Full-time and part-time.
**Program Entrance Requirements** Clinical experience, minimum overall college GPA of 3.0, transcript of college record, written essay, 3 letters of recommendation, nursing research course, prerequisite course work, statistics course, GRE or MAT.
**Advanced Placement** Credit given for nursing courses completed elsewhere dependent upon specific evaluations.
**Degree Requirements** 50 total credit hours, thesis or project.

# ARIZONA

## Arizona State University at the Downtown Phoenix Campus
### College of Nursing
### Phoenix, Arizona

***https://campus.asu.edu/downtown***
Founded in 2006

**DEGREES • BSN • DNP • MS • MS/MPH**
**Nursing Program Faculty** 119 (44% with doctorates).
**Baccalaureate Enrollment** 1,085 **Women** 88% **Men** 12% **Minority** 31% **International** 1% **Part-time** 18%
**Graduate Enrollment** 363 **Women** 91% **Men** 9% **Minority** 7% **Part-time** 46%
**Distance Learning Courses** Available.
**Nursing Student Activities** Nursing Honor Society, Sigma Theta Tau, Student Nurses' Association, nursing club.
**Nursing Student Resources** Academic advising; academic or career counseling; assistance for students with disabilities; bookstore; campus computer network; career placement assistance; computer lab; computer-assisted instruction; daycare for children of students; e-mail services; employment services for current students; housing assistance; interactive nursing skills videos; Internet; learning resource lab; library services; nursing audiovisuals; paid internships; placement services for program completers; remedial services; resume preparation assistance; skills, simulation, or other laboratory; tutoring; unpaid internships.
**Library Facilities** 77,814 volumes in health, 7,501 volumes in nursing; 755 periodical subscriptions health-care related.

### BACCALAUREATE PROGRAMS
**Degree** BSN
**Available Programs** Accelerated Baccalaureate; Accelerated Baccalaureate for Second Degree; Accelerated RN Baccalaureate; Baccalaureate for Second Degree; Generic Baccalaureate; RN Baccalaureate.
**Site Options** Phoenix, AZ; Scottsdale, AZ.
**Study Options** Full-time.
**Online Degree Options** Yes.
**Program Entrance Requirements** Minimum overall college GPA of 3.5, transcript of college record, CPR certification, health exam, health insurance, high school biology, high school chemistry, high school foreign language, 4 years high school math, 3 years high school science, high school transcript, immunizations, minimum high school GPA of 3.5, minimum high school rank 25%, minimum GPA in nursing prerequisites of 3.75, professional liability insurance/malpractice insurance, prerequisite course work. Transfer students are accepted. *Application deadline:* 2/1 (fall), 9/1 (spring), 2/1 (summer). *Application fee:* $65.
**Financial Aid** 70% of baccalaureate students in nursing programs received some form of financial aid in 2012–13.
**Contact** Sara Sullivan, Senior Student Support Specialist, College of Nursing, Arizona State University at the Downtown Phoenix Campus, 502 East Monroe Street, Suite C 250, Phoenix, AZ 85004-4431. *Telephone:* 602-496-0887. *Fax:* 602-496-0705. *E-mail:* sara.sullivan@asu.edu.

### GRADUATE PROGRAMS
**Financial Aid** 75% of graduate students in nursing programs received some form of financial aid in 2012–13.
**Contact** Ms. Eula Bradley, Manager, Graduate Student Success, College of Nursing, Arizona State University at the Downtown Phoenix Campus, 550 North 3rd Street, Phoenix, AZ 85004. *Telephone:* 602-496-0703. *E-mail:* eula.bradley@asu.edu.

**MASTER'S DEGREE PROGRAM**
**Degrees** MS; MS/MPH
**Available Programs** Master's.
**Concentrations Available** *Clinical nurse specialist programs in:* acute care, adult health, community health, pediatric, psychiatric/mental health.

*Nurse practitioner programs in:* acute care, adult health, family health, neonatal health, pediatric, psychiatric/mental health,women's health.
**Site Options** Phoenix, AZ.
**Study Options** Full-time and part-time.
**Program Entrance Requirements** Clinical experience, minimum overall college GPA of 3.0, transcript of college record, immunizations, interview, 3 letters of recommendation, physical assessment course, prerequisite course work, resume, statistics course, GRE.
**Advanced Placement** Credit given for nursing courses completed elsewhere dependent upon specific evaluations.
**Degree Requirements** 40 total credit hours, thesis or project.

**POST-MASTER'S PROGRAM**
**Areas of Study** *Clinical nurse specialist programs in:* acute care, adult health, community health, pediatric, psychiatric/mental health. *Nurse practitioner programs in:* acute care, adult health, family health, neonatal health, pediatric, psychiatric/mental health,women's health.

**DOCTORAL DEGREE PROGRAM**
**Degree** DNP
**Available Programs** Doctorate.
**Areas of Study** Advanced practice nursing.
**Site Options** Phoenix, AZ.

### CONTINUING EDUCATION PROGRAM
**Contact** Amy Fitzgerald, RN, Assistant Director, College of Nursing, Arizona State University at the Downtown Phoenix Campus, 550 North 3rd Street, Phoenix, AZ 85004. *Telephone:* 602-496-2175. *E-mail:* Amy.Fitzgerald@asu.edu.

## Brookline College
### Baccalaureate Nursing Program
### Phoenix, Arizona

*http://brooklinecollege.edu/*
Founded in 1979

**DEGREE • BSN**

### BACCALAUREATE PROGRAMS
**Degree** BSN
**Available Programs** Accelerated Baccalaureate for Second Degree; Generic Baccalaureate.
**Contact** Phoenix Campus, Baccalaureate Nursing Program, Brookline College, 2445 West Dunlap Avenue, Suite 100, Phoenix, AZ 85021-5820. *Telephone:* 602-242-6265. *Fax:* 602-973-2572.

## Chamberlain College of Nursing
### Chamberlain College of Nursing
### Phoenix, Arizona

*http://www.chamberlain.edu/nursing-schools/phoenix-arizona*

**DEGREES • BSN • MSN**
**Distance Learning Courses** Available.

### BACCALAUREATE PROGRAMS
**Degree** BSN
**Available Programs** Accelerated Baccalaureate; Accelerated Baccalaureate for Second Degree; RN Baccalaureate.
**Contact** *Telephone:* 888-556-8226.

### GRADUATE PROGRAMS
**Contact** *Telephone:* 888-556-8226.

**MASTER'S DEGREE PROGRAM**
**Degree** MSN
**Available Programs** Master's.

## Grand Canyon University
### College of Nursing and Health Sciences
### Phoenix, Arizona

*http://www.gcu.edu/*
Founded in 1949

**DEGREES • BSN • MS • MSN/MBA**
**Nursing Program Faculty** 122 (3% with doctorates).
**Baccalaureate Enrollment** 1,067 **Women** 90% **Men** 10% **International** .01% **Part-time** 58%
**Graduate Enrollment** 297 **Women** 93% **Men** 7% **Part-time** 89%
**Distance Learning Courses** Available.
**Nursing Student Activities** Sigma Theta Tau, Student Nurses' Association.
**Nursing Student Resources** Academic advising; academic or career counseling; assistance for students with disabilities; bookstore; campus computer network; career placement assistance; computer lab; computer-assisted instruction; e-mail services; employment services for current students; housing assistance; Internet; learning resource lab; library services; nursing audiovisuals; other; paid internships; remedial services; resume preparation assistance; skills, simulation, or other laboratory; tutoring; unpaid internships.
**Library Facilities** 158,587 volumes (9,663 in health); 57,802 periodical subscriptions (177 health-care related).

### BACCALAUREATE PROGRAMS
**Degree** BSN
**Available Programs** ADN to Baccalaureate; RN Baccalaureate.
**Site Options** Phoenix, AZ; Tucson, AZ; Albuquerque, NM.
**Study Options** Full-time.
**Online Degree Options** Yes.
**Program Entrance Requirements** Minimum overall college GPA of 3.0, transcript of college record, CPR certification, health exam, health insurance, high school transcript, immunizations, minimum GPA in nursing prerequisites of 3.0, prerequisite course work. Transfer students are accepted. *Application deadline:* 5/15 (fall), 9/15 (spring), 1/15 (summer).
**Advanced Placement** Credit by examination available. Credit given for nursing courses completed elsewhere dependent upon specific evaluations.
**Contact** *Telephone:* 602-639-6429.

### GRADUATE PROGRAMS
**Contact** *Telephone:* 602-639-7982.

**MASTER'S DEGREE PROGRAM**
**Degrees** MS; MSN/MBA
**Available Programs** Master's.
**Concentrations Available** Nursing administration; nursing education. *Clinical nurse specialist programs in:* adult health. *Nurse practitioner programs in:* acute care, family health.
**Site Options** Phoenix, AZ; Tucson, AZ.
**Study Options** Full-time and part-time.
**Online Degree Options** Yes.
**Program Entrance Requirements** Clinical experience, computer literacy, minimum overall college GPA of 3.0, transcript of college record, CPR certification, written essay, immunizations, interview, nursing research course, physical assessment course, professional liability insurance/malpractice insurance, prerequisite course work, resume, statistics course. *Application deadline:* Applications may be processed on a rolling basis for some programs.
**Advanced Placement** Credit given for nursing courses completed elsewhere dependent upon specific evaluations.
**Degree Requirements** 52 total credit hours, thesis or project.

**POST-MASTER'S PROGRAM**
**Areas of Study** Nursing education. *Clinical nurse specialist programs in:* adult health. *Nurse practitioner programs in:* acute care, family health.

### CONTINUING EDUCATION PROGRAM
**Contact** *Telephone:* 602-639-7982. *Fax:* 602-639-7982.

# Northern Arizona University
## School of Nursing
## Flagstaff, Arizona

***http://www.nau.edu/chhs/nursing/***
Founded in 1899

**DEGREES • BSN • DNP • MS**

**Nursing Program Faculty** 80 (30% with doctorates).
**Baccalaureate Enrollment** 1,200 **Women** 88% **Men** 12% **Minority** 20% **International** 1% **Part-time** 50%
**Graduate Enrollment** 120 **Women** 96% **Men** 4% **Minority** 20% **Part-time** 65%
**Distance Learning Courses** Available.
**Nursing Student Activities** Sigma Theta Tau, Student Nurses' Association.
**Nursing Student Resources** Academic advising; academic or career counseling; assistance for students with disabilities; bookstore; campus computer network; computer lab; computer-assisted instruction; e-mail services; interactive nursing skills videos; Internet; learning resource lab; library services; nursing audiovisuals; remedial services; skills, simulation, or other laboratory; tutoring.
**Library Facilities** 892,809 volumes; 59,863 periodical subscriptions.

### BACCALAUREATE PROGRAMS

**Degree** BSN
**Available Programs** ADN to Baccalaureate; Accelerated Baccalaureate for Second Degree; Generic Baccalaureate; RN Baccalaureate.
**Site Options** Yuma, AZ; Tucson, AZ; St. Michaels/Window Rock, AZ.
**Study Options** Full-time.
**Online Degree Options** Yes.
**Program Entrance Requirements** Transcript of college record, CPR certification, health exam, health insurance, high school transcript, immunizations, 2 letters of recommendation, minimum GPA in nursing prerequisites of 2.75, professional liability insurance/malpractice insurance, prerequisite course work. Transfer students are accepted. *Application deadline:* 3/15 (fall), 10/15 (spring).
**Advanced Placement** Credit given for nursing courses completed elsewhere dependent upon specific evaluations.
**Financial Aid** 75% of baccalaureate students in nursing programs received some form of financial aid in 2012–13. *Gift aid (need-based):* Federal Pell, FSEOG, state, private, college/university gift aid from institutional funds, Federal Nursing, TEACH Grants, tribal grants, LEAP Grants. *Loans:* Federal Nursing Student Loans, Federal Direct (Subsidized and Unsubsidized Stafford PLUS), Perkins, state, college/university. *Work-study:* Federal Work-Study, part-time campus jobs. *Financial aid application deadline (priority):* 2/1.
**Contact** Mr. Gregg Schneider, Senior Academic Advisor, School of Nursing, Northern Arizona University, Box 15035, Flagstaff, AZ 86011. *Telephone:* 928-523-6717. *Fax:* 928-523-7171. *E-mail:* gregg.schneider@nau.edu.

### GRADUATE PROGRAMS

**Financial Aid** 75% of graduate students in nursing programs received some form of financial aid in 2012–13. Career-related internships or fieldwork, Federal Work-Study, scholarships, traineeships, tuition waivers, and unspecified assistantships available.
**Contact** Dr. Barbara Tomlinson, Graduate Program Coordinator, School of Nursing, Northern Arizona University, Box 15035, Flagstaff, AZ 86011. *Telephone:* 928-523-3536. *Fax:* 928-523-7171. *E-mail:* barbara.tomlinson@nau.edu.

#### MASTER'S DEGREE PROGRAM

**Degree** MS
**Available Programs** Master's.
**Concentrations Available** *Nurse practitioner programs in:* family health.
**Site Options** Yuma, AZ; Tucson, AZ; St. Michaels/Window Rock, AZ.
**Study Options** Full-time and part-time.
**Online Degree Options** Yes (online only).
**Program Entrance Requirements** Clinical experience, computer literacy, minimum overall college GPA of 3.0, transcript of college record, CPR certification, written essay, immunizations, 3 letters of recommendation, nursing research course, physical assessment course, professional liability insurance/malpractice insurance, prerequisite course work, resume, statistics course, GRE General Test or minimum GPA of 3.0. *Application deadline:* 10/15 (fall), 1/15 (spring), 7/15 (summer).
**Advanced Placement** Credit given for nursing courses completed elsewhere dependent upon specific evaluations.
**Degree Requirements** 40 total credit hours, thesis or project.

#### POST-MASTER'S PROGRAM

**Areas of Study** *Nurse practitioner programs in:* family health.

#### DOCTORAL DEGREE PROGRAM

**Degree** DNP
**Available Programs** Doctorate.
**Areas of Study** Clinical practice, health policy.
**Site Options** Yuma, AZ; Tucson, AZ; St. Michaels/Window Rock, AZ.
**Online Degree Options** Yes (online only).
**Program Entrance Requirements** Clinical experience, minimum overall college GPA of 3.0, interview by faculty committee, 3 letters of recommendation, MSN or equivalent, statistics course, vita. *Application deadline:* Applications may be processed on a rolling basis for some programs.
**Degree Requirements** 31 total credit hours, dissertation.

# The University of Arizona
## College of Nursing
## Tucson, Arizona

***http://www.nursing.arizona.edu/***
Founded in 1885

**DEGREES • BSN • MSN • PHD**

**Nursing Program Faculty** 96 (51% with doctorates).
**Baccalaureate Enrollment** 213 **Women** 90.1% **Men** 9.9% **Minority** 30.5%
**Graduate Enrollment** 555 **Women** 86.8% **Men** 13.2% **Minority** 27.3% **Part-time** 18%
**Distance Learning Courses** Available.
**Nursing Student Activities** Nursing Honor Society, Sigma Theta Tau, Student Nurses' Association, nursing club.
**Nursing Student Resources** Academic advising; academic or career counseling; assistance for students with disabilities; bookstore; campus computer network; career placement assistance; computer lab; computer-assisted instruction; e-mail services; externships; housing assistance; interactive nursing skills videos; Internet; learning resource lab; library services; nursing audiovisuals; other; placement services for program completers; remedial services; resume preparation assistance; skills, simulation, or other laboratory; tutoring.
**Library Facilities** 112,500 volumes in health, 5,400 volumes in nursing; 10,785 periodical subscriptions health-care related.

### BACCALAUREATE PROGRAMS

**Degree** BSN
**Available Programs** Generic Baccalaureate.
**Study Options** Full-time.
**Program Entrance Requirements** Minimum overall college GPA of 3.0, transcript of college record, CPR certification, written essay, health insurance, high school transcript, immunizations, interview, minimum GPA in nursing prerequisites of 3.0, prerequisite course work. Transfer students are accepted. *Application deadline:* 2/1 (fall), 9/1 (spring).
**Advanced Placement** Credit by examination available. Credit given for nursing courses completed elsewhere dependent upon specific evaluations.
**Expenses (2013–14)** *Tuition, state resident:* full-time $13,888; part-time $754 per unit. *Tuition, nonresident:* full-time $28,070; part-time $1169 per unit. *International tuition:* $28,070 full-time. *Room and board:* room only: $9714 per academic year. *Required fees:* full-time $1018; part-time $93 per credit; part-time $509 per term.
**Financial Aid** 82% of baccalaureate students in nursing programs received some form of financial aid in 2012–13. *Gift aid (need-based):* Federal Pell, FSEOG, state, private, college/university gift aid from institutional funds, Federal Nursing. *Loans:* Federal Nursing Student Loans, Federal Direct (Subsidized and Unsubsidized Stafford PLUS), Perkins, college/university. *Work-study:* Federal Work-Study, part-time campus jobs. *Financial aid application deadline:* Continuous.
**Contact** Mr. Thomas M. Dickson, Director for Student Affairs, College of Nursing, The University of Arizona, 1305 North Martin, PO Box 210203, Tucson, AZ 85721-0203. *Telephone:* 520-626-3808. *Fax:* 520-626-6424. *E-mail:* tdickson@nursing.arizona.edu.

## GRADUATE PROGRAMS

**Expenses (2013–14)** *Tuition, state resident:* full-time $15,548; part-time $1031 per unit. *Tuition, nonresident:* full-time $31,420; part-time $1746 per unit. *International tuition:* $31,420 full-time. *Required fees:* full-time $572; part-time $57 per credit; part-time $227 per term.
**Financial Aid** 72% of graduate students in nursing programs received some form of financial aid in 2012–13. 11 research assistantships with full tuition reimbursements available (averaging $18,220 per year), 5 teaching assistantships (averaging $18,327 per year) were awarded; career-related internships or fieldwork, institutionally sponsored loans, scholarships, traineeships, tuition waivers (full), and unspecified assistantships also available. *Financial aid application deadline:* 6/1.
**Contact** Graduate Support Services, Senior, College of Nursing, The University of Arizona, 1305 North Martin, PO Box 210203, Tucson, AZ 85721-0203. *Telephone:* 520-626-3808. *Fax:* 520-626-6424. *E-mail:* advanced@nursing.arizona.edu.

### MASTER'S DEGREE PROGRAM

**Degree** MSN
**Available Programs** Accelerated Master's; Accelerated Master's for Non-Nursing College Graduates; RN to Master's.
**Site Options** Phoenix, AZ.
**Study Options** Full-time.
**Online Degree Options** Yes.
**Program Entrance Requirements** Minimum overall college GPA of 3.0, transcript of college record, CPR certification, written essay, immunizations, interview, prerequisite course work, statistics course. *Application deadline:* 1/15 (fall). *Application fee:* $75.
**Advanced Placement** Credit given for nursing courses completed elsewhere dependent upon specific evaluations.
**Degree Requirements** 56 total credit hours, thesis or project, comprehensive exam.

### POST-MASTER'S PROGRAM

**Areas of Study** *Nurse practitioner programs in:* acute care, adult health, family health, gerontology, pediatric, psychiatric/mental health.

### DOCTORAL DEGREE PROGRAM

**Degree** PhD
**Available Programs** Doctorate; Post-Baccalaureate Doctorate.
**Areas of Study** Addiction/substance abuse, advanced practice nursing, aging, bio-behavioral research, biology of health and illness, clinical practice, clinical research, community health, critical care, faculty preparation, family health, gerontology, health policy, health promotion/disease prevention, health-care systems, human health and illness, illness and transition, individualized study, information systems, neuro-behavior, nursing research, nursing science, oncology, palliative care, urban health,women's health.
**Online Degree Options** Yes (online only).
**Program Entrance Requirements** Minimum overall college GPA of 3.0, interview by faculty committee, interview, 3 letters of recommendation, statistics course, vita. *Application deadline:* 12/15 (fall). *Application fee:* $75.
**Degree Requirements** 64 total credit hours, dissertation, oral exam, written exam, residency.

### POSTDOCTORAL PROGRAM

**Postdoctoral Program Contact** Mr. Thomas Matthew Dickson, Director of Student Affairs, College of Nursing, The University of Arizona, 1305 North Martin, PO Box 210203, Tucson, AZ 85721-0203. *Telephone:* 520-626-3808. *E-mail:* tdickson@email.arizona.edu.

# University of Phoenix–Online Campus

**Online Campus**
**Phoenix, Arizona**

***http://www.uopxonline.com/***
Founded in 1989

**DEGREES • BSN • MSN • MSN/MBA • MSN/MHA • PHD**
**Nursing Program Faculty** 444 (29% with doctorates).
**Baccalaureate Enrollment** 5,644 **Women** 92.2% **Men** 7.8% **Minority** 18.1%
**Graduate Enrollment** 5,878 **Women** 92.5% **Men** 7.5% **Minority** 23%
**Distance Learning Courses** Available.
**Nursing Student Activities** Sigma Theta Tau.
**Nursing Student Resources** Academic advising; academic or career counseling; assistance for students with disabilities; bookstore; campus computer network; computer lab; computer-assisted instruction; e-mail services; interactive nursing skills videos; Internet; learning resource lab; library services; nursing audiovisuals; remedial services; skills, simulation, or other laboratory; tutoring.
**Library Facilities** 16,781 periodical subscriptions (1,300 health-care related).

## BACCALAUREATE PROGRAMS

**Degree** BSN
**Available Programs** Accelerated Baccalaureate.
**Study Options** Full-time.
**Online Degree Options** Yes.
**Program Entrance Requirements** Transcript of college record, CPR certification, immunizations, 1 letter of recommendation, RN licensure. Transfer students are accepted. *Application deadline:* Applications may be processed on a rolling basis for some programs.
**Advanced Placement** Credit by examination available. Credit given for nursing courses completed elsewhere dependent upon specific evaluations.
**Contact** *Telephone:* 602-387-7000.

## GRADUATE PROGRAMS

**Contact** *Telephone:* 602-387-7000.

### MASTER'S DEGREE PROGRAM

**Degrees** MSN; MSN/MBA; MSN/MHA
**Available Programs** Master's; Master's for Nurses with Non-Nursing Degrees.
**Concentrations Available** Health-care administration; nursing administration; nursing education. *Nurse practitioner programs in:* family health.
**Study Options** Full-time.
**Online Degree Options** Yes.
**Program Entrance Requirements** Clinical experience, computer literacy, minimum overall college GPA of 3.0, transcript of college record, CPR certification. *Application deadline:* Applications may be processed on a rolling basis for some programs.
**Advanced Placement** Credit given for nursing courses completed elsewhere dependent upon specific evaluations.
**Degree Requirements** 39 total credit hours, thesis or project.

### POST-MASTER'S PROGRAM

**Areas of Study** *Nurse practitioner programs in:* family health.

### DOCTORAL DEGREE PROGRAM

**Degree** PhD
**Available Programs** Doctorate.
**Areas of Study** Nursing administration, nursing education.
**Online Degree Options** Yes (online only).
**Program Entrance Requirements** Minimum overall college GPA of 3.0, MSN or equivalent. *Application deadline:* Applications may be processed on a rolling basis for some programs. *Application fee:* $45.
**Degree Requirements** 62 total credit hours, dissertation, residency.

## CONTINUING EDUCATION PROGRAM

**Contact** *Telephone:* 602-387-7000.

# University of Phoenix–Phoenix Campus

**College of Nursing**
**Tempe, Arizona**

***http://www.phoenix.edu/campus-locations/az/phoenix-main-campus/phoenix-main-campus.html***
Founded in 1976

**DEGREES • BSN • MSN • MSN/MBA • MSN/MHA**
**Nursing Program Faculty** 38 (32% with doctorates).
**Baccalaureate Enrollment** 239 **Women** 89.5% **Men** 10.5% **Minority** 23.4%
**Graduate Enrollment** 148 **Women** 91.9% **Men** 8.1% **Minority** 14.86%
**Nursing Student Activities** Sigma Theta Tau.
**Nursing Student Resources** Academic advising; academic or career counseling; assistance for students with disabilities; bookstore; campus

computer network; computer lab; computer-assisted instruction; interactive nursing skills videos; Internet; learning resource lab; library services; nursing audiovisuals; skills, simulation, or other laboratory; tutoring.
**Library Facilities** 16,781 periodical subscriptions (1,300 health-care related).

### BACCALAUREATE PROGRAMS

**Degree** BSN
**Available Programs** Accelerated Baccalaureate; LPN to Baccalaureate.
**Site Options** Scottsdale, AZ; Mesa, AZ; Chandler, AZ.
**Study Options** Full-time.
**Online Degree Options** Yes.
**Program Entrance Requirements** Transcript of college record, CPR certification, immunizations, 1 letter of recommendation, RN licensure. Transfer students are accepted. *Application deadline:* Applications may be processed on a rolling basis for some programs.
**Advanced Placement** Credit by examination available. Credit given for nursing courses completed elsewhere dependent upon specific evaluations.
**Contact** *Telephone:* 480-804-7600.

### GRADUATE PROGRAMS

**Contact** *Telephone:* 480-804-7600.

**MASTER'S DEGREE PROGRAM**
**Degrees** MSN; MSN/MBA; MSN/MHA
**Available Programs** Master's.
**Concentrations Available** Health-care administration; nursing administration; nursing education. *Nurse practitioner programs in:* family health.
**Site Options** Scottsdale, AZ; Mesa, AZ; Chandler, AZ.
**Study Options** Full-time.
**Online Degree Options** Yes.
**Program Entrance Requirements** Clinical experience, computer literacy, minimum overall college GPA of 2.5, transcript of college record. *Application deadline:* Applications may be processed on a rolling basis for some programs. *Application fee:* $45.
**Advanced Placement** Credit given for nursing courses completed elsewhere dependent upon specific evaluations.
**Degree Requirements** 39 total credit hours, thesis or project.

**POST-MASTER'S PROGRAM**
**Areas of Study** *Nurse practitioner programs in:* family health.

### CONTINUING EDUCATION PROGRAM

**Contact** *Telephone:* 480-557-2279. *Fax:* 480-557-2338.

## University of Phoenix–Southern Arizona Campus

**College of Social Sciences**
**Tucson, Arizona**

***http://www.phoenix.edu/campus-locations/az/southern-arizona-campus/southern-arizona-campus.html***
Founded in 1979

**DEGREES • BSN • MSN**
**Nursing Program Faculty** 19 (32% with doctorates).
**Baccalaureate Enrollment** 67 **Women** 85.1% **Men** 14.9% **Minority** 33.8%
**Graduate Enrollment** 97 **Women** 80.4% **Men** 19.6% **Minority** 18.56%
**Nursing Student Activities** Sigma Theta Tau.
**Nursing Student Resources** Academic advising; academic or career counseling; assistance for students with disabilities; bookstore; campus computer network; computer lab; computer-assisted instruction; e-mail services; interactive nursing skills videos; Internet; learning resource lab; library services; nursing audiovisuals; remedial services; skills, simulation, or other laboratory; tutoring.
**Library Facilities** 16,781 periodical subscriptions (1,300 health-care related).

### BACCALAUREATE PROGRAMS

**Degree** BSN
**Available Programs** Accelerated Baccalaureate; LPN to Baccalaureate.
**Site Options** Sierra Vista, AZ; Yuma, AZ; Nogales, AZ.
**Study Options** Full-time.
**Online Degree Options** Yes.
**Program Entrance Requirements** Transcript of college record, CPR certification, immunizations, 1 letter of recommendation, RN licensure. Transfer students are accepted. *Application deadline:* Applications may be processed on a rolling basis for some programs.
**Advanced Placement** Credit by examination available. Credit given for nursing courses completed elsewhere dependent upon specific evaluations.
**Contact** *Telephone:* 520-881-6512.

### GRADUATE PROGRAMS

**Contact** *Telephone:* 520-881-6512.

**MASTER'S DEGREE PROGRAM**
**Degree** MSN
**Available Programs** Master's.
**Concentrations Available** Health-care administration; nursing administration; nursing education. *Nurse practitioner programs in:* family health.
**Site Options** Sierra Vista, AZ; Yuma, AZ; Nogales, AZ.
**Study Options** Full-time.
**Online Degree Options** Yes.
**Program Entrance Requirements** Clinical experience, computer literacy, minimum overall college GPA of 2.5, transcript of college record. *Application deadline:* Applications may be processed on a rolling basis for some programs. *Application fee:* $45.
**Advanced Placement** Credit given for nursing courses completed elsewhere dependent upon specific evaluations.
**Degree Requirements** 39 total credit hours, thesis or project.

**POST-MASTER'S PROGRAM**
**Areas of Study** *Nurse practitioner programs in:* family health.

### CONTINUING EDUCATION PROGRAM

**Contact** *Telephone:* 520-881-6512.

# ARKANSAS

## Arkansas State University

**Department of Nursing**
**Jonesboro, State University, Arkansas**

***http://www.astate.edu/***
Founded in 1909

**DEGREES • BSN • DNP • MSN**
**Nursing Program Faculty** 91 (17% with doctorates).
**Baccalaureate Enrollment** 303 **Women** 82% **Men** 18% **Minority** 12% **International** 1% **Part-time** 35%
**Graduate Enrollment** 202 **Women** 55% **Men** 45% **Minority** 15% **Part-time** 50%
**Distance Learning Courses** Available.
**Nursing Student Activities** Sigma Theta Tau, Student Nurses' Association.
**Nursing Student Resources** Academic advising; academic or career counseling; assistance for students with disabilities; bookstore; campus computer network; computer lab; computer-assisted instruction; daycare for children of students; e-mail services; housing assistance; Internet; learning resource lab; library services; nursing audiovisuals; resume preparation assistance; skills, simulation, or other laboratory; tutoring.
**Library Facilities** 1.1 million volumes; 33,889 periodical subscriptions.

### BACCALAUREATE PROGRAMS

**Degree** BSN
**Available Programs** Accelerated Baccalaureate for Second Degree; Generic Baccalaureate; LPN to Baccalaureate; RN Baccalaureate.
**Site Options** Mountain Home, AR; Beebe, AR; West Memphis, AR.
**Study Options** Full-time.
**Online Degree Options** Yes.
**Program Entrance Requirements** Minimum overall college GPA of 2.8, transcript of college record, CPR certification, written essay, immu-

nizations, 3 letters of recommendation, professional liability insurance/malpractice insurance, prerequisite course work. Transfer students are accepted. *Application deadline:* 6/15 (fall).
**Advanced Placement** Credit by examination available. Credit given for nursing courses completed elsewhere dependent upon specific evaluations.
**Expenses (2013–14)** *Tuition, state resident:* full-time $5792; part-time $181 per credit hour. *Tuition, nonresident:* full-time $11,584. *International tuition:* $11,584 full-time. *Room and board:* $3195; room only: $1850 per academic year. *Required fees:* full-time $2486; part-time $76 per credit; part-time $35 per term.
**Contact** Jenafer Wray, Nursing Advisor, Department of Nursing, Arkansas State University, PO Box 910, State University, AR 72467. *Telephone:* 870-972-3074. *Fax:* 870-972-2954. *E-mail:* jwray@astate.edu.

## GRADUATE PROGRAMS

**Expenses (2013–14)** *Tuition, state resident:* full-time $4140; part-time $230 per credit hour. *Tuition, nonresident:* full-time $8280; part-time $460 per credit hour. *International tuition:* $8280 full-time. *Room and board:* $3830; room only: $2630 per academic year. *Required fees:* full-time $1924; part-time $103 per credit; part-time $35 per term.
**Contact** Dr. Angela Schmidt, MSN Program Director, Department of Nursing, Arkansas State University, PO Box 910, MSN Program, State University, AR 72467. *Telephone:* 870-972-3701. *Fax:* 870-972-2954. *E-mail:* aschmidt@astate.edu.

### MASTER'S DEGREE PROGRAM

**Degree** MSN
**Available Programs** Master's.
**Concentrations Available** Nurse anesthesia; nursing administration; nursing education. *Clinical nurse specialist programs in:* adult health. *Nurse practitioner programs in:* primary care.
**Study Options** Full-time and part-time.
**Program Entrance Requirements** Clinical experience, minimum overall college GPA of 2.75, transcript of college record, CPR certification, written essay, immunizations, physical assessment course, professional liability insurance/malpractice insurance, statistics course. *Application deadline:* 4/15 (fall), 10/15 (spring). *Application fee:* $30.
**Degree Requirements** 45 total credit hours, thesis or project, comprehensive exam.

### POST-MASTER'S PROGRAM

**Areas of Study** Nursing education. *Nurse practitioner programs in:* primary care.

### DOCTORAL DEGREE PROGRAM

**Degree** DNP
**Available Programs** Doctorate.
**Online Degree Options** Yes (online only).
**Program Entrance Requirements** Clinical experience, minimum overall college GPA of 3.0, interview, MSN or equivalent, statistics course, vita. *Application deadline:* 10/1 (spring).
**Degree Requirements** 41 total credit hours.

# Arkansas Tech University

**Program in Nursing**
**Russellville, Arkansas**

*https://www.atu.edu/nursing/*
Founded in 1909

## DEGREES • BSN • MSN

**Nursing Program Faculty** 27 (20% with doctorates).
**Baccalaureate Enrollment** 248 **Women** 87% **Men** 13% **Minority** 11% **International** 4% **Part-time** 14%
**Graduate Enrollment** 23 **Women** 87% **Men** 13% **Part-time** 50%
**Distance Learning Courses** Available.
**Nursing Student Activities** Nursing Honor Society, Sigma Theta Tau, Student Nurses' Association.
**Nursing Student Resources** Academic advising; academic or career counseling; assistance for students with disabilities; bookstore; campus computer network; career placement assistance; computer lab; computer-assisted instruction; e-mail services; employment services for current students; housing assistance; interactive nursing skills videos; Internet; learning resource lab; library services; nursing audiovisuals; other; paid internships; placement services for program completers; remedial services; resume preparation assistance; skills, simulation, or other laboratory; tutoring.
**Library Facilities** 299,283 volumes (16,900 in health, 2,100 in nursing); 756 periodical subscriptions (130 health-care related).

## BACCALAUREATE PROGRAMS

**Degree** BSN
**Available Programs** ADN to Baccalaureate; Baccalaureate for Second Degree; Generic Baccalaureate; LPN to Baccalaureate; RN Baccalaureate.
**Site Options** Russellville, AR.
**Study Options** Full-time and part-time.
**Online Degree Options** Yes.
**Program Entrance Requirements** Transcript of college record, CPR certification, health exam, immunizations, minimum GPA in nursing prerequisites of 3.0, professional liability insurance/malpractice insurance, prerequisite course work. Transfer students are accepted. *Application deadline:* 3/1 (fall), 10/1 (spring).
**Advanced Placement** Credit by examination available. Credit given for nursing courses completed elsewhere dependent upon specific evaluations.
**Expenses (2012–13)** *Tuition, state resident:* full-time $5610; part-time $187 per credit hour. *Tuition, nonresident:* full-time $11,220; part-time $374 per credit hour. *International tuition:* $11,400 full-time. *Room and board:* $6000; room only: $3600 per academic year. *Required fees:* full-time $918; part-time $50 per credit; part-time $318 per term.
**Financial Aid** 80% of baccalaureate students in nursing programs received some form of financial aid in 2011–12. *Gift aid (need-based):* Federal Pell, FSEOG, state, private. *Loans:* Federal Direct (Subsidized and Unsubsidized Stafford PLUS), Perkins. *Work-study:* Federal Work-Study, part-time campus jobs. *Financial aid application deadline (priority):* 4/15.
**Contact** Dr. Rebecca F. Burris, Professor and Department Chair, Program in Nursing, Arkansas Tech University, 402 West O Street, Russellville, AR 72801. *Telephone:* 479-968-0383. *Fax:* 479-968-0219. *E-mail:* rburris@atu.edu.

## GRADUATE PROGRAMS

**Expenses (2012–13)** *Tuition, state resident:* full-time $5160; part-time $215 per credit hour. *Tuition, nonresident:* full-time $10,320; part-time $430 per credit hour. *International tuition:* $10,350 full-time. *Required fees:* full-time $780; part-time $50 per credit; part-time $318 per term.
**Financial Aid** 75% of graduate students in nursing programs received some form of financial aid in 2011–12.
**Contact** Dr. Mary Gunter, Dean of Graduate College, Program in Nursing, Arkansas Tech University, Tomlinson Graduate College, Russellville, AR 72801. *Telephone:* 479-968-0398. *E-mail:* mgunter@atu.edu.

### MASTER'S DEGREE PROGRAM

**Degree** MSN
**Available Programs** Master's; Master's for Nurses with Non-Nursing Degrees; RN to Master's.
**Concentrations Available** Nursing administration.
**Site Options** Russellville, AR.
**Study Options** Full-time and part-time.
**Program Entrance Requirements** Clinical experience, computer literacy, minimum overall college GPA of 3.0, transcript of college record, statistics course. *Application deadline:* 5/1 (fall). Applications may be processed on a rolling basis for some programs. *Application fee:* $25.
**Advanced Placement** Credit given for nursing courses completed elsewhere dependent upon specific evaluations.
**Degree Requirements** 39 total credit hours, thesis or project.

# Harding University

**College of Nursing**
**Searcy, Arkansas**

*http://www.harding.edu/nursing*
Founded in 1924

## DEGREE • BSN

**Nursing Program Faculty** 19 (25% with doctorates).
**Baccalaureate Enrollment** 97 **Women** 80% **Men** 20% **Minority** 1% **International** 1% **Part-time** 12%
**Nursing Student Activities** Nursing Honor Society, Sigma Theta Tau, Student Nurses' Association.

**Nursing Student Resources** Academic advising; academic or career counseling; assistance for students with disabilities; bookstore; campus computer network; career placement assistance; computer lab; computer-assisted instruction; e-mail services; employment services for current students; externships; housing assistance; interactive nursing skills videos; Internet; learning resource lab; library services; nursing audiovisuals; placement services for program completers; remedial services; resume preparation assistance; skills, simulation, or other laboratory; tutoring.
**Library Facilities** 325,134 volumes (5,000 in health, 1,729 in nursing); 75,942 periodical subscriptions (120 health-care related).

## BACCALAUREATE PROGRAMS

**Degree** BSN
**Available Programs** ADN to Baccalaureate; Generic Baccalaureate; LPN to Baccalaureate; LPN to RN Baccalaureate; RN Baccalaureate.
**Site Options** Searcy, AR.
**Study Options** Full-time and part-time.
**Program Entrance Requirements** Minimum overall college GPA of 2.0, transcript of college record, CPR certification, health exam, high school transcript, immunizations, 3 letters of recommendation, minimum GPA in nursing prerequisites of 2.5, prerequisite course work. Transfer students are accepted. *Application deadline:* 3/1 (fall), 10/1 (spring).
**Advanced Placement** Credit by examination available. Credit given for nursing courses completed elsewhere dependent upon specific evaluations.
**Expenses (2013–14)** *Tuition:* full-time $16,170; part-time $8084 per credit. *International tuition:* $161,710 full-time. *Room and board:* $6366; room only: $1601 per academic year. *Required fees:* full-time $2000.
**Financial Aid** 95% of baccalaureate students in nursing programs received some form of financial aid in 2012–13.
**Contact** Ms. Jeanne L. Castleberry, Assistant to the Dean, College of Nursing, Harding University, Box 12265, 914 East Market Avenue, Searcy, AR 72149-2265. *Telephone:* 501-279-4682. *Fax:* 501-305-8902. *E-mail:* nursing@harding.edu.

## CONTINUING EDUCATION PROGRAM

**Contact** Dr. Cathleen M. Shultz, Dean and Professor, College of Nursing, Harding University, Carr College of Nursing, Box 12265, Searcy, AR 72149-5615. *Telephone:* 501-279-4476. *Fax:* 501-279-4669. *E-mail:* nursing@harding.edu.

# Henderson State University

### Department of Nursing
### Arkadelphia, Arkansas

*http://www.hsu.edu/nursing/*
Founded in 1890

**DEGREE • BSN**
**Nursing Program Faculty** 7 (29% with doctorates).
**Baccalaureate Enrollment** 43 **Women** 79% **Men** 21% **Minority** 28% **International** 2%
**Nursing Student Activities** Sigma Theta Tau, Student Nurses' Association, nursing club.
**Nursing Student Resources** Academic advising; academic or career counseling; assistance for students with disabilities; bookstore; campus computer network; career placement assistance; computer lab; computer-assisted instruction; e-mail services; employment services for current students; housing assistance; interactive nursing skills videos; Internet; learning resource lab; library services; nursing audiovisuals; remedial services; resume preparation assistance; skills, simulation, or other laboratory; tutoring.
**Library Facilities** 270,989 volumes (1,000 in health, 200 in nursing); 40 periodical subscriptions health-care related.

## BACCALAUREATE PROGRAMS

**Degree** BSN
**Available Programs** ADN to Baccalaureate; Generic Baccalaureate; LPN to Baccalaureate.
**Study Options** Full-time.
**Program Entrance Requirements** Minimum overall college GPA of 2.5, transcript of college record, CPR certification, written essay, immunizations, minimum GPA in nursing prerequisites of 2.50, prerequisite course work. Transfer students are accepted. *Application deadline:* 2/15 (fall). *Application fee:* $57.
**Advanced Placement** Credit given for nursing courses completed elsewhere dependent upon specific evaluations.
**Financial Aid** 80% of baccalaureate students in nursing programs received some form of financial aid in 2012–13. *Gift aid (need-based):* Federal Pell, FSEOG, state, private. *Loans:* Federal Direct (Subsidized and Unsubsidized Stafford PLUS), Perkins. *Work-study:* Federal Work-Study, part-time campus jobs. *Financial aid application deadline (priority):* 6/1.
**Contact** Dr. Barbara J. Landrum, Professor and Department Chair, Department of Nursing, Henderson State University, Box 7803, 1100 Henderson Street, Arkadelphia, AR 71999-0001. *Telephone:* 870-230-5508. *Fax:* 870-230-5390. *E-mail:* landrub@hsu.edu.

# Southern Arkansas University–Magnolia

### Department of Nursing
### Magnolia, Arkansas

*http://web.saumag.edu/nursing/*
Founded in 1909

**DEGREE • BSN**
**Nursing Program Faculty** 13 (23% with doctorates).
**Baccalaureate Enrollment** 51 **Women** 90% **Men** 10% **Minority** 15% **Part-time** 58%
**Distance Learning Courses** Available.
**Nursing Student Activities** Student Nurses' Association.
**Nursing Student Resources** Academic advising; academic or career counseling; assistance for students with disabilities; bookstore; campus computer network; career placement assistance; computer lab; computer-assisted instruction; e-mail services; employment services for current students; housing assistance; interactive nursing skills videos; Internet; learning resource lab; library services; nursing audiovisuals; remedial services; resume preparation assistance; skills, simulation, or other laboratory; tutoring.
**Library Facilities** 185,522 volumes (800 in health, 200 in nursing); 2,896 periodical subscriptions (2,000 health-care related).

## BACCALAUREATE PROGRAMS

**Degree** BSN
**Available Programs** ADN to Baccalaureate; Generic Baccalaureate; RN Baccalaureate.
**Study Options** Full-time.
**Online Degree Options** Yes.
**Program Entrance Requirements** Minimum overall college GPA of 2.5, transcript of college record, CPR certification, high school chemistry, immunizations, minimum GPA in nursing prerequisites of 2.5, prerequisite course work. Transfer students are accepted. *Application deadline:* 2/28 (fall). Applications may be processed on a rolling basis for some programs.
**Advanced Placement** Credit given for nursing courses completed elsewhere dependent upon specific evaluations.
**Contact** *Telephone:* 870-235-4331. *Fax:* 870-235-5058.

# University of Arkansas

### Eleanor Mann School of Nursing
### Fayetteville, Arkansas

*http://nurs.uark.edu/*
Founded in 1871

**DEGREES • BSN • MSN**
**Nursing Program Faculty** 25 (26% with doctorates).
**Baccalaureate Enrollment** 220 **Women** 95% **Men** 5% **Minority** 7%
**Graduate Enrollment** 20
**Nursing Student Activities** Sigma Theta Tau, Student Nurses' Association.
**Nursing Student Resources** Academic advising; academic or career counseling; assistance for students with disabilities; bookstore; campus computer network; career placement assistance; computer lab; computer-assisted instruction; e-mail services; employment services for current students; housing assistance; interactive nursing skills videos; Internet; learning resource lab; library services; nursing audiovisuals; other; placement services for program completers; remedial services; resume preparation assistance; skills, simulation, or other laboratory; tutoring.

**Library Facilities** 1.9 million volumes (60,000 in health, 20,000 in nursing); 27,518 periodical subscriptions (130,000 health-care related).

### BACCALAUREATE PROGRAMS

**Degree** BSN
**Available Programs** Generic Baccalaureate; LPN to Baccalaureate; LPN to RN Baccalaureate; RN Baccalaureate.
**Study Options** Full-time and part-time.
**Program Entrance Requirements** Minimum overall college GPA of 2.75, transcript of college record, CPR certification, health insurance, immunizations, minimum GPA in nursing prerequisites of 2.75, professional liability insurance/malpractice insurance, prerequisite course work. Transfer students are accepted.
**Advanced Placement** Credit by examination available. Credit given for nursing courses completed elsewhere dependent upon specific evaluations.
**Contact** *Telephone:* 479-575-3907. *Fax:* 479-575-3218.

### GRADUATE PROGRAMS

**Contact** *Telephone:* 479-575-3907. *Fax:* 479-575-3218.

**MASTER'S DEGREE PROGRAM**
**Degree** MSN
**Available Programs** Master's.
**Concentrations Available** Nursing education. *Clinical nurse specialist programs in:* acute care, medical-surgical.
**Study Options** Full-time and part-time.
**Online Degree Options** Yes.
**Program Entrance Requirements** Computer literacy, minimum overall college GPA of 3.0, transcript of college record, CPR certification, immunizations, nursing research course, physical assessment course, statistics course.
**Degree Requirements** 42 total credit hours, thesis or project, comprehensive exam.

### CONTINUING EDUCATION PROGRAM

**Contact** *Telephone:* 479-575-3907. *Fax:* 479-575-3218.

## University of Arkansas at Little Rock

**BSN Programs**
**Little Rock, Arkansas**

*http://ualr.edu/*
Founded in 1927

**DEGREE • BSN**

### BACCALAUREATE PROGRAMS

**Degree** BSN
**Available Programs** RN Baccalaureate.
**Contact** *Telephone:* 501-569-8081.

## University of Arkansas at Monticello

**School of Nursing**
**Monticello, Arkansas**

*http://www.uamont.edu/Nursing/*
Founded in 1909

**DEGREE • BSN**

**Nursing Program Faculty** 10
**Baccalaureate Enrollment** 46 **Women** 87% **Men** 13% **Minority** 23% **International** .01%
**Distance Learning Courses** Available.
**Nursing Student Activities** Sigma Theta Tau, Student Nurses' Association.
**Nursing Student Resources** Academic advising; academic or career counseling; assistance for students with disabilities; bookstore; campus computer network; computer lab; computer-assisted instruction; e-mail services; interactive nursing skills videos; Internet; learning resource lab; library services; nursing audiovisuals; resume preparation assistance; skills, simulation, or other laboratory; tutoring.
**Library Facilities** 241,822 volumes (3,888 in health, 539 in nursing); 956 periodical subscriptions (5,015 health-care related).

### BACCALAUREATE PROGRAMS

**Degree** BSN
**Available Programs** ADN to Baccalaureate; Generic Baccalaureate; LPN to Baccalaureate; RN Baccalaureate.
**Study Options** Full-time.
**Program Entrance Requirements** Minimum overall college GPA, transcript of college record, CPR certification, immunizations, minimum GPA in nursing prerequisites of 2.5, prerequisite course work. Transfer students are accepted. *Application deadline:* 3/1 (spring).
**Advanced Placement** Credit by examination available. Credit given for nursing courses completed elsewhere dependent upon specific evaluations.
**Expenses (2013–14)** *Tuition, state resident:* full-time $4650; part-time $137 per credit hour. *Tuition, nonresident:* full-time $6570; part-time $193 per credit hour. *International tuition:* $6570 full-time. *Room and board:* $7410; room only: $4400 per academic year. *Required fees:* full-time $119.
**Financial Aid** 83% of baccalaureate students in nursing programs received some form of financial aid in 2012–13.
**Contact** Dr. Laura K. Evans, Dean, School of Nursing, University of Arkansas at Monticello, 124 University Place, PO Box 3606, Monticello, AR 71656. *Telephone:* 870-460-1069. *Fax:* 870-460-1969. *E-mail:* evansl@uamont.edu.

## University of Arkansas at Pine Bluff

**Department of Nursing**
**Pine Bluff, Arkansas**

*http://www.uapb.edu/*
Founded in 1873

**DEGREE • BSN**

**Nursing Program Faculty** 5 (40% with doctorates).
**Baccalaureate Enrollment** 20 **Women** 95% **Men** 5% **Minority** 100% **International** 20%
**Nursing Student Activities** Student Nurses' Association.
**Nursing Student Resources** Academic advising; academic or career counseling; assistance for students with disabilities; bookstore; campus computer network; career placement assistance; computer lab; computer-assisted instruction; e-mail services; housing assistance; interactive nursing skills videos; Internet; learning resource lab; library services; nursing audiovisuals; remedial services; resume preparation assistance; skills, simulation, or other laboratory; tutoring.
**Library Facilities** 187,582 volumes (2,600 in health, 1,550 in nursing); 3,041 periodical subscriptions (60 health-care related).

### BACCALAUREATE PROGRAMS

**Degree** BSN
**Available Programs** Generic Baccalaureate.
**Study Options** Full-time and part-time.
**Program Entrance Requirements** Minimum overall college GPA of 2.5, transcript of college record, CPR certification, written essay, health exam, immunizations, 3 letters of recommendation, minimum GPA in nursing prerequisites of 2.5, professional liability insurance/malpractice insurance, prerequisite course work. Transfer students are accepted.
**Advanced Placement** Credit by examination available. Credit given for nursing courses completed elsewhere dependent upon specific evaluations.
**Contact** *Telephone:* 870-575-8220. *Fax:* 870-575-8229.

# University of Arkansas for Medical Sciences
## College of Nursing
## Little Rock, Arkansas

***http://www.nursing.uams.edu/***
Founded in 1879

**DEGREES • BSN • DNP • MN SC • PHD**
**Nursing Program Faculty** 85 (38% with doctorates).
**Baccalaureate Enrollment** 384 **Women** 83.07% **Men** 16.93% **Minority** 13.02%
**Graduate Enrollment** 262 **Women** 85.5% **Men** 14.5% **Minority** 15.27%
**Distance Learning Courses** Available.
**Nursing Student Activities** Nursing Honor Society, Sigma Theta Tau, Student Nurses' Association.
**Nursing Student Resources** Academic advising; academic or career counseling; assistance for students with disabilities; bookstore; campus computer network; computer lab; computer-assisted instruction; e-mail services; externships; interactive nursing skills videos; Internet; learning resource lab; library services; nursing audiovisuals; remedial services; skills, simulation, or other laboratory; tutoring.
**Library Facilities** 183,975 volumes (183,975 in health); 1,567 periodical subscriptions (1,567 health-care related).

### BACCALAUREATE PROGRAMS
**Degree** BSN
**Available Programs** ADN to Baccalaureate; Accelerated RN Baccalaureate; Baccalaureate for Second Degree; Generic Baccalaureate; LPN to Baccalaureate; RN Baccalaureate.
**Site Options** Fayetteville, AR; El Dorado, AR; Texarkana, AR; Helena, AR; Jonesboro, AR; Hope, AR.
**Study Options** Full-time.
**Online Degree Options** Yes.
**Program Entrance Requirements** Minimum overall college GPA of 2.5, transcript of college record, CPR certification, health insurance, immunizations, interview, minimum high school GPA of 2.5, minimum GPA in nursing prerequisites of 2.5, prerequisite course work. Transfer students are accepted. *Application deadline:* 2/1 (summer). *Application fee:* $60.
**Advanced Placement** Credit by examination available. Credit given for nursing courses completed elsewhere dependent upon specific evaluations.
**Expenses (2012–13)** *Tuition, state resident:* full-time $2844; part-time $237 per credit hour. *Tuition, nonresident:* full-time $7080; part-time $590 per credit hour. *International tuition:* $7080 full-time.
**Financial Aid** 90% of baccalaureate students in nursing programs received some form of financial aid in 2011–12.
**Contact** Dr. Donna Middaugh, Associate Dean for Academic Programs, College of Nursing, University of Arkansas for Medical Sciences, 4301 West Markham, #529, Little Rock, AR 72205-7199. *Telephone:* 501-686-5374. *Fax:* 501-686-8350. *E-mail:* middaughdonnaj@uams.edu.

### GRADUATE PROGRAMS
**Expenses (2012–13)** *Tuition, state resident:* full-time $3078; part-time $342 per credit hour. *Tuition, nonresident:* full-time $7080; part-time $590 per credit hour. *International tuition:* $7080 full-time.
**Financial Aid** 90% of graduate students in nursing programs received some form of financial aid in 2011–12. Career-related internships or fieldwork and traineeships available. Aid available to part-time students.
**Contact** Dr. Donna Middaugh, Associate Dean for Academic Programs, College of Nursing, University of Arkansas for Medical Sciences, 4301 West Markham, #529, Little Rock, AR 72205-7199. *Telephone:* 501-686-8349. *Fax:* 501-686-8350. *E-mail:* middaughdonnaj@uams.edu.

#### MASTER'S DEGREE PROGRAM
**Degree** MN Sc
**Available Programs** Master's; Master's for Nurses with Non-Nursing Degrees; RN to Master's.
**Concentrations Available** Nursing administration; nursing education. *Clinical nurse specialist programs in:* acute care, adult health, pediatric. *Nurse practitioner programs in:* acute care, family health, pediatric, psychiatric/mental health.
**Site Options** Fayetteville, AR; El Dorado, AR; Texarkana, AR; Helena, AR; Jonesboro, AR.
**Study Options** Full-time and part-time.
**Program Entrance Requirements** Clinical experience, minimum overall college GPA of 2.85, transcript of college record, CPR certification, immunizations, physical assessment course, professional liability insurance/malpractice insurance, statistics course. *Application deadline:* 4/1 (fall), 9/1 (spring). *Application fee:* $60.
**Advanced Placement** Credit given for nursing courses completed elsewhere dependent upon specific evaluations.
**Degree Requirements** 39 total credit hours, thesis or project, comprehensive exam.

#### DOCTORAL DEGREE PROGRAM
**Degree** DNP
**Available Programs** Doctorate.
**Areas of Study** Clinical practice.
**Program Entrance Requirements** Minimum overall college GPA of 3.4, clinical experience, interview, interview by faculty committee, 3 letters of recommendation, MSN or equivalent, statistics course. *Application deadline:* 3/1 (spring). *Application fee:* $60.
**Degree Requirements** 29 total credit hours, oral exam, written exam.

**Degree** PhD
**Available Programs** Doctorate; Post-Baccalaureate Doctorate.
**Areas of Study** Advanced practice nursing, clinical practice, gerontology, health-care systems, nursing administration, nursing education, nursing research, nursing science, oncology.
**Program Entrance Requirements** Minimum overall college GPA of 3.65, interview by faculty committee, interview, 4 letters of recommendation, MSN or equivalent, scholarly papers, statistics course, writing sample, GRE. *Application deadline:* 3/1 (spring). *Application fee:* $60.
**Degree Requirements** 60 total credit hours, dissertation, oral exam, written exam.

#### POSTDOCTORAL PROGRAM
**Areas of Study** Aging, cancer care, gerontology, nursing research, nursing science.
**Postdoctoral Program Contact** Dr. Jean McSweeney, Postdoctoral Contact, College of Nursing, University of Arkansas for Medical Sciences, 4301 West Markham, #529, Little Rock, AR 72205-7199. *Telephone:* 501-686-5374. *Fax:* 501-686-8350. *E-mail:* mcsweeneyjeanc@uams.edu.

### CONTINUING EDUCATION PROGRAM
**Contact** Dr. Lorraine Frazier, Dean and Professor, College of Nursing, University of Arkansas for Medical Sciences, 4301 West Markham, #529, Little Rock, AR 72205-7199. *Telephone:* 501-686-5374. *Fax:* 501-686-8350. *E-mail:* lfrazier@uams.edu.

# University of Arkansas–Fort Smith
## Carol McKelvey Moore School of Nursing
## Fort Smith, Arkansas

***http://uafs.edu/***
Founded in 1928

**DEGREE • BSN**
**Nursing Program Faculty** 18
**Baccalaureate Enrollment** 20 **Women** 60% **Men** 40% **Minority** 5%
**Distance Learning Courses** Available.
**Nursing Student Activities** Student Nurses' Association.
**Nursing Student Resources** Academic advising; academic or career counseling; assistance for students with disabilities; bookstore; campus computer network; career placement assistance; computer lab; computer-assisted instruction; e-mail services; housing assistance; interactive nursing skills videos; Internet; learning resource lab; library services; nursing audiovisuals; remedial services; resume preparation assistance; skills, simulation, or other laboratory; tutoring.
**Library Facilities** 164,876 volumes (2,231 in health, 1,183 in nursing); 23,000 periodical subscriptions (5,350 health-care related).

### BACCALAUREATE PROGRAMS
**Degree** BSN
**Available Programs** ADN to Baccalaureate; Generic Baccalaureate.
**Study Options** Full-time.
**Online Degree Options** Yes (online only).

**Program Entrance Requirements** Minimum overall college GPA of 2.5, transcript of college record, CPR certification, health exam, health insurance, immunizations, interview, minimum GPA in nursing prerequisites of 2.5, prerequisite course work. Transfer students are accepted.
**Advanced Placement** Credit given for nursing courses completed elsewhere dependent upon specific evaluations.
**Contact** *Telephone:* 479-788-7840. *Fax:* 479-788-7869.

## University of Central Arkansas
### Department of Nursing
### Conway, Arkansas

*http://www.uca.edu/nursing/*
Founded in 1907

**DEGREES • BSN • MSN**
**Nursing Program Faculty** 32 (28% with doctorates).
**Baccalaureate Enrollment** 245 **Women** 84.9% **Men** 15.1% **Minority** 12.65% **International** 2.04% **Part-time** 23.67%
**Graduate Enrollment** 136 **Women** 95.59% **Men** 4.41% **Minority** 11.76% **International** .74% **Part-time** 95.59%
**Distance Learning Courses** Available.
**Nursing Student Activities** Sigma Theta Tau, Student Nurses' Association.
**Nursing Student Resources** Academic advising; academic or career counseling; assistance for students with disabilities; bookstore; campus computer network; career placement assistance; computer lab; computer-assisted instruction; e-mail services; employment services for current students; externships; housing assistance; interactive nursing skills videos; Internet; learning resource lab; library services; nursing audiovisuals; paid internships; placement services for program completers; remedial services; resume preparation assistance; skills, simulation, or other laboratory; tutoring; unpaid internships.
**Library Facilities** 585,928 volumes; 49,556 periodical subscriptions.

#### BACCALAUREATE PROGRAMS
**Degree** BSN
**Available Programs** ADN to Baccalaureate; Generic Baccalaureate; LPN to Baccalaureate; LPN to RN Baccalaureate; RN Baccalaureate.
**Study Options** Full-time and part-time.
**Program Entrance Requirements** Minimum overall college GPA of 2.5, transcript of college record, health exam, health insurance, immunizations, minimum GPA in nursing prerequisites, prerequisite course work. Transfer students are accepted. *Application deadline:* 3/1 (fall). *Application fee:* $50.
**Advanced Placement** Credit given for nursing courses completed elsewhere dependent upon specific evaluations.
**Contact** *Telephone:* 501-450-5526. *Fax:* 501-450-5560.

#### GRADUATE PROGRAMS
**Contact** *Telephone:* 501-450-5532. *Fax:* 501-450-5560.

**MASTER'S DEGREE PROGRAM**
**Degree** MSN
**Available Programs** Master's; RN to Master's.
**Concentrations Available** Nursing education. *Clinical nurse specialist programs in:* medical-surgical. *Nurse practitioner programs in:* adult health, family health.
**Site Options** Russelville, AR; Pine Bluff, AR; Fort Smith, AR.
**Study Options** Full-time and part-time.
**Online Degree Options** Yes (online only).
**Program Entrance Requirements** Clinical experience, minimum overall college GPA of 2.7, transcript of college record, CPR certification, immunizations, professional liability insurance/malpractice insurance, prerequisite course work, resume, statistics course, GRE General Test. *Application deadline:* 4/1 (fall), 8/1 (spring). *Application fee:* $50.
**Degree Requirements** 39 total credit hours, comprehensive exam.

**POST-MASTER'S PROGRAM**
**Areas of Study** Nursing education. *Clinical nurse specialist programs in:* medical-surgical. *Nurse practitioner programs in:* adult health, family health.

# CALIFORNIA

## American University of Health Sciences
### School of Nursing
### Signal Hill, California

*http://www.auhs.edu/*
**DEGREE • BSN**

#### BACCALAUREATE PROGRAMS
**Degree** BSN
**Available Programs** Accelerated Baccalaureate; Generic Baccalaureate.
**Program Entrance Requirements** Minimum overall college GPA of 2.5, written essay, interview, 2 letters of recommendation, prerequisite course work.
**Contact** School of Nursing, School of Nursing, American University of Health Sciences, 1600 East Hill Street, Building #1, Signal Hill, CA 90755. *Telephone:* 562-988-2278. *E-mail:* bsninfo@auhs.edu.

## Azusa Pacific University
### School of Nursing
### Azusa, California

*http://www.apu.edu/nursing/*
Founded in 1899

**DEGREES • BSN • MSN • PHD**
**Nursing Program Faculty** 77 (22% with doctorates).
**Baccalaureate Enrollment** 236 **Women** 90% **Men** 10% **Minority** 44% **International** 11% **Part-time** 2%
**Graduate Enrollment** 110 **Women** 89% **Men** 11% **Minority** 37%
**Nursing Student Activities** Sigma Theta Tau, Student Nurses' Association, nursing club.
**Nursing Student Resources** Academic advising; academic or career counseling; bookstore; campus computer network; career placement assistance; computer lab; computer-assisted instruction; e-mail services; employment services for current students; housing assistance; interactive nursing skills videos; Internet; learning resource lab; library services; nursing audiovisuals; remedial services; resume preparation assistance; skills, simulation, or other laboratory; tutoring.
**Library Facilities** 254,337 volumes (14,206 in health, 4,712 in nursing); 56,262 periodical subscriptions (432 health-care related).

#### BACCALAUREATE PROGRAMS
**Degree** BSN
**Available Programs** ADN to Baccalaureate; Accelerated Baccalaureate; Accelerated RN Baccalaureate; Generic Baccalaureate.
**Study Options** Full-time and part-time.
**Program Entrance Requirements** Minimum overall college GPA of 3.0, transcript of college record, CPR certification, written essay, health exam, high school biology, high school chemistry, 2 years high school math, high school transcript, immunizations, 3 letters of recommendation, minimum high school GPA of 3.0, minimum GPA in nursing prerequisites of 3.0. Transfer students are accepted.
**Advanced Placement** Credit by examination available. Credit given for nursing courses completed elsewhere dependent upon specific evaluations.
**Contact** *Telephone:* 626-815-6000 Ext. 5501. *Fax:* 626-815-5414.

#### GRADUATE PROGRAMS
**Contact** *Telephone:* 626-815-5386. *Fax:* 626-815-5414.

**MASTER'S DEGREE PROGRAM**
**Degree** MSN
**Available Programs** Accelerated Master's for Non-Nursing College Graduates; Accelerated Master's for Nurses with Non-Nursing Degrees; Master's.
**Concentrations Available** Nursing administration; nursing education. *Clinical nurse specialist programs in:* adult health, medical-surgical, parent-child, pediatric, school health. *Nurse practitioner programs in:* adult health, family health, pediatric, primary care.
**Study Options** Full-time and part-time.

**Program Entrance Requirements** Clinical experience, computer literacy, minimum overall college GPA of 3.0, transcript of college record, CPR certification, written essay, immunizations, 3 letters of recommendation, nursing research course, physical assessment course, professional liability insurance/malpractice insurance, prerequisite course work, resume, statistics course.
**Advanced Placement** Credit by examination available. Credit given for nursing courses completed elsewhere dependent upon specific evaluations.
**Degree Requirements** 42 total credit hours, thesis or project, comprehensive exam.

### POST-MASTER'S PROGRAM

**Areas of Study** Nursing administration; nursing education. *Clinical nurse specialist programs in:* adult health, medical-surgical, parent-child, pediatric, school health. *Nurse practitioner programs in:* adult health, family health, pediatric, primary care.

### DOCTORAL DEGREE PROGRAM

**Degree** PhD
**Available Programs** Doctorate.
**Areas of Study** Community health, family health, nursing education.
**Program Entrance Requirements** Clinical experience, minimum overall college GPA of 3.5, interview by faculty committee, interview, 3 letters of recommendation, MSN or equivalent, scholarly papers, statistics course, vita, writing sample.
**Degree Requirements** 64 total credit hours, dissertation, oral exam, written exam.

### CONTINUING EDUCATION PROGRAM

**Contact** *Telephone:* 626-815-5385. *Fax:* 626-815-5414.

## Biola University
### Department of Nursing
### La Mirada, California

*http://www.biola.edu/*
Founded in 1908

**DEGREE • BSN**
**Nursing Program Faculty** 18 (28% with doctorates).
**Baccalaureate Enrollment** 118 **Women** 91% **Men** 9% **Minority** 44% **International** 1%
**Nursing Student Activities** Student Nurses' Association.
**Nursing Student Resources** Academic advising; academic or career counseling; assistance for students with disabilities; bookstore; campus computer network; career placement assistance; computer lab; computer-assisted instruction; e-mail services; employment services for current students; housing assistance; Internet; learning resource lab; library services; nursing audiovisuals; placement services for program completers; remedial services; resume preparation assistance; skills, simulation, or other laboratory; tutoring.
**Library Facilities** 545,611 volumes (20,000 in health, 10,000 in nursing); 994 periodical subscriptions (750 health-care related).

### BACCALAUREATE PROGRAMS

**Degree** BSN
**Available Programs** ADN to Baccalaureate; Generic Baccalaureate; LPN to Baccalaureate; RN Baccalaureate.
**Study Options** Full-time.
**Program Entrance Requirements** Minimum overall college GPA of 3.0, transcript of college record, written essay, high school chemistry, 2 years high school math, high school transcript, interview, 2 letters of recommendation, minimum high school GPA of 3.5, minimum GPA in nursing prerequisites of 3.0, prerequisite course work. *Application deadline:* 1/15 (fall). *Application fee:* $50.
**Advanced Placement** Credit given for nursing courses completed elsewhere dependent upon specific evaluations.
**Expenses (2013–14)** *Tuition:* full-time $32,142; part-time $1340 per unit. *International tuition:* $32,142 full-time. *Room and board:* $9596; room only: $5228 per academic year. *Required fees:* full-time $600; part-time $300 per term.
**Financial Aid** 94% of baccalaureate students in nursing programs received some form of financial aid in 2012–13.
**Contact** Ms. Shannon Gramatky, Nursing Department Advisor, Department of Nursing, Biola University, 13800 Biola Avenue, La Mirada, CA 90639. *Telephone:* 562-903-4850. *Fax:* 562-903-4803. *E-mail:* shannon.gramatky@biola.edu.

## Brandman University
### School of Nursing and Health Professions
### Irvine, California

*http://www.brandman.edu/*
Founded in 2009

**DEGREES • BSN • DNP • MS**

### BACCALAUREATE PROGRAMS

**Degree** BSN
**Available Programs** RN Baccalaureate.
**Program Entrance Requirements** Minimum overall college GPA of 2.0, transcript of college record, prerequisite course work. *Application deadline:* 8/1 (fall), 12/1 (winter).
**Contact** *Telephone:* 800-581-4100. *Fax:* 949-754-1335.

### GRADUATE PROGRAMS

**Contact** *Telephone:* 800-581-4100. *Fax:* 949-754-1335.

### MASTER'S DEGREE PROGRAM

**Degree** MS
**Available Programs** Master's.
**Concentrations Available** Nursing administration.
**Online Degree Options** Yes.
**Program Entrance Requirements** Transcript of college record, 3 letters of recommendation, resume. *Application deadline:* 8/1 (fall), 12/1 (winter).

### DOCTORAL DEGREE PROGRAM

**Degree** DNP
**Available Programs** Doctorate; Post-Baccalaureate Doctorate.
**Areas of Study** Family health, gerontology, maternity-newborn.
**Program Entrance Requirements** 3 letters of recommendation. *Application deadline:* 12/1 (winter).

### CONTINUING EDUCATION PROGRAM

**Contact** *Telephone:* 800-581-4100. *Fax:* 949-754-1335.

## California Baptist University
### School of Nursing
### Riverside, California

*http://www.calbaptist.edu/nursing*
Founded in 1950

**DEGREES • BSN • MSN**
**Nursing Program Faculty** 26 (4% with doctorates).
**Baccalaureate Enrollment** 180 **Women** 87.78% **Men** 12.22% **Minority** 33.89% **International** 1.67%
**Graduate Enrollment** 16 **Women** 87.5% **Men** 12.5% **Minority** 56.25%
**Nursing Student Activities** Student Nurses' Association.
**Nursing Student Resources** Academic advising; academic or career counseling; bookstore; campus computer network; career placement assistance; computer lab; e-mail services; employment services for current students; interactive nursing skills videos; Internet; learning resource lab; library services; nursing audiovisuals; resume preparation assistance; skills, simulation, or other laboratory; tutoring.
**Library Facilities** 232,039 volumes (335 in health, 236 in nursing); 24,506 periodical subscriptions (286 health-care related).

### BACCALAUREATE PROGRAMS

**Degree** BSN
**Available Programs** ADN to Baccalaureate; Generic Baccalaureate; RN Baccalaureate.
**Site Options** Corona, CA; San Bernardino, CA; Fullerton, CA.
**Study Options** Full-time.
**Program Entrance Requirements** Minimum overall college GPA of 2.7, transcript of college record, CPR certification, written essay, health exam, health insurance, immunizations, 2 letters of recommendation, minimum GPA in nursing prerequisites of 2.7, professional liability insurance/malpractice insurance, prerequisite course work. Transfer stu-

dents are accepted. *Application deadline:* 3/11 (fall), 8/31 (spring). *Application fee:* $50.
**Contact** *Telephone:* 951-343-4336.

## GRADUATE PROGRAMS

**Contact** *Telephone:* 951-343-4336. *Fax:* 951-343-4703.

### MASTER'S DEGREE PROGRAM

**Degree** MSN
**Available Programs** Accelerated Master's for Non-Nursing College Graduates; Master's.
**Concentrations Available** Clinical nurse leader; nursing education. *Clinical nurse specialist programs in:* adult health.
**Study Options** Part-time.
**Program Entrance Requirements** Computer literacy, minimum overall college GPA of 3.25, transcript of college record, CPR certification, written essay, immunizations, interview, 3 letters of recommendation, professional liability insurance/malpractice insurance, prerequisite course work, resume, statistics course. *Application deadline:* Applications may be processed on a rolling basis for some programs. *Application fee:* $45.
**Degree Requirements** 42 total credit hours, thesis or project, comprehensive exam.

# California State University, Bakersfield

## Program in Nursing
## Bakersfield, California

*http://www.csub.edu/nursing*
Founded in 1970

**DEGREE • BSN**
**Nursing Program Faculty** 24 (15% with doctorates).
**Baccalaureate Enrollment** 208 **Women** 86% **Men** 14% **Minority** 60% **International** 4% **Part-time** 6%
**Distance Learning Courses** Available.
**Nursing Student Activities** Nursing Honor Society, Sigma Theta Tau, Student Nurses' Association, nursing club.
**Nursing Student Resources** Academic advising; academic or career counseling; assistance for students with disabilities; bookstore; campus computer network; career placement assistance; computer lab; computer-assisted instruction; daycare for children of students; e-mail services; employment services for current students; externships; housing assistance; interactive nursing skills videos; Internet; learning resource lab; library services; nursing audiovisuals; paid internships; placement services for program completers; remedial services; resume preparation assistance; skills, simulation, or other laboratory; tutoring; unpaid internships.
**Library Facilities** 20,000 volumes in health, 1,850 volumes in nursing; 255 periodical subscriptions health-care related.

## BACCALAUREATE PROGRAMS

**Degree** BSN
**Available Programs** ADN to Baccalaureate; Generic Baccalaureate.
**Site Options** Visalia, CA; Lancaster, CA.
**Study Options** Full-time.
**Program Entrance Requirements** Minimum overall college GPA of 2.0, transcript of college record, CPR certification, health exam, health insurance, high school transcript, immunizations, interview, minimum GPA in nursing prerequisites of 2.8, professional liability insurance/malpractice insurance, prerequisite course work. Transfer students are accepted. *Application deadline:* 4/30 (fall), 12/31 (spring). *Application fee:* $25.
**Advanced Placement** Credit by examination available. Credit given for nursing courses completed elsewhere dependent upon specific evaluations.
**Contact** *Telephone:* 661-654-2508. *Fax:* 661-654-6347.

## CONTINUING EDUCATION PROGRAM

**Contact** *Telephone:* 661-654-2446. *Fax:* 661-664-2447.

# California State University Channel Islands

## Nursing Program
## Camarillo, California

*http://www.csuci.edu/*
Founded in 2002

**DEGREE • BSN**
**Nursing Program Faculty** 13 (20% with doctorates).
**Baccalaureate Enrollment** 120
**Nursing Student Activities** Student Nurses' Association.
**Nursing Student Resources** Academic advising; academic or career counseling; assistance for students with disabilities; bookstore; campus computer network; career placement assistance; computer lab; e-mail services; housing assistance; interactive nursing skills videos; Internet; learning resource lab; library services; nursing audiovisuals; remedial services; skills, simulation, or other laboratory; tutoring.

## BACCALAUREATE PROGRAMS

**Degree** BSN
**Available Programs** Generic Baccalaureate; RN Baccalaureate.
**Contact** *Telephone:* 805-437-3307.

# California State University, Chico

## School of Nursing
## Chico, California

*http://www.csuchico.edu/nurs/*
Founded in 1887

**DEGREES • BSN • MSN**
**Nursing Program Faculty** 36 (20% with doctorates).
**Baccalaureate Enrollment** 220 **Women** 85% **Men** 15% **Minority** 35%
**Graduate Enrollment** 21 **Women** 85% **Men** 15% **Minority** 25% **Part-time** 100%
**Distance Learning Courses** Available.
**Nursing Student Activities** Sigma Theta Tau, Student Nurses' Association, nursing club.
**Nursing Student Resources** Academic advising; academic or career counseling; assistance for students with disabilities; bookstore; campus computer network; career placement assistance; computer lab; computer-assisted instruction; daycare for children of students; e-mail services; employment services for current students; externships; housing assistance; interactive nursing skills videos; Internet; learning resource lab; library services; nursing audiovisuals; paid internships; placement services for program completers; remedial services; resume preparation assistance; skills, simulation, or other laboratory; tutoring; unpaid internships.
**Library Facilities** 924,410 volumes (17,727 in health, 1,467 in nursing); 22,000 periodical subscriptions (133 health-care related).

## BACCALAUREATE PROGRAMS

**Degree** BSN
**Available Programs** ADN to Baccalaureate; Baccalaureate for Second Degree; Generic Baccalaureate; LPN to RN Baccalaureate; RN Baccalaureate.
**Study Options** Full-time.
**Program Entrance Requirements** Minimum overall college GPA of 3.0, transcript of college record, CPR certification, health insurance, immunizations, minimum GPA in nursing prerequisites of 3.0, prerequisite course work. Transfer students are accepted. *Application deadline:* 3/1 (fall), 11/1 (spring). *Application fee:* $50.
**Advanced Placement** Credit by examination available. Credit given for nursing courses completed elsewhere dependent upon specific evaluations.
**Expenses (2013–14)** *Tuition, state resident:* full-time $5472; part-time $1587 per semester. *Tuition, nonresident:* full-time $15,900. *Room and board:* $11,000; room only: $6800 per academic year. *Required fees:* full-time $1500; part-time $750 per term.
**Financial Aid** 75% of baccalaureate students in nursing programs received some form of financial aid in 2012–13. *Gift aid (need-based):* Federal Pell, FSEOG, state, private, college/university gift aid from institutional funds, United Negro College Fund. *Loans:* Federal Direct (Subsidized and Unsubsidized Stafford PLUS), Perkins, college/university.

*Work-study:* Federal Work-Study. *Financial aid application deadline:* Continuous.
**Contact** Dr. Carol L. Huston, Director, School of Nursing, California State University, Chico, Holt Hall 369, Chico, CA 95929-0200. *Telephone:* 530-898-5891. *Fax:* 530-898-4363. *E-mail:* chuston@csuchico.edu.

## GRADUATE PROGRAMS

**Expenses (2013–14)** *Tuition, state resident:* full-time $8238; part-time $2703 per semester. *Tuition, nonresident:* full-time $17,166; part-time $4935 per semester. *Room and board:* $11,000; room only: $7000 per academic year. *Required fees:* full-time $4119.
**Financial Aid** 25% of graduate students in nursing programs received some form of financial aid in 2012–13. Career-related internships or fieldwork and scholarships available. *Financial aid application deadline:* 3/1.
**Contact** Jennifer Lillibridge, Graduate Coordinator, School of Nursing, California State University, Chico, 400 West 1st Street, Chico, CA 95929-0200. *Telephone:* 530-898-5891. *Fax:* 530-898-6709. *E-mail:* jlillibridge@csuchico.edu.

### MASTER'S DEGREE PROGRAM

**Degree** MSN
**Available Programs** Master's.
**Concentrations Available** Nursing administration; nursing education.
**Study Options** Part-time.
**Online Degree Options** Yes (online only).
**Program Entrance Requirements** Clinical experience, minimum overall college GPA of 3.0, transcript of college record, CPR certification, written essay, immunizations, prerequisite course work, statistics course, GRE. *Application deadline:* 3/1 (fall), 3/1 (spring).
**Advanced Placement** Credit given for nursing courses completed elsewhere dependent upon specific evaluations.
**Degree Requirements** 30 total credit hours, thesis or project.

## CONTINUING EDUCATION PROGRAM

**Contact** Dr. Carol L. Huston, Director, School of Nursing, School of Nursing, California State University, Chico, Holt Hall 369, Chico, CA 95929-0200. *Telephone:* 530-898-5891. *Fax:* 530-898-6709. *E-mail:* chuston@csuchico.edu.

# California State University, Dominguez Hills

## Program in Nursing
## Carson, California

***http://www.csudh.edu/cps/son***
Founded in 1960

**DEGREES • BSN • MSN**
**Nursing Program Faculty** 79 (34% with doctorates).
**Baccalaureate Enrollment** 725 **Women** 91% **Men** 9% **Minority** 37% **Part-time** 81%
**Graduate Enrollment** 456 **Women** 91% **Men** 9% **Minority** 28% **Part-time** 95%
**Distance Learning Courses** Available.
**Nursing Student Activities** Nursing Honor Society, Sigma Theta Tau, nursing club.
**Nursing Student Resources** Academic advising; academic or career counseling; assistance for students with disabilities; bookstore; campus computer network; career placement assistance; computer lab; computer-assisted instruction; daycare for children of students; e-mail services; housing assistance; interactive nursing skills videos; Internet; learning resource lab; library services; nursing audiovisuals; remedial services; skills, simulation, or other laboratory; tutoring.
**Library Facilities** 454,476 volumes (10,000 in nursing); 656 periodical subscriptions (215 health-care related).

## BACCALAUREATE PROGRAMS

**Degree** BSN
**Available Programs** Baccalaureate for Second Degree; RN Baccalaureate.
**Site Options** Ventura, CA; Santa Monica, CA; Whittier, CA.
**Online Degree Options** Yes.
**Program Entrance Requirements** Minimum overall college GPA of 2.0, transcript of college record, minimum GPA in nursing prerequisites of 2.0, prerequisite course work, RN licensure. Transfer students are accepted. *Application fee:* $55.
**Contact** *Telephone:* 310-243-2005. *Fax:* 310-516-3542.

## GRADUATE PROGRAMS

**Contact** *Telephone:* 310-243-2522. *Fax:* 310-516-3542.

### MASTER'S DEGREE PROGRAM

**Degree** MSN
**Available Programs** Master's; Master's for Non-Nursing College Graduates; Master's for Nurses with Non-Nursing Degrees.
**Concentrations Available** Clinical nurse leader; nursing administration; nursing education. *Clinical nurse specialist programs in:* gerontology, parent-child. *Nurse practitioner programs in:* family health.
**Site Options** Whittier, CA.
**Study Options** Full-time and part-time.
**Online Degree Options** Yes (online only).
**Program Entrance Requirements** Minimum overall college GPA of 3.0, transcript of college record, written essay, nursing research course, physical assessment course, prerequisite course work, resume, statistics course. *Application deadline:* 4/1 (fall), 11/1 (spring). Applications may be processed on a rolling basis for some programs. *Application fee:* $55.
**Advanced Placement** Credit given for nursing courses completed elsewhere dependent upon specific evaluations.
**Degree Requirements** 45 total credit hours, comprehensive exam.

### POST-MASTER'S PROGRAM

**Areas of Study** Nursing administration; nursing education. *Clinical nurse specialist programs in:* gerontology, parent-child. *Nurse practitioner programs in:* family health.

# California State University, East Bay

## Department of Nursing and Health Sciences
## Hayward, California

***http://www20.csueastbay.edu/csci/departments/nursing/***
Founded in 1957

**DEGREE • BS**
**Nursing Program Faculty** 53 (23% with doctorates).
**Baccalaureate Enrollment** 494 **Women** 80% **Men** 20% **Minority** 40% **International** 5% **Part-time** 10%
**Distance Learning Courses** Available.
**Nursing Student Activities** Sigma Theta Tau, Student Nurses' Association.
**Nursing Student Resources** Academic advising; academic or career counseling; assistance for students with disabilities; bookstore; campus computer network; career placement assistance; computer lab; computer-assisted instruction; e-mail services; employment services for current students; externships; interactive nursing skills videos; Internet; learning resource lab; library services; nursing audiovisuals; other; paid internships; placement services for program completers; remedial services; resume preparation assistance; skills, simulation, or other laboratory; tutoring; unpaid internships.

## BACCALAUREATE PROGRAMS

**Degree** BS
**Available Programs** ADN to Baccalaureate; Generic Baccalaureate.
**Site Options** Concord, CA.
**Study Options** Full-time.
**Program Entrance Requirements** Transcript of college record, CPR certification, health exam, health insurance, immunizations, minimum GPA in nursing prerequisites of 3.0, prerequisite course work. Transfer students are accepted. *Application deadline:* 11/30 (fall).
**Advanced Placement** Credit given for nursing courses completed elsewhere dependent upon specific evaluations.
**Expenses (2012–13)** *Tuition, state resident:* full-time $6500. *Tuition, nonresident:* full-time $15,500. *International tuition:* $15,500 full-time.
**Financial Aid** ***Gift aid (need-based):*** Federal Pell, FSEOG, state, private, college/university gift aid from institutional funds. *Loans:* Federal Direct (Subsidized and Unsubsidized Stafford PLUS), Perkins, college/university. *Work-study:* Federal Work-Study. *Financial aid application deadline (priority):* 3/2.
**Contact** Lara Dungan, Admissions Coordinator/Advisor, Department of Nursing and Health Sciences, California State University, East Bay,

25800 Carlos Bee Boulevard, Hayward, CA 94542. *Telephone:* 510-885-3481. *Fax:* 510-885-2156. *E-mail:* lara.dungan@csueastbay.edu.

# California State University, Fresno

## Department of Nursing
## Fresno, California

*http://www.csufresno.edu/chhs/depts_programs/nursing/*
Founded in 1911

**DEGREES • BSN • DNP • MSN**
**Nursing Program Faculty** 55 (30% with doctorates).
**Baccalaureate Enrollment** 450 **Women** 80% **Men** 20% **Minority** 49% **Part-time** 5%
**Graduate Enrollment** 270 **Women** 86% **Men** 14% **Minority** 53% **International** 4% **Part-time** 36%
**Distance Learning Courses** Available.
**Nursing Student Activities** Sigma Theta Tau, Student Nurses' Association.
**Nursing Student Resources** Academic advising; academic or career counseling; assistance for students with disabilities; bookstore; campus computer network; career placement assistance; computer lab; computer-assisted instruction; daycare for children of students; e-mail services; externships; housing assistance; interactive nursing skills videos; Internet; learning resource lab; library services; nursing audiovisuals; paid internships; placement services for program completers; remedial services; skills, simulation, or other laboratory; tutoring.
**Library Facilities** 28,197 volumes in health, 1,287 volumes in nursing; 1,700 periodical subscriptions health-care related.

### BACCALAUREATE PROGRAMS

**Degree** BSN
**Available Programs** ADN to Baccalaureate; Generic Baccalaureate.
**Study Options** Full-time.
**Program Entrance Requirements** Minimum overall college GPA of 3.0, transcript of college record, CPR certification, health exam, immunizations, minimum GPA in nursing prerequisites of 3.0, professional liability insurance/malpractice insurance, prerequisite course work. Transfer students are accepted. *Application deadline:* 3/31 (fall), 8/31 (spring).
**Advanced Placement** Credit by examination available. Credit given for nursing courses completed elsewhere dependent upon specific evaluations.
**Expenses (2013–14)** *Tuition, state resident:* full-time $6287; part-time $3989 per semester.
**Financial Aid** 65% of baccalaureate students in nursing programs received some form of financial aid in 2012–13. *Gift aid (need-based):* Federal Pell, FSEOG, state, private, college/university gift aid from institutional funds. *Loans:* Federal Nursing Student Loans, Federal Direct (Subsidized and Unsubsidized Stafford PLUS), Perkins, college/university, alternative loans. *Work-study:* Federal Work-Study. *Financial aid application deadline (priority):* 3/2.
**Contact** Dr. Mary Barakzai, Chair, Department of Nursing, California State University, Fresno, 2345 East San Ramon Avenue, MH25, Fresno, CA 93740-8031. *Telephone:* 559-278-2041. *Fax:* 559-278-6360. *E-mail:* maryb@csufresno.edu.

### GRADUATE PROGRAMS

**Expenses (2013–14)** *Tuition, state resident:* full-time $7553; part-time $2360 per semester.
**Financial Aid** 30% of graduate students in nursing programs received some form of financial aid in 2012–13. 2 teaching assistantships were awarded; career-related internships or fieldwork, Federal Work-Study, scholarships, and traineeships also available. Aid available to part-time students. *Financial aid application deadline:* 3/1.
**Contact** Dr. Ndidi Griffin, Graduate Coordinator, Department of Nursing, California State University, Fresno, 2345 East San Ramon Avenue, MH25, Fresno, CA 93740-8031. *Telephone:* 559-278-6697. *Fax:* 559-278-6360. *E-mail:* ndidig@csufresno.edu.

#### MASTER'S DEGREE PROGRAM

**Degree** MSN
**Available Programs** Accelerated Master's; Master's.
**Concentrations Available** Nursing education. *Clinical nurse specialist programs in:* adult health, gerontology, pediatric. *Nurse practitioner programs in:* family health, pediatric.
**Study Options** Full-time.
**Program Entrance Requirements** Clinical experience, computer literacy, minimum overall college GPA of 3.0, transcript of college record, CPR certification, written essay, 3 letters of recommendation, nursing research course, physical assessment course, professional liability insurance/malpractice insurance, prerequisite course work, resume, statistics course, GRE General Test. *Application deadline:* 4/1 (fall).
**Advanced Placement** Credit given for nursing courses completed elsewhere dependent upon specific evaluations.
**Degree Requirements** 40 total credit hours, thesis or project.

#### POST-MASTER'S PROGRAM

**Areas of Study** *Nurse practitioner programs in:* family health, pediatric.

#### DOCTORAL DEGREE PROGRAM

**Degree** DNP
**Available Programs** Doctorate.
**Online Degree Options** Yes (online only).
**Program Entrance Requirements** Clinical experience, minimum overall college GPA of 3.0, interview by faculty committee, 3 letters of recommendation, MSN or equivalent, vita, writing sample. *Application deadline:* 1/31 (fall).
**Degree Requirements** 37 total credit hours, oral exam.

### CONTINUING EDUCATION PROGRAM

**Contact** Dr. Scott Moore, Interim Associate Vice President, Department of Nursing, California State University, Fresno, 5005 North Maple Avenue, ED76, Fresno, CA 93740-0076. *Telephone:* 559-278-2691. *Fax:* 559-278-0333. *E-mail:* scottm@csufresno.edu.

# California State University, Fullerton

## Department of Nursing
## Fullerton, California

*http://www.fullerton.edu/*
Founded in 1957

**DEGREES • BSN • DNP • MSN**
**Nursing Program Faculty** 71 (28% with doctorates).
**Baccalaureate Enrollment** 464 **Women** 83.2% **Men** 16.8% **Minority** 60.8% **International** 4.3% **Part-time** 69%
**Graduate Enrollment** 372 **Women** 84.9% **Men** 15.1% **Minority** 44.9% **International** 1.1% **Part-time** 46.5%
**Distance Learning Courses** Available.
**Nursing Student Activities** Nursing Honor Society, Sigma Theta Tau, Student Nurses' Association.
**Nursing Student Resources** Academic advising; academic or career counseling; assistance for students with disabilities; bookstore; campus computer network; computer lab; computer-assisted instruction; daycare for children of students; e-mail services; housing assistance; Internet; learning resource lab; library services; resume preparation assistance; skills, simulation, or other laboratory; tutoring.
**Library Facilities** 1.3 million volumes (17,340 in health, 837 in nursing); 55,756 periodical subscriptions (8,145 health-care related).

### BACCALAUREATE PROGRAMS

**Degree** BSN
**Available Programs** ADN to Baccalaureate; Baccalaureate for Second Degree; Generic Baccalaureate; LPN to Baccalaureate; RN Baccalaureate.
**Site Options** Los Angeles, CA; Riverside, CA; Mission Viejo, CA.
**Study Options** Full-time.
**Program Entrance Requirements** Minimum overall college GPA, transcript of college record, minimum GPA in nursing prerequisites, prerequisite course work. *Application deadline:* 2/15 (fall).
**Advanced Placement** Credit given for nursing courses completed elsewhere dependent upon specific evaluations.
**Expenses (2012–13)** *Tuition, state resident:* full-time $3313.
**Financial Aid** 50% of baccalaureate students in nursing programs received some form of financial aid in 2011–12. *Gift aid (need-based):* Federal Pell, FSEOG, state, private, college/university gift aid from institutional funds, Federal Nursing. *Loans:* Federal Direct (Subsidized and Unsubsidized Stafford PLUS), Perkins, college/university, private loans. *Work-study:* Federal Work-Study. *Financial aid application deadline (priority):* 3/2.

**Contact** Nursing Advisor, Department of Nursing, California State University, Fullerton, EC-182, PO Box 6868, Fullerton, CA 92834-6868. *Telephone:* 657-278-3217. *Fax:* 657-278-2096. *E-mail:* nursingadvising@fullerton.edu.

## GRADUATE PROGRAMS

**Expenses (2012–13)** *Tuition, state resident:* full-time $4006; part-time $2461 per semester.

**Financial Aid** 44% of graduate students in nursing programs received some form of financial aid in 2011–12.

**Contact** Ms. Mary Lehn-Mooney, Advisor, Department of Nursing, California State University, Fullerton, EC 190, 800 North State College Boulevard, Fullerton, CA 92834-6868. *Telephone:* 714-278-3217. *Fax:* 714-278-2096. *E-mail:* mlehn-mooney@fullerton.edu.

### MASTER'S DEGREE PROGRAM

**Degree** MSN

**Available Programs** Master's; Master's for Non-Nursing College Graduates.

**Concentrations Available** Nurse anesthesia; nurse-midwifery; nursing administration; nursing education. *Clinical nurse specialist programs in:* school health. *Nurse practitioner programs in:*women's health.

**Study Options** Full-time and part-time.

**Online Degree Options** Yes.

**Program Entrance Requirements** Clinical experience, minimum overall college GPA of 3.0, transcript of college record, CPR certification, written essay, immunizations, interview, 3 letters of recommendation, nursing research course, professional liability insurance/malpractice insurance, prerequisite course work, statistics course. *Application deadline:* 11/30 (fall). Applications may be processed on a rolling basis for some programs. *Application fee:* $55.

**Advanced Placement** Credit given for nursing courses completed elsewhere dependent upon specific evaluations.

**Degree Requirements** 71 total credit hours, thesis or project, comprehensive exam.

### DOCTORAL DEGREE PROGRAM

**Degree** DNP

**Available Programs** Doctorate; Doctorate for Nurses with Non-Nursing Degrees; Post-Baccalaureate Doctorate.

**Areas of Study** Advanced practice nursing, clinical practice, community health, critical care, family health, nursing administration, nursing education, nursing research, nursing science,women's health.

**Program Entrance Requirements** Clinical experience, minimum overall college GPA of 3.5, interview, 3 letters of recommendation, MSN or equivalent, statistics course, writing sample. *Application deadline:* 12/15 (fall). *Application fee:* $55.

**Degree Requirements** 36 total credit hours, dissertation, written exam.

# California State University, Long Beach

## School of Nursing
## Long Beach, California

***http://www.csulb.edu/colleges/chhs/departments/nursing/***

Founded in 1949

## DEGREES • BSN • MSN • MSN/MHA

**Nursing Program Faculty** 76 (40% with doctorates).

**Baccalaureate Enrollment** 539 **Women** 79.2% **Men** 20.8% **Minority** 73.6% **International** .01% **Part-time** 10%

**Graduate Enrollment** 484 **Women** 86.4% **Men** 13.6% **Minority** 71.7% **International** .02% **Part-time** 50%

**Nursing Student Activities** Nursing Honor Society, Sigma Theta Tau, Student Nurses' Association.

**Nursing Student Resources** Academic advising; academic or career counseling; assistance for students with disabilities; bookstore; e-mail services; interactive nursing skills videos; Internet; learning resource lab; library services; nursing audiovisuals; remedial services; resume preparation assistance; skills, simulation, or other laboratory; tutoring; unpaid internships.

**Library Facilities** 2 million volumes; 99,416 periodical subscriptions.

## BACCALAUREATE PROGRAMS

**Degree** BSN

**Available Programs** ADN to Baccalaureate; Accelerated Baccalaureate; Baccalaureate for Second Degree; Generic Baccalaureate; LPN to Baccalaureate.

**Site Options** Huntington Beach, CA.

**Study Options** Full-time.

**Program Entrance Requirements** Transcript of college record, CPR certification, health exam, health insurance, immunizations, interview, minimum GPA in nursing prerequisites of 3.0, professional liability insurance/malpractice insurance, prerequisite course work. Transfer students are accepted. *Application deadline:* 2/15 (fall), 9/15 (spring). *Application fee:* $55.

**Advanced Placement** Credit given for nursing courses completed elsewhere dependent upon specific evaluations.

**Expenses (2012–13)** *Tuition, state resident:* full-time $6700; part-time $4230 per semester. *Tuition, nonresident:* full-time $15,666; part-time $8694 per semester. *International tuition:* $15,666 full-time. *Room and board:* $11,000; room only: $8200 per academic year. *Required fees:* full-time $3000; part-time $300 per credit; part-time $1500 per term.

**Financial Aid** 75% of baccalaureate students in nursing programs received some form of financial aid in 2011–12. *Gift aid (need-based):* Federal Pell, FSEOG, state, private, college/university gift aid from institutional funds. *Loans:* Federal Direct (Subsidized and Unsubsidized Stafford PLUS), Perkins. *Work-study:* Federal Work-Study. *Financial aid application deadline (priority):* 3/2.

**Contact** Dr. Beth R. Keely, Assistant Director, Undergraduate Nursing Programs, School of Nursing, California State University, Long Beach, 1250 Bellflower Boulevard, Long Beach, CA 90840. *Telephone:* 562-985-4478. *Fax:* 562-985-2382. *E-mail:* bkeely@csulb.edu.

## GRADUATE PROGRAMS

**Expenses (2012–13)** *Tuition, state resident:* full-time $8124; part-time $5034 per semester. *Tuition, nonresident:* full-time $12,588; part-time $9498 per semester. *International tuition:* $12,588 full-time. *Room and board:* $10,658; room only: $8208 per academic year. *Required fees:* full-time $3000; part-time $372 per credit; part-time $1500 per term.

**Financial Aid** 25% of graduate students in nursing programs received some form of financial aid in 2011–12. Federal Work-Study, institutionally sponsored loans, and scholarships available. *Financial aid application deadline:* 3/2.

**Contact** Alison Kliachko-Trafas, Administrative Assistant, School of Nursing, California State University, Long Beach, 1250 Bellflower Boulevard, Long Beach, CA 90840. *Telephone:* 562-985-4473. *Fax:* 562-985-2382. *E-mail:* akliachk@csulb.edu.

### MASTER'S DEGREE PROGRAM

**Degrees** MSN; MSN/MHA

**Available Programs** Accelerated Master's; Master's; Master's for Non-Nursing College Graduates.

**Concentrations Available** Health-care administration; nursing administration; nursing education. *Clinical nurse specialist programs in:* adult health. *Nurse practitioner programs in:* adult health, family health, gerontology, pediatric, psychiatric/mental health,women's health.

**Site Options** Long Beach, CA; Huntington Beach, CA.

**Study Options** Full-time and part-time.

**Program Entrance Requirements** Clinical experience, minimum overall college GPA of 2.75, transcript of college record, written essay, 3 letters of recommendation, physical assessment course, prerequisite course work, resume, statistics course. *Application deadline:* 3/15 (fall), 10/15 (spring). *Application fee:* $55.

**Advanced Placement** Credit given for nursing courses completed elsewhere dependent upon specific evaluations.

**Degree Requirements** 37 total credit hours, thesis or project, comprehensive exam.

### POST-MASTER'S PROGRAM

**Areas of Study** Nursing administration. *Clinical nurse specialist programs in:* adult health. *Nurse practitioner programs in:* adult health, family health, gerontology, pediatric, psychiatric/mental health,women's health.

# California State University, Los Angeles

### School of Nursing
### Los Angeles, California

*http://web.calstatela.edu/academic/hhs/nursing/*
Founded in 1947

**DEGREES • BSN • MSN**
**Nursing Program Faculty** 31 (39% with doctorates).
**Baccalaureate Enrollment** 300
**Graduate Enrollment** 100
**Nursing Student Resources** Academic advising.
**Library Facilities** 2 million volumes; 140 periodical subscriptions.

## BACCALAUREATE PROGRAMS

**Degree** BSN
**Available Programs** Generic Baccalaureate; LPN to RN Baccalaureate; RN Baccalaureate.
**Study Options** Full-time.
**Program Entrance Requirements** Minimum overall college GPA of 2.75, CPR certification, health exam, health insurance, high school biology, immunizations, minimum GPA in nursing prerequisites of 2.75, professional liability insurance/malpractice insurance, prerequisite course work. Transfer students are accepted. *Application deadline:* 12/1 (fall).
**Advanced Placement** Credit given for nursing courses completed elsewhere dependent upon specific evaluations.
**Contact** *Telephone:* 323-343-4700. *Fax:* 323-343-6454.

## GRADUATE PROGRAMS

**Contact** *Telephone:* 323-343-4700. *Fax:* 323-343-6454.

### MASTER'S DEGREE PROGRAM

**Degree** MSN
**Available Programs** Accelerated Master's for Nurses with Non-Nursing Degrees; Accelerated RN to Master's; Master's; Master's for Non-Nursing College Graduates.
**Concentrations Available** Nursing administration; nursing education. *Clinical nurse specialist programs in:* psychiatric/mental health. *Nurse practitioner programs in:* acute care, adult health, family health, pediatric, primary care, psychiatric/mental health.
**Study Options** Full-time and part-time.
**Program Entrance Requirements** Clinical experience, minimum overall college GPA of 3.0, transcript of college record, written essay, immunizations, letters of recommendation, nursing research course, physical assessment course, professional liability insurance/malpractice insurance, resume, statistics course. *Application deadline:* 11/15 (fall), 5/15 (spring).
**Advanced Placement** Credit given for nursing courses completed elsewhere dependent upon specific evaluations.
**Degree Requirements** 45 total credit hours, comprehensive exam.

### POST-MASTER'S PROGRAM

**Areas of Study** *Nurse practitioner programs in:* acute care, adult health, family health, pediatric, primary care.

# California State University, Northridge

### Nursing Program
### Northridge, California

*http://www.csun.edu/~nursing/*
Founded in 1958

**DEGREE • BSN**
**Nursing Program Faculty** 18 (3.6% with doctorates).
**Baccalaureate Enrollment** 140 **Women** 92% **Men** 8% **Minority** 60% **International** 12% **Part-time** 66%
**Nursing Student Activities** Sigma Theta Tau, Student Nurses' Association.
**Nursing Student Resources** Academic advising; academic or career counseling; assistance for students with disabilities; bookstore; campus computer network; career placement assistance; computer lab; computer-assisted instruction; daycare for children of students; e-mail services; housing assistance; interactive nursing skills videos; Internet; learning resource lab; library services; nursing audiovisuals; remedial services; resume preparation assistance; skills, simulation, or other laboratory; tutoring.
**Library Facilities** 61,848 volumes in health, 1,401 volumes in nursing; 303 periodical subscriptions health-care related.

## BACCALAUREATE PROGRAMS

**Degree** BSN
**Available Programs** ADN to Baccalaureate; Accelerated Baccalaureate.
**Site Options** Panorama City, CA; Ventura , CA; Antelope Valley, CA.
**Study Options** Full-time and part-time.
**Program Entrance Requirements** Minimum overall college GPA of 3.0, transcript of college record, CPR certification, written essay, health exam, health insurance, immunizations, interview, 3 letters of recommendation, minimum GPA in nursing prerequisites of 3.0, professional liability insurance/malpractice insurance, prerequisite course work, RN licensure. Transfer students are accepted. *Application deadline:* 11/30 (fall), 11/30 (summer). *Application fee:* $55.
**Advanced Placement** Credit by examination available. Credit given for nursing courses completed elsewhere dependent upon specific evaluations.
**Expenses (2012–13)** *Tuition, state resident:* full-time $7002; part-time $4494 per semester. *Tuition, nonresident:* full-time $11,466; part-time $6726 per semester. *International tuition:* $11,466 full-time. *Room and board:* $11,511; room only: $6771 per academic year. *Required fees:* full-time $1032; part-time $516 per term.
**Financial Aid** 90% of baccalaureate students in nursing programs received some form of financial aid in 2011–12. *Gift aid (need-based):* Federal Pell, FSEOG, state, private, college/university gift aid from institutional funds. *Loans:* Perkins. *Work-study:* Federal Work-Study. *Financial aid application deadline (priority):* 3/2.
**Contact** Department of Nursing, Nursing Program, California State University, Northridge, 18111 Nordhoff Street, Northridge, CA 91330-8285. *Telephone:* 818-677-3101. *Fax:* 818-677-2045. *E-mail:* absn@csun.edu.

# California State University, Sacramento

### School of Nursing
### Sacramento, California

*http://www.hhs.csus.edu/nrs*
Founded in 1947

**DEGREES • BSN • MS**
**Nursing Program Faculty** 64 (50% with doctorates).
**Baccalaureate Enrollment** 286 **Women** 89% **Men** 11%
**Graduate Enrollment** 180 **Women** 95% **Men** 5% **Part-time** 100%
**Distance Learning Courses** Available.
**Nursing Student Activities** Sigma Theta Tau, Student Nurses' Association.
**Nursing Student Resources** Academic advising; academic or career counseling; assistance for students with disabilities; bookstore; campus computer network; computer lab; computer-assisted instruction; daycare for children of students; e-mail services; externships; housing assistance; interactive nursing skills videos; Internet; learning resource lab; library services; nursing audiovisuals; paid internships; placement services for program completers; remedial services; resume preparation assistance; skills, simulation, or other laboratory; tutoring.
**Library Facilities** 33,000 volumes in health; 327 periodical subscriptions health-care related.

## BACCALAUREATE PROGRAMS

**Degree** BSN
**Available Programs** ADN to Baccalaureate; Baccalaureate for Second Degree; Generic Baccalaureate; LPN to RN Baccalaureate.
**Study Options** Full-time.
**Program Entrance Requirements** Transcript of college record, CPR certification, health exam, health insurance, high school biology, high school math, immunizations, minimum GPA in nursing prerequisites of 3.3, professional liability insurance/malpractice insurance, prerequisite course work. Transfer students are accepted. *Application deadline:* 3/1 (fall), 10/1 (spring).

**Advanced Placement** Credit by examination available. Credit given for nursing courses completed elsewhere dependent upon specific evaluations.
**Contact** *Telephone:* 916-278-6525.

### GRADUATE PROGRAMS

**Contact** *Fax:* 916-278-6311.

**MASTER'S DEGREE PROGRAM**
**Degree** MS
**Available Programs** Master's.
**Concentrations Available** Nursing administration; nursing education. *Nurse practitioner programs in:* family health, primary care.
**Study Options** Part-time.
**Program Entrance Requirements** Clinical experience, computer literacy, minimum overall college GPA of 3.0, transcript of college record, CPR certification, immunizations, nursing research course, professional liability insurance/malpractice insurance, prerequisite course work, statistics course, GRE. *Application deadline:* 11/30 (fall).
**Advanced Placement** Credit given for nursing courses completed elsewhere dependent upon specific evaluations.
**Degree Requirements** 33 total credit hours, comprehensive exam.

## California State University, San Bernardino

**Department of Nursing**
**San Bernardino, California**

*https://www.csusb.edu/*
Founded in 1965

**DEGREES • BSN • MSN**
**Nursing Program Faculty** 42 (19% with doctorates).
**Baccalaureate Enrollment** 457 **Women** 81% **Men** 19% **Minority** 59%
**Graduate Enrollment** 19 **Women** 89% **Men** 11% **Minority** 47%
**Distance Learning Courses** Available.
**Nursing Student Activities** Sigma Theta Tau, Student Nurses' Association.
**Nursing Student Resources** Academic advising; academic or career counseling; assistance for students with disabilities; bookstore; campus computer network; computer lab; computer-assisted instruction; daycare for children of students; e-mail services; Internet; learning resource lab; library services; nursing audiovisuals; remedial services; skills, simulation, or other laboratory.
**Library Facilities** 731,259 volumes (1,500 in health, 1,000 in nursing); 2,028 periodical subscriptions (5,000 health-care related).

### BACCALAUREATE PROGRAMS

**Degree** BSN
**Available Programs** Generic Baccalaureate; LPN to Baccalaureate; RN Baccalaureate.
**Site Options** Palm Desert, CA.
**Study Options** Full-time.
**Program Entrance Requirements** Minimum overall college GPA of 2.5, transcript of college record, 3 letters of recommendation, minimum GPA in nursing prerequisites of 2.5, prerequisite course work. Transfer students are accepted. *Application deadline:* 3/1 (fall), 10/1 (winter).
**Advanced Placement** Credit given for nursing courses completed elsewhere dependent upon specific evaluations.
**Contact** *Telephone:* 909-537-5381.

### GRADUATE PROGRAMS

**Contact** *Telephone:* 909-537-7241.

**MASTER'S DEGREE PROGRAM**
**Degree** MSN
**Available Programs** Master's.
**Concentrations Available** Nursing administration; nursing education. *Clinical nurse specialist programs in:* community health.
**Study Options** Full-time and part-time.
**Program Entrance Requirements** Clinical experience, minimum overall college GPA of 3.0, transcript of college record, letters of recommendation, prerequisite course work, resume, statistics course. *Application deadline:* 6/10 (fall).
**Advanced Placement** Credit given for nursing courses completed elsewhere dependent upon specific evaluations.
**Degree Requirements** 65 total credit hours, thesis or project, comprehensive exam.

## California State University, San Marcos

**School of Nursing**
**San Marcos, California**

*http://www.csusm.edu/*
Founded in 1990

**DEGREE • BSN**
**Nursing Student Activities** Student Nurses' Association.
**Library Facilities** 406,748 volumes; 43,681 periodical subscriptions.

### BACCALAUREATE PROGRAMS

**Degree** BSN
**Available Programs** Accelerated Baccalaureate; Generic Baccalaureate.
**Contact** *Telephone:* 706-750-7550. *Fax:* 706-750-3646.

## California State University, Stanislaus

**Department of Nursing**
**Turlock, California**

*http://www.csustan.edu/academics/CHHS/Nursing.html*
Founded in 1957

**DEGREE • BSN**
**Nursing Program Faculty** 17 (24% with doctorates).
**Baccalaureate Enrollment** 164 **Women** 88% **Men** 12% **Minority** 42% **Part-time** 30%
**Nursing Student Activities** Sigma Theta Tau, Student Nurses' Association.
**Nursing Student Resources** Academic advising; academic or career counseling; assistance for students with disabilities; bookstore; campus computer network; career placement assistance; computer lab; computer-assisted instruction; daycare for children of students; e-mail services; employment services for current students; externships; interactive nursing skills videos; Internet; learning resource lab; library services; nursing audiovisuals; resume preparation assistance; skills, simulation, or other laboratory; tutoring.
**Library Facilities** 502,279 volumes (12,642 in health, 1,338 in nursing); 62,850 periodical subscriptions (93 health-care related).

### BACCALAUREATE PROGRAMS

**Degree** BSN
**Available Programs** ADN to Baccalaureate; Generic Baccalaureate; LPN to Baccalaureate.
**Study Options** Full-time.
**Program Entrance Requirements** Minimum overall college GPA of 3.0, transcript of college record, CPR certification, health exam, immunizations, minimum GPA in nursing prerequisites of 3.0, professional liability insurance/malpractice insurance, prerequisite course work. Transfer students are accepted.
**Advanced Placement** Credit given for nursing courses completed elsewhere dependent upon specific evaluations.
**Contact** *Telephone:* 209-667-3141. *Fax:* 209-667-3690.

## Charles Drew University of Medicine and Science

**School of Nursing**
**Los Angeles, California**

Founded in 1966

**DEGREE • MSN**
**Library Facilities** 84,336 volumes; 36,693 periodical subscriptions.

## GRADUATE PROGRAMS

**Contact** School of Nursing, School of Nursing, Charles Drew University of Medicine and Science, 1731 East 120th Street, Los Angeles, CA 90059. *Telephone:* 323-568-3301. *E-mail:* mmdson@cdrewu.edu.

**MASTER'S DEGREE PROGRAM**
**Degree** MSN
**Available Programs** Accelerated Master's for Nurses with Non-Nursing Degrees; Master's.
**Program Entrance Requirements** Minimum overall college GPA of 3.0, written essay, 3 letters of recommendation, resume. *Application fee:* $100.

# Concordia University

### Bachelor of Science in Nursing Program
### Irvine, California

Founded in 1972
**DEGREE • BSN**
**Library Facilities** 81,602 volumes; 31,209 periodical subscriptions.

## BACCALAUREATE PROGRAMS

**Degree** BSN
**Available Programs** Accelerated Baccalaureate for Second Degree; RN Baccalaureate.
**Program Entrance Requirements** Transcript of college record, prerequisite course work, RN licensure.
**Contact** *Telephone:* 949-854-8002 Ext. 1144.

# Dominican University of California

### Program in Nursing
### San Rafael, California

*http://www.dominican.edu/*
Founded in 1890
**DEGREES • BSN • MSN**
**Nursing Program Faculty** 53 (23% with doctorates).
**Baccalaureate Enrollment** 497 **Women** 88% **Men** 12% **Minority** 55% **International** 1% **Part-time** 17%
**Graduate Enrollment** 30 **Women** 87% **Men** 13% **Minority** 23% **Part-time** 50%
**Nursing Student Activities** Sigma Theta Tau, Student Nurses' Association, nursing club.
**Nursing Student Resources** Academic advising; academic or career counseling; assistance for students with disabilities; bookstore; campus computer network; career placement assistance; computer lab; computer-assisted instruction; e-mail services; employment services for current students; housing assistance; interactive nursing skills videos; Internet; learning resource lab; library services; nursing audiovisuals; remedial services; resume preparation assistance; skills, simulation, or other laboratory; tutoring; unpaid internships.
**Library Facilities** 114,625 volumes (1,200 in health, 1,000 in nursing); 93,144 periodical subscriptions (1,300 health-care related).

## BACCALAUREATE PROGRAMS

**Degree** BSN
**Available Programs** Baccalaureate for Second Degree; Generic Baccalaureate; RN Baccalaureate.
**Study Options** Full-time and part-time.
**Program Entrance Requirements** Minimum overall college GPA of 3.0, transcript of college record, CPR certification, written essay, health exam, health insurance, high school biology, high school chemistry, 2 years high school math, high school transcript, immunizations, 1 letter of recommendation, minimum high school GPA of 3.0, minimum GPA in nursing prerequisites of 3.0, prerequisite course work. Transfer students are accepted. *Application deadline:* 2/1 (fall), 9/1 (spring). Applications may be processed on a rolling basis for some programs. *Application fee:* $40.
**Advanced Placement** Credit given for nursing courses completed elsewhere dependent upon specific evaluations.
**Contact** *Telephone:* 415-485-3204. *Fax:* 415-485-3214.

## GRADUATE PROGRAMS

**Contact** *Telephone:* 415-458-3748.

**MASTER'S DEGREE PROGRAM**
**Degree** MSN
**Available Programs** Master's; Master's for Nurses with Non-Nursing Degrees; RN to Master's.
**Concentrations Available** Clinical nurse leader.
**Study Options** Full-time and part-time.
**Program Entrance Requirements** Clinical experience, minimum overall college GPA of 3.0, transcript of college record, CPR certification, written essay, interview, 2 letters of recommendation, nursing research course, prerequisite course work, resume, statistics course. *Application deadline:* 6/15 (fall), 11/15 (spring). Applications may be processed on a rolling basis for some programs. *Application fee:* $40.
**Advanced Placement** Credit given for nursing courses completed elsewhere dependent upon specific evaluations.
**Degree Requirements** 32 total credit hours, thesis or project.

## CONTINUING EDUCATION PROGRAM

**Contact** *Telephone:* 415-458-3748.

# Fresno Pacific University

### RN to BSN Program
### Fresno, California

Founded in 1944
**DEGREE • BSN**
**Library Facilities** 197,032 volumes; 16,000 periodical subscriptions.

## BACCALAUREATE PROGRAMS

**Degree** BSN
**Available Programs** RN Baccalaureate.
**Contact** *Telephone:* 559-453-2000.

# Holy Names University

### Department of Nursing
### Oakland, California

*http://www.hnu.edu/*
Founded in 1868
**DEGREES • BSN • MSN • MSN/MBA**
**Nursing Program Faculty** 44 (8% with doctorates).
**Baccalaureate Enrollment** 68 **Women** 90% **Men** 10% **Minority** 52% **International** 1% **Part-time** 100%
**Graduate Enrollment** 70 **Women** 85% **Men** 15% **Minority** 60% **International** 2% **Part-time** 10%
**Distance Learning Courses** Available.
**Nursing Student Activities** Nursing Honor Society, Sigma Theta Tau, nursing club.
**Nursing Student Resources** Academic advising; academic or career counseling; assistance for students with disabilities; bookstore; campus computer network; career placement assistance; computer lab; computer-assisted instruction; e-mail services; employment services for current students; externships; housing assistance; interactive nursing skills videos; Internet; learning resource lab; library services; nursing audiovisuals; placement services for program completers; remedial services; resume preparation assistance; skills, simulation, or other laboratory; tutoring.
**Library Facilities** 86,954 volumes (500 in health, 200 in nursing); 27,803 periodical subscriptions (200 health-care related).

## BACCALAUREATE PROGRAMS

**Degree** BSN
**Available Programs** LPN to RN Baccalaureate; RN Baccalaureate.
**Site Options** Stanford, CA.
**Study Options** Full-time and part-time.
**Program Entrance Requirements** Minimum overall college GPA of 2.75, transcript of college record, written essay, prerequisite course work, RN licensure. Transfer students are accepted. *Application deadline:* Applications may be processed on a rolling basis for some programs. *Application fee:* $50.
**Advanced Placement** Credit given for nursing courses completed elsewhere dependent upon specific evaluations.

**Financial Aid** 95% of baccalaureate students in nursing programs received some form of financial aid in 2011–12.
**Contact** Ms. Nancy Flinn, Admission Counselor, Department of Nursing, Holy Names University, 3500 Mountain Boulevard, Oakland, CA 94619-1699. *Telephone:* 510-436-1325. *Fax:* 510-436-1376. *E-mail:* flinn@hnu.edu.

## GRADUATE PROGRAMS

**Financial Aid** 95% of graduate students in nursing programs received some form of financial aid in 2011–12. Scholarships available. Aid available to part-time students. *Financial aid application deadline:* 3/2.
**Contact** Ms. Lisa Marie Gibson, Admission Counselor, Department of Nursing, Holy Names University, 3500 Mountain Boulevard, Oakland, CA 94619-1699. *Telephone:* 510-436-1317. *Fax:* 510-436-1376. *E-mail:* lgibson@hnu.edu.

### MASTER'S DEGREE PROGRAM

**Degrees** MSN; MSN/MBA
**Available Programs** Master's; Master's for Nurses with Non-Nursing Degrees.
**Concentrations Available** Nursing administration; nursing education. *Nurse practitioner programs in:* family health.
**Site Options** Arroyo Grande.
**Study Options** Full-time and part-time.
**Program Entrance Requirements** Minimum overall college GPA of 2.8, transcript of college record, written essay, 2 letters of recommendation, resume. *Application deadline:* Applications may be processed on a rolling basis for some programs. *Application fee:* $65.
**Degree Requirements** 45 total credit hours, thesis or project.

### POST-MASTER'S PROGRAM

**Areas of Study** Nursing administration; nursing education. *Nurse practitioner programs in:* family health.

# Loma Linda University

## School of Nursing
## Loma Linda, California

***http://www.llu.edu/nursing***
Founded in 1905

**DEGREES • BS • DNP • MS**
**Nursing Program Faculty** 47 (55% with doctorates).
**Baccalaureate Enrollment** 496 **Women** 81% **Men** 19% **Minority** 62% **International** 19% **Part-time** 22%
**Graduate Enrollment** 191 **Women** 98% **Men** 2% **Minority** 40% **International** 8% **Part-time** 73%
**Nursing Student Activities** Nursing Honor Society, Sigma Theta Tau, Student Nurses' Association, nursing club.
**Nursing Student Resources** Academic advising; academic or career counseling; assistance for students with disabilities; bookstore; campus computer network; computer lab; computer-assisted instruction; e-mail services; employment services for current students; externships; housing assistance; interactive nursing skills videos; Internet; learning resource lab; library services; nursing audiovisuals; paid internships; remedial services; resume preparation assistance; skills, simulation, or other laboratory; tutoring.
**Library Facilities** 338,418 volumes (73,702 in health, 4,965 in nursing); 1,671 periodical subscriptions (6,516 health-care related).

## BACCALAUREATE PROGRAMS

**Degree** BS
**Available Programs** ADN to Baccalaureate; Accelerated Baccalaureate for Second Degree; Accelerated RN Baccalaureate; Baccalaureate for Second Degree; Generic Baccalaureate; LPN to Baccalaureate; RN Baccalaureate.
**Study Options** Full-time and part-time.
**Program Entrance Requirements** Minimum overall college GPA of 3.0, transcript of college record, CPR certification, written essay, health exam, high school transcript, immunizations, interview, 3 letters of recommendation, minimum GPA in nursing prerequisites of 3.0, prerequisite course work. Transfer students are accepted. *Application deadline:* 3/31 (fall), 8/15 (winter), 11/1 (spring). Applications may be processed on a rolling basis for some programs. *Application fee:* $120.
**Advanced Placement** Credit by examination available. Credit given for nursing courses completed elsewhere dependent upon specific evaluations.
**Expenses (2013–14)** *Tuition:* full-time $28,080; part-time $585 per quarter hour. *International tuition:* $28,080 full-time. *Room and board:* room only: $2685 per academic year. *Required fees:* full-time $3850; part-time $1283 per term.
**Financial Aid** 95% of baccalaureate students in nursing programs received some form of financial aid in 2012–13.
**Contact** Mrs. Heather Krause, Director of Admissions, Marketing, and Recruitment, School of Nursing, Loma Linda University, 11262 Campus Street, Loma Linda, CA 92350. *Telephone:* 909-558-4923. *Fax:* 909-558-0175. *E-mail:* hkrause@llu.edu.

## GRADUATE PROGRAMS

**Expenses (2013–14)** *Tuition:* part-time $715 per quarter hour. *Room and board:* room only: $2685 per academic year. *Required fees:* part-time $715 per credit.
**Financial Aid** 26% of graduate students in nursing programs received some form of financial aid in 2012–13.
**Contact** Mr. K.C. Larsen, Assistant Director of Admissions, Marketing, and Recruitment, School of Nursing, Loma Linda University, 11262 Campus Street, Loma Linda, CA 92350. *Telephone:* 909-558-4923. *E-mail:* graduatenursing@llu.edu.

### MASTER'S DEGREE PROGRAM

**Degree** MS
**Available Programs** Master's; RN to Master's.
**Concentrations Available** Health-care administration; nurse anesthesia; nursing administration; nursing education. *Clinical nurse specialist programs in:* adult health, family health, maternity-newborn, medical-surgical, parent-child, pediatric, perinatal. *Nurse practitioner programs in:* adult health, family health, gerontology, neonatal health, pediatric, primary care, psychiatric/mental health.
**Study Options** Full-time and part-time.
**Program Entrance Requirements** Clinical experience, minimum overall college GPA of 3.0, transcript of college record, written essay, immunizations, interview, 3 letters of recommendation, nursing research course, prerequisite course work, resume, statistics course. *Application fee:* $60.
**Advanced Placement** Credit given for nursing courses completed elsewhere dependent upon specific evaluations.
**Degree Requirements** Comprehensive exam.

### POST-MASTER'S PROGRAM

**Areas of Study** *Clinical nurse specialist programs in:* adult health, family health, maternity-newborn, medical-surgical, parent-child, pediatric, perinatal. *Nurse practitioner programs in:* adult health, family health, gerontology, neonatal health, pediatric, primary care, psychiatric/mental health.

### DOCTORAL DEGREE PROGRAM

**Degree** DNP
**Available Programs** Doctorate.
**Areas of Study** Addiction/substance abuse, advanced practice nursing, aging, clinical nurse leader, clinical practice, clinical research, community health, critical care, ethics, faculty preparation, family health, gerontology, health policy, health promotion/disease prevention, health-care systems, human health and illness, individualized study, maternity-newborn, neuro-behavior, nurse case management, nursing administration, nursing education, nursing policy, nursing research, nursing science, oncology, palliative care,women's health.
**Program Entrance Requirements** Clinical experience, minimum overall college GPA of 3.2, interview by faculty committee, interview, 3 letters of recommendation, MSN or equivalent, scholarly papers, statistics course, vita, writing sample. *Application deadline:* 2/1 (summer). Applications may be processed on a rolling basis for some programs. *Application fee:* $60.
**Degree Requirements** 65 total credit hours, dissertation, written exam.

# Mount St. Mary's College

## Department of Nursing
## Los Angeles, California

***http://www.msmc.la.edu/index.asp***
Founded in 1925

**DEGREES • BSN • BSC PN • MSN**
**Nursing Program Faculty** 112 (10% with doctorates).
**Baccalaureate Enrollment** 326 **Women** 87% **Men** 13% **Minority** 80%

**Graduate Enrollment** 51 **Women** 91% **Men** 9% **Minority** 54%
**Distance Learning Courses** Available.
**Nursing Student Activities** Nursing Honor Society, Student Nurses' Association, nursing club.
**Nursing Student Resources** Academic advising; academic or career counseling; assistance for students with disabilities; bookstore; campus computer network; career placement assistance; computer lab; computer-assisted instruction; daycare for children of students; e-mail services; employment services for current students; housing assistance; interactive nursing skills videos; Internet; learning resource lab; library services; nursing audiovisuals; remedial services; resume preparation assistance; skills, simulation, or other laboratory; tutoring.
**Library Facilities** 150,000 volumes (4,000 in health, 1,000 in nursing); 150,000 periodical subscriptions (150 health-care related).

## BACCALAUREATE PROGRAMS

**Degrees** BSN; BSc PN
**Available Programs** ADN to Baccalaureate; Accelerated Baccalaureate; Generic Baccalaureate.
**Study Options** Full-time.
**Program Entrance Requirements** Minimum overall college GPA of 2.7, transcript of college record, CPR certification, written essay, health exam, high school chemistry, high school transcript, immunizations, 1 letter of recommendation, minimum GPA in nursing prerequisites of 2.5, professional liability insurance/malpractice insurance, prerequisite course work. Transfer students are accepted. *Application deadline:* 2/1 (fall). *Application fee:* $20.
**Advanced Placement** Credit by examination available. Credit given for nursing courses completed elsewhere dependent upon specific evaluations.
**Contact** *Telephone:* 310-954-4279. *Fax:* 310-954-4229.

## GRADUATE PROGRAMS

**Contact** *Telephone:* 213-477-2980. *Fax:* 213-477-2639.

### MASTER'S DEGREE PROGRAM

**Degree** MSN
**Available Programs** Master's; RN to Master's.
**Concentrations Available** Nursing administration; nursing education. *Clinical nurse specialist programs in:* adult health, community health.
**Study Options** Full-time and part-time.
**Program Entrance Requirements** Minimum overall college GPA of 3.0, transcript of college record, CPR certification, written essay, immunizations, interview, professional liability insurance/malpractice insurance, statistics course. *Application deadline:* Applications may be processed on a rolling basis for some programs. *Application fee:* $50.
**Advanced Placement** Credit given for nursing courses completed elsewhere dependent upon specific evaluations.
**Degree Requirements** 39 total credit hours, thesis or project.

# National University

## Department of Nursing
## La Jolla, California

***http://www.nu.edu***
Founded in 1971

**DEGREES • BSN • MSN**
**Nursing Program Faculty** 167 (10% with doctorates).
**Baccalaureate Enrollment** 734 **Women** 80% **Men** 20% **Minority** 45%
**Graduate Enrollment** 21 **Women** 43% **Men** 57% **Minority** 52%
**Distance Learning Courses** Available.
**Nursing Student Activities** Nursing Honor Society, Student Nurses' Association.
**Nursing Student Resources** Academic advising; academic or career counseling; assistance for students with disabilities; bookstore; campus computer network; computer lab; Internet; library services; nursing audiovisuals; other; remedial services; resume preparation assistance; skills, simulation, or other laboratory; tutoring.
**Library Facilities** 371,040 volumes (5,000 in health, 2,500 in nursing); 39,475 periodical subscriptions (1,400 health-care related).

## BACCALAUREATE PROGRAMS

**Degree** BSN
**Available Programs** Baccalaureate for Second Degree; Generic Baccalaureate; LPN to Baccalaureate; RN Baccalaureate.
**Site Options** Fresno, CA; Los Angeles, CA.
**Study Options** Full-time.
**Program Entrance Requirements** Minimum overall college GPA of 2.75, transcript of college record, CPR certification, written essay, health exam, health insurance, immunizations, minimum GPA in nursing prerequisites of 2.75, professional liability insurance/malpractice insurance, prerequisite course work. Transfer students are accepted. *Application deadline:* 4/17 (fall), 7/18 (winter), 10/16 (spring), 1/16 (summer). Applications may be processed on a rolling basis for some programs. *Application fee:* $60.
**Advanced Placement** Credit given for nursing courses completed elsewhere dependent upon specific evaluations.
**Expenses (2013–14)** *Tuition:* full-time $12,096; part-time $336 per unit. *Required fees:* full-time $2025.
**Financial Aid** 76% of baccalaureate students in nursing programs received some form of financial aid in 2012–13.
**Contact** Mr. Jalal Omar, Enrollment Counselor, Nursing, Department of Nursing, National University, 16875 West Bernardo Drive, San Diego, CA 92127. *Telephone:* 800-628-8648 Ext. 3906. *Fax:* 858-521-3995. *E-mail:* jomar@nu.edu.

## GRADUATE PROGRAMS

**Expenses (2013–14)** *Tuition:* full-time $13,824; part-time $384 per unit. *Required fees:* full-time $11,869; part-time $330 per credit.
**Financial Aid** 92% of graduate students in nursing programs received some form of financial aid in 2012–13. Institutionally sponsored loans, scholarships, and tuition waivers (full and partial) available. Aid available to part-time students.
**Contact** Mr. Jalal Omar, Enrollment Counselor, Nursing, Department of Nursing, National University, 16875 W Bernardo Dr, Suite 150, San Diego, CA 92127. *Telephone:* 858-521-3906. *Fax:* 858-521-3995. *E-mail:* jomar@nu.edu.

### MASTER'S DEGREE PROGRAM

**Degree** MSN
**Available Programs** RN to Master's.
**Concentrations Available** Nurse anesthesia; nursing administration; nursing informatics. *Clinical nurse specialist programs in:* forensic nursing.
**Site Options** Fresno, CA.
**Study Options** Full-time.
**Program Entrance Requirements** Clinical experience, computer literacy, minimum overall college GPA of 3.0, transcript of college record, CPR certification, written essay, immunizations, interview, 3 letters of recommendation, nursing research course, physical assessment course, professional liability insurance/malpractice insurance, prerequisite course work, statistics course. *Application deadline:* Applications may be processed on a rolling basis for some programs. *Application fee:* $60.
**Advanced Placement** Credit given for nursing courses completed elsewhere dependent upon specific evaluations.
**Degree Requirements** 59 total credit hours, thesis or project.

### DOCTORAL DEGREE PROGRAM

**Program Entrance Requirements** *Application deadline:* Applications may be processed on a rolling basis for some programs. *Application fee:* $60.

# Pacific Union College

## Department of Nursing
## Angwin, California

***http://www.puc.edu***
Founded in 1882

**DEGREE • BSN**
**Nursing Program Faculty** 16 (14% with doctorates).
**Baccalaureate Enrollment** 56 **Women** 77% **Men** 23% **Minority** 39% **Part-time** 59%
**Nursing Student Activities** Student Nurses' Association.
**Nursing Student Resources** Academic advising; academic or career counseling; assistance for students with disabilities; bookstore; campus computer network; career placement assistance; computer lab; daycare for children of students; e-mail services; employment services for current students; externships; housing assistance; Internet; learning resource lab; library services; nursing audiovisuals; skills, simulation, or other laboratory; tutoring.
**Library Facilities** 125 volumes in health, 75 volumes in nursing; 109 periodical subscriptions health-care related.

## BACCALAUREATE PROGRAMS

**Degree** BSN
**Available Programs** ADN to Baccalaureate.
**Site Options** Napa, CA.
**Study Options** Full-time and part-time.
**Program Entrance Requirements** Transcript of college record, CPR certification, health exam, health insurance, immunizations, interview, 2 letters of recommendation, minimum GPA in nursing prerequisites of 2.0, professional liability insurance/malpractice insurance, prerequisite course work, RN licensure. Transfer students are accepted.
**Advanced Placement** Credit given for nursing courses completed elsewhere dependent upon specific evaluations.
**Contact** *Telephone:* 707-965-7618. *Fax:* 707-965-6499.

## CONTINUING EDUCATION PROGRAM

**Contact** *Telephone:* 707-965-7262. *Fax:* 707-965-6499.

# Point Loma Nazarene University

### School of Nursing
### San Diego, California

***http://www.pointloma.edu/experience/academics/schools-departments/school-nursing***
Founded in 1902

**DEGREES • BSN • MSN**
**Nursing Program Faculty** 28 (40% with doctorates).
**Baccalaureate Enrollment** 170 **Women** 90% **Men** 10% **Minority** 23% **International** 1% **Part-time** 2%
**Graduate Enrollment** 43 **Women** 92% **Men** 8% **Minority** 45% **Part-time** 5%
**Nursing Student Activities** Sigma Theta Tau, Student Nurses' Association.
**Nursing Student Resources** Academic advising; academic or career counseling; bookstore; campus computer network; computer lab; computer-assisted instruction; daycare for children of students; e-mail services; employment services for current students; externships; housing assistance; interactive nursing skills videos; Internet; learning resource lab; library services; nursing audiovisuals; paid internships; resume preparation assistance; skills, simulation, or other laboratory; tutoring; unpaid internships.

## BACCALAUREATE PROGRAMS

**Degree** BSN
**Available Programs** ADN to Baccalaureate; Generic Baccalaureate; LPN to RN Baccalaureate; RN Baccalaureate.
**Site Options** San Diego, CA.
**Study Options** Full-time.
**Program Entrance Requirements** Minimum overall college GPA of 2.7, transcript of college record, CPR certification, written essay, health exam, health insurance, 2 years high school math, immunizations, 1 letter of recommendation, minimum GPA in nursing prerequisites of 2.7, prerequisite course work. Transfer students are accepted. *Application deadline:* 2/1 (fall), 2/1 (winter).
**Advanced Placement** Credit by examination available. Credit given for nursing courses completed elsewhere dependent upon specific evaluations.
**Contact** *Telephone:* 619-849-7055. *Fax:* 619-849-2672.

## GRADUATE PROGRAMS

**Contact** *Telephone:* 619-849-2863. *Fax:* 619-849-2672.

### MASTER'S DEGREE PROGRAM

**Degree** MSN
**Available Programs** Master's; RN to Master's.
**Concentrations Available** Nursing education. *Clinical nurse specialist programs in:* family health, gerontology, medical-surgical, psychiatric/mental health.
**Site Options** San Diego, CA.
**Study Options** Full-time and part-time.
**Program Entrance Requirements** Clinical experience, computer literacy, minimum overall college GPA of 3.0, transcript of college record, CPR certification, written essay, immunizations, interview, 3 letters of recommendation, professional liability insurance/malpractice insurance, resume. *Application deadline:* 8/1 (fall), 12/1 (winter), 8/1 (summer). *Application fee:* $40.
**Degree Requirements** 43 total credit hours, thesis or project.

### POST-MASTER'S PROGRAM

**Areas of Study** Nursing education. *Clinical nurse specialist programs in:* family health, gerontology, medical-surgical, psychiatric/mental health.

## CONTINUING EDUCATION PROGRAM

**Contact** *Telephone:* 619-849-7055. *Fax:* 619-849-2672.

# Samuel Merritt University

### School of Nursing
### Oakland, California

***http://www.samuelmerritt.edu/nursing***
Founded in 1909

**DEGREES • BSN • DNP • MSN**
**Nursing Program Faculty** 179 (27% with doctorates).
**Baccalaureate Enrollment** 497 **Women** 85% **Men** 15% **Minority** 58% **International** 1% **Part-time** 3%
**Graduate Enrollment** 429 **Women** 79% **Men** 21% **Minority** 62% **Part-time** 16%
**Distance Learning Courses** Available.
**Nursing Student Activities** Sigma Theta Tau, Student Nurses' Association.
**Nursing Student Resources** Academic advising; academic or career counseling; assistance for students with disabilities; bookstore; campus computer network; computer lab; computer-assisted instruction; e-mail services; housing assistance; interactive nursing skills videos; Internet; learning resource lab; library services; nursing audiovisuals; remedial services; skills, simulation, or other laboratory; tutoring; unpaid internships.
**Library Facilities** 34,729 volumes (26,596 in health, 15,718 in nursing); 9,188 periodical subscriptions (18,514 health-care related).

## BACCALAUREATE PROGRAMS

**Degree** BSN
**Available Programs** Accelerated Baccalaureate; Generic Baccalaureate.
**Site Options** Sacramento, CA; San Mateo, CA.
**Study Options** Full-time and part-time.
**Program Entrance Requirements** Minimum overall college GPA of 3.0, transcript of college record, CPR certification, written essay, health exam, health insurance, immunizations, 1 letter of recommendation, prerequisite course work. Transfer students are accepted. *Application deadline:* 3/1 (fall), 7/1 (spring), 9/1 (summer). *Application fee:* $50.
**Advanced Placement** Credit by examination available. Credit given for nursing courses completed elsewhere dependent upon specific evaluations.
**Expenses (2013–14)** *Tuition:* full-time $41,330; part-time $1742 per credit. *International tuition:* $41,330 full-time. *Required fees:* full-time $1206.
**Financial Aid** 68% of baccalaureate students in nursing programs received some form of financial aid in 2012–13.
**Contact** Mr. Timothy Cranford, Dean of Admission, School of Nursing, Samuel Merritt University, 3100 Telegraph Avenue, Office of Admissions, Oakland, CA 94609. *Telephone:* 510-869-1508. *Fax:* 510-869-6525. *E-mail:* admission@samuelmerritt.edu.

## GRADUATE PROGRAMS

**Expenses (2013–14)** *Tuition:* full-time $36,305; part-time $1171 per credit. *International tuition:* $36,305 full-time. *Required fees:* full-time $434.
**Financial Aid** 81% of graduate students in nursing programs received some form of financial aid in 2012–13. Career-related internships or fieldwork, Federal Work-Study, scholarships, and traineeships available. Aid available to part-time students. *Financial aid application deadline:* 3/2.
**Contact** Mr. Timothy Cranford, Dean of Admission, School of Nursing, Samuel Merritt University, 3100 Telegraph Avenue, Office of Admissions, Oakland, CA 94609. *Telephone:* 510-869-1508. *Fax:* 510-869-6525. *E-mail:* tcranford@samuelmerritt.edu.

### MASTER'S DEGREE PROGRAM

**Degree** MSN
**Available Programs** Master's; Master's for Non-Nursing College Graduates; Master's for Nurses with Non-Nursing Degrees.

**Concentrations Available** Nurse anesthesia; nurse case management. *Nurse practitioner programs in:* family health.
**Site Options** Sacramento, CA.
**Study Options** Full-time and part-time.
**Program Entrance Requirements** Computer literacy, minimum overall college GPA of 3.0, transcript of college record, CPR certification, written essay, immunizations, interview, 2 letters of recommendation, prerequisite course work, statistics course. *Application deadline:* 11/1 (fall), 7/1 (spring). *Application fee:* $50.
**Advanced Placement** Credit by examination available. Credit given for nursing courses completed elsewhere dependent upon specific evaluations.
**Degree Requirements** 49 total credit hours, thesis or project, comprehensive exam.

**POST-MASTER'S PROGRAM**
**Areas of Study** Nurse anesthesia; nurse case management. *Nurse practitioner programs in:* family health.

**DOCTORAL DEGREE PROGRAM**
**Degree** DNP
**Available Programs** Doctorate; Post-Baccalaureate Doctorate.
**Program Entrance Requirements** Minimum overall college GPA of 3.0, interview by faculty committee, 3 letters of recommendation, MSN or equivalent, scholarly papers, statistics course, writing sample. *Application deadline:* 8/1 (spring). *Application fee:* $50.
**Degree Requirements** 36 total credit hours.

# San Diego State University
## School of Nursing
## San Diego, California

*http://www.nursing.sdsu.edu/*
Founded in 1897
**DEGREES • BSN • MSN**
**Nursing Program Faculty** 65 (30% with doctorates).
**Baccalaureate Enrollment** 419 **Women** 85% **Men** 15% **Minority** 50% **International** 1% **Part-time** 2%
**Graduate Enrollment** 96 **Women** 95% **Men** 5% **Minority** 10% **Part-time** 77%
**Distance Learning Courses** Available.
**Nursing Student Activities** Sigma Theta Tau, Student Nurses' Association.
**Nursing Student Resources** Academic advising; academic or career counseling; assistance for students with disabilities; bookstore; campus computer network; career placement assistance; computer lab; daycare for children of students; e-mail services; housing assistance; Internet; learning resource lab; library services; nursing audiovisuals; paid internships; placement services for program completers; remedial services; resume preparation assistance; skills, simulation, or other laboratory; unpaid internships.
**Library Facilities** 2.2 million volumes (36,000 in health, 14,000 in nursing); 75,661 periodical subscriptions (335 health-care related).

### BACCALAUREATE PROGRAMS
**Degree** BSN
**Available Programs** ADN to Baccalaureate; Generic Baccalaureate; RN Baccalaureate.
**Study Options** Full-time and part-time.
**Program Entrance Requirements** Minimum overall college GPA of 2.8, transcript of college record, high school transcript, minimum GPA in nursing prerequisites of 2.8, prerequisite course work. Transfer students are accepted. *Application deadline:* 11/30 (fall). Applications may be processed on a rolling basis for some programs.
**Advanced Placement** Credit by examination available. Credit given for nursing courses completed elsewhere dependent upon specific evaluations.
**Contact** *Telephone:* 619-594-2540. *Fax:* 619-594-2765.

### GRADUATE PROGRAMS
**Contact** *Telephone:* 619-594-2766. *Fax:* 619-594-2765.

**MASTER'S DEGREE PROGRAM**
**Degree** MSN
**Available Programs** Master's.
**Concentrations Available** Nurse-midwifery; nursing administration; nursing education. *Clinical nurse specialist programs in:* adult health, community health, critical care, gerontology, maternity-newborn, school health,women's health. *Nurse practitioner programs in:* acute care, adult health, gerontology,women's health.
**Study Options** Full-time and part-time.
**Program Entrance Requirements** Clinical experience, minimum overall college GPA of 3.0, transcript of college record, written essay, 3 letters of recommendation, nursing research course, physical assessment course, professional liability insurance/malpractice insurance, resume, statistics course, GRE General Test. *Application deadline:* 2/1 (fall), 2/1 (spring). Applications may be processed on a rolling basis for some programs.
**Advanced Placement** Credit by examination available. Credit given for nursing courses completed elsewhere dependent upon specific evaluations.
**Degree Requirements** 39 total credit hours, thesis or project, comprehensive exam.

**POST-MASTER'S PROGRAM**
**Areas of Study** Nurse-midwifery.

### CONTINUING EDUCATION PROGRAM
**Contact** *Telephone:* 619-594-2766. *Fax:* 619-594-2765.

# San Francisco State University
## School of Nursing
## San Francisco, California

*http://www.nursing.sfsu.edu/*
Founded in 1899
**DEGREES • BSN • MSN**
**Nursing Program Faculty** 40 (50% with doctorates).
**Baccalaureate Enrollment** 250 **Women** 88% **Men** 12% **Minority** 53% **International** 2% **Part-time** 5%
**Graduate Enrollment** 180 **Women** 80% **Men** 20% **Minority** 80% **International** 10% **Part-time** 20%
**Nursing Student Activities** Sigma Theta Tau, Student Nurses' Association.
**Nursing Student Resources** Academic advising; academic or career counseling; assistance for students with disabilities; bookstore; campus computer network; career placement assistance; computer lab; computer-assisted instruction; daycare for children of students; e-mail services; employment services for current students; externships; housing assistance; interactive nursing skills videos; Internet; learning resource lab; library services; nursing audiovisuals; other; placement services for program completers; remedial services; resume preparation assistance; skills, simulation, or other laboratory; tutoring.
**Library Facilities** 11,000 volumes in health, 1,500 volumes in nursing; 200 periodical subscriptions health-care related.

### BACCALAUREATE PROGRAMS
**Degree** BSN
**Available Programs** ADN to Baccalaureate; Accelerated LPN to Baccalaureate; Generic Baccalaureate; RN Baccalaureate.
**Study Options** Full-time.
**Program Entrance Requirements** Minimum overall college GPA of 2.5, transcript of college record, CPR certification, health exam, health insurance, immunizations, minimum GPA in nursing prerequisites of 2.5, professional liability insurance/malpractice insurance, prerequisite course work. Transfer students are accepted.
**Advanced Placement** Credit by examination available. Credit given for nursing courses completed elsewhere dependent upon specific evaluations.
**Contact** *Telephone:* 415-338-2315 Ext. 1. *Fax:* 415-338-0555.

### GRADUATE PROGRAMS
**Contact** *Telephone:* 415-338-1802. *Fax:* 415-338-0555.

**MASTER'S DEGREE PROGRAM**
**Degree** MSN
**Available Programs** Accelerated Master's for Non-Nursing College Graduates; Accelerated Master's for Nurses with Non-Nursing Degrees; Master's; Master's for Non-Nursing College Graduates; Master's for Nurses with Non-Nursing Degrees.

**Concentrations Available** Nurse case management; nursing administration. *Clinical nurse specialist programs in:* adult health, perinatal, public health. *Nurse practitioner programs in:* family health.
**Study Options** Full-time and part-time.
**Program Entrance Requirements** Minimum overall college GPA of 3.0, transcript of college record, CPR certification, written essay, immunizations, 3 letters of recommendation, nursing research course, professional liability insurance/malpractice insurance, resume, statistics course.
**Advanced Placement** Credit by examination available. Credit given for nursing courses completed elsewhere dependent upon specific evaluations.
**Degree Requirements** 36 total credit hours, thesis or project.

**POST-MASTER'S PROGRAM**
**Areas of Study** Nursing administration. *Nurse practitioner programs in:* family health.

### CONTINUING EDUCATION PROGRAM
**Contact** *Telephone:* 415-405-3660. *Fax:* 415-338-0555.

## San Jose State University
### The Valley Foundation School of Nursing
### San Jose, California

*http://www.sjsu.edu/nursing*
Founded in 1857

**DEGREES • BS • MS**
**Nursing Program Faculty** 46 (41% with doctorates).
**Baccalaureate Enrollment** 415 **Women** 83% **Men** 17% **Minority** 32%
**Graduate Enrollment** 38 **Women** 87% **Men** 13% **Minority** 61%
**Nursing Student Activities** Sigma Theta Tau, Student Nurses' Association, nursing club.
**Nursing Student Resources** Academic advising; academic or career counseling; assistance for students with disabilities; bookstore; campus computer network; career placement assistance; computer lab; computer-assisted instruction; daycare for children of students; e-mail services; employment services for current students; housing assistance; interactive nursing skills videos; Internet; library services; nursing audiovisuals; remedial services; resume preparation assistance; skills, simulation, or other laboratory; tutoring.
**Library Facilities** 1.3 million volumes (280 in health, 250 in nursing); 109,730 periodical subscriptions (80 health-care related).

### BACCALAUREATE PROGRAMS
**Degree** BS
**Available Programs** Generic Baccalaureate; RPN to Baccalaureate.
**Study Options** Full-time.
**Program Entrance Requirements** Transcript of college record, health exam, health insurance, high school biology, high school chemistry, high school foreign language, 3 years high school math, 3 years high school science, immunizations, minimum high school GPA of 3.0, minimum GPA in nursing prerequisites of 3.0, professional liability insurance/malpractice insurance, prerequisite course work. Transfer students are accepted. *Application deadline:* 4/1 (fall), 10/1 (spring). *Application fee:* $150.
**Expenses (2013–14)** *Tuition, state resident:* full-time $2736; part-time $1587 per unit. *International tuition:* $5790 full-time. *Room and board:* $12,484; room only: $7594 per academic year. *Required fees:* full-time $1910; part-time $955 per credit; part-time $955 per term.
**Financial Aid** 85% of baccalaureate students in nursing programs received some form of financial aid in 2012–13. *Gift aid (need-based):* Federal Pell, FSEOG, state, private, college/university gift aid from institutional funds. *Loans:* Federal Direct (Subsidized and Unsubsidized Stafford PLUS), Perkins. *Work-study:* Federal Work-Study. *Financial aid application deadline:* 6/15(priority: 3/2).
**Contact** Ms. Trudy Miller, Administrative Support Assistant, The Valley Foundation School of Nursing, San Jose State University, One Washington Square, San Jose, CA 95192-0057. *Telephone:* 408-924-3176. *Fax:* 408-924-3135. *E-mail:* trudy.miller@sjsu.edu.

### GRADUATE PROGRAMS
**Expenses (2013–14)** *Tuition, area resident:* full-time $5909; part-time $3477 per unit. *Room and board:* $20,374; room only: $15,484 per academic year. *Required fees:* full-time $1910; part-time $1910 per credit.
**Financial Aid** 40% of graduate students in nursing programs received some form of financial aid in 2012–13.
**Contact** Dr. Daryl Canham, Graduate Coordinator, The Valley Foundation School of Nursing, San Jose State University, One Washington Square, San Jose, CA 95192-0057. *Telephone:* 408-924-1323. *Fax:* 408-924-3135. *E-mail:* daryl.canham@sjsu.edu.

**MASTER'S DEGREE PROGRAM**
**Degree** MS
**Available Programs** Master's.
**Concentrations Available** Health-care administration; nursing administration; nursing education; nursing informatics. *Nurse practitioner programs in:* family health.
**Study Options** Full-time and part-time.
**Program Entrance Requirements** Minimum overall college GPA of 3.0, transcript of college record, CPR certification, written essay, immunizations, 3 letters of recommendation, nursing research course, physical assessment course, professional liability insurance/malpractice insurance, resume, statistics course. *Application deadline:* 4/1 (fall), 11/1 (spring). *Application fee:* $150.
**Degree Requirements** 36 total credit hours, thesis or project.

**POST-MASTER'S PROGRAM**
**Areas of Study** Nursing education.

## Sonoma State University
### Department of Nursing
### Rohnert Park, California

*http://www.sonoma.edu/nursing*
Founded in 1960

**DEGREE • BSN**
**Library Facilities** 647,168 volumes; 116,888 periodical subscriptions.

### BACCALAUREATE PROGRAMS
**Degree** BSN
**Available Programs** Generic Baccalaureate.
**Study Options** Full-time.
**Program Entrance Requirements** Written essay, health exam, high school biology, high school chemistry, high school foreign language, 3 years high school math, 2 years high school science, high school transcript, immunizations, minimum high school GPA of 3.5. Transfer students are accepted. *Application deadline:* 2/28 (fall).
**Contact** Nursing Department, Department of Nursing, Sonoma State University, 1801 East Cotati Avenue, Rohnert Park, CA 94928. *Telephone:* 707-664-2465. *Fax:* 707-664-2653. *E-mail:* nursing@sonoma.edu.

## University of California, Davis
### The Betty Irene Moore School of Nursing
### Davis, California

*http://www.ucdmc.ucdavis.edu/nursing/*
Founded in 1905

**DEGREES • MS • MSN/MS • PHD**
**Nursing Program Faculty** 19 (79% with doctorates).
**Graduate Enrollment** 94 **Women** 83% **Men** 17% **Minority** 30% **International** 3%
**Distance Learning Courses** Available.
**Nursing Student Activities** Sigma Theta Tau.
**Nursing Student Resources** Academic advising; academic or career counseling; assistance for students with disabilities; bookstore; campus computer network; career placement assistance; computer lab; computer-assisted instruction; e-mail services; employment services for current students; Internet; learning resource lab; library services; remedial services; resume preparation assistance; skills, simulation, or other laboratory; tutoring.
**Library Facilities** 26,350 volumes in health, 1,750 volumes in nursing; 104,999 periodical subscriptions (789 health-care related).

### GRADUATE PROGRAMS
**Expenses (2013–14)** *Tuition, state resident:* full-time $23,318. *Tuition, nonresident:* full-time $35,563. *International tuition:* $35,563 full-time. *Room and board:* $11,591; room only: $8010 per academic year. *Required fees:* full-time $2135.

**Financial Aid** 100% of graduate students in nursing programs received some form of financial aid in 2012–13.
**Contact** Anna Libonati, Student Affairs Officer, The Betty Irene Moore School of Nursing, University of California, Davis, School of Nursing, 4610 X Street, Suite 4202, Sacramento, CA 95817. *Telephone:* 916-734-2145. *Fax:* 916-734-3257. *E-mail:* BettyIreneMooreSON@ucdmc.ucdavis.edu.

### MASTER'S DEGREE PROGRAM

**Degrees** MS; MSN/MS
**Available Programs** Master's.
**Concentrations Available** *Nurse practitioner programs in:* family health.
**Study Options** Full-time.
**Program Entrance Requirements** Minimum overall college GPA of 3.0, transcript of college record, CPR certification, written essay, immunizations, interview, 3 letters of recommendation, prerequisite course work. *Application deadline:* 9/1 (fall). *Application fee:* $80.
**Degree Requirements** 60 total credit hours, thesis or project.

### DOCTORAL DEGREE PROGRAM

**Degree** PhD
**Available Programs** Doctorate; Doctorate for Nurses with Non-Nursing Degrees; Post-Baccalaureate Doctorate.
**Areas of Study** Health policy, nursing education, nursing research, nursing science.
**Program Entrance Requirements** Minimum overall college GPA of 3.0, interview, 3 letters of recommendation, writing sample. *Application deadline:* 1/15 (fall). *Application fee:* $80.
**Degree Requirements** 144 total credit hours, dissertation.

### POSTDOCTORAL PROGRAM

**Areas of Study** Individualized study, nursing research, nursing science.
**Postdoctoral Program Contact** Lisa Reevesman, Academic Personnel Coordinator, The Betty Irene Moore School of Nursing, University of California, Davis, School of Nursing, 4610 X Street, Suite 4202, Sacramento, CA 95817. *Telephone:* 916-734-4737. *Fax:* 916-734-3257. *E-mail:* lisa.reevesman@ucdmc.ucdavis.edu.

### CONTINUING EDUCATION PROGRAM

**Contact** Ms. Janice Carpenter, Telehealth Education Manager, The Betty Irene Moore School of Nursing, University of California, Davis, 4610 X Street, Suite 2301, Sacramento, CA 95817. *Telephone:* 916-734-1414. *Fax:* 916-734-3580. *E-mail:* janice.carpenter@ucdmc.ucdavis.edu.

## University of California, Irvine

### Program in Nursing Science
### Irvine, California

***http://www.nursing.uci.edu/***
Founded in 1965

**DEGREES • BS • MS • PHD**

**Nursing Program Faculty** 59 (29% with doctorates).
**Baccalaureate Enrollment** 155 **Women** 88% **Men** 12% **Minority** 76%
**Graduate Enrollment** 33 **Women** 91% **Men** 9% **Minority** 56%
**Nursing Student Activities** Student Nurses' Association, nursing club.
**Nursing Student Resources** Academic advising; academic or career counseling; assistance for students with disabilities; bookstore; campus computer network; computer lab; computer-assisted instruction; daycare for children of students; e-mail services; employment services for current students; housing assistance; interactive nursing skills videos; Internet; learning resource lab; library services; nursing audiovisuals; skills, simulation, or other laboratory; tutoring.
**Library Facilities** 3.2 million volumes (342,244 in health, 3,296 in nursing); 132,134 periodical subscriptions (12,346 health-care related).

### BACCALAUREATE PROGRAMS

**Degree** BS
**Available Programs** Baccalaureate for Second Degree; Generic Baccalaureate.
**Study Options** Full-time.
**Program Entrance Requirements** Written essay, high school biology, high school chemistry, 2 years high school science. Transfer students are accepted. *Application deadline:* 11/30 (fall). *Application fee:* $70.
**Financial Aid** ***Gift aid (need-based):*** Federal Pell, FSEOG, state, private, college/university gift aid from institutional funds. *Loans:* Federal Direct (Subsidized and Unsubsidized Stafford PLUS), Perkins, college/university, private loans. *Work-study:* Federal Work-Study, part-time campus jobs. *Financial aid application deadline:* 6/28(priority: 3/2).
**Contact** Baccalaureate Program, Program in Nursing Science, University of California, Irvine, 106 Berk Hall, Building 802, Irvine, CA 92697-3959. *Telephone:* 949-824-1514. *Fax:* 949-824-0060.

### GRADUATE PROGRAMS

**Contact** Masters Program, Program in Nursing Science, University of California, Irvine, 106 Berk Hall, Irvine, CA 92697-3959. *Telephone:* 949-824-1514. *Fax:* 949-824-0060. *E-mail:* gsnao@uci.edu.

### MASTER'S DEGREE PROGRAM

**Degree** MS
**Available Programs** Master's.
**Concentrations Available** *Nurse practitioner programs in:* adult health, family health, gerontology.
**Study Options** Full-time.
**Program Entrance Requirements** Clinical experience, transcript of college record, written essay, interview, 3 letters of recommendation, nursing research course, physical assessment course, resume, statistics course. *Application deadline:* 3/1 (fall). *Application fee:* $80.
**Degree Requirements** 72 total credit hours, comprehensive exam.

### POST-MASTER'S PROGRAM

**Areas of Study** *Nurse practitioner programs in:* adult health, family health, gerontology.

### DOCTORAL DEGREE PROGRAM

**Degree** PhD
**Available Programs** Doctorate.
**Areas of Study** Addiction/substance abuse, advanced practice nursing, aging, bio-behavioral research, biology of health and illness, clinical practice, clinical research, community health, critical care, ethics, faculty preparation, family health, forensic nursing, gerontology, health policy, health promotion/disease prevention, health-care systems, human health and illness, illness and transition, individualized study, information systems, maternity-newborn, neuro-behavior, nurse case management, nursing administration, nursing education, nursing policy, nursing research, nursing science, oncology, palliative care,women's health.
**Program Entrance Requirements** Interview by faculty committee, 3 letters of recommendation, statistics course, vita, writing sample. *Application deadline:* 3/1 (fall). *Application fee:* $80.
**Degree Requirements** 44 total credit hours, dissertation, oral exam.

### CONTINUING EDUCATION PROGRAM

**Contact** Continuing Education - Post-Graduate Certificate, Program in Nursing Science, University of California, Irvine, 106 Berk Hall, Irvine, CA 92697-3959. *Telephone:* 949-824-1514. *Fax:* 949-824-0060. *E-mail:* gsnao@uci.edu.

## University of California, Los Angeles

### School of Nursing
### Los Angeles, California

***http://www.nursing.ucla.edu***
Founded in 1919

**DEGREES • BS • MSN • MSN/MBA • PHD**

**Nursing Program Faculty** 87 (54% with doctorates).
**Baccalaureate Enrollment** 195 **Women** 89% **Men** 11% **Minority** 71%
**Graduate Enrollment** 406 **Women** 87% **Men** 13% **Minority** 49% **International** 4%
**Nursing Student Activities** Nursing Honor Society, Sigma Theta Tau, Student Nurses' Association, nursing club.
**Nursing Student Resources** Academic advising; academic or career counseling; assistance for students with disabilities; bookstore; campus computer network; computer lab; daycare for children of students; e-mail services; housing assistance; Internet; library services; nursing audiovisuals; skills, simulation, or other laboratory.
**Library Facilities** 9 million volumes (760,000 in health, 8,000 in nursing); 38,975 periodical subscriptions (600,000 health-care related).

### BACCALAUREATE PROGRAMS

**Degree** BS

**Available Programs** Generic Baccalaureate.
**Study Options** Full-time.
**Program Entrance Requirements** Transcript of college record, written essay, high school transcript, 2 letters of recommendation, minimum high school GPA, prerequisite course work. Transfer students are accepted. *Application deadline:* 11/30 (fall). *Application fee:* $60.
**Expenses (2013–14)** *Tuition, state resident:* full-time $14,392. *Tuition, nonresident:* full-time $37,270. *International tuition:* $37,270 full-time. *Room and board:* $14,454; room only: $10,446 per academic year.
**Financial Aid** 78% of baccalaureate students in nursing programs received some form of financial aid in 2012–13. *Gift aid (need-based):* Federal Pell, FSEOG, state, private, college/university gift aid from institutional funds, United Negro College Fund, Federal Nursing. *Loans:* Federal Nursing Student Loans, Federal Direct (Subsidized and Unsubsidized Stafford PLUS), Perkins, state, college/university. *Work-study:* Federal Work-Study, part-time campus jobs. *Financial aid application deadline (priority):* 3/2.
**Contact** Ms. Rhonda Flenoy-Younger, Director of Recruitment, Outreach, and Admissions, School of Nursing, University of California, Los Angeles, Box 951702, Los Angeles, CA 90095-1702. *Telephone:* 310-825-9193. *Fax:* 310-206-7433. *E-mail:* rflenoy@sonnet.ucla.edu.

## GRADUATE PROGRAMS

**Expenses (2013–14)** *Tuition, state resident:* full-time $23,646. *Tuition, nonresident:* full-time $35,891. *International tuition:* $35,891 full-time.
**Financial Aid** 89% of graduate students in nursing programs received some form of financial aid in 2012–13. 244 fellowships with full and partial tuition reimbursements available, 14 research assistantships with full and partial tuition reimbursements available, 44 teaching assistantships with full and partial tuition reimbursements available were awarded; Federal Work-Study, scholarships, tuition waivers (full and partial), and unspecified assistantships also available. *Financial aid application deadline:* 3/2.
**Contact** Ms. Rhonda Flenoy-Younger, Director of Recruitment, Outreach, and Admissions, School of Nursing, University of California, Los Angeles, Box 951702, Los Angeles, CA 90095-1702. *Telephone:* 310-825-9193. *Fax:* 310-267-0330. *E-mail:* rflenoy@sonnet.ucla.edu.

### MASTER'S DEGREE PROGRAM

**Degrees** MSN; MSN/MBA
**Available Programs** Master's; Master's for Non-Nursing College Graduates.
**Concentrations Available** Clinical nurse leader; nursing administration. *Clinical nurse specialist programs in:* acute care, pediatric. *Nurse practitioner programs in:* acute care, adult health, family health, gerontology, occupational health, pediatric.
**Study Options** Full-time.
**Program Entrance Requirements** Minimum overall college GPA of 3.0, transcript of college record, written essay, 3 letters of recommendation, nursing research course, physical assessment course, prerequisite course work, resume, statistics course. *Application deadline:* 12/1 (fall). *Application fee:* $80.
**Degree Requirements** 72 total credit hours, comprehensive exam.

### POST-MASTER'S PROGRAM

**Areas of Study** Nursing administration. *Clinical nurse specialist programs in:* acute care, pediatric. *Nurse practitioner programs in:* acute care, adult health, family health, gerontology, occupational health, pediatric.

### DOCTORAL DEGREE PROGRAM

**Degree** PhD
**Available Programs** Doctorate; Post-Baccalaureate Doctorate.
**Areas of Study** Addiction/substance abuse, advanced practice nursing, aging, bio-behavioral research, biology of health and illness, clinical practice, community health, critical care, family health, gerontology, health policy, health promotion/disease prevention, health-care systems, human health and illness, illness and transition, neuro-behavior, nursing administration, nursing research, nursing science, oncology,women's health.
**Program Entrance Requirements** Minimum overall college GPA of 3.5, interview, 3 letters of recommendation, scholarly papers, statistics course, vita, writing sample. *Application deadline:* 12/1 (fall). *Application fee:* $80.
**Degree Requirements** 127 total credit hours, dissertation, oral exam, written exam, residency.

### POSTDOCTORAL PROGRAM

**Areas of Study** Addiction/substance abuse, adolescent health, aging, cancer care, gerontology, health promotion/disease prevention, nursing research, vulnerable population,women's health.
**Postdoctoral Program Contact** Dr. Sally Maliski, Associate Dean for Academic Affairs, School of Nursing, University of California, Los Angeles, Box 951702, Los Angeles, CA 90095-1702. *Telephone:* 310-206-2825. *Fax:* 310-206-7433. *E-mail:* smaliski@sonnet.ucla.edu.

## CONTINUING EDUCATION PROGRAM

**Contact** Ms. Salpy Akaragian, Education Specialist, School of Nursing, University of California, Los Angeles, Box 951701, Los Angeles, CA 90095-1701. *Telephone:* 310-206-9581. *E-mail:* nssa@mednet.ucla.edu.

# University of California, San Francisco

## School of Nursing
## San Francisco, California

*http://www.nurseweb.ucsf.edu/*
Founded in 1864

## DEGREES • MS • PHD

**Nursing Program Faculty** 151 (72% with doctorates).
**Graduate Enrollment** 721 **Women** 87% **Men** 13% **Minority** 30% **International** 10% **Part-time** 1%
**Distance Learning Courses** Available.
**Nursing Student Activities** Nursing Honor Society, Sigma Theta Tau, Student Nurses' Association, nursing club.
**Nursing Student Resources** Academic advising; academic or career counseling; assistance for students with disabilities; bookstore; campus computer network; career placement assistance; computer lab; computer-assisted instruction; daycare for children of students; e-mail services; employment services for current students; housing assistance; interactive nursing skills videos; Internet; learning resource lab; library services; nursing audiovisuals; other; paid internships; placement services for program completers; remedial services; resume preparation assistance; skills, simulation, or other laboratory; tutoring; unpaid internships.
**Library Facilities** 856,169 volumes in health, 131,046 volumes in nursing; 3,270 periodical subscriptions health-care related.

## GRADUATE PROGRAMS

**Contact** *Telephone:* 415-476-1435. *Fax:* 415-476-9707.

### MASTER'S DEGREE PROGRAM

**Degree** MS
**Available Programs** Master's; Master's for Non-Nursing College Graduates; Master's for Nurses with Non-Nursing Degrees.
**Concentrations Available** Nurse-midwifery; nursing administration. *Clinical nurse specialist programs in:* cardiovascular, community health, critical care, gerontology, occupational health, oncology, pediatric, perinatal, psychiatric/mental health. *Nurse practitioner programs in:* acute care, adult health, family health, gerontology, neonatal health, occupational health, pediatric, psychiatric/mental health.
**Study Options** Full-time.
**Program Entrance Requirements** Clinical experience, computer literacy, minimum overall college GPA of 3.0, transcript of college record, written essay, immunizations, 4 letters of recommendation, statistics course, GRE General Test. *Application deadline:* 2/1 (fall). *Application fee:* $60.
**Advanced Placement** Credit given for nursing courses completed elsewhere dependent upon specific evaluations.
**Degree Requirements** 44 total credit hours, comprehensive exam.

### POST-MASTER'S PROGRAM

**Areas of Study** *Clinical nurse specialist programs in:* cardiovascular, community health, critical care, gerontology, occupational health, oncology, pediatric, perinatal, psychiatric/mental health. *Nurse practitioner programs in:* acute care, adult health, family health, gerontology, neonatal health, occupational health, pediatric, psychiatric/mental health.

### DOCTORAL DEGREE PROGRAM

**Degree** PhD
**Available Programs** Doctorate; Post-Baccalaureate Doctorate.
**Areas of Study** Addiction/substance abuse, aging, bio-behavioral research, biology of health and illness, community health, critical care,

ethics, family health, gerontology, health policy, health promotion/disease prevention, health-care systems, human health and illness, illness and transition, individualized study, information systems, maternity-newborn, nursing administration, nursing policy, nursing research, nursing science, oncology, urban health,women's health.

**Program Entrance Requirements** Minimum overall college GPA of 3.0, 4 letters of recommendation, statistics course, writing sample, GRE General Test. *Application deadline:* 12/15 (fall). *Application fee:* $60.

**Degree Requirements** Dissertation, oral exam, written exam, residency.

### POSTDOCTORAL PROGRAM

**Areas of Study** Individualized study.

**Postdoctoral Program Contact***Telephone:* 415-476-1435. *Fax:* 415-476-9707.

## University of Phoenix–Bay Area Campus

### College of Nursing
### San Jose, California

### DEGREES • BSN • MSN • MSN/MBA • MSN/MHA

**Nursing Program Faculty** 12 (58% with doctorates).

**Baccalaureate Enrollment** 39 **Women** 92.3% **Men** 7.7% **Minority** 35.9%

**Graduate Enrollment** 22 **Women** 86.4% **Men** 13.6% **Minority** 40.91%

**Nursing Student Activities** Sigma Theta Tau.

**Nursing Student Resources** Academic advising; academic or career counseling; assistance for students with disabilities; bookstore; campus computer network; computer lab; computer-assisted instruction; e-mail services; interactive nursing skills videos; Internet; learning resource lab; library services; nursing audiovisuals; remedial services; skills, simulation, or other laboratory; tutoring.

**Library Facilities** 16,781 periodical subscriptions (1,300 health-care related).

### BACCALAUREATE PROGRAMS

**Degree** BSN

**Available Programs** Accelerated Baccalaureate.

**Site Options** Oakland, CA; San Francisco, CA; Novato, CA.

**Study Options** Full-time.

**Program Entrance Requirements** Transcript of college record, CPR certification, immunizations, 1 letter of recommendation, RN licensure. Transfer students are accepted. *Application deadline:* Applications may be processed on a rolling basis for some programs.

**Advanced Placement** Credit by examination available. Credit given for nursing courses completed elsewhere dependent upon specific evaluations.

**Contact** *Telephone:* 877-416-4100.

### GRADUATE PROGRAMS

**Contact** *Telephone:* 877-416-4100.

### MASTER'S DEGREE PROGRAM

**Degrees** MSN; MSN/MBA; MSN/MHA

**Available Programs** Master's.

**Concentrations Available** Health-care administration; nursing administration; nursing education.

**Site Options** Oakland, CA; San Francisco, CA; Novato, CA.

**Study Options** Full-time.

**Program Entrance Requirements** Clinical experience, computer literacy, minimum overall college GPA of 2.5, transcript of college record. *Application deadline:* Applications may be processed on a rolling basis for some programs. *Application fee:* $45.

**Advanced Placement** Credit given for nursing courses completed elsewhere dependent upon specific evaluations.

**Degree Requirements** 39 total credit hours, thesis or project.

## University of Phoenix–Central Valley Campus

### College of Health and Human Services
### Fresno, California

Founded in 2004

### DEGREE • BSN

**Nursing Program Faculty** 8 (13% with doctorates).

**Baccalaureate Enrollment** 53 **Women** 94.3% **Men** 5.7% **Minority** 30.2%

**Nursing Student Activities** Sigma Theta Tau.

**Nursing Student Resources** Academic advising; academic or career counseling; bookstore; campus computer network; computer lab; computer-assisted instruction; e-mail services; interactive nursing skills videos; Internet; learning resource lab; library services; nursing audiovisuals; remedial services; skills, simulation, or other laboratory; tutoring.

**Library Facilities** 1,300 periodical subscriptions health-care related.

### BACCALAUREATE PROGRAMS

**Degree** BSN

**Available Programs** RN Baccalaureate.

**Site Options** Fresno, CA; Visalia, CA; Bakersfield, CA.

**Study Options** Full-time.

**Program Entrance Requirements** Transcript of college record, CPR certification, immunizations, 1 letter of recommendation, RN licensure. Transfer students are accepted.

**Advanced Placement** Credit by examination available. Credit given for nursing courses completed elsewhere dependent upon specific evaluations.

**Contact** *Telephone:* 661-663-0300. *Fax:* 661-633-2711.

## University of Phoenix–Sacramento Valley Campus

### College of Nursing
### Sacramento, California

Founded in 1993

### DEGREES • BSN • MSN • MSN/MHA

**Nursing Program Faculty** 29 (28% with doctorates).

**Baccalaureate Enrollment** 250 **Women** 88.8% **Men** 11.2% **Minority** 32%

**Graduate Enrollment** 53 **Women** 90.6% **Men** 9.4% **Minority** 15.09%

**Nursing Student Activities** Sigma Theta Tau.

**Nursing Student Resources** Academic advising; academic or career counseling; assistance for students with disabilities; bookstore; campus computer network; computer lab; computer-assisted instruction; e-mail services; interactive nursing skills videos; Internet; learning resource lab; library services; nursing audiovisuals; skills, simulation, or other laboratory; tutoring.

**Library Facilities** 16,781 periodical subscriptions (1,300 health-care related).

### BACCALAUREATE PROGRAMS

**Degree** BSN

**Available Programs** Accelerated Baccalaureate; LPN to Baccalaureate.

**Site Options** Lathrop, CA; Modesto, CA; Fairfield, CA.

**Study Options** Full-time.

**Online Degree Options** Yes.

**Program Entrance Requirements** Transcript of college record, CPR certification, immunizations, 1 letter of recommendation, RN licensure. Transfer students are accepted. *Application deadline:* Applications may be processed on a rolling basis for some programs.

**Advanced Placement** Credit by examination available. Credit given for nursing courses completed elsewhere dependent upon specific evaluations.

**Contact** *Telephone:* 800-266-2107.

### GRADUATE PROGRAMS

**Contact** *Telephone:* 800-266-2107.

### MASTER'S DEGREE PROGRAM

**Degrees** MSN; MSN/MHA

**Available Programs** Accelerated Master's.
**Concentrations Available** Health-care administration; nursing administration; nursing education. *Nurse practitioner programs in:* family health.
**Site Options** Lathrop, CA; Modesto, CA; Fairfield, CA.
**Study Options** Full-time and part-time.
**Program Entrance Requirements** Clinical experience, computer literacy, minimum overall college GPA of 2.5, transcript of college record. *Application deadline:* Applications may be processed on a rolling basis for some programs. *Application fee:* $45.
**Advanced Placement** Credit given for nursing courses completed elsewhere dependent upon specific evaluations.
**Degree Requirements** 39 total credit hours, thesis or project.

**POST-MASTER'S PROGRAM**
**Areas of Study** *Nurse practitioner programs in:* family health.

### CONTINUING EDUCATION PROGRAM
**Contact** *Telephone:* 800-266-2107.

## University of Phoenix–San Diego Campus
### College of Nursing
### San Diego, California

Founded in 1988
**DEGREES • BSN • MSN • MSN/ED D**
**Nursing Program Faculty** 30 (37% with doctorates).
**Baccalaureate Enrollment** 103 **Women** 81.6% **Men** 18.4% **Minority** 29.1%
**Graduate Enrollment** 46 **Women** 89.1% **Men** 10.9% **Minority** 58.7%
**Nursing Student Activities** Sigma Theta Tau.
**Nursing Student Resources** Academic advising; academic or career counseling; assistance for students with disabilities; bookstore; campus computer network; computer lab; computer-assisted instruction; e-mail services; interactive nursing skills videos; Internet; learning resource lab; library services; nursing audiovisuals; skills, simulation, or other laboratory; tutoring.
**Library Facilities** 16,781 periodical subscriptions (1,300 health-care related).

### BACCALAUREATE PROGRAMS
**Degree** BSN
**Available Programs** Accelerated Baccalaureate.
**Site Options** Chula Vista, CA; Imperial, CA; Palm Desert, CA.
**Study Options** Full-time.
**Program Entrance Requirements** Transcript of college record, CPR certification, immunizations, 1 letter of recommendation, RN licensure. Transfer students are accepted. *Application deadline:* Applications may be processed on a rolling basis for some programs.
**Advanced Placement** Credit by examination available. Credit given for nursing courses completed elsewhere dependent upon specific evaluations.
**Contact** *Telephone:* 888-867-4636.

### GRADUATE PROGRAMS
**Contact** *Telephone:* 888-867-4636.

**MASTER'S DEGREE PROGRAM**
**Degrees** MSN; MSN/Ed D
**Available Programs** Master's.
**Concentrations Available** Health-care administration; nursing administration; nursing education.
**Site Options** Chula Vista, CA; Imperial, CA; Palm Desert, CA.
**Study Options** Full-time.
**Program Entrance Requirements** Clinical experience, computer literacy, minimum overall college GPA of 2.5, transcript of college record. *Application deadline:* Applications may be processed on a rolling basis for some programs. *Application fee:* $45.
**Advanced Placement** Credit given for nursing courses completed elsewhere dependent upon specific evaluations.
**Degree Requirements** 39 total credit hours, thesis or project.

## University of Phoenix–Southern California Campus
### College of Nursing
### Costa Mesa, California

Founded in 1980
**DEGREES • BSN • MSN • MSN/MBA • MSN/MHA**
**Nursing Program Faculty** 109 (23% with doctorates).
**Baccalaureate Enrollment** 563 **Women** 89.2% **Men** 10.8% **Minority** 36.8%
**Graduate Enrollment** 379 **Women** 90.2% **Men** 9.8% **Minority** 40.9%
**Nursing Student Activities** Sigma Theta Tau.
**Nursing Student Resources** Academic advising; academic or career counseling; assistance for students with disabilities; bookstore; campus computer network; computer lab; computer-assisted instruction; e-mail services; interactive nursing skills videos; Internet; learning resource lab; library services; nursing audiovisuals; remedial services; skills, simulation, or other laboratory; tutoring.
**Library Facilities** 16,781 periodical subscriptions (1,300 health-care related).

### BACCALAUREATE PROGRAMS
**Degree** BSN
**Available Programs** Accelerated Baccalaureate.
**Site Options** Diamond Bar, CA; La Marada, CA; Lancaster, CA.
**Study Options** Full-time.
**Program Entrance Requirements** Transcript of college record, CPR certification, immunizations, 1 letter of recommendation, RN licensure. Transfer students are accepted. *Application deadline:* Applications may be processed on a rolling basis for some programs.
**Advanced Placement** Credit by examination available. Credit given for nursing courses completed elsewhere dependent upon specific evaluations.
**Contact** *Telephone:* 800-697-8223.

### GRADUATE PROGRAMS
**Contact** *Telephone:* 800-697-8223.

**MASTER'S DEGREE PROGRAM**
**Degrees** MSN; MSN/MBA; MSN/MHA
**Available Programs** Master's.
**Concentrations Available** Health-care administration; nursing administration; nursing education. *Nurse practitioner programs in:* family health.
**Site Options** Diamond Bar, CA; La Marada, CA; Lancaster, CA.
**Study Options** Full-time.
**Program Entrance Requirements** Clinical experience, computer literacy, minimum overall college GPA of 2.5, transcript of college record, 1 letter of recommendation. *Application deadline:* Applications may be processed on a rolling basis for some programs. *Application fee:* $45.
**Advanced Placement** Credit given for nursing courses completed elsewhere dependent upon specific evaluations.
**Degree Requirements** 39 total credit hours, thesis or project.

**POST-MASTER'S PROGRAM**
**Areas of Study** *Nurse practitioner programs in:* family health.

### CONTINUING EDUCATION PROGRAM
**Contact** *Telephone:* 714-338-1720.

## University of San Diego
### Hahn School of Nursing and Health Science
### San Diego, California

***http://www.sandiego.edu/nursing***
Founded in 1949
**DEGREES • DNP • MSN • PHD**
**Nursing Program Faculty** 66 (90% with doctorates).
**Graduate Enrollment** 371 **Women** 86% **Men** 14% **Minority** 39% **International** 1% **Part-time** 25%
**Nursing Student Activities** Nursing Honor Society, Sigma Theta Tau, Student Nurses' Association.

**Nursing Student Resources** Academic advising; academic or career counseling; assistance for students with disabilities; bookstore; campus computer network; career placement assistance; computer lab; computer-assisted instruction; daycare for children of students; e-mail services; employment services for current students; externships; interactive nursing skills videos; Internet; learning resource lab; library services; nursing audiovisuals; resume preparation assistance; skills, simulation, or other laboratory; tutoring.

**Library Facilities** 1 million volumes (47,500 in health, 24,600 in nursing); 38,368 periodical subscriptions (2,200 health-care related).

## GRADUATE PROGRAMS

**Expenses (2013–14)** *Tuition:* full-time $24,000; part-time $1320 per credit hour. *International tuition:* $24,000 full-time. *Required fees:* full-time $500; part-time $250 per credit.

**Financial Aid** 90% of graduate students in nursing programs received some form of financial aid in 2012–13. Scholarships and traineeships available. Aid available to part-time students. *Financial aid application deadline:* 4/1.

**Contact** Ms. Cathleen Mumper, Director of Student Services and Admissions Officer, Hahn School of Nursing and Health Science, University of San Diego, 5998 Alcala Park, San Diego, CA 92110-2492. *Telephone:* 619-260-4548. *Fax:* 619-260-6814. *E-mail:* cmm@sandiego.edu.

### MASTER'S DEGREE PROGRAM

**Degree** MSN

**Available Programs** Accelerated Master's for Non-Nursing College Graduates; Master's.

**Concentrations Available** Clinical nurse leader; nursing administration; nursing education; nursing informatics. *Clinical nurse specialist programs in:* acute care, adult health, critical care, medical-surgical, palliative care. *Nurse practitioner programs in:* adult health, family health, gerontology, pediatric, primary care, psychiatric/mental health.

**Study Options** Full-time and part-time.

**Program Entrance Requirements** Clinical experience, computer literacy, minimum overall college GPA of 3.0, transcript of college record, CPR certification, written essay, immunizations, interview, 3 letters of recommendation, prerequisite course work, resume, statistics course, GRE General Test (for entry-level nursing). *Application deadline:* 3/1 (fall), 11/1 (spring). *Application fee:* $45.

**Advanced Placement** Credit by examination available. Credit given for nursing courses completed elsewhere dependent upon specific evaluations.

**Degree Requirements** 31–52 total credits, depending on specialty.

### DOCTORAL DEGREE PROGRAM

**Degree** DNP

**Available Programs** Doctorate, Post-Baccalaureate Doctorate.

**Areas of Study** Addiction/substance abuse, advanced practice nursing, aging, bio-behavioral research, biology of health and illness, clinical practice, community health, ethics, faculty preparation, family health, gerontology, health policy, health promotion/disease prevention, health-care systems, human health and illness, illness and transition, information systems, maternity-newborn, nursing education,women's health.

**Program Entrance Requirements** Minimum overall college GPA of 3.5, clinical experience, interview, 3 letters of recommendation, MSN or equivalent, vita, writing sample. *Application deadline:* 3/1 (fall).

**Degree Requirements** Residency.

**Degree** PhD

**Available Programs** Doctorate; Post-Baccalaureate Doctorate.

**Areas of Study** Addiction/substance abuse, advanced practice nursing, aging, bio-behavioral research, clinical practice, community health, critical care, ethics, faculty preparation, family health, gerontology, health policy, health promotion/disease prevention, health-care systems, human health and illness, illness and transition, individualized study, information systems, maternity-newborn, nurse case management, nursing administration, nursing education, nursing policy, nursing research, nursing science, oncology, palliative care, urban health,women's health.

**Program Entrance Requirements** Clinical experience, minimum overall college GPA of 3.5, interview by faculty committee, interview, 3 letters of recommendation, MSN or equivalent, statistics course, vita, writing sample. *Application deadline:* 2/1 (fall). *Application fee:* $45.

**Degree Requirements** 48 total credit hours, dissertation, residency.

# University of San Francisco

## School of Nursing
## San Francisco, California

***http://www.usfca.edu/nursing/***

Founded in 1855

**DEGREES • BSN • DNP • MSN**

**Nursing Program Faculty** 112 (75% with doctorates).

**Baccalaureate Enrollment** 756 **Women** 86% **Men** 14% **Minority** 57% **International** 1% **Part-time** 1%

**Graduate Enrollment** 378 **Women** 84% **Men** 16% **Minority** 40% **Part-time** 5%

**Distance Learning Courses** Available.

**Nursing Student Activities** Nursing Honor Society, Sigma Theta Tau, Student Nurses' Association, nursing club.

**Nursing Student Resources** Academic advising; academic or career counseling; assistance for students with disabilities; bookstore; campus computer network; career placement assistance; computer lab; computer-assisted instruction; e-mail services; employment services for current students; housing assistance; interactive nursing skills videos; Internet; learning resource lab; library services; nursing audiovisuals; remedial services; resume preparation assistance; skills, simulation, or other laboratory; tutoring; unpaid internships.

**Library Facilities** 1.1 million volumes; 5,560 periodical subscriptions (200 health-care related).

## BACCALAUREATE PROGRAMS

**Degree** BSN

**Available Programs** Generic Baccalaureate.

**Study Options** Full-time.

**Online Degree Options** Yes.

**Program Entrance Requirements** Minimum overall college GPA of 3.0, transcript of college record, written essay, health insurance, high school biology, high school chemistry, 3 years high school math, 2 years high school science, high school transcript, immunizations, 2 letters of recommendation, minimum high school GPA of 3.9, prerequisite course work. Transfer students are accepted. *Application deadline:* 1/15 (fall), 12/15 (winter). *Application fee:* $55.

**Advanced Placement** Credit given for nursing courses completed elsewhere dependent upon specific evaluations.

**Contact** *Telephone:* 800-422-6563. *Fax:* 415-422-6877.

## GRADUATE PROGRAMS

**Contact** *Telephone:* 415-422-6681. *Fax:* 415-422-6877.

### MASTER'S DEGREE PROGRAM

**Degree** MSN

**Available Programs** Accelerated AD/RN to Master's; Accelerated Master's for Non-Nursing College Graduates; Master's for Nurses with Non-Nursing Degrees; RN to Master's.

**Concentrations Available** Clinical nurse leader.

**Site Options** San Jose, CA; San Ramon, CA; Santa Rosa, CA.

**Study Options** Full-time.

**Online Degree Options** Yes.

**Program Entrance Requirements** Clinical experience, minimum overall college GPA of 3.5, transcript of college record, written essay, 2 letters of recommendation, prerequisite course work, resume, statistics course. *Application deadline:* 6/15 (fall), 10/15 (spring), 2/15 (summer). *Application fee:* $55.

**Advanced Placement** Credit given for nursing courses completed elsewhere dependent upon specific evaluations.

**Degree Requirements** 40 total credit hours, thesis or project, comprehensive exam.

### POST-MASTER'S PROGRAM

**Areas of Study** Clinical nurse leader.

### DOCTORAL DEGREE PROGRAM

**Degree** DNP

**Available Programs** Doctorate; Post-Baccalaureate Doctorate.

**Areas of Study** Advanced practice nursing, family health, health-care systems.

**Program Entrance Requirements** Clinical experience, minimum overall college GPA of 3.0, 3 letters of recommendation, vita, writing sample. *Application deadline:* 6/15 (fall), 10/15 (spring). *Application fee:* $55.

**Degree Requirements** Dissertation, oral exam, residency.

## Vanguard University of Southern California

### Nursing Program
### Costa Mesa, California

Founded in 1920

**DEGREE • BSN**
**Baccalaureate Enrollment** 75
**Library Facilities** 164,333 volumes; 17,342 periodical subscriptions.

#### BACCALAUREATE PROGRAMS

**Degree** BSN
**Available Programs** RN Baccalaureate.
**Contact** *Telephone:* 714-668-6130 Ext. 3902. *Fax:* 714-668-6194.

## West Coast University

### Nursing Programs
### North Hollywood, California

Founded in 1909

**DEGREE • BSN**

#### BACCALAUREATE PROGRAMS

**Degree** BSN
**Available Programs** Accelerated RN Baccalaureate; RN Baccalaureate.
**Contact** *Telephone:* 866-508-2684.

## Western University of Health Sciences

### College of Graduate Nursing
### Pomona, California

***http://www.westernu.edu/nursing-visitor***
Founded in 1975

**DEGREES • DNP • MSN**
**Nursing Program Faculty** 25 (65% with doctorates).
**Graduate Enrollment** 285 **Women** 85% **Men** 15% **Minority** 54% **International** 1% **Part-time** 5%
**Distance Learning Courses** Available.
**Nursing Student Activities** Nursing Honor Society, Sigma Theta Tau, Student Nurses' Association, nursing club.
**Nursing Student Resources** Academic advising; academic or career counseling; assistance for students with disabilities; bookstore; campus computer network; career placement assistance; computer lab; computer-assisted instruction; e-mail services; interactive nursing skills videos; Internet; learning resource lab; library services; nursing audiovisuals; other; remedial services; resume preparation assistance; skills, simulation, or other laboratory; tutoring.
**Library Facilities** 17,171 volumes in health, 322 volumes in nursing; 5,000 periodical subscriptions health-care related.

#### GRADUATE PROGRAMS

**Contact** *Telephone:* 909-469-5255. *Fax:* 909-469-5521.

**MASTER'S DEGREE PROGRAM**
**Degree** MSN
**Available Programs** Accelerated AD/RN to Master's; Accelerated Master's; Accelerated Master's for Non-Nursing College Graduates; Master's.
**Concentrations Available** Clinical nurse leader; nursing administration. *Nurse practitioner programs in:* family health.
**Study Options** Full-time and part-time.
**Online Degree Options** Yes (online only).
**Program Entrance Requirements** Computer literacy, minimum overall college GPA of 3.0, transcript of college record, CPR certification, written essay, immunizations, interview, 3 letters of recommendation, prerequisite course work, resume, statistics course. *Application deadline:* 3/1 (fall). Applications may be processed on a rolling basis for some programs. *Application fee:* $60.
**Advanced Placement** Credit given for nursing courses completed elsewhere dependent upon specific evaluations.
**Degree Requirements** 50 total credit hours, thesis or project.

**POST-MASTER'S PROGRAM**
**Areas of Study** *Nurse practitioner programs in:* family health.

**DOCTORAL DEGREE PROGRAM**
**Degree** DNP
**Available Programs** Doctorate.
**Online Degree Options** Yes (online only).
**Program Entrance Requirements** Minimum overall college GPA of 3.0, 3 letters of recommendation, MSN or equivalent, scholarly papers, statistics course, vita, writing sample. *Application deadline:* 3/1 (fall). Applications may be processed on a rolling basis for some programs. *Application fee:* $60.
**Degree Requirements** 30 total credit hours, dissertation.

# COLORADO

## Adams State University

### Nursing Program
### Alamosa, Colorado

Founded in 1921

**DEGREE • BSN**
**Nursing Program Faculty** 10 (10% with doctorates).
**Baccalaureate Enrollment** 67 **Women** 89% **Men** 11% **Minority** 48% **International** 1% **Part-time** 39%
**Nursing Student Activities** Nursing Honor Society, Sigma Theta Tau, Student Nurses' Association.
**Nursing Student Resources** Academic advising; academic or career counseling; assistance for students with disabilities; bookstore; campus computer network; computer lab; computer-assisted instruction; daycare for children of students; e-mail services; employment services for current students; housing assistance; interactive nursing skills videos; Internet; learning resource lab; library services; nursing audiovisuals; remedial services; resume preparation assistance; skills, simulation, or other laboratory; tutoring; unpaid internships.
**Library Facilities** 127,024 volumes (565 in health, 565 in nursing); 338 periodical subscriptions (200 health-care related).

#### BACCALAUREATE PROGRAMS

**Degree** BSN
**Available Programs** Generic Baccalaureate; RN Baccalaureate.
**Site Options** Salida, CO; Trinidad, CO.
**Study Options** Full-time.
**Program Entrance Requirements** Minimum overall college GPA of 3.0, transcript of college record, written essay, immunizations, interview, 2 letters of recommendation, minimum GPA in nursing prerequisites of 3.0, prerequisite course work. Transfer students are accepted. *Application deadline:* 8/1 (fall).
**Advanced Placement** Credit by examination available. Credit given for nursing courses completed elsewhere dependent upon specific evaluations.
**Contact** *Telephone:* 719-587-8134. *Fax:* 719-587-7522.

## American Sentinel University

### RN to Bachelor of Science Nursing
### Aurora, Colorado

***http://www.americansentinel.edu***
Founded in 1988

**DEGREES • BSN • MSN**
**Distance Learning Courses** Available.

#### BACCALAUREATE PROGRAMS

**Degree** BSN

**Available Programs** RN Baccalaureate.
**Program Entrance Requirements** Transcript of college record, RN licensure.
**Contact** *Telephone:* 866-922-5690.

### GRADUATE PROGRAMS

**Contact** *Telephone:* 866-922-5690.

**MASTER'S DEGREE PROGRAM**
**Degree** MSN
**Available Programs** Master's.
**Concentrations Available** Nurse case management; nursing administration; nursing education; nursing informatics.
**Program Entrance Requirements** Transcript of college record.
**Degree Requirements** 36 total credit hours.

## Aspen University

### Graduate School of Health Professions and Studies
### Denver, Colorado

*http://www.aspen.edu*
Founded in 1987

**DEGREE • MSN**
**Nursing Program Faculty** 4 (100% with doctorates).
**Graduate Enrollment** 206
**Distance Learning Courses** Available.
**Nursing Student Resources** Academic advising; computer-assisted instruction.

### GRADUATE PROGRAMS

**Contact** Enrollment Office, Graduate School of Health Professions and Studies, Aspen University, 720 South Colorado Boulevard, Suite 1150N, Denver, CO 80246. *Telephone:* 800-373-7814. *E-mail:* enrollment@aspen.edu.

**MASTER'S DEGREE PROGRAM**
**Degree** MSN
**Available Programs** Master's; RN to Master's.
**Concentrations Available** Nursing administration; nursing education.
**Study Options** Full-time and part-time.
**Online Degree Options** Yes (online only).
**Program Entrance Requirements** Clinical experience, minimum overall college GPA of 3.0, transcript of college record, written essay, resume. *Application deadline:* Applications may be processed on a rolling basis for some programs.
**Advanced Placement** Credit given for nursing courses completed elsewhere dependent upon specific evaluations.
**Degree Requirements** 36 total credit hours, thesis or project, comprehensive exam.

## Colorado Christian University

### Nursing Programs
### Lakewood, Colorado

Founded in 1914

**DEGREE • BSN**

### BACCALAUREATE PROGRAMS

**Degree** BSN
**Available Programs** Generic Baccalaureate; RN Baccalaureate.
**Online Degree Options** Yes.
**Contact** College of Adult and Graduate Studies, Nursing Programs, Colorado Christian University, 8787 West Alameda Avenue, Lakewood, CO 80226. *Telephone:* 303-963-3311. *E-mail:* agsadmission@ccu.edu.

## Colorado Mesa University

### Department of Nursing and Radiologic Sciences
### Grand Junction, Colorado

*http://www.coloradomesa.edu/healthsciences/index.html*
Founded in 1925

**DEGREE • BSN**
**Nursing Program Faculty** 40 (7% with doctorates).
**Baccalaureate Enrollment** 190 **Women** 88% **Men** 12% **Minority** 11% **International** 4% **Part-time** 8%
**Distance Learning Courses** Available.
**Nursing Student Activities** Sigma Theta Tau, Student Nurses' Association.
**Nursing Student Resources** Academic advising; academic or career counseling; assistance for students with disabilities; bookstore; campus computer network; career placement assistance; computer lab; computer-assisted instruction; daycare for children of students; e-mail services; employment services for current students; housing assistance; interactive nursing skills videos; Internet; learning resource lab; library services; nursing audiovisuals; placement services for program completers; resume preparation assistance; skills, simulation, or other laboratory; tutoring; unpaid internships.
**Library Facilities** 545,373 volumes (7,500 in health, 6,576 in nursing); 76,724 periodical subscriptions (100 health-care related).

### BACCALAUREATE PROGRAMS

**Degree** BSN
**Available Programs** ADN to Baccalaureate; Generic Baccalaureate; LPN to Baccalaureate; LPN to RN Baccalaureate; RN Baccalaureate.
**Study Options** Full-time and part-time.
**Online Degree Options** Yes.
**Program Entrance Requirements** Minimum overall college GPA of 2.0, transcript of college record, CPR certification, health exam, immunizations, minimum GPA in nursing prerequisites of 2.0, professional liability insurance/malpractice insurance, prerequisite course work. Transfer students are accepted. *Application deadline:* 3/1 (fall), 10/1 (spring).
**Advanced Placement** Credit by examination available. Credit given for nursing courses completed elsewhere dependent upon specific evaluations.
**Contact** *Telephone:* 970-248-1840. *Fax:* 970-248-1133.

## Colorado State University–Pueblo

### Department of Nursing
### Pueblo, Colorado

Founded in 1933

**DEGREES • BSN • MS**
**Nursing Program Faculty** 30 (10% with doctorates).
**Baccalaureate Enrollment** 134 **Women** 90% **Men** 10% **Minority** 42% **International** 1% **Part-time** 2%
**Graduate Enrollment** 26 **Women** 73% **Men** 27% **Minority** 50% **Part-time** 92%
**Nursing Student Activities** Sigma Theta Tau, Student Nurses' Association.
**Nursing Student Resources** Academic advising; academic or career counseling; assistance for students with disabilities; bookstore; campus computer network; computer lab; computer-assisted instruction; daycare for children of students; e-mail services; employment services for current students; housing assistance; Internet; learning resource lab; library services; nursing audiovisuals; remedial services; resume preparation assistance; skills, simulation, or other laboratory; tutoring.
**Library Facilities** 274,890 volumes (2,891 in health, 1,168 in nursing); 14,672 periodical subscriptions (101 health-care related).

### BACCALAUREATE PROGRAMS

**Degree** BSN
**Available Programs** ADN to Baccalaureate; Accelerated Baccalaureate for Second Degree; Accelerated RN Baccalaureate; Baccalaureate for Second Degree; Generic Baccalaureate; LPN to Baccalaureate; LPN to RN Baccalaureate; RN Baccalaureate.
**Study Options** Full-time.

**Program Entrance Requirements** Minimum overall college GPA of 2.75, transcript of college record, CPR certification, health exam, immunizations, minimum GPA in nursing prerequisites of 2.75, professional liability insurance/malpractice insurance, prerequisite course work. Transfer students are accepted. *Application deadline:* 5/25 (fall), 10/1 (summer). *Application fee:* $25.
**Advanced Placement** Credit by examination available. Credit given for nursing courses completed elsewhere dependent upon specific evaluations.
**Contact** *Telephone:* 719-549-2422. *Fax:* 719-549-2113.

## GRADUATE PROGRAMS

**Contact** *Telephone:* 719-549-2502. *Fax:* 719-549-2949.

### MASTER'S DEGREE PROGRAM

**Degree** MS
**Available Programs** Master's.
**Concentrations Available** Nursing education. *Clinical nurse specialist programs in:* acute care, psychiatric/mental health. *Nurse practitioner programs in:* acute care, family health, pediatric.
**Study Options** Full-time and part-time.
**Program Entrance Requirements** Clinical experience, computer literacy, minimum overall college GPA of 3.0, transcript of college record, CPR certification, written essay, immunizations, 3 letters of recommendation, nursing research course, professional liability insurance/malpractice insurance, prerequisite course work, resume, statistics course. *Application deadline:* 5/25 (fall). *Application fee:* $35.
**Advanced Placement** Credit given for nursing courses completed elsewhere dependent upon specific evaluations.
**Degree Requirements** 46 total credit hours, thesis or project, comprehensive exam.

### POST-MASTER'S PROGRAM

**Areas of Study** Nursing education. *Clinical nurse specialist programs in:* acute care, psychiatric/mental health. *Nurse practitioner programs in:* acute care, family health, pediatric.

# Denver School of Nursing

## Denver School of Nursing
## Denver, Colorado

### DEGREE • BSN

**Nursing Program Faculty** 78 (5% with doctorates).
**Baccalaureate Enrollment** 270 **Women** 80% **Men** 20% **Minority** 15%
**Distance Learning Courses** Available.
**Nursing Student Activities** Student Nurses' Association.
**Nursing Student Resources** Academic advising; academic or career counseling; assistance for students with disabilities; bookstore; campus computer network; career placement assistance; computer lab; computer-assisted instruction; e-mail services; employment services for current students; externships; interactive nursing skills videos; Internet; learning resource lab; library services; nursing audiovisuals; placement services for program completers; remedial services; resume preparation assistance; skills, simulation, or other laboratory; tutoring; unpaid internships.
**Library Facilities** 1,000 volumes in health, 1,000 volumes in nursing; 26,000 periodical subscriptions health-care related.

## BACCALAUREATE PROGRAMS

**Degree** BSN
**Available Programs** ADN to Baccalaureate; Accelerated Baccalaureate; Accelerated Baccalaureate for Second Degree; Generic Baccalaureate; LPN to RN Baccalaureate; RN Baccalaureate.
**Site Options** Denver, CO.
**Study Options** Full-time.
**Program Entrance Requirements** Transcript of college record, CPR certification, written essay, health exam, health insurance, immunizations, interview, 3 letters of recommendation, minimum high school GPA of 2.0, minimum GPA in nursing prerequisites of 2.0, prerequisite course work. Transfer students are accepted. *Application deadline:* 4/1 (fall), 7/1 (winter), 10/1 (spring), 1/1 (summer). Applications may be processed on a rolling basis for some programs. *Application fee:* $50.
**Advanced Placement** Credit given for nursing courses completed elsewhere dependent upon specific evaluations.
**Financial Aid** 60% of baccalaureate students in nursing programs received some form of financial aid in 2012–13.
**Contact** Mr. Jeff Johnson, Director of Admissions, Denver School of Nursing, 1401 Nineteenth Street, Denver, CO 80202. *Telephone:* 303-292-0015 Ext. 3611. *Fax:* 720-974-0290. *E-mail:* j.johnson@denverschoolofnursing.edu.

# Metropolitan State University of Denver

## Department of Health Professions
## Denver, Colorado

*http://www.mscd.edu/*
Founded in 1963

### DEGREE • BSN

**Nursing Program Faculty** 19 (10% with doctorates).
**Baccalaureate Enrollment** 124 **Women** 89% **Men** 11% **Minority** 17%
**International** 2% **Part-time** 63%
**Distance Learning Courses** Available.
**Nursing Student Activities** Nursing club.
**Nursing Student Resources** Academic advising; academic or career counseling; assistance for students with disabilities; bookstore; campus computer network; computer lab; computer-assisted instruction; daycare for children of students; e-mail services; interactive nursing skills videos; Internet; library services; nursing audiovisuals; remedial services; resume preparation assistance; skills, simulation, or other laboratory.
**Library Facilities** 607,971 volumes (21,503 in health); 2,380 periodical subscriptions (204 health-care related).

## BACCALAUREATE PROGRAMS

**Degree** BSN
**Available Programs** ADN to Baccalaureate; Accelerated Baccalaureate for Second Degree.
**Study Options** Full-time and part-time.
**Program Entrance Requirements** Transcript of college record, CPR certification, written essay, immunizations, minimum GPA in nursing prerequisites of 2.5, professional liability insurance/malpractice insurance, prerequisite course work, RN licensure. Transfer students are accepted. *Application deadline:* 4/15 (spring). *Application fee:* $25.
**Advanced Placement** Credit given for nursing courses completed elsewhere dependent upon specific evaluations.
**Expenses (2012–13)** *Tuition, area resident:* full-time $2152; part-time $1076 per semester. *Tuition, nonresident:* full-time $7993; part-time $3996 per semester. *Required fees:* full-time $1037; part-time $518 per term.
**Financial Aid** 35% of baccalaureate students in nursing programs received some form of financial aid in 2011–12.
**Contact** M. Linda Stroup, Associate Chair of the Nursing Department. *Telephone:* 303-556-4391. *Fax:* 303-556-5165. *E-mail:* lstroup@msudenver.edu.

# Platt College

## School of Nursing
## Aurora, Colorado

*http://www.plattcolorado.edu/*
Founded in 1986

### DEGREE • BSN

**Nursing Program Faculty** 8 (2% with doctorates).
**Baccalaureate Enrollment** 134 **Women** 90% **Men** 10% **Minority** 2.5%
**Nursing Student Activities** Student Nurses' Association.
**Nursing Student Resources** Academic advising; academic or career counseling; assistance for students with disabilities; campus computer network; career placement assistance; housing assistance; Internet; learning resource lab; library services; nursing audiovisuals; resume preparation assistance; skills, simulation, or other laboratory; tutoring; unpaid internships.
**Library Facilities** 1,000 volumes in health, 888 volumes in nursing; 12 periodical subscriptions health-care related.

## BACCALAUREATE PROGRAMS

**Degree** BSN
**Available Programs** Accelerated Baccalaureate.
**Study Options** Full-time.

**Program Entrance Requirements** Transcript of college record, CPR certification, written essay, health exam, health insurance, high school transcript, interview, letters of recommendation, minimum GPA in nursing prerequisites. Transfer students are accepted. *Application deadline:* 7/15 (fall), 11/15 (winter), 2/15 (spring), 5/15 (summer). Applications may be processed on a rolling basis for some programs. *Application fee:* $50.
**Advanced Placement** Credit by examination available. Credit given for nursing courses completed elsewhere dependent upon specific evaluations.
**Contact** *Telephone:* 303-369-5151.

# Regis University

## School of Nursing
## Denver, Colorado

Founded in 1877

**DEGREES • BSN • MS**

**Nursing Program Faculty** 18 (55% with doctorates).
**Distance Learning Courses** Available.
**Nursing Student Activities** Nursing Honor Society, Sigma Theta Tau, Student Nurses' Association.
**Nursing Student Resources** Academic advising; academic or career counseling; assistance for students with disabilities; bookstore; campus computer network; computer lab; computer-assisted instruction; e-mail services; interactive nursing skills videos; Internet; learning resource lab; library services; nursing audiovisuals; resume preparation assistance; skills, simulation, or other laboratory; tutoring; unpaid internships.
**Library Facilities** 618,544 volumes; 35,000 periodical subscriptions.

### BACCALAUREATE PROGRAMS

**Degree** BSN
**Available Programs** Accelerated Baccalaureate; Generic Baccalaureate; RN Baccalaureate.
**Site Options** Cheyenne, WY.
**Study Options** Full-time.
**Program Entrance Requirements** Minimum overall college GPA of 2.5, transcript of college record, written essay, 2 letters of recommendation, prerequisite course work. Transfer students are accepted.
**Advanced Placement** Credit by examination available.
**Contact** *Telephone:* 303-964-5178. *Fax:* 303-964-5400.

### GRADUATE PROGRAMS

**Contact** *Telephone:* 303-458-3534. *Fax:* 303-964-5400.

#### MASTER'S DEGREE PROGRAM

**Degree** MS
**Available Programs** Master's; RN to Master's.
**Concentrations Available** Health-care administration; nursing administration; nursing education. *Nurse practitioner programs in:* family health, neonatal health.
**Study Options** Full-time and part-time.
**Online Degree Options** Yes.
**Program Entrance Requirements** Minimum overall college GPA of 2.75, transcript of college record, written essay, 3 letters of recommendation, prerequisite course work, statistics course.
**Advanced Placement** Credit by examination available.
**Degree Requirements** 42 total credit hours, thesis or project.

# University of Colorado Colorado Springs

## Beth-El College of Nursing and Health Sciences
## Colorado Springs, Colorado

*http://www.uccs.edu/~bethel/*
Founded in 1965

**DEGREES • BSN • DNP • MSN**

**Nursing Program Faculty** 43 (32% with doctorates).
**Baccalaureate Enrollment** 332 **Women** 92% **Men** 8% **Minority** 6.5% **Part-time** 5%
**Graduate Enrollment** 155 **Women** 94% **Men** 6% **Minority** 8% **Part-time** 38%
**Distance Learning Courses** Available.
**Nursing Student Activities** Nursing Honor Society, Sigma Theta Tau, Student Nurses' Association, nursing club.
**Nursing Student Resources** Academic advising; academic or career counseling; assistance for students with disabilities; bookstore; campus computer network; career placement assistance; computer lab; computer-assisted instruction; daycare for children of students; e-mail services; employment services for current students; externships; housing assistance; interactive nursing skills videos; Internet; learning resource lab; library services; nursing audiovisuals; resume preparation assistance; skills, simulation, or other laboratory; tutoring; unpaid internships.
**Library Facilities** 421,567 volumes (10,454 in health, 1,040 in nursing); 4,765 periodical subscriptions (331 health-care related).

### BACCALAUREATE PROGRAMS

**Degree** BSN
**Available Programs** Accelerated Baccalaureate for Second Degree; Generic Baccalaureate; RN Baccalaureate.
**Study Options** Full-time.
**Online Degree Options** Yes.
**Program Entrance Requirements** Minimum overall college GPA of 3.3, transcript of college record, CPR certification, health insurance, high school biology, high school chemistry, high school foreign language, 3 years high school math, 1 year of high school science, high school transcript, immunizations, minimum high school GPA of 3.3, minimum GPA in nursing prerequisites of 3.0. Transfer students are accepted. *Application deadline:* Applications may be processed on a rolling basis for some programs. *Application fee:* $50.
**Advanced Placement** Credit given for nursing courses completed elsewhere dependent upon specific evaluations.
**Contact** *Telephone:* 719-255-3867. *Fax:* 719-255-3645.

### GRADUATE PROGRAMS

**Contact** *Telephone:* 719-255-4424. *Fax:* 719-255-4496.

#### MASTER'S DEGREE PROGRAM

**Degree** MSN
**Available Programs** Master's.
**Concentrations Available** *Clinical nurse specialist programs in:* adult health. *Nurse practitioner programs in:* adult health, family health.
**Study Options** Full-time and part-time.
**Online Degree Options** Yes (online only).
**Program Entrance Requirements** Clinical experience, computer literacy, minimum overall college GPA of 3.0, transcript of college record, CPR certification, immunizations, 4 letters of recommendation, nursing research course, physical assessment course, professional liability insurance/malpractice insurance, prerequisite course work, resume, statistics course. *Application deadline:* 7/1 (fall), 11/1 (spring). *Application fee:* $60.
**Advanced Placement** Credit given for nursing courses completed elsewhere dependent upon specific evaluations.
**Degree Requirements** 47 total credit hours, thesis or project, comprehensive exam.

#### POST-MASTER'S PROGRAM

**Areas of Study** Nursing education. *Clinical nurse specialist programs in:* adult health. *Nurse practitioner programs in:* adult health, family health.

#### DOCTORAL DEGREE PROGRAM

**Degree** DNP
**Available Programs** Doctorate.
**Areas of Study** Forensic nursing, gerontology, individualized study.
**Online Degree Options** Yes (online only).
**Program Entrance Requirements** Clinical experience, minimum overall college GPA of 3.3, interview, 3 letters of recommendation, MSN or equivalent, statistics course, vita. *Application deadline:* 3/1 (summer). *Application fee:* $60.
**Degree Requirements** 36 total credit hours, written exam, residency.

### CONTINUING EDUCATION PROGRAM

**Contact** *Telephone:* 719-255-4651. *Fax:* 719-255-4284.

# University of Colorado Denver
## College of Nursing
## Aurora, Colorado

*http://www.nursing.ucdenver.edu/*
Founded in 1912

### DEGREES • BS • DNP • MS • PHD

**Nursing Program Faculty** 87 (57% with doctorates).
**Baccalaureate Enrollment** 487 **Women** 86.25% **Men** 13.75% **Minority** 21.97% **International** .41% **Part-time** 13.9%
**Graduate Enrollment** 466 **Women** 92.92% **Men** 7.08% **Minority** 13.73% **International** 1.07% **Part-time** 30.9%
**Distance Learning Courses** Available.
**Nursing Student Activities** Nursing Honor Society, Sigma Theta Tau, Student Nurses' Association, nursing club.
**Nursing Student Resources** Academic advising; academic or career counseling; assistance for students with disabilities; bookstore; campus computer network; computer lab; computer-assisted instruction; e-mail services; housing assistance; interactive nursing skills videos; Internet; learning resource lab; library services; nursing audiovisuals; resume preparation assistance; skills, simulation, or other laboratory; tutoring.
**Library Facilities** 653,885 volumes (107,073 in health, 4,552 in nursing); 75,585 periodical subscriptions (8,948 health-care related).

### BACCALAUREATE PROGRAMS

**Degree** BS
**Available Programs** Accelerated Baccalaureate; Generic Baccalaureate; RN Baccalaureate.
**Study Options** Full-time and part-time.
**Online Degree Options** Yes.
**Program Entrance Requirements** Minimum overall college GPA of 3.0, transcript of college record, CPR certification, written essay, health exam, health insurance, immunizations, interview, minimum GPA in nursing prerequisites of 2.0, professional liability insurance/malpractice insurance, prerequisite course work. Transfer students are accepted. *Application deadline:* 6/15 (spring), 10/15 (summer). *Application fee:* $65.
**Expenses (2012–13)** *Tuition, state resident:* part-time $340 per credit hour. *Tuition, nonresident:* part-time $819 per credit hour.
**Contact** Pre-Admissions Advising, College of Nursing, University of Colorado Denver, 13120 East 19th Avenue, Campus Box C288-6, Aurora, CO 80045. *Telephone:* 303-724-1812. *Fax:* 303-724-1710. *E-mail:* nursing.admissions@ucdenver.edu.

### GRADUATE PROGRAMS

**Expenses (2012–13)** *Tuition, state resident:* part-time $490 per credit hour. *Tuition, nonresident:* part-time $990 per credit hour.
**Financial Aid** Fellowships, research assistantships, teaching assistantships, Federal Work-Study, institutionally sponsored loans, scholarships, traineeships, and unspecified assistantships available.
**Contact** Pre-Admissions Advising, College of Nursing, University of Colorado Denver, 13120 East 19th Avenue, Box C288-6, Aurora, CO 80045. *Telephone:* 303-724-1812. *Fax:* 303-724-1710. *E-mail:* nursing.admissions@ucdenver.edu.

#### MASTER'S DEGREE PROGRAM

**Degree** MS
**Available Programs** Master's.
**Concentrations Available** Nurse-midwifery; nursing administration; nursing informatics. *Clinical nurse specialist programs in:* adult health. *Nurse practitioner programs in:* adult health, family health, pediatric, psychiatric/mental health,women's health.
**Study Options** Full-time and part-time.
**Online Degree Options** Yes.
**Program Entrance Requirements** Computer literacy, minimum overall college GPA of 3.0, transcript of college record, written essay, immunizations, 4 letters of recommendation, nursing research course, prerequisite course work, resume, statistics course, GRE if cumulative undergraduate GPA is less than 3.0. *Application deadline:* 7/1 (fall), 2/1 (spring). *Application fee:* $50.
**Degree Requirements** 30 total credit hours, thesis or project, comprehensive exam.

#### POST-MASTER'S PROGRAM

**Areas of Study** Nurse-midwifery; nursing administration; nursing informatics. *Clinical nurse specialist programs in:* adult health. *Nurse practitioner programs in:* adult health, family health, pediatric, psychiatric/mental health,women's health.

#### DOCTORAL DEGREE PROGRAM

**Degree** DNP
**Available Programs** Doctorate.
**Areas of Study** Advanced practice nursing, clinical nurse specialist--general, nurse anesthesia, nurse-midwifery.
**Online Degree Options** Yes (online only).
**Program Entrance Requirements** Minimum overall college GPA of 3.0, essay, interview, letters of recommendation, MSN or equivalent, vita. *Application deadline:* 2/1 (fall), 7/1 (spring). *Application fee:* $65.
**Degree Requirements** 41 total credit hours, Capstone project.

**Degree** PhD
**Available Programs** Doctorate.
**Areas of Study** Bio-behavioral research, health-care systems.
**Program Entrance Requirements** Minimum overall college GPA of 3.0, interview by faculty committee, interview, 4 letters of recommendation, MSN or equivalent, statistics course, vita, writing sample, GRE. *Application deadline:* 3/1 (fall). *Application fee:* $50.
**Degree Requirements** 72 total credit hours, dissertation, oral exam, written exam.

#### POSTDOCTORAL PROGRAM

**Postdoctoral Program Contact** Pre-Admissions Advising, College of Nursing, University of Colorado Denver, 13120 East 19th Avenue, Campus Box C288-6, Aurora, CO 80045. *Telephone:* 303-724-1812. *Fax:* 303-724-1710. *E-mail:* nursing.admissions@ucdenver.edu.

### CONTINUING EDUCATION PROGRAM

**Contact** Office of Lifelong Learning, College of Nursing, University of Colorado Denver, 13120 East 19th Avenue, Box C288-8, Aurora, CO 80045. *Telephone:* 303-724-1372. *E-mail:* professional.development@ucdenver.edu.

# University of Northern Colorado
## School of Nursing
## Greeley, Colorado

*http://www.unco.edu/nhs/nursing/*
Founded in 1890

### DEGREES • BS • MS • PHD

**Nursing Program Faculty** 52 (60% with doctorates).
**Baccalaureate Enrollment** 216 **Women** 94% **Men** 6% **Minority** 18%
**Graduate Enrollment** 57 **Women** 98% **Men** 2% **Minority** 10% **Part-time** 60%
**Distance Learning Courses** Available.
**Nursing Student Activities** Sigma Theta Tau, Student Nurses' Association.
**Nursing Student Resources** Academic advising; academic or career counseling; assistance for students with disabilities; bookstore; campus computer network; career placement assistance; computer lab; computer-assisted instruction; e-mail services; employment services for current students; housing assistance; interactive nursing skills videos; Internet; learning resource lab; library services; nursing audiovisuals; paid internships; placement services for program completers; resume preparation assistance; skills, simulation, or other laboratory; tutoring.
**Library Facilities** 1.2 million volumes (43,602 in health, 25,700 in nursing); 43,646 periodical subscriptions (140 health-care related).

### BACCALAUREATE PROGRAMS

**Degree** BS
**Available Programs** Accelerated Baccalaureate; Generic Baccalaureate; RN Baccalaureate.
**Site Options** Greeley, CO.
**Study Options** Full-time.
**Program Entrance Requirements** Minimum overall college GPA of 3.0, transcript of college record, CPR certification, health exam, immunizations, 2 letters of recommendation, minimum GPA in nursing prerequisites of 3.0, professional liability insurance/malpractice insurance, prerequisite course work. Transfer students are accepted.
**Advanced Placement** Credit given for nursing courses completed elsewhere dependent upon specific evaluations.
**Contact** *Telephone:* 970-351-2293. *Fax:* 970-351-1707.

## GRADUATE PROGRAMS

**Contact** *Telephone:* 970-351-2293. *Fax:* 970-351-1707.

### MASTER'S DEGREE PROGRAM

**Degree** MS
**Available Programs** Master's.
**Concentrations Available** Nursing education. *Clinical nurse specialist programs in:* family health. *Nurse practitioner programs in:* family health.
**Site Options** Greeley, CO.
**Study Options** Full-time and part-time.
**Online Degree Options** Yes (online only).
**Program Entrance Requirements** Clinical experience, minimum overall college GPA of 3.0, transcript of college record, CPR certification, immunizations, 2 letters of recommendation, GRE General Test.
**Advanced Placement** Credit given for nursing courses completed elsewhere dependent upon specific evaluations.
**Degree Requirements** 45 total credit hours, thesis or project, comprehensive exam.

### POST-MASTER'S PROGRAM

**Areas of Study** Nursing education. *Nurse practitioner programs in:* family health.

### DOCTORAL DEGREE PROGRAM

**Degree** PhD
**Available Programs** Doctorate.
**Areas of Study** Nursing education.
**Site Options** Greeley, CO.
**Online Degree Options** Yes (online only).
**Program Entrance Requirements** Clinical experience, minimum overall college GPA of 3.0, 2 letters of recommendation, MSN or equivalent, vita, writing sample, GRE General Test.
**Degree Requirements** 60 total credit hours, dissertation.

# CONNECTICUT

## Central Connecticut State University

### Department of Nursing
### New Britain, Connecticut

Founded in 1849

**DEGREE • BSN**

**Nursing Program Faculty** 4 (100% with doctorates).
**Nursing Student Activities** Sigma Theta Tau, nursing club.
**Nursing Student Resources** Academic advising; academic or career counseling; assistance for students with disabilities; bookstore; campus computer network; career placement assistance; computer lab; computer-assisted instruction; e-mail services; employment services for current students; externships; Internet; learning resource lab; library services; nursing audiovisuals; resume preparation assistance; skills, simulation, or other laboratory; tutoring.
**Library Facilities** 734,780 volumes; 55,879 periodical subscriptions.

### BACCALAUREATE PROGRAMS

**Degree** BSN
**Available Programs** Generic Baccalaureate; RN Baccalaureate.
**Site Options** New Britain, CT.
**Study Options** Full-time and part-time.
**Program Entrance Requirements** Minimum overall college GPA of 2.7, CPR certification, health exam, high school transcript, immunizations, minimum GPA in nursing prerequisites of 2.7, prerequisite course work. Transfer students are accepted.
**Advanced Placement** Credit given for nursing courses completed elsewhere dependent upon specific evaluations.
**Contact** *Telephone:* 860-832-2147. *Fax:* 860-832-2188.

## Fairfield University

### School of Nursing
### Fairfield, Connecticut

*http://www.fairfield.edu/son/*
Founded in 1942

**DEGREES • BSN • DNP • MSN**

**Nursing Program Faculty** 52 (84% with doctorates).
**Baccalaureate Enrollment** 399 **Women** 93.4% **Men** 6.6% **Minority** 8.8% **Part-time** 15%
**Graduate Enrollment** 184 **Women** 86.4% **Men** 13.6% **Minority** 6.5% **International** .5% **Part-time** 85.3%
**Distance Learning Courses** Available.
**Nursing Student Activities** Nursing Honor Society, Sigma Theta Tau, Student Nurses' Association.
**Nursing Student Resources** Academic advising; academic or career counseling; assistance for students with disabilities; bookstore; campus computer network; career placement assistance; computer lab; computer-assisted instruction; daycare for children of students; e-mail services; housing assistance; interactive nursing skills videos; Internet; learning resource lab; library services; nursing audiovisuals; placement services for program completers; resume preparation assistance; skills, simulation, or other laboratory; tutoring; unpaid internships.
**Library Facilities** 375,927 volumes (9,855 in health, 4,937 in nursing); 60,156 periodical subscriptions (6,904 health-care related).

### BACCALAUREATE PROGRAMS

**Degree** BSN
**Available Programs** Accelerated Baccalaureate for Second Degree; Generic Baccalaureate; RN Baccalaureate.
**Study Options** Full-time and part-time.
**Program Entrance Requirements** Minimum overall college GPA, transcript of college record, written essay, health exam, health insurance, high school biology, high school chemistry, high school foreign language, 3 years high school math, 3 years high school science, high school transcript, immunizations, interview, letters of recommendation, minimum high school GPA of 3.0, minimum GPA in nursing prerequisites, prerequisite course work. *Application deadline:* 1/15 (fall). *Application fee:* $60.
**Advanced Placement** Credit given for nursing courses completed elsewhere dependent upon specific evaluations.
**Expenses (2013–14)** *Tuition:* full-time $42,320; part-time $725 per hour. *International tuition:* $42,320 full-time. *Room and board:* $12,930 per academic year. *Required fees:* full-time $600.
**Financial Aid** 88% of baccalaureate students in nursing programs received some form of financial aid in 2012–13. *Gift aid (need-based):* Federal Pell, FSEOG, state, private, college/university gift aid from institutional funds. *Loans:* Federal Nursing Student Loans, Federal Direct (Subsidized and Unsubsidized Stafford PLUS), Perkins, alternative loans. *Work-study:* Federal Work-Study. *Financial aid application deadline:* 2/15.
**Contact** Theresa Quell, Assistant Dean and Undergrad Director, School of Nursing, Fairfield University, 1073 North Benson Road, School of Nuring, Fairfield, CT 06824-5171. *Telephone:* 203-254-4000 Ext. 2704. *E-mail:* tquell@fairfield.edu.

### GRADUATE PROGRAMS

**Expenses (2013–14)** *Tuition:* part-time $800 per hour. *Room and board:* $6465; room only: $5422 per academic year.
**Financial Aid** 10% of graduate students in nursing programs received some form of financial aid in 2012–13. Unspecified assistantships available.
**Contact** Meredith Kazer, Associate Dean of School of Nursing, School of Nursing, Fairfield University, 1073 North Benson Road, School of Nuring, Fairfield, CT 06824-5171. *Telephone:* 203-254-4000 Ext. 2719. *E-mail:* mkazer@fairfield.edu.

### MASTER'S DEGREE PROGRAM

**Degree** MSN
**Available Programs** Master's; Master's for Nurses with Non-Nursing Degrees.
**Concentrations Available** Clinical nurse leader. *Nurse practitioner programs in:* family health, psychiatric/mental health.
**Site Options** Danbury, CT.
**Study Options** Full-time and part-time.
**Program Entrance Requirements** Computer literacy, minimum overall college GPA of 3.0, transcript of college record, CPR certification,

written essay, immunizations, interview, 2 letters of recommendation, professional liability insurance/malpractice insurance, resume. *Application deadline:* Applications may be processed on a rolling basis for some programs. *Application fee:* $60.
**Advanced Placement** Credit given for nursing courses completed elsewhere dependent upon specific evaluations.
**Degree Requirements** 38 total credit hours.

### DOCTORAL DEGREE PROGRAM

**Degree** DNP
**Available Programs** Doctorate; Post-Baccalaureate Doctorate.
**Areas of Study** Advanced practice nursing, family health.
**Program Entrance Requirements** Minimum overall college GPA of 3.2, interview by faculty committee, interview, 2 letters of recommendation, vita, writing sample, GRE (nurse anesthesia applicants only). *Application deadline:* Applications may be processed on a rolling basis for some programs. *Application fee:* $60.
**Degree Requirements** 34 total credit hours, residency.

### CONTINUING EDUCATION PROGRAM

**Contact** Carole A. Pomarico, Adult Program Director, School of Nursing, Fairfield University, 1073 North Benson Road, Fairfield, CT 06824-5171. *Telephone:* 203-254-4000 Ext. 2711. *Fax:* 203-254-4126. *E-mail:* capomarico@fairfield.edu.

# Quinnipiac University

## School of Nursing
## Hamden, Connecticut

***http://www.quinnipiac.edu/nursing***
Founded in 1929

### DEGREES • BSN • DNP • MSN

**Nursing Program Faculty** 80 (90% with doctorates).
**Baccalaureate Enrollment** 526 **Women** 97% **Men** 3% **Minority** 7% **International** 2%
**Graduate Enrollment** 122 **Women** 98% **Men** 2% **Minority** 6% **International** 1% **Part-time** 60%
**Nursing Student Activities** Sigma Theta Tau, Student Nurses' Association.
**Nursing Student Resources** Academic advising; academic or career counseling; bookstore; campus computer network; career placement assistance; computer lab; computer-assisted instruction; e-mail services; employment services for current students; externships; housing assistance; interactive nursing skills videos; Internet; learning resource lab; library services; nursing audiovisuals; paid internships; placement services for program completers; resume preparation assistance; skills, simulation, or other laboratory; tutoring; unpaid internships.
**Library Facilities** 311,000 volumes (1,700 in nursing); 44,700 periodical subscriptions.

### BACCALAUREATE PROGRAMS

**Degree** BSN
**Available Programs** Accelerated Baccalaureate for Second Degree; Generic Baccalaureate; RN Baccalaureate.
**Site Options** North Haven, CT.
**Study Options** Full-time.
**Program Entrance Requirements** Minimum overall college GPA of 3.0, transcript of college record, written essay, health exam, high school biology, high school chemistry, 4 years high school math, 4 years high school science, high school transcript, immunizations, 1 letter of recommendation, minimum high school GPA of 3.0, minimum high school rank 35%, minimum GPA in nursing prerequisites of 3.0. Transfer students are accepted. *Application deadline:* 11/15 (fall), 12/1 (spring). Applications may be processed on a rolling basis for some programs. *Application fee:* $45.
**Advanced Placement** Credit given for nursing courses completed elsewhere dependent upon specific evaluations.
**Expenses (2013–14)** *Tuition:* full-time $37,380; part-time $900 per credit. *International tuition:* $37,380 full-time. *Room and board:* $14,250 per academic year. *Required fees:* full-time $1500; part-time $37 per credit.
**Financial Aid** 82% of baccalaureate students in nursing programs received some form of financial aid in 2012–13. *Gift aid (need-based):* Federal Pell, FSEOG, state, private, college/university gift aid from institutional funds. *Loans:* Federal Direct (Subsidized and Unsubsidized Stafford PLUS), Perkins. *Work-study:* Federal Work-Study, part-time campus jobs. *Financial aid application deadline (priority):* 3/1.
**Contact** Ms. Carla Knowlton, Director of Undergraduate Admissions, School of Nursing, Quinnipiac University, 275 Mount Carmel Avenue, Hamden, CT 06518. *Telephone:* 203-582-8600. *Fax:* 203-582-8906. *E-mail:* admissions@quinnipiac.edu.

### GRADUATE PROGRAMS

**Expenses (2013–14)** *Tuition:* full-time $28,640; part-time $895 per credit. *International tuition:* $28,640 full-time. *Required fees:* part-time $37 per credit.
**Financial Aid** 30% of graduate students in nursing programs received some form of financial aid in 2012–13.
**Contact** Ms. Kristin Parent, Senior Associate Director of Graduate Admissions, School of Nursing, Quinnipiac University, 275 Mount Carmel Avenue, Hamden, CT 06518. *Telephone:* 203-582-8672. *Fax:* 203-582-3443. *E-mail:* graduate@quinnipiac.edu.

### MASTER'S DEGREE PROGRAM

**Degree** MSN
**Available Programs** Master's.
**Concentrations Available** *Nurse practitioner programs in:* adult health, family health.
**Site Options** North Haven, CT.
**Study Options** Full-time and part-time.
**Program Entrance Requirements** Clinical experience, minimum overall college GPA of 3.0, transcript of college record, written essay, 2 letters of recommendation. *Application deadline:* 6/1 (fall). Applications may be processed on a rolling basis for some programs. *Application fee:* $45.
**Degree Requirements** 43 total credit hours.

### POST-MASTER'S PROGRAM

**Areas of Study** *Nurse practitioner programs in:* adult health, family health.

### DOCTORAL DEGREE PROGRAM

**Degree** DNP
**Available Programs** Doctorate; Post-Baccalaureate Doctorate.
**Areas of Study** Advanced practice nursing.
**Site Options** North Haven, CT.
**Program Entrance Requirements** Minimum overall college GPA of 3.0, interview, 2 letters of recommendation, vita, writing sample. *Application deadline:* 6/1 (fall). Applications may be processed on a rolling basis for some programs. *Application fee:* $45.
**Degree Requirements** 75 total credit hours, residency.

***See display on next page and full description on page 486.***

# Sacred Heart University

## Program in Nursing
## Fairfield, Connecticut

***http://www.sacredheart.edu/nursing.cfm***
Founded in 1963

### DEGREES • BSN • DNP • MSN

**Nursing Program Faculty** 77
**Baccalaureate Enrollment** 410 **Women** 94% **Men** 6% **Minority** 8% **Part-time** 30%
**Graduate Enrollment** 767 **Women** 75% **Men** 25% **Minority** 10% **International** .01% **Part-time** 100%
**Distance Learning Courses** Available.
**Nursing Student Activities** Nursing Honor Society, Sigma Theta Tau, Student Nurses' Association.
**Nursing Student Resources** Academic advising; academic or career counseling; assistance for students with disabilities; bookstore; campus computer network; career placement assistance; computer lab; computer-assisted instruction; e-mail services; employment services for current students; externships; housing assistance; interactive nursing skills videos; Internet; learning resource lab; library services; nursing audiovisuals; paid internships; placement services for program completers; remedial services; resume preparation assistance; skills, simulation, or other laboratory; tutoring; unpaid internships.
**Library Facilities** 132,062 volumes (5,000 in health, 649 in nursing); 39,306 periodical subscriptions (328 health-care related).

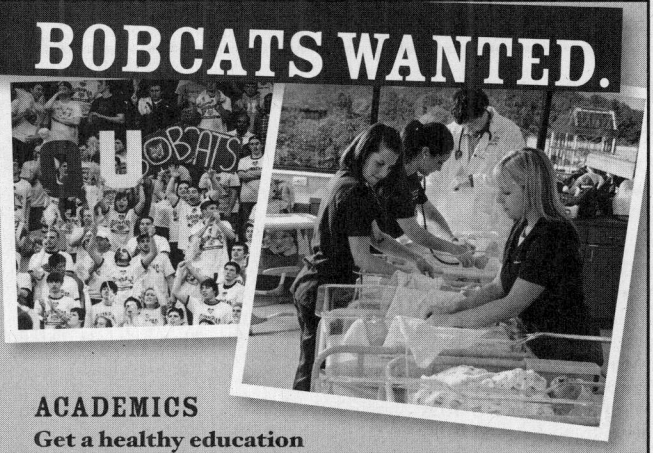

## BACCALAUREATE PROGRAMS

**Degree** BSN
**Available Programs** Generic Baccalaureate; RN Baccalaureate.
**Study Options** Full-time.
**Program Entrance Requirements** Minimum overall college GPA of 2.8, transcript of college record, written essay, high school biology, high school chemistry, 3 years high school math, 3 years high school science, high school transcript, interview, 1 letter of recommendation, minimum high school GPA of 3.3, minimum GPA in nursing prerequisites of 3.0. Transfer students are accepted. *Application deadline:* Applications may be processed on a rolling basis for some programs. *Application fee:* $70.
**Advanced Placement** Credit given for nursing courses completed elsewhere dependent upon specific evaluations.
**Expenses (2012–13)** *Tuition:* full-time $33,780; part-time $515 per credit. *International tuition:* $33,780 full-time. *Room and board:* $13,230; room only: $9380 per academic year. *Required fees:* full-time $1990.
**Financial Aid** 78% of baccalaureate students in nursing programs received some form of financial aid in 2011–12.
**Contact** Ms. Cori Nevers, Executive Director of International Admissions/Director of Admissions for the College of Health Professions, Program in Nursing, Sacred Heart University, 5151 Park Avenue, Fairfield, CT 06825-1000. *Telephone:* 203-767-0386. *E-mail:* NeversC@sacredheart.edu.

## GRADUATE PROGRAMS

**Expenses (2012–13)** *Tuition:* part-time $580 per credit.
**Financial Aid** 38% of graduate students in nursing programs received some form of financial aid in 2011–12.
**Contact** Ms. Kathy Dilks, Associate Dean of Graduate Admissions, Program in Nursing, Sacred Heart University, 5151 Park Avenue, Fairfield, CT 06825-1000. *Telephone:* 203-396-8259. *E-mail:* dilksk@sacredheart.edu.

### MASTER'S DEGREE PROGRAM

**Degree** MSN
**Available Programs** Master's; RN to Master's.
**Concentrations Available** Clinical nurse leader; nursing administration; nursing education. *Nurse practitioner programs in:* family health.
**Study Options** Full-time and part-time.
**Online Degree Options** Yes.
**Program Entrance Requirements** Clinical experience, minimum overall college GPA of 3.0, transcript of college record, written essay, interview, 2 letters of recommendation, prerequisite course work, statistics course. *Application deadline:* 2/15 (fall). Applications may be processed on a rolling basis for some programs. *Application fee:* $60.
**Advanced Placement** Credit given for nursing courses completed elsewhere dependent upon specific evaluations.
**Degree Requirements** 38 total credit hours, thesis or project.

### POST-MASTER'S PROGRAM

**Areas of Study** *Nurse practitioner programs in:* family health.

### DOCTORAL DEGREE PROGRAM

**Degree** DNP
**Available Programs** Doctorate.
**Areas of Study** Clinical practice, nursing administration.
**Program Entrance Requirements** Minimum overall college GPA of 3.2, interview by faculty committee, 2 letters of recommendation, MSN or equivalent, scholarly papers, statistics course, writing sample. *Application deadline:* 4/1 (fall). *Application fee:* $60.
**Degree Requirements** 39 total credit hours, dissertation.

# St. Vincent's College

## Nursing Program
## Bridgeport, Connecticut

Founded in 1991

**DEGREE • BSN**

## BACCALAUREATE PROGRAMS

**Degree** BSN
**Available Programs** Accelerated Baccalaureate.
**Online Degree Options** Yes (online only).
**Contact** Sharon Makowski, Associate Professor/Chair, Nursing, RN to BSN Completion Program, Nursing Program, St. Vincent's College, 2800

Main Street, Bridgeport, CT 06606. *Telephone:* 203-576-5478. *E-mail:* smakowski@stvincentscollege.edu.

# Southern Connecticut State University

## Department of Nursing
## New Haven, Connecticut

***http://www.southernct.edu/nursing/***
Founded in 1893

**DEGREES • BS • EDD • MSN**
**Nursing Program Faculty** 45 (65% with doctorates).
**Baccalaureate Enrollment** 220 **Women** 85% **Men** 15% **Minority** 20% **Part-time** 5%
**Graduate Enrollment** 40 **Women** 97% **Men** 3% **Part-time** 97%
**Distance Learning Courses** Available.
**Nursing Student Activities** Nursing Honor Society, Sigma Theta Tau, Student Nurses' Association.
**Nursing Student Resources** Academic advising; academic or career counseling; assistance for students with disabilities; bookstore; campus computer network; career placement assistance; computer lab; daycare for children of students; e-mail services; employment services for current students; housing assistance; Internet; learning resource lab; library services; nursing audiovisuals; resume preparation assistance; skills, simulation, or other laboratory; tutoring.
**Library Facilities** 428,990 volumes (35,540 in health, 2,279 in nursing); 59,264 periodical subscriptions (318 health-care related).

### BACCALAUREATE PROGRAMS

**Degree** BS
**Available Programs** ADN to Baccalaureate; Accelerated Baccalaureate; Generic Baccalaureate; RN Baccalaureate.
**Study Options** Full-time and part-time.
**Program Entrance Requirements** Minimum overall college GPA of 2.8, transcript of college record, CPR certification, health exam, high school transcript, immunizations, minimum GPA in nursing prerequisites, prerequisite course work. Transfer students are accepted. *Application deadline:* 2/1 (spring).
**Advanced Placement** Credit given for nursing courses completed elsewhere dependent upon specific evaluations.
**Contact** *Telephone:* 203-392-6475. *Fax:* 203-392-6493.

### GRADUATE PROGRAMS

**Contact** *Telephone:* 203-392-6480. *Fax:* 203-392-6493.

#### MASTER'S DEGREE PROGRAM

**Degree** MSN
**Available Programs** Master's; RN to Master's.
**Concentrations Available** Clinical nurse leader; nursing education. *Nurse practitioner programs in:* family health.
**Study Options** Full-time and part-time.
**Program Entrance Requirements** Clinical experience, minimum overall college GPA of 3.0, transcript of college record, CPR certification, immunizations, interview, 2 letters of recommendation, nursing research course, physical assessment course, professional liability insurance/malpractice insurance, prerequisite course work, resume, statistics course, GRE, MAT. *Application deadline:* 10/1 (fall), 3/1 (spring). Applications may be processed on a rolling basis for some programs.
**Advanced Placement** Credit given for nursing courses completed elsewhere dependent upon specific evaluations.
**Degree Requirements** 42 total credit hours, thesis or project.

#### POST-MASTER'S PROGRAM

**Areas of Study** Nursing education. *Nurse practitioner programs in:* family health.

#### DOCTORAL DEGREE PROGRAM

**Degree** EdD
**Available Programs** Doctorate.
**Areas of Study** Nursing education.
**Online Degree Options** Yes (online only).
**Program Entrance Requirements** Minimum overall college GPA of 3.0, interview, 2 letters of recommendation, MSN or equivalent, vita, writing sample. *Application deadline:* 3/1 (spring).
**Degree Requirements** 51 total credit hours, dissertation, written exam, residency.

# University of Connecticut

## School of Nursing
## Storrs, Connecticut

***http://www.nursing.uconn.edu/***
Founded in 1881

**DEGREES • BS • DNP • MS • PHD**
**Nursing Program Faculty** 118 (76% with doctorates).
**Baccalaureate Enrollment** 602 **Women** 85% **Men** 15% **Minority** 25%
**Graduate Enrollment** 196 **Women** 95% **Men** 5% **Minority** 16% **International** .5% **Part-time** 56%
**Distance Learning Courses** Available.
**Nursing Student Activities** Nursing Honor Society, Sigma Theta Tau, Student Nurses' Association, nursing club.
**Nursing Student Resources** Academic advising; academic or career counseling; assistance for students with disabilities; bookstore; campus computer network; career placement assistance; computer lab; e-mail services; housing assistance; interactive nursing skills videos; Internet; learning resource lab; library services; nursing audiovisuals; remedial services; resume preparation assistance; skills, simulation, or other laboratory; tutoring; unpaid internships.
**Library Facilities** 3.5 million volumes (46,250 in health, 1,170 in nursing); 87,556 periodical subscriptions (7,648 health-care related).

### BACCALAUREATE PROGRAMS

**Degree** BS
**Available Programs** Accelerated Baccalaureate for Second Degree; Generic Baccalaureate.
**Site Options** Groton, CT; Waterbury, CT; Stamford, CT.
**Study Options** Full-time and part-time.
**Program Entrance Requirements** Minimum overall college GPA of 3.3, transcript of college record, written essay, health exam, health insurance, high school chemistry, high school foreign language, 3 years high school math, 2 years high school science, high school transcript, immunizations, 3 letters of recommendation, minimum high school GPA of 3.0, minimum GPA in nursing prerequisites of 3.0, prerequisite course work. Transfer students are accepted. *Application deadline:* 1/15 (fall). *Application fee:* $70.
**Advanced Placement** Credit by examination available. Credit given for nursing courses completed elsewhere dependent upon specific evaluations.
**Expenses (2013–14)** *Tuition, state resident:* full-time $9256; part-time $386 per credit. *Tuition, nonresident:* full-time $28,204; part-time $1175 per credit. *International tuition:* $28,204 full-time. *Room and board:* $11,722; room only: $6278 per academic year. *Required fees:* full-time $2766; part-time $515 per credit.
**Financial Aid** 77% of baccalaureate students in nursing programs received some form of financial aid in 2012–13. *Gift aid (need-based):* Federal Pell, FSEOG, state, private, college/university gift aid from institutional funds. *Loans:* Federal Nursing Student Loans, Federal Direct (Subsidized and Unsubsidized Stafford PLUS), Perkins, state. *Work-study:* Federal Work-Study, part-time campus jobs. *Financial aid application deadline (priority):* 3/1.
**Contact** Ms. Dorine Nagy, Admissions Coordinator, School of Nursing, University of Connecticut, 231 Glenbrook Road, Unit 4026, Storrs, CT 06269-4026. *Telephone:* 860-486-1937. *Fax:* 860-486-0906. *E-mail:* Dorine.Nagy@uconn.edu.

### GRADUATE PROGRAMS

**Expenses (2013–14)** *Tuition, state resident:* full-time $9256; part-time $636 per credit. *Tuition, nonresident:* full-time $28,204; part-time $1652 per credit. *International tuition:* $28,204 full-time. *Room and board:* $11,722; room only: $6278 per academic year. *Required fees:* full-time $2766; part-time $472 per credit.
**Financial Aid** 24% of graduate students in nursing programs received some form of financial aid in 2012–13. 9 research assistantships with full tuition reimbursements available, 12 teaching assistantships with full tuition reimbursements available were awarded; fellowships, Federal Work-Study, scholarships, and unspecified assistantships also available. *Financial aid application deadline:* 2/1.
**Contact** Ms. Dorine Nagy, Graduate Program Contact, School of Nursing, University of Connecticut, 231 Glenbrook Road, Unit 4026,

Storrs, CT 06269-4026. *Telephone:* 860-486-1937. *Fax:* 860-486-0906. *E-mail:* Dorine.Nagy@uconn.edu.

**MASTER'S DEGREE PROGRAM**

**Degree** MS

**Available Programs** Master's; RN to Master's.

**Concentrations Available** Clinical nurse leader. *Clinical nurse specialist programs in:* acute care, maternity-newborn. *Nurse practitioner programs in:* acute care, family health, neonatal health, primary care.

**Study Options** Full-time and part-time.

**Program Entrance Requirements** Clinical experience, computer literacy, minimum overall college GPA of 3.0, transcript of college record, interview, 3 letters of recommendation, nursing research course, physical assessment course, resume, statistics course. *Application deadline:* 5/1 (fall). Applications may be processed on a rolling basis for some programs. *Application fee:* $75.

**Advanced Placement** Credit given for nursing courses completed elsewhere dependent upon specific evaluations.

**Degree Requirements** 24 total credit hours, comprehensive exam.

**POST-MASTER'S PROGRAM**

**Areas of Study** *Clinical nurse specialist programs in:* maternity-newborn. *Nurse practitioner programs in:* acute care, neonatal health, primary care.

**DOCTORAL DEGREE PROGRAM**

**Degree** DNP

**Available Programs** Doctorate, Post-Baccalaureate Doctorate.

**Areas of Study** Advanced practice nursing, nursing policy.

**Program Entrance Requirements** Minimum overall college GPA of 3.25, clinical experience, interview, interview by faculty committee, 3 letters of recommendation, statistics course, vita, writing sample. *Application deadline:* 2/1 (fall). Applications may be processed on a rolling basis for some programs. *Application fee:* $75.

**Degree Requirements** 38 total credit hours, dissertation, oral exam, written exam.

**Degree** PhD

**Available Programs** Doctorate; Post-Baccalaureate Doctorate.

**Areas of Study** Nursing research, nursing science.

**Program Entrance Requirements** Minimum overall college GPA of 3.25, interview by faculty committee, interview, 3 letters of recommendation, statistics course, vita, writing sample. *Application deadline:* 2/1 (fall). *Application fee:* $75.

**Degree Requirements** 59 total credit hours, dissertation, oral exam, written exam.

**POSTDOCTORAL PROGRAM**

**Postdoctoral Program Contact** Dr. Jacqueline McGrath, Associate Dean for Research and Scholarship, School of Nursing, University of Connecticut, School of Nursing, 231 Glenbrook Road, U-4026, Storrs, CT 06269-4026. *Telephone:* 860-486-0537. *Fax:* 860-486-9085. *E-mail:* Jacqueline.Mcgrath@uconn.edu.

## CONTINUING EDUCATION PROGRAM

**Contact** Ms. Elise Bennett, School of Nursing, University of Connecticut, School of Nursing, 231 Glenbrook Road, U-4026, Storrs, CT 06269-4026. *Telephone:* 860-486-8321. *Fax:* 860-486-0001. *E-mail:* Elise.Bennett@uconn.edu.

# University of Hartford

## College of Education, Nursing, and Health Professions

## West Hartford, Connecticut

***http://www.hartford.edu/enhp***

Founded in 1877

**DEGREES • BSN • MSN**

**Nursing Program Faculty** 5 (80% with doctorates).

**Baccalaureate Enrollment** 73 **Women** 88% **Men** 12% **Minority** 40% **Part-time** 100%

**Graduate Enrollment** 159 **Women** 94% **Men** 6% **Minority** 17% **International** 2% **Part-time** 100%

**Distance Learning Courses** Available.

**Nursing Student Activities** Nursing Honor Society, Sigma Theta Tau.

**Nursing Student Resources** Academic advising; academic or career counseling; assistance for students with disabilities; bookstore; campus computer network; computer lab; e-mail services; interactive nursing skills videos; Internet; library services; nursing audiovisuals; resume preparation assistance; skills, simulation, or other laboratory; tutoring.

**Library Facilities** 590,724 volumes; 49,600 periodical subscriptions.

## BACCALAUREATE PROGRAMS

**Degree** BSN

**Available Programs** ADN to Baccalaureate; RN Baccalaureate.

**Study Options** Part-time.

**Program Entrance Requirements** Transcript of college record, professional liability insurance/malpractice insurance, prerequisite course work, RN licensure. Transfer students are accepted. *Application deadline:* Applications may be processed on a rolling basis for some programs. *Application fee:* $35.

**Advanced Placement** Credit by examination available. Credit given for nursing courses completed elsewhere dependent upon specific evaluations.

**Expenses (2013–14)** *Tuition:* part-time $480 per credit hour.

**Financial Aid** 50% of baccalaureate students in nursing programs received some form of financial aid in 2012–13.

**Contact** Kim Groot, Nursing Faculty, College of Education, Nursing, and Health Professions, University of Hartford, 200 Bloomfield Avenue, West Hartford, CT 06117-1599. *Telephone:* 860-768-5408. *Fax:* 860-768-5043. *E-mail:* groot@hartford.edu.

## GRADUATE PROGRAMS

**Expenses (2013–14)** *Tuition:* part-time $495 per credit.

**Financial Aid** 50% of graduate students in nursing programs received some form of financial aid in 2012–13. 4 research assistantships (averaging $4,500 per year) were awarded; teaching assistantships, institutionally sponsored loans and unspecified assistantships also available. *Financial aid application deadline:* 6/1.

**Contact** Susan Eichar, Associate Professor of Nursing, College of Education, Nursing, and Health Professions, University of Hartford, 200 Bloomfield Avenue, West Hartford, CT 06117-1599. *Telephone:* 860-768-4214. *Fax:* 860-768-5346. *E-mail:* seichar@hartford.edu.

**MASTER'S DEGREE PROGRAM**

**Degree** MSN

**Available Programs** Master's; Master's for Nurses with Non-Nursing Degrees.

**Concentrations Available** Nursing administration; nursing education. *Clinical nurse specialist programs in:* public health.

**Study Options** Part-time.

**Program Entrance Requirements** Clinical experience, minimum overall college GPA of 3.0, transcript of college record, written essay, immunizations, 2 letters of recommendation, nursing research course, physical assessment course, professional liability insurance/malpractice insurance, resume. *Application deadline:* 4/15 (fall), 11/15 (spring). *Application fee:* $50.

**Advanced Placement** Credit given for nursing courses completed elsewhere dependent upon specific evaluations.

**Degree Requirements** 34 total credit hours, thesis or project.

**POST-MASTER'S PROGRAM**

**Areas of Study** Nursing education.

**DOCTORAL DEGREE PROGRAM**

**Program Entrance Requirements** MAT.

## CONTINUING EDUCATION PROGRAM

**Contact** Dr. Susan Eichar, Associate Professor, Department of Health Sciences and Nursing, College of Education, Nursing, and Health Professions, University of Hartford, 200 Bloomfield Avenue, West Hartford, CT 06117-1599. *Telephone:* 860-768-4214. *Fax:* 860-768-5346. *E-mail:* seichar@hartford.edu.

# University of Saint Joseph

## Department of Nursing
## West Hartford, Connecticut

*http://www.usj.edu/*
Founded in 1932

**DEGREES • BS • MS**

**Nursing Program Faculty** 23 (44% with doctorates).

**Baccalaureate Enrollment** 250 **Women** 100% **Minority** 21% **International** 4% **Part-time** 38%

**Graduate Enrollment** 120 **Women** 92% **Men** 8% **Minority** 35% **International** 1% **Part-time** 66%

**Distance Learning Courses** Available.

**Nursing Student Activities** Sigma Theta Tau, Student Nurses' Association, nursing club.

**Nursing Student Resources** Academic advising; academic or career counseling; assistance for students with disabilities; bookstore; campus computer network; career placement assistance; computer lab; computer-assisted instruction; daycare for children of students; e-mail services; employment services for current students; externships; housing assistance; interactive nursing skills videos; Internet; learning resource lab; library services; nursing audiovisuals; paid internships; placement services for program completers; remedial services; resume preparation assistance; skills, simulation, or other laboratory; tutoring; unpaid internships.

**Library Facilities** 92,813 volumes (7,058 in health, 1,949 in nursing); 11,208 periodical subscriptions (1,495 health-care related).

### BACCALAUREATE PROGRAMS

**Degree** BS

**Available Programs** Baccalaureate for Second Degree; Generic Baccalaureate; RN Baccalaureate.

**Site Options** Middletown, CT.

**Study Options** Full-time.

**Program Entrance Requirements** Minimum overall college GPA of 2.8, transcript of college record, CPR certification, written essay, health exam, health insurance, high school biology, high school chemistry, high school transcript, immunizations, minimum high school GPA, minimum GPA in nursing prerequisites of 2.8, prerequisite course work. Transfer students are accepted. *Application deadline:* 4/1 (fall), 12/1 (spring). Applications may be processed on a rolling basis for some programs. *Application fee:* $50.

**Advanced Placement** Credit given for nursing courses completed elsewhere dependent upon specific evaluations.

**Contact** *Telephone:* 860-231-5304.

### GRADUATE PROGRAMS

**Contact** *Telephone:* 860-231-5352. *Fax:* 860-231-8396.

#### MASTER'S DEGREE PROGRAM

**Degree** MS

**Available Programs** Master's; Master's for Nurses with Non-Nursing Degrees.

**Concentrations Available** Nursing education. *Nurse practitioner programs in:* family health, psychiatric/mental health.

**Site Options** Middletown, CT.

**Study Options** Full-time and part-time.

**Program Entrance Requirements** Clinical experience, minimum overall college GPA of 3.0, transcript of college record, CPR certification, written essay, immunizations, interview, 2 letters of recommendation, professional liability insurance/malpractice insurance, resume. *Application deadline:* Applications may be processed on a rolling basis for some programs. *Application fee:* $50.

**Advanced Placement** Credit given for nursing courses completed elsewhere dependent upon specific evaluations.

**Degree Requirements** 44 total credit hours, comprehensive exam.

#### POST-MASTER'S PROGRAM

**Areas of Study** *Nurse practitioner programs in:* psychiatric/mental health.

# Western Connecticut State University

## Department of Nursing
## Danbury, Connecticut

*http://www.wcsu.edu/*
Founded in 1903

**DEGREES • BS • MS**

**Nursing Program Faculty** 18 (50% with doctorates).

**Baccalaureate Enrollment** 160 **Women** 95% **Men** 5% **Minority** 20%

**Graduate Enrollment** 35 **Women** 100% **Minority** 2% **Part-time** 100%

**Distance Learning Courses** Available.

**Nursing Student Activities** Sigma Theta Tau, Student Nurses' Association.

**Nursing Student Resources** Academic advising; academic or career counseling; assistance for students with disabilities; bookstore; campus computer network; career placement assistance; computer lab; computer-assisted instruction; daycare for children of students; e-mail services; employment services for current students; externships; housing assistance; interactive nursing skills videos; Internet; learning resource lab; library services; nursing audiovisuals; paid internships; remedial services; resume preparation assistance; skills, simulation, or other laboratory; tutoring.

**Library Facilities** 213,314 volumes; 1,089 periodical subscriptions.

### BACCALAUREATE PROGRAMS

**Degree** BS

**Available Programs** Generic Baccalaureate; RN Baccalaureate.

**Site Options** Waterbury, CT.

**Study Options** Full-time.

**Program Entrance Requirements** Minimum overall college GPA of 2.5, transcript of college record, CPR certification, health exam, health insurance, high school biology, high school chemistry, high school foreign language, 3 years high school math, 2 years high school science, high school transcript, immunizations, minimum GPA in nursing prerequisites of 2.5, prerequisite course work. Transfer students are accepted. *Application deadline:* Applications may be processed on a rolling basis for some programs. *Application fee:* $60.

**Advanced Placement** Credit by examination available. Credit given for nursing courses completed elsewhere dependent upon specific evaluations.

**Contact** *Telephone:* 203-837-8556. *Fax:* 203-837-8550.

### GRADUATE PROGRAMS

**Contact** *Telephone:* 203-837-8556. *Fax:* 203-837-8550.

#### MASTER'S DEGREE PROGRAM

**Degree** MS

**Available Programs** Master's.

**Concentrations Available** *Clinical nurse specialist programs in:* adult health. *Nurse practitioner programs in:* adult health.

**Study Options** Part-time.

**Program Entrance Requirements** Clinical experience, computer literacy, minimum overall college GPA of 3.0, transcript of college record, CPR certification, immunizations, interview, 2 letters of recommendation, nursing research course, physical assessment course, professional liability insurance/malpractice insurance, prerequisite course work, resume, statistics course. *Application deadline:* Applications may be processed on a rolling basis for some programs. *Application fee:* $60.

**Advanced Placement** Credit by examination available. Credit given for nursing courses completed elsewhere dependent upon specific evaluations.

**Degree Requirements** 36 total credit hours, thesis or project.

#### POST-MASTER'S PROGRAM

**Areas of Study** *Clinical nurse specialist programs in:* adult health. *Nurse practitioner programs in:* adult health.

## Yale University
### School of Nursing
### New Haven, Connecticut

*http://www.nursing.yale.edu/*
Founded in 1701

**DEGREES • DNP • MSN • MSN/MDIV • MSN/MPH • PHD**
**Nursing Program Faculty** 60 (70% with doctorates).
**Graduate Enrollment** 338 **Women** 90% **Men** 10% **Minority** 24% **International** 5% **Part-time** 18%
**Distance Learning Courses** Available.
**Nursing Student Activities** Nursing Honor Society, Sigma Theta Tau.
**Nursing Student Resources** Academic advising; academic or career counseling; assistance for students with disabilities; bookstore; campus computer network; career placement assistance; computer lab; computer-assisted instruction; daycare for children of students; e-mail services; employment services for current students; housing assistance; interactive nursing skills videos; Internet; learning resource lab; library services; nursing audiovisuals; placement services for program completers; remedial services; resume preparation assistance; skills, simulation, or other laboratory; tutoring; unpaid internships.
**Library Facilities** 15 million volumes (400,000 in health); 450,000 periodical subscriptions (2,900 health-care related).

#### GRADUATE PROGRAMS

**Financial Aid** 90% of graduate students in nursing programs received some form of financial aid in 2012–13. 239 fellowships (averaging $5,905 per year), 13 research assistantships with tuition reimbursements available (averaging $28,450 per year) were awarded; Federal Work-Study, scholarships, and traineeships also available. Aid available to part-time students. *Financial aid application deadline:* 2/1.
**Contact** Ms. Melissa Pucci, Director of Admissions, School of Nursing, Yale University, PO Box 27399, West Haven, CT 06516. *Telephone:* 203-737-1793. *Fax:* 203-737-5409. *E-mail:* melissa.pucci@yale.edu.

#### MASTER'S DEGREE PROGRAM
**Degrees** MSN; MSN/MDIV; MSN/MPH
**Available Programs** Master's; Master's for Non-Nursing College Graduates; Master's for Nurses with Non-Nursing Degrees.
**Concentrations Available** Nurse-midwifery. *Nurse practitioner programs in:* acute care, family health, pediatric, psychiatric/mental health.
**Study Options** Full-time.
**Program Entrance Requirements** Minimum overall college GPA of 3.0, transcript of college record, CPR certification, written essay, immunizations, interview, 3 letters of recommendation, resume, GRE General Test. *Application deadline:* 11/1 (fall). *Application fee:* $100.
**Advanced Placement** Credit by examination available. Credit given for nursing courses completed elsewhere dependent upon specific evaluations.
**Degree Requirements** 40 total credit hours.

#### POST-MASTER'S PROGRAM
**Areas of Study** *Nurse practitioner programs in:* acute care, family health, pediatric, psychiatric/mental health.

#### DOCTORAL DEGREE PROGRAM
**Degree** DNP
**Available Programs** Doctorate.
**Areas of Study** Health policy, health-care systems, nursing administration, nursing policy.
**Online Degree Options** Yes (online only).
**Program Entrance Requirements** Clinical experience, minimum overall college GPA of 3.0, interview by faculty committee, interview, 3 letters of recommendation, MSN or equivalent, vita, GRE General Test. *Application deadline:* 3/1 (fall). *Application fee:* $100.
**Degree Requirements** 40 total credit hours.
**Degree** PhD
**Available Programs** Doctorate.
**Areas of Study** Aging, critical care, family health, gerontology, health policy, health promotion/disease prevention, health-care systems, human health and illness, maternity-newborn, neuro-behavior, nursing policy, nursing research, oncology.
**Program Entrance Requirements** Minimum overall college GPA of 3.0, clinical experience, interview, interview by faculty committee, 3 letters of recommendation, MSN or equivalent, statistics course, vita, writing sample. *Application deadline:* 1/2 (fall). *Application fee:* $100.
**Degree Requirements** 60 total credit hours, dissertation, oral exam, written exam.

#### POSTDOCTORAL PROGRAM
**Areas of Study** Adolescent health, chronic illness.
**Postdoctoral Program Contact** Ms. Sarah Zaino, Assistant Director, Research Activities, School of Nursing, Yale University, PO Box 27399, West Haven, CT 06516. *Telephone:* 203-737-2420. *Fax:* 203-737-4480. *E-mail:* sarah.zaino@yale.edu.

# DELAWARE

## Delaware State University
### Department of Nursing
### Dover, Delaware

*http://www.desu.edu/department-nursing*
Founded in 1891

**DEGREES • BSN • MS**
**Nursing Program Faculty** 11
**Baccalaureate Enrollment** 72 **Women** 93% **Men** 7%
**Nursing Student Activities** Sigma Theta Tau, Student Nurses' Association.
**Nursing Student Resources** Academic advising; assistance for students with disabilities; bookstore; campus computer network; computer lab; daycare for children of students; e-mail services; interactive nursing skills videos; library services; nursing audiovisuals; skills, simulation, or other laboratory.
**Library Facilities** 190,613 volumes; 74,881 periodical subscriptions.

#### BACCALAUREATE PROGRAMS
**Degree** BSN
**Available Programs** Generic Baccalaureate; LPN to Baccalaureate; RN Baccalaureate.
**Study Options** Full-time and part-time.
**Program Entrance Requirements** CPR certification, health exam, high school biology, high school chemistry, high school transcript, immunizations, minimum high school GPA of 2.0, professional liability insurance/malpractice insurance, prerequisite course work. Transfer students are accepted. *Application deadline:* 2/25 (winter).
**Contact** *Telephone:* 302-857-6700.

#### GRADUATE PROGRAMS
**Contact** *Telephone:* 302-857-6700.

#### MASTER'S DEGREE PROGRAM
**Degree** MS
**Available Programs** Master's.
**Concentrations Available** Nursing education. *Clinical nurse specialist programs in:* public health.
**Study Options** Full-time.
**Program Entrance Requirements** Clinical experience, minimum overall college GPA of 3.0, transcript of college record, CPR certification, written essay, immunizations, 3 letters of recommendation, professional liability insurance/malpractice insurance, resume. *Application deadline:* 2/1 (winter). *Application fee:* $35.
**Advanced Placement** Credit given for nursing courses completed elsewhere dependent upon specific evaluations.
**Degree Requirements** 39 total credit hours, thesis or project.

## University of Delaware
### School of Nursing
### Newark, Delaware

*http://www.udel.edu/nursing/*
Founded in 1743

**DEGREES • BSN • MSN • PHD**
**Nursing Program Faculty** 37 (70% with doctorates).
**Baccalaureate Enrollment** 635 **Women** 93% **Men** 7% **Minority** 16%

**Graduate Enrollment** 159 **Women** 94% **Men** 6% **Minority** 18% **Part-time** 94%
**Distance Learning Courses** Available.
**Nursing Student Activities** Sigma Theta Tau, Student Nurses' Association.
**Nursing Student Resources** Academic advising; academic or career counseling; assistance for students with disabilities; bookstore; campus computer network; career placement assistance; computer lab; computer-assisted instruction; e-mail services; employment services for current students; externships; housing assistance; interactive nursing skills videos; Internet; learning resource lab; library services; nursing audiovisuals; paid internships; resume preparation assistance; skills, simulation, or other laboratory; tutoring.
**Library Facilities** 2.8 million volumes (2.7 million in health, 40,000 in nursing); 42,000 periodical subscriptions (240 health-care related).

## BACCALAUREATE PROGRAMS

**Degree** BSN
**Available Programs** Accelerated Baccalaureate for Second Degree; Generic Baccalaureate; RN Baccalaureate.
**Study Options** Full-time.
**Online Degree Options** Yes.
**Program Entrance Requirements** Written essay, high school biology, high school chemistry, high school foreign language, 3 years high school math, 4 years high school science, high school transcript, 1 letter of recommendation, minimum high school GPA of 3.0. Transfer students are accepted. *Application deadline:* 1/15 (fall). *Application fee:* $75.
**Advanced Placement** Credit given for nursing courses completed elsewhere dependent upon specific evaluations.
**Expenses (2013–14)** *Tuition, state resident:* full-time $10,580; part-time $441 per credit. *Tuition, nonresident:* full-time $28,400; part-time $1183 per credit. *International tuition:* $28,400 full-time. *Room and board:* $11,200; room only: $6810 per academic year. *Required fees:* full-time $1532; part-time $30 per credit.
**Financial Aid** 71% of baccalaureate students in nursing programs received some form of financial aid in 2012–13. *Gift aid (need-based):* Federal Pell, FSEOG, state, private, college/university gift aid from institutional funds. *Loans:* Federal Nursing Student Loans, Federal Direct (Subsidized and Unsubsidized Stafford PLUS), Perkins. *Work-study:* Federal Work-Study, part-time campus jobs. *Financial aid application deadline:* 3/15(priority: 2/1).
**Contact** Ms. Anne DeCaire, Nursing Recruiter, School of Nursing, University of Delaware, 385 McDowell Hall, Newark, DE 19716. *Telephone:* 302-831-0442. *Fax:* 302-831-2382. *E-mail:* aderb@udel.edu.

## GRADUATE PROGRAMS

**Expenses (2013–14)** *Tuition, state resident:* full-time $6390; part-time $710 per credit. *Tuition, nonresident:* full-time $6390; part-time $710 per credit. *International tuition:* $6390 full-time. *Required fees:* full-time $842.
**Financial Aid** 100% of graduate students in nursing programs received some form of financial aid in 2012–13. Research assistantships with tuition reimbursements available (averaging $15,000 per year); scholarships, traineeships, tuition waivers (full), and unspecified assistantships also available. Aid available to part-time students. *Financial aid application deadline:* 7/1.
**Contact** Ms. Joanne Marra, Office Coordinator, School of Nursing, University of Delaware, 349 McDowell Hall, Newark, DE 19716. *Telephone:* 302-831-8386. *Fax:* 302-831-2382. *E-mail:* udgradnursing@udel.edu.

### MASTER'S DEGREE PROGRAM

**Degree** MSN
**Available Programs** Master's; RN to Master's.
**Concentrations Available** Health-care administration. *Clinical nurse specialist programs in:* adult health, pediatric. *Nurse practitioner programs in:* adult health, family health.
**Study Options** Full-time and part-time.
**Online Degree Options** Yes.
**Program Entrance Requirements** Clinical experience, minimum overall college GPA of 3.0, transcript of college record, CPR certification, written essay, immunizations, interview, 3 letters of recommendation, resume. *Application deadline:* 3/1 (fall), 10/1 (spring). *Application fee:* $75.
**Advanced Placement** Credit given for nursing courses completed elsewhere dependent upon specific evaluations.
**Degree Requirements** 46 total credit hours.

### POST-MASTER'S PROGRAM

**Areas of Study** Health-care administration. *Clinical nurse specialist programs in:* adult health, pediatric. *Nurse practitioner programs in:* adult health, family health.

### DOCTORAL DEGREE PROGRAM

**Degree** PhD
**Available Programs** Doctorate.
**Areas of Study** Advanced practice nursing, aging, bio-behavioral research, community health, faculty preparation, gerontology, health policy, health promotion/disease prevention, illness and transition, individualized study, nursing education, nursing research, nursing science, oncology.
**Program Entrance Requirements** Clinical experience, minimum overall college GPA of 3.5, interview by faculty committee, 3 letters of recommendation, MSN or equivalent, statistics course, vita, writing sample. *Application deadline:* 2/1 (fall). *Application fee:* $75.
**Degree Requirements** 50 total credit hours, dissertation, oral exam, written exam, residency.

## CONTINUING EDUCATION PROGRAM

**Contact** Dr. Dayle Thorpe, Division of Professional and Continuing Studies, School of Nursing, University of Delaware, 201 Clayton Hall, Newark, DE 19716. *Telephone:* 302-831-7600. *Fax:* 302-831-0701. *E-mail:* continuing-ed@udel.edu.

# Wesley College
## Nursing Program
## Dover, Delaware

***http://www.wesley.edu/***
Founded in 1873

**DEGREES • BSN • MSN**
**Nursing Program Faculty** 12 (80% with doctorates).
**Baccalaureate Enrollment** 210 **Women** 85% **Men** 15% **Minority** 35% **International** 1% **Part-time** 2%
**Graduate Enrollment** 87 **Women** 90% **Men** 10% **Minority** 25% **Part-time** 10%
**Distance Learning Courses** Available.
**Nursing Student Activities** Sigma Theta Tau, Student Nurses' Association.
**Nursing Student Resources** Academic advising; academic or career counseling; assistance for students with disabilities; bookstore; campus computer network; career placement assistance; computer lab; computer-assisted instruction; e-mail services; employment services for current students; externships; housing assistance; interactive nursing skills videos; Internet; learning resource lab; library services; nursing audiovisuals; placement services for program completers; remedial services; resume preparation assistance; skills, simulation, or other laboratory; tutoring; unpaid internships.
**Library Facilities** 104,636 volumes (15,000 in health, 1,500 in nursing); 252 periodical subscriptions (40 health-care related).

## BACCALAUREATE PROGRAMS

**Degree** BSN
**Available Programs** Generic Baccalaureate; International Nurse to Baccalaureate; LPN to Baccalaureate.
**Study Options** Full-time and part-time.
**Program Entrance Requirements** Minimum overall college GPA of 2.75, transcript of college record, CPR certification, written essay, health exam, health insurance, high school biology, high school chemistry, 2 years high school math, 2 years high school science, high school transcript, immunizations, minimum high school GPA of 2.75, minimum GPA in nursing prerequisites of 2.5, professional liability insurance/malpractice insurance. Transfer students are accepted. *Application deadline:* Applications may be processed on a rolling basis for some programs. *Application fee:* $25.
**Advanced Placement** Credit by examination available. Credit given for nursing courses completed elsewhere dependent upon specific evaluations.
**Contact** *Telephone:* 302-736-2511. *Fax:* 302-736-2548.

## GRADUATE PROGRAMS

**Contact** *Telephone:* 302-736-2512. *Fax:* 302-736-2548.

**MASTER'S DEGREE PROGRAM**
**Degree** MSN
**Available Programs** Accelerated AD/RN to Master's; Accelerated RN to Master's; Master's; RN to Master's.
**Concentrations Available** *Clinical nurse specialist programs in:* community health,women's health. *Nurse practitioner programs in:*women's health.
**Site Options** New Castle, DE.
**Study Options** Full-time and part-time.
**Program Entrance Requirements** Clinical experience, computer literacy, minimum overall college GPA of 3.0, transcript of college record, interview, 2 letters of recommendation, professional liability insurance/malpractice insurance, resume, statistics course, GRE or MAT. *Application deadline:* Applications may be processed on a rolling basis for some programs. *Application fee:* $35.
**Advanced Placement** Credit by examination available. Credit given for nursing courses completed elsewhere dependent upon specific evaluations.
**Degree Requirements** 39 total credit hours, thesis or project.

**POST-MASTER'S PROGRAM**
**Areas of Study** Nursing education. *Clinical nurse specialist programs in:*women's health.

## CONTINUING EDUCATION PROGRAM

**Contact** *Telephone:* 302-736-2512. *Fax:* 302-736-2548.

# Wilmington University

## College of Health Professions
## New Castle, Delaware

*http://www.wilmu.edu/health/index.aspx*
Founded in 1967

**DEGREES • BSN • MSN • MSN/MBA • MSN/MS**
**Nursing Program Faculty** 13 (50% with doctorates).
**Baccalaureate Enrollment** 620 **Women** 95% **Men** 5% **Minority** 8% **Part-time** 88%
**Graduate Enrollment** 253 **Women** 97% **Men** 3% **Minority** 11% **Part-time** 50%
**Distance Learning Courses** Available.
**Nursing Student Activities** Sigma Theta Tau.
**Nursing Student Resources** Academic advising; academic or career counseling; assistance for students with disabilities; bookstore; campus computer network; career placement assistance; computer lab; computer-assisted instruction; e-mail services; employment services for current students; housing assistance; interactive nursing skills videos; learning resource lab; library services; nursing audiovisuals; remedial services; resume preparation assistance; skills, simulation, or other laboratory; tutoring.
**Library Facilities** 98,713 volumes (6,000 in health, 3,500 in nursing); 425 periodical subscriptions (60 health-care related).

## BACCALAUREATE PROGRAMS

**Degree** BSN
**Available Programs** Accelerated RN Baccalaureate; International Nurse to Baccalaureate; RN Baccalaureate.
**Site Options** Georgetown, DE; New Castle, DE; Dover, DE.
**Online Degree Options** Yes.
**Program Entrance Requirements** Transfer students are accepted. *Application deadline:* 8/31 (fall), 1/1 (spring), 5/1 (summer). Applications may be processed on a rolling basis for some programs. *Application fee:* $35.
**Contact** *Telephone:* 302-356-6915. *Fax:* 302-322-7081.

## GRADUATE PROGRAMS

**Contact** *Telephone:* 302-295-1121.

**MASTER'S DEGREE PROGRAM**
**Degrees** MSN; MSN/MBA; MSN/MS
**Available Programs** Accelerated AD/RN to Master's; Accelerated Master's for Nurses with Non-Nursing Degrees; Master's.
**Concentrations Available** Legal nurse consultant; nursing administration; nursing education. *Nurse practitioner programs in:* adult health, family health, gerontology.
**Site Options** Georgetown, DE; New Castle, DE.
**Study Options** Full-time and part-time.
**Online Degree Options** Yes.
**Program Entrance Requirements** Minimum overall college GPA of 3.0, transcript of college record, prerequisite course work. *Application deadline:* Applications may be processed on a rolling basis for some programs. *Application fee:* $35.
**Advanced Placement** Credit given for nursing courses completed elsewhere dependent upon specific evaluations.
**Degree Requirements** 36 total credit hours, thesis or project.

**POST-MASTER'S PROGRAM**
**Areas of Study** Legal nurse consultant; nursing administration; nursing education. *Nurse practitioner programs in:* adult health, family health, gerontology.

# DISTRICT OF COLUMBIA

# The Catholic University of America

## School of Nursing
## Washington, District of Columbia

*http://www.cua.edu/*
Founded in 1887

**DEGREES • BSN • MA/MSM • MSN • PHD**
**Nursing Program Faculty** 47 (43% with doctorates).
**Baccalaureate Enrollment** 286 **Women** 94% **Men** 6% **Minority** 16% **International** 1% **Part-time** 1%
**Graduate Enrollment** 102 **Women** 96% **Men** 4% **Minority** 35% **International** 1% **Part-time** 69%
**Distance Learning Courses** Available.
**Nursing Student Activities** Nursing Honor Society, Sigma Theta Tau, Student Nurses' Association, nursing club.
**Nursing Student Resources** Academic advising; academic or career counseling; assistance for students with disabilities; bookstore; campus computer network; career placement assistance; computer lab; computer-assisted instruction; e-mail services; interactive nursing skills videos; Internet; learning resource lab; library services; nursing audiovisuals; remedial services; resume preparation assistance; skills, simulation, or other laboratory; tutoring.
**Library Facilities** 1.7 million volumes (39,000 in health, 17,500 in nursing); 8,418 periodical subscriptions (250 health-care related).

## BACCALAUREATE PROGRAMS

**Degree** BSN
**Available Programs** Accelerated Baccalaureate; Accelerated Baccalaureate for Second Degree; Generic Baccalaureate.
**Study Options** Full-time and part-time.
**Program Entrance Requirements** Minimum overall college GPA of 3.0, transcript of college record, written essay, health exam, health insurance, high school chemistry, 3 years high school math, high school transcript, immunizations, 1 letter of recommendation, minimum high school GPA of 3.0, minimum GPA in nursing prerequisites of 2.75, prerequisite course work. *Application deadline:* 7/15 (fall), 11/15 (spring), 2/28 (summer). *Application fee:* $55.
**Contact** *Telephone:* 202-319-6457. *Fax:* 202-319-6485.

## GRADUATE PROGRAMS

**Contact** *Telephone:* 202-319-5403. *Fax:* 202-319-5403.

**MASTER'S DEGREE PROGRAM**
**Degrees** MA/MSM; MSN
**Available Programs** Master's.
**Concentrations Available** *Clinical nurse specialist programs in:* adult health, community health. *Nurse practitioner programs in:* acute care, adult health, family health, pediatric.
**Site Options** Washington, DC.
**Study Options** Full-time and part-time.
**Program Entrance Requirements** Clinical experience, minimum overall college GPA of 3.0, transcript of college record, written essay, immunizations, 3 letters of recommendation, professional liability insurance/malpractice insurance, prerequisite course work, statistics course, GRE General Test. *Application deadline:* 8/1 (fall), 12/1

(spring). Applications may be processed on a rolling basis for some programs. *Application fee:* $55.
**Advanced Placement** Credit given for nursing courses completed elsewhere dependent upon specific evaluations.
**Degree Requirements** 44 total credit hours, comprehensive exam.

### POST-MASTER'S PROGRAM
**Areas of Study** *Clinical nurse specialist programs in:* adult health, community health. *Nurse practitioner programs in:* acute care, adult health, family health, pediatric.

### DOCTORAL DEGREE PROGRAM
**Degree** PhD
**Available Programs** Doctorate; Post-Baccalaureate Doctorate.
**Areas of Study** Advanced practice nursing, clinical practice, community health, ethics, gerontology, human health and illness, nursing research, nursing science,women's health.
**Online Degree Options** Yes.
**Program Entrance Requirements** Clinical experience, minimum overall college GPA of 3.5, interview by faculty committee, interview, 3 letters of recommendation, MSN or equivalent, scholarly papers, statistics course, writing sample, GRE General Test. *Application deadline:* 8/1 (fall), 12/1 (spring). Applications may be processed on a rolling basis for some programs. *Application fee:* $55.
**Degree Requirements** 70 total credit hours, dissertation, oral exam, written exam, residency.

# Georgetown University
## School of Nursing and Health Studies
## Washington, District of Columbia

***http://nhs.georgetown.edu/***
Founded in 1789

### DEGREES • BSN • DNP • MS
**Nursing Program Faculty** 222 (54% with doctorates).
**Baccalaureate Enrollment** 184 **Women** 94.1% **Men** 5.9% **Minority** 16.3% **International** 1%
**Graduate Enrollment** 935 **Women** 93.7% **Men** 6.3% **Minority** 23.7% **International** 2.67% **Part-time** 80%
**Distance Learning Courses** Available.
**Nursing Student Activities** Nursing Honor Society, Sigma Theta Tau, Student Nurses' Association.
**Nursing Student Resources** Academic advising; academic or career counseling; assistance for students with disabilities; bookstore; campus computer network; career placement assistance; computer lab; computer-assisted instruction; e-mail services; employment services for current students; externships; housing assistance; interactive nursing skills videos; Internet; learning resource lab; library services; nursing audiovisuals; placement services for program completers; resume preparation assistance; skills, simulation, or other laboratory; tutoring; unpaid internships.

### BACCALAUREATE PROGRAMS
**Degree** BSN
**Available Programs** Accelerated Baccalaureate for Second Degree; Generic Baccalaureate.
**Study Options** Full-time.
**Program Entrance Requirements** CPR certification, written essay, health exam, health insurance, 3 years high school math, 4 years high school science, high school transcript, immunizations, interview, 2 letters of recommendation. Transfer students are accepted. *Application deadline:* 1/10 (fall). *Application fee:* $65.
**Expenses (2013–14)** *Tuition:* full-time $44,280. *International tuition:* $44,280 full-time.
**Financial Aid** 70% of baccalaureate students in nursing programs received some form of financial aid in 2012–13. *Gift aid (need-based):* Federal Pell, FSEOG, state, private, college/university gift aid from institutional funds. *Loans:* Federal Nursing Student Loans, Federal Direct (Subsidized and Unsubsidized Stafford PLUS), Perkins, alternative loans. *Work-study:* Federal Work-Study. *Financial aid application deadline:* 2/1.
**Contact** Office of Undergraduate Admissions, School of Nursing and Health Studies, Georgetown University, 37th and O Street NW, Washington, DC 20057. *Telephone:* 202-687-3600.

### GRADUATE PROGRAMS
**Expenses (2013–14)** *Tuition:* part-time $1756 per credit hour.
**Financial Aid** 70% of graduate students in nursing programs received some form of financial aid in 2012–13. Scholarships and traineeships available.
**Contact** Office of Graduate Admissions, School of Nursing and Health Studies, Georgetown University, 37th and O Street NW, Washington, DC 20057. *Telephone:* 202-687-5568.

### MASTER'S DEGREE PROGRAM
**Degree** MS
**Available Programs** Master's.
**Concentrations Available** Health-care administration; nurse anesthesia; nurse-midwifery. *Nurse practitioner programs in:* acute care, family health,women's health.
**Study Options** Full-time and part-time.
**Online Degree Options** Yes (online only).
**Program Entrance Requirements** Clinical experience, minimum overall college GPA of 3.0, transcript of college record, CPR certification, written essay, immunizations, interview, 3 letters of recommendation, resume, statistics course, GRE General Test or MAT.
**Advanced Placement** Credit given for nursing courses completed elsewhere dependent upon specific evaluations.
**Degree Requirements** Thesis or project.

### DOCTORAL DEGREE PROGRAM
**Degree** DNP
**Available Programs** Doctorate.
**Program Entrance Requirements** Clinical experience, minimum overall college GPA of 3.3, interview by faculty committee, 3 letters of recommendation, MSN or equivalent, vita. *Application deadline:* 4/15 (fall). Applications may be processed on a rolling basis for some programs.
**Degree Requirements** 38 total credit hours.

# The George Washington University
## School of Nursing
## Washington, District of Columbia

Founded in 1821

### DEGREES • BSN • DNP • MSN
**Distance Learning Courses** Available.
**Nursing Student Activities** Sigma Theta Tau.
**Nursing Student Resources** Academic advising; academic or career counseling; bookstore; campus computer network; computer lab; computer-assisted instruction; e-mail services; interactive nursing skills videos; Internet; learning resource lab; library services; nursing audiovisuals; skills, simulation, or other laboratory.

### BACCALAUREATE PROGRAMS
**Degree** BSN
**Available Programs** Accelerated Baccalaureate for Second Degree.
**Study Options** Full-time.
**Program Entrance Requirements** Minimum overall college GPA of 2.8, transcript of college record, CPR certification, written essay, health exam, health insurance, immunizations, 2 letters of recommendation, minimum GPA in nursing prerequisites of 3.0, prerequisite course work. *Application deadline:* 6/15 (fall). *Application fee:* $60.
**Contact** *Telephone:* 202-994-7901. *Fax:* 202-994-2777.

### GRADUATE PROGRAMS
**Contact** *Telephone:* 202-994-7901. *Fax:* 202-994-2777.

### MASTER'S DEGREE PROGRAM
**Degree** MSN
**Available Programs** Master's.
**Concentrations Available** Clinical nurse leader; health-care administration; nursing administration. *Nurse practitioner programs in:* adult health, family health.

### POST-MASTER'S PROGRAM
**Areas of Study** *Nurse practitioner programs in:* adult health, family health.

### DOCTORAL DEGREE PROGRAM
**Degree** DNP
**Available Programs** Doctorate.

# Howard University
## Division of Nursing
## Washington, District of Columbia

***http://huhealthcare.com/education/schools-and-academics/nursing-allied-health/division-of-nursing***
Founded in 1867

**DEGREES • BSN • MSN**
**Nursing Program Faculty** 29 (62% with doctorates).
**Baccalaureate Enrollment** 253 **Women** 90% **Men** 10% **Minority** 99% **International** 4% **Part-time** 10%
**Graduate Enrollment** 40 **Women** 87% **Men** 13% **Minority** 100% **International** 10% **Part-time** 45%
**Distance Learning Courses** Available.
**Nursing Student Activities** Nursing Honor Society, Sigma Theta Tau, Student Nurses' Association, nursing club.
**Nursing Student Resources** Academic advising; academic or career counseling; assistance for students with disabilities; bookstore; campus computer network; career placement assistance; computer lab; computer-assisted instruction; e-mail services; externships; housing assistance; interactive nursing skills videos; Internet; learning resource lab; library services; nursing audiovisuals; paid internships; placement services for program completers; remedial services; resume preparation assistance; skills, simulation, or other laboratory; tutoring.
**Library Facilities** 2.5 million volumes (219,448 in health, 4,500 in nursing); 26,382 periodical subscriptions (5,247 health-care related).

### BACCALAUREATE PROGRAMS

**Degree** BSN
**Available Programs** Generic Baccalaureate; LPN to Baccalaureate; RN Baccalaureate.
**Study Options** Full-time and part-time.
**Online Degree Options** Yes.
**Program Entrance Requirements** Minimum overall college GPA of 2.8, transcript of college record, written essay, health exam, high school biology, high school chemistry, high school foreign language, 3 years high school math, 2 years high school science, high school transcript, immunizations, 2 letters of recommendation, minimum high school GPA of 2.5, minimum high school rank 50%, minimum GPA in nursing prerequisites of 2.5, prerequisite course work. Transfer students are accepted. *Application deadline:* 2/15 (fall), 11/1 (spring), 4/1 (summer). Applications may be processed on a rolling basis for some programs. *Application fee:* $45.
**Expenses (2013–14)** *Tuition:* full-time $21,450; part-time $895 per credit. *Room and board:* $6522; room only: $4608 per academic year. *Required fees:* full-time $1433; part-time $717 per term.
**Financial Aid** 92% of baccalaureate students in nursing programs received some form of financial aid in 2012–13. *Gift aid (need-based):* Federal Pell, FSEOG, state, private, college/university gift aid from institutional funds, Federal Nursing. *Loans:* Federal Nursing Student Loans, Federal Direct (Subsidized and Unsubsidized Stafford PLUS), Perkins, state, college/university. *Work-study:* Federal Work-Study, part-time campus jobs. *Financial aid application deadline:* 8/15(priority: 2/1).
**Contact** Miss Melissa L. Weir, Interim Chairperson, Undergraduate Program, Division of Nursing, Howard University, 516 Bryant Street NW, Annex 1, Washington, DC 20059. *Telephone:* 202-806-7854. *Fax:* 202-806-5085. *E-mail:* melissa.weir@howard.edu.

### GRADUATE PROGRAMS

**Expenses (2013–14)** *Tuition:* full-time $32,378; part-time $1700 per credit hour. *Room and board:* $6522; room only: $4608 per academic year. *Required fees:* full-time $2533; part-time $1267 per term.
**Financial Aid** 16% of graduate students in nursing programs received some form of financial aid in 2012–13. Teaching assistantships (averaging $16,000 per year); career-related internships or fieldwork, institutionally sponsored loans, and scholarships also available. *Financial aid application deadline:* 4/1.
**Contact** Dr. Tammi L. Damas, Interim Chairperson, Graduate Program, Division of Nursing, Howard University, 516 Bryant Street NW, Annex 1, Washington, DC 20059. *Telephone:* 202-806-7460. *Fax:* 202-806-5085. *E-mail:* Tammi.damas@howard.edu.

#### MASTER'S DEGREE PROGRAM

**Degree** MSN
**Available Programs** Master's.
**Concentrations Available** Nursing education. *Nurse practitioner programs in:* family health.
**Study Options** Full-time and part-time.
**Program Entrance Requirements** Clinical experience, minimum overall college GPA of 3.0, transcript of college record, written essay, interview, 3 letters of recommendation, resume, statistics course. *Application deadline:* Applications may be processed on a rolling basis for some programs. *Application fee:* $45.
**Advanced Placement** Credit given for nursing courses completed elsewhere dependent upon specific evaluations.
**Degree Requirements** 46 total credit hours, thesis or project.

#### POST-MASTER'S PROGRAM

**Areas of Study** Nursing education. *Nurse practitioner programs in:* family health.

# Trinity Washington University
## Nursing Program
## Washington, District of Columbia

Founded in 1897

**DEGREE • BSN**
**Nursing Program Faculty** 9 (4% with doctorates).
**Baccalaureate Enrollment** 80
**Nursing Student Activities** Sigma Theta Tau, Student Nurses' Association.
**Nursing Student Resources** Academic advising; academic or career counseling; assistance for students with disabilities; bookstore; campus computer network; career placement assistance; computer lab; computer-assisted instruction; e-mail services; employment services for current students; housing assistance; Internet; learning resource lab; library services; nursing audiovisuals; paid internships; remedial services; resume preparation assistance; skills, simulation, or other laboratory; tutoring; unpaid internships.
**Library Facilities** 207,000 volumes (1,200 in health, 200 in nursing); 498 periodical subscriptions (40 health-care related).

### BACCALAUREATE PROGRAMS

**Degree** BSN
**Available Programs** Generic Baccalaureate; RN Baccalaureate.
**Study Options** Full-time and part-time.
**Program Entrance Requirements** Transcript of college record, CPR certification, written essay, health exam, health insurance, high school transcript, immunizations, interview, 1 letter of recommendation, minimum GPA in nursing prerequisites of 2.0, professional liability insurance/malpractice insurance, prerequisite course work, RN licensure. Transfer students are accepted. *Application deadline:* Applications may be processed on a rolling basis for some programs.
**Advanced Placement** Credit by examination available. Credit given for nursing courses completed elsewhere dependent upon specific evaluations.
**Contact** *Telephone:* 202-884-9245. *Fax:* 202-884-9308.

# University of the District of Columbia
## Nursing Education Program
## Washington, District of Columbia

Founded in 1976

**DEGREE • BSN**
**Nursing Program Faculty** 6 (3% with doctorates).
**Baccalaureate Enrollment** 40 **Women** 97% **Men** 3% **Minority** 98% **International** 50% **Part-time** 50%
**Nursing Student Activities** Student Nurses' Association.
**Nursing Student Resources** Academic advising; academic or career counseling; assistance for students with disabilities; bookstore; campus computer network; career placement assistance; computer lab; computer-assisted instruction; daycare for children of students; e-mail services; employment services for current students; Internet; learning resource lab; library services; nursing audiovisuals; remedial services; resume preparation assistance; skills, simulation, or other laboratory; tutoring.

**Library Facilities** 554,412 volumes (500 in health, 250 in nursing); 647 periodical subscriptions (75 health-care related).

## BACCALAUREATE PROGRAMS

**Degree** BSN
**Available Programs** RN Baccalaureate.
**Site Options** Washington, DC.
**Study Options** Full-time and part-time.
**Program Entrance Requirements** Minimum overall college GPA of 2.7, transcript of college record, CPR certification, written essay, health exam, health insurance, immunizations, 2 letters of recommendation, minimum GPA in nursing prerequisites of 2.7, professional liability insurance/malpractice insurance, prerequisite course work, RN licensure. Transfer students are accepted. *Application deadline:* 6/15 (fall), 11/15 (spring), 4/15 (summer).
**Advanced Placement** Credit by examination available. Credit given for nursing courses completed elsewhere dependent upon specific evaluations.
**Contact** *Telephone:* 202-274-5916. *Fax:* 202-274-5952.

# FLORIDA

## Adventist University of Health Sciences

### Department of Nursing
### Orlando, Florida

Founded in 1913

**DEGREE • BSN**
**Nursing Program Faculty** 21 (23% with doctorates).
**Baccalaureate Enrollment** 562
**Distance Learning Courses** Available.
**Nursing Student Activities** Nursing Honor Society, Student Nurses' Association.
**Nursing Student Resources** Academic advising; academic or career counseling; bookstore; campus computer network; computer lab; computer-assisted instruction; e-mail services; interactive nursing skills videos; Internet; learning resource lab; library services; nursing audiovisuals; skills, simulation, or other laboratory; tutoring.
**Library Facilities** 77,755 volumes; 220 periodical subscriptions.

## BACCALAUREATE PROGRAMS

**Degree** BSN
**Available Programs** Generic Baccalaureate; RN Baccalaureate.
**Study Options** Full-time and part-time.
**Online Degree Options** Yes (online only).
**Program Entrance Requirements** Minimum overall college GPA of 3.0, transcript of college record, CPR certification, written essay, health exam, high school transcript, immunizations, 2 letters of recommendation, minimum high school GPA of 3.0, prerequisite course work, RN licensure. Transfer students are accepted. *Application deadline:* 4/15 (fall).
**Advanced Placement** Credit by examination available. Credit given for nursing courses completed elsewhere dependent upon specific evaluations.
**Contact** *Telephone:* 407-303-5762. *Fax:* 407-303-1872.

## Barry University

### Division of Nursing
### Miami Shores, Florida

***http://www.barry.edu/nursing***
Founded in 1940

**DEGREES • BSN • MSN • MSN/MBA • PHD**
**Nursing Program Faculty** 30 (50% with doctorates).
**Baccalaureate Enrollment** 431 **Women** 87% **Men** 13% **Minority** 51% **International** 2% **Part-time** 20%
**Graduate Enrollment** 161 **Women** 93% **Men** 7% **Minority** 51% **International** 1% **Part-time** 99%
**Nursing Student Activities** Sigma Theta Tau, Student Nurses' Association.
**Nursing Student Resources** Academic advising; academic or career counseling; assistance for students with disabilities; bookstore; campus computer network; career placement assistance; computer lab; computer-assisted instruction; e-mail services; employment services for current students; housing assistance; interactive nursing skills videos; Internet; learning resource lab; library services; nursing audiovisuals; paid internships; remedial services; resume preparation assistance; skills, simulation, or other laboratory; tutoring.
**Library Facilities** 352,609 volumes (15,000 in health, 8,500 in nursing); 400 periodical subscriptions health-care related.

## BACCALAUREATE PROGRAMS

**Degree** BSN
**Available Programs** ADN to Baccalaureate; Accelerated Baccalaureate; Accelerated Baccalaureate for Second Degree; Baccalaureate for Second Degree; Generic Baccalaureate; LPN to Baccalaureate; LPN to RN Baccalaureate; RN Baccalaureate.
**Site Options** Kendall, FL.
**Study Options** Full-time and part-time.
**Program Entrance Requirements** Minimum overall college GPA of 3.0, transcript of college record, CPR certification, health exam, health insurance, high school biology, high school chemistry, high school math, high school science, high school transcript, immunizations, 2 letters of recommendation, minimum high school GPA of 3.0, minimum GPA in nursing prerequisites of 3.0, professional liability insurance/malpractice insurance. Transfer students are accepted. *Application deadline:* Applications may be processed on a rolling basis for some programs. *Application fee:* $30.
**Advanced Placement** Credit given for nursing courses completed elsewhere dependent upon specific evaluations.
**Expenses (2012–13)** *Tuition:* full-time $28,160; part-time $845 per credit.
**Financial Aid** 90% of baccalaureate students in nursing programs received some form of financial aid in 2011–12. *Gift aid (need-based):* Federal Pell, FSEOG, state, private, college/university gift aid from institutional funds, Federal Nursing. *Loans:* Federal Nursing Student Loans, Perkins, college/university, alternative loans. *Work-study:* Federal Work-Study, part-time campus jobs. *Financial aid application deadline:* Continuous.
**Contact** Ms. Rosanne Sonshine, Recruiter and Clinical Coordinator, Division of Nursing, Barry University, 11300 NE Second Avenue, Miami Shores, FL 33161-6695. *Telephone:* 305-899-3813. *Fax:* 305-899-3831. *E-mail:* rsonshine@mail.barry.edu.

## GRADUATE PROGRAMS

**Expenses (2012–13)** *Tuition:* part-time $935 per credit.
**Financial Aid** 90% of graduate students in nursing programs received some form of financial aid in 2011–12. 3 research assistantships (averaging $5,000 per year), 3 teaching assistantships (averaging $5,000 per year) were awarded; scholarships and tuition waivers (full) also available. *Financial aid application deadline:* 5/1.
**Contact** Ms. Kelley Eddington, Operations Manager, Division of Nursing, Barry University, 11300 NE Second Avenue, Miami Shores, FL 33161-6695. *Telephone:* 305-899-3814. *Fax:* 305-899-3831. *E-mail:* keddington@mail.barry.edu.

### MASTER'S DEGREE PROGRAM

**Degrees** MSN; MSN/MBA
**Available Programs** Master's.
**Concentrations Available** Nursing administration; nursing education. *Nurse practitioner programs in:* acute care, family health.
**Site Options** Kendall, FL.
**Study Options** Part-time.
**Program Entrance Requirements** Clinical experience, computer literacy, minimum overall college GPA of 3.0, transcript of college record, written essay, 2 letters of recommendation, nursing research course, professional liability insurance/malpractice insurance, statistics course, GRE General Test or MAT. *Application deadline:* Applications may be processed on a rolling basis for some programs.
**Advanced Placement** Credit given for nursing courses completed elsewhere dependent upon specific evaluations.
**Degree Requirements** 45 total credit hours.

### POST-MASTER'S PROGRAM

**Areas of Study** Nursing administration; nursing education. *Nurse practitioner programs in:* acute care, family health.

**DOCTORAL DEGREE PROGRAM**
**Degree** PhD
**Available Programs** Doctorate.
**Areas of Study** Nursing research, nursing science.
**Site Options** Orlando, FL; Kendall, FL; Palm Beach, FL.
**Program Entrance Requirements** Clinical experience, minimum overall college GPA of 3.0, interview, 2 letters of recommendation, MSN or equivalent, statistics course, writing sample, GRE General Test or MAT. *Application deadline:* Applications may be processed on a rolling basis for some programs.
**Degree Requirements** 45 total credit hours, dissertation, written exam, residency.

# Bethune-Cookman University
## School of Nursing
## Daytona Beach, Florida

*http://www.cookman.edu/academics/schools/sn/index.html*
Founded in 1904
**DEGREE • BSN**
**Nursing Program Faculty** 11 (2% with doctorates).
**Baccalaureate Enrollment** 137 **Women** 93% **Men** 7% **Minority** 95% **International** 2%
**Nursing Student Activities** Nursing Honor Society, Student Nurses' Association.
**Nursing Student Resources** Academic advising; bookstore; campus computer network; computer lab; computer-assisted instruction; e-mail services; interactive nursing skills videos; Internet; learning resource lab; library services; nursing audiovisuals; resume preparation assistance; skills, simulation, or other laboratory; tutoring; unpaid internships.
**Library Facilities** 149,194 volumes; 91 periodical subscriptions.

### BACCALAUREATE PROGRAMS
**Degree** BSN
**Available Programs** Generic Baccalaureate; RN Baccalaureate.
**Study Options** Full-time.
**Program Entrance Requirements** Minimum overall college GPA of 2.8, transcript of college record, CPR certification, written essay, health exam, high school transcript, immunizations, interview, 2 letters of recommendation, minimum GPA in nursing prerequisites of 2.8, prerequisite course work. Transfer students are accepted.
**Advanced Placement** Credit by examination available. Credit given for nursing courses completed elsewhere dependent upon specific evaluations.
**Contact** *Telephone:* 386-481-2000.

# Broward College
## Nursing Program
## Fort Lauderdale, Florida

Founded in 1960
**DEGREE • BSN**

### BACCALAUREATE PROGRAMS
**Degree** BSN
**Available Programs** RN Baccalaureate.
**Program Entrance Requirements** Minimum overall college GPA of 2.5, RN licensure.
**Contact** RN-BSN Program Office, Nursing Program, Broward College, Building 9, Room 200, 3501 Davie Road, Davie, FL 33314. *Telephone:* 954-201-4880. *E-mail:* bsn@broward.edu.

# Edison State College
## Bachelor of Science in Nursing Program
## Fort Myers, Florida

Founded in 1962
**DEGREE • BSN**
**Library Facilities** 181,085 volumes.

### BACCALAUREATE PROGRAMS
**Degree** BSN
**Available Programs** RN Baccalaureate.
**Program Entrance Requirements** Minimum overall college GPA of 2.0, transcript of college record, prerequisite course work, RN licensure. *Application deadline:* 8/1 (fall), 12/1 (spring), 4/1 (summer).
**Contact** Admissions Office, Bachelor of Science in Nursing Program, Edison State College, 8099 College Parkway, Fort Myers, FL 33919. *Telephone:* 800-749-2322. *E-mail:* admissions@edison.edu.

# Florida Agricultural and Mechanical University
## School of Nursing
## Tallahassee, Florida

*http://www.famu.edu/index.cfm?a=nursing*
Founded in 1887
**DEGREES • BSN • MSN • PHD**
**Nursing Program Faculty** 28 (18% with doctorates).
**Baccalaureate Enrollment** 161 **Women** 90% **Men** 10% **Minority** 98%
**Graduate Enrollment** 17 **Women** 83% **Men** 17% **Minority** 76% **Part-time** 12%
**Nursing Student Activities** Sigma Theta Tau, Student Nurses' Association.
**Nursing Student Resources** Academic advising; academic or career counseling; bookstore; campus computer network; career placement assistance; computer lab; computer-assisted instruction; daycare for children of students; e-mail services; employment services for current students; externships; interactive nursing skills videos; Internet; library services; nursing audiovisuals; placement services for program completers; remedial services; resume preparation assistance; skills, simulation, or other laboratory; tutoring.
**Library Facilities** 1.1 million volumes (5,000 in health, 4,091 in nursing); 201,405 periodical subscriptions (385 health-care related).

### BACCALAUREATE PROGRAMS
**Degree** BSN
**Available Programs** Generic Baccalaureate.
**Study Options** Part-time.
**Program Entrance Requirements** CPR certification, health exam, immunizations, 3 letters of recommendation, minimum high school GPA of 2.5, prerequisite course work. Transfer students are accepted.
**Contact** *Telephone:* 850-599-3458. *Fax:* 850-599-3508.

### GRADUATE PROGRAMS
**Contact** *Telephone:* 850-599-3017. *Fax:* 850-599-3508.

**MASTER'S DEGREE PROGRAM**
**Degree** MSN
**Available Programs** Master's.
**Concentrations Available** *Nurse practitioner programs in:* adult health, gerontology,women's health.
**Study Options** Full-time and part-time.
**Program Entrance Requirements** Clinical experience, minimum overall college GPA of 3.0, CPR certification, immunizations, interview, nursing research course, physical assessment course, professional liability insurance/malpractice insurance, statistics course.
**Degree Requirements** 42 total credit hours, thesis or project.

**POST-MASTER'S PROGRAM**
**Areas of Study** *Nurse practitioner programs in:* adult health, gerontology,women's health.

**DOCTORAL DEGREE PROGRAM**
**Degree** PhD
**Program Entrance Requirements** Minimum overall college GPA of 3.5, 3 letters of recommendation, MSN or equivalent.
**Degree Requirements** 90 total credit hours, dissertation, oral exam, written exam.

### CONTINUING EDUCATION PROGRAM
**Contact** *Telephone:* 850-599-3017. *Fax:* 850-599-3508.

# Florida Atlantic University
## Christine E. Lynn College of Nursing
## Boca Raton, Florida

***http://nursing.fau.edu/***
Founded in 1961

**DEGREES • BSN • DNP • MSN**
**Nursing Program Faculty** 61 (70% with doctorates).
**Baccalaureate Enrollment** 531 **Women** 90% **Men** 10% **Minority** 42% **International** 2% **Part-time** 54%
**Graduate Enrollment** 395 **Women** 92% **Men** 8% **Minority** 48% **International** 5% **Part-time** 58%
**Distance Learning Courses** Available.
**Nursing Student Activities** Sigma Theta Tau, Student Nurses' Association, nursing club.
**Nursing Student Resources** Academic advising; academic or career counseling; assistance for students with disabilities; bookstore; campus computer network; computer lab; computer-assisted instruction; e-mail services; housing assistance; interactive nursing skills videos; Internet; learning resource lab; library services; nursing audiovisuals; remedial services; skills, simulation, or other laboratory; tutoring.
**Library Facilities** 1.3 million volumes (28,670 in health, 5,749 in nursing); 12,811 periodical subscriptions (903 health-care related).

### BACCALAUREATE PROGRAMS

**Degree** BSN
**Available Programs** Accelerated Baccalaureate for Second Degree; Generic Baccalaureate; RN Baccalaureate.
**Site Options** Davie, FL; Fort Pierce, FL.
**Study Options** Full-time.
**Online Degree Options** Yes (online only).
**Program Entrance Requirements** Minimum overall college GPA of 3.0, transcript of college record, CPR certification, health exam, health insurance, high school transcript, immunizations, interview, minimum GPA in nursing prerequisites of 2.0, prerequisite course work. Transfer students are accepted. *Application deadline:* 1/15 (winter). *Application fee:* $30.
**Expenses (2013–14)** *Tuition, area resident:* full-time $3152; part-time $105 per credit hour. *Tuition, state resident:* full-time $3152; part-time $200 per credit hour. *Tuition, nonresident:* full-time $17,915; part-time $597 per credit hour. *International tuition:* $17,915 full-time. *Room and board:* $10,940; room only: $7404 per academic year. *Required fees:* full-time $2834; part-time $94 per credit.
**Financial Aid** 80% of baccalaureate students in nursing programs received some form of financial aid in 2012–13. *Gift aid (need-based):* Federal Pell, FSEOG, state, private, college/university gift aid from institutional funds, Federal Nursing. *Loans:* Federal Direct (Subsidized and Unsubsidized Stafford PLUS), Perkins, college/university. *Work-study:* Federal Work-Study, part-time campus jobs. *Financial aid application deadline (priority):* 3/1.
**Contact** Dr. Nancey Lee France, Assistant Dean of Undergraduate Programs, Christine E. Lynn College of Nursing, Florida Atlantic University, 777 Glades Road, Boca Raton, FL 33431. *Telephone:* 561-297-2535. *Fax:* 561-297-3652. *E-mail:* nfrance@fau.edu.

### GRADUATE PROGRAMS

**Expenses (2013–14)** *Tuition, area resident:* full-time $5466; part-time $304 per credit hour. *Tuition, state resident:* full-time $5467; part-time $304 per credit hour. *Tuition, nonresident:* full-time $16,695; part-time $928 per credit hour. *International tuition:* $16,695 full-time. *Room and board:* $10,940; room only: $7404 per academic year. *Required fees:* full-time $3889; part-time $216 per credit.
**Financial Aid** 20% of graduate students in nursing programs received some form of financial aid in 2012–13. Research assistantships with partial tuition reimbursements available, teaching assistantships with partial tuition reimbursements available, career-related internships or fieldwork, Federal Work-Study, institutionally sponsored loans, scholarships, and traineeships available. Aid available to part-time students.
**Contact** Dr. Shirley Gordon, Masters Program Director, Christine E. Lynn College of Nursing, Florida Atlantic University, 777 Glades Road, Boca Raton, FL 33431. *Telephone:* 561-297-3389. *Fax:* 561-297-3652. *E-mail:* sgordon@fau.edu.

#### MASTER'S DEGREE PROGRAM

**Degree** MSN
**Available Programs** Master's.
**Concentrations Available** Clinical nurse leader; nursing administration; nursing education. *Nurse practitioner programs in:* adult health, family health, gerontology, primary care.
**Site Options** Davie, FL; Fort Pierce, FL.
**Study Options** Full-time and part-time.
**Online Degree Options** Yes.
**Program Entrance Requirements** Minimum overall college GPA of 3.0, transcript of college record, CPR certification, written essay, immunizations, interview, 2 letters of recommendation, nursing research course, physical assessment course, professional liability insurance/malpractice insurance, prerequisite course work, resume, statistics course, GRE General Test. *Application deadline:* 6/1 (fall), 10/1 (spring), 2/1 (summer). *Application fee:* $30.
**Advanced Placement** Credit given for nursing courses completed elsewhere dependent upon specific evaluations.
**Degree Requirements** 39 total credit hours.

#### POST-MASTER'S PROGRAM

**Areas of Study** Clinical nurse leader; nursing administration; nursing education. *Nurse practitioner programs in:* adult health, family health, gerontology, primary care.

#### DOCTORAL DEGREE PROGRAM

**Degree** DNP
**Available Programs** Doctorate; Post-Baccalaureate Doctorate.
**Areas of Study** Advanced practice nursing, aging, family health, gerontology, health-care systems, nursing administration.
**Program Entrance Requirements** Minimum overall college GPA of 3.5, interview by faculty committee, interview, 3 letters of recommendation, scholarly papers, statistics course, vita, writing sample, GRE General Test. *Application deadline:* 11/1 (fall), 3/1 (spring). *Application fee:* $30.
**Degree Requirements** 83 total credit hours, written exam, residency.

# Florida Gulf Coast University
## School of Nursing
## Fort Myers, Florida

***http://www.fgcu.edu/chp/nursing/***
Founded in 1991

**DEGREES • BSN • MSN**
**Nursing Program Faculty** 17 (57% with doctorates).
**Baccalaureate Enrollment** 141 **Women** 89% **Men** 11% **Minority** 20.5% **Part-time** 15%
**Graduate Enrollment** 75 **Women** 88% **Men** 12% **Minority** 12% **Part-time** 10%
**Nursing Student Activities** Sigma Theta Tau, Student Nurses' Association.
**Nursing Student Resources** Academic advising; academic or career counseling; assistance for students with disabilities; bookstore; campus computer network; career placement assistance; computer lab; computer-assisted instruction; e-mail services; employment services for current students; Internet; learning resource lab; library services; nursing audiovisuals; skills, simulation, or other laboratory; tutoring.
**Library Facilities** 396,625 volumes (13,943 in health, 6,742 in nursing); 94,274 periodical subscriptions (471 health-care related).

### BACCALAUREATE PROGRAMS

**Degree** BSN
**Available Programs** Generic Baccalaureate.
**Study Options** Full-time.
**Program Entrance Requirements** Minimum overall college GPA of 3.0, transcript of college record, CPR certification, health insurance, high school foreign language, immunizations, professional liability insurance/malpractice insurance, prerequisite course work. Transfer students are accepted. *Application deadline:* 2/1 (fall), 5/15 (spring).
**Advanced Placement** Credit given for nursing courses completed elsewhere dependent upon specific evaluations.
**Contact** *Telephone:* 239-590-7454. *Fax:* 239-590-7474.

### GRADUATE PROGRAMS

**Contact** *Telephone:* 239-590-7505. *Fax:* 239-590-7474.

#### MASTER'S DEGREE PROGRAM

**Degree** MSN
**Available Programs** Master's.

**Concentrations Available** Nurse anesthesia. *Nurse practitioner programs in:* acute care, adult health, family health.
**Study Options** Full-time and part-time.
**Program Entrance Requirements** Clinical experience, minimum overall college GPA of 3.0, transcript of college record, interview, physical assessment course, resume, statistics course.
**Advanced Placement** Credit given for nursing courses completed elsewhere dependent upon specific evaluations.

**POST-MASTER'S PROGRAM**
**Areas of Study** *Nurse practitioner programs in:* acute care, family health.

### CONTINUING EDUCATION PROGRAM
**Contact** *Telephone:* 239-590-7513. *Fax:* 239-590-7474.

## Florida International University
### Nursing Program
### Miami, Florida

***http://www.fiu.edu/***
Founded in 1965

**DEGREES • BSN • DNP • MSN • PHD**
**Nursing Program Faculty** 105 (45% with doctorates).
**Baccalaureate Enrollment** 648 **Women** 73% **Men** 27% **Minority** 89% **International** 4% **Part-time** 44%
**Graduate Enrollment** 531 **Women** 66% **Men** 34% **Minority** 75% **International** 8% **Part-time** 62%
**Distance Learning Courses** Available.
**Nursing Student Activities** Sigma Theta Tau, Student Nurses' Association.
**Nursing Student Resources** Academic advising; academic or career counseling; assistance for students with disabilities; bookstore; campus computer network; career placement assistance; computer lab; computer-assisted instruction; daycare for children of students; e-mail services; externships; housing assistance; interactive nursing skills videos; Internet; learning resource lab; library services; nursing audiovisuals; paid internships; remedial services; resume preparation assistance; skills, simulation, or other laboratory; tutoring.
**Library Facilities** 2 million volumes (35,000 in health, 3,800 in nursing); 149,685 periodical subscriptions (1,700 health-care related).

### BACCALAUREATE PROGRAMS
**Degree** BSN
**Available Programs** Accelerated Baccalaureate for Second Degree; Generic Baccalaureate; RN Baccalaureate.
**Site Options** North Miami, FL.
**Study Options** Full-time.
**Online Degree Options** Yes.
**Program Entrance Requirements** Minimum overall college GPA of 3.25, transcript of college record, CPR certification, written essay, health exam, health insurance, high school foreign language, high school transcript, immunizations, minimum GPA in nursing prerequisites of 3.25, prerequisite course work. Transfer students are accepted. *Application deadline:* 3/15 (fall). *Application fee:* $30.
**Advanced Placement** Credit by examination available. Credit given for nursing courses completed elsewhere dependent upon specific evaluations.
**Expenses (2013–14)** *Tuition, state resident:* full-time $6892; part-time $1540 per semester. *Tuition, nonresident:* full-time $24,994; part-time $5582 per semester. *Room and board:* $16,000; room only: $14,000 per academic year. *Required fees:* full-time $2025; part-time $1357 per credit; part-time $455 per term.
**Financial Aid** 75% of baccalaureate students in nursing programs received some form of financial aid in 2012–13.
**Contact** Diane M. Loffredo, Director for Admissions and Student Services, Nursing Program, Florida International University, 11200 SW 8th Street, Modesto A. Maidique Campus, HLS 2, RM 482, Miami, FL 33199. *Telephone:* 305-348-7717. *Fax:* 305-348-7764. *E-mail:* dloffred@fiu.edu.

### GRADUATE PROGRAMS
**Expenses (2013–14)** *Tuition, state resident:* full-time $10,489; part-time $2343 per semester. *Tuition, nonresident:* full-time $20,811; part-time $4648 per semester. *Room and board:* $16,000; room only: $14,000 per academic year. *Required fees:* full-time $1817; part-time $1217 per credit; part-time $486 per term.
**Financial Aid** 38% of graduate students in nursing programs received some form of financial aid in 2012–13. Institutionally sponsored loans and scholarships available. *Financial aid application deadline:* 3/1.
**Contact** Diane M. Loffredo, Director for Admissions and Student Services, Nursing Program, Florida International University, 11200 SW 8th Street, Modesto A. Maidique Campus, HLS 2, RM 482, Miami, FL 33199. *Telephone:* 305-348-7717. *Fax:* 305-348-7764. *E-mail:* dloffred@fiu.edu.

**MASTER'S DEGREE PROGRAM**
**Degree** MSN
**Available Programs** Accelerated AD/RN to Master's; Master's; Master's for Nurses with Non-Nursing Degrees.
**Concentrations Available** Nurse anesthesia; nursing administration; nursing education. *Nurse practitioner programs in:* adult health, family health, pediatric.
**Study Options** Full-time and part-time.
**Program Entrance Requirements** Clinical experience, computer literacy, minimum overall college GPA of 3.0, transcript of college record, CPR certification, written essay, immunizations, interview, 3 letters of recommendation, nursing research course, physical assessment course, professional liability insurance/malpractice insurance, prerequisite course work, resume, statistics course. *Application deadline:* 3/1 (fall). *Application fee:* $30.
**Advanced Placement** Credit given for nursing courses completed elsewhere dependent upon specific evaluations.
**Degree Requirements** 43 total credit hours.

**POST-MASTER'S PROGRAM**
**Areas of Study** Nursing administration; nursing education. *Nurse practitioner programs in:* adult health, family health, pediatric.

**DOCTORAL DEGREE PROGRAM**
**Degree** DNP
**Available Programs** Doctorate.
**Areas of Study** Clinical practice, faculty preparation, family health, gerontology, health policy, health-care systems, individualized study, nursing education, nursing policy, nursing research, nursing science.
**Program Entrance Requirements** Minimum overall college GPA of 3.25, clinical experience, interview by faculty committee, 3 letters of recommendation, MSN or equivalent, statistics course, writing sample. *Application deadline:* 6/1 (fall), 10/1 (spring). Applications may be processed on a rolling basis for some programs. *Application fee:* $30.
**Degree Requirements** 36 total credit hours, oral exam, written exam.

**Degree** PhD
**Available Programs** Doctorate.
**Areas of Study** Faculty preparation, health policy, health-care systems, individualized study, nursing administration, nursing education, nursing policy, nursing research, nursing science.
**Program Entrance Requirements** Minimum overall college GPA of 3.3, interview by faculty committee, 3 letters of recommendation, MSN or equivalent, statistics course, writing sample, GRE. *Application deadline:* 6/1 (fall), 10/1 (spring), 3/1 (summer). Applications may be processed on a rolling basis for some programs. *Application fee:* $30.
**Degree Requirements** 60 total credit hours, dissertation, oral exam, written exam.

## Florida Southern College
### School of Nursing & Health Sciences
### Lakeland, Florida

***http://www.flsouthern.edu/KCMS/Nursing-Health-Sciences.aspx***
Founded in 1885

**DEGREES • BSN • MSN • MSN/MBA**
**Nursing Program Faculty** 12 (75% with doctorates).
**Baccalaureate Enrollment** 149
**Graduate Enrollment** 89
**Nursing Student Activities** Nursing Honor Society, Sigma Theta Tau, Student Nurses' Association.
**Nursing Student Resources** Academic advising; academic or career counseling; assistance for students with disabilities; bookstore; campus computer network; career placement assistance; computer lab; computer-assisted instruction; e-mail services; externships; interactive nursing

skills videos; Internet; learning resource lab; library services; nursing audiovisuals; paid internships; placement services for program completers; remedial services; resume preparation assistance; skills, simulation, or other laboratory; tutoring.
**Library Facilities** 153,456 volumes (4,000 in health, 3,500 in nursing); 119,861 periodical subscriptions (40 health-care related).

## BACCALAUREATE PROGRAMS

**Degree** BSN
**Available Programs** Accelerated Baccalaureate; Accelerated Baccalaureate for Second Degree; Baccalaureate for Second Degree; Generic Baccalaureate; RN Baccalaureate.
**Study Options** Full-time.
**Program Entrance Requirements** Minimum overall college GPA of 3.2, transcript of college record, CPR certification, written essay, health exam, health insurance, immunizations, minimum high school GPA of 3.2, minimum GPA in nursing prerequisites of 3.0, prerequisite course work. Transfer students are accepted. *Application deadline:* 5/1 (fall). Applications may be processed on a rolling basis for some programs.
**Advanced Placement** Credit by examination available. Credit given for nursing courses completed elsewhere dependent upon specific evaluations.
**Expenses (2012–13)** *Tuition:* full-time $26,600; part-time $750 per credit hour. *Room and board:* $9100 per academic year.
**Contact** Dr. John Welton, Dean, School of Nursing & Health Sciences, Florida Southern College, 111 Lake Hollingsworth Drive, Lakeland, FL 33801. *Telephone:* 863-680-3951. *Fax:* 863-680-3860. *E-mail:* jwelton@flsouthern.edu.

## GRADUATE PROGRAMS

**Expenses (2012–13)** *Tuition:* part-time $460 per credit hour.
**Contact** Dr. Beverley Brown, Graduate Program Director, School of Nursing & Health Sciences, Florida Southern College, 111 Lake Hollingsworth Drive, Lakeland, FL 33801. *Telephone:* 863-680-3951. *Fax:* 863-680-3860. *E-mail:* bbrown@flsouthern.edu.

### MASTER'S DEGREE PROGRAM

**Degrees** MSN; MSN/MBA
**Available Programs** Master's; Master's for Nurses with Non-Nursing Degrees.
**Concentrations Available** Nursing administration; nursing education. *Clinical nurse specialist programs in:* adult health, gerontology. *Nurse practitioner programs in:* adult health, primary care.
**Study Options** Full-time and part-time.
**Program Entrance Requirements** Clinical experience, computer literacy, minimum overall college GPA of 3.0, transcript of college record, CPR certification, written essay, immunizations, 3 letters of recommendation, nursing research course, physical assessment course, professional liability insurance/malpractice insurance, prerequisite course work, resume, statistics course. *Application deadline:* 6/1 (fall), 11/1 (spring). *Application fee:* $30.
**Advanced Placement** Credit given for nursing courses completed elsewhere dependent upon specific evaluations.
**Degree Requirements** 42 total credit hours, thesis or project.

### POST-MASTER'S PROGRAM

**Areas of Study** Nursing administration; nursing education. *Clinical nurse specialist programs in:* adult health, gerontology. *Nurse practitioner programs in:* adult health, primary care.

# Florida State College at Jacksonville

## Nursing Department
## Jacksonville, Florida

Founded in 1963

### DEGREE • BSN

**Nursing Program Faculty** 4 (100% with doctorates).
**Baccalaureate Enrollment** 81 **Women** 98% **Men** 2% **Minority** 56%
**Distance Learning Courses** Available.
**Nursing Student Activities** Student Nurses' Association.
**Nursing Student Resources** Academic advising; academic or career counseling; assistance for students with disabilities; bookstore; campus computer network; career placement assistance; computer lab; computer-assisted instruction; daycare for children of students; e-mail services; employment services for current students; interactive nursing skills videos; Internet; learning resource lab; library services; nursing audiovisuals; resume preparation assistance; skills, simulation, or other laboratory; tutoring.
**Library Facilities** 211,361 volumes (50,000 in health, 5,000 in nursing); 3,299 periodical subscriptions (148 health-care related).

## BACCALAUREATE PROGRAMS

**Degree** BSN
**Available Programs** RN Baccalaureate.
**Study Options** Part-time.
**Program Entrance Requirements** Minimum overall college GPA of 2.0, transcript of college record, CPR certification, written essay, health exam, high school transcript, immunizations, 1 letter of recommendation, minimum GPA in nursing prerequisites of 2.0, professional liability insurance/malpractice insurance, prerequisite course work, RN licensure. Transfer students are accepted. *Application deadline:* 6/1 (fall), 10/1 (winter), 2/1 (spring). *Application fee:* $25.
**Advanced Placement** Credit given for nursing courses completed elsewhere dependent upon specific evaluations.
**Expenses (2013–14)** *Tuition, state resident:* part-time $115 per credit hour. *Tuition, nonresident:* part-time $399 per credit hour. *International tuition:* $399 full-time.
**Financial Aid** 54% of baccalaureate students in nursing programs received some form of financial aid in 2012–13. *Loans:* college/university. *Work-study:* Federal Work-Study.
**Contact** Dr. Mary Kathleen Ebener, Associate Dean of Nursing for BSN Program, Nursing Department, Florida State College at Jacksonville, North Campus, 4501 Capper Road, Jacksonville, FL 32218. *Telephone:* 904-713-6015. *Fax:* 904-713-4850. *E-mail:* mebener@fscj.edu.

# Florida State University

## College of Nursing
## Tallahassee, Florida

*http://www.nursing.fsu.edu/*
Founded in 1851

### DEGREES • BSN • DNP • MSN

**Nursing Program Faculty** 29 (90% with doctorates).
**Baccalaureate Enrollment** 226 **Women** 89% **Men** 11% **Minority** 29% **International** 1% **Part-time** 5%
**Graduate Enrollment** 81 **Women** 98% **Men** 2% **Minority** 5% **Part-time** 55%
**Distance Learning Courses** Available.
**Nursing Student Activities** Sigma Theta Tau, Student Nurses' Association.
**Nursing Student Resources** Academic advising; academic or career counseling; assistance for students with disabilities; campus computer network; computer lab; e-mail services; interactive nursing skills videos; Internet; learning resource lab; nursing audiovisuals; skills, simulation, or other laboratory; unpaid internships.
**Library Facilities** 3 million volumes; 83,241 periodical subscriptions.

## BACCALAUREATE PROGRAMS

**Degree** BSN
**Available Programs** Accelerated Baccalaureate; Generic Baccalaureate.
**Study Options** Full-time.
**Program Entrance Requirements** Minimum overall college GPA of 3.0, transcript of college record, CPR certification, health exam, health insurance, high school biology, high school chemistry, high school foreign language, 3 years high school math, immunizations, minimum high school GPA of 3.7, minimum GPA in nursing prerequisites of 3.0, prerequisite course work. Transfer students are accepted. *Application deadline:* 2/1 (fall). *Application fee:* $20.
**Advanced Placement** Credit given for nursing courses completed elsewhere dependent upon specific evaluations.
**Expenses (2013–14)** *Tuition, state resident:* full-time $3152; part-time $105 per credit hour. *Tuition, nonresident:* full-time $17,580; part-time $586 per credit hour. *International tuition:* $17,580 full-time. *Room and board:* $9912; room only: $5980 per academic year. *Required fees:* full-time $3000; part-time $100 per credit.
**Financial Aid** 96% of baccalaureate students in nursing programs received some form of financial aid in 2012–13. *Gift aid (need-based):* Federal Pell, FSEOG, state, private, college/university gift aid from institutional funds, Academic Competitiveness Grants, National SMART Grants. *Loans:* Federal Direct (Subsidized and Unsubsidized Stafford

PLUS), Perkins, college/university. *Work-study:* Federal Work-Study, part-time campus jobs. *Financial aid application deadline:* Continuous.

**Contact** Mr. Carlos Urrutia, Director of Student Services, College of Nursing, Florida State University, 98 Varsity Way, 103 SCN, Tallahassee, FL 32306-4310. *Telephone:* 850-644-5638. *Fax:* 850-645-7249. *E-mail:* currutia@admin.fsu.edu.

## GRADUATE PROGRAMS

**Expenses (2013–14)** *Tuition, state resident:* part-time $404 per credit hour. *Tuition, nonresident:* full-time $10,048; part-time $1005 per credit hour. *International tuition:* $10,048 full-time. *Room and board:* $9912; room only: $5980 per academic year. *Required fees:* full-time $2274; part-time $76 per credit.

**Financial Aid** 91% of graduate students in nursing programs received some form of financial aid in 2012–13. Fellowships with partial tuition reimbursements available (averaging $6,300 per year), research assistantships with partial tuition reimbursements available (averaging $3,000 per year), 3 teaching assistantships with partial tuition reimbursements available (averaging $3,000 per year) were awarded; career-related internships or fieldwork, Federal Work-Study, institutionally sponsored loans, scholarships, traineeships, and tuition waivers (partial) also available. *Financial aid application deadline:* 4/15.

**Contact** Mr. Carlos Urrutia, Director of Student Services, College of Nursing, Florida State University, 98 Varsity Way, 103 SCN, Tallahassee, FL 32306-4310. *Telephone:* 850-644-5638. *Fax:* 850-645-7249. *E-mail:* currutia@admin.fsu.edu.

### MASTER'S DEGREE PROGRAM

**Degree** MSN

**Available Programs** Master's.

**Concentrations Available** Nursing administration; nursing education.

**Study Options** Full-time and part-time.

**Online Degree Options** Yes (online only).

**Program Entrance Requirements** Minimum overall college GPA of 3.0, transcript of college record, CPR certification, immunizations, interview, 2 letters of recommendation, resume, GRE General Test, MAT. *Application deadline:* 7/1 (fall). *Application fee:* $20.

**Advanced Placement** Credit given for nursing courses completed elsewhere dependent upon specific evaluations.

**Degree Requirements** 38 total credit hours.

### POST-MASTER'S PROGRAM

**Areas of Study** Nursing administration; nursing education.

### DOCTORAL DEGREE PROGRAM

**Degree** DNP

**Available Programs** Doctorate; Post-Baccalaureate Doctorate.

**Areas of Study** Advanced practice nursing, health-care systems.

**Site Options** Panama City, FL; Sarasota, FL.

**Program Entrance Requirements** Minimum overall college GPA of 3.0, interview by faculty committee, interview, 2 letters of recommendation, GRE General Test, MAT. *Application deadline:* 4/15 (fall).

**Degree Requirements** 90 total credit hours, residency.

# Indian River State College

## Bachelor of Science in Nursing Program
## Fort Pierce, Florida

Founded in 1960

## DEGREE • BSN

**Library Facilities** 73,566 volumes; 205 periodical subscriptions.

## BACCALAUREATE PROGRAMS

**Degree** BSN

**Available Programs** RN Baccalaureate.

**Contact** *Telephone:* 772-462-7415.

# Jacksonville University

## School of Nursing
## Jacksonville, Florida

***http://www.jacksonvilleu.com/?loc=logo***
Founded in 1934

## DEGREES • BSN • DNP • MSN • MSN/MBA

**Nursing Program Faculty** 62 (42% with doctorates).

**Baccalaureate Enrollment** 1,351 **Women** 90% **Men** 10% **Minority** 40% **International** .5% **Part-time** 15%

**Graduate Enrollment** 356 **Women** 97% **Men** 3% **Minority** 9% **Part-time** 80%

**Distance Learning Courses** Available.

**Nursing Student Activities** Nursing Honor Society, Sigma Theta Tau, Student Nurses' Association.

**Nursing Student Resources** Academic advising; academic or career counseling; assistance for students with disabilities; bookstore; campus computer network; career placement assistance; computer lab; computer-assisted instruction; e-mail services; employment services for current students; interactive nursing skills videos; Internet; learning resource lab; library services; nursing audiovisuals; remedial services; resume preparation assistance; skills, simulation, or other laboratory; tutoring.

**Library Facilities** 4,821 volumes in health, 1,762 volumes in nursing; 6,150 periodical subscriptions health-care related.

## BACCALAUREATE PROGRAMS

**Degree** BSN

**Available Programs** ADN to Baccalaureate; Accelerated Baccalaureate; Accelerated Baccalaureate for Second Degree; Baccalaureate for Second Degree; Generic Baccalaureate.

**Site Options** Jacksonville, FL.

**Study Options** Full-time.

**Online Degree Options** Yes.

**Program Entrance Requirements** Minimum overall college GPA of 2.5, transcript of college record, CPR certification, written essay, health exam, health insurance, high school biology, high school chemistry, high school transcript, immunizations, interview, 3 letters of recommendation, minimum high school GPA of 3.5, minimum GPA in nursing prerequisites of 2.0, prerequisite course work. Transfer students are accepted. *Application deadline:* 4/1 (fall), 12/1 (summer). *Application fee:* $15.

**Advanced Placement** Credit given for nursing courses completed elsewhere dependent upon specific evaluations.

**Expenses (2013–14)** *Tuition:* full-time $29,000; part-time $993 per credit hour. *International tuition:* $29,000 full-time.

**Financial Aid** 92% of baccalaureate students in nursing programs received some form of financial aid in 2012–13. *Gift aid (need-based):* Federal Pell, FSEOG, state, private, college/university gift aid from institutional funds. *Loans:* Federal Direct (Subsidized and Unsubsidized Stafford PLUS), Perkins. *Work-study:* Federal Work-Study. *Financial aid application deadline (priority):* 3/31.

**Contact** Mrs. Stephanie Bloom, Director of Enrollment and Program Development, School of Nursing, Jacksonville University, 2800 University Boulevard North, Jacksonville, FL 32211. *Telephone:* 904-256-7286. *Fax:* 904-256-7287. *E-mail:* slbloom@ju.edu.

## GRADUATE PROGRAMS

**Expenses (2013–14)** *Tuition:* full-time $12,000; part-time $500 per credit hour.

**Financial Aid** 59% of graduate students in nursing programs received some form of financial aid in 2012–13.

**Contact** Ms. Marie Peoples, Graduate Program Advisor, School of Nursing, Jacksonville University, 2800 University Boulevard North, Jacksonville, FL 32211. *Telephone:* 904-256-7034. *Fax:* 904-256-7133. *E-mail:* mpeople1@ju.edu.

### MASTER'S DEGREE PROGRAM

**Degrees** MSN; MSN/MBA

**Available Programs** Master's.

**Concentrations Available** Nursing administration; nursing education. *Nurse practitioner programs in:* family health.

**Site Options** Jacksonville, FL.

**Study Options** Full-time and part-time.

**Online Degree Options** Yes.

**Program Entrance Requirements** Clinical experience, minimum overall college GPA of 3.0, transcript of college record, CPR certification, written essay, immunizations, interview, 3 letters of recommendation, physical assessment course, professional liability

insurance/malpractice insurance, prerequisite course work, resume, statistics course. *Application deadline:* 4/30 (fall). Applications may be processed on a rolling basis for some programs. *Application fee:* $50.
**Advanced Placement** Credit given for nursing courses completed elsewhere dependent upon specific evaluations.
**Degree Requirements** 30 total credit hours.

### POST-MASTER'S PROGRAM
**Areas of Study** *Nurse practitioner programs in:* family health.

### DOCTORAL DEGREE PROGRAM
**Degree** DNP
**Available Programs** Doctorate.
**Areas of Study** Advanced practice nursing, nursing administration.
**Site Options** Jacksonville, FL.
**Program Entrance Requirements** Clinical experience, minimum overall college GPA of 3.3, interview by faculty committee, 3 letters of recommendation, MSN or equivalent, statistics course, vita, writing sample. *Application deadline:* Applications may be processed on a rolling basis for some programs. *Application fee:* $50.
**Degree Requirements** 39 total credit hours, residency.

# Kaplan University Online
## The School of Nursing Online
## Fort Lauderdale, Florida

**DEGREES • BSN • MSN**

### BACCALAUREATE PROGRAMS
**Degree** BSN
**Available Programs** Generic Baccalaureate.
**Contact** *Telephone:* 866-527-5268.

### GRADUATE PROGRAMS
**Contact** *Telephone:* 866-527-5268.

### MASTER'S DEGREE PROGRAM
**Degree** MSN
**Available Programs** Master's; RN to Master's.
**Concentrations Available** Health-care administration; nursing education; nursing informatics. *Nurse practitioner programs in:* adult health, family health.

# Keiser University
## Nursing Programs
## Fort Lauderdale, Florida

Founded in 1977

**DEGREES • BSN • MSN**

### BACCALAUREATE PROGRAMS
**Degree** BSN
**Available Programs** RN Baccalaureate.
**Contact** Fort Lauderdale campus, Nursing Programs, Keiser University, 1500 Northwest 49th Street, Fort Lauderdale, FL 33309. *Telephone:* 954-776-4456. *Fax:* 954-771-4894.

### GRADUATE PROGRAMS
**Contact** Fort Lauderdale campus, Nursing Programs, Keiser University, 1500 Northwest 49th Street, Fort Lauderdale, FL 33309. *Telephone:* 954-776-4456. *Fax:* 954-771-4894.

### MASTER'S DEGREE PROGRAM
**Degree** MSN
**Available Programs** Master's.
**Program Entrance Requirements** Minimum overall college GPA of 2.7.
**Degree Requirements** 33 total credit hours.

# Keiser University
## Nursing Programs
## Fort Myers, Florida

**DEGREES • BSN • MSN**

### BACCALAUREATE PROGRAMS
**Degree** BSN
**Available Programs** RN Baccalaureate.
**Contact** Ft. Myers campus, Nursing Programs, Keiser University, 9100 Forum Corporate Parkway, Ft. Myers, FL 33905. *Telephone:* 239-277-1336. *Fax:* 239-277-1259.

### GRADUATE PROGRAMS
**Contact** Ft. Myers campus, Nursing Programs, Keiser University, 9100 Forum Corporate Parkway, Ft. Myers, FL 33905. *Telephone:* 239-277-1336. *Fax:* 239-277-1259.

### MASTER'S DEGREE PROGRAM
**Degree** MSN
**Available Programs** Master's.
**Program Entrance Requirements** Minimum overall college GPA of 2.7.
**Degree Requirements** 33 total credit hours.

# Keiser University
## Nursing Programs
## Jacksonville, Florida

**DEGREES • BSN • MSN**

### BACCALAUREATE PROGRAMS
**Degree** BSN
**Available Programs** RN Baccalaureate.
**Contact** Jacksonville campus, Nursing Programs, Keiser University, 6430 Southpoint Parkway, Jacksonville, FL 32216. *Telephone:* 904-296-3440. *Fax:* 904-296-3407.

### GRADUATE PROGRAMS
**Contact** Jacksonville campus, Nursing Programs, Keiser University, 6430 Southpoint Parkway, Jacksonville, FL 32216. *Telephone:* 904-296-3440. *Fax:* 904-296-3407.

### MASTER'S DEGREE PROGRAM
**Degree** MSN
**Available Programs** Master's.
**Program Entrance Requirements** Minimum overall college GPA of 2.7.
**Degree Requirements** 33 total credit hours.

# Keiser University
## Nursing Programs
## Lakeland, Florida

**DEGREES • BSN • MSN**

### BACCALAUREATE PROGRAMS
**Degree** BSN
**Available Programs** RN Baccalaureate.
**Contact** Lakeland campus, Nursing Programs, Keiser University, 2400 Interstate Drive, Lakeland, FL 33805. *Telephone:* 863-682-6020. *Fax:* 863-688-6196.

### GRADUATE PROGRAMS
**Contact** Lakeland campus, Nursing Programs, Keiser University, 2400 Interstate Drive, Lakeland, FL 33805. *Telephone:* 863-682-6020. *Fax:* 863-688-6196.

### MASTER'S DEGREE PROGRAM
**Degree** MSN
**Available Programs** Master's.

**Program Entrance Requirements** Minimum overall college GPA of 2.7.
**Degree Requirements** 33 total credit hours.

## Keiser University
### Nursing Programs
### Melbourne, Florida

Founded in 1989

**DEGREES • BSN • MSN**

#### BACCALAUREATE PROGRAMS

**Degree** BSN
**Available Programs** RN Baccalaureate.
**Contact** Melbourne campus, Nursing Programs, Keiser University, 900 South Babcock Street, Melbourne, FL 32901. *Telephone:* 321-409-4800. *Fax:* 321-725-3766.

#### GRADUATE PROGRAMS

**Contact** Melbourne campus, Nursing Programs, Keiser University, 900 South Babcock Street, Melbourne, FL 32901. *Telephone:* 321-409-4800. *Fax:* 321-725-3766.

**MASTER'S DEGREE PROGRAM**
**Degree** MSN
**Available Programs** Master's.
**Program Entrance Requirements** Minimum overall college GPA of 2.7.
**Degree Requirements** 33 total credit hours.

## Keiser University
### Nursing Programs
### Miami, Florida

**DEGREES • BSN • MSN**

#### BACCALAUREATE PROGRAMS

**Degree** BSN
**Available Programs** RN Baccalaureate.
**Contact** Miami campus, Nursing Programs, Keiser University, 2101 NW 117th Avenue, Miami, FL 33172. *Telephone:* 305-596-2226. *Fax:* 305-596-7077.

#### GRADUATE PROGRAMS

**Contact** Miami campus, Nursing Programs, Keiser University, 2101 NW 117th Avenue, Miami, FL 33172. *Telephone:* 305-596-2226. *Fax:* 305-596-7077.

**MASTER'S DEGREE PROGRAM**
**Degree** MSN
**Available Programs** Master's.
**Program Entrance Requirements** Minimum overall college GPA of 2.7.
**Degree Requirements** 33 total credit hours.

## Keiser University
### Nursing Programs
### Orlando, Florida

**DEGREES • BSN • MSN**

#### BACCALAUREATE PROGRAMS

**Degree** BSN
**Available Programs** RN Baccalaureate.
**Contact** Orlando campus, Nursing Programs, Keiser University, 5600 Lake Underhill Road, Orlando, FL 32807. *Telephone:* 407-273-5800. *Fax:* 407-381-1233.

#### GRADUATE PROGRAMS

**Contact** Orland campus, Nursing Programs, Keiser University, 5600 Lake Underhill Road, Orlando, FL 32807. *Telephone:* 407-273-5800. *Fax:* 407-381-1233.

**MASTER'S DEGREE PROGRAM**
**Degree** MSN
**Available Programs** Master's.
**Program Entrance Requirements** Minimum overall college GPA of 2.7.
**Degree Requirements** 33 total credit hours.

## Keiser University
### Nursing Programs
### Port St. Lucie, Florida

Founded in 1999

**DEGREES • BSN • MSN**

#### BACCALAUREATE PROGRAMS

**Degree** BSN
**Available Programs** RN Baccalaureate.
**Contact** Port St. Lucie campus, Nursing Programs, Keiser University, 10330 South U.S. 1, Port St. Lucie, FL 34952. *Telephone:* 772-398-9990. *Fax:* 772-335-9619.

#### GRADUATE PROGRAMS

**Contact** Port St. Lucie campus, Nursing Programs, Keiser University, 10330 South U.S. 1, Port St. Lucie, FL 34952. *Telephone:* 772-398-9990. *Fax:* 772-335-9619.

**MASTER'S DEGREE PROGRAM**
**Degree** MSN
**Available Programs** Master's.
**Program Entrance Requirements** Minimum overall college GPA of 2.7.
**Degree Requirements** 33 total credit hours.

## Keiser University
### Nursing Programs
### Sarasota, Florida

Founded in 1995

**DEGREES • BSN • MSN**

#### BACCALAUREATE PROGRAMS

**Degree** BSN
**Available Programs** RN Baccalaureate.
**Contact** Sarasota campus, Nursing Programs, Keiser University, 6151 Lake Osprey Drive, Sarasota, FL 34240. *Telephone:* 941-907-3900. *Fax:* 941-907-2016.

#### GRADUATE PROGRAMS

**Contact** Sarasota campus, Nursing Programs, Keiser University, 6151 Lake Osprey Drive, Sarasota, FL 34240. *Telephone:* 941-907-3900. *Fax:* 941-907-2016.

**MASTER'S DEGREE PROGRAM**
**Degree** MSN
**Available Programs** Master's.
**Program Entrance Requirements** Minimum overall college GPA of 2.7.
**Degree Requirements** 33 total credit hours.

## Keiser University

### Nursing Programs
### Tallahassee, Florida

Founded in 1992

**DEGREES • BSN • MSN**

#### BACCALAUREATE PROGRAMS

**Degree** BSN
**Available Programs** RN Baccalaureate.
**Contact** Tallahassee campus, Nursing Programs, Keiser University, 1700 Halstead Boulevard, Building 2, Tallahassee, FL 32309. *Telephone:* 850-906-9494. *Fax:* 850-906-9497.

#### GRADUATE PROGRAMS

**Contact** Tallahassee campus, Nursing Programs, Keiser University, 1700 Halstead Boulevard, Building 2, Tallahassee, FL 32309. *Telephone:* 850-906-9494. *Fax:* 850-906-9497.

**MASTER'S DEGREE PROGRAM**
**Degree** MSN
**Available Programs** Master's.
**Program Entrance Requirements** Minimum overall college GPA of 2.7.
**Degree Requirements** 33 total credit hours.

## Keiser University

### Nursing Programs
### Tampa, Florida

**DEGREES • BSN • MSN**

#### BACCALAUREATE PROGRAMS

**Degree** BSN
**Available Programs** RN Baccalaureate.
**Contact** Tampa campus, Nursing Programs, Keiser University, 5002 West Waters Avenue, Tampa, FL 33634. *Telephone:* 813-885-4900. *Fax:* 813-885-4911.

#### GRADUATE PROGRAMS

**Contact** Tampa campus, Nursing Programs, Keiser University, 5002 West Waters Avenue, Tampa, FL 33634. *Telephone:* 813-885-4900. *Fax:* 813-885-4911.

**MASTER'S DEGREE PROGRAM**
**Degree** MSN
**Available Programs** Master's.
**Program Entrance Requirements** Minimum overall college GPA of 2.7.
**Degree Requirements** 33 total credit hours.

## Miami Dade College

### School of Nursing
### Miami, Florida

***http://mdc.edu***
Founded in 1960

**DEGREE • BSN**
**Nursing Program Faculty** 14 (73% with doctorates).
**Baccalaureate Enrollment** 578 **Women** 88% **Men** 12% **Minority** 94% **International** 3% **Part-time** 92%
**Distance Learning Courses** Available.
**Nursing Student Activities** Nursing Honor Society, Student Nurses' Association.
**Nursing Student Resources** Academic advising; academic or career counseling; assistance for students with disabilities; bookstore; campus computer network; computer lab; computer-assisted instruction; e-mail services; interactive nursing skills videos; Internet; learning resource lab; library services; nursing audiovisuals; remedial services; resume preparation assistance; skills, simulation, or other laboratory; tutoring.
**Library Facilities** 367,687 volumes (14,000 in health, 3,580 in nursing); 750 periodical subscriptions (14,090 health-care related).

#### BACCALAUREATE PROGRAMS

**Degree** BSN
**Available Programs** RN Baccalaureate.
**Site Options** Miami, FL.
**Program Entrance Requirements** CPR certification, health exam, immunizations, minimum GPA in nursing prerequisites of 2.5, prerequisite course work, RN licensure. Transfer students are accepted. *Application deadline:* 5/1 (fall), 9/1 (spring). *Application fee:* $200.
**Expenses (2012–13)** *Tuition, state resident:* full-time $3304; part-time $92 per credit hour. *Tuition, nonresident:* full-time $16,156; part-time $449 per credit hour. *International tuition:* $16,156 full-time. *Required fees:* full-time $1157; part-time $32 per credit; part-time $385 per term.
**Financial Aid** 63% of baccalaureate students in nursing programs received some form of financial aid in 2011–12. *Gift aid (need-based):* Federal Pell, FSEOG, state, private, college/university gift aid from institutional funds. *Loans:* Perkins. *Work-study:* Federal Work-Study, part-time campus jobs. *Financial aid application deadline (priority):* 2/15.
**Contact** Amy Pettigrew, Dean, Benjamn Len School of Nursing, School of Nursing, Miami Dade College, 950 NW 20th Street, Miami, FL 33127. *Telephone:* 305-237-4039. *E-mail:* apettigr@mdc.edu.

## Northwest Florida State College

### RN to BSN Degree Program
### Niceville, Florida

***http://www.nwfsc.edu/RNtoBSN/***
Founded in 1963

**DEGREE • BSN**
**Nursing Program Faculty** 7 (2% with doctorates).
**Baccalaureate Enrollment** 99
**Distance Learning Courses** Available.
**Nursing Student Activities** Student Nurses' Association, nursing club.
**Nursing Student Resources** Academic advising; academic or career counseling; assistance for students with disabilities; bookstore; campus computer network; career placement assistance; computer lab; computer-assisted instruction; daycare for children of students; employment services for current students; interactive nursing skills videos; Internet; learning resource lab; library services; nursing audiovisuals; placement services for program completers; remedial services; resume preparation assistance; skills, simulation, or other laboratory; tutoring; unpaid internships.
**Library Facilities** 106,383 volumes (1,880 in health, 1,048 in nursing); 399 periodical subscriptions (70 health-care related).

#### BACCALAUREATE PROGRAMS

**Degree** BSN
**Available Programs** ADN to Baccalaureate; Accelerated RN Baccalaureate; RN Baccalaureate.
**Study Options** Full-time and part-time.
**Program Entrance Requirements** Transcript of college record, CPR certification, health exam, immunizations, minimum GPA in nursing prerequisites of 2.75, RN licensure. Transfer students are accepted. *Application deadline:* 7/1 (fall), 11/1 (spring), 3/15 (summer). Applications may be processed on a rolling basis for some programs.
**Advanced Placement** Credit given for nursing courses completed elsewhere dependent upon specific evaluations.
**Expenses (2013–14)** *Tuition, state resident:* part-time $121 per credit. *Tuition, nonresident:* part-time $449 per credit.
**Contact** Dr. Beth C. Norton, Director, Bachelor of Science in Nursing, RN to BSN Degree Program, Northwest Florida State College, 100 College Boulevard, Niceville, FL 32578. *Telephone:* 850-729-6473. *Fax:* 850-729-6484. *E-mail:* nortonb@nwfsc.edu.

# Nova Southeastern University
## College of Health Care Sciences
## Fort Lauderdale, Florida

*http://www.nova.edu/nursing*
Founded in 1964

**DEGREES • BSN • MSN**
**Distance Learning Courses** Available.
**Nursing Student Activities** Sigma Theta Tau, Student Nurses' Association.
**Nursing Student Resources** Academic advising; academic or career counseling; assistance for students with disabilities; bookstore; campus computer network; career placement assistance; computer lab; computer-assisted instruction; e-mail services; employment services for current students; housing assistance; interactive nursing skills videos; Internet; learning resource lab; library services; placement services for program completers; resume preparation assistance; skills, simulation, or other laboratory; tutoring.
**Library Facilities** 1 million volumes; 197,340 periodical subscriptions.

### BACCALAUREATE PROGRAMS
**Degree** BSN
**Available Programs** Generic Baccalaureate; RN Baccalaureate.
**Site Options** Fort Myers, FL; Kendall, FL.
**Study Options** Full-time.
**Online Degree Options** Yes.
**Program Entrance Requirements** Minimum overall college GPA of 3.0, transcript of college record, health insurance, immunizations, interview, minimum GPA in nursing prerequisites of 2.75, prerequisite course work. *Application deadline:* 4/1 (fall), 10/1 (winter). *Application fee:* $50.
**Expenses (2012–13)** *Tuition:* full-time $23,450. *International tuition:* $24,500 full-time. *Room and board:* $7530 per academic year. *Required fees:* full-time $1045.
**Contact** Dr. Mary Botter, Associate Dean (Entry Level Nursing), College of Health Care Sciences, Nova Southeastern University, 3200 South University Drive, Fort Lauderdale, FL 33328. *Telephone:* 800-338-4723. *Fax:* 954-262-8000 Ext. 7184. *E-mail:* aalvarez1@nova.edu.

### GRADUATE PROGRAMS
**Expenses (2012–13)** *Tuition:* part-time $550 per credit. *International tuition:* $550 full-time. *Room and board:* $14,050 per academic year. *Required fees:* full-time $1045; part-time $300 per term.
**Financial Aid** 2 research assistantships (averaging $4,200 per year), 3 teaching assistantships (averaging $10,200 per year) were awarded; institutionally sponsored loans and unspecified assistantships also available.
**Contact** Dr. Diane Whitehead, Associate Dean, College of Health Care Sciences, Nova Southeastern University, 3200 South University Drive, Fort Lauderdale, FL 33328. *Telephone:* 954-262-1101. *Fax:* 877-640-0218. *E-mail:* keatta@nova.edu.

**MASTER'S DEGREE PROGRAM**
**Degree** MSN
**Available Programs** Master's; RN to Master's.
**Concentrations Available** Nursing administration; nursing education; nursing informatics.
**Study Options** Full-time and part-time.
**Online Degree Options** Yes (online only).
**Program Entrance Requirements** Minimum overall college GPA of 3.0, transcript of college record, written essay, immunizations, 2 letters of recommendation, statistics course, GRE General Test. *Application deadline:* 8/1 (fall), 12/1 (winter). *Application fee:* $50.
**Degree Requirements** 36 total credit hours, thesis or project.

**DOCTORAL DEGREE PROGRAM**
**Program Entrance Requirements** GRE General Test.

# Palm Beach Atlantic University
## School of Nursing
## West Palm Beach, Florida

Founded in 1968

**DEGREE • BSN**
**Nursing Student Activities** Student Nurses' Association.
**Library Facilities** 265,745 volumes; 28,841 periodical subscriptions.

### BACCALAUREATE PROGRAMS
**Degree** BSN
**Available Programs** RN Baccalaureate.
**Program Entrance Requirements** RN licensure.
**Contact** *Telephone:* 561-803-2825. *Fax:* 561-803-2828.

# Polk State College
## RN to BSN Program
## Winter Haven, Florida

Founded in 1964

**DEGREE • BSN**
**Library Facilities** 162,767 volumes; 217 periodical subscriptions.

### BACCALAUREATE PROGRAMS
**Degree** BSN
**Available Programs** RN Baccalaureate.
**Contact** Annette Hutcherson, Nursing Program Director, RN to BSN Program, Polk State College, 999 Avenue H, NE, Winter Haven, FL 33881. *Telephone:* 863-297-1039. *E-mail:* ahutcherson@polk.edu.

# Remington College of Nursing
## Remington College of Nursing
## Lake Mary, Florida

**DEGREE • BSN**
**Nursing Program Faculty** 23 (8% with doctorates).
**Baccalaureate Enrollment** 77 **Women** 86% **Men** 14% **Minority** 49% **International** 4% **Part-time** 1%
**Distance Learning Courses** Available.
**Nursing Student Activities** Student Nurses' Association.
**Nursing Student Resources** Academic advising; academic or career counseling; assistance for students with disabilities; campus computer network; career placement assistance; computer-assisted instruction; e-mail services; interactive nursing skills videos; Internet; learning resource lab; library services; nursing audiovisuals; other; remedial services; resume preparation assistance; skills, simulation, or other laboratory; tutoring.
**Library Facilities** 990 volumes in health, 880 volumes in nursing; 905 periodical subscriptions health-care related.

### BACCALAUREATE PROGRAMS
**Degree** BSN
**Available Programs** Accelerated Baccalaureate for Second Degree.
**Study Options** Full-time.
**Program Entrance Requirements** Minimum overall college GPA of 2.5, transcript of college record, CPR certification, written essay, health exam, health insurance, immunizations, interview, 2 letters of recommendation, prerequisite course work. *Application deadline:* 12/1 (winter), 4/1 (summer). Applications may be processed on a rolling basis for some programs. *Application fee:* $50.
**Advanced Placement** Credit given for nursing courses completed elsewhere dependent upon specific evaluations.
**Contact** *Telephone:* 800-294-4434.

# St. Petersburg College
## Department of Nursing
## St. Petersburg, Florida

*http://www.spcollege.edu/*
Founded in 1927

**DEGREE • BSN**
**Nursing Program Faculty** 27 (56% with doctorates).
**Baccalaureate Enrollment** 688 **Women** 85% **Men** 15% **Minority** 28% **International** 1%
**Distance Learning Courses** Available.
**Nursing Student Activities** Sigma Theta Tau, Student Nurses' Association.

**Nursing Student Resources** Academic advising; academic or career counseling; assistance for students with disabilities; bookstore; campus computer network; computer lab; computer-assisted instruction; e-mail services; employment services for current students; interactive nursing skills videos; Internet; learning resource lab; library services; nursing audiovisuals; placement services for program completers; remedial services; resume preparation assistance; skills, simulation, or other laboratory; tutoring; unpaid internships.
**Library Facilities** 241,761 volumes (1,390 in health, 484 in nursing); 1,987 periodical subscriptions (77 health-care related).

### BACCALAUREATE PROGRAMS

**Degree** BSN
**Available Programs** ADN to Baccalaureate; RN Baccalaureate.
**Site Options** Pinellas Park, FL.
**Online Degree Options** Yes.
**Program Entrance Requirements** Minimum overall college GPA of 2.0, transcript of college record, high school transcript, prerequisite course work, RN licensure. Transfer students are accepted. *Application deadline:* 7/13 (fall), 11/9 (spring). *Application fee:* $40.
**Expenses (2012–13)** *Tuition, state resident:* full-time $5879; part-time $117 per credit hour. *Tuition, nonresident:* full-time $18,002; part-time $420 per credit hour. *Required fees:* full-time $3000; part-time $1000 per term.
**Financial Aid** 45% of baccalaureate students in nursing programs received some form of financial aid in 2011–12. *Gift aid (need-based):* Federal Pell, FSEOG, state, private, college/university gift aid from institutional funds. *Loans:* college/university. *Work-study:* Federal Work-Study. *Financial aid application deadline (priority):* 4/15.
**Contact** Dr. Susan Anita Baker, Dean, Department of Nursing, St. Petersburg College, PO Box 13489, St. Petersburg, FL 33733. *Telephone:* 727-341-3640. *Fax:* 727-341-3646. *E-mail:* baker.susan@spcollege.edu.

### CONTINUING EDUCATION PROGRAM

**Contact** Denise Kerwin, Program Director, Department of Nursing, St. Petersburg College, PO Box 13489, St. Petersburg, FL 33733. *Telephone:* 727-341-3374. *Fax:* 727-341-4197. *E-mail:* kerwin.denise@spcollege.edu.

## State College of Florida Manatee-Sarasota

**Nursing Degree Program**
**Bradenton, Florida**

Founded in 1957

**DEGREE • BSN**

**Library Facilities** 65,386 volumes; 378 periodical subscriptions.

### BACCALAUREATE PROGRAMS

**Degree** BSN
**Available Programs** RN Baccalaureate.
**Program Entrance Requirements** Prerequisite course work, RN licensure. *Application deadline:* 3/1 (summer).
**Contact** Admissions, Nursing Degree Program, State College of Florida Manatee-Sarasota, 5840 26th Street West, Bradenton, FL 34206. *Telephone:* 941-752-5050. *Fax:* 941-727-6380. *E-mail:* admissions@scf.edu.

## University of Central Florida

**College of Nursing**
**Orlando, Florida**

*http://www.nursing.ucf.edu/*
Founded in 1963

**DEGREES • BSN • DNP • MSN • PHD**

**Nursing Program Faculty** 56 (43% with doctorates).
**Baccalaureate Enrollment** 1,530 **Women** 88% **Men** 12% **Minority** 26% **Part-time** 32%
**Graduate Enrollment** 350 **Women** 88% **Men** 12% **Minority** 27% **Part-time** 75%
**Distance Learning Courses** Available.
**Nursing Student Activities** Nursing Honor Society, Sigma Theta Tau, Student Nurses' Association.
**Nursing Student Resources** Academic advising; academic or career counseling; assistance for students with disabilities; bookstore; campus computer network; career placement assistance; computer lab; computer-assisted instruction; daycare for children of students; e-mail services; employment services for current students; externships; housing assistance; interactive nursing skills videos; Internet; learning resource lab; library services; nursing audiovisuals; paid internships; remedial services; resume preparation assistance; skills, simulation, or other laboratory; tutoring.
**Library Facilities** 2.5 million volumes (38,944 in health, 2,848 in nursing); 44,976 periodical subscriptions (360 health-care related).

### BACCALAUREATE PROGRAMS

**Degree** BSN
**Available Programs** ADN to Baccalaureate; Accelerated Baccalaureate for Second Degree; Generic Baccalaureate; RN Baccalaureate.
**Site Options** Daytona Beach, FL; Leesburg, FL; Cocoa Beach, FL.
**Study Options** Full-time and part-time.
**Online Degree Options** Yes.
**Program Entrance Requirements** Minimum overall college GPA of 3.0, transcript of college record, CPR certification, health exam, health insurance, high school foreign language, high school math, high school transcript, immunizations, minimum high school GPA of 3.0, minimum GPA in nursing prerequisites, prerequisite course work. Transfer students are accepted.
**Advanced Placement** Credit given for nursing courses completed elsewhere dependent upon specific evaluations.
**Expenses (2013–14)** *Tuition, area resident:* full-time $3700; part-time $105 per credit hour. *Tuition, state resident:* full-time $3700; part-time $150 per credit hour. *Tuition, nonresident:* full-time $18,480; part-time $616 per credit hour. *Room and board:* $9600; room only: $6000 per academic year. *Required fees:* full-time $3150; part-time $105 per credit.
**Financial Aid** 30% of baccalaureate students in nursing programs received some form of financial aid in 2012–13.
**Contact** Dr. Kelly Allred, Undergraduate Program Coordinator, College of Nursing, University of Central Florida, 12201 Research Parkway, Suite 300, Orlando, FL 32826. *Telephone:* 407-823-2744. *Fax:* 407-823-5675. *E-mail:* ucfnurse@mail.ucf.edu.

### GRADUATE PROGRAMS

**Expenses (2013–14)** *Tuition, state resident:* part-time $288 per credit hour. *Tuition, nonresident:* part-time $1073 per credit hour. *Required fees:* part-time $80 per credit.
**Financial Aid** 70% of graduate students in nursing programs received some form of financial aid in 2012–13.
**Contact** Dr. Susan Chase, Associate Dean for Graduate Affairs, College of Nursing, University of Central Florida, PO Box 162210, Orlando, FL 32816-2210. *Telephone:* 407-823-3079. *Fax:* 407-823-5675. *E-mail:* susan.chase@ucf.edu.

#### MASTER'S DEGREE PROGRAM

**Degree** MSN
**Available Programs** Master's; RN to Master's.
**Concentrations Available** Nursing administration; nursing education. *Clinical nurse specialist programs in:* acute care. *Nurse practitioner programs in:* adult health, family health.
**Study Options** Full-time and part-time.
**Program Entrance Requirements** Clinical experience, minimum overall college GPA of 3.0, transcript of college record, CPR certification, written essay, immunizations, 3 letters of recommendation, physical assessment course, resume, statistics course.
**Advanced Placement** Credit given for nursing courses completed elsewhere dependent upon specific evaluations.
**Degree Requirements** 47 total credit hours, thesis or project.

#### POST-MASTER'S PROGRAM

**Areas of Study** *Clinical nurse specialist programs in:* acute care. *Nurse practitioner programs in:* adult health, family health.

#### DOCTORAL DEGREE PROGRAM

**Degree** DNP
**Available Programs** Doctorate.
**Areas of Study** Advanced practice nursing, family health, nursing administration.
**Online Degree Options** Yes.
**Program Entrance Requirements** Minimum overall college GPA of 3.5, 3 letters of recommendation, statistics course, vita.

**Degree Requirements** 43-86 total credit hours, project.

**Degree** PhD
**Available Programs** Doctorate; Doctorate for Nurses with Non-Nursing Degrees.
**Areas of Study** Clinical practice, health policy, health-care systems, individualized study, information systems, nursing research.
**Program Entrance Requirements** Minimum overall college GPA of 3.5, interview by faculty committee, 3 letters of recommendation, MSN or equivalent, statistics course, vita.
**Degree Requirements** 57 total credit hours, dissertation.

# University of Florida
## College of Nursing
## Gainesville, Florida

*http://www.nursing.ufl.edu/*
Founded in 1853

**DEGREES • BSN • MSN • MSN/PHD • PHD**
**Nursing Program Faculty** 62 (50% with doctorates).
**Baccalaureate Enrollment** 374 **Women** 94% **Men** 6% **Minority** 23% **International** 1%
**Graduate Enrollment** 364 **Women** 97% **Men** 3% **Minority** 17% **International** 1% **Part-time** 56%
**Distance Learning Courses** Available.
**Nursing Student Activities** Nursing Honor Society, Sigma Theta Tau, Student Nurses' Association.
**Nursing Student Resources** Academic advising; academic or career counseling; assistance for students with disabilities; bookstore; campus computer network; career placement assistance; computer lab; computer-assisted instruction; daycare for children of students; e-mail services; employment services for current students; housing assistance; interactive nursing skills videos; Internet; learning resource lab; library services; nursing audiovisuals; placement services for program completers; remedial services; resume preparation assistance; skills, simulation, or other laboratory; tutoring.
**Library Facilities** 4.8 million volumes (260,000 in health, 3,000 in nursing); 141,195 periodical subscriptions (200 health-care related).

### BACCALAUREATE PROGRAMS

**Degree** BSN
**Available Programs** Accelerated Baccalaureate for Second Degree; Generic Baccalaureate.
**Study Options** Full-time.
**Program Entrance Requirements** Minimum overall college GPA of 2.8, transcript of college record, CPR certification, written essay, health exam, health insurance, high school biology, high school chemistry, high school foreign language, high school transcript, immunizations, 2 letters of recommendation, minimum GPA in nursing prerequisites of 2.8, prerequisite course work. Transfer students are accepted. *Application deadline:* 3/15 (fall), 1/15 (summer). *Application fee:* $30.
**Advanced Placement** Credit by examination available. Credit given for nursing courses completed elsewhere dependent upon specific evaluations.
**Contact** *Telephone:* 352-273-6383. *Fax:* 352-273-6440.

### GRADUATE PROGRAMS

**Contact** *Telephone:* 352-273-6331. *Fax:* 352-273-6440.

**MASTER'S DEGREE PROGRAM**
**Degrees** MSN; MSN/PhD
**Available Programs** Master's.
**Concentrations Available** Clinical nurse leader; nurse-midwifery. *Clinical nurse specialist programs in:* psychiatric/mental health, public health. *Nurse practitioner programs in:* acute care, adult health, family health, neonatal health, pediatric, psychiatric/mental health.
**Site Options** Jacksonville, FL.
**Study Options** Full-time and part-time.
**Online Degree Options** Yes.
**Program Entrance Requirements** Minimum overall college GPA of 3.0, transcript of college record, CPR certification, written essay, immunizations, 2 letters of recommendation, resume, GRE General Test. *Application deadline:* 3/15 (fall). Applications may be processed on a rolling basis for some programs. *Application fee:* $30.
**Advanced Placement** Credit given for nursing courses completed elsewhere dependent upon specific evaluations.
**Degree Requirements** 46 total credit hours, comprehensive exam.

**POST-MASTER'S PROGRAM**
**Areas of Study** Clinical nurse leader; nurse-midwifery. *Clinical nurse specialist programs in:* psychiatric/mental health, public health. *Nurse practitioner programs in:* acute care, adult health, family health, neonatal health, pediatric, psychiatric/mental health.

**DOCTORAL DEGREE PROGRAM**
**Degree** PhD
**Available Programs** Doctorate; Post-Baccalaureate Doctorate.
**Areas of Study** Aging, bio-behavioral research, health policy, nursing policy, nursing science, oncology,women's health.
**Site Options** Jacksonville, FL.
**Online Degree Options** Yes.
**Program Entrance Requirements** Minimum overall college GPA of 3.5, 3 letters of recommendation, MSN or equivalent, vita, writing sample, GRE General Test. *Application deadline:* 3/15 (fall). Applications may be processed on a rolling basis for some programs. *Application fee:* $30.
**Degree Requirements** 62 total credit hours, dissertation.

# University of Miami
## School of Nursing and Health Studies
## Coral Gables, Florida

*http://www.miami.edu/sonhs*
Founded in 1925

**DEGREES • BSN • MSN • PHD**
**Nursing Program Faculty** 75 (52% with doctorates).
**Baccalaureate Enrollment** 324 **Women** 88.31% **Men** 11.69% **Minority** 64.62% **International** 1.23% **Part-time** 9.85%
**Graduate Enrollment** 270 **Women** 76.03% **Men** 23.97% **Minority** 67.36% **International** 6.61% **Part-time** 42.15%
**Distance Learning Courses** Available.
**Nursing Student Activities** Nursing Honor Society, Sigma Theta Tau, Student Nurses' Association.
**Nursing Student Resources** Academic advising; academic or career counseling; assistance for students with disabilities; bookstore; campus computer network; career placement assistance; computer lab; computer-assisted instruction; e-mail services; employment services for current students; externships; housing assistance; interactive nursing skills videos; Internet; learning resource lab; library services; nursing audiovisuals; placement services for program completers; remedial services; resume preparation assistance; skills, simulation, or other laboratory; tutoring; unpaid internships.
**Library Facilities** 3.6 million volumes (89,472 in health, 1,720 in nursing); 81,066 periodical subscriptions.

### BACCALAUREATE PROGRAMS

**Degree** BSN
**Available Programs** Accelerated Baccalaureate for Second Degree; Generic Baccalaureate; RN Baccalaureate.
**Study Options** Full-time.
**Program Entrance Requirements** Minimum overall college GPA of 3.5, transcript of college record, CPR certification, written essay, health exam, health insurance, immunizations, 2 letters of recommendation, minimum GPA in nursing prerequisites of 3.3, prerequisite course work. Transfer students are accepted. *Application deadline:* 3/1 (fall). Applications may be processed on a rolling basis for some programs. *Application fee:* $65.
**Expenses (2013–14)** *Tuition:* full-time $41,580; part-time $1730 per credit. *International tuition:* $41,580 full-time. *Room and board:* $15,404; room only: $10,442 per academic year. *Required fees:* full-time $2312; part-time $187 per term.
**Financial Aid** 90% of baccalaureate students in nursing programs received some form of financial aid in 2012–13.
**Contact** Ms. Deborah Paris, Assistant Dean for Student Services, School of Nursing and Health Studies, University of Miami, PO Box 248153-3850, Coral Gables, FL 33124-3850. *Telephone:* 305-284-4199. *Fax:* 305-284-4827. *E-mail:* dparis@miami.edu.

### GRADUATE PROGRAMS

**Expenses (2013–14)** *Tuition:* part-time $1730 per credit.
**Financial Aid** 1 fellowship (averaging $36,000 per year), 6 research assistantships (averaging $36,000 per year), 4 teaching assistantships

(averaging $36,000 per year) were awarded; Federal Work-Study, institutionally sponsored loans, scholarships, and unspecified assistantships also available.
**Contact** Ms. Deborah Paris, Assistant Dean for Student Services, School of Nursing and Health Studies, University of Miami, PO Box 248153, M. Christine Schwartz Center, Coral Gables, FL 33124-3850. *Telephone:* 305-284-4099. *Fax:* 305-284-5686. *E-mail:* dparis@miami.edu.

### MASTER'S DEGREE PROGRAM
**Degree** MSN
**Available Programs** Master's.
**Concentrations Available** Nurse anesthesia. *Nurse practitioner programs in:* acute care, adult health, family health, gerontology.
**Study Options** Full-time and part-time.
**Program Entrance Requirements** Clinical experience, minimum overall college GPA of 3.0, transcript of college record, CPR certification, written essay, immunizations, interview, 3 letters of recommendation, resume, statistics course, GRE General Test. *Application deadline:* 4/1 (fall), 10/15 (spring). Applications may be processed on a rolling basis for some programs. *Application fee:* $65.
**Degree Requirements** 30 total credit hours, comprehensive exam.

### POST-MASTER'S PROGRAM
**Areas of Study** *Nurse practitioner programs in:* acute care, adult health, family health, gerontology, psychiatric/mental health.

### DOCTORAL DEGREE PROGRAM
**Degree** PhD
**Available Programs** Doctorate; Post-Baccalaureate Doctorate.
**Areas of Study** Clinical research, ethics, health policy, health promotion/disease prevention, health-care systems, human health and illness, nursing policy, nursing research, nursing science.
**Program Entrance Requirements** Minimum overall college GPA of 3.0, interview, 3 letters of recommendation, MSN or equivalent, statistics course, vita, writing sample, GRE General Test. *Application deadline:* 10/15 (spring). Applications may be processed on a rolling basis for some programs. *Application fee:* $65.
**Degree Requirements** 40 total credit hours, dissertation, oral exam, written exam, residency.

## CONTINUING EDUCATION PROGRAM
**Contact** Ms. Deborah Paris, Assistant Dean, School of Nursing and Health Studies, University of Miami, PO Box 248153, M. Christine Schwartz Center, Room 152, Coral Gables, FL 33124-3850. *Telephone:* 305-284-4325. *Fax:* 305-284-4827. *E-mail:* dparis@miami.edu.

# University of North Florida
## School of Nursing
## Jacksonville, Florida

*http://www.unf.edu/brooks/nursing/*
Founded in 1965

**DEGREES • BSN • MSN**
**Nursing Program Faculty** 19 (50% with doctorates).
**Baccalaureate Enrollment** 279 **Women** 85% **Men** 15% **Minority** 20% **International** 1% **Part-time** 27%
**Graduate Enrollment** 35 **Women** 86% **Men** 14% **Minority** 6% **Part-time** 70%
**Nursing Student Activities** Sigma Theta Tau, Student Nurses' Association.
**Nursing Student Resources** Academic advising; academic or career counseling; assistance for students with disabilities; bookstore; campus computer network; career placement assistance; computer lab; computer-assisted instruction; e-mail services; interactive nursing skills videos; Internet; learning resource lab; library services; nursing audiovisuals; resume preparation assistance; skills, simulation, or other laboratory.
**Library Facilities** 864,706 volumes (30,466 in health, 3,000 in nursing); 37,919 periodical subscriptions (200 health-care related).

## BACCALAUREATE PROGRAMS
**Degree** BSN
**Available Programs** Accelerated Baccalaureate for Second Degree; Generic Baccalaureate; RN Baccalaureate.
**Study Options** Full-time.
**Program Entrance Requirements** Minimum overall college GPA of 2.7, CPR certification, written essay, health exam, immunizations, interview, minimum high school GPA, minimum GPA in nursing prerequisites of 3.0, professional liability insurance/malpractice insurance, prerequisite course work. Transfer students are accepted.
**Advanced Placement** Credit given for nursing courses completed elsewhere dependent upon specific evaluations.
**Contact** *Telephone:* 904-620-2418.

## GRADUATE PROGRAMS
**Contact** *Telephone:* 904-620-2684. *Fax:* 904-620-2848.

### MASTER'S DEGREE PROGRAM
**Degree** MSN
**Available Programs** Master's; RN to Master's.
**Concentrations Available** *Clinical nurse specialist programs in:* adult health, cardiovascular, community health, critical care, gerontology, maternity-newborn, medical-surgical, pediatric, psychiatric/mental health,women's health. *Nurse practitioner programs in:* family health, primary care.
**Study Options** Full-time and part-time.
**Program Entrance Requirements** Clinical experience, computer literacy, minimum overall college GPA of 3.0, transcript of college record, CPR certification, written essay, immunizations, 2 letters of recommendation, nursing research course, physical assessment course, professional liability insurance/malpractice insurance, resume, statistics course.
**Advanced Placement** Credit given for nursing courses completed elsewhere dependent upon specific evaluations.
**Degree Requirements** 43 total credit hours, thesis or project.

### POST-MASTER'S PROGRAM
**Areas of Study** *Nurse practitioner programs in:* family health, primary care.

# University of Phoenix–North Florida Campus
## College of Nursing
## Jacksonville, Florida

Founded in 1976

**DEGREES • BSN • MSN • MSN/ED D • MSN/MHA**
**Nursing Program Faculty** 7 (29% with doctorates).
**Baccalaureate Enrollment** 13 **Women** 92.3% **Men** 7.7% **Minority** 38.5%
**Graduate Enrollment** 10 **Women** 100% **Minority** 20%
**Nursing Student Activities** Sigma Theta Tau.
**Nursing Student Resources** Academic advising; academic or career counseling; assistance for students with disabilities; bookstore; campus computer network; computer lab; computer-assisted instruction; e-mail services; interactive nursing skills videos; Internet; learning resource lab; library services; nursing audiovisuals; remedial services; skills, simulation, or other laboratory; tutoring.
**Library Facilities** 1,300 periodical subscriptions health-care related.

## BACCALAUREATE PROGRAMS
**Degree** BSN
**Available Programs** Accelerated Baccalaureate.
**Site Options** Orange Park, FL.
**Study Options** Full-time.
**Program Entrance Requirements** Transcript of college record, CPR certification, immunizations, 1 letter of recommendation, RN licensure. Transfer students are accepted. *Application deadline:* Applications may be processed on a rolling basis for some programs.
**Advanced Placement** Credit by examination available. Credit given for nursing courses completed elsewhere dependent upon specific evaluations.
**Contact** *Telephone:* 904-636-6645.

## GRADUATE PROGRAMS
**Contact** *Telephone:* 904-636-6645.

### MASTER'S DEGREE PROGRAM
**Degrees** MSN; MSN/Ed D; MSN/MHA
**Available Programs** Master's.
**Concentrations Available** Health-care administration; nursing administration; nursing education.
**Site Options** Orange Park, FL.

**Study Options** Full-time.
**Program Entrance Requirements** Clinical experience, computer literacy, minimum overall college GPA of 2.5, transcript of college record. *Application deadline:* Applications may be processed on a rolling basis for some programs. *Application fee:* $45.
**Advanced Placement** Credit given for nursing courses completed elsewhere dependent upon specific evaluations.
**Degree Requirements** 39 total credit hours, thesis or project.

# University of Phoenix–South Florida Campus
## College of Nursing
## Miramar, Florida

### DEGREES • BSN • MSN • MSN/MBA • MSN/MHA
**Nursing Program Faculty** 24 (21% with doctorates).
**Baccalaureate Enrollment** 135 **Women** 96.3% **Men** 3.7% **Minority** 38.5%
**Graduate Enrollment** 102 **Women** 91.2% **Men** 8.8% **Minority** 41.18%
**Nursing Student Activities** Sigma Theta Tau.
**Nursing Student Resources** Academic advising; academic or career counseling; assistance for students with disabilities; bookstore; campus computer network; computer lab; computer-assisted instruction; e-mail services; interactive nursing skills videos; Internet; learning resource lab; library services; nursing audiovisuals; skills, simulation, or other laboratory; tutoring.
**Library Facilities** 16,781 periodical subscriptions (1,300 health-care related).

### BACCALAUREATE PROGRAMS
**Degree** BSN
**Available Programs** RN Baccalaureate.
**Site Options** Palm Beach Gardens, FL; Ft. Lauderdale, FL; Miramar, FL.
**Study Options** Full-time.
**Online Degree Options** Yes.
**Program Entrance Requirements** Transcript of college record, CPR certification, immunizations, 1 letter of recommendation, RN licensure. Transfer students are accepted. *Application deadline:* Applications may be processed on a rolling basis for some programs.
**Advanced Placement** Credit by examination available. Credit given for nursing courses completed elsewhere dependent upon specific evaluations.
**Contact** *Telephone:* 954-382-5303.

### GRADUATE PROGRAMS
**Contact** *Telephone:* 954-382-5303.

**MASTER'S DEGREE PROGRAM**
**Degrees** MSN; MSN/MBA; MSN/MHA
**Available Programs** Master's.
**Concentrations Available** Health-care administration; nursing administration; nursing education.
**Site Options** Palm Beach Gardens, FL; Ft. Lauderdale, FL; Miramar, FL.
**Study Options** Full-time.
**Online Degree Options** Yes.
**Program Entrance Requirements** Clinical experience, computer literacy, minimum overall college GPA of 2.5, transcript of college record. *Application deadline:* Applications may be processed on a rolling basis for some programs. *Application fee:* $45.
**Advanced Placement** Credit given for nursing courses completed elsewhere dependent upon specific evaluations.
**Degree Requirements** 39 total credit hours, thesis or project.

# University of Phoenix–West Florida Campus
## College of Nursing
## Temple Terrace, Florida

### DEGREE • BSN
**Nursing Program Faculty** 5 (60% with doctorates).
**Baccalaureate Enrollment** 8 **Women** 87.5% **Men** 12.5% **Minority** 12.5%
**Nursing Student Activities** Sigma Theta Tau.
**Nursing Student Resources** Academic advising; academic or career counseling; assistance for students with disabilities; bookstore; campus computer network; computer lab; computer-assisted instruction; e-mail services; interactive nursing skills videos; Internet; learning resource lab; library services; nursing audiovisuals; remedial services; skills, simulation, or other laboratory; tutoring.
**Library Facilities** 16,781 periodical subscriptions (1,300 health-care related).

### BACCALAUREATE PROGRAMS
**Degree** BSN
**Available Programs** Accelerated Baccalaureate.
**Site Options** Tampa, FL; Clearwater, FL; Sarasota, FL.
**Study Options** Full-time.
**Online Degree Options** Yes.
**Program Entrance Requirements** Transcript of college record, CPR certification, immunizations, 1 letter of recommendation, RN licensure. Transfer students are accepted. *Application deadline:* Applications may be processed on a rolling basis for some programs.
**Advanced Placement** Credit by examination available. Credit given for nursing courses completed elsewhere dependent upon specific evaluations.
**Contact** *Telephone:* 813-626-7911.

# University of South Florida
## College of Nursing
## Tampa, Florida

***http://www.hsc.usf.edu/nursing***
Founded in 1956

### DEGREES • BS • DNP • MS • MS/MPH • PHD
**Nursing Program Faculty** 77 (63% with doctorates).
**Baccalaureate Enrollment** 939 **Women** 88% **Men** 12% **Minority** 33% **International** 4% **Part-time** 65%
**Graduate Enrollment** 921 **Women** 88% **Men** 12% **Minority** 35% **International** 4% **Part-time** 85%
**Distance Learning Courses** Available.
**Nursing Student Activities** Sigma Theta Tau, Student Nurses' Association.
**Nursing Student Resources** Academic advising; academic or career counseling; assistance for students with disabilities; bookstore; campus computer network; career placement assistance; computer lab; computer-assisted instruction; daycare for children of students; e-mail services; employment services for current students; housing assistance; interactive nursing skills videos; Internet; learning resource lab; library services; nursing audiovisuals; remedial services; resume preparation assistance; skills, simulation, or other laboratory; tutoring.
**Library Facilities** 2.2 million volumes (106,028 in health, 4,000 in nursing); 83,938 periodical subscriptions (1,750 health-care related).

### BACCALAUREATE PROGRAMS
**Degree** BS
**Available Programs** ADN to Baccalaureate; Accelerated Baccalaureate for Second Degree; Generic Baccalaureate.
**Study Options** Full-time.
**Online Degree Options** Yes.
**Program Entrance Requirements** Minimum overall college GPA of 3.2, transcript of college record, CPR certification, written essay, health insurance, immunizations, prerequisite course work. Transfer students are accepted. *Application deadline:* 6/15 (fall), 3/15 (summer). *Application fee:* $30.
**Expenses (2013–14)** *Tuition, state resident:* full-time $9504; part-time $211 per credit hour. *Tuition, nonresident:* full-time $25,875; part-time $575 per credit hour. *International tuition:* $25,875 full-time. *Room and board:* $13,875; room only: $8082 per academic year. *Required fees:* full-time $2795; part-time $66 per credit; part-time $1040 per term.
**Financial Aid** 66% of baccalaureate students in nursing programs received some form of financial aid in 2012–13.
**Contact** Ms. Joylynn Grier, Coordinator, Undergraduate Admissions, College of Nursing, University of South Florida, 12901 Bruce B. Downs Boulevard, MDC Box 22, Tampa, FL 33612. *Telephone:* 813-974-2191. *Fax:* 813-974-3118. *E-mail:* nurstudent@health.usf.edu.

## GRADUATE PROGRAMS

**Expenses (2013–14)** *Tuition, state resident:* full-time $15,531; part-time $431 per credit hour. *Tuition, nonresident:* full-time $31,578; part-time $877 per credit hour. *International tuition:* $31,578 full-time. *Room and board:* $14,675; room only: $8548 per academic year. *Required fees:* full-time $2161; part-time $84 per credit; part-time $840 per term.

**Financial Aid** 34% of graduate students in nursing programs received some form of financial aid in 2012–13. 7 research assistantships with tuition reimbursements available (averaging $18,935 per year), 29 teaching assistantships with tuition reimbursements available (averaging $30,814 per year) were awarded; tuition waivers (partial) and unspecified assistantships also available. *Financial aid application deadline:* 2/1.

**Contact** Mr. Mark Freeman, Admissions Recruiter Advisor, College of Nursing, University of South Florida, 12901 Bruce B. Downs Boulevard, MDC Box 22, Tampa, FL 33612. *Telephone:* 813-974-2952. *Fax:* 813-974-5418. *E-mail:* nurstudent@health.usf.edu.

### MASTER'S DEGREE PROGRAM

**Degrees** MS; MS/MPH

**Available Programs** Master's; Master's for Nurses with Non-Nursing Degrees; RN to Master's.

**Concentrations Available** Nurse anesthesia; nursing education. *Nurse practitioner programs in:* acute care, adult health, family health, gerontology, occupational health, oncology, pediatric.

**Study Options** Full-time and part-time.

**Program Entrance Requirements** Computer literacy, minimum overall college GPA of 3.0, transcript of college record, CPR certification, immunizations, interview, 3 letters of recommendation, resume, GRE General Test. *Application deadline:* 2/15 (fall), 10/15 (spring). *Application fee:* $30.

**Advanced Placement** Credit given for nursing courses completed elsewhere dependent upon specific evaluations.

**Degree Requirements** 45 total credit hours, comprehensive exam.

### DOCTORAL DEGREE PROGRAM

**Degree** DNP

**Available Programs** Doctorate, Post-Baccalaureate Doctorate.

**Areas of Study** Adult gerontology, advanced practice nursing, dual oncology/adult gerontology, dual occupational health/adult gerontology, family health, pediatrics.

**Program Entrance Requirements** Minimum overall college GPA of 3.0, interview, interview by faculty committee, letters of recommendation, MSN or equivalent, statistics course, vita, writing sample. *Application deadline:* 2/1 (fall). Deadline varies for each admission cycle.

**Degree Requirements** 30-91 total credit hours, final project, residency.

**Degree** PhD

**Available Programs** Doctorate; Post-Baccalaureate Doctorate.

**Areas of Study** Family health, gerontology, nursing education, oncology.

**Program Entrance Requirements** Minimum overall college GPA of 3.0, interview, 3 letters of recommendation, MSN or equivalent, vita, writing sample, GRE General Test (recommended). *Application deadline:* 12/15 (fall). *Application fee:* $30.

**Degree Requirements** 60 total credit hours, dissertation, oral exam, written exam.

## CONTINUING EDUCATION PROGRAM

**Contact** Dr. Deborah Sutherland, Associate Vice President, College of Nursing, University of South Florida, 124 South Franklin Street, Tampa, FL 33602. *Telephone:* 813-224-7840. *E-mail:* dsutherl@health.usf.edu.

# The University of Tampa

**Department of Nursing**
**Tampa, Florida**

***http://www.ut.edu/nursing***
Founded in 1931

**DEGREES • BSN • MSN**

**Nursing Program Faculty** 28 (36% with doctorates).

**Baccalaureate Enrollment** 149 **Women** 90% **Men** 10% **Minority** 18% **International** .7% **Part-time** .7%

**Graduate Enrollment** 142 **Women** 89% **Men** 11% **Minority** 30% **Part-time** 80%

**Nursing Student Activities** Sigma Theta Tau, Student Nurses' Association.

**Nursing Student Resources** Academic advising; academic or career counseling; assistance for students with disabilities; bookstore; campus computer network; career placement assistance; computer lab; computer-assisted instruction; e-mail services; employment services for current students; externships; housing assistance; interactive nursing skills videos; Internet; learning resource lab; library services; nursing audiovisuals; paid internships; placement services for program completers; remedial services; resume preparation assistance; skills, simulation, or other laboratory; tutoring; unpaid internships.

**Library Facilities** 243,334 volumes (252,152 in health, 3,025 in nursing); 56,220 periodical subscriptions (10,870 health-care related).

## BACCALAUREATE PROGRAMS

**Degree** BSN

**Available Programs** ADN to Baccalaureate; Generic Baccalaureate; RN Baccalaureate.

**Study Options** Full-time.

**Program Entrance Requirements** Minimum overall college GPA of 3.25, transcript of college record, CPR certification, written essay, health exam, health insurance, high school transcript, immunizations, 1 letter of recommendation, minimum GPA in nursing prerequisites, professional liability insurance/malpractice insurance, prerequisite course work. Transfer students are accepted. *Application deadline:* 10/15 (spring). *Application fee:* $40.

**Expenses (2013–14)** *Tuition:* full-time $25,772; part-time $510 per credit hour. *Room and board:* $9388; room only: $4500 per academic year.

**Financial Aid** 85% of baccalaureate students in nursing programs received some form of financial aid in 2012–13.

**Contact** Admissions Office, Department of Nursing, The University of Tampa, 401 West Kennedy Boulevard, Box F, Tampa, FL 33606. *Telephone:* 813-253-6211. *Fax:* 813-258-7398. *E-mail:* admissions@ut.edu.

## GRADUATE PROGRAMS

**Expenses (2013–14)** *Tuition:* part-time $546 per credit hour.

**Financial Aid** 80% of graduate students in nursing programs received some form of financial aid in 2012–13.

**Contact** Graduate Studies Office, Department of Nursing, The University of Tampa, 401 West Kennedy Boulevard, Tampa, FL 33606. *Telephone:* 813-258-7409. *Fax:* 813-259-5403. *E-mail:* utgrad@ut.edu.

### MASTER'S DEGREE PROGRAM

**Degree** MSN

**Available Programs** Master's; RN to Master's.

**Concentrations Available** *Nurse practitioner programs in:* adult health, family health, gerontology.

**Study Options** Full-time and part-time.

**Program Entrance Requirements** Computer literacy, minimum overall college GPA of 3.0, transcript of college record, CPR certification, written essay, immunizations, 2 letters of recommendation, nursing research course, physical assessment course, professional liability insurance/malpractice insurance, prerequisite course work, resume, statistics course. *Application deadline:* Applications may be processed on a rolling basis for some programs. *Application fee:* $40.

**Advanced Placement** Credit given for nursing courses completed elsewhere dependent upon specific evaluations.

**Degree Requirements** 48 total credit hours, comprehensive exam.

### POST-MASTER'S PROGRAM

**Areas of Study** *Nurse practitioner programs in:* adult health, family health, gerontology.

## CONTINUING EDUCATION PROGRAM

**Contact** Dr. Susan Garbutt, Clinical Simulation Coordinator, Department of Nursing, The University of Tampa, 401 West Kennedy Boulevard, Box 10-F, Tampa, FL 33606-1490. *Telephone:* 813-257-3295. *Fax:* 813-258-7214. *E-mail:* sgarbutt@ut.edu.

## University of West Florida

### Department of Nursing
### Pensacola, Florida

*http://www.uwf.edu/nursing*
Founded in 1963

**DEGREES • BSN • MSN**
**Nursing Program Faculty** 13 (64% with doctorates).
**Baccalaureate Enrollment** 133 **Women** 73% **Men** 27% **Minority** 14% **International** 10% **Part-time** 60%
**Graduate Enrollment** 30 **Women** 87% **Men** 13% **Minority** 14% **International** 1% **Part-time** 60%
**Distance Learning Courses** Available.
**Nursing Student Activities** Sigma Theta Tau, Student Nurses' Association.
**Nursing Student Resources** Academic advising; academic or career counseling; assistance for students with disabilities; bookstore; campus computer network; computer lab; computer-assisted instruction; daycare for children of students; e-mail services; employment services for current students; housing assistance; interactive nursing skills videos; Internet; learning resource lab; library services; nursing audiovisuals; remedial services; resume preparation assistance; skills, simulation, or other laboratory; tutoring; unpaid internships.
**Library Facilities** 976,188 volumes (3,500 in health, 1,300 in nursing); 11,851 periodical subscriptions (54 health-care related).

### BACCALAUREATE PROGRAMS

**Degree** BSN
**Available Programs** ADN to Baccalaureate; Generic Baccalaureate; RN Baccalaureate.
**Study Options** Full-time.
**Program Entrance Requirements** Minimum overall college GPA of 3.0, transcript of college record, CPR certification, health exam, health insurance, immunizations, prerequisite course work. Transfer students are accepted. *Application deadline:* 3/1 (fall).
**Expenses (2013–14)** *Tuition, state resident:* full-time $6567; part-time $850 per course. *Tuition, nonresident:* full-time $9822.
**Financial Aid** 70% of baccalaureate students in nursing programs received some form of financial aid in 2012–13. *Gift aid (need-based):* Federal Pell, FSEOG, state, private, college/university gift aid from institutional funds. *Loans:* Federal Direct (Subsidized and Unsubsidized Stafford PLUS), Perkins. *Work-study:* Federal Work-Study, part-time campus jobs. *Financial aid application deadline:* Continuous.
**Contact** Mrs. Genia Taylor, Nursing Advisor, Department of Nursing, University of West Florida, 11000 University Parkway, Bldg. 37, Pensacola, FL 32514. *Telephone:* 850-473-7757. *Fax:* 850-473-7769. *E-mail:* etaylor3@uwf.edu.

### GRADUATE PROGRAMS

**Expenses (2013–14)** *Tuition, area resident:* full-time $7453; part-time $415 per contact hour.
**Contact** Dr. Angela Blackburn, Assistant Professor, Department of Nursing, University of West Florida, 11000 University Parkway, Building 37, Pensacola, FL 32514. *Telephone:* 850-473-7760. *Fax:* 850-473-7769. *E-mail:* ablackburn@uwf.edu.

#### MASTER'S DEGREE PROGRAM

**Degree** MSN
**Available Programs** Master's.
**Concentrations Available** Nursing administration; nursing education.
**Study Options** Full-time and part-time.
**Online Degree Options** Yes (online only).
**Program Entrance Requirements** Clinical experience, computer literacy, minimum overall college GPA of 3.0, transcript of college record, CPR certification, immunizations, 3 letters of recommendation, professional liability insurance/malpractice insurance, resume. *Application deadline:* 6/1 (fall), 10/1 (spring), 3/1 (summer). Applications may be processed on a rolling basis for some programs.
**Advanced Placement** Credit given for nursing courses completed elsewhere dependent upon specific evaluations.
**Degree Requirements** 39 total credit hours, thesis or project.

# GEORGIA

## Albany State University

### College of Sciences and Health Professions
### Albany, Georgia

*http://www.asurams.edu/*
Founded in 1903

**DEGREES • BSN • MSN**
**Nursing Program Faculty** 19 (37% with doctorates).
**Baccalaureate Enrollment** 90 **Women** 93% **Men** 7% **Minority** 96% **Part-time** 26%
**Graduate Enrollment** 90 **Women** 90% **Men** 10% **Minority** 49% **International** 3% **Part-time** 40%
**Distance Learning Courses** Available.
**Nursing Student Activities** Nursing Honor Society, Student Nurses' Association, nursing club.
**Nursing Student Resources** Academic advising; academic or career counseling; assistance for students with disabilities; bookstore; campus computer network; career placement assistance; computer lab; computer-assisted instruction; e-mail services; interactive nursing skills videos; Internet; learning resource lab; library services; nursing audiovisuals; paid internships; placement services for program completers; remedial services; resume preparation assistance; skills, simulation, or other laboratory; tutoring; unpaid internships.
**Library Facilities** 201,063 volumes (15,075 in health, 7,032 in nursing); 327 periodical subscriptions (75 health-care related).

### BACCALAUREATE PROGRAMS

**Degree** BSN
**Available Programs** ADN to Baccalaureate; Accelerated Baccalaureate for Second Degree; Generic Baccalaureate.
**Study Options** Full-time.
**Online Degree Options** Yes.
**Program Entrance Requirements** Minimum overall college GPA of 2.75, transcript of college record, CPR certification, health exam, health insurance, high school biology, high school foreign language, 4 years high school math, 3 years high school science, high school transcript, immunizations, minimum GPA in nursing prerequisites of 2.75, professional liability insurance/malpractice insurance, prerequisite course work. Transfer students are accepted. *Application deadline:* 7/1 (fall), 11/1 (spring), 4/1 (summer). Applications may be processed on a rolling basis for some programs. *Application fee:* $20.
**Advanced Placement** Credit given for nursing courses completed elsewhere dependent upon specific evaluations.
**Expenses (2013–14)** *Tuition, state resident:* full-time $4624; part-time $151 per credit hour. *Tuition, nonresident:* full-time $16,826; part-time $561 per credit hour. *Room and board:* $7646; room only: $4708 per academic year. *Required fees:* full-time $1400; part-time $758 per credit.
**Financial Aid** 92% of baccalaureate students in nursing programs received some form of financial aid in 2012–13.
**Contact** Dr. Cathy H. Williams, Chair, Department of Nursing, College of Sciences and Health Professions, Albany State University, 504 College Drive, Albany, GA 31705. *Telephone:* 229-430-4728. *Fax:* 229-434-7118. *E-mail:* cathy.williams@asurams.edu.

### GRADUATE PROGRAMS

**Expenses (2013–14)** *Tuition, state resident:* full-time $4528; part-time $189 per credit hour. *Tuition, nonresident:* full-time $18,106; part-time $755 per credit hour. *Room and board:* $8738; room only: $5800 per academic year. *Required fees:* full-time $1400; part-time $379 per credit.
**Financial Aid** 70% of graduate students in nursing programs received some form of financial aid in 2012–13. Scholarships and traineeships available. *Financial aid application deadline:* 4/15.
**Contact** Dr. Cathy H. Williams, Chair, Department of Nursing, College of Sciences and Health Professions, Albany State University, 504 College Drive, Albany, GA 31705. *Telephone:* 229-430-4728. *Fax:* 229-434-7118. *E-mail:* cathy.williams@asurams.edu.

#### MASTER'S DEGREE PROGRAM

**Degree** MSN
**Available Programs** Master's; RN to Master's.
**Concentrations Available** Nursing education. *Nurse practitioner programs in:* family health.
**Study Options** Full-time and part-time.
**Online Degree Options** Yes (online only).

**Program Entrance Requirements** Clinical experience, computer literacy, minimum overall college GPA of 3.0, transcript of college record, CPR certification, immunizations, 2 letters of recommendation, nursing research course, physical assessment course, professional liability insurance/malpractice insurance, prerequisite course work, resume, statistics course, GRE or MAT. *Application deadline:* 7/1 (fall), 11/1 (spring), 4/1 (summer). Applications may be processed on a rolling basis for some programs. *Application fee:* $20.
**Advanced Placement** Credit given for nursing courses completed elsewhere dependent upon specific evaluations.
**Degree Requirements** 36 total credit hours, thesis or project, comprehensive exam.

**POST-MASTER'S PROGRAM**
**Areas of Study** Nursing education. *Nurse practitioner programs in:* family health.

# Armstrong Atlantic State University
## Program in Nursing
## Savannah, Georgia

***http://www.armstrong.edu/Health_professions/nursing/nursing_welcome***
Founded in 1935

**DEGREES • BSN • MSN**
**Nursing Program Faculty** 53 (19% with doctorates).
**Baccalaureate Enrollment** 350 **Women** 85% **Men** 15% **Minority** 35% **International** 2% **Part-time** 10%
**Graduate Enrollment** 45 **Women** 89% **Men** 11% **Minority** 33% **Part-time** 75%
**Distance Learning Courses** Available.
**Nursing Student Activities** Nursing Honor Society, Sigma Theta Tau, Student Nurses' Association.
**Nursing Student Resources** Academic advising; academic or career counseling; assistance for students with disabilities; bookstore; campus computer network; career placement assistance; computer lab; computer-assisted instruction; e-mail services; employment services for current students; externships; housing assistance; interactive nursing skills videos; Internet; learning resource lab; library services; nursing audiovisuals; remedial services; resume preparation assistance; skills, simulation, or other laboratory; tutoring.
**Library Facilities** 254,777 volumes (8,500 in nursing); 496 periodical subscriptions (200 health-care related).

### BACCALAUREATE PROGRAMS
**Degree** BSN
**Available Programs** ADN to Baccalaureate; Accelerated Baccalaureate for Second Degree; Generic Baccalaureate; LPN to Baccalaureate; RN Baccalaureate.
**Study Options** Full-time and part-time.
**Program Entrance Requirements** Minimum overall college GPA of 3.0, transcript of college record, CPR certification, health exam, health insurance, immunizations, minimum GPA in nursing prerequisites of 3.0, professional liability insurance/malpractice insurance, prerequisite course work. Transfer students are accepted. *Application deadline:* 2/28 (fall), 10/15 (spring). *Application fee:* $25.
**Advanced Placement** Credit by examination available. Credit given for nursing courses completed elsewhere dependent upon specific evaluations.
**Financial Aid** 90% of baccalaureate students in nursing programs received some form of financial aid in 2012–13.
**Contact** Ms. Kristy Gose, Administrative Assistant, Program in Nursing, Armstrong Atlantic State University, 11935 Abercorn Street, Savannah, GA 31419-1997. *Telephone:* 912-344-2575. *Fax:* 912-344-3481. *E-mail:* kristy.gose@armstrong.edu.

### GRADUATE PROGRAMS
**Financial Aid** 85% of graduate students in nursing programs received some form of financial aid in 2012–13. Research assistantships with full tuition reimbursements available (averaging $5,000 per year); Federal Work-Study, scholarships, and unspecified assistantships also available. Aid available to part-time students. *Financial aid application deadline:* 3/1.
**Contact** Dr. Anita Nivens, Graduate Program Coordinator, Program in Nursing, Armstrong Atlantic State University, 11935 Abercorn Street, Savannah, GA 31419-1997. *Telephone:* 912-344-2724. *Fax:* 912-344-3481. *E-mail:* anita.nivens@armstrong.edu.

**MASTER'S DEGREE PROGRAM**
**Degree** MSN
**Available Programs** Master's.
**Concentrations Available** *Nurse practitioner programs in:* acute care, adult health.
**Study Options** Full-time and part-time.
**Program Entrance Requirements** Clinical experience, computer literacy, minimum overall college GPA of 3.0, transcript of college record, CPR certification, written essay, immunizations, interview, 3 letters of recommendation, nursing research course, physical assessment course, professional liability insurance/malpractice insurance, prerequisite course work, statistics course, GRE General Test or MAT. *Application deadline:* 5/15 (fall), 11/15 (spring).
**Advanced Placement** Credit by examination available. Credit given for nursing courses completed elsewhere dependent upon specific evaluations.
**Degree Requirements** 36 total credit hours, thesis or project.

**POST-MASTER'S PROGRAM**
**Areas of Study** *Nurse practitioner programs in:* acute care, adult health.

# Brenau University
## College of Health and Science
## Gainesville, Georgia

Founded in 1878

**DEGREES • BSN • DNP • MSN**
**Nursing Program Faculty** 15 (65% with doctorates).
**Baccalaureate Enrollment** 300 **Women** 95% **Men** 5% **Minority** 40% **International** 10% **Part-time** 50%
**Graduate Enrollment** 100 **Women** 95% **Men** 5% **Minority** 40% **Part-time** 100%
**Distance Learning Courses** Available.
**Nursing Student Activities** Sigma Theta Tau, Student Nurses' Association.
**Nursing Student Resources** Academic advising; academic or career counseling; assistance for students with disabilities; bookstore; campus computer network; career placement assistance; computer lab; computer-assisted instruction; e-mail services; housing assistance; interactive nursing skills videos; Internet; learning resource lab; library services; nursing audiovisuals; remedial services; skills, simulation, or other laboratory; tutoring.
**Library Facilities** 86,590 volumes (6,000 in health, 5,000 in nursing); 20,128 periodical subscriptions (500 health-care related).

### BACCALAUREATE PROGRAMS
**Degree** BSN
**Available Programs** ADN to Baccalaureate; Generic Baccalaureate; RN Baccalaureate.
**Study Options** Full-time and part-time.
**Online Degree Options** Yes.
**Program Entrance Requirements** Minimum overall college GPA of 2.75, transcript of college record, high school biology, high school chemistry, high school foreign language, 2 years high school math, 1 year of high school science, high school transcript, minimum high school GPA of 2.75, minimum GPA in nursing prerequisites of 2.5. Transfer students are accepted. *Application deadline:* 7/15 (spring), 11/15 (summer). *Application fee:* $35.
**Advanced Placement** Credit by examination available. Credit given for nursing courses completed elsewhere dependent upon specific evaluations.
**Contact** *Telephone:* 770-534-6100. *Fax:* 770-538-4306.

### GRADUATE PROGRAMS
**Contact** *Telephone:* 770-534-6125. *Fax:* 770-534-4666.

**MASTER'S DEGREE PROGRAM**
**Degree** MSN
**Available Programs** Accelerated AD/RN to Master's; Accelerated RN to Master's; Master's; RN to Master's.

**Concentrations Available** Clinical nurse leader; nursing education. *Nurse practitioner programs in:* family health.
**Site Options** Atlanta, GA.
**Study Options** Part-time.
**Program Entrance Requirements** Clinical experience, minimum overall college GPA of 3.0, transcript of college record, CPR certification, written essay, immunizations, 2 letters of recommendation, nursing research course, physical assessment course, prerequisite course work, statistics course, GRE General Test or MAT (for some programs). *Application deadline:* Applications may be processed on a rolling basis for some programs.
**Degree Requirements** Thesis or project.

**POST-MASTER'S PROGRAM**
**Areas of Study** *Nurse practitioner programs in:* family health.

**DOCTORAL DEGREE PROGRAM**
**Degree** DNP
**Available Programs** Doctorate.
**Site Options** Atlanta, GA.
**Program Entrance Requirements** Clinical experience, minimum overall college GPA of 3.0, letters of recommendation, MSN or equivalent, statistics course, vita, writing sample.

# Clayton State University
## Department of Nursing
## Morrow, Georgia

***http://www.clayton.edu/health/Nursing***
Founded in 1969

### DEGREES • BSN • MSN
**Nursing Program Faculty** 42 (35% with doctorates).
**Baccalaureate Enrollment** 258 **Women** 85.7% **Men** 14.3% **Minority** 69% **International** 14.3% **Part-time** 38%
**Graduate Enrollment** 25 **Women** 96% **Men** 4% **Minority** 76% **International** 4% **Part-time** 64%
**Distance Learning Courses** Available.
**Nursing Student Activities** Nursing Honor Society, Sigma Theta Tau, Student Nurses' Association.
**Nursing Student Resources** Academic advising; academic or career counseling; assistance for students with disabilities; bookstore; campus computer network; career placement assistance; computer lab; computer-assisted instruction; e-mail services; employment services for current students; externships; housing assistance; interactive nursing skills videos; Internet; learning resource lab; library services; nursing audiovisuals; paid internships; placement services for program completers; remedial services; resume preparation assistance; skills, simulation, or other laboratory; tutoring.
**Library Facilities** 148,798 volumes (3,450 in health, 1,800 in nursing); 618 periodical subscriptions (151 health-care related).

### BACCALAUREATE PROGRAMS
**Degree** BSN
**Available Programs** Generic Baccalaureate; RN Baccalaureate.
**Study Options** Full-time.
**Online Degree Options** Yes.
**Program Entrance Requirements** Minimum overall college GPA of 2.5, transcript of college record, CPR certification, health exam, health insurance, immunizations, interview, minimum GPA in nursing prerequisites of 2.5, professional liability insurance/malpractice insurance, prerequisite course work. Transfer students are accepted. *Application deadline:* 2/15 (fall), 9/15 (spring). *Application fee:* $25.
**Expenses (2012–13)** *Tuition, state resident:* full-time $3610; part-time $150 per credit hour. *Tuition, nonresident:* full-time $13,113; part-time $547 per credit hour. *International tuition:* $13,113 full-time. *Room and board:* $8862; room only: $5574 per academic year. *Required fees:* full-time $1404.
**Financial Aid** 61% of baccalaureate students in nursing programs received some form of financial aid in 2011–12. *Gift aid (need-based):* Federal Pell, FSEOG, state, private, college/university gift aid from institutional funds, Federal Nursing. *Loans:* Federal Direct (Subsidized and Unsubsidized Stafford PLUS), state. *Work-study:* Federal Work-Study. *Financial aid application deadline (priority):* 7/15.
**Contact** Dr. Sue E. Odom, Director of the Undergraduate Nursing Program, Department of Nursing, Clayton State University, 2000 Clayton State Boulevard, Morrow, GA 30260. *Telephone:* 678-466-4959. *Fax:* 678-466-4999. *E-mail:* sueodom@clayton.edu.

### GRADUATE PROGRAMS
**Expenses (2012–13)** *Tuition, state resident:* part-time $385 per credit hour. *Tuition, nonresident:* part-time $385 per credit hour. *Room and board:* $8862; room only: $5574 per academic year.
**Financial Aid** 3.8% of graduate students in nursing programs received some form of financial aid in 2011–12.
**Contact** Dr. Betty Lane, Director of the MSN Program, Department of Nursing, Clayton State University, 2000 Clayton State Boulevard, Morrow, GA 30260. *Telephone:* 678-466-4953. *Fax:* 678-466-4999. *E-mail:* bettylane@clayton.edu.

**MASTER'S DEGREE PROGRAM**
**Degree** MSN
**Available Programs** Master's; RN to Master's.
**Concentrations Available** Nursing administration; nursing education.
**Study Options** Full-time and part-time.
**Online Degree Options** Yes (online only).
**Program Entrance Requirements** Computer literacy, minimum overall college GPA of 3.0, transcript of college record, CPR certification, written essay, immunizations, interview, 3 letters of recommendation, professional liability insurance/malpractice insurance. *Application deadline:* 7/1 (fall), 11/1 (spring), 3/1 (summer). Applications may be processed on a rolling basis for some programs. *Application fee:* $25.
**Advanced Placement** Credit given for nursing courses completed elsewhere dependent upon specific evaluations.
**Degree Requirements** 36 total credit hours, thesis or project.

# College of Coastal Georgia
## Department of Nursing and Health Sciences
## Brunswick, Georgia

***http://www.ccga.edu/Academics/SchoolNursing/***
Founded in 1961

### DEGREE • BSN
**Nursing Program Faculty** 16 (31% with doctorates).
**Baccalaureate Enrollment** 168 **Women** 85% **Men** 15% **Minority** 20% **Part-time** 11%
**Distance Learning Courses** Available.
**Nursing Student Activities** Student Nurses' Association.
**Nursing Student Resources** Academic advising; academic or career counseling; assistance for students with disabilities; bookstore; campus computer network; career placement assistance; computer lab; computer-assisted instruction; e-mail services; employment services for current students; externships; housing assistance; interactive nursing skills videos; Internet; learning resource lab; library services; nursing audiovisuals; placement services for program completers; remedial services; resume preparation assistance; skills, simulation, or other laboratory; tutoring; unpaid internships.
**Library Facilities** 15.3 million volumes (1,730 in health, 282 in nursing); 330 periodical subscriptions (48 health-care related).

### BACCALAUREATE PROGRAMS
**Degree** BSN
**Available Programs** RN Baccalaureate.
**Study Options** Full-time.
**Online Degree Options** Yes.
**Program Entrance Requirements** Minimum overall college GPA of 2.8, transcript of college record, CPR certification, health exam, health insurance, immunizations, minimum GPA in nursing prerequisites of 2.8, professional liability insurance/malpractice insurance, prerequisite course work. Transfer students are accepted. *Application deadline:* 2/15 (fall).
**Expenses (2013–14)** *Tuition, state resident:* full-time $2918; part-time $97 per credit hour. *Tuition, nonresident:* full-time $10,776; part-time $359 per credit hour. *Room and board:* $13,764 per academic year. *Required fees:* full-time $1320.
**Financial Aid** 98% of baccalaureate students in nursing programs received some form of financial aid in 2012–13. *Gift aid (need-based):* Federal Pell, FSEOG, state, private, college/university gift aid from institutional funds. *Work-study:* Federal Work-Study. *Financial aid application deadline (priority):* 7/1.
**Contact** Dr. Patricia Kraft, Southeast Georgia Health System Distinguished Dean of Nursing and Health Sciences, Department of Nursing and Health Sciences, College of Coastal Georgia, One College

Drive, Brunswick, GA 31520. *Telephone:* 912-279-5860. *Fax:* 912-279-5912. *E-mail:* pkraft@ccga.edu.

# Columbus State University

## Nursing Program
## Columbus, Georgia

*http://nursing.columbusstate.edu/*
Founded in 1958

### DEGREE • BSN

**Nursing Program Faculty** 31 (12% with doctorates).
**Baccalaureate Enrollment** 187 **Women** 91% **Men** 9% **Minority** 42% **International** 6% **Part-time** 3%
**Distance Learning Courses** Available.
**Nursing Student Activities** Sigma Theta Tau, Student Nurses' Association.
**Nursing Student Resources** Academic advising; academic or career counseling; assistance for students with disabilities; bookstore; campus computer network; career placement assistance; computer lab; computer-assisted instruction; e-mail services; housing assistance; interactive nursing skills videos; Internet; learning resource lab; library services; nursing audiovisuals; remedial services; resume preparation assistance; skills, simulation, or other laboratory; tutoring.
**Library Facilities** 376,614 volumes (284 in health, 260 in nursing); 1,392 periodical subscriptions (81 health-care related).

### BACCALAUREATE PROGRAMS

**Degree** BSN
**Available Programs** Generic Baccalaureate; RN Baccalaureate.
**Study Options** Full-time.
**Online Degree Options** Yes.
**Program Entrance Requirements** Minimum overall college GPA of 2.75, transcript of college record, CPR certification, health exam, health insurance, immunizations, 3 letters of recommendation, minimum GPA in nursing prerequisites of 2.75, professional liability insurance/malpractice insurance, prerequisite course work. *Application deadline:* 2/28 (fall).
**Advanced Placement** Credit given for nursing courses completed elsewhere dependent upon specific evaluations.
**Contact** *Telephone:* 706-568-5050. *Fax:* 706-569-3101.

# Emory University

## Nell Hodgson Woodruff School of Nursing
## Atlanta, Georgia

*http://www.nursing.emory.edu/*
Founded in 1836

### DEGREES • BSN • MSN • MSN/MPH • PHD

**Nursing Program Faculty** 102 (86% with doctorates).
**Baccalaureate Enrollment** 298 **Women** 92% **Men** 8% **Minority** 44% **International** 3%
**Graduate Enrollment** 172 **Women** 92% **Men** 8% **Minority** 22% **International** 1% **Part-time** 17%
**Nursing Student Activities** Sigma Theta Tau, Student Nurses' Association.
**Nursing Student Resources** Academic advising; academic or career counseling; assistance for students with disabilities; bookstore; campus computer network; career placement assistance; computer lab; computer-assisted instruction; daycare for children of students; e-mail services; employment services for current students; externships; housing assistance; interactive nursing skills videos; Internet; learning resource lab; library services; nursing audiovisuals; other; resume preparation assistance; skills, simulation, or other laboratory; tutoring; unpaid internships.
**Library Facilities** 3.9 million volumes (250,000 in health); 1,800 periodical subscriptions health-care related.

### BACCALAUREATE PROGRAMS

**Degree** BSN
**Available Programs** Accelerated Baccalaureate for Second Degree; Baccalaureate for Second Degree; Generic Baccalaureate.
**Study Options** Full-time.
**Program Entrance Requirements** Minimum overall college GPA of 3.0, transcript of college record, written essay, 3 letters of recommendation, minimum GPA in nursing prerequisites of 3.0, prerequisite course work. Transfer students are accepted. *Application deadline:* 1/15 (fall), 12/1 (summer). *Application fee:* $50.
**Advanced Placement** Credit given for nursing courses completed elsewhere dependent upon specific evaluations.
**Expenses (2013–14)** *Tuition:* full-time $39,000; part-time $1625 per credit hour. *International tuition:* $39,000 full-time. *Room and board:* $10,460; room only: $7360 per academic year. *Required fees:* full-time $608.
**Financial Aid** 98% of baccalaureate students in nursing programs received some form of financial aid in 2012–13. *Gift aid (need-based):* Federal Pell, FSEOG, private, college/university gift aid from institutional funds. *Loans:* Federal Nursing Student Loans, Federal Direct (Subsidized and Unsubsidized Stafford PLUS), Perkins, state, college/university, alternative loans. *Work-study:* Federal Work-Study, part-time campus jobs. *Financial aid application deadline:* 3/1(priority: 2/15).
**Contact** Mrs. Katie Kennedy, Office of Enrollment and Student Affairs, Nell Hodgson Woodruff School of Nursing, Emory University, 1520 Clifton Road NE, Atlanta, GA 30322. *Telephone:* 404-727-7980. *Fax:* 404-727-8509. *E-mail:* admit@nursing.emory.edu.

### GRADUATE PROGRAMS

**Expenses (2013–14)** *Tuition:* full-time $58,500; part-time $1625 per credit hour. *International tuition:* $58,500 full-time. *Room and board:* $11,892; room only: $9792 per academic year. *Required fees:* full-time $534; part-time $534 per term.
**Financial Aid** 98% of graduate students in nursing programs received some form of financial aid in 2012–13. 14 fellowships (averaging $28,000 per year) were awarded; career-related internships or fieldwork, Federal Work-Study, institutionally sponsored loans, and scholarships also available. Aid available to part-time students. *Financial aid application deadline:* 3/1.
**Contact** Mrs. Katie Kennedy, Office of Enrollment and Student Affairs, Nell Hodgson Woodruff School of Nursing, Emory University, 1520 Clifton Road NE, Atlanta, GA 30322. *Telephone:* 404-727-7980. *Fax:* 404-727-8509. *E-mail:* admit@nursing.emory.edu.

#### MASTER'S DEGREE PROGRAM

**Degrees** MSN; MSN/MPH
**Available Programs** Master's.
**Concentrations Available** Nurse-midwifery. *Nurse practitioner programs in:* acute care, adult health, family health, pediatric, primary care,women's health.
**Study Options** Full-time and part-time.
**Program Entrance Requirements** Clinical experience, minimum overall college GPA of 3.0, transcript of college record, written essay, interview, 3 letters of recommendation, physical assessment course, prerequisite course work, resume, statistics course, GRE General Test or MAT. *Application deadline:* 1/15 (fall), 10/1 (spring), 1/15 (summer). Applications may be processed on a rolling basis for some programs. *Application fee:* $50.
**Advanced Placement** Credit given for nursing courses completed elsewhere dependent upon specific evaluations.
**Degree Requirements** 64 total credit hours.

#### POST-MASTER'S PROGRAM

**Areas of Study** Nurse-midwifery. *Nurse practitioner programs in:* acute care, adult health, family health, pediatric, primary care,women's health.

#### DOCTORAL DEGREE PROGRAM

**Degree** PhD
**Available Programs** Doctorate; Post-Baccalaureate Doctorate.
**Areas of Study** Aging, biology of health and illness, ethics, faculty preparation, gerontology, health policy, human health and illness, illness and transition, individualized study, neuro-behavior, nursing policy, nursing research, nursing science,women's health.
**Program Entrance Requirements** Minimum overall college GPA of 3.0, interview by faculty committee, 3 letters of recommendation, MSN or equivalent, statistics course, vita, writing sample. *Application deadline:* 1/3 (fall). Applications may be processed on a rolling basis for some programs.
**Degree Requirements** 50 total credit hours, dissertation, oral exam, written exam, residency.

**POSTDOCTORAL PROGRAM**
**Postdoctoral Program Contact** Ms. Teresa Fosque, Senior Business Manager, Nell Hodgson Woodruff School of Nursing, Emory University, 1520 Clifton Road NE, Atlanta, GA 30322. *E-mail:* tfosque@emory.edu.

# Georgia College & State University

## College of Health Sciences
## Milledgeville, Georgia

***http://www.gcsu.edu/nursing***
Founded in 1889

**DEGREES • BSN • DNP • MSN**
**Nursing Program Faculty** 20 (50% with doctorates).
**Baccalaureate Enrollment** 230 **Women** 89% **Men** 11% **Minority** 7% **International** 1% **Part-time** 30%
**Graduate Enrollment** 87 **Women** 88% **Men** 12% **Minority** 4% **Part-time** 20%
**Distance Learning Courses** Available.
**Nursing Student Activities** Nursing Honor Society, Sigma Theta Tau, Student Nurses' Association.
**Nursing Student Resources** Academic advising; academic or career counseling; assistance for students with disabilities; bookstore; campus computer network; career placement assistance; computer lab; computer-assisted instruction; e-mail services; employment services for current students; housing assistance; interactive nursing skills videos; Internet; learning resource lab; library services; nursing audiovisuals; remedial services; resume preparation assistance; skills, simulation, or other laboratory; tutoring; unpaid internships.
**Library Facilities** 210,609 volumes (3,095 in health, 1,465 in nursing); 43,000 periodical subscriptions (315 health-care related).

### BACCALAUREATE PROGRAMS

**Degree** BSN
**Available Programs** Generic Baccalaureate; RN Baccalaureate.
**Study Options** Full-time.
**Online Degree Options** Yes.
**Program Entrance Requirements** Minimum overall college GPA of 2.75, transcript of college record, CPR certification, health exam, health insurance, high school foreign language, 4 years high school math, 4 years high school science, high school transcript, immunizations, minimum high school GPA of 2.5, minimum GPA in nursing prerequisites of 2.75, professional liability insurance/malpractice insurance, prerequisite course work. Transfer students are accepted. *Application deadline:* 2/1 (fall), 7/15 (spring). *Application fee:* $10.
**Advanced Placement** Credit by examination available.
**Expenses (2013–14)** *Tuition, state resident:* full-time $8790. *Tuition, nonresident:* full-time $26,690. *Room and board:* $9258 per academic year. *Required fees:* full-time $2700.
**Financial Aid** 94% of baccalaureate students in nursing programs received some form of financial aid in 2012–13. *Gift aid (need-based):* Federal Pell, FSEOG, state, college/university gift aid from institutional funds. *Loans:* Federal Direct (Subsidized and Unsubsidized Stafford PLUS), Perkins. *Work-study:* Federal Work-Study. *Financial aid application deadline (priority):* 3/1.
**Contact** Ms. Tamette Farrington, Pre-Nursing Advisor, College of Health Sciences, Georgia College & State University, Campus Box 115, Milledgeville, GA 31061. *Telephone:* 478-445-2634. *E-mail:* tamette.farrington@gcsu.edu.

### GRADUATE PROGRAMS

**Expenses (2013–14)** *Tuition, state resident:* full-time $7310. *Tuition, nonresident:* full-time $7310. *Required fees:* full-time $2700.
**Financial Aid** 51% of graduate students in nursing programs received some form of financial aid in 2012–13. 31 research assistantships with tuition reimbursements available were awarded; career-related internships or fieldwork and unspecified assistantships also available. Aid available to part-time students.
**Contact** Dr. Debby MacmiIllan, Assistant Director, Graduate Programs, College of Health Sciences, Georgia College & State University, Macon Graduate Center, 433 Cherry Street, Macon, GA 31204. *Telephone:* 478-752-1074. *E-mail:* debby.macmillan@gcsu.edu.

**MASTER'S DEGREE PROGRAM**
**Degree** MSN
**Available Programs** Master's.
**Concentrations Available** *Nurse practitioner programs in:* family health.
**Site Options** Macon, GA.
**Study Options** Full-time and part-time.
**Online Degree Options** Yes (online only).
**Program Entrance Requirements** Clinical experience, computer literacy, minimum overall college GPA of 2.75, transcript of college record, CPR certification, written essay, immunizations, interview, 2 letters of recommendation, nursing research course, physical assessment course, professional liability insurance/malpractice insurance, statistics course, GRE, GMAT or MAT. *Application deadline:* 1/15 (summer).
**Advanced Placement** Credit given for nursing courses completed elsewhere dependent upon specific evaluations.
**Degree Requirements** 36 total credit hours, thesis or project, comprehensive exam.

**POST-MASTER'S PROGRAM**
**Areas of Study** *Nurse practitioner programs in:* family health.

**DOCTORAL DEGREE PROGRAM**
**Degree** DNP
**Available Programs** Doctorate.
**Site Options** Macon, GA.
**Online Degree Options** Yes (online only).
**Program Entrance Requirements** Clinical experience, minimum overall college GPA of 3.2, interview by faculty committee, 2 letters of recommendation, MSN or equivalent, statistics course, vita, writing sample. *Application deadline:* 1/15 (spring). *Application fee:* $10.
**Degree Requirements** 37 total credit hours.

# Georgia Regents University

## School of Nursing
## Augusta, Georgia

***http://www.gru.edu/nursing/***
Founded in 1828

**DEGREES • BSN • DNP • MSN • PHD**
**Nursing Program Faculty** 61 (47% with doctorates).
**Baccalaureate Enrollment** 162
**Graduate Enrollment** 396
**Distance Learning Courses** Available.
**Nursing Student Activities** Nursing Honor Society, Sigma Theta Tau, Student Nurses' Association, nursing club.
**Nursing Student Resources** Academic advising; academic or career counseling; assistance for students with disabilities; bookstore; campus computer network; career placement assistance; computer lab; computer-assisted instruction; daycare for children of students; e-mail services; employment services for current students; externships; housing assistance; interactive nursing skills videos; Internet; learning resource lab; library services; nursing audiovisuals; paid internships; remedial services; skills, simulation, or other laboratory; tutoring.
**Library Facilities** 178,650 volumes in health, 14,650 volumes in nursing; 1,307 periodical subscriptions health-care related.

### BACCALAUREATE PROGRAMS

**Degree** BSN
**Available Programs** Generic Baccalaureate.
**Site Options** Athens, GA.
**Study Options** Full-time.
**Program Entrance Requirements** Minimum overall college GPA of 2.8, transcript of college record, CPR certification, written essay, health insurance, immunizations, 2 letters of recommendation, prerequisite course work. Transfer students are accepted. *Application deadline:* 2/15 (fall). *Application fee:* $50.
**Contact** Office of Academic Admissions, School of Nursing, Georgia Regents University, AA-170 Kelly Building, Augusta, GA 30912. *Telephone:* 706-721-2725. *Fax:* 706-721-0186. *E-mail:* admissions@georgiahealth.edu.

### GRADUATE PROGRAMS

**Contact** Director, Academic Admissions, School of Nursing, Georgia Regents University, AA-170 Kelly Building, Augusta, GA 30912. *Telephone:* 706-721-2725. *Fax:* 706-721-0186. *E-mail:* admissions@georgiahealth.edu.

### MASTER'S DEGREE PROGRAM
**Degree** MSN
**Available Programs** Accelerated Master's for Non-Nursing College Graduates; Master's.
**Concentrations Available** Clinical nurse leader; nurse anesthesia. *Nurse practitioner programs in:* family health, pediatric.
**Site Options** Columbus, GA; Athens, GA.
**Study Options** Full-time and part-time.
**Online Degree Options** Yes.
**Program Entrance Requirements** Clinical experience, computer literacy, minimum overall college GPA of 3.0, transcript of college record, CPR certification, written essay, immunizations, interview, 3 letters of recommendation, professional liability insurance/malpractice insurance, prerequisite course work, resume, statistics course. *Application fee:* $50.
**Degree Requirements** Thesis or project.

### POST-MASTER'S PROGRAM
**Areas of Study** *Nurse practitioner programs in:* family health, pediatric, psychiatric/mental health.

### DOCTORAL DEGREE PROGRAM
**Degree** DNP
**Available Programs** Doctorate, Post-Baccalaureate Doctorate.
**Areas of Study** Advanced practice nursing.
**Online Degree Options** Yes.
**Program Entrance Requirements** Minimum overall college GPA of 3.3, clinical experience, interview, interview by faculty committee, 3 letters of recommendation, statistics course, vita, writing sample. *Application deadline:* 2/1 (fall). *Application fee:* $50.
**Degree Requirements** Capstone project.

**Degree** PhD
**Available Programs** Doctorate; Post-Baccalaureate Doctorate.
**Areas of Study** Bio-behavioral research, nursing research.
**Site Options** Columbus, GA; Athens, GA.
**Program Entrance Requirements** Clinical experience, minimum overall college GPA of 3.2, interview by faculty committee, interview, 3 letters of recommendation, MSN or equivalent, scholarly papers, statistics course, vita, writing sample. *Application fee:* $50.
**Degree Requirements** Dissertation, oral exam, written exam.

# Georgia Southern University
## School of Nursing
## Statesboro, Georgia

*http://chhs.georgiasouthern.edu/nursing/*
Founded in 1906

### DEGREES • BSN • DNP • MSN
**Nursing Program Faculty** 36 (18% with doctorates).
**Baccalaureate Enrollment** 267 **Women** 86.5% **Men** 13.5% **Minority** 15.3% **International** .4% **Part-time** 24.7%
**Graduate Enrollment** 64 **Women** 94% **Men** 6% **Minority** 27% **Part-time** 1.5%
**Distance Learning Courses** Available.
**Nursing Student Activities** Sigma Theta Tau, Student Nurses' Association.
**Nursing Student Resources** Academic advising; academic or career counseling; assistance for students with disabilities; bookstore; campus computer network; career placement assistance; computer lab; computer-assisted instruction; daycare for children of students; e-mail services; employment services for current students; housing assistance; interactive nursing skills videos; Internet; learning resource lab; library services; nursing audiovisuals; placement services for program completers; resume preparation assistance; skills, simulation, or other laboratory; tutoring.
**Library Facilities** 631,881 volumes (25,000 in health, 12,000 in nursing); 42,688 periodical subscriptions (20,000 health-care related).

## BACCALAUREATE PROGRAMS
**Degree** BSN
**Available Programs** ADN to Baccalaureate; Generic Baccalaureate; LPN to RN Baccalaureate.
**Study Options** Full-time.
**Online Degree Options** Yes.
**Program Entrance Requirements** Minimum overall college GPA of 3.0, transcript of college record, CPR certification, written essay, health exam, health insurance, high school biology, high school chemistry, high school foreign language, 2 years high school math, 4 years high school science, high school transcript, immunizations, minimum GPA in nursing prerequisites of 3.0, professional liability insurance/malpractice insurance, prerequisite course work. Transfer students are accepted. *Application deadline:* 2/4 (fall), 8/5 (spring).
**Advanced Placement** Credit by examination available. Credit given for nursing courses completed elsewhere dependent upon specific evaluations.
**Expenses (2013–14)** *Tuition, state resident:* full-time $2487; part-time $166 per credit hour. *Tuition, nonresident:* full-time $8778; part-time $585 per credit hour. *International tuition:* $8778 full-time. *Room and board:* $8933; room only: $3130 per academic year. *Required fees:* full-time $1046.
**Financial Aid** 94% of baccalaureate students in nursing programs received some form of financial aid in 2012–13.
**Contact** Dr. Melissa Garno, BSN Program Director, School of Nursing, Georgia Southern University, PO Box 8158, Statesboro, GA 30460-8158. *Telephone:* 912-478-5454. *Fax:* 912-478-1159. *E-mail:* mel@georgiasouthern.edu.

## GRADUATE PROGRAMS
**Expenses (2013–14)** *Tuition, state resident:* full-time $3834; part-time $320 per credit hour. *Tuition, nonresident:* full-time $13,523; part-time $1127 per credit hour. *International tuition:* $13,523 full-time. *Room and board:* room only: $3130 per academic year. *Required fees:* full-time $1046.
**Financial Aid** 39% of graduate students in nursing programs received some form of financial aid in 2012–13. Research assistantships with partial tuition reimbursements available (averaging $7,200 per year), teaching assistantships with partial tuition reimbursements available (averaging $7,200 per year) were awarded; career-related internships or fieldwork, Federal Work-Study, scholarships, traineeships, tuition waivers (partial), and unspecified assistantships also available. Aid available to part-time students. *Financial aid application deadline:* 4/15.
**Contact** Dr. Deborah Allen, Director, Graduate Program, School of Nursing, Georgia Southern University, PO Box 8158, Statesboro, GA 30460-8158. *Telephone:* 912-478-0017. *Fax:* 912-478-1679. *E-mail:* debbieallen@georgiasouthern.edu.

### MASTER'S DEGREE PROGRAM
**Degree** MSN
**Available Programs** Master's; RN to Master's.
**Concentrations Available** *Clinical nurse specialist programs in:* community health. *Nurse practitioner programs in:* family health.
**Study Options** Full-time and part-time.
**Program Entrance Requirements** Clinical experience, computer literacy, minimum overall college GPA of 3.0, transcript of college record, CPR certification, immunizations, interview, 3 letters of recommendation, professional liability insurance/malpractice insurance, prerequisite course work, statistics course, GRE General Test or MAT. *Application deadline:* 3/15 (fall).
**Advanced Placement** Credit given for nursing courses completed elsewhere dependent upon specific evaluations.
**Degree Requirements** 48 total credit hours, comprehensive exam.

### POST-MASTER'S PROGRAM
**Areas of Study** *Clinical nurse specialist programs in:* community health. *Nurse practitioner programs in:* family health.

### DOCTORAL DEGREE PROGRAM
**Degree** DNP
**Available Programs** Doctorate.
**Areas of Study** Advanced practice nursing, nursing science.
**Online Degree Options** Yes (online only).
**Program Entrance Requirements** Minimum overall college GPA of 3.0, interview by faculty committee, 3 letters of recommendation, MSN or equivalent, vita, writing sample, GRE, MAT. *Application deadline:* 3/1 (fall).
**Degree Requirements** 40 total credit hours, oral exam, written exam.

## Georgia Southwestern State University

### School of Nursing
### Americus, Georgia

*http://www.gsw.edu/*
Founded in 1906

**DEGREES • BSN • MSN**

**Nursing Program Faculty** 15 (33% with doctorates).
**Baccalaureate Enrollment** 330 **Women** 86% **Men** 14% **Minority** 33% **International** 8% **Part-time** 35%
**Graduate Enrollment** 21 **Women** 95% **Men** 5% **Part-time** 50%
**Distance Learning Courses** Available.
**Nursing Student Activities** Sigma Theta Tau, Student Nurses' Association.
**Nursing Student Resources** Academic advising; academic or career counseling; assistance for students with disabilities; bookstore; campus computer network; career placement assistance; computer lab; computer-assisted instruction; e-mail services; employment services for current students; interactive nursing skills videos; Internet; learning resource lab; library services; nursing audiovisuals; placement services for program completers; remedial services; resume preparation assistance; skills, simulation, or other laboratory; tutoring.
**Library Facilities** 787,018 volumes (627 in health, 528 in nursing); 237 periodical subscriptions (141 health-care related).

#### BACCALAUREATE PROGRAMS

**Degree** BSN
**Available Programs** Baccalaureate for Second Degree; Generic Baccalaureate; LPN to RN Baccalaureate; RN Baccalaureate.
**Study Options** Full-time.
**Online Degree Options** Yes.
**Program Entrance Requirements** Minimum overall college GPA of 2.8, transcript of college record, CPR certification, written essay, health exam, health insurance, high school foreign language, 4 years high school math, 4 years high school science, high school transcript, immunizations, 2 letters of recommendation, minimum high school GPA of 2.8, minimum GPA in nursing prerequisites of 2.8, professional liability insurance/malpractice insurance, prerequisite course work, RN licensure. Transfer students are accepted. *Application deadline:* 2/15 (fall), 1/15 (summer).
**Expenses (2013–14)** *Tuition, area resident:* full-time $6264; part-time $174 per credit hour. *Tuition, state resident:* full-time $6264; part-time $174. *Tuition, nonresident:* full-time $24,984; part-time $561 per credit hour. *International tuition:* $24,984 full-time. *Room and board:* $9951; room only: $5340 per academic year. *Required fees:* full-time $2004; part-time $650 per term.
**Financial Aid** 91% of baccalaureate students in nursing programs received some form of financial aid in 2012–13. *Gift aid (need-based):* Federal Pell, FSEOG, state, private, college/university gift aid from institutional funds. *Loans:* Federal Direct (Subsidized and Unsubsidized Stafford PLUS), Perkins, state, college/university. *Work-study:* Federal Work-Study, part-time campus jobs. *Financial aid application deadline:* 6/15(priority: 4/15).
**Contact** Dr. Sandra Daniel, Dean and Professor, School of Nursing, Georgia Southwestern State University, 800 Georgia Southwestern State University Drive, Americus, GA 31709. *Telephone:* 229-931-2280. *Fax:* 229-931-2288. *E-mail:* sandra.daniel@gsw.edu.

#### GRADUATE PROGRAMS

**Expenses (2013–14)** *Tuition, area resident:* part-time $385 per credit hour. *Tuition, state resident:* part-time $385. *Tuition, nonresident:* part-time $385 per credit hour. *Room and board:* $9951; room only: $5340 per academic year. *Required fees:* part-time $325 per term.
**Contact** Dr. Sandra Daniel, Dean, School of Nursing, Georgia Southwestern State University, 800 Georgia Southwestern State University Drive, Americus, GA 31709. *Telephone:* 912-931-2275. *Fax:* 912-931-2288. *E-mail:* Sandra.Daniel@gsw.edu.

##### MASTER'S DEGREE PROGRAM

**Degree** MSN
**Available Programs** Master's.
**Concentrations Available** Nursing administration; nursing education; nursing informatics.
**Study Options** Full-time and part-time.
**Online Degree Options** Yes (online only).
**Program Entrance Requirements** Clinical experience, computer literacy, minimum overall college GPA of 3.0, transcript of college record, CPR certification, written essay, immunizations, interview, 3 letters of recommendation, nursing research course, physical assessment course, professional liability insurance/malpractice insurance, prerequisite course work, resume, statistics course. *Application deadline:* Applications may be processed on a rolling basis for some programs. *Application fee:* $25.
**Degree Requirements** 36 total credit hours, thesis or project, comprehensive exam.

## Georgia State University

### Byrdine F. Lewis School of Nursing and Health Professions
### Atlanta, Georgia

*http://snhp.gsu.edu/*
Founded in 1913

**DEGREES • BS • MSN • PHD**

**Nursing Program Faculty** 60 (40% with doctorates).
**Baccalaureate Enrollment** 297 **Women** 86% **Men** 14% **Minority** 35% **International** 5% **Part-time** 5%
**Graduate Enrollment** 300 **Women** 90% **Men** 10% **Minority** 31% **International** 2% **Part-time** 90%
**Distance Learning Courses** Available.
**Nursing Student Activities** Sigma Theta Tau, Student Nurses' Association.
**Nursing Student Resources** Academic advising; academic or career counseling; assistance for students with disabilities; bookstore; campus computer network; career placement assistance; computer lab; computer-assisted instruction; e-mail services; interactive nursing skills videos; Internet; learning resource lab; library services; nursing audiovisuals; remedial services; resume preparation assistance; skills, simulation, or other laboratory; tutoring.
**Library Facilities** 1.7 million volumes (52,835 in health, 20,856 in nursing); 18,639 periodical subscriptions (725 health-care related).

#### BACCALAUREATE PROGRAMS

**Degree** BS
**Available Programs** Accelerated RN Baccalaureate; Generic Baccalaureate.
**Study Options** Full-time and part-time.
**Program Entrance Requirements** Minimum overall college GPA of 3.5, transcript of college record, CPR certification, written essay, health exam, immunizations, 2 letters of recommendation, minimum GPA in nursing prerequisites of 3.0, professional liability insurance/malpractice insurance, prerequisite course work. Transfer students are accepted. *Application deadline:* 3/1 (fall), 10/1 (spring).
**Advanced Placement** Credit given for nursing courses completed elsewhere dependent upon specific evaluations.
**Expenses (2012–13)** *Tuition, state resident:* full-time $7034; part-time $251 per credit hour. *Tuition, nonresident:* full-time $24,030; part-time $858 per credit hour. *International tuition:* $24,030 full-time. *Room and board:* $11,046; room only: $5661 per academic year. *Required fees:* full-time $1064; part-time $312 per credit; part-time $642 per term.
**Financial Aid** 90% of baccalaureate students in nursing programs received some form of financial aid in 2011–12.
**Contact** Ms. Denisa Hightower, Admissions Counselor, Byrdine F. Lewis School of Nursing and Health Professions, Georgia State University, College of Health and Human Sciences, Office of Academic Assistance, Atlanta, GA 30303-3083. *Telephone:* 404-413-1000. *Fax:* 404-413-1001. *E-mail:* dhightower@gsu.edu.

#### GRADUATE PROGRAMS

**Expenses (2012–13)** *Tuition, state resident:* full-time $9234; part-time $342 per credit hour. *Tuition, nonresident:* full-time $32,562; part-time $1206 per credit hour. *International tuition:* $32,562 full-time. *Required fees:* full-time $1064; part-time $312 per credit; part-time $642 per term.
**Financial Aid** 50% of graduate students in nursing programs received some form of financial aid in 2011–12. 3 research assistantships with full and partial tuition reimbursements available (averaging $1,666 per year), 25 teaching assistantships with full and partial tuition reimbursements available (averaging $1,920 per year) were awarded; scholarships, tuition waivers (full and partial), and unspecified assistantships also available. Aid available to part-time students. *Financial aid application deadline:* 8/1.

**Contact** Ms. Barbara Smith, Admissions Counselor, Byrdine F. Lewis School of Nursing and Health Professions, Georgia State University, College of Health and Human Sciences, PO Box 3995, Atlanta, GA 30302-3995. *Telephone:* 404-413-1007. *Fax:* 404-413-1001. *E-mail:* alhbbs@langate.gsu.edu.

### MASTER'S DEGREE PROGRAM

**Degree** MSN
**Available Programs** Master's; RN to Master's.
**Concentrations Available** Nursing administration; nursing informatics. *Clinical nurse specialist programs in:* adult health, pediatric, perinatal, psychiatric/mental health,women's health. *Nurse practitioner programs in:* adult health, family health, pediatric, psychiatric/mental health,women's health.
**Site Options** Alpharetta, GA.
**Study Options** Full-time and part-time.
**Program Entrance Requirements** Clinical experience, computer literacy, minimum overall college GPA of 3.0, transcript of college record, CPR certification, written essay, interview, 2 letters of recommendation, professional liability insurance/malpractice insurance. *Application deadline:* 3/1 (fall), 10/15 (spring), 3/1 (summer). *Application fee:* $50.
**Advanced Placement** Credit given for nursing courses completed elsewhere dependent upon specific evaluations.
**Degree Requirements** 48 total credit hours.

### POST-MASTER'S PROGRAM

**Areas of Study** *Clinical nurse specialist programs in:* adult health, pediatric, perinatal, psychiatric/mental health,women's health. *Nurse practitioner programs in:* adult health, family health, pediatric, psychiatric/mental health,women's health.

### DOCTORAL DEGREE PROGRAM

**Degree** PhD
**Available Programs** Doctorate; Post-Baccalaureate Doctorate.
**Areas of Study** Bio-behavioral research, health promotion/disease prevention, individualized study, nursing research, nursing science.
**Site Options** Alpharetta, GA.
**Program Entrance Requirements** Minimum overall college GPA of 3.0, interview by faculty committee, interview, 3 letters of recommendation, MSN or equivalent, statistics course, vita, GRE. *Application deadline:* 3/1 (fall). *Application fee:* $50.
**Degree Requirements** 60 total credit hours, dissertation, written exam, residency.

# Gordon State College

## Division of Nursing and Health Sciences
## Barnesville, Georgia

*https://www.gordonstate.edu/nhs/*
Founded in 1852

**DEGREE • BSN**
**Nursing Program Faculty** 2 (50% with doctorates).
**Baccalaureate Enrollment** 26
**Nursing Student Activities** Student Nurses' Association.
**Nursing Student Resources** Academic advising; academic or career counseling; assistance for students with disabilities; bookstore; campus computer network; computer lab; computer-assisted instruction; e-mail services; employment services for current students; externships; interactive nursing skills videos; Internet; learning resource lab; library services; nursing audiovisuals; remedial services; skills, simulation, or other laboratory; tutoring.
**Library Facilities** 150,062 volumes (15 in nursing); 55,588 periodical subscriptions.

### BACCALAUREATE PROGRAMS

**Degree** BSN
**Available Programs** RN Baccalaureate.
**Program Entrance Requirements** Transcript of college record.
**Contact** *Telephone:* 678-359-5085. *Fax:* 678-359-5064.

# Kennesaw State University

## School of Nursing
## Kennesaw, Georgia

*http://www.kennesaw.edu/*
Founded in 1963

**DEGREES • BSN • MSN**
**Distance Learning Courses** Available.
**Nursing Student Activities** Sigma Theta Tau, Student Nurses' Association.
**Nursing Student Resources** Academic advising; academic or career counseling; assistance for students with disabilities; bookstore; campus computer network; career placement assistance; computer lab; computer-assisted instruction; e-mail services; employment services for current students; externships; housing assistance; interactive nursing skills videos; Internet; learning resource lab; library services; nursing audiovisuals; paid internships; placement services for program completers; remedial services; resume preparation assistance; skills, simulation, or other laboratory; tutoring.
**Library Facilities** 573,000 volumes (20,000 in health, 10,000 in nursing); 55,000 periodical subscriptions (503 health-care related).

### BACCALAUREATE PROGRAMS

**Degree** BSN
**Available Programs** ADN to Baccalaureate; Accelerated Baccalaureate; Accelerated Baccalaureate for Second Degree; Baccalaureate for Second Degree; Generic Baccalaureate; RN Baccalaureate.
**Site Options** Rome, GA; Jasper, GA.
**Study Options** Full-time and part-time.
**Program Entrance Requirements** Minimum overall college GPA of 2.7, transcript of college record, CPR certification, health exam, health insurance, 2 years high school math, 2 years high school science, high school transcript, immunizations, interview, 1 letter of recommendation, minimum high school GPA of 2.5, minimum GPA in nursing prerequisites of 2.7, professional liability insurance/malpractice insurance, prerequisite course work. Transfer students are accepted.
**Advanced Placement** Credit by examination available. Credit given for nursing courses completed elsewhere dependent upon specific evaluations.
**Contact** *Telephone:* 770-499-3211. *Fax:* 770-423-6627.

### GRADUATE PROGRAMS

**Contact** *Telephone:* 770-423-6061. *Fax:* 770-423-6627.

### MASTER'S DEGREE PROGRAM

**Degree** MSN
**Available Programs** Master's.
**Concentrations Available** *Clinical nurse specialist programs in:* adult health. *Nurse practitioner programs in:* adult health, family health, primary care.
**Study Options** Full-time.
**Program Entrance Requirements** Clinical experience, minimum overall college GPA of 3.0, transcript of college record, CPR certification, written essay, immunizations, 2 letters of recommendation, nursing research course, physical assessment course, professional liability insurance/malpractice insurance, prerequisite course work, resume.
**Advanced Placement** Credit given for nursing courses completed elsewhere dependent upon specific evaluations.
**Degree Requirements** 40 total credit hours, thesis or project.

### CONTINUING EDUCATION PROGRAM

**Contact** *Telephone:* 770-423-6064. *Fax:* 770-423-6627.

# LaGrange College

## Department of Nursing
## LaGrange, Georgia

*http://www.lagrange.edu/*
Founded in 1831

**DEGREE • BSN**
**Nursing Program Faculty** 7 (20% with doctorates).
**Baccalaureate Enrollment** 96 **Women** 85% **Men** 15% **Minority** 20%
**Nursing Student Activities** Nursing Honor Society, Student Nurses' Association.

**Nursing Student Resources** Academic advising; academic or career counseling; assistance for students with disabilities; bookstore; campus computer network; career placement assistance; computer lab; computer-assisted instruction; e-mail services; employment services for current students; externships; interactive nursing skills videos; Internet; learning resource lab; library services; nursing audiovisuals; paid internships; placement services for program completers; remedial services; resume preparation assistance; skills, simulation, or other laboratory; tutoring; unpaid internships.
**Library Facilities** 402,389 volumes (19,000 in health, 10,000 in nursing); 493 periodical subscriptions (100 health-care related).

### BACCALAUREATE PROGRAMS

**Degree** BSN
**Available Programs** Generic Baccalaureate; RN Baccalaureate.
**Study Options** Full-time.
**Program Entrance Requirements** Minimum overall college GPA of 2.5, transcript of college record, CPR certification, written essay, health exam, health insurance, immunizations, interview, 2 letters of recommendation, minimum GPA in nursing prerequisites of 2.5, professional liability insurance/malpractice insurance, prerequisite course work. Transfer students are accepted. *Application deadline:* 4/15 (fall).
**Advanced Placement** Credit given for nursing courses completed elsewhere dependent upon specific evaluations.
**Expenses (2013–14)** *Tuition:* full-time $18,000. *Room and board:* $16,000 per academic year.
**Financial Aid** 95% of baccalaureate students in nursing programs received some form of financial aid in 2012–13. *Gift aid (need-based):* Federal Pell, FSEOG, private, college/university gift aid from institutional funds. *Loans:* Federal Direct (Subsidized and Unsubsidized Stafford PLUS), Perkins. *Work-study:* Federal Work-Study, part-time campus jobs. *Financial aid application deadline (priority):* 3/1.
**Contact** Dr. Celia G. Hay, Chair, Department of Nursing, LaGrange College, 601 Broad Street, LaGrange, GA 30240-2999. *Telephone:* 706-880-8220. *Fax:* 706-880-8029. *E-mail:* chay@lagrange.edu.

## Mercer University Georgia Baptist College of Nursing

### Mercer University Georgia Baptist College of Nursing
### Atlanta, Georgia

***http://www.mercer.edu/nursing***

**DEGREES • BSN • DNP • MSN • PHD**

**Nursing Program Faculty** 31 (58% with doctorates).
**Baccalaureate Enrollment** 298 **Women** 92% **Men** 8% **Minority** 38% **International** 1% **Part-time** 6%
**Graduate Enrollment** 95 **Women** 95% **Men** 5% **Minority** 43% **International** 2% **Part-time** 36%
**Nursing Student Activities** Sigma Theta Tau, Student Nurses' Association, nursing club.
**Nursing Student Resources** Academic advising; academic or career counseling; assistance for students with disabilities; bookstore; campus computer network; career placement assistance; computer lab; computer-assisted instruction; e-mail services; employment services for current students; housing assistance; interactive nursing skills videos; Internet; learning resource lab; library services; nursing audiovisuals; placement services for program completers; remedial services; resume preparation assistance; skills, simulation, or other laboratory; tutoring.
**Library Facilities** 4,072 volumes in health, 2,805 volumes in nursing; 218 periodical subscriptions health-care related.

### BACCALAUREATE PROGRAMS

**Degree** BSN
**Available Programs** Generic Baccalaureate; RN Baccalaureate.
**Study Options** Full-time.
**Program Entrance Requirements** Transcript of college record, written essay, health exam, health insurance, high school biology, high school foreign language, 3 years high school math, 3 years high school science, high school transcript, immunizations, prerequisite course work. Transfer students are accepted. *Application deadline:* 5/1 (fall). Applications may be processed on a rolling basis for some programs. *Application fee:* $50.
**Advanced Placement** Credit by examination available. Credit given for nursing courses completed elsewhere dependent upon specific evaluations.
**Expenses (2012–13)** *Tuition:* full-time $21,100; part-time $875 per credit hour. *International tuition:* $21,100 full-time. *Room and board:* room only: $9660 per academic year. *Required fees:* full-time $1461; part-time $1106 per term.
**Financial Aid** 90% of baccalaureate students in nursing programs received some form of financial aid in 2011–12.
**Contact** Mrs. Lynn Vines, Director of Admissions, Mercer University Georgia Baptist College of Nursing, 3001 Mercer University Drive, Atlanta, GA 30341. *Telephone:* 678-547-6700. *Fax:* 678-547-6794. *E-mail:* vines_ml@mercer.edu.

### GRADUATE PROGRAMS

**Expenses (2012–13)** *Tuition:* full-time $19,764; part-time $1098 per credit hour. *International tuition:* $19,764 full-time. *Room and board:* room only: $9660 per academic year. *Required fees:* full-time $1210; part-time $735 per term.
**Financial Aid** 90% of graduate students in nursing programs received some form of financial aid in 2011–12.
**Contact** Dr. Virginia Dare Domico, Associate Dean for Graduate Programs, Mercer University Georgia Baptist College of Nursing, 3001 Mercer University Drive, Atlanta, GA 30341. *Telephone:* 678-547-6741. *Fax:* 678-547-6777. *E-mail:* domico_vd@mercer.edu.

#### MASTER'S DEGREE PROGRAM

**Degree** MSN
**Available Programs** Master's.
**Concentrations Available** Nursing education. *Clinical nurse specialist programs in:* acute care, adult health, critical care, gerontology, pediatric. *Nurse practitioner programs in:* family health.
**Study Options** Full-time and part-time.
**Program Entrance Requirements** Clinical experience, computer literacy, minimum overall college GPA of 3.0, transcript of college record, CPR certification, written essay, immunizations, interview, 3 letters of recommendation, nursing research course, physical assessment course, statistics course. *Application deadline:* 7/1 (fall), 11/1 (spring), 4/15 (summer). Applications may be processed on a rolling basis for some programs. *Application fee:* $50.
**Advanced Placement** Credit given for nursing courses completed elsewhere dependent upon specific evaluations.
**Degree Requirements** 38 total credit hours, thesis or project.

#### POST-MASTER'S PROGRAM

**Areas of Study** Nursing education.

#### DOCTORAL DEGREE PROGRAM

**Degree** DNP
**Available Programs** Doctorate.
**Areas of Study** Clinical research, health policy, nursing policy.
**Online Degree Options** Yes (online only).
**Program Entrance Requirements** Minimum overall college GPA of 3.5, clinical experience, interview, 3 letters of recommendation, MSN or equivalent, scholarly papers, statistics course, vita, writing sample. *Application deadline:* 5/15 (fall). Applications may be processed on a rolling basis for some programs. *Application fee:* $50.
**Degree Requirements** 41 total credit hours, oral exam, residency.

**Degree** PhD
**Available Programs** Doctorate.
**Areas of Study** Clinical practice, ethics, nursing education.
**Online Degree Options** Yes (online only).
**Program Entrance Requirements** Minimum overall college GPA of 3.5, interview, 3 letters of recommendation, MSN or equivalent, scholarly papers, statistics course, vita, writing sample. *Application deadline:* 3/15 (fall). Applications may be processed on a rolling basis for some programs. *Application fee:* $50.
**Degree Requirements** 58 total credit hours, dissertation, oral exam, written exam.

## Middle Georgia State College

### School of Nursing and Health Sciences
### Cochran, Georgia

***http://www.maconstate.edu***
Founded in 1884

**DEGREE • BSN**

**Nursing Program Faculty** 30 (7% with doctorates).

**Baccalaureate Enrollment** 104 **Women** 88% **Men** 12% **Minority** 21% **International** 2%
**Nursing Student Activities** Student Nurses' Association.
**Nursing Student Resources** Academic advising; academic or career counseling; assistance for students with disabilities; bookstore; campus computer network; career placement assistance; computer lab; computer-assisted instruction; e-mail services; interactive nursing skills videos; Internet; learning resource lab; library services; nursing audiovisuals; remedial services; resume preparation assistance; skills, simulation, or other laboratory; tutoring.
**Library Facilities** 105,568 volumes (4,000 in health, 920 in nursing); 220 periodical subscriptions (90 health-care related).

## BACCALAUREATE PROGRAMS

**Degree** BSN
**Available Programs** ADN to Baccalaureate; Generic Baccalaureate.
**Study Options** Full-time and part-time.
**Program Entrance Requirements** Minimum overall college GPA of 2.0, transcript of college record, CPR certification, health exam, health insurance, immunizations, minimum GPA in nursing prerequisites of 2.5, professional liability insurance/malpractice insurance, prerequisite course work. Transfer students are accepted. *Application deadline:* 2/15 (fall).
**Contact** *Telephone:* 478-471-2761. *Fax:* 478-471-2983.

# Piedmont College
## School of Nursing
## Demorest, Georgia

***http://www.piedmont.edu/pc/index.php/nursing-home***
Founded in 1897

### DEGREE • BSN

**Nursing Program Faculty** 8 (25% with doctorates).
**Baccalaureate Enrollment** 60 **Women** 99% **Men** 1% **Minority** 10% **International** 1% **Part-time** 20%
**Distance Learning Courses** Available.
**Nursing Student Activities** Nursing Honor Society, Student Nurses' Association.
**Nursing Student Resources** Academic advising; academic or career counseling; assistance for students with disabilities; bookstore; campus computer network; career placement assistance; computer lab; computer-assisted instruction; e-mail services; externships; housing assistance; interactive nursing skills videos; Internet; learning resource lab; library services; nursing audiovisuals; other; paid internships; resume preparation assistance; skills, simulation, or other laboratory; tutoring.
**Library Facilities** 311,722 volumes (3,000 in health, 500 in nursing); 290 periodical subscriptions (75 health-care related).

## BACCALAUREATE PROGRAMS

**Degree** BSN
**Available Programs** Generic Baccalaureate; LPN to Baccalaureate; RN Baccalaureate.
**Study Options** Full-time.
**Program Entrance Requirements** Transcript of college record, CPR certification, health exam, health insurance, high school foreign language, 2 years high school math, 3 years high school science, high school transcript, immunizations, minimum GPA in nursing prerequisites of 3.0, professional liability insurance/malpractice insurance, prerequisite course work. Transfer students are accepted. *Application deadline:* 10/15 (fall).
**Advanced Placement** Credit given for nursing courses completed elsewhere dependent upon specific evaluations.
**Contact** *Telephone:* 706-776-0116. *Fax:* 706-778-0701.

# Shorter University
## School of Nursing
## Rome, Georgia

***http://su.shorter.edu/nursing/***
Founded in 1873

### DEGREE • BSN

**Nursing Program Faculty** 10 (10% with doctorates).
**Baccalaureate Enrollment** 62 **Women** 75% **Men** 25% **Minority** 10% **International** 5%
**Nursing Student Activities** Student Nurses' Association, nursing club.
**Nursing Student Resources** Academic advising; academic or career counseling; assistance for students with disabilities; bookstore; campus computer network; computer lab; e-mail services; housing assistance; interactive nursing skills videos; Internet; learning resource lab; library services; nursing audiovisuals; resume preparation assistance; skills, simulation, or other laboratory; tutoring.
**Library Facilities** 144,475 volumes; 8,511 periodical subscriptions.

## BACCALAUREATE PROGRAMS

**Degree** BSN
**Available Programs** Generic Baccalaureate.
**Site Options** Rome, GA.
**Study Options** Full-time.
**Program Entrance Requirements** Minimum overall college GPA of 3.0, transcript of college record, CPR certification, written essay, health exam, health insurance, immunizations, interview, letters of recommendation, minimum GPA in nursing prerequisites of 3.0, professional liability insurance/malpractice insurance, prerequisite course work. Transfer students are accepted. *Application deadline:* 3/1 (fall). *Application fee:* $25.
**Expenses (2013–14)** *Tuition:* full-time $14,760. *Required fees:* full-time $800.
**Financial Aid** 60% of baccalaureate students in nursing programs received some form of financial aid in 2012–13. *Gift aid (need-based):* Federal Pell, FSEOG, state, private, college/university gift aid from institutional funds. *Loans:* Federal Direct (Subsidized and Unsubsidized Stafford PLUS), Perkins, state. *Work-study:* Federal Work-Study, part-time campus jobs. *Financial aid application deadline (priority):* 4/1.
**Contact** April Allen, Administrative Assistant to the Dean, School of Nursing, Shorter University, 315 Shorter Avenue, Rome, GA 30165. *Telephone:* 706-233-7464. *Fax:* 706-291-4283. *E-mail:* aallen@shorter.edu.

# Thomas University
## Division of Nursing
## Thomasville, Georgia

***http://www.thomasu.edu/nursing.htm***
Founded in 1950

### DEGREES • BSN • MSN • MSN/MBA

**Nursing Program Faculty** 10 (60% with doctorates).
**Baccalaureate Enrollment** 88 **Women** 85% **Men** 15% **Minority** 30%
**Graduate Enrollment** 42 **Women** 90% **Men** 10% **Minority** 40% **Part-time** 50%
**Distance Learning Courses** Available.
**Nursing Student Activities** Nursing Honor Society, Sigma Theta Tau.
**Nursing Student Resources** Academic advising; academic or career counseling; assistance for students with disabilities; bookstore; campus computer network; career placement assistance; computer lab; computer-assisted instruction; e-mail services; housing assistance; interactive nursing skills videos; Internet; learning resource lab; library services; nursing audiovisuals; remedial services; resume preparation assistance; skills, simulation, or other laboratory; tutoring.
**Library Facilities** 41,467 volumes (1,200 in health, 400 in nursing); 451 periodical subscriptions (150 health-care related).

## BACCALAUREATE PROGRAMS

**Degree** BSN
**Available Programs** ADN to Baccalaureate; Accelerated RN Baccalaureate; International Nurse to Baccalaureate; RN Baccalaureate.
**Site Options** Tallahassee, FL; Moultrie, GA.
**Study Options** Full-time and part-time.
**Program Entrance Requirements** Minimum overall college GPA of 2.5, transcript of college record, CPR certification, health exam, health insurance, immunizations, minimum GPA in nursing prerequisites of 2.5, professional liability insurance/malpractice insurance, prerequisite course work, RN licensure. Transfer students are accepted. *Application deadline:* 8/1 (fall), 12/1 (spring), 4/15 (summer). Applications may be processed on a rolling basis for some programs. *Application fee:* $35.
**Advanced Placement** Credit by examination available. Credit given for nursing courses completed elsewhere dependent upon specific evaluations.
**Financial Aid** 90% of baccalaureate students in nursing programs received some form of financial aid in 2011–12. *Gift aid (need-based):* Federal Pell, FSEOG, state, private, college/university gift aid from institutional funds. *Loans:* Federal Direct (Subsidized and Unsubsidized

Stafford PLUS), state, alternative loans. *Work-study:* Federal Work-Study. *Financial aid application deadline (priority):* 5/1.
**Contact** Kerri Knight, Director of Admissions, Division of Nursing, Thomas University, 1501 Millpond Road, Thomasville, GA 31792. *Fax:* 229-226-1653. *E-mail:* kknight@thomasu.edu.

### GRADUATE PROGRAMS

**Financial Aid** 50% of graduate students in nursing programs received some form of financial aid in 2011–12.
**Contact** Kerri Knight, Admissions Representative, Division of Nursing, Thomas University, 1501 Millpond Road, Thomasville, GA 31792. *Fax:* 229-226-1653. *E-mail:* kknight@thomasu.edu.

#### MASTER'S DEGREE PROGRAM

**Degrees** MSN; MSN/MBA
**Available Programs** Accelerated Master's; Master's; RN to Master's.
**Concentrations Available** Health-care administration; nursing administration; nursing education.
**Study Options** Full-time and part-time.
**Program Entrance Requirements** Computer literacy, minimum overall college GPA of 3.0, transcript of college record, CPR certification, written essay, immunizations, 3 letters of recommendation, professional liability insurance/malpractice insurance, resume, statistics course. *Application deadline:* 8/1 (fall), 12/1 (spring), 4/15 (summer). Applications may be processed on a rolling basis for some programs. *Application fee:* $50.
**Advanced Placement** Credit given for nursing courses completed elsewhere dependent upon specific evaluations.
**Degree Requirements** 36 total credit hours, thesis or project.

#### POST-MASTER'S PROGRAM

**Areas of Study** Health-care administration; nursing administration; nursing education.

## University of North Georgia

### Department of Nursing
### Dahlonega, Georgia

*http://www.northgeorgia.edu/*
Founded in 1873

**DEGREES • BSN • MS**
**Nursing Program Faculty** 42 (17% with doctorates).
**Baccalaureate Enrollment** 70 **Women** 90% **Men** 10% **Minority** 12% **International** 4% **Part-time** 40%
**Graduate Enrollment** 50 **Women** 90% **Men** 10% **Minority** 10% **International** 2% **Part-time** 5%
**Distance Learning Courses** Available.
**Nursing Student Activities** Nursing Honor Society, Sigma Theta Tau, Student Nurses' Association.
**Nursing Student Resources** Academic advising; academic or career counseling; assistance for students with disabilities; bookstore; campus computer network; career placement assistance; computer lab; computer-assisted instruction; e-mail services; externships; interactive nursing skills videos; Internet; learning resource lab; library services; nursing audiovisuals; remedial services; resume preparation assistance; skills, simulation, or other laboratory; tutoring.
**Library Facilities** 275,898 volumes (6,875 in health, 619 in nursing); 9,000 periodical subscriptions (2,377 health-care related).

### BACCALAUREATE PROGRAMS

**Degree** BSN
**Available Programs** ADN to Baccalaureate.
**Study Options** Full-time and part-time.
**Online Degree Options** Yes (online only).
**Program Entrance Requirements** Minimum overall college GPA of 2.75, transcript of college record, CPR certification, health exam, health insurance, high school biology, high school chemistry, high school foreign language, 3 years high school math, 2 years high school science, high school transcript, immunizations, 2 letters of recommendation, professional liability insurance/malpractice insurance, prerequisite course work, RN licensure. Transfer students are accepted. *Application deadline:* 2/1 (fall). *Application fee:* $25.
**Contact** *Telephone:* 706-864-1937. *Fax:* 706-864-1845.

### GRADUATE PROGRAMS

**Contact** *Telephone:* 706-864-1489. *Fax:* 706-864-1845.

#### MASTER'S DEGREE PROGRAM

**Degree** MS
**Available Programs** Master's.
**Concentrations Available** Nursing education. *Nurse practitioner programs in:* family health.
**Study Options** Full-time and part-time.
**Program Entrance Requirements** Clinical experience, computer literacy, minimum overall college GPA of 2.75, transcript of college record, CPR certification, written essay, immunizations, 3 letters of recommendation, nursing research course, physical assessment course, professional liability insurance/malpractice insurance, prerequisite course work. *Application deadline:* 2/28 (spring). *Application fee:* $25.
**Degree Requirements** 46 total credit hours, thesis or project, comprehensive exam.

#### POST-MASTER'S PROGRAM

**Areas of Study** Nursing education. *Nurse practitioner programs in:* family health.

## University of Phoenix–Atlanta Campus

### College of Health and Human Services
### Sandy Springs, Georgia

**Nursing Student Activities** Sigma Theta Tau.
**Nursing Student Resources** Academic advising; academic or career counseling; assistance for students with disabilities; bookstore; campus computer network; computer lab; computer-assisted instruction; e-mail services; interactive nursing skills videos; Internet; learning resource lab; library services; nursing audiovisuals; remedial services; skills, simulation, or other laboratory; tutoring.
**Library Facilities** 16,781 periodical subscriptions (1,300 health-care related).

## University of West Georgia

### School of Nursing
### Carrollton, Georgia

*http://nursing.westga.edu/*
Founded in 1933

**DEGREES • BSN • EDD • MSN**
**Nursing Program Faculty** 42 (36% with doctorates).
**Baccalaureate Enrollment** 357 **Women** 89% **Men** 11% **Minority** 38% **International** 1% **Part-time** 65%
**Graduate Enrollment** 120 **Women** 94% **Men** 6% **Minority** 30% **International** .8% **Part-time** 24%
**Distance Learning Courses** Available.
**Nursing Student Activities** Sigma Theta Tau, Student Nurses' Association.
**Nursing Student Resources** Academic advising; academic or career counseling; assistance for students with disabilities; bookstore; campus computer network; career placement assistance; computer lab; computer-assisted instruction; e-mail services; employment services for current students; externships; housing assistance; interactive nursing skills videos; Internet; learning resource lab; library services; nursing audiovisuals; remedial services; resume preparation assistance; skills, simulation, or other laboratory; tutoring.
**Library Facilities** 572,251 volumes (9,420 in health, 526 in nursing); 84,316 periodical subscriptions (32 health-care related).

### BACCALAUREATE PROGRAMS

**Degree** BSN
**Available Programs** Accelerated RN Baccalaureate; Generic Baccalaureate.
**Site Options** Newnan, GA.
**Study Options** Full-time and part-time.
**Program Entrance Requirements** Minimum overall college GPA of 2.75, transcript of college record, CPR certification, health exam, health insurance, immunizations, minimum GPA in nursing prerequisites of 2.75, professional liability insurance/malpractice insurance, prerequisite course work. Transfer students are accepted. *Application deadline:* 2/1 (summer). *Application fee:* $40.

**Expenses (2013–14)** *Tuition, state resident:* full-time $3416; part-time $166 per credit hour. *Tuition, nonresident:* full-time $9707; part-time $585 per credit hour. *Room and board:* $5290; room only: $2500 per academic year. *Required fees:* full-time $677; part-time $225 per term.
**Financial Aid** 69% of baccalaureate students in nursing programs received some form of financial aid in 2012–13. *Gift aid (need-based):* Federal Pell, FSEOG, state, private, college/university gift aid from institutional funds. *Loans:* Federal Direct (Subsidized and Unsubsidized Stafford PLUS), Perkins. *Work-study:* Federal Work-Study, part-time campus jobs. *Financial aid application deadline (priority):* 4/1.
**Contact** Dr. Cynthia D. Epps, Associate Dean and Undergraduate Program Coordinator, School of Nursing, University of West Georgia, 1601 Maple Street, Carrollton, GA 30118. *Telephone:* 678-839-6552. *Fax:* 678-839-6553. *E-mail:* cepps@westga.edu.

## GRADUATE PROGRAMS

**Expenses (2013–14)** *Tuition, state resident:* full-time $2888; part-time $282 per credit hour. *Tuition, nonresident:* full-time $2888; part-time $282 per credit hour. *Room and board:* $5290; room only: $2500 per academic year. *Required fees:* full-time $100; part-time $50 per term.
**Financial Aid** 26% of graduate students in nursing programs received some form of financial aid in 2012–13.
**Contact** Dr. Laurie Jowers Ware, Associate Dean and Director of Graduate Program, School of Nursing, University of West Georgia, 1601 Maple Street, Carrollton, GA 30118. *Telephone:* 678-839-6552. *Fax:* 678-839-6553. *E-mail:* lware@westga.edu.

### MASTER'S DEGREE PROGRAM

**Degree** MSN
**Available Programs** Master's.
**Concentrations Available** Clinical nurse leader; nursing administration; nursing education.
**Study Options** Full-time and part-time.
**Online Degree Options** Yes (online only).
**Program Entrance Requirements** Clinical experience, computer literacy, minimum overall college GPA of 3.0, transcript of college record, CPR certification, immunizations, 2 letters of recommendation, nursing research course, professional liability insurance/malpractice insurance, prerequisite course work, resume, statistics course. *Application deadline:* 6/1 (fall). *Application fee:* $40.
**Degree Requirements** 36 total credit hours, thesis or project.

### POST-MASTER'S PROGRAM

**Areas of Study** Clinical nurse leader; nursing administration; nursing education.

### DOCTORAL DEGREE PROGRAM

**Degree** EdD
**Available Programs** Doctorate.
**Areas of Study** Nursing education.
**Online Degree Options** Yes (online only).
**Program Entrance Requirements** Minimum overall college GPA of 3.0, 3 letters of recommendation, MSN or equivalent, statistics course, vita, writing sample. *Application deadline:* 2/1 (fall). *Application fee:* $40.
**Degree Requirements** 60 total credit hours, dissertation, oral exam, written exam.

# Valdosta State University

## College of Nursing
## Valdosta, Georgia

***http://www.valdosta.edu/nursing/***
Founded in 1906

### DEGREES • BSN • MSN

**Nursing Program Faculty** 23 (52% with doctorates).
**Baccalaureate Enrollment** 183 **Women** 87% **Men** 13% **Minority** 21% **International** 1% **Part-time** 7%
**Graduate Enrollment** 25 **Women** 99% **Men** 1% **Minority** 15% **International** 1% **Part-time** 49%
**Nursing Student Activities** Sigma Theta Tau, Student Nurses' Association.
**Nursing Student Resources** Academic advising; academic or career counseling; assistance for students with disabilities; bookstore; campus computer network; career placement assistance; computer lab; computer-assisted instruction; e-mail services; employment services for current students; externships; housing assistance; Internet; learning resource lab; library services; nursing audiovisuals; placement services for program completers; resume preparation assistance; skills, simulation, or other laboratory; tutoring; unpaid internships.
**Library Facilities** 728,261 volumes (21,688 in health); 2,558 periodical subscriptions (75 health-care related).

## BACCALAUREATE PROGRAMS

**Degree** BSN
**Available Programs** Generic Baccalaureate; RN Baccalaureate.
**Study Options** Full-time.
**Program Entrance Requirements** Minimum overall college GPA of 2.8, transcript of college record, CPR certification, health exam, health insurance, immunizations, minimum GPA in nursing prerequisites of 2.8, professional liability insurance/malpractice insurance, prerequisite course work. Transfer students are accepted.
**Advanced Placement** Credit given for nursing courses completed elsewhere dependent upon specific evaluations.
**Contact** *Telephone:* 229-333-5959. *Fax:* 229-333-7300.

## GRADUATE PROGRAMS

**Contact** *Telephone:* 229-333-5959. *Fax:* 229-333-7300.

### MASTER'S DEGREE PROGRAM

**Degree** MSN
**Available Programs** Master's; RN to Master's.
**Concentrations Available** Nurse case management; nursing administration; nursing education. *Clinical nurse specialist programs in:* adult health, family health, psychiatric/mental health.
**Study Options** Full-time and part-time.
**Program Entrance Requirements** Minimum overall college GPA of 2.8, transcript of college record, CPR certification, immunizations, 3 letters of recommendation, physical assessment course, professional liability insurance/malpractice insurance, statistics course, GRE General Test.
**Advanced Placement** Credit given for nursing courses completed elsewhere dependent upon specific evaluations.
**Degree Requirements** 36 total credit hours, thesis or project, comprehensive exam.

## CONTINUING EDUCATION PROGRAM

**Contact** *Telephone:* 229-333-5960.

# GUAM

# University of Guam

## School of Nursing and Health Sciences
## Mangilao, Guam

***http://www.uog.edu/***
Founded in 1952

### DEGREE • BSN

**Nursing Program Faculty** 10 (30% with doctorates).
**Baccalaureate Enrollment** 175 **Women** 97% **Men** 3% **International** 2%
**Nursing Student Activities** Student Nurses' Association.
**Nursing Student Resources** Academic advising; academic or career counseling; assistance for students with disabilities; bookstore; campus computer network; career placement assistance; computer lab; daycare for children of students; e-mail services; employment services for current students; interactive nursing skills videos; Internet; learning resource lab; library services; nursing audiovisuals; remedial services; skills, simulation, or other laboratory; tutoring.
**Library Facilities** 315,478 volumes (5,246 in health, 982 in nursing); 28,845 periodical subscriptions (53 health-care related).

## BACCALAUREATE PROGRAMS

**Degree** BSN
**Available Programs** ADN to Baccalaureate; Generic Baccalaureate; RN Baccalaureate.
**Study Options** Full-time and part-time.

**Program Entrance Requirements** Transcript of college record, CPR certification, written essay, health exam, high school biology, high school chemistry, 1 year of high school math, 1 year of high school science, high school transcript, immunizations, interview, minimum high school GPA of 2.5, minimum GPA in nursing prerequisites of 2.7, prerequisite course work. Transfer students are accepted.
**Advanced Placement** Credit by examination available. Credit given for nursing courses completed elsewhere dependent upon specific evaluations.
**Contact** *Telephone:* 671-735-2210. *Fax:* 671-734-4245.

# HAWAII

## Chaminade University of Honolulu

### Nursing Program
### Honolulu, Hawaii

***http://www.chaminade.edu/nursing***
Founded in 1955

**DEGREE • BSN**
**Nursing Program Faculty** 11 (36% with doctorates).
**Baccalaureate Enrollment** 280 **Women** 74% **Men** 26% **Minority** 87% **International** 1%
**Nursing Student Activities** Nursing Honor Society, Sigma Theta Tau, Student Nurses' Association, nursing club.
**Nursing Student Resources** Academic advising; academic or career counseling; assistance for students with disabilities; bookstore; campus computer network; computer lab; computer-assisted instruction; e-mail services; employment services for current students; interactive nursing skills videos; Internet; learning resource lab; library services; nursing audiovisuals; paid internships; remedial services; resume preparation assistance; skills, simulation, or other laboratory; tutoring.
**Library Facilities** 78,000 volumes; 6,730 periodical subscriptions.

#### BACCALAUREATE PROGRAMS

**Degree** BSN
**Available Programs** Generic Baccalaureate.
**Study Options** Full-time.
**Program Entrance Requirements** Minimum overall college GPA of 2.75, transcript of college record, written essay, high school chemistry, 4 years high school math, high school transcript, 2 letters of recommendation, minimum high school GPA of 2.75. Transfer students are accepted. *Application deadline:* 2/1 (fall). *Application fee:* $25.
**Financial Aid** ***Gift aid (need-based):*** Federal Pell, FSEOG, state, private, college/university gift aid from institutional funds. *Loans:* Federal Direct (Subsidized and Unsubsidized Stafford PLUS), alternative loans. *Work-study:* Federal Work-Study. *Financial aid application deadline:* Continuous.
**Contact** Dr. Stephanie Genz, Nursing Program Assistant, Nursing Program, Chaminade University of Honolulu, 3140 Waialae Avenue, Henry Hall 110, Honolulu, HI 96816. *Telephone:* 808-735-4813. *E-mail:* ashley.wiswell@chaminade.edu.

## Hawaii Pacific University

### College of Nursing and Health Sciences
### Honolulu, Hawaii

***http://www.hpu.edu/***
Founded in 1965

**DEGREES • BSN • MSN • MSN/MBA**
**Nursing Program Faculty** 102 (16% with doctorates).
**Baccalaureate Enrollment** 1,279 **Women** 82% **Men** 18% **Minority** 74% **International** 2% **Part-time** 26%
**Graduate Enrollment** 65 **Women** 81% **Men** 19% **Minority** 90% **International** 20% **Part-time** 22%
**Distance Learning Courses** Available.
**Nursing Student Activities** Nursing Honor Society, Sigma Theta Tau, Student Nurses' Association.
**Nursing Student Resources** Academic advising; academic or career counseling; assistance for students with disabilities; bookstore; campus computer network; career placement assistance; computer lab; computer-assisted instruction; e-mail services; employment services for current students; externships; housing assistance; Internet; learning resource lab; library services; paid internships; placement services for program completers; resume preparation assistance; skills, simulation, or other laboratory; tutoring.
**Library Facilities** 175,000 volumes (5,314 in health, 1,996 in nursing); 45,000 periodical subscriptions (7,243 health-care related).

#### BACCALAUREATE PROGRAMS

**Degree** BSN
**Available Programs** Generic Baccalaureate; International Nurse to Baccalaureate; LPN to Baccalaureate; RN Baccalaureate.
**Site Options** Kaneohe, HI; Honolulu, HI.
**Study Options** Full-time and part-time.
**Program Entrance Requirements** Minimum overall college GPA of 2.75, transcript of college record, CPR certification, health exam, health insurance, immunizations, minimum GPA in nursing prerequisites of 2.75, prerequisite course work. Transfer students are accepted. *Application deadline:* Applications may be processed on a rolling basis for some programs. *Application fee:* $50.
**Advanced Placement** Credit given for nursing courses completed elsewhere dependent upon specific evaluations.
**Expenses (2012–13)** *Tuition:* full-time $18,500; part-time $617 per credit. *International tuition:* $18,500 full-time. *Room and board:* $12,482 per academic year. *Required fees:* full-time $100.
**Financial Aid** 79% of baccalaureate students in nursing programs received some form of financial aid in 2011–12. *Gift aid (need-based):* Federal Pell, FSEOG, state, private, college/university gift aid from institutional funds, Federal Nursing. *Loans:* Federal Nursing Student Loans, Federal Direct (Subsidized and Unsubsidized Stafford PLUS), Perkins. *Work-study:* Federal Work-Study. *Financial aid application deadline (priority):* 3/1.
**Contact** Miss Sara Sato, Director of Admissions, College of Nursing and Health Sciences, Hawai`i Pacific University, 1164 Bishop Street, Honolulu, HI 96813. *Telephone:* 808-544-0238. *Fax:* 808-544-1136. *E-mail:* ssato@hpu.edu.

#### GRADUATE PROGRAMS

**Expenses (2012–13)** *Tuition:* full-time $13,590; part-time $755 per credit hour. *International tuition:* $13,590 full-time. *Required fees:* full-time $100.
**Financial Aid** 60% of graduate students in nursing programs received some form of financial aid in 2011–12. Career-related internships or fieldwork, Federal Work-Study, scholarships, traineeships, and tuition waivers available. *Financial aid application deadline:* 3/1.
**Contact** Dr. Diane Knight, Chair, Department of Graduate and Post-Baccalaureate Nursing Programs, College of Nursing and Health Sciences, Hawai`i Pacific University, 45-045 Kamehameha Highway, Kaneohe, HI 96744-5297. *Telephone:* 808-236-3552. *Fax:* 808-236-3524. *E-mail:* dknight@hpu.edu.

#### MASTER'S DEGREE PROGRAM

**Degrees** MSN; MSN/MBA
**Available Programs** Master's; RN to Master's.
**Concentrations Available** Nursing education. *Clinical nurse specialist programs in:* community health. *Nurse practitioner programs in:* family health.
**Site Options** Kaneohe, HI.
**Study Options** Full-time and part-time.
**Program Entrance Requirements** Clinical experience, minimum overall college GPA of 3.0, transcript of college record, written essay, 2 letters of recommendation, nursing research course, prerequisite course work, statistics course. *Application deadline:* Applications may be processed on a rolling basis for some programs. *Application fee:* $50.
**Advanced Placement** Credit given for nursing courses completed elsewhere dependent upon specific evaluations.
**Degree Requirements** 48 total credit hours, thesis or project.

#### POST-MASTER'S PROGRAM

**Areas of Study** Nursing education. *Nurse practitioner programs in:* family health.

# University of Hawaii at Hilo
## Department in Nursing
## Hilo, Hawaii

*http://www.uhh.hawaii.edu/*
Founded in 1970

**DEGREE • BSN**
**Nursing Program Faculty** 10 (50% with doctorates).
**Baccalaureate Enrollment** 78 **Women** 83% **Men** 17% **Minority** 68% **International** 1% **Part-time** 18%
**Distance Learning Courses** Available.
**Nursing Student Activities** Nursing Honor Society, Sigma Theta Tau, Student Nurses' Association.
**Nursing Student Resources** Academic advising; academic or career counseling; assistance for students with disabilities; bookstore; campus computer network; career placement assistance; computer lab; computer-assisted instruction; e-mail services; employment services for current students; externships; housing assistance; interactive nursing skills videos; Internet; learning resource lab; library services; nursing audiovisuals; paid internships; remedial services; resume preparation assistance; skills, simulation, or other laboratory; tutoring.
**Library Facilities** 250,000 volumes (680 in health, 284 in nursing); 2,500 periodical subscriptions (15,000 health-care related).

### BACCALAUREATE PROGRAMS
**Degree** BSN
**Available Programs** ADN to Baccalaureate; Generic Baccalaureate; RN Baccalaureate.
**Site Options** Kona, HI; Lihue, HI; Kahalui, HI.
**Study Options** Full-time.
**Program Entrance Requirements** Minimum overall college GPA of 2.7, transcript of college record, CPR certification, written essay, health exam, health insurance, high school biology, high school chemistry, high school foreign language, 1 year of high school math, 3 years high school science, high school transcript, immunizations, 2 letters of recommendation, minimum high school GPA of 3.0, minimum GPA in nursing prerequisites of 2.7, professional liability insurance/malpractice insurance, prerequisite course work. *Application deadline:* 1/15 (fall).
**Contact** *Telephone:* 808-974-7760. *Fax:* 808-974-7665.

# University of Hawaii at Manoa
## School of Nursing and Dental Hygiene
## Honolulu, Hawaii

*http://www.nursing.hawaii.edu/*
Founded in 1907

**DEGREES • BSN • MS • MSN/MBA • PHD**
**Nursing Program Faculty** 97 (35% with doctorates).
**Baccalaureate Enrollment** 336 **Women** 77% **Men** 23% **Minority** 83% **International** 3% **Part-time** 56%
**Graduate Enrollment** 170 **Women** 88% **Men** 12% **Minority** 60% **International** 2% **Part-time** 66%
**Distance Learning Courses** Available.
**Nursing Student Activities** Nursing Honor Society, Sigma Theta Tau, Student Nurses' Association, nursing club.
**Nursing Student Resources** Academic advising; academic or career counseling; assistance for students with disabilities; bookstore; computer lab; computer-assisted instruction; e-mail services; employment services for current students; housing assistance; Internet; learning resource lab; library services; nursing audiovisuals; resume preparation assistance; skills, simulation, or other laboratory.
**Library Facilities** 3.4 million volumes; 58,434 periodical subscriptions.

### BACCALAUREATE PROGRAMS
**Degree** BSN
**Available Programs** ADN to Baccalaureate; Generic Baccalaureate; RN Baccalaureate.
**Study Options** Full-time and part-time.
**Program Entrance Requirements** Minimum overall college GPA of 2.5, transcript of college record, CPR certification, health exam, health insurance, immunizations, minimum GPA in nursing prerequisites of 2.5, prerequisite course work. Transfer students are accepted. *Application deadline:* 3/1 (fall), 10/1 (spring). *Application fee:* $50.
**Advanced Placement** Credit by examination available. Credit given for nursing courses completed elsewhere dependent upon specific evaluations.
**Contact** *Telephone:* 808-956-8939. *Fax:* 808-956-5977.

### GRADUATE PROGRAMS
**Contact** *Telephone:* 808-956-3519. *Fax:* 808-956-5977.

#### MASTER'S DEGREE PROGRAM
**Degrees** MS; MSN/MBA
**Available Programs** Accelerated Master's; Master's; Master's for Non-Nursing College Graduates; RN to Master's.
**Concentrations Available** Nursing administration; nursing education. *Clinical nurse specialist programs in:* psychiatric/mental health. *Nurse practitioner programs in:* adult health, community health, family health, gerontology, pediatric.
**Site Options** Kahului, HI; Lihue, HI; Kailua Kona, HI.
**Study Options** Full-time and part-time.
**Online Degree Options** Yes.
**Program Entrance Requirements** Minimum overall college GPA of 3.0, transcript of college record, CPR certification, written essay, immunizations, interview, 2 letters of recommendation, resume, statistics course. *Application deadline:* 3/1 (fall). *Application fee:* $60.
**Advanced Placement** Credit given for nursing courses completed elsewhere dependent upon specific evaluations.
**Degree Requirements** 52 total credit hours.

#### POST-MASTER'S PROGRAM
**Areas of Study** Nursing administration; nursing education. *Clinical nurse specialist programs in:* psychiatric/mental health. *Nurse practitioner programs in:* adult health, community health, family health, gerontology, pediatric.

#### DOCTORAL DEGREE PROGRAM
**Degree** PhD
**Available Programs** Doctorate.
**Areas of Study** Faculty preparation, nursing education, nursing research, nursing science.
**Site Options** Kahului, HI; Lihue, HI; Kailua Kona, HI.
**Online Degree Options** Yes (online only).
**Program Entrance Requirements** Clinical experience, minimum overall college GPA of 3.0, interview by faculty committee, interview, 3 letters of recommendation, MSN or equivalent, scholarly papers, statistics course, vita, writing sample. *Application deadline:* 2/1 (fall).
**Degree Requirements** 46 total credit hours, dissertation, oral exam, residency.

# University of Phoenix–Hawaii Campus
## College of Nursing
## Honolulu, Hawaii

**DEGREES • BSN • MSN • MSN/ED D**
**Nursing Program Faculty** 26 (15% with doctorates).
**Baccalaureate Enrollment** 70 **Women** 90% **Men** 10% **Minority** 40%
**Graduate Enrollment** 14 **Women** 71.4% **Men** 28.6% **Minority** 57.14%
**Nursing Student Activities** Sigma Theta Tau.
**Nursing Student Resources** Academic advising; academic or career counseling; assistance for students with disabilities; bookstore; campus computer network; computer lab; computer-assisted instruction; e-mail services; interactive nursing skills videos; Internet; learning resource lab; library services; nursing audiovisuals; remedial services; skills, simulation, or other laboratory; tutoring.
**Library Facilities** 16,781 periodical subscriptions (1,300 health-care related).

### BACCALAUREATE PROGRAMS
**Degree** BSN
**Available Programs** Accelerated Baccalaureate; LPN to Baccalaureate.
**Site Options** Kaneohe, HI; Mililani, HI; Kapolei, HI.
**Study Options** Full-time.
**Program Entrance Requirements** Transcript of college record, CPR certification, immunizations, 1 letter of recommendation, RN licensure. Transfer students are accepted. *Application deadline:* Applications may be processed on a rolling basis for some programs.

**Advanced Placement** Credit by examination available. Credit given for nursing courses completed elsewhere dependent upon specific evaluations.
**Contact** *Telephone:* 808-536-2686.

### GRADUATE PROGRAMS

**Contact** *Telephone:* 808-536-2686.

#### MASTER'S DEGREE PROGRAM

**Degrees** MSN; MSN/Ed D
**Available Programs** Master's.
**Concentrations Available** Health-care administration; nursing administration; nursing education. *Nurse practitioner programs in:* family health.
**Site Options** Kaneohe, HI; Mililani, HI; Kapolei, HI.
**Study Options** Full-time.
**Program Entrance Requirements** Clinical experience, computer literacy, minimum overall college GPA of 2.5, transcript of college record. *Application deadline:* Applications may be processed on a rolling basis for some programs. *Application fee:* $45.
**Advanced Placement** Credit given for nursing courses completed elsewhere dependent upon specific evaluations.
**Degree Requirements** 39 total credit hours, thesis or project.

# IDAHO

## Boise State University

**Department of Nursing**
**Boise, Idaho**

*http://hs.boisestate.edu/nursing/*
Founded in 1932

**DEGREES • BS • MSN • MSN/MS**

**Nursing Program Faculty** 55 (25% with doctorates).
**Baccalaureate Enrollment** 540 **Women** 75% **Men** 25% **Minority** 1% **International** 1%
**Graduate Enrollment** 12
**Distance Learning Courses** Available.
**Nursing Student Activities** Nursing Honor Society, Sigma Theta Tau, Student Nurses' Association.
**Nursing Student Resources** Academic advising; academic or career counseling; assistance for students with disabilities; bookstore; campus computer network; career placement assistance; computer lab; computer-assisted instruction; daycare for children of students; e-mail services; employment services for current students; housing assistance; interactive nursing skills videos; Internet; learning resource lab; library services; nursing audiovisuals; placement services for program completers; remedial services; resume preparation assistance; skills, simulation, or other laboratory; tutoring.
**Library Facilities** 1 million volumes (27,919 in health, 2,617 in nursing); 96,687 periodical subscriptions (158 health-care related).

### BACCALAUREATE PROGRAMS

**Degree** BS
**Available Programs** Accelerated RN Baccalaureate; Generic Baccalaureate; LPN to Baccalaureate; RN Baccalaureate.
**Site Options** Nampa, ID.
**Study Options** Full-time.
**Online Degree Options** Yes.
**Program Entrance Requirements** Transcript of college record, immunizations, minimum GPA in nursing prerequisites of 3.0, professional liability insurance/malpractice insurance, prerequisite course work. Transfer students are accepted. *Application deadline:* 3/1 (fall), 10/1 (spring). *Application fee:* $20.
**Advanced Placement** Credit by examination available. Credit given for nursing courses completed elsewhere dependent upon specific evaluations.
**Contact** *Telephone:* 208-426-4143. *Fax:* 208-426-1370.

### GRADUATE PROGRAMS

**Contact** *Telephone:* 208-426-4143.

#### MASTER'S DEGREE PROGRAM

**Degrees** MSN; MSN/MS
**Available Programs** Master's.
**Concentrations Available** Clinical nurse leader; health-care administration; nurse case management; nursing administration; nursing education.
**Study Options** Part-time.
**Program Entrance Requirements** Minimum overall college GPA of 3.0, transcript of college record, CPR certification, written essay, letters of recommendation, nursing research course, professional liability insurance/malpractice insurance, prerequisite course work, resume, statistics course. *Application deadline:* 3/31 (spring).
**Degree Requirements** 39 total credit hours, thesis or project.

## Brigham Young University–Idaho

**Department of Nursing**
**Rexburg, Idaho**

*http://www.byui.edu*
Founded in 1888

**DEGREE • BSN**

### BACCALAUREATE PROGRAMS

**Degree** BSN
**Available Programs** RN Baccalaureate.
**Program Entrance Requirements** RN licensure. Transfer students are accepted. *Application deadline:* 6/1 (fall), 10/1 (winter), 2/1 (spring).
**Contact** *Telephone:* 208-496-4555. *Fax:* 208-496-4553.

## Idaho State University

**Department of Nursing**
**Pocatello, Idaho**

*http://www.isu.edu/nursing*
Founded in 1901

**DEGREES • BS • DNP • MS • PHD**

**Nursing Program Faculty** 16 (44% with doctorates).
**Baccalaureate Enrollment** 159 **Women** 74% **Men** 26%
**Graduate Enrollment** 65 **Women** 88% **Men** 12% **Minority** 6% **Part-time** 26%
**Distance Learning Courses** Available.
**Nursing Student Activities** Sigma Theta Tau, Student Nurses' Association.
**Nursing Student Resources** Academic advising; academic or career counseling; assistance for students with disabilities; bookstore; campus computer network; computer lab; computer-assisted instruction; daycare for children of students; e-mail services; employment services for current students; housing assistance; interactive nursing skills videos; Internet; learning resource lab; library services; nursing audiovisuals; resume preparation assistance; skills, simulation, or other laboratory; tutoring.
**Library Facilities** 6 million volumes (35,948 in health, 1,775 in nursing); 3,981 periodical subscriptions (5,312 health-care related).

### BACCALAUREATE PROGRAMS

**Degree** BS
**Available Programs** ADN to Baccalaureate; Accelerated Baccalaureate for Second Degree; Generic Baccalaureate; LPN to RN Baccalaureate.
**Site Options** Meridian, ID; Idaho Falls, ID.
**Study Options** Full-time.
**Program Entrance Requirements** Minimum overall college GPA, transcript of college record, CPR certification, health exam, health insurance, high school transcript, immunizations, minimum high school GPA of 2.0, minimum GPA in nursing prerequisites of 3.0, professional liability insurance/malpractice insurance, prerequisite course work. Transfer students are accepted. *Application deadline:* 9/15 (spring). *Application fee:* $50.
**Advanced Placement** Credit given for nursing courses completed elsewhere dependent upon specific evaluations.
**Contact** Dr. Sandie Nadelson, Associate Director of Undergraduate Studies, School of Nursing, Department of Nursing, Idaho State University, 921 South 8th Avenue, Stop 8101, Pocatello, ID 83209-8101. *Telephone:* 208-282-2854. *Fax:* 208-236-4476. *E-mail:* nadesand@isu.edu.

## GRADUATE PROGRAMS

**Financial Aid** 1 research assistantship (averaging $9,401 per year), 4 teaching assistantships (averaging $10,841 per year) were awarded; career-related internships or fieldwork, Federal Work-Study, institutionally sponsored loans, scholarships, tuition waivers (full and partial), and unspecified assistantships also available.

**Contact** Dr. Karen Neill, Associate Director of Graduate Studies, School of Nursing, Department of Nursing, Idaho State University, 921 South 8th Avenue, Stop 8101, Pocatello, ID 83209-8101. *Telephone:* 208-282-2102. *Fax:* 208-282-4476. *E-mail:* nielkare@isu.edu.

### MASTER'S DEGREE PROGRAM

**Degree** MS
**Available Programs** Master's.
**Concentrations Available** Nursing administration; nursing education.
**Study Options** Full-time and part-time.
**Online Degree Options** Yes (online only).
**Program Entrance Requirements** Minimum overall college GPA of 3.0, transcript of college record, CPR certification, written essay, immunizations, interview, 3 letters of recommendation, professional liability insurance/malpractice insurance, prerequisite course work, resume, statistics course, GRE General Test. *Application deadline:* Applications may be processed on a rolling basis for some programs. *Application fee:* $55.
**Advanced Placement** Credit given for nursing courses completed elsewhere dependent upon specific evaluations.
**Degree Requirements** 43 total credit hours, comprehensive exam.

### POST-MASTER'S PROGRAM

**Areas of Study** Nursing administration; nursing education.

### DOCTORAL DEGREE PROGRAM

**Degree** DNP
**Available Programs** Doctorate; Post-Baccalaureate Doctorate.
**Areas of Study** Adult gerontology, family nurse.
**Online Degree Options** Yes (online only).
**Program Entrance Requirements** Minimum overall college GPA of 3.0, 3 letters of recommendation, statistics course, vita, writing sample. *Application deadline:* Applications may be processed on a rolling basis for some programs. *Application fee:* $55.
**Degree Requirements** 76 total credit hours, oral exam, written exam.

**Degree** PhD
**Available Programs** Doctorate, Post-Baccalaureate Doctorate.
**Areas of Study** Nursing science.
**Online Degree Options** Yes (online only).
**Program Entrance Requirements** Minimum overall college GPA of 3.0, interview by faculty committee, 3 letters of recommendation, statistics course, vita, writing sample. *Application deadline:* Applications are processed on a rolling basis. *Application fee:* $55.
**Degree Requirements** 59 total credit hours, dissertation, written exam.

# Lewis-Clark State College

**Division of Nursing and Health Sciences**
**Lewiston, Idaho**

*http://www.lcsc.edu/nursing/*
Founded in 1893

## DEGREE • BSN

**Nursing Program Faculty** 32 (16% with doctorates).
**Baccalaureate Enrollment** 193 **Women** 83% **Men** 17% **Minority** 10% **International** 5% **Part-time** 21%
**Distance Learning Courses** Available.
**Nursing Student Activities** Student Nurses' Association.
**Nursing Student Resources** Academic advising; academic or career counseling; assistance for students with disabilities; bookstore; campus computer network; career placement assistance; computer lab; computer-assisted instruction; daycare for children of students; e-mail services; housing assistance; interactive nursing skills videos; Internet; learning resource lab; library services; nursing audiovisuals; remedial services; resume preparation assistance; skills, simulation, or other laboratory; tutoring; unpaid internships.
**Library Facilities** 19,920 volumes in health, 5,101 volumes in nursing; 12,058 periodical subscriptions health-care related.

## BACCALAUREATE PROGRAMS

**Degree** BSN
**Available Programs** ADN to Baccalaureate; Generic Baccalaureate; LPN to Baccalaureate; LPN to RN Baccalaureate.
**Site Options** Coeur d'Alene, ID.
**Study Options** Full-time.
**Program Entrance Requirements** Minimum overall college GPA of 2.5, transcript of college record, CPR certification, health insurance, immunizations, minimum GPA in nursing prerequisites of 2.5, prerequisite course work. Transfer students are accepted. *Application deadline:* 2/15 (fall), 9/30 (spring). *Application fee:* $35.
**Advanced Placement** Credit given for nursing courses completed elsewhere dependent upon specific evaluations.
**Expenses (2012–13)** *Tuition, state resident:* full-time $2781; part-time $285 per credit. *Tuition, nonresident:* full-time $7738. *International tuition:* $7738 full-time. *Room and board:* $5950; room only: $3200 per academic year. *Required fees:* full-time $340.
**Financial Aid** 75% of baccalaureate students in nursing programs received some form of financial aid in 2011–12.
**Contact** Advising Center, Division of Nursing and Health Sciences, Lewis-Clark State College, 500 8th Avenue, Lewiston, ID 83501. *Telephone:* 208-792-2688. *Fax:* 208-792-2062. *E-mail:* nhs@lcsc.edu.

# Northwest Nazarene University

**School of Health and Science**
**Nampa, Idaho**

*http://www.nnu.edu/*
Founded in 1913

## DEGREES • BSN • MSN

**Nursing Program Faculty** 26 (27% with doctorates).
**Baccalaureate Enrollment** 120 **Women** 88% **Men** 12% **Minority** 12% **International** 3% **Part-time** 1%
**Graduate Enrollment** 17 **Women** 100%
**Distance Learning Courses** Available.
**Nursing Student Activities** Student Nurses' Association.
**Nursing Student Resources** Academic advising; academic or career counseling; assistance for students with disabilities; bookstore; campus computer network; career placement assistance; computer lab; computer-assisted instruction; e-mail services; housing assistance; interactive nursing skills videos; Internet; learning resource lab; library services; nursing audiovisuals; remedial services; resume preparation assistance; skills, simulation, or other laboratory; tutoring; unpaid internships.
**Library Facilities** 141,947 volumes (1,500 in health, 950 in nursing); 548 periodical subscriptions (218 health-care related).

## BACCALAUREATE PROGRAMS

**Degree** BSN
**Available Programs** Generic Baccalaureate.
**Study Options** Full-time.
**Program Entrance Requirements** Transcript of college record, CPR certification, health exam, health insurance, high school chemistry, immunizations, minimum GPA in nursing prerequisites of 2.75, professional liability insurance/malpractice insurance, prerequisite course work. Transfer students are accepted. *Application deadline:* 4/15 (fall).
**Advanced Placement** Credit given for nursing courses completed elsewhere dependent upon specific evaluations.
**Expenses (2012–13)** *Tuition:* full-time $24,790; part-time $1074 per credit. *Room and board:* $6400 per academic year. *Required fees:* full-time $660.
**Financial Aid** 90% of baccalaureate students in nursing programs received some form of financial aid in 2011–12.
**Contact** Dr. Barbara A. Lester, Chair, Department of Nursing, School of Health and Science, Northwest Nazarene University, 623 South University Boulevard, Nampa, ID 83686. *Telephone:* 208-467-8650. *Fax:* 208-467-8651. *E-mail:* nursing@nnu.edu.

## GRADUATE PROGRAMS

**Financial Aid** 90% of graduate students in nursing programs received some form of financial aid in 2011–12.
**Contact** Mrs. Kathy L. Hanson, Program Administrator, School of Health and Science, Northwest Nazarene University, 623 South University Boulevard, Nampa, ID 83686. *Telephone:* 208-467-8642. *Fax:* 208-467-8651. *E-mail:* klhanson@nnu.edu.

**MASTER'S DEGREE PROGRAM**
**Degree** MSN
**Available Programs** Master's; RN to Master's.
**Concentrations Available** Nursing education.
**Study Options** Full-time.
**Online Degree Options** Yes (online only).
**Program Entrance Requirements** Computer literacy, minimum overall college GPA of 3.0, transcript of college record, nursing research course, prerequisite course work, resume, statistics course. *Application deadline:* 7/31 (fall). Applications may be processed on a rolling basis for some programs. *Application fee:* $50.
**Degree Requirements** 36 total credit hours, thesis or project.

# ILLINOIS

## Aurora University
### School of Nursing
### Aurora, Illinois

*http://www.aurora.edu/*
Founded in 1893

**DEGREES • BSN • MSN**
**Nursing Program Faculty** 23 (17% with doctorates).
**Baccalaureate Enrollment** 291 **Women** 92% **Men** 8% **Minority** 29% **Part-time** 41%
**Graduate Enrollment** 30 **Women** 93% **Men** 7% **Minority** 40% **Part-time** 93%
**Distance Learning Courses** Available.
**Nursing Student Activities** Sigma Theta Tau, Student Nurses' Association, nursing club.
**Nursing Student Resources** Academic advising; academic or career counseling; assistance for students with disabilities; bookstore; campus computer network; career placement assistance; computer lab; computer-assisted instruction; e-mail services; externships; interactive nursing skills videos; Internet; learning resource lab; library services; nursing audiovisuals; remedial services; resume preparation assistance; skills, simulation, or other laboratory; tutoring.
**Library Facilities** 95,869 volumes (4,908 in health, 620 in nursing); 30,124 periodical subscriptions (1,700 health-care related).

### BACCALAUREATE PROGRAMS

**Degree** BSN
**Available Programs** Generic Baccalaureate; RN Baccalaureate.
**Site Options** Winfield, IL; Williams Bay, WI; Aurora, IL.
**Study Options** Full-time.
**Online Degree Options** Yes.
**Program Entrance Requirements** Minimum overall college GPA of 2.75, transcript of college record, CPR certification, written essay, health exam, health insurance, immunizations, interview, minimum GPA in nursing prerequisites of 2.75, prerequisite course work. Transfer students are accepted. *Application deadline:* 1/15 (fall). *Application fee:* $25.
**Advanced Placement** Credit given for nursing courses completed elsewhere dependent upon specific evaluations.
**Expenses (2012–13)** *Tuition:* full-time $19,900; part-time $590 per credit hour. *International tuition:* $19,900 full-time. *Room and board:* $8714 per academic year. *Required fees:* full-time $200.
**Financial Aid** 85% of baccalaureate students in nursing programs received some form of financial aid in 2011–12. *Gift aid (need-based):* Federal Pell, FSEOG, state, private, college/university gift aid from institutional funds. *Loans:* Federal Direct (Subsidized and Unsubsidized Stafford PLUS), Perkins, college/university, alternative loans. *Work-study:* Federal Work-Study, part-time campus jobs. *Financial aid application deadline (priority):* 1/1.
**Contact** Dr. Carmella M. Moran, Director and Associate Professor of Nursing, School of Nursing, Aurora University, 347 South Gladstone Avenue, Aurora, IL 60506-4892. *Telephone:* 630-844-5130. *Fax:* 630-844-7822. *E-mail:* cmoran@aurora.edu.

### GRADUATE PROGRAMS

**Expenses (2012–13)** *Tuition:* part-time $640 per credit hour.
**Financial Aid** 75% of graduate students in nursing programs received some form of financial aid in 2011–12.
**Contact** Dr. Barbara Lockwood, Coordinator, MSN Program, School of Nursing, Aurora University, 347 South Gladstone Avenue, Aurora, IL 60506-4892. *Telephone:* 630-844-5139. *Fax:* 630-844-7822. *E-mail:* lockwood@aurora.edu.

**MASTER'S DEGREE PROGRAM**
**Degree** MSN
**Available Programs** Master's.
**Concentrations Available** Nursing administration; nursing education.
**Site Options** Aurora, IL.
**Study Options** Part-time.
**Program Entrance Requirements** Clinical experience, computer literacy, minimum overall college GPA of 3.0, transcript of college record, CPR certification, written essay, immunizations, interview, 3 letters of recommendation, nursing research course, physical assessment course, professional liability insurance/malpractice insurance, resume, statistics course. *Application deadline:* 7/15 (fall), 10/15 (spring). Applications may be processed on a rolling basis for some programs. *Application fee:* $25.
**Degree Requirements** 36 total credit hours, thesis or project.

## Benedictine University
### Department of Nursing
### Lisle, Illinois

*http://www.ben.edu/nursing*
Founded in 1887

**DEGREES • BSN • MSN**
**Nursing Program Faculty** 30 (80% with doctorates).
**Baccalaureate Enrollment** 157 **Women** 95% **Men** 5% **Minority** 25% **International** 1%
**Graduate Enrollment** 322 **Women** 96% **Men** 4% **Minority** 37%
**Distance Learning Courses** Available.
**Nursing Student Activities** Nursing Honor Society, Sigma Theta Tau.
**Nursing Student Resources** Academic advising; academic or career counseling; assistance for students with disabilities; bookstore; campus computer network; career placement assistance; computer lab; computer-assisted instruction; e-mail services; interactive nursing skills videos; Internet; learning resource lab; library services; nursing audiovisuals; placement services for program completers; remedial services; resume preparation assistance; skills, simulation, or other laboratory; tutoring.
**Library Facilities** 240,500 volumes (1,350 in health, 850 in nursing); 64,586 periodical subscriptions (291 health-care related).

### BACCALAUREATE PROGRAMS

**Degree** BSN
**Available Programs** Accelerated RN Baccalaureate.
**Site Options** Springfield, IL; Glen Ellyn, IL; River Grove, IL.
**Study Options** Full-time.
**Program Entrance Requirements** Minimum overall college GPA of 2.5, transcript of college record, 1 letter of recommendation, RN licensure. Transfer students are accepted. *Application deadline:* 7/1 (fall), 11/1 (winter), 2/1 (spring), 5/1 (summer). Applications may be processed on a rolling basis for some programs.
**Advanced Placement** Credit given for nursing courses completed elsewhere dependent upon specific evaluations.
**Contact** *Telephone:* 630-829-1152. *Fax:* 630-829-1154.

### GRADUATE PROGRAMS

**Contact** *Telephone:* 866-295-3104 Ext. 5411. *Fax:* 866-789-5608.

**MASTER'S DEGREE PROGRAM**
**Degree** MSN
**Available Programs** Accelerated Master's; Master's.
**Study Options** Full-time and part-time.
**Online Degree Options** Yes (online only).
**Program Entrance Requirements** Minimum overall college GPA of 3.0, transcript of college record, written essay, 1 letter of recommendation, resume. *Application deadline:* Applications may be processed on a rolling basis for some programs.
**Advanced Placement** Credit given for nursing courses completed elsewhere dependent upon specific evaluations.
**Degree Requirements** 36 total credit hours, thesis or project.

# Blessing–Rieman College of Nursing

## Blessing–Rieman College of Nursing
## Quincy, Illinois

*http://www.brcn.edu/*

**DEGREES • BSN • MSN**

**Nursing Program Faculty** 29 (21% with doctorates).
**Baccalaureate Enrollment** 300 **Women** 85% **Men** 15% **Minority** 5% **International** 1% **Part-time** 8%
**Graduate Enrollment** 8 **Women** 90% **Men** 10% **Minority** 2% **Part-time** 100%
**Distance Learning Courses** Available.
**Nursing Student Activities** Nursing Honor Society, Sigma Theta Tau, Student Nurses' Association.
**Nursing Student Resources** Academic advising; academic or career counseling; bookstore; campus computer network; computer lab; computer-assisted instruction; daycare for children of students; e-mail services; employment services for current students; externships; interactive nursing skills videos; Internet; learning resource lab; library services; nursing audiovisuals; paid internships; resume preparation assistance; skills, simulation, or other laboratory; tutoring.
**Library Facilities** 3,752 volumes in health, 3,752 volumes in nursing; 125 periodical subscriptions health-care related.

### BACCALAUREATE PROGRAMS

**Degree** BSN
**Available Programs** ADN to Baccalaureate; Accelerated Baccalaureate for Second Degree; Generic Baccalaureate; RN Baccalaureate.
**Study Options** Full-time and part-time.
**Online Degree Options** Yes.
**Program Entrance Requirements** Minimum overall college GPA of 2.7, transcript of college record, CPR certification, health insurance, high school biology, high school chemistry, 2 years high school math, 2 years high school science, high school transcript, immunizations, minimum high school GPA of 3.0, minimum GPA in nursing prerequisites of 2.7, prerequisite course work. Transfer students are accepted. *Application deadline:* Applications may be processed on a rolling basis for some programs.
**Advanced Placement** Credit by examination available. Credit given for nursing courses completed elsewhere dependent upon specific evaluations.
**Expenses (2013–14)** *Tuition:* full-time $19,782; part-time $659 per credit hour. *Room and board:* room only: $2982 per academic year. *Required fees:* full-time $450; part-time $450 per credit.
**Financial Aid** 90% of baccalaureate students in nursing programs received some form of financial aid in 2012–13.
**Contact** Mrs. Heather Mutter, Admission Counselor, Blessing–Rieman College of Nursing, Broadway at 11th Street, PO Box 7005, Quincy, IL 62305-7005. *Telephone:* 217-228-5520 Ext. 6949. *Fax:* 217-223-4661. *E-mail:* admissions@brcn.edu.

### GRADUATE PROGRAMS

**Expenses (2013–14)** *Tuition:* part-time $500 per credit hour.
**Contact** Mrs. Heather Mutter, Admissions Counselor, Blessing–Rieman College of Nursing, Broadway at 11th Street, PO Box 7005, Quincy, IL 62305-7005. *Telephone:* 217-228-5520 Ext. 6949. *Fax:* 217-223-4661. *E-mail:* admissions@brcn.edu.

### MASTER'S DEGREE PROGRAM

**Degree** MSN
**Available Programs** Master's; RN to Master's.
**Concentrations Available** Nursing administration; nursing education.
**Study Options** Part-time.
**Program Entrance Requirements** Clinical experience, computer literacy, minimum overall college GPA of 3.0, transcript of college record, CPR certification, written essay, immunizations, letters of recommendation, nursing research course, physical assessment course, professional liability insurance/malpractice insurance, resume, statistics course. *Application deadline:* 4/15 (spring). Applications may be processed on a rolling basis for some programs.
**Advanced Placement** Credit given for nursing courses completed elsewhere dependent upon specific evaluations.
**Degree Requirements** 44 total credit hours, thesis or project.

# Bradley University

## Department of Nursing
## Peoria, Illinois

*http://www.bradley.edu/academic/departments/nursing/*
Founded in 1897

**DEGREES • BSN • BSC PN • MSN**

**Nursing Program Faculty** 66 (12% with doctorates).
**Baccalaureate Enrollment** 349 **Women** 95% **Men** 5% **Minority** 16% **Part-time** 1%
**Graduate Enrollment** 13 **Women** 92% **Men** 8% **Minority** 2% **International** 1% **Part-time** 92%
**Nursing Student Activities** Sigma Theta Tau, Student Nurses' Association.
**Nursing Student Resources** Academic advising; academic or career counseling; assistance for students with disabilities; bookstore; campus computer network; career placement assistance; computer lab; computer-assisted instruction; e-mail services; employment services for current students; externships; housing assistance; Internet; learning resource lab; library services; nursing audiovisuals; placement services for program completers; remedial services; resume preparation assistance; skills, simulation, or other laboratory; tutoring.
**Library Facilities** 511,000 volumes (11,612 in health, 2,383 in nursing); 41,689 periodical subscriptions (205 health-care related).

### BACCALAUREATE PROGRAMS

**Degrees** BSN; BSc PN
**Available Programs** ADN to Baccalaureate; Accelerated Baccalaureate for Second Degree; Baccalaureate for Second Degree; Generic Baccalaureate; LPN to Baccalaureate; RN Baccalaureate.
**Study Options** Full-time.
**Program Entrance Requirements** Written essay, high school biology, high school chemistry, 3 years high school math, 3 years high school science, high school transcript, immunizations, 1 letter of recommendation, minimum high school GPA of 3.25. Transfer students are accepted. *Application deadline:* Applications may be processed on a rolling basis for some programs.
**Financial Aid** 93% of baccalaureate students in nursing programs received some form of financial aid in 2012–13. *Gift aid (need-based):* Federal Pell, FSEOG, state, private, college/university gift aid from institutional funds. *Loans:* Federal Nursing Student Loans, Federal Direct (Subsidized and Unsubsidized Stafford PLUS), Perkins. *Work-study:* Federal Work-Study. *Financial aid application deadline (priority):* 3/1.
**Contact** Mr. Justin Ball, Director of Admissions, Department of Nursing, Bradley University, 1501 West Bradley Avenue, Peoria, IL 61625. *Telephone:* 309-677-1000. *Fax:* 309-677-2797. *E-mail:* admissions@bradley.edu.

### GRADUATE PROGRAMS

**Financial Aid** 80% of graduate students in nursing programs received some form of financial aid in 2012–13. Research assistantships, scholarships, tuition waivers (partial), and unspecified assistantships available. *Financial aid application deadline:* 4/1.
**Contact** Dr. Deborah Erickson, Graduate Coordinator, Department of Nursing, Bradley University, 1501 West Bradley Avenue, Burgess Hall 312, Peoria, IL 61625. *Telephone:* 309-677-4974. *Fax:* 309-677-2527. *E-mail:* erickson@bradley.edu.

### MASTER'S DEGREE PROGRAM

**Degree** MSN
**Available Programs** Master's; RN to Master's.
**Concentrations Available** Nursing administration; nursing education.
**Study Options** Full-time and part-time.
**Program Entrance Requirements** Clinical experience, minimum overall college GPA of 3.0, transcript of college record, interview, 3 letters of recommendation, nursing research course, physical assessment course, resume, statistics course, GRE General Test or MAT. *Application deadline:* Applications may be processed on a rolling basis for some programs.
**Advanced Placement** Credit given for nursing courses completed elsewhere dependent upon specific evaluations.
**Degree Requirements** 36 total credit hours, thesis or project, comprehensive exam.

# Chicago State University

## Department of Nursing
## Chicago, Illinois

*http://www.csu.edu/*
Founded in 1867

**DEGREE • BSN**

**Nursing Program Faculty** 23 (60% with doctorates).
**Baccalaureate Enrollment** 372 **Women** 90% **Men** 10% **Minority** 97% **International** 15% **Part-time** 24%
**Nursing Student Activities** Nursing Honor Society, Student Nurses' Association.
**Nursing Student Resources** Academic advising; academic or career counseling; assistance for students with disabilities; bookstore; campus computer network; computer lab; computer-assisted instruction; daycare for children of students; e-mail services; employment services for current students; externships; interactive nursing skills videos; Internet; learning resource lab; library services; nursing audiovisuals; remedial services; resume preparation assistance; skills, simulation, or other laboratory; tutoring; unpaid internships.
**Library Facilities** 426,691 volumes; 1,654 periodical subscriptions.

### BACCALAUREATE PROGRAMS

**Degree** BSN
**Available Programs** Generic Baccalaureate; LPN to Baccalaureate; RN Baccalaureate.
**Study Options** Full-time.
**Program Entrance Requirements** Minimum overall college GPA of 2.5, transcript of college record, written essay, health exam, health insurance, 3 years high school math, 3 years high school science, high school transcript, immunizations, interview, 3 letters of recommendation, minimum GPA in nursing prerequisites of 2.5, professional liability insurance/malpractice insurance, prerequisite course work. Transfer students are accepted.
**Advanced Placement** Credit by examination available.
**Contact** *Telephone:* 773-995-3992. *Fax:* 773-821-2438.

# DePaul University

## School of Nursing
## Chicago, Illinois

*http://csh.depaul.edu/departments/nursing/Pages/default.aspx*
Founded in 1898

**DEGREES • DNP • MS**

**Nursing Program Faculty** 81 (25% with doctorates).
**Graduate Enrollment** 371 **Women** 85% **Men** 15% **Minority** 29% **International** 1% **Part-time** 11%
**Nursing Student Activities** Sigma Theta Tau, Student Nurses' Association.
**Nursing Student Resources** Academic advising; academic or career counseling; assistance for students with disabilities; bookstore; campus computer network; career placement assistance; computer lab; computer-assisted instruction; e-mail services; employment services for current students; housing assistance; interactive nursing skills videos; Internet; learning resource lab; library services; nursing audiovisuals; resume preparation assistance; skills, simulation, or other laboratory; tutoring.
**Library Facilities** 928,933 volumes (27,000 in health, 5,800 in nursing); 30,348 periodical subscriptions (1,800 health-care related).

### GRADUATE PROGRAMS

**Financial Aid** 82% of graduate students in nursing programs received some form of financial aid in 2012–13. 6 fellowships (averaging $1,500 per year) were awarded; traineeships also available.
**Contact** The Office of Graduate Admission, School of Nursing, DePaul University, DePaul University, 2400 North Sheffield Avenue, Chicago, IL 60614. *Telephone:* 773-325-7315. *Fax:* 312-476-3244. *E-mail:* GradDePaul@depaul.edu.

### MASTER'S DEGREE PROGRAM

**Degree** MS
**Available Programs** Master's; Master's for Non-Nursing College Graduates.
**Concentrations Available** Nurse anesthesia. *Nurse practitioner programs in:* adult health, family health.
**Site Options** North Chicago, IL.
**Study Options** Full-time and part-time.
**Program Entrance Requirements** Computer literacy, minimum overall college GPA of 3.0, transcript of college record, CPR certification, written essay, immunizations, interview, 2 letters of recommendation, professional liability insurance/malpractice insurance, prerequisite course work, resume, GRE (if bachelor's GPA less than 3.2). *Application deadline:* 1/15 (fall), 6/15 (winter). Applications may be processed on a rolling basis for some programs. *Application fee:* $40.
**Advanced Placement** Credit given for nursing courses completed elsewhere dependent upon specific evaluations.
**Degree Requirements** 107 total credit hours, thesis or project.

### POST-MASTER'S PROGRAM

**Areas of Study** Nurse anesthesia. *Nurse practitioner programs in:* adult health, family health.

### DOCTORAL DEGREE PROGRAM

**Degree** DNP
**Available Programs** Doctorate; Post-Baccalaureate Doctorate.
**Areas of Study** Advanced practice nursing.
**Program Entrance Requirements** Clinical experience, minimum overall college GPA of 3.5, interview by faculty committee, interview, 2 letters of recommendation, vita, GRE. *Application deadline:* 3/15 (fall). *Application fee:* $40.
**Degree Requirements** 100 total credit hours.

# Eastern Illinois University

## Nursing Program
## Charleston, Illinois

*http://www.eiu.edu/nursing*
Founded in 1895

**DEGREE • BSN**

**Nursing Program Faculty** 5 (100% with doctorates).
**Baccalaureate Enrollment** 55 **Women** 65% **Men** 35% **Minority** 45% **Part-time** 80%
**Distance Learning Courses** Available.
**Nursing Student Resources** Academic advising; academic or career counseling; assistance for students with disabilities; bookstore; campus computer network; computer lab; computer-assisted instruction; e-mail services; interactive nursing skills videos; Internet; library services; nursing audiovisuals; remedial services; resume preparation assistance; skills, simulation, or other laboratory; tutoring.
**Library Facilities** 1.1 million volumes (500 in nursing); 46,047 periodical subscriptions (50 health-care related).

### BACCALAUREATE PROGRAMS

**Degree** BSN
**Available Programs** ADN to Baccalaureate.
**Study Options** Full-time and part-time.
**Online Degree Options** Yes (online only).
**Program Entrance Requirements** Minimum overall college GPA of 2.5, transcript of college record, CPR certification, written essay, health exam, health insurance, high school transcript, immunizations, 2 letters of recommendation, professional liability insurance/malpractice insurance, prerequisite course work, RN licensure. *Application deadline:* 11/15 (fall), 7/15 (summer). *Application fee:* $30.
**Advanced Placement** Credit given for nursing courses completed elsewhere dependent upon specific evaluations.
**Contact** *Telephone:* 217-581-7049. *Fax:* 217-581-7050.

# Elmhurst College

## Deicke Center for Nursing Education
## Elmhurst, Illinois

Founded in 1871

**DEGREES • BS • MS • MSN/MBA**

**Nursing Program Faculty** 13 (55% with doctorates).
**Baccalaureate Enrollment** 195
**Graduate Enrollment** 34

**Nursing Student Activities** Sigma Theta Tau, Student Nurses' Association.
**Nursing Student Resources** Academic advising; academic or career counseling; assistance for students with disabilities; bookstore; campus computer network; career placement assistance; computer lab; daycare for children of students; e-mail services; employment services for current students; housing assistance; Internet; learning resource lab; library services; nursing audiovisuals; remedial services; resume preparation assistance; skills, simulation, or other laboratory; tutoring.
**Library Facilities** 230,055 volumes (6,000 in health); 1,859 periodical subscriptions (80 health-care related).

## BACCALAUREATE PROGRAMS

**Degree** BS
**Available Programs** Generic Baccalaureate; RN Baccalaureate.
**Study Options** Full-time.
**Program Entrance Requirements** Minimum overall college GPA of 2.75, transcript of college record, CPR certification, written essay, health insurance, immunizations, 2 letters of recommendation, minimum GPA in nursing prerequisites of 2.75, prerequisite course work. Transfer students are accepted. *Application deadline:* 6/1 (fall).
**Advanced Placement** Credit given for nursing courses completed elsewhere dependent upon specific evaluations.
**Contact** *Telephone:* 630-617-3344. *Fax:* 630-617-3237.

## GRADUATE PROGRAMS

**Contact** *Fax:* 630-617-3514.

### MASTER'S DEGREE PROGRAM

**Degrees** MS; MSN/MBA
**Available Programs** Master's.
**Concentrations Available** Clinical nurse leader; nursing education.
**Study Options** Full-time.
**Program Entrance Requirements** Clinical experience, computer literacy, transcript of college record, CPR certification, written essay, immunizations, interview, 3 letters of recommendation, nursing research course, physical assessment course, prerequisite course work, resume, statistics course. *Application deadline:* Applications may be processed on a rolling basis for some programs.
**Degree Requirements** 33 total credit hours.

# Governors State University
## College of Health and Human Services
## University Park, Illinois

***http://www.govst.edu/***
Founded in 1969

**DEGREES • BS • MS**
**Nursing Program Faculty** 7 (85% with doctorates).
**Baccalaureate Enrollment** 31 **Women** 98% **Men** 2% **Minority** 92% **International** 1% **Part-time** 100%
**Graduate Enrollment** 72 **Women** 97% **Men** 3% **Minority** 89% **International** 6% **Part-time** 4%
**Nursing Student Activities** Sigma Theta Tau.
**Nursing Student Resources** Academic advising; assistance for students with disabilities; bookstore; campus computer network; computer lab; daycare for children of students; e-mail services; Internet; learning resource lab; library services; nursing audiovisuals; tutoring.
**Library Facilities** 465,000 volumes; 51,000 periodical subscriptions.

## BACCALAUREATE PROGRAMS

**Degree** BS
**Available Programs** RN Baccalaureate.
**Study Options** Part-time.
**Program Entrance Requirements** Transcript of college record, CPR certification, health exam, health insurance, immunizations, minimum GPA in nursing prerequisites of 2.0, professional liability insurance/malpractice insurance, prerequisite course work, RN licensure. Transfer students are accepted.
**Contact** *Telephone:* 708-534-4053. *Fax:* 708-534-2197.

## GRADUATE PROGRAMS

**Contact** *Telephone:* 708-534-4053. *Fax:* 708-534-2197.

### MASTER'S DEGREE PROGRAM

**Degree** MS
**Available Programs** Master's.
**Concentrations Available** *Clinical nurse specialist programs in:* adult health.
**Study Options** Full-time and part-time.
**Program Entrance Requirements** Clinical experience, computer literacy, minimum overall college GPA of 3.0, transcript of college record, CPR certification, written essay, immunizations, nursing research course, physical assessment course, professional liability insurance/malpractice insurance, prerequisite course work, statistics course.
**Degree Requirements** 42 total credit hours, comprehensive exam.

### POST-MASTER'S PROGRAM

**Areas of Study** Nursing education.

# Illinois State University
## Mennonite College of Nursing
## Normal, Illinois

***http://www.mcn.illinoisstate.edu/***
Founded in 1857

**DEGREES • BSN • DNP • MSN • PHD**
**Nursing Program Faculty** 77 (21% with doctorates).
**Baccalaureate Enrollment** 398 **Women** 89% **Men** 11% **Minority** 11% **Part-time** 5%
**Graduate Enrollment** 115 **Women** 93% **Men** 7% **Minority** 3% **International** 1% **Part-time** 86%
**Distance Learning Courses** Available.
**Nursing Student Activities** Nursing Honor Society, Sigma Theta Tau, Student Nurses' Association.
**Nursing Student Resources** Academic advising; academic or career counseling; assistance for students with disabilities; bookstore; campus computer network; career placement assistance; computer lab; computer-assisted instruction; daycare for children of students; e-mail services; employment services for current students; interactive nursing skills videos; Internet; learning resource lab; library services; nursing audiovisuals; remedial services; resume preparation assistance; skills, simulation, or other laboratory; tutoring.
**Library Facilities** 1.6 million volumes (28,392 in health, 2,850 in nursing); 83,375 periodical subscriptions (420 health-care related).

## BACCALAUREATE PROGRAMS

**Degree** BSN
**Available Programs** Accelerated Baccalaureate for Second Degree; Generic Baccalaureate; RN Baccalaureate.
**Site Options** Normal, IL.
**Study Options** Full-time and part-time.
**Online Degree Options** Yes.
**Program Entrance Requirements** Minimum overall college GPA of 2.5, transcript of college record, CPR certification, written essay, health exam, health insurance, immunizations, minimum GPA in nursing prerequisites of 2.0, prerequisite course work. Transfer students are accepted. *Application deadline:* 1/15 (fall), 6/15 (spring), 6/15 (summer). *Application fee:* $50.
**Advanced Placement** Credit given for nursing courses completed elsewhere dependent upon specific evaluations.
**Expenses (2013–14)** *Tuition, state resident:* full-time $13,009; part-time $342 per credit hour. *Tuition, nonresident:* full-time $19,190; part-time $590 per credit hour. *Room and board:* $9624 per academic year. *Required fees:* full-time $1492; part-time $77 per credit; part-time $168 per term.
**Financial Aid** 81% of baccalaureate students in nursing programs received some form of financial aid in 2012–13.
**Contact** Ms. Nancy Diller, Academic Advisor, Mennonite College of Nursing, Illinois State University, Campus Box 5810, Uptown Crossing, Suite C, Normal, IL 61790-5810. *Telephone:* 309-438-7400. *Fax:* 309-438-7711. *E-mail:* njakubc@ilstu.edu.

## GRADUATE PROGRAMS

**Expenses (2013–14)** *Tuition, state resident:* full-time $5175; part-time $345 per credit hour. *Tuition, nonresident:* full-time $10,740; part-time $716 per credit hour. *International tuition:* $12,007 full-time. *Required fees:* full-time $1157; part-time $77 per credit.
**Financial Aid** 66% of graduate students in nursing programs received some form of financial aid in 2012–13.

**Contact** Ms. Melissa K. Moody, Academic Advisor, Mennonite College of Nursing, Illinois State University, Campus Box 5810, Uptown Crossing Office, Suite C, Normal, IL 61790-5810. *Telephone:* 309-438-7035. *Fax:* 309-438-7711. *E-mail:* mkmoody@ilstu.edu.

**MASTER'S DEGREE PROGRAM**
**Degree** MSN
**Available Programs** Master's.
**Concentrations Available** Clinical nurse leader; nursing administration. *Nurse practitioner programs in:* family health.
**Site Options** Normal, IL.
**Study Options** Full-time and part-time.
**Online Degree Options** Yes (online only).
**Program Entrance Requirements** Minimum overall college GPA of 3.0, transcript of college record, CPR certification, written essay, immunizations, interview, 3 letters of recommendation, nursing research course, physical assessment course, prerequisite course work, resume, statistics course. *Application deadline:* 2/1 (fall). *Application fee:* $50.
**Advanced Placement** Credit given for nursing courses completed elsewhere dependent upon specific evaluations.
**Degree Requirements** 44 total credit hours, comprehensive exam.

**POST-MASTER'S PROGRAM**
**Areas of Study** *Nurse practitioner programs in:* family health.

**DOCTORAL DEGREE PROGRAM**
**Degree** DNP
**Available Programs** Doctorate.
**Areas of Study** Nursing administration.
**Online Degree Options** Yes (online only).
**Program Entrance Requirements** Minimum overall college GPA of 3.0, 3 letters of recommendation, MSN or equivalent, vita. *Application deadline:* 2/1 (spring). Applications may be processed on a rolling basis for some programs. *Application fee:* $50.
**Degree Requirements** 34 total credit hours, dissertation.

**Degree** PhD
**Available Programs** Doctorate.
**Areas of Study** Aging.
**Site Options** Normal, IL.
**Program Entrance Requirements** Minimum overall college GPA of 3.0, interview by faculty committee, interview, 3 letters of recommendation, MSN or equivalent, statistics course, vita. *Application deadline:* 2/1 (fall). *Application fee:* $50.
**Degree Requirements** 66 total credit hours, dissertation, oral exam, written exam, residency.

# Illinois Wesleyan University

## School of Nursing
## Bloomington, Illinois

***http://www2.iwu.edu/nursing/***
Founded in 1850

**DEGREE • BSN**
**Nursing Program Faculty** 26 (35% with doctorates).
**Baccalaureate Enrollment** 161 **Women** 91% **Men** 9% **Minority** 17%
**Nursing Student Activities** Nursing Honor Society, Sigma Theta Tau, Student Nurses' Association, nursing club.
**Nursing Student Resources** Academic advising; academic or career counseling; assistance for students with disabilities; bookstore; campus computer network; career placement assistance; computer lab; computer-assisted instruction; e-mail services; employment services for current students; externships; housing assistance; interactive nursing skills videos; Internet; learning resource lab; library services; nursing audiovisuals; paid internships; placement services for program completers; resume preparation assistance; skills, simulation, or other laboratory; tutoring; unpaid internships.
**Library Facilities** 9,957 volumes in health, 7,940 volumes in nursing; 115 periodical subscriptions health-care related.

**BACCALAUREATE PROGRAMS**
**Degree** BSN
**Available Programs** Generic Baccalaureate.
**Study Options** Full-time and part-time.
**Program Entrance Requirements** Minimum overall college GPA of 3.0, transcript of college record, written essay, health exam, health insurance, high school biology, high school chemistry, 2 years high school math, 2 years high school science, high school transcript, immunizations, interview, minimum high school GPA of 3.0, minimum high school rank 25%, minimum GPA in nursing prerequisites of 3.0. Transfer students are accepted. *Application deadline:* Applications may be processed on a rolling basis for some programs.
**Expenses (2013–14)** *Tuition:* full-time $39,136; part-time $4892 per unit. *International tuition:* $39,136 full-time. *Room and board:* $9136; room only: $5752 per academic year. *Required fees:* full-time $180; part-time $90 per term.
**Financial Aid** 96% of baccalaureate students in nursing programs received some form of financial aid in 2012–13. *Gift aid (need-based):* Federal Pell, FSEOG, state, private, college/university gift aid from institutional funds. *Loans:* Federal Nursing Student Loans, Federal Direct (Subsidized and Unsubsidized Stafford PLUS), Perkins, college/university. *Work-study:* Federal Work-Study, part-time campus jobs. *Financial aid application deadline (priority):* 3/1.
**Contact** Dr. Victoria N. Folse, Director and Associate Professor, School of Nursing, Illinois Wesleyan University, PO Box 2900, Bloomington, IL 61702-2900. *Telephone:* 309-556-3051. *Fax:* 309-556-3043. *E-mail:* vfolse@iwu.edu.

# Lakeview College of Nursing

## Lakeview College of Nursing
## Danville, Illinois

***http://www.lakeviewcol.edu/***
Founded in 1987

**DEGREE • BSN**
**Nursing Program Faculty** 24 (4% with doctorates).
**Baccalaureate Enrollment** 284 **Women** 87% **Men** 13% **Minority** 20% **Part-time** 8%
**Nursing Student Activities** Nursing Honor Society, Sigma Theta Tau, Student Nurses' Association.
**Nursing Student Resources** Academic advising; academic or career counseling; assistance for students with disabilities; bookstore; campus computer network; career placement assistance; computer lab; Internet; library services; nursing audiovisuals; resume preparation assistance; skills, simulation, or other laboratory; tutoring.
**Library Facilities** 2,000 volumes in health; 41 periodical subscriptions health-care related.

**BACCALAUREATE PROGRAMS**
**Degree** BSN
**Available Programs** Accelerated RN Baccalaureate; Generic Baccalaureate; RN Baccalaureate.
**Site Options** Charleston, IL.
**Study Options** Full-time and part-time.
**Program Entrance Requirements** Minimum overall college GPA of 2.5, transcript of college record, CPR certification, written essay, health exam, immunizations, 2 letters of recommendation, prerequisite course work. Transfer students are accepted. *Application deadline:* 4/1 (fall), 10/1 (spring). *Application fee:* $100.
**Advanced Placement** Credit given for nursing courses completed elsewhere dependent upon specific evaluations.
**Expenses (2013–14)** *Tuition:* full-time $12,800.
**Financial Aid** 52% of baccalaureate students in nursing programs received some form of financial aid in 2012–13. *Gift aid (need-based):* Federal Pell, state, private, college/university gift aid from institutional funds. *Loans:* Federal Direct (Subsidized and Unsubsidized Stafford PLUS). *Financial aid application deadline:* Continuous.
**Contact** Mrs. Connie Young, Director of Enrollment/Registrar, Lakeview College of Nursing, 903 North Logan Avenue, Danville, IL 61832. *Telephone:* 217-709-0931. *Fax:* 217-709-0953. *E-mail:* cyoung@lakeviewcol.edu.

# Lewis University

## Program in Nursing
## Romeoville, Illinois

***http://www.lewisu.edu/academics/nursing/index.htm***
Founded in 1932

**DEGREES • BSN • DNP • MSN • MSN/MBA**
**Nursing Program Faculty** 44 (23% with doctorates).

**Baccalaureate Enrollment** 636 **Women** 90% **Men** 10% **Minority** 31% **International** 9% **Part-time** 69%
**Graduate Enrollment** 289 **Women** 95% **Men** 5% **Minority** 28% **International** 28% **Part-time** 89%
**Distance Learning Courses** Available.
**Nursing Student Activities** Sigma Theta Tau, Student Nurses' Association.
**Nursing Student Resources** Academic advising; academic or career counseling; assistance for students with disabilities; bookstore; campus computer network; career placement assistance; computer lab; computer-assisted instruction; e-mail services; employment services for current students; externships; interactive nursing skills videos; Internet; learning resource lab; library services; nursing audiovisuals; other; placement services for program completers; remedial services; resume preparation assistance; skills, simulation, or other laboratory; tutoring.
**Library Facilities** 169,371 volumes (3,100 in health, 2,038 in nursing); 47,529 periodical subscriptions (90 health-care related).

## BACCALAUREATE PROGRAMS

**Degree** BSN
**Available Programs** Accelerated Baccalaureate for Second Degree; Accelerated RN Baccalaureate; Generic Baccalaureate.
**Site Options** Oak Brook, IL; Tinley Park, IL; Hickory Hills, IL; Shorewood, IL.
**Study Options** Full-time.
**Program Entrance Requirements** Minimum overall college GPA of 2.75, transcript of college record, CPR certification, health exam, health insurance, high school biology, high school chemistry, 3 years high school math, high school transcript, immunizations, minimum high school GPA of 2.75, minimum GPA in nursing prerequisites of 2.75, prerequisite course work. Transfer students are accepted. *Application deadline:* Applications may be processed on a rolling basis for some programs. *Application fee:* $40.
**Advanced Placement** Credit given for nursing courses completed elsewhere dependent upon specific evaluations.
**Expenses (2013–14)** *Tuition:* full-time $26,780; part-time $790 per credit. *International tuition:* $26,780 full-time. *Room and board:* $4800; room only: $3250 per academic year. *Required fees:* full-time $400; part-time $200 per term.
**Financial Aid** 80% of baccalaureate students in nursing programs received some form of financial aid in 2012–13. *Gift aid (need-based):* Federal Pell, FSEOG, state, private, college/university gift aid from institutional funds, Federal Nursing. *Loans:* Federal Direct (Subsidized and Unsubsidized Stafford PLUS), Perkins. *Work-study:* Federal Work-Study, part-time campus jobs. *Financial aid application deadline:* 5/1.
**Contact** Dr. Peggy Rice, Dean and Professor, Program in Nursing, Lewis University, One University Parkway, Romeoville, IL 60446. *Telephone:* 815-836-5245. *Fax:* 815-838-8306. *E-mail:* ricepe@lewisu.edu.

## GRADUATE PROGRAMS

**Expenses (2013–14)** *Tuition:* part-time $750 per credit hour. *Room and board:* $10,330; room only: $7360 per academic year.
**Financial Aid** 85% of graduate students in nursing programs received some form of financial aid in 2012–13. Federal Work-Study, scholarships, tuition waivers (full and partial), and unspecified assistantships available. *Financial aid application deadline:* 5/1.
**Contact** Dr. Suling Li, Associate Dean for Faculty Scholarship and Director of Graduate Studies, Program in Nursing, Lewis University, One University Parkway, Unit 1215, Romeoville, IL 60446. *Telephone:* 815-836-5878 Ext. 815. *Fax:* 815-836-5806. *E-mail:* lisu@lewisu.edu.

### MASTER'S DEGREE PROGRAM

**Degrees** MSN; MSN/MBA
**Available Programs** Accelerated Master's; Accelerated Master's for Nurses with Non-Nursing Degrees; Accelerated RN to Master's; Master's; RN to Master's.
**Concentrations Available** Nursing administration; nursing education. *Clinical nurse specialist programs in:* adult health, gerontology. *Nurse practitioner programs in:* adult health, family health, gerontology.
**Site Options** Oak Brook, IL; Tinley Park, IL; Hickory Hills, IL; Shorewood, IL.
**Study Options** Full-time and part-time.
**Online Degree Options** Yes.
**Program Entrance Requirements** Minimum overall college GPA of 3.0, transcript of college record, CPR certification, written essay, immunizations, 2 letters of recommendation, nursing research course, prerequisite course work, resume, statistics course. *Application deadline:* 4/1 (fall), 11/15 (spring). Applications may be processed on a rolling basis for some programs. *Application fee:* $40.
**Advanced Placement** Credit given for nursing courses completed elsewhere dependent upon specific evaluations.
**Degree Requirements** 40 total credit hours, thesis or project.

### POST-MASTER'S PROGRAM

**Areas of Study** Nursing administration; nursing education. *Clinical nurse specialist programs in:* adult health, gerontology. *Nurse practitioner programs in:* adult health, family health, gerontology.

### DOCTORAL DEGREE PROGRAM

**Degree** DNP
**Available Programs** Doctorate.
**Areas of Study** Health-care systems.
**Online Degree Options** Yes (online only).
**Program Entrance Requirements** Clinical experience, minimum overall college GPA of 3.25, letters of recommendation, MSN or equivalent, statistics course, vita, writing sample. *Application deadline:* 4/1 (fall), 11/15 (spring). Applications may be processed on a rolling basis for some programs. *Application fee:* $40.
**Degree Requirements** 30 total credit hours, residency.

## CONTINUING EDUCATION PROGRAM

**Contact** Ms. Nanci Peek, Coordinator of Continuing Education, Program in Nursing, Lewis University, One University Parkway, Romeoville, IL 60446. *Telephone:* 815-836-5720. *Fax:* 815-838-8306. *E-mail:* peekna@lewisu.edu.

# Loyola University Chicago
## Marcella Niehoff School of Nursing
## Maywood, Illinois

*http://www.luc.edu/nursing/*
Founded in 1870

**DEGREES • BSN • DNP • MSN • MSN/MBA • PHD**
**Nursing Program Faculty** 52 (82% with doctorates).
**Baccalaureate Enrollment** 863 **Women** 94.6% **Men** 5.4% **Minority** 19.8% **Part-time** 15.6%
**Graduate Enrollment** 329 **Women** 92.4% **Men** 7.6% **Minority** 20% **Part-time** 90.2%
**Distance Learning Courses** Available.
**Nursing Student Activities** Nursing Honor Society, Sigma Theta Tau, Student Nurses' Association.
**Nursing Student Resources** Academic advising; academic or career counseling; assistance for students with disabilities; bookstore; campus computer network; computer lab; computer-assisted instruction; e-mail services; interactive nursing skills videos; Internet; learning resource lab; library services; nursing audiovisuals; remedial services; resume preparation assistance; skills, simulation, or other laboratory; tutoring.
**Library Facilities** 1.4 million volumes (36,709 in health, 6,316 in nursing); 52,535 periodical subscriptions (2,630 health-care related).

## BACCALAUREATE PROGRAMS

**Degree** BSN
**Available Programs** Accelerated Baccalaureate for Second Degree; Generic Baccalaureate; RN Baccalaureate.
**Site Options** Chicago, IL; Maywood, IL.
**Study Options** Full-time.
**Program Entrance Requirements** Transcript of college record, CPR certification, written essay, health exam, health insurance, high school biology, high school chemistry, 2 years high school math, high school transcript, immunizations, 2 letters of recommendation, minimum high school GPA of 3.0, minimum high school rank 25%, prerequisite course work. *Application deadline:* 3/1 (fall). Applications may be processed on a rolling basis for some programs.
**Expenses (2013–14)** *Tuition:* full-time $18,150; part-time $770 per semester. *Room and board:* $11,325; room only: $9000 per academic year. *Required fees:* full-time $3000.
**Financial Aid** 96% of baccalaureate students in nursing programs received some form of financial aid in 2012–13. *Gift aid (need-based):* Federal Pell, FSEOG, state, private, college/university gift aid from institutional funds. *Loans:* Federal Nursing Student Loans, Federal Direct (Subsidized and Unsubsidized Stafford PLUS), Perkins. *Work-study:* Federal Work-Study. *Financial aid application deadline:* Continuous.
**Contact** Ms. Janet Campbell, Director, Undergraduate Student Affairs, Marcella Niehoff School of Nursing, Loyola University Chicago, 1032 West Sheridan Road, BVM Hall, 8th Floor, Chicago, IL 60660.

*Telephone:* 773-508-3241. *Fax:* 773-508-2918. *E-mail:* jcampbell2@luc.edu.

## GRADUATE PROGRAMS

**Expenses (2013–14)** *Tuition:* part-time $970 per credit hour. *Required fees:* part-time $525 per term.
**Financial Aid** 1 fellowship, 4 research assistantships, 1 teaching assistantship were awarded; career-related internships or fieldwork, Federal Work-Study, institutionally sponsored loans, traineeships, and unspecified assistantships also available.
**Contact** Ms. Amy Weatherford, Enrollment Advisor, Marcella Niehoff School of Nursing, Loyola University Chicago, 2160 South 1st Avenue, 125-4524, Maywood, IL 60153. *Telephone:* 708-216-3751. *Fax:* 708-216-9555. *E-mail:* aweatherford@luc.edu.

### MASTER'S DEGREE PROGRAM

**Degrees** MSN; MSN/MBA
**Available Programs** Master's; RN to Master's.
**Concentrations Available** Nursing administration; nursing informatics. *Clinical nurse specialist programs in:* acute care, adult health, critical care, oncology. *Nurse practitioner programs in:* acute care, adult health, family health, primary care,women's health.
**Site Options** Chicago, IL; Maywood, IL.
**Study Options** Full-time and part-time.
**Online Degree Options** Yes (online only).
**Program Entrance Requirements** Clinical experience, minimum overall college GPA of 3.0, transcript of college record, CPR certification, written essay, immunizations, 3 letters of recommendation, physical assessment course, professional liability insurance/malpractice insurance, resume, statistics course. *Application deadline:* 7/1 (fall), 11/15 (spring), 3/15 (summer). Applications may be processed on a rolling basis for some programs.
**Advanced Placement** Credit given for nursing courses completed elsewhere dependent upon specific evaluations.
**Degree Requirements** 48 total credit hours, comprehensive exam.

### POST-MASTER'S PROGRAM

**Areas of Study** Nursing administration; nursing informatics. *Clinical nurse specialist programs in:* acute care, adult health, critical care, oncology. *Nurse practitioner programs in:* acute care, adult health, family health, primary care,women's health.

### DOCTORAL DEGREE PROGRAM

**Degree** DNP
**Available Programs** Doctorate, Post-Baccalaureate Doctorate.
**Areas of Study** Advanced practice nursing.
**Program Entrance Requirements** Minimum overall college GPA of 3.0, clinical experience, interview, interview by faculty committee, 3 letters of recommendation, MSN or equivalent, vita. *Application deadline:* 7/15 (fall). Applications may be processed on a rolling basis for some programs.
**Degree Requirements** 39 total credit hours.

**Degree** PhD
**Available Programs** Doctorate; Post-Baccalaureate Doctorate.
**Areas of Study** Nursing research, nursing science.
**Site Options** Chicago, IL; Maywood, IL.
**Program Entrance Requirements** Minimum overall college GPA of 3.0, interview by faculty committee, interview, 3 letters of recommendation, MSN or equivalent, statistics course, vita, writing sample, GRE General Test. *Application deadline:* 7/1 (fall). Applications may be processed on a rolling basis for some programs.
**Degree Requirements** 45 total credit hours, dissertation, oral exam, written exam.

# MacMurray College

## Department of Nursing
## Jacksonville, Illinois

***http://www.mac.edu/index.asp***
Founded in 1846

### DEGREE • BSN

**Nursing Program Faculty** 9 (44% with doctorates).
**Baccalaureate Enrollment** 112 **Women** 90% **Men** 10% **Minority** 6% **Part-time** 8%
**Distance Learning Courses** Available.
**Nursing Student Activities** Sigma Theta Tau, nursing club.
**Nursing Student Resources** Academic advising; academic or career counseling; bookstore; campus computer network; career placement assistance; computer lab; computer-assisted instruction; e-mail services; Internet; learning resource lab; library services; nursing audiovisuals; resume preparation assistance; skills, simulation, or other laboratory; tutoring.
**Library Facilities** 150,000 volumes (1,800 in health, 1,300 in nursing); 125 periodical subscriptions (50 health-care related).

## BACCALAUREATE PROGRAMS

**Degree** BSN
**Available Programs** ADN to Baccalaureate; Generic Baccalaureate; LPN to RN Baccalaureate.
**Study Options** Full-time and part-time.
**Program Entrance Requirements** Minimum overall college GPA of 2.5, transcript of college record, CPR certification, health exam, health insurance, high school chemistry, high school transcript, immunizations, minimum high school GPA of 2.5, minimum GPA in nursing prerequisites of 2.5. Transfer students are accepted. *Application deadline:* 3/1 (fall).
**Advanced Placement** Credit by examination available.
**Expenses (2013–14)** *Tuition:* full-time $21,900; part-time $700 per credit hour. *Room and board:* $7850 per academic year. *Required fees:* full-time $675; part-time $440 per credit.
**Financial Aid** 98% of baccalaureate students in nursing programs received some form of financial aid in 2012–13.
**Contact** Director of Admissions, Department of Nursing, MacMurray College, 447 East College Avenue, Jacksonville, IL 62650. *Telephone:* 800-252-7485. *Fax:* 217-291-0702. *E-mail:* admissions@mac.edu.

# McKendree University

## Department of Nursing
## Lebanon, Illinois

***http://www.mckendree.edu/nursing***
Founded in 1828

### DEGREES • BSN • MSN • MSN/MBA

**Nursing Program Faculty** 24 (33% with doctorates).
**Baccalaureate Enrollment** 323 **Women** 96% **Men** 4% **Minority** 12% **Part-time** 76%
**Graduate Enrollment** 122 **Women** 96% **Men** 4% **Minority** 13% **Part-time** 81%
**Distance Learning Courses** Available.
**Nursing Student Activities** Nursing Honor Society.
**Nursing Student Resources** Academic advising; academic or career counseling; assistance for students with disabilities; bookstore; campus computer network; career placement assistance; computer lab; computer-assisted instruction; e-mail services; interactive nursing skills videos; Internet; learning resource lab; library services; nursing audiovisuals; resume preparation assistance; tutoring.
**Library Facilities** 112,000 volumes (4,450 in health, 2,880 in nursing); 1,500 periodical subscriptions (80 health-care related).

## BACCALAUREATE PROGRAMS

**Degree** BSN
**Available Programs** ADN to Baccalaureate.
**Site Options** Louisville, KY; Radcliff, KY.
**Study Options** Full-time and part-time.
**Online Degree Options** Yes.
**Program Entrance Requirements** Minimum overall college GPA of 2.0, transcript of college record, CPR certification, health exam, high school transcript, immunizations, prerequisite course work, RN licensure. Transfer students are accepted. *Application deadline:* Applications may be processed on a rolling basis for some programs.
**Advanced Placement** Credit given for nursing courses completed elsewhere dependent upon specific evaluations.
**Expenses (2013–14)** *Tuition:* part-time $305 per credit hour.
**Financial Aid** 50% of baccalaureate students in nursing programs received some form of financial aid in 2012–13. *Gift aid (need-based):* Federal Pell, FSEOG, state, private, college/university gift aid from institutional funds. *Loans:* Federal Direct (Subsidized and Unsubsidized Stafford PLUS), Perkins. *Work-study:* Federal Work-Study, part-time campus jobs. *Financial aid application deadline (priority):* 5/31.
**Contact** Kim Eichelberger, Director of Nursing Admissions, Department of Nursing, McKendree University, 701 College Road, Lebanon, IL

62254. *Telephone:* 800-232-7228 Ext. 6411. *Fax:* 618-537-6259. *E-mail:* kaeichelberger@mckendree.edu.

## GRADUATE PROGRAMS

**Expenses (2013–14)** *Tuition:* part-time $410 per credit hour.

**Financial Aid** 11% of graduate students in nursing programs received some form of financial aid in 2012–13.

**Contact** Michelle Koester, MSN Admissions, Department of Nursing, McKendree University, 701 College Road, Lebanon, IL 62254. *Telephone:* 502-266-6696. *Fax:* 502-267-4340. *E-mail:* makoester@mckendree.edu.

### MASTER'S DEGREE PROGRAM

**Degrees** MSN; MSN/MBA

**Available Programs** Master's; RN to Master's.

**Concentrations Available** Nursing administration; nursing education.

**Site Options** Louisville, KY.

**Study Options** Full-time and part-time.

**Online Degree Options** Yes.

**Program Entrance Requirements** Minimum overall college GPA of 3.0, transcript of college record, CPR certification, written essay, immunizations, interview, resume. *Application deadline:* Applications may be processed on a rolling basis for some programs.

**Advanced Placement** Credit given for nursing courses completed elsewhere dependent upon specific evaluations.

**Degree Requirements** 38 total credit hours, thesis or project.

### POST-MASTER'S PROGRAM

**Areas of Study** Nursing administration; nursing education.

# Methodist College

## Methodist College
## Peoria, Illinois

### DEGREE • BSN

**Nursing Program Faculty** 44 (13% with doctorates).

**Baccalaureate Enrollment** 522 **Women** 87% **Men** 13% **Minority** 16% **Part-time** 12%

**Distance Learning Courses** Available.

**Nursing Student Activities** Nursing Honor Society, Student Nurses' Association.

**Nursing Student Resources** Academic advising; academic or career counseling; assistance for students with disabilities; bookstore; campus computer network; career placement assistance; computer lab; computer-assisted instruction; daycare for children of students; e-mail services; employment services for current students; externships; housing assistance; interactive nursing skills videos; Internet; learning resource lab; library services; nursing audiovisuals; remedial services; resume preparation assistance; skills, simulation, or other laboratory; tutoring; unpaid internships.

**Library Facilities** 2,425 volumes in health, 1,175 volumes in nursing; 880 periodical subscriptions health-care related.

## BACCALAUREATE PROGRAMS

**Degree** BSN

**Available Programs** Accelerated Baccalaureate for Second Degree; Baccalaureate for Second Degree; Generic Baccalaureate; RN Baccalaureate.

**Study Options** Full-time and part-time.

**Online Degree Options** Yes (online only).

**Program Entrance Requirements** Transcript of college record, CPR certification, health exam, high school transcript, immunizations, minimum high school GPA of 2.5, minimum GPA in nursing prerequisites of 3.0, professional liability insurance/malpractice insurance. Transfer students are accepted. *Application deadline:* 4/15 (fall), 9/15 (spring). *Application fee:* $35.

**Advanced Placement** Credit by examination available. Credit given for nursing courses completed elsewhere dependent upon specific evaluations.

**Contact** *Telephone:* 309-672-5513. *Fax:* 309-671-8303.

# Millikin University

## School of Nursing
## Decatur, Illinois

***http://www.millikin.edu/academics/cps/nursing/pages/default.aspx***

Founded in 1901

### DEGREES • BSN • DNP • MSN

**Nursing Program Faculty** 25 (54% with doctorates).

**Baccalaureate Enrollment** 236 **Women** 86% **Men** 14% **Minority** 22% **International** 1% **Part-time** 2%

**Graduate Enrollment** 66 **Women** 71% **Men** 29% **Minority** 11% **Part-time** 38%

**Distance Learning Courses** Available.

**Nursing Student Activities** Nursing Honor Society, Sigma Theta Tau, Student Nurses' Association, nursing club.

**Nursing Student Resources** Academic advising; academic or career counseling; assistance for students with disabilities; bookstore; campus computer network; career placement assistance; computer lab; computer-assisted instruction; e-mail services; employment services for current students; housing assistance; interactive nursing skills videos; Internet; learning resource lab; library services; nursing audiovisuals; other; placement services for program completers; remedial services; resume preparation assistance; skills, simulation, or other laboratory; tutoring; unpaid internships.

**Library Facilities** 220,402 volumes (10,000 in health, 6,000 in nursing); 237 periodical subscriptions (64 health-care related).

## BACCALAUREATE PROGRAMS

**Degree** BSN

**Available Programs** Baccalaureate for Second Degree; Generic Baccalaureate; RN Baccalaureate.

**Study Options** Full-time and part-time.

**Program Entrance Requirements** Minimum overall college GPA of 2.5, transcript of college record, CPR certification, written essay, health exam, high school biology, high school chemistry, 2 years high school math, 2 years high school science, high school transcript, immunizations, 2 letters of recommendation, minimum high school GPA of 3.0, minimum high school rank 75%, minimum GPA in nursing prerequisites of 2.5. Transfer students are accepted. *Application deadline:* Applications may be processed on a rolling basis for some programs.

**Advanced Placement** Credit given for nursing courses completed elsewhere dependent upon specific evaluations.

**Expenses (2013–14)** *Tuition:* full-time $27,852; part-time $931 per credit hour. *Room and board:* $9210; room only: $5000 per academic year. *Required fees:* full-time $792; part-time $22 per credit.

**Financial Aid** 98% of baccalaureate students in nursing programs received some form of financial aid in 2012–13.

**Contact** Ms. Kim Wenthe, Administrative Assistant, School of Nursing, Millikin University, 1184 West Main Street, Decatur, IL 62522. *Telephone:* 217-424-6348. *Fax:* 217-420-6731. *E-mail:* kwenthe@mail.millikin.edu.

## GRADUATE PROGRAMS

**Expenses (2013–14)** *Tuition:* full-time $25,200; part-time $700 per credit hour. *Room and board:* room only: $6604 per academic year.

**Financial Aid** 82% of graduate students in nursing programs received some form of financial aid in 2012–13.

**Contact** Ms. Marianne G. Taylor, Administrative Assistant II, School of Nursing, Millikin University, 1184 West Main Street, Decatur, IL 62522. *Telephone:* 800-373-7733 Ext. 5034. *Fax:* 217-424-5034. *E-mail:* mgtaylor@mail.millikin.edu.

### MASTER'S DEGREE PROGRAM

**Degree** MSN

**Available Programs** Accelerated Master's for Non-Nursing College Graduates; Master's.

**Concentrations Available** Clinical nurse leader; nurse anesthesia; nursing education.

**Study Options** Full-time and part-time.

**Program Entrance Requirements** Clinical experience, computer literacy, minimum overall college GPA of 3.0, transcript of college record, CPR certification, written essay, immunizations, interview, 3 letters of recommendation, nursing research course, professional liability insurance/malpractice insurance, prerequisite course work, resume, statistics course. *Application deadline:* Applications may be processed on a rolling basis for some programs.

**Advanced Placement** Credit given for nursing courses completed elsewhere dependent upon specific evaluations.
**Degree Requirements** 37–83 credit hours, thesis or project.

### DOCTORAL DEGREE PROGRAM

**Degree** DNP
**Available Programs** Doctorate; Post-Baccalaureate Doctorate.
**Areas of Study** Advanced practice nursing, biology of health and illness, clinical practice, health policy, health promotion/disease prevention, health-care systems, human health and illness, illness and transition, information systems, nursing science.
**Program Entrance Requirements** Clinical experience, minimum overall college GPA of 3.0, interview by faculty committee, 3 letters of recommendation, MSN or equivalent, statistics course, vita, writing sample. *Application deadline:* 7/1 (fall).
**Degree Requirements** 23–88 total credit hours, residency.

# Northern Illinois University

## School of Nursing and Health Studies
## De Kalb, Illinois

*http://www.chhs.niu.edu/nuhs/*
Founded in 1895

**DEGREES • BS • MS • MSN/MPH**

**Nursing Program Faculty** 43 (44% with doctorates).
**Baccalaureate Enrollment** 469 **Women** 92% **Men** 8% **Minority** 20% **Part-time** 23%
**Graduate Enrollment** 164 **Women** 96% **Men** 4% **Minority** 23% **Part-time** 96%
**Distance Learning Courses** Available.
**Nursing Student Activities** Nursing Honor Society, Sigma Theta Tau, Student Nurses' Association, nursing club.
**Nursing Student Resources** Academic advising; academic or career counseling; assistance for students with disabilities; bookstore; campus computer network; career placement assistance; computer lab; computer-assisted instruction; daycare for children of students; e-mail services; employment services for current students; externships; housing assistance; interactive nursing skills videos; Internet; learning resource lab; library services; nursing audiovisuals; paid internships; placement services for program completers; remedial services; resume preparation assistance; skills, simulation, or other laboratory; tutoring; unpaid internships.
**Library Facilities** 3.6 million volumes (39,869 in health, 7,600 in nursing); 56,250 periodical subscriptions (676 health-care related).

### BACCALAUREATE PROGRAMS

**Degree** BS
**Available Programs** ADN to Baccalaureate; Generic Baccalaureate; RN Baccalaureate.
**Site Options** Rockford, IL; Palatine, IL; Aurora, IL.
**Study Options** Full-time and part-time.
**Program Entrance Requirements** Transcript of college record, CPR certification, health exam, health insurance, high school transcript, immunizations, minimum high school GPA of 3.25, minimum high school rank 50%, minimum GPA in nursing prerequisites of 2.5, professional liability insurance/malpractice insurance. Transfer students are accepted.
**Advanced Placement** Credit given for nursing courses completed elsewhere dependent upon specific evaluations.
**Contact** *Telephone:* 815-753-0665. *Fax:* 815-753-0814.

### GRADUATE PROGRAMS

**Contact** *Telephone:* 815-753-6551. *Fax:* 815-753-0814.

### MASTER'S DEGREE PROGRAM

**Degrees** MS; MSN/MPH
**Available Programs** Master's.
**Concentrations Available** Nursing education. *Clinical nurse specialist programs in:* adult health, community health. *Nurse practitioner programs in:* adult health, family health.
**Study Options** Full-time and part-time.
**Program Entrance Requirements** Minimum overall college GPA of 3.0, transcript of college record, CPR certification, written essay, immunizations, 2 letters of recommendation, nursing research course, physical assessment course, professional liability insurance/malpractice insurance, statistics course.
**Degree Requirements** 48 total credit hours.

### POST-MASTER'S PROGRAM

**Areas of Study** Nursing education. *Nurse practitioner programs in:* family health.

# North Park University

## School of Nursing
## Chicago, Illinois

*http://www.northpark.edu/nursing/*
Founded in 1891

**DEGREES • BS • MS • MSN/MA • MSN/MBA • MSN/MM**

**Nursing Program Faculty** 35 (63% with doctorates).
**Baccalaureate Enrollment** 278 **Women** 88.4% **Men** 11.6% **Minority** 57% **International** 4% **Part-time** 36%
**Graduate Enrollment** 189 **Women** 95% **Men** 5% **Minority** 76% **International** 7% **Part-time** 80%
**Nursing Student Activities** Sigma Theta Tau, Student Nurses' Association.
**Nursing Student Resources** Academic advising; academic or career counseling; assistance for students with disabilities; bookstore; campus computer network; career placement assistance; computer lab; computer-assisted instruction; e-mail services; employment services for current students; interactive nursing skills videos; Internet; learning resource lab; library services; nursing audiovisuals; remedial services; skills, simulation, or other laboratory; tutoring.
**Library Facilities** 260,685 volumes (3,959 in health, 1,791 in nursing); 1,178 periodical subscriptions (239 health-care related).

### BACCALAUREATE PROGRAMS

**Degree** BS
**Available Programs** Generic Baccalaureate; RN Baccalaureate.
**Site Options** Evanston, IL; Arlington Heights, IL; Grayslake, IL.
**Study Options** Full-time.
**Program Entrance Requirements** Minimum overall college GPA of 2.75, transcript of college record, CPR certification, health exam, health insurance, immunizations, 1 letter of recommendation, minimum GPA in nursing prerequisites of 2.75, prerequisite course work. Transfer students are accepted.
**Contact** *Telephone:* 773-244-5516.

### GRADUATE PROGRAMS

**Contact** *Telephone:* 773-244-5508. *Fax:* 773-279-7082.

### MASTER'S DEGREE PROGRAM

**Degrees** MS; MSN/MA; MSN/MBA; MSN/MM
**Available Programs** Master's; RN to Master's.
**Concentrations Available** Nursing administration. *Clinical nurse specialist programs in:* community health. *Nurse practitioner programs in:* adult health, family health.
**Site Options** Arlington Heights, IL; Grayslake, IL.
**Study Options** Full-time and part-time.
**Program Entrance Requirements** Clinical experience, minimum overall college GPA of 3.0, transcript of college record, CPR certification, immunizations, 2 letters of recommendation, nursing research course, physical assessment course, professional liability insurance/malpractice insurance, prerequisite course work, resume, statistics course.
**Degree Requirements** 37 total credit hours.

### POST-MASTER'S PROGRAM

**Areas of Study** *Nurse practitioner programs in:* adult health, family health.

# Olivet Nazarene University

## Division of Nursing
## Bourbonnais, Illinois

*http://www.olivet.edu/*
Founded in 1907

**DEGREES • BSN • MSN**

**Nursing Program Faculty** 76 (24% with doctorates).

**Baccalaureate Enrollment** 759 **Women** 88% **Men** 12% **Minority** 30% **Part-time** 33%

**Graduate Enrollment** 339 **Women** 93% **Men** 7% **Minority** 44% **Part-time** 65%

**Nursing Student Activities** Sigma Theta Tau, Student Nurses' Association.

**Nursing Student Resources** Academic advising; academic or career counseling; assistance for students with disabilities; bookstore; campus computer network; career placement assistance; computer lab; computer-assisted instruction; e-mail services; employment services for current students; externships; housing assistance; interactive nursing skills videos; Internet; learning resource lab; library services; nursing audiovisuals; placement services for program completers; remedial services; resume preparation assistance; skills, simulation, or other laboratory; tutoring.

**Library Facilities** 160,039 volumes (4,280 in health, 1,394 in nursing); 925 periodical subscriptions (4,445 health-care related).

## BACCALAUREATE PROGRAMS

**Degree** BSN

**Available Programs** Accelerated Baccalaureate; Generic Baccalaureate; RN Baccalaureate.

**Site Options** Oak Brook, IL; Rolling Meadows, IL.

**Study Options** Full-time.

**Program Entrance Requirements** Minimum overall college GPA of 2.75, transcript of college record, CPR certification, health exam, health insurance, high school biology, high school chemistry, 2 years high school science, high school transcript, immunizations, minimum GPA in nursing prerequisites of 2.75, prerequisite course work. Transfer students are accepted. *Application deadline:* Applications may be processed on a rolling basis for some programs.

**Expenses (2013–14)** *Tuition:* full-time $27,250; part-time $757 per credit hour. *Room and board:* $7900 per academic year. *Required fees:* full-time $420.

**Financial Aid** 91% of baccalaureate students in nursing programs received some form of financial aid in 2012–13. *Gift aid (need-based):* Federal Pell, FSEOG, state, private, college/university gift aid from institutional funds. *Loans:* Federal Direct (Subsidized and Unsubsidized Stafford PLUS), Perkins, private loans. *Work-study:* Federal Work-Study, part-time campus jobs. *Financial aid application deadline (priority):* 3/1.

**Contact** Mrs. Susan Wolff, Director of Admissions, Division of Nursing, Olivet Nazarene University, One University Avenue, Bourbonnais, IL 60914-2345. *Telephone:* 815-939-5203. *Fax:* 815-935-4998. *E-mail:* swolff@olivet.edu.

## GRADUATE PROGRAMS

**Expenses (2013–14)** *Tuition:* full-time $21,350. *Required fees:* full-time $50.

**Financial Aid** 81% of graduate students in nursing programs received some form of financial aid in 2012–13.

**Contact** Dr. Rhoberta Haley, Division of Nursing, Olivet Nazarene University, One University Avenue, Bourbonnais, IL 60914-2345. *Telephone:* 815-939-5186. *Fax:* 815-935-4991. *E-mail:* rjhaley@olivet.edu.

### MASTER'S DEGREE PROGRAM

**Degree** MSN

**Available Programs** Master's.

**Concentrations Available** *Nurse practitioner programs in:* family health.

**Site Options** Rolling Meadows, IL.

**Study Options** Full-time.

**Online Degree Options** Yes.

**Program Entrance Requirements** Computer literacy, minimum overall college GPA of 2.75, transcript of college record, nursing research course, statistics course. *Application deadline:* Applications may be processed on a rolling basis for some programs. *Application fee:* $50.

**Degree Requirements** 34 total credit hours, thesis or project.

## CONTINUING EDUCATION PROGRAM

**Contact** Dr. Pamela Lee, Professor of Nursing, Division of Nursing, Olivet Nazarene University, One University Avenue, Bourbonnais, IL 60914. *Telephone:* 815-939-5316. *Fax:* 815-939-5383. *E-mail:* plee@olivet.edu.

# Quincy University

### Blessing–Rieman College of Nursing
### Quincy, Illinois

*http://www.quincy.edu/*

***See description of programs under Blessing–Rieman College of Nursing (Quincy, Illinois).***

# Resurrection University

### Resurrection University
### Chicago, Illinois

Founded in 1982

**DEGREES • BSN • MSN**

**Nursing Program Faculty** 20 (20% with doctorates).

**Baccalaureate Enrollment** 237 **Women** 82.7% **Men** 17.3% **Minority** 64.5% **Part-time** 21.5%

**Graduate Enrollment** 20 **Women** 98% **Men** 2% **Minority** 52% **Part-time** 100%

**Distance Learning Courses** Available.

**Nursing Student Activities** Student Nurses' Association.

**Nursing Student Resources** Academic advising; academic or career counseling; bookstore; campus computer network; career placement assistance; computer lab; computer-assisted instruction; e-mail services; employment services for current students; externships; Internet; learning resource lab; library services; nursing audiovisuals; resume preparation assistance; skills, simulation, or other laboratory; tutoring.

**Library Facilities** 3,084 volumes (2,400 in health, 1,100 in nursing); 7,060 periodical subscriptions (300 health-care related).

## BACCALAUREATE PROGRAMS

**Degree** BSN

**Available Programs** ADN to Baccalaureate; Accelerated Baccalaureate; Accelerated Baccalaureate for Second Degree; Accelerated RN Baccalaureate; Baccalaureate for Second Degree; RN Baccalaureate.

**Study Options** Full-time and part-time.

**Program Entrance Requirements** Minimum overall college GPA of 2.75, transcript of college record, CPR certification, written essay, health exam, health insurance, immunizations, 1 letter of recommendation, minimum GPA in nursing prerequisites of 2.75, prerequisite course work. Transfer students are accepted. *Application deadline:* 2/1 (fall), 9/15 (spring), 2/1 (summer). Applications may be processed on a rolling basis for some programs. *Application fee:* $30.

**Advanced Placement** Credit by examination available. Credit given for nursing courses completed elsewhere dependent upon specific evaluations.

**Contact** *Telephone:* 708-763-6532. *Fax:* 708-763-1531.

## GRADUATE PROGRAMS

**Contact** *Telephone:* 708-763-6532. *Fax:* 708-763-1531.

### MASTER'S DEGREE PROGRAM

**Degree** MSN

**Available Programs** Accelerated Master's for Nurses with Non-Nursing Degrees; Master's; Master's for Nurses with Non-Nursing Degrees; RN to Master's.

**Concentrations Available** Clinical nurse leader; health-care administration; nursing administration; nursing education.

**Study Options** Part-time.

**Program Entrance Requirements** Computer literacy, minimum overall college GPA of 3.0, transcript of college record, CPR certification, written essay, immunizations, 3 letters of recommendation, resume. *Application deadline:* 7/1 (fall). Applications may be processed on a rolling basis for some programs. *Application fee:* $30.

**Advanced Placement** Credit given for nursing courses completed elsewhere dependent upon specific evaluations.

**Degree Requirements** 32 total credit hours, thesis or project.

### POST-MASTER'S PROGRAM

**Areas of Study** Clinical nurse leader; health-care administration; nursing administration; nursing education.

# Rockford University
## Department of Nursing
## Rockford, Illinois

*http://www.rockford.edu/*
Founded in 1847

### DEGREE • BSN

**Nursing Program Faculty** 7
**Baccalaureate Enrollment** 101 **Women** 94% **Men** 6% **Minority** 22% **Part-time** 7%
**Nursing Student Activities** Student Nurses' Association.
**Nursing Student Resources** Academic advising; academic or career counseling; assistance for students with disabilities; bookstore; campus computer network; career placement assistance; computer lab; computer-assisted instruction; e-mail services; employment services for current students; externships; housing assistance; interactive nursing skills videos; Internet; learning resource lab; library services; nursing audiovisuals; paid internships; placement services for program completers; remedial services; resume preparation assistance; skills, simulation, or other laboratory; tutoring.
**Library Facilities** 137,000 volumes (655 in health, 600 in nursing); 23,000 periodical subscriptions (55 health-care related).

### BACCALAUREATE PROGRAMS

**Degree** BSN
**Available Programs** ADN to Baccalaureate; Generic Baccalaureate; RN Baccalaureate.
**Study Options** Full-time.
**Program Entrance Requirements** Minimum overall college GPA of 2.75, transcript of college record, CPR certification, health exam, health insurance, high school biology, high school chemistry, 4 years high school math, 2 years high school science, high school transcript, immunizations, minimum high school GPA of 2.75, minimum high school rank 50%, minimum GPA in nursing prerequisites of 2.75, prerequisite course work. Transfer students are accepted. *Application deadline:* 3/1 (fall), 9/1 (spring).
**Advanced Placement** Credit given for nursing courses completed elsewhere dependent upon specific evaluations.
**Contact** *Telephone:* 815-226-4050.

# Rush University
## College of Nursing
## Chicago, Illinois

*http://www.rushu.rush.edu/nursing*
Founded in 1969

### DEGREES • MSN • PHD

**Nursing Program Faculty** 90 (69% with doctorates).
**Graduate Enrollment** 700 **Women** 91% **Men** 9% **Minority** 16% **Part-time** 68%
**Distance Learning Courses** Available.
**Nursing Student Activities** Nursing Honor Society, Sigma Theta Tau, Student Nurses' Association.
**Nursing Student Resources** Academic advising; academic or career counseling; assistance for students with disabilities; bookstore; campus computer network; computer lab; computer-assisted instruction; e-mail services; employment services for current students; housing assistance; interactive nursing skills videos; Internet; learning resource lab; library services; nursing audiovisuals; remedial services; resume preparation assistance; skills, simulation, or other laboratory; tutoring; unpaid internships.
**Library Facilities** 120,042 volumes; 1,100 periodical subscriptions (5,228 health-care related).

### GRADUATE PROGRAMS

**Contact** *Telephone:* 312-942-7100. *Fax:* 312-942-3043.

#### MASTER'S DEGREE PROGRAM

**Degree** MSN
**Available Programs** Master's; Master's for Nurses with Non-Nursing Degrees.
**Concentrations Available** Clinical nurse leader; nurse anesthesia. *Clinical nurse specialist programs in:* adult health, community health, critical care, gerontology, pediatric, public health. *Nurse practitioner programs in:* acute care, adult health, family health, gerontology, neonatal health, pediatric, psychiatric/mental health.
**Study Options** Full-time and part-time.
**Online Degree Options** Yes.
**Program Entrance Requirements** Minimum overall college GPA of 3.0, transcript of college record, CPR certification, written essay, immunizations, interview, 3 letters of recommendation, resume, GRE General Test (waived if cumulative GPA is 3.25 or greater or nursing GPA is 3.0 or greater). *Application deadline:* 2/1 (fall), 6/1 (winter). *Application fee:* $65.
**Advanced Placement** Credit given for nursing courses completed elsewhere dependent upon specific evaluations.
**Degree Requirements** 68 total credit hours, thesis or project.

#### POST-MASTER'S PROGRAM

**Areas of Study** *Clinical nurse specialist programs in:* adult health, community health, gerontology, pediatric, public health. *Nurse practitioner programs in:* adult health, family health, gerontology, neonatal health, pediatric, psychiatric/mental health.

#### DOCTORAL DEGREE PROGRAM

**Degree** PhD
**Available Programs** Doctorate; Post-Baccalaureate Doctorate.
**Areas of Study** Addiction/substance abuse, advanced practice nursing, aging, bio-behavioral research, biology of health and illness, clinical practice, community health, critical care, family health, gerontology, health policy, health promotion/disease prevention, health-care systems, human health and illness, illness and transition, maternity-newborn, neuro-behavior, nursing research, nursing science, oncology, urban health,women's health.
**Online Degree Options** Yes (online only).
**Program Entrance Requirements** Minimum overall college GPA of 3.0, interview by faculty committee, interview, 3 letters of recommendation, statistics course, vita, GRE General Test (waived for DNP if cumulative GPA is 3.25 or greater, nursing GPA is 3.0 or greater, or a completed graduate program GPA is 3.5 or greater). *Application deadline:* 2/1 (fall). Applications may be processed on a rolling basis for some programs. *Application fee:* $65.
**Degree Requirements** 56 total credit hours, dissertation, residency.

#### POSTDOCTORAL PROGRAM

**Postdoctoral Program Contact***Telephone:* 312-942-6955. *Fax:* 312-942-3043.

### CONTINUING EDUCATION PROGRAM

**Contact** *Telephone:* 312-942-7013. *Fax:* 312-942-3043.

# Saint Anthony College of Nursing
## Saint Anthony College of Nursing
## Rockford, Illinois

*http://www.sacn.edu/*
Founded in 1915

### DEGREES • BSN • MSN

**Nursing Program Faculty** 17 (23% with doctorates).
**Baccalaureate Enrollment** 178 **Women** 93% **Men** 7% **Minority** 30% **Part-time** 24%
**Graduate Enrollment** 25 **Women** 96% **Men** 4% **Minority** 8% **Part-time** 100%
**Nursing Student Activities** Nursing Honor Society, Student Nurses' Association.
**Nursing Student Resources** Academic advising; academic or career counseling; campus computer network; computer lab; computer-assisted instruction; e-mail services; interactive nursing skills videos; Internet; learning resource lab; library services; nursing audiovisuals; skills, simulation, or other laboratory; tutoring.
**Library Facilities** 1,258 volumes (1,751 in health, 1,385 in nursing); 3,136 periodical subscriptions (60 health-care related).

### BACCALAUREATE PROGRAMS

**Degree** BSN
**Available Programs** Baccalaureate for Second Degree; Generic Baccalaureate; RN Baccalaureate.
**Site Options** Freeport, IL.
**Study Options** Full-time and part-time.

**Program Entrance Requirements** Minimum overall college GPA of 2.5, transcript of college record, CPR certification, written essay, health exam, health insurance, immunizations, interview, 3 letters of recommendation, minimum GPA in nursing prerequisites of 2.7, prerequisite course work. Transfer students are accepted. *Application deadline:* 2/15 (fall), 9/15 (spring). *Application fee:* $50.

**Advanced Placement** Credit by examination available. Credit given for nursing courses completed elsewhere dependent upon specific evaluations.

**Contact** *Telephone:* 815-227-2141. *Fax:* 815-227-2730.

## GRADUATE PROGRAMS

**Contact** *Telephone:* 815-395-5476. *Fax:* 815-395-2275.

### MASTER'S DEGREE PROGRAM

**Degree** MSN

**Available Programs** Master's.

**Concentrations Available** Clinical nurse leader; nursing education. *Clinical nurse specialist programs in:* adult health. *Nurse practitioner programs in:* family health.

**Study Options** Part-time.

**Program Entrance Requirements** Minimum overall college GPA of 2.7, transcript of college record, CPR certification, written essay, immunizations, interview, 3 letters of recommendation, professional liability insurance/malpractice insurance, prerequisite course work, resume, statistics course. *Application deadline:* 4/1 (fall). *Application fee:* $50.

**Advanced Placement** Credit given for nursing courses completed elsewhere dependent upon specific evaluations.

**Degree Requirements** 48 total credit hours, thesis or project.

### POST-MASTER'S PROGRAM

**Areas of Study** Nursing education.

***See display below and full description on page 488.***

# Saint Francis Medical Center College of Nursing

## Baccalaureate Nursing Program
## Peoria, Illinois

*http://www.sfmccon.edu/*
Founded in 1986

**DEGREES • BSN • DNP • MSN**

**Nursing Program Faculty** 52 (15% with doctorates).
**Baccalaureate Enrollment** 420 **Women** 89% **Men** 11% **Minority** 11% **Part-time** 13%
**Graduate Enrollment** 281 **Women** 91% **Men** 9% **Minority** 1% **Part-time** 95%
**Distance Learning Courses** Available.
**Nursing Student Activities** Sigma Theta Tau, Student Nurses' Association.
**Nursing Student Resources** Academic advising; academic or career counseling; campus computer network; computer lab; computer-assisted instruction; e-mail services; housing assistance; interactive nursing skills videos; Internet; learning resource lab; library services; nursing audiovisuals; skills, simulation, or other laboratory; tutoring.
**Library Facilities** 6,790 volumes (2,045 in nursing); 139 periodical subscriptions (124 health-care related).

## BACCALAUREATE PROGRAMS

**Degree** BSN
**Available Programs** Generic Baccalaureate; RN Baccalaureate.
**Study Options** Full-time and part-time.
**Program Entrance Requirements** Transcript of college record, CPR certification, written essay, health exam, high school transcript, immunizations, minimum GPA in nursing prerequisites of 2.5, professional liability insurance/malpractice insurance, prerequisite course work. Transfer students are accepted. *Application deadline:* 9/15 (fall), 2/15 (spring). *Application fee:* $50.
**Advanced Placement** Credit given for nursing courses completed elsewhere dependent upon specific evaluations.
**Expenses (2013–14)** *Tuition:* full-time $16,368; part-time $528 per credit hour. *International tuition:* $16,368 full-time. *Room and board:* room only: $3300 per academic year. *Required fees:* full-time $596.

**Financial Aid** 89% of baccalaureate students in nursing programs received some form of financial aid in 2012–13. *Gift aid (need-based):* Federal Pell, state, private, college/university gift aid from institutional funds. *Loans:* Federal Direct (Subsidized and Unsubsidized Stafford PLUS), college/university. *Financial aid application deadline (priority):* 3/1.
**Contact** Ms. Janice E. Farquharson, Director of Admissions/Registrar, Baccalaureate Nursing Program, Saint Francis Medical Center College of Nursing, 511 NE Greenleaf Street, Peoria, IL 61603. *Telephone:* 309-624-8980. *Fax:* 309-624-8973. *E-mail:* janice.farquharson@osfhealthcare.org.

### GRADUATE PROGRAMS

**Expenses (2013–14)** *Tuition:* full-time $6336; part-time $528 per credit hour. *International tuition:* $6336 full-time. *Required fees:* full-time $436.
**Financial Aid** 70% of graduate students in nursing programs received some form of financial aid in 2012–13.
**Contact** Dr. Janice F. Boundy, Associate Dean of Graduate Program, Baccalaureate Nursing Program, Saint Francis Medical Center College of Nursing, 511 NE Greenleaf Street, Peoria, IL 61603. *Telephone:* 309-655-2230. *Fax:* 309-655-3648. *E-mail:* janice.f.boundy@osfhealthcare.org.

#### MASTER'S DEGREE PROGRAM

**Degree** MSN
**Available Programs** Accelerated RN to Master's; Master's.
**Concentrations Available** Clinical nurse leader; nursing administration; nursing education. *Clinical nurse specialist programs in:* family health, gerontology. *Nurse practitioner programs in:* family health, neonatal health, psychiatric/mental health.
**Study Options** Full-time and part-time.
**Online Degree Options** Yes (online only).
**Program Entrance Requirements** Clinical experience, computer literacy, minimum overall college GPA of 2.8, transcript of college record, CPR certification, written essay, immunizations, interview, 3 letters of recommendation, nursing research course, physical assessment course, professional liability insurance/malpractice insurance, prerequisite course work, resume, statistics course. *Application deadline:* Applications may be processed on a rolling basis for some programs. *Application fee:* $50.
**Advanced Placement** Credit given for nursing courses completed elsewhere dependent upon specific evaluations.
**Degree Requirements** 45 total credit hours, thesis or project.

#### POST-MASTER'S PROGRAM

**Areas of Study** Nursing education. *Clinical nurse specialist programs in:* family health, gerontology.

#### DOCTORAL DEGREE PROGRAM

**Degree** DNP
**Available Programs** Doctorate.
**Areas of Study** Clinical practice, nursing administration.
**Online Degree Options** Yes (online only).
**Program Entrance Requirements** Clinical experience, minimum overall college GPA of 3.2, 3 letters of recommendation, scholarly papers, statistics course, vita, writing sample. *Application deadline:* Applications may be processed on a rolling basis for some programs. *Application fee:* $50.
**Degree Requirements** 39 total credit hours, oral exam, residency.

## St. John's College

**Department of Nursing**
**Springfield, Illinois**

*http://www.stjohnscollegespringfield.edu/*
Founded in 1886

### DEGREE • BSN

**Nursing Program Faculty** 15 (13% with doctorates).
**Baccalaureate Enrollment** 81 **Women** 93% **Men** 7% **Minority** 4% **International** 1% **Part-time** 5%
**Nursing Student Activities** Student Nurses' Association.
**Nursing Student Resources** Academic advising; computer lab; daycare for children of students; interactive nursing skills videos; Internet; library services; resume preparation assistance; skills, simulation, or other laboratory.

### BACCALAUREATE PROGRAMS

**Degree** BSN
**Available Programs** Generic Baccalaureate.
**Study Options** Full-time and part-time.
**Program Entrance Requirements** Transcript of college record, CPR certification, health exam, high school transcript, immunizations, 2 letters of recommendation, minimum GPA in nursing prerequisites of 2.4, professional liability insurance/malpractice insurance, prerequisite course work. Transfer students are accepted.
**Advanced Placement** Credit given for nursing courses completed elsewhere dependent upon specific evaluations.
**Contact** *Telephone:* 217-525-5628. *Fax:* 217-757-6870.

## Saint Xavier University

**School of Nursing**
**Chicago, Illinois**

*http://www.sxu.edu/academics/colleges_schools/son/*
Founded in 1847

### DEGREES • BSN • MSN • MSN/MBA

**Nursing Program Faculty** 33 (57% with doctorates).
**Baccalaureate Enrollment** 593 **Women** 85% **Men** 15% **Minority** 40% **International** .2% **Part-time** 11%
**Graduate Enrollment** 250 **Women** 94% **Men** 6% **Minority** 30% **Part-time** 34%
**Distance Learning Courses** Available.
**Nursing Student Activities** Nursing Honor Society, Sigma Theta Tau, Student Nurses' Association.
**Nursing Student Resources** Academic advising; academic or career counseling; assistance for students with disabilities; bookstore; campus computer network; career placement assistance; computer lab; computer-assisted instruction; e-mail services; employment services for current students; externships; housing assistance; interactive nursing skills videos; Internet; learning resource lab; library services; nursing audiovisuals; other; placement services for program completers; remedial services; resume preparation assistance; skills, simulation, or other laboratory; tutoring; unpaid internships.
**Library Facilities** 179,000 volumes (2,170 in health, 1,650 in nursing); 35,000 periodical subscriptions (9,260 health-care related).

### BACCALAUREATE PROGRAMS

**Degree** BSN
**Available Programs** Accelerated Baccalaureate for Second Degree; Generic Baccalaureate; LPN to RN Baccalaureate.
**Site Options** Chicago, IL.
**Study Options** Full-time.
**Program Entrance Requirements** Minimum overall college GPA of 2.75, transcript of college record, CPR certification, written essay, health exam, health insurance, high school biology, high school chemistry, high school foreign language, 3 years high school math, 4 years high school science, high school transcript, immunizations, minimum high school GPA of 2.75, minimum GPA in nursing prerequisites of 2.75, prerequisite course work. Transfer students are accepted. *Application deadline:* 5/1 (fall), 11/1 (spring). Applications may be processed on a rolling basis for some programs.
**Advanced Placement** Credit by examination available. Credit given for nursing courses completed elsewhere dependent upon specific evaluations.
**Expenses (2013–14)** *Tuition:* full-time $28,150; part-time $650 per credit hour. *International tuition:* $28,150 full-time. *Room and board:* $9920; room only: $5900 per academic year. *Required fees:* full-time $1100; part-time $395 per term.
**Financial Aid** 98% of baccalaureate students in nursing programs received some form of financial aid in 2012–13.
**Contact** Mr. Brian Hotzfield, Director, Undergraduate Admission, School of Nursing, Saint Xavier University, 3700 West 103rd Street, Chicago, IL 60655. *Telephone:* 773-298-3050. *Fax:* 773-298-3076. *E-mail:* admission@sxu.edu.

### GRADUATE PROGRAMS

**Expenses (2013–14)** *Tuition:* full-time $10,260; part-time $855 per credit hour. *International tuition:* $10,260 full-time. *Room and board:* $11,280; room only: $8500 per academic year. *Required fees:* full-time $450; part-time $225 per term.
**Financial Aid** 66% of graduate students in nursing programs received some form of financial aid in 2012–13. Available to part-time students.

**Contact** Brian Condon, Associate Director, Graduate Admission, School of Nursing, Saint Xavier University, 3700 West 103rd Street, Chicago, IL 60655. *Telephone:* 773-298-3053. *Fax:* 773-298-3951. *E-mail:* graduateadmission@sxu.edu.

**MASTER'S DEGREE PROGRAM**
**Degrees** MSN; MSN/MBA
**Available Programs** Master's.
**Concentrations Available** Clinical nurse leader; nursing administration. *Nurse practitioner programs in:* family health.
**Site Options** Chicago, IL.
**Study Options** Full-time and part-time.
**Online Degree Options** Yes.
**Program Entrance Requirements** Minimum overall college GPA of 3.0, transcript of college record, written essay, 2 letters of recommendation, prerequisite course work, GRE General Test or MAT. *Application deadline:* 4/1 (fall). Applications may be processed on a rolling basis for some programs.
**Advanced Placement** Credit given for nursing courses completed elsewhere dependent upon specific evaluations.
**Degree Requirements** 36 total credit hours, thesis or project.

**POST-MASTER'S PROGRAM**
**Areas of Study** Nursing education. *Nurse practitioner programs in:* family health.

### CONTINUING EDUCATION PROGRAM
**Contact** Darlene O'Callaghan, Assistant Dean, Special Initiatives, School of Nursing, Saint Xavier University, 3700 West 103rd Street, Chicago, IL 60655. *Telephone:* 773-298-3742. *Fax:* 773-298-3704. *E-mail:* ocallaghan@sxu.edu.

## Southern Illinois University Edwardsville
### School of Nursing
### Edwardsville, Illinois

***http://www.siue.edu/nursing***
Founded in 1957

### DEGREES • BS • DNP • MS
**Nursing Program Faculty** 87 (38% with doctorates).
**Baccalaureate Enrollment** 713 **Women** 83% **Men** 17% **Minority** 11% **International** 2% **Part-time** 27%
**Graduate Enrollment** 263 **Women** 86% **Men** 14% **Minority** 10% **International** 2% **Part-time** 69%
**Distance Learning Courses** Available.
**Nursing Student Activities** Sigma Theta Tau, Student Nurses' Association, nursing club.
**Nursing Student Resources** Academic advising; academic or career counseling; assistance for students with disabilities; bookstore; campus computer network; career placement assistance; computer lab; computer-assisted instruction; daycare for children of students; e-mail services; employment services for current students; externships; housing assistance; interactive nursing skills videos; Internet; learning resource lab; library services; nursing audiovisuals; placement services for program completers; remedial services; resume preparation assistance; skills, simulation, or other laboratory; tutoring.
**Library Facilities** 1.4 million volumes; 32,858 periodical subscriptions.

### BACCALAUREATE PROGRAMS
**Degree** BS
**Available Programs** ADN to Baccalaureate; Accelerated Baccalaureate; Generic Baccalaureate.
**Site Options** Carbondale, IL.
**Study Options** Full-time.
**Program Entrance Requirements** Minimum overall college GPA of 2.5, transcript of college record, minimum GPA in nursing prerequisites of 2.7, prerequisite course work. Transfer students are accepted. *Application deadline:* 3/1 (fall).
**Advanced Placement** Credit given for nursing courses completed elsewhere dependent upon specific evaluations.
**Expenses (2012–13)** *Tuition, state resident:* full-time $6948; part-time $232 per credit hour. *Tuition, nonresident:* full-time $17,370; part-time $579 per credit hour. *International tuition:* $17,370 full-time. *Room and board:* $8281; room only: $5270 per academic year. *Required fees:* full-time $3700.
**Financial Aid** ***Gift aid (need-based):*** Federal Pell, FSEOG, state, private, college/university gift aid from institutional funds, Federal Nursing. *Loans:* Federal Nursing Student Loans, Federal Direct (Subsidized and Unsubsidized Stafford PLUS), Perkins, college/university, alternative loans. *Work-study:* Federal Work-Study, part-time campus jobs. *Financial aid application deadline (priority):* 3/1.
**Contact** Mrs. Karen Montgomery, Coordinator, Academic Advising, School of Nursing, Southern Illinois University Edwardsville, Box 1066, Edwardsville, IL 62026-1066. *Telephone:* 618-650-3956. *Fax:* 618-650-3854. *E-mail:* kmontgo@siue.edu.

### GRADUATE PROGRAMS
**Expenses (2012–13)** *Tuition, state resident:* full-time $4878; part-time $271 per credit hour. *Tuition, nonresident:* full-time $12,195; part-time $678 per credit hour. *International tuition:* $12,195 full-time. *Room and board:* $8281; room only: $5270 per academic year. *Required fees:* full-time $1600.
**Financial Aid** Fellowships (averaging $8,370 per year), 1 research assistantship (averaging $9,585 per year), 4 teaching assistantships (averaging $9,585 per year) were awarded; institutionally sponsored loans, scholarships, and unspecified assistantships also available.
**Contact** Dr. Kathy Ketchum, Assistant Dean, Graduate Programs, School of Nursing, Southern Illinois University Edwardsville, Alumni Hall, Room 2107, Edwardsville, IL 62026-1066. *Telephone:* 618-650-3956. *Fax:* 618-650-3854. *E-mail:* kketchu@siue.edu.

**MASTER'S DEGREE PROGRAM**
**Degree** MS
**Available Programs** Master's.
**Concentrations Available** Health-care administration; nurse anesthesia; nursing education. *Nurse practitioner programs in:* family health.
**Site Options** Springfield, IL.
**Study Options** Full-time and part-time.
**Program Entrance Requirements** Clinical experience, minimum overall college GPA of 3.0, transcript of college record, written essay, interview, 3 letters of recommendation, prerequisite course work, statistics course. *Application deadline:* 3/1 (fall), 6/1 (summer).
**Advanced Placement** Credit given for nursing courses completed elsewhere dependent upon specific evaluations.
**Degree Requirements** 35 total credit hours, thesis or project.

**POST-MASTER'S PROGRAM**
**Areas of Study** Health-care administration; nurse anesthesia; nursing education. *Nurse practitioner programs in:* family health.

**DOCTORAL DEGREE PROGRAM**
**Degree** DNP
**Available Programs** Doctorate.
**Program Entrance Requirements** Clinical experience, minimum overall college GPA of 3.0, interview by faculty committee, 3 letters of recommendation, MSN or equivalent, statistics course, vita, writing sample. *Application deadline:* 3/1 (fall).
**Degree Requirements** 36 total credit hours, written exam.

### CONTINUING EDUCATION PROGRAM
**Contact** Dr. Karen Kelly, Associate Professor and Director Continuing Education, School of Nursing, Southern Illinois University Edwardsville, Box 1066, Edwardsville, IL 62026-1066. *Telephone:* 618-650-3908. *Fax:* 618-650-3854. *E-mail:* kkelly@siue.edu.

## Trinity Christian College
### Department of Nursing
### Palos Heights, Illinois

***http://www.trnty.edu/academics/nursing/nursing.html***
Founded in 1959

### DEGREE • BSN
**Nursing Program Faculty** 8 (37% with doctorates).
**Baccalaureate Enrollment** 200 **Women** 94.5% **Men** 5.5% **Minority** 14% **International** 3% **Part-time** 3%
**Distance Learning Courses** Available.
**Nursing Student Activities** Student Nurses' Association.
**Nursing Student Resources** Academic advising; academic or career counseling; assistance for students with disabilities; bookstore; campus

computer network; career placement assistance; computer lab; computer-assisted instruction; e-mail services; interactive nursing skills videos; Internet; learning resource lab; library services; nursing audiovisuals; resume preparation assistance; skills, simulation, or other laboratory; tutoring; unpaid internships.

**Library Facilities** 71,226 volumes (2,500 in health, 500 in nursing); 44,165 periodical subscriptions (100 health-care related).

### BACCALAUREATE PROGRAMS

**Degree** BSN

**Available Programs** ADN to Baccalaureate; Generic Baccalaureate.

**Study Options** Full-time.

**Program Entrance Requirements** Minimum overall college GPA of 2.5, transcript of college record, CPR certification, health exam, health insurance, high school biology, 3 years high school math, 2 years high school science, high school transcript, immunizations, minimum high school GPA of 2.0, minimum GPA in nursing prerequisites of 2.5, prerequisite course work. Transfer students are accepted. *Application deadline:* 8/15 (fall).

**Advanced Placement** Credit given for nursing courses completed elsewhere dependent upon specific evaluations.

**Financial Aid** 90% of baccalaureate students in nursing programs received some form of financial aid in 2012–13.

**Contact** Admissions Office, Department of Nursing, Trinity Christian College, 6601 West College Drive, Palos Heights, IL 60463. *Telephone:* 866-874-6463. *Fax:* 708-385-5665. *E-mail:* admissions@trnty.edu.

## Trinity College of Nursing and Health Sciences

### Trinity College of Nursing and Health Sciences
### Rock Island, Illinois

*http://www.trinitycollegeqc.edu/*
Founded in 1994

**DEGREE • BSN**

**Nursing Program Faculty** 15 (20% with doctorates).

**Baccalaureate Enrollment** 76 **Women** 92% **Men** 8% **Minority** 13% **Part-time** 67%

**Distance Learning Courses** Available.

**Nursing Student Activities** Nursing Honor Society.

**Nursing Student Resources** Academic advising; academic or career counseling; assistance for students with disabilities; bookstore; campus computer network; career placement assistance; computer lab; computer-assisted instruction; daycare for children of students; e-mail services; interactive nursing skills videos; Internet; library services; nursing audiovisuals; placement services for program completers; remedial services; resume preparation assistance; skills, simulation, or other laboratory; tutoring.

**Library Facilities** 8,500 volumes (6,000 in health, 3,400 in nursing); 791 periodical subscriptions (746 health-care related).

### BACCALAUREATE PROGRAMS

**Degree** BSN

**Available Programs** ADN to Baccalaureate; Accelerated Baccalaureate; Accelerated Baccalaureate for Second Degree; Generic Baccalaureate; RN Baccalaureate.

**Study Options** Full-time.

**Program Entrance Requirements** Minimum overall college GPA of 2.75, transcript of college record, prerequisite course work. Transfer students are accepted. *Application deadline:* 12/20 (fall). Applications may be processed on a rolling basis for some programs. *Application fee:* $50.

**Advanced Placement** Credit given for nursing courses completed elsewhere dependent upon specific evaluations.

**Contact** *Telephone:* 309-779-7708. *Fax:* 309-779-7798.

## University of Illinois at Chicago

### College of Nursing
### Chicago, Illinois

*http://www.uic.edu/nursing*
Founded in 1946

**DEGREES • BSN • MS • MS/MBA • MS/MPH • PHD**

**Nursing Program Faculty** 200 (75% with doctorates).
**Baccalaureate Enrollment** 411 **Women** 84% **Men** 16% **Minority** 21% **International** 2% **Part-time** 25%
**Graduate Enrollment** 932 **Women** 91% **Men** 9% **Minority** 13% **International** 3% **Part-time** 62%
**Distance Learning Courses** Available.
**Nursing Student Activities** Sigma Theta Tau, Student Nurses' Association.
**Nursing Student Resources** Academic advising; academic or career counseling; assistance for students with disabilities; bookstore; campus computer network; computer lab; computer-assisted instruction; daycare for children of students; e-mail services; employment services for current students; externships; Internet; learning resource lab; library services; nursing audiovisuals; resume preparation assistance; skills, simulation, or other laboratory; tutoring.
**Library Facilities** 500,000 volumes in health; 5,100 periodical subscriptions health-care related.

### BACCALAUREATE PROGRAMS

**Degree** BSN
**Available Programs** ADN to Baccalaureate; Baccalaureate for Second Degree; Generic Baccalaureate; RN Baccalaureate.
**Site Options** Urbana, IL.
**Study Options** Full-time and part-time.
**Online Degree Options** Yes.
**Program Entrance Requirements** Minimum overall college GPA of 2.75, transcript of college record, written essay, immunizations, 2 letters of recommendation, minimum GPA in nursing prerequisites of 2.5, prerequisite course work. Transfer students are accepted. *Application deadline:* 1/15 (fall).
**Contact** Mr. Michael Behlke, Admissions Coordinator, College of Nursing, University of Illinois at Chicago, MC 802, 845 South Damen Avenue, Chicago, IL 60612. *Telephone:* 312-996-9645. *Fax:* 312-996-8066. *E-mail:* mbehlke@uic.edu.

### GRADUATE PROGRAMS

**Financial Aid** 3 fellowships were awarded; research assistantships, teaching assistantships, career-related internships or fieldwork, Federal Work-Study, institutionally sponsored loans, scholarships, traineeships, tuition waivers (full and partial), and unspecified assistantships also available.
**Contact** Mr. Michael Spielman, Admissions Coordinator, College of Nursing, University of Illinois at Chicago, MC 802, 845 South Damen Avenue, Chicago, IL 60612. *Telephone:* 312-413-1550. *Fax:* 312-996-8066. *E-mail:* mspiel2@uic.edu.

#### MASTER'S DEGREE PROGRAM

**Degrees** MS; MS/MBA; MS/MPH
**Available Programs** Master's; Master's for Non-Nursing College Graduates; Master's for Nurses with Non-Nursing Degrees.
**Concentrations Available** Health-care administration; nurse-midwifery; nursing administration; nursing informatics. *Clinical nurse specialist programs in:* acute care, adult health, cardiovascular, community health, family health, gerontology, maternity-newborn, medical-surgical, occupational health, pediatric, perinatal, psychiatric/mental health, public health, school health,women's health. *Nurse practitioner programs in:* acute care, adult health, family health, gerontology, occupational health, pediatric, psychiatric/mental health, school health,women's health.
**Site Options** Peoria, IL; Urbana, IL; Rockford, IL.
**Study Options** Full-time and part-time.
**Program Entrance Requirements** Clinical experience, computer literacy, minimum overall college GPA of 3.0, transcript of college record, CPR certification, written essay, immunizations, interview, 3 letters of recommendation, nursing research course, physical assessment course, prerequisite course work, resume, statistics course, GRE General Test. *Application deadline:* 2/1 (fall).
**Advanced Placement** Credit given for nursing courses completed elsewhere dependent upon specific evaluations.
**Degree Requirements** Thesis or project.

### POST-MASTER'S PROGRAM

**Areas of Study** Health-care administration; nurse-midwifery; nursing administration; nursing education; nursing informatics. *Clinical nurse specialist programs in:* acute care, adult health, cardiovascular, family health, forensic nursing, gerontology, medical-surgical, occupational health, palliative care, pediatric, psychiatric/mental health, public health, school health,women's health. *Nurse practitioner programs in:* acute care, adult health, family health, gerontology, occupational health, pediatric, psychiatric/mental health, school health,women's health.

### DOCTORAL DEGREE PROGRAM

**Degree** PhD
**Available Programs** Doctorate; Post-Baccalaureate Doctorate.
**Areas of Study** Advanced practice nursing, aging, bio-behavioral research, clinical practice, community health, faculty preparation, family health, forensic nursing, gerontology, health policy, health-care systems, individualized study, information systems, maternity-newborn, nursing administration, nursing policy, nursing research, nursing science,women's health.
**Site Options** Peoria, IL; Urbana, IL; Rockford, IL.
**Program Entrance Requirements** Minimum overall college GPA of 3.0, interview by faculty committee, interview, 3 letters of recommendation, MSN or equivalent, statistics course, vita, writing sample, GRE General Test.
**Degree Requirements** 96 total credit hours, dissertation.

### POSTDOCTORAL PROGRAM

**Areas of Study** Individualized study, information systems, nursing informatics, nursing interventions, nursing research, nursing science, vulnerable population.
**Postdoctoral Program Contact** Dr. Linda D. Scott, Associate Dean for Academic Affairs, College of Nursing, University of Illinois at Chicago, 845 South Damen Avenue (MS 802), Chicago, IL 60612. *Telephone:* 312-413-1505. *Fax:* 312-996-8066. *E-mail:* ldscott@uic.edu.

### CONTINUING EDUCATION PROGRAM

**Contact** Prof. Susan M. Ohlson, Clinical Instructor, College of Nursing, University of Illinois at Chicago, 845 South Damen Avenue (MC 802), Chicago, IL 60612. *Telephone:* 312-413-2978. *E-mail:* sohlso1@uic.edu.

## University of St. Francis

**Leach College of Nursing**
**Joliet, Illinois**

***https://www.stfrancis.edu/academics/college-of-nursing***
Founded in 1920

**DEGREES • BSN • DNP • MSN**

**Nursing Program Faculty** 52 (29% with doctorates).
**Baccalaureate Enrollment** 476 **Women** 89% **Men** 11% **Minority** 18% **International** .4% **Part-time** 23%
**Graduate Enrollment** 391 **Women** 90% **Men** 10% **Minority** 26% **International** 1% **Part-time** 77%
**Distance Learning Courses** Available.
**Nursing Student Activities** Nursing Honor Society, Sigma Theta Tau, Student Nurses' Association, nursing club.
**Nursing Student Resources** Academic advising; academic or career counseling; assistance for students with disabilities; bookstore; campus computer network; career placement assistance; computer lab; computer-assisted instruction; e-mail services; employment services for current students; externships; housing assistance; interactive nursing skills videos; Internet; learning resource lab; library services; nursing audiovisuals; remedial services; resume preparation assistance; skills, simulation, or other laboratory; tutoring.
**Library Facilities** 135,000 volumes (3,120 in health, 3,106 in nursing); 15,250 periodical subscriptions (71 health-care related).

### BACCALAUREATE PROGRAMS

**Degree** BSN
**Available Programs** Accelerated RN Baccalaureate; Generic Baccalaureate.
**Study Options** Full-time and part-time.
**Online Degree Options** Yes.
**Program Entrance Requirements** Minimum overall college GPA of 2.75, transcript of college record, health exam, high school biology, high school chemistry, 3 years high school math, 2 years high school science, high school transcript, immunizations, minimum high school GPA of 2.5, minimum high school rank 50%, minimum GPA in nursing prerequisites of 2.75, prerequisite course work. Transfer students are accepted. *Application deadline:* Applications may be processed on a rolling basis for some programs.
**Advanced Placement** Credit by examination available. Credit given for nursing courses completed elsewhere dependent upon specific evaluations.
**Expenses (2013–14)** *Tuition:* full-time $27,400; part-time $825 per credit. *International tuition:* $27,400 full-time. *Room and board:* $8520 per academic year. *Required fees:* full-time $570; part-time $125 per term.
**Financial Aid** 87% of baccalaureate students in nursing programs received some form of financial aid in 2012–13. *Gift aid (need-based):* Federal Pell, FSEOG, state, private, college/university gift aid from institutional funds, Federal Nursing. *Loans:* Federal Direct (Subsidized and Unsubsidized Stafford PLUS), Perkins, alternative loans. *Work-study:* Federal Work-Study, part-time campus jobs. *Financial aid application deadline (priority):* 2/15.
**Contact** Cynthia Lambert, Director, Undergraduate Admissions, Leach College of Nursing, University of St. Francis, 500 Wilcox Street, Joliet, IL 60435. *Telephone:* 800-735-7500. *Fax:* 815-740-5078. *E-mail:* clambert@stfrancis.edu.

### GRADUATE PROGRAMS

**Expenses (2013–14)** *Tuition:* part-time $710 per credit. *Required fees:* part-time $125 per term.
**Financial Aid** 68% of graduate students in nursing programs received some form of financial aid in 2012–13.
**Contact** Ms. Sandee Sloka, Director, Graduate/Degree Completion Admissions, Leach College of Nursing, University of St. Francis, 500 Wilcox Street, Joliet, IL 60435. *Telephone:* 800-735-7500. *Fax:* 815-740-3431. *E-mail:* ssloka@stfrancis.edu.

### MASTER'S DEGREE PROGRAM

**Degree** MSN
**Available Programs** Master's; Master's for Nurses with Non-Nursing Degrees.
**Concentrations Available** Nursing administration; nursing education. *Nurse practitioner programs in:* family health, psychiatric/mental health.
**Site Options** Albuquerque, NM.
**Study Options** Part-time.
**Online Degree Options** Yes.
**Program Entrance Requirements** Clinical experience, computer literacy, minimum overall college GPA of 3.0, transcript of college record, CPR certification, written essay, immunizations, interview, 3 letters of recommendation, nursing research course, physical assessment course, professional liability insurance/malpractice insurance, prerequisite course work, resume, statistics course. *Application deadline:* Applications may be processed on a rolling basis for some programs.
**Advanced Placement** Credit given for nursing courses completed elsewhere dependent upon specific evaluations.
**Degree Requirements** 47 total credit hours.

### POST-MASTER'S PROGRAM

**Areas of Study** *Nurse practitioner programs in:* family health, psychiatric/mental health.

### DOCTORAL DEGREE PROGRAM

**Degree** DNP
**Available Programs** Doctorate.
**Areas of Study** Nursing education.
**Online Degree Options** Yes (online only).
**Program Entrance Requirements** Minimum overall college GPA of 3.0, interview, 2 letters of recommendation, MSN or equivalent, statistics course, vita. *Application deadline:* Applications may be processed on a rolling basis for some programs.
**Degree Requirements** 40 total credit hours, residency.

## Western Illinois University

**School of Nursing**
**Macomb, Illinois**

***http://www.wiu.edu/nursing***
Founded in 1899

**DEGREE • BSN**

**Nursing Program Faculty** 14 (40% with doctorates).

**Baccalaureate Enrollment** 75 **Women** 75% **Men** 25% **Minority** 12% **International** 5% **Part-time** 1%
**Distance Learning Courses** Available.
**Nursing Student Activities** Nursing Honor Society, Student Nurses' Association.
**Nursing Student Resources** Academic advising; academic or career counseling; assistance for students with disabilities; bookstore; campus computer network; career placement assistance; computer lab; computer-assisted instruction; daycare for children of students; e-mail services; housing assistance; interactive nursing skills videos; Internet; learning resource lab; library services; nursing audiovisuals; resume preparation assistance; skills, simulation, or other laboratory; tutoring.
**Library Facilities** 994,880 volumes; 7,098 periodical subscriptions.

### BACCALAUREATE PROGRAMS

**Degree** BSN
**Available Programs** Baccalaureate for Second Degree; Generic Baccalaureate; RN Baccalaureate.
**Site Options** Moline, IL.
**Study Options** Full-time.
**Online Degree Options** Yes.
**Program Entrance Requirements** Minimum overall college GPA of 3.0, transcript of college record, CPR certification, written essay, health exam, immunizations, 2 letters of recommendation, minimum high school GPA of 2.75, minimum GPA in nursing prerequisites of 3.0, professional liability insurance/malpractice insurance, prerequisite course work. Transfer students are accepted. *Application deadline:* 3/1 (fall).
**Advanced Placement** Credit given for nursing courses completed elsewhere dependent upon specific evaluations.
**Expenses (2013–14)** *Tuition, state resident:* full-time $6274; part-time $280 per credit hour. *Tuition, nonresident:* full-time $10,086; part-time $420 per credit hour. *International tuition:* $10,086 full-time. *Room and board:* $9190; room only: $5630 per academic year. *Required fees:* full-time $2028; part-time $84 per credit; part-time $1014 per term.
**Financial Aid** 90% of baccalaureate students in nursing programs received some form of financial aid in 2012–13. *Gift aid (need-based):* Federal Pell, FSEOG, state, private, college/university gift aid from institutional funds. *Loans:* Federal Direct (Subsidized and Unsubsidized Stafford PLUS), Perkins, college/university. *Work-study:* Federal Work-Study, part-time campus jobs. *Financial aid application deadline (priority):* 2/15.
**Contact** Mr. Theo E. Schultz, Academic Advisor, School of Nursing, Western Illinois University, 1 University Circle, Macomb, IL 61455. *Telephone:* 309-298-2571. *Fax:* 309-298-3190. *E-mail:* t-schultz@wiu.ecu.

# INDIANA

## Anderson University
### School of Nursing
### Anderson, Indiana

***http://www.anderson.edu/academics/nursing***
Founded in 1917

**DEGREES • BSN • MSN • MSN/MBA**
**Nursing Program Faculty** 21 (5% with doctorates).
**Baccalaureate Enrollment** 153 **Women** 95% **Men** 5% **Minority** 3% **International** 2% **Part-time** 9%
**Graduate Enrollment** 31 **Women** 87% **Men** 13% **Minority** 5%
**Distance Learning Courses** Available.
**Nursing Student Activities** Sigma Theta Tau, Student Nurses' Association.
**Nursing Student Resources** Academic advising; academic or career counseling; assistance for students with disabilities; bookstore; campus computer network; career placement assistance; computer lab; computer-assisted instruction; e-mail services; housing assistance; interactive nursing skills videos; Internet; learning resource lab; library services; nursing audiovisuals; placement services for program completers; remedial services; resume preparation assistance; skills, simulation, or other laboratory; tutoring.
**Library Facilities** 303,170 volumes (570 in health, 565 in nursing); 457 periodical subscriptions (54 health-care related).

### BACCALAUREATE PROGRAMS

**Degree** BSN
**Available Programs** Generic Baccalaureate; RN Baccalaureate.
**Site Options** Indianapolis, IN.
**Study Options** Full-time and part-time.
**Program Entrance Requirements** Minimum overall college GPA of 3.0, transcript of college record, CPR certification, health exam, high school biology, high school chemistry, 2 years high school math, 3 years high school science, high school transcript, immunizations, minimum high school GPA of 3.5, minimum high school rank 33%, minimum GPA in nursing prerequisites of 3.0, professional liability insurance/malpractice insurance, prerequisite course work. Transfer students are accepted. *Application deadline:* 5/31 (spring), 8/30 (summer).
**Advanced Placement** Credit given for nursing courses completed elsewhere dependent upon specific evaluations.
**Expenses (2013–14)** *Tuition:* full-time $26,120; part-time $13,060 per semester. *International tuition:* $26,120 full-time. *Room and board:* $9110; room only: $5830 per academic year. *Required fees:* full-time $464.
**Financial Aid** 98% of baccalaureate students in nursing programs received some form of financial aid in 2012–13.
**Contact** Dr. Karen S. Williams, Dean, School of Nursing, School of Nursing, Anderson University, 1100 East 5th Street, Anderson, IN 46012-3495. *Telephone:* 765-641-4385. *Fax:* 765-641-3095. *E-mail:* kswilliams@anderson.edu.

### GRADUATE PROGRAMS

**Expenses (2013–14)** *Tuition:* full-time $21,100; part-time $440 per credit hour. *International tuition:* $21,100 full-time. *Required fees:* full-time $184.
**Financial Aid** 90% of graduate students in nursing programs received some form of financial aid in 2012–13.
**Contact** Mrs. Lynn Schmidt, Graduate Coordinator and Assistant Professor, School of Nursing, Anderson University, 1100 East 5th Street, Anderson, IN 46012-3495. *Telephone:* 765-641-4388. *Fax:* 765-641-3095. *E-mail:* lmschmidt@anderson.edu.

#### MASTER'S DEGREE PROGRAM

**Degrees** MSN; MSN/MBA
**Available Programs** Master's; RN to Master's.
**Concentrations Available** Nursing administration; nursing education; nursing informatics.
**Site Options** Indianapolis, IN.
**Study Options** Full-time and part-time.
**Program Entrance Requirements** Clinical experience, minimum overall college GPA of 2.75, transcript of college record, CPR certification, written essay, immunizations, 3 letters of recommendation, professional liability insurance/malpractice insurance. *Application deadline:* Applications may be processed on a rolling basis for some programs. *Application fee:* $50.
**Degree Requirements** 55 total credit hours, thesis or project.

#### POST-MASTER'S PROGRAM

**Areas of Study** Nursing administration; nursing education; nursing informatics.

## Ball State University
### School of Nursing
### Muncie, Indiana

***http://www.bsu.edu/nursing***
Founded in 1918

**DEGREES • BS • DNP • MS**
**Nursing Program Faculty** 54 (28% with doctorates).
**Baccalaureate Enrollment** 401 **Women** 89% **Men** 11% **Minority** 5% **International** .25% **Part-time** 1%
**Graduate Enrollment** 421 **Women** 93% **Men** 7% **Minority** 8% **Part-time** 100%
**Distance Learning Courses** Available.
**Nursing Student Activities** Nursing Honor Society, Sigma Theta Tau, Student Nurses' Association.
**Nursing Student Resources** Academic advising; academic or career counseling; assistance for students with disabilities; bookstore; campus computer network; career placement assistance; computer lab; computer-assisted instruction; e-mail services; employment services for current students; housing assistance; interactive nursing skills videos; Internet;

learning resource lab; library services; nursing audiovisuals; placement services for program completers; remedial services; resume preparation assistance; skills, simulation, or other laboratory; tutoring.
**Library Facilities** 1 million volumes (16,885 in health, 9,221 in nursing); 2,551 periodical subscriptions (3,713 health-care related).

## BACCALAUREATE PROGRAMS

**Degree** BS
**Available Programs** Accelerated Baccalaureate; Accelerated Baccalaureate for Second Degree; Baccalaureate for Second Degree; Generic Baccalaureate; LPN to Baccalaureate; LPN to RN Baccalaureate; RN Baccalaureate.
**Study Options** Full-time.
**Program Entrance Requirements** Minimum overall college GPA of 3.00, transcript of college record, CPR certification, health exam, immunizations, minimum GPA in nursing prerequisites of 3.0, prerequisite course work. Transfer students are accepted. *Application deadline:* 8/28 (fall), 1/21 (spring).
**Expenses (2013–14)** *Tuition, state resident:* full-time $7024; part-time $277 per credit hour. *Tuition, nonresident:* full-time $22,168; part-time $926 per credit hour. *Room and board:* $4251 per academic year. *Required fees:* full-time $2454.
**Financial Aid** 90% of baccalaureate students in nursing programs received some form of financial aid in 2012–13. *Gift aid (need-based):* Federal Pell, FSEOG, state, private, college/university gift aid from institutional funds. *Loans:* Federal Direct (Subsidized and Unsubsidized Stafford PLUS), Perkins. *Work-study:* Federal Work-Study, part-time campus jobs. *Financial aid application deadline (priority):* 3/10.
**Contact** Dr. Linda Siktberg, Director, School of Nursing, Ball State University, CN 418, Muncie, IN 47306. *Telephone:* 765-285-5570. *Fax:* 765-285-2169. *E-mail:* lsiktber@bsu.edu.

## GRADUATE PROGRAMS

**Expenses (2013–14)** *Tuition, state resident:* part-time $307 per credit hour. *Tuition, nonresident:* part-time $528 per credit hour. *Required fees:* part-time $362 per credit.
**Financial Aid** Research assistantships; career-related internships or fieldwork available.
**Contact** Mrs. Shantelle Estes, Advisor, Graduate Programs, School of Nursing, Ball State University, CN 418, Muncie, IN 47306. *Telephone:* 765-285-9130. *Fax:* 765-285-2169. *E-mail:* smestes@bsu.edu.

### MASTER'S DEGREE PROGRAM

**Degree** MS
**Available Programs** Master's; RN to Master's.
**Concentrations Available** Nursing administration; nursing education. *Nurse practitioner programs in:* adult health, family health.
**Study Options** Part-time.
**Online Degree Options** Yes (online only).
**Program Entrance Requirements** Computer literacy, minimum overall college GPA of 2.8, transcript of college record, CPR certification, written essay, immunizations, 1 letter of recommendation, nursing research course, physical assessment course, prerequisite course work, statistics course. *Application deadline:* 1/14 (fall), 8/9 (spring), 1/14 (summer). *Application fee:* $50.
**Advanced Placement** Credit given for nursing courses completed elsewhere dependent upon specific evaluations.
**Degree Requirements** 50 total credit hours.

### POST-MASTER'S PROGRAM

**Areas of Study** Nursing education.

### DOCTORAL DEGREE PROGRAM

**Degree** DNP
**Available Programs** Doctorate.
**Areas of Study** Advanced practice nursing.
**Online Degree Options** Yes (online only).
**Program Entrance Requirements** Clinical experience, minimum overall college GPA of 3.2, interview by faculty committee, letters of recommendation, MSN or equivalent, statistics course, writing sample. *Application deadline:* 6/1 (spring). *Application fee:* $50.
**Degree Requirements** 48 total credit hours, residency.

# Bethel College
## School of Nursing
## Mishawaka, Indiana

***http://www.bethelcollege.edu/***
Founded in 1947

**DEGREES • BSN • MSN**
**Nursing Program Faculty** 37 (20% with doctorates).
**Baccalaureate Enrollment** 152 **Women** 88% **Men** 12% **Minority** 7.8% **International** 1.3% **Part-time** 34%
**Graduate Enrollment** 24 **Women** 96% **Men** 4% **Minority** 12.5% **Part-time** 100%
**Nursing Student Activities** Sigma Theta Tau, Student Nurses' Association.
**Nursing Student Resources** Academic advising; academic or career counseling; assistance for students with disabilities; bookstore; campus computer network; career placement assistance; computer lab; computer-assisted instruction; e-mail services; employment services for current students; housing assistance; interactive nursing skills videos; Internet; learning resource lab; library services; nursing audiovisuals; remedial services; resume preparation assistance; skills, simulation, or other laboratory; tutoring.
**Library Facilities** 146,563 volumes (3,000 in health, 2,050 in nursing); 2,678 periodical subscriptions (175 health-care related).

## BACCALAUREATE PROGRAMS

**Degree** BSN
**Available Programs** ADN to Baccalaureate; Generic Baccalaureate; RN Baccalaureate.
**Site Options** Winona Lake, IN; Mishawaka, IN; St. Joseph, MI.
**Study Options** Full-time and part-time.
**Program Entrance Requirements** Minimum overall college GPA of 2.5, transcript of college record, CPR certification, written essay, health exam, health insurance, high school chemistry, high school transcript, immunizations, 1 letter of recommendation, minimum high school GPA of 2.5, minimum GPA in nursing prerequisites of 2.5, prerequisite course work. Transfer students are accepted. *Application deadline:* 8/1 (fall). Applications may be processed on a rolling basis for some programs. *Application fee:* $25.
**Advanced Placement** Credit by examination available. Credit given for nursing courses completed elsewhere dependent upon specific evaluations.
**Expenses (2012–13)** *Tuition:* full-time $23,930; part-time $600 per credit hour. *International tuition:* $23,932 full-time. *Room and board:* $3485; room only: $1700 per academic year. *Required fees:* full-time $600; part-time $300 per term.
**Financial Aid** 77% of baccalaureate students in nursing programs received some form of financial aid in 2011–12. *Gift aid (need-based):* Federal Pell, FSEOG, state, private, college/university gift aid from institutional funds, Federal Nursing. *Loans:* Federal Nursing Student Loans, Federal Direct (Subsidized and Unsubsidized Stafford PLUS), Perkins, college/university. *Work-study:* Federal Work-Study. *Financial aid application deadline:* 3/10(priority: 3/1).
**Contact** Dr. Deborah R. Gillum, Dean of Nursing, School of Nursing, Bethel College, 1001 Bethel Circle, Mishawaka, IN 46545. *Telephone:* 574-807-7015. *Fax:* 574-257-2683. *E-mail:* gillumd@bethelcollege.edu.

## GRADUATE PROGRAMS

**Expenses (2012–13)** *Tuition:* part-time $400 per credit hour.
**Financial Aid** 95% of graduate students in nursing programs received some form of financial aid in 2011–12.
**Contact** Dr. Karon Schwartz, Graduate Nursing Program Director, School of Nursing, Bethel College, 1001 Bethel Circle, Mishawaka, IN 46545. *Telephone:* 574-257-3382. *Fax:* 574-257-7616. *E-mail:* schwark@bethelcollege.edu.

### MASTER'S DEGREE PROGRAM

**Degree** MSN
**Available Programs** Master's.
**Concentrations Available** Nursing administration; nursing education.
**Site Options** Mishawaka, IN.
**Study Options** Part-time.
**Program Entrance Requirements** Clinical experience, minimum overall college GPA of 3.0, transcript of college record, CPR certification, immunizations, 3 letters of recommendation, nursing research course, physical assessment course, statistics course. *Application*

*deadline:* 8/1 (fall). Applications may be processed on a rolling basis for some programs. *Application fee:* $25.
**Advanced Placement** Credit given for nursing courses completed elsewhere dependent upon specific evaluations.
**Degree Requirements** 36 total credit hours, thesis or project.

**POST-MASTER'S PROGRAM**
**Areas of Study** Nursing administration; nursing education.

# Goshen College
## Department of Nursing
## Goshen, Indiana

***http://www.goshen.edu/***
Founded in 1894
**DEGREES • BSN • MSN**
**Nursing Program Faculty** 12
**Baccalaureate Enrollment** 130 **Women** 95% **Men** 5% **Minority** 23% **International** 3%
**Graduate Enrollment** 44 **Women** 89% **Men** 11% **Minority** 6%
**Nursing Student Activities** Nursing Honor Society, Sigma Theta Tau, Student Nurses' Association.
**Nursing Student Resources** Academic advising; academic or career counseling; assistance for students with disabilities; bookstore; campus computer network; career placement assistance; computer lab; computer-assisted instruction; daycare for children of students; e-mail services; employment services for current students; externships; housing assistance; interactive nursing skills videos; Internet; learning resource lab; library services; nursing audiovisuals; placement services for program completers; remedial services; resume preparation assistance; skills, simulation, or other laboratory; tutoring.
**Library Facilities** 135,000 volumes (80 in health, 80 in nursing); 400 periodical subscriptions (68 health-care related).

### BACCALAUREATE PROGRAMS
**Degree** BSN
**Available Programs** Generic Baccalaureate; RN Baccalaureate.
**Site Options** Elkhart, IN.
**Study Options** Full-time and part-time.
**Program Entrance Requirements** Minimum overall college GPA of 2.7, transcript of college record, CPR certification, written essay, health exam, health insurance, high school chemistry, high school foreign language, 2 years high school math, high school science, high school transcript, immunizations, 2 letters of recommendation, minimum high school GPA of 2.7, minimum high school rank 50%. Transfer students are accepted. *Application deadline:* 8/15 (fall), 12/17 (winter), 3/1 (spring).
**Advanced Placement** Credit by examination available. Credit given for nursing courses completed elsewhere dependent upon specific evaluations.
**Expenses (2013–14)** *Tuition:* full-time $28,500; part-time $1190 per credit hour. *Room and board:* $9460; room only: $5060 per academic year. *Required fees:* full-time $375.
**Financial Aid** 98% of baccalaureate students in nursing programs received some form of financial aid in 2012–13.
**Contact** Admissions, Department of Nursing, Goshen College, 1700 South Main Street, Goshen, IN 46526. *Telephone:* 574-535-7535. *Fax:* 574-535-7609. *E-mail:* admissions@goshen.edu.

### GRADUATE PROGRAMS
**Expenses (2013–14)** *Tuition:* part-time $600 per credit.
**Financial Aid** 25% of graduate students in nursing programs received some form of financial aid in 2012–13.
**Contact** Dr. Brenda Srof, Director, Masters in Nursing, Department of Nursing, Goshen College, 1700 South Main Street, Goshen, IN 46526. *Telephone:* 574-535-7375. *Fax:* 575-535-7375. *E-mail:* brendajs@goshen.edu.

**MASTER'S DEGREE PROGRAM**
**Degree** MSN
**Available Programs** Master's.
**Concentrations Available** *Nurse practitioner programs in:* family health.
**Study Options** Part-time.
**Program Entrance Requirements** Clinical experience, computer literacy, minimum overall college GPA of 3.0, transcript of college record, CPR certification, written essay, immunizations, interview, letters of recommendation, prerequisite course work, resume, statistics course. *Application deadline:* 3/15 (fall). *Application fee:* $50.
**Degree Requirements** 48 total credit hours.

# Huntington University
## Department of Nursing
## Huntington, Indiana

***http://www.huntington.edu/nursing/***
Founded in 1897
**DEGREE • BSN**
**Nursing Program Faculty** 6 (17% with doctorates).
**Baccalaureate Enrollment** 42 **Women** 90% **Men** 10% **Minority** 15% **International** 4%
**Nursing Student Activities** Nursing club.
**Nursing Student Resources** Academic advising; academic or career counseling; assistance for students with disabilities; bookstore; campus computer network; career placement assistance; computer lab; computer-assisted instruction; daycare for children of students; e-mail services; employment services for current students; housing assistance; interactive nursing skills videos; Internet; learning resource lab; library services; nursing audiovisuals; other; remedial services; resume preparation assistance; skills, simulation, or other laboratory; tutoring; unpaid internships.
**Library Facilities** 235,824 volumes (1,544 in health, 100 in nursing); 51,338 periodical subscriptions (114 health-care related).

### BACCALAUREATE PROGRAMS
**Degree** BSN
**Available Programs** ADN to Baccalaureate; Generic Baccalaureate; RN Baccalaureate.
**Study Options** Full-time.
**Program Entrance Requirements** Minimum overall college GPA of 2.75, transcript of college record, CPR certification, health exam, high school biology, high school chemistry, 2 years high school math, 2 years high school science, high school transcript, immunizations, interview, minimum high school GPA of 2.3, minimum high school rank 33%, minimum GPA in nursing prerequisites of 2.5, professional liability insurance/malpractice insurance, prerequisite course work. Transfer students are accepted. *Application deadline:* 3/31 (fall). *Application fee:* $20.
**Contact** *Telephone:* 260-359-4360. *Fax:* 260-359-4133.

# Indiana State University
## Department of Nursing
## Terre Haute, Indiana

***http://www.indstate.edu/nursing/***
Founded in 1865
**DEGREES • BS • DNP • MS**
**Nursing Program Faculty** 64 (27% with doctorates).
**Baccalaureate Enrollment** 1,196 **Women** 89% **Men** 11% **Minority** 24% **International** 1% **Part-time** 29%
**Graduate Enrollment** 268 **Women** 85% **Men** 15% **Minority** 13% **International** 1% **Part-time** 100%
**Distance Learning Courses** Available.
**Nursing Student Activities** Sigma Theta Tau, Student Nurses' Association.
**Nursing Student Resources** Academic advising; academic or career counseling; assistance for students with disabilities; bookstore; campus computer network; career placement assistance; computer lab; computer-assisted instruction; daycare for children of students; e-mail services; employment services for current students; externships; housing assistance; interactive nursing skills videos; Internet; learning resource lab; library services; nursing audiovisuals; paid internships; placement services for program completers; remedial services; resume preparation assistance; skills, simulation, or other laboratory; tutoring; unpaid internships.
**Library Facilities** 12,140 volumes in health, 2,677 volumes in nursing; 9,170 periodical subscriptions health-care related.

### BACCALAUREATE PROGRAMS
**Degree** BS

**Available Programs** Accelerated Baccalaureate for Second Degree; Generic Baccalaureate; LPN to Baccalaureate; RN Baccalaureate.

**Study Options** Full-time and part-time.

**Online Degree Options** Yes.

**Program Entrance Requirements** Minimum overall college GPA of 2.75, transcript of college record, CPR certification, health exam, high school chemistry, high school foreign language, 3 years high school math, 3 years high school science, high school transcript, immunizations, minimum high school GPA of 2.5, minimum high school rank 40%, minimum GPA in nursing prerequisites of 2.75, prerequisite course work. Transfer students are accepted. *Application deadline:* 6/1 (fall), 11/1 (spring).

**Advanced Placement** Credit by examination available. Credit given for nursing courses completed elsewhere dependent upon specific evaluations.

**Expenses (2013–14)** *Tuition, state resident:* full-time $8056; part-time $292 per credit hour. *Tuition, nonresident:* full-time $17,792; part-time $630 per credit hour. *International tuition:* $17,792 full-time. *Room and board:* $9010 per academic year. *Required fees:* full-time $300.

**Financial Aid** 35% of baccalaureate students in nursing programs received some form of financial aid in 2012–13.

**Contact** Office of Student Affairs, Department of Nursing, Indiana State University, College of Nursing, Health, and Human Services, 749 Chestnut Street, Terre Haute, IN 47809. *Telephone:* 812-237-2316. *Fax:* 812-237-8022.

## GRADUATE PROGRAMS

**Expenses (2013–14)** *Tuition, state resident:* part-time $373 per credit hour. *Tuition, nonresident:* part-time $466 per credit hour. *Required fees:* part-time $600 per term.

**Financial Aid** 55% of graduate students in nursing programs received some form of financial aid in 2012–13. 5 research assistantships with partial tuition reimbursements available (averaging $7,500 per year) were awarded; teaching assistantships with partial tuition reimbursements available, career-related internships or fieldwork and Federal Work-Study also available. Aid available to part-time students. *Financial aid application deadline:* 3/1.

**Contact** Dr. Susan Eley, Chairperson, Advanced Practice Nursing, Department of Nursing, Indiana State University, Landsbaum Center for Health Education, 1433 No. 6 1/2 Street, Terre Haute, IN 47807. *Telephone:* 812-237-7916. *Fax:* 812-237-8939. *E-mail:* susan.eley@indstate.edu.

### MASTER'S DEGREE PROGRAM

**Degree** MS

**Available Programs** Master's.

**Concentrations Available** Nursing administration; nursing education. *Nurse practitioner programs in:* family health.

**Study Options** Full-time and part-time.

**Online Degree Options** Yes (online only).

**Program Entrance Requirements** Clinical experience, minimum overall college GPA of 3.0, transcript of college record, CPR certification, written essay, immunizations, 3 letters of recommendation, prerequisite course work. *Application deadline:* 2/1 (fall), 9/1 (spring). *Application fee:* $35.

**Advanced Placement** Credit given for nursing courses completed elsewhere dependent upon specific evaluations.

**Degree Requirements** 48 total credit hours, thesis or project.

### POST-MASTER'S PROGRAM

**Areas of Study** Nursing education. *Nurse practitioner programs in:* family health.

### DOCTORAL DEGREE PROGRAM

**Degree** DNP

**Available Programs** Doctorate.

**Areas of Study** Advanced practice nursing.

**Online Degree Options** Yes (online only).

**Program Entrance Requirements** Clinical experience, minimum overall college GPA of 3.0, 3 letters of recommendation, MSN or equivalent, statistics course, writing sample. *Application deadline:* Applications may be processed on a rolling basis for some programs. *Application fee:* $35.

**Degree Requirements** 39 total credit hours.

## CONTINUING EDUCATION PROGRAM

**Contact** Ms. Esther Acree, Department of Nursing, Indiana State University, 749 Chestnut Street, Terre Haute, IN 47809. *Telephone:* 812-237-2320. *E-mail:* esther.acree@indstate.edu.

# Indiana University Bloomington

## Department of Nursing–Bloomington Division
## Bloomington, Indiana

Founded in 1820

### DEGREE • BSN

**Nursing Program Faculty** 25 (3.5% with doctorates).

**Baccalaureate Enrollment** 187 **Women** 97% **Men** 3% **Minority** 1%

**Distance Learning Courses** Available.

**Nursing Student Activities** Nursing Honor Society, Sigma Theta Tau, Student Nurses' Association.

**Nursing Student Resources** Academic advising; academic or career counseling; assistance for students with disabilities; campus computer network; computer lab; computer-assisted instruction; e-mail services; employment services for current students; interactive nursing skills videos; Internet; learning resource lab; library services; nursing audiovisuals; remedial services; resume preparation assistance; skills, simulation, or other laboratory; tutoring.

**Library Facilities** 9.1 million volumes (8,500 in nursing); 1,000 periodical subscriptions health-care related.

## BACCALAUREATE PROGRAMS

**Degree** BSN

**Available Programs** Baccalaureate for Second Degree; Generic Baccalaureate; RN Baccalaureate.

**Site Options** Columbus , IN; Bedford, IN; Bloomington , IN.

**Study Options** Full-time.

**Program Entrance Requirements** Minimum overall college GPA of 2.5, transcript of college record, CPR certification, written essay, health exam, health insurance, high school chemistry, 3 years high school math, high school transcript, immunizations, interview, minimum GPA in nursing prerequisites of 2.7, prerequisite course work. Transfer students are accepted. *Application deadline:* 3/15 (fall).

**Advanced Placement** Credit by examination available. Credit given for nursing courses completed elsewhere dependent upon specific evaluations.

**Financial Aid** 50% of baccalaureate students in nursing programs received some form of financial aid in 2012–13.

**Contact** Mrs. Deborah Hrisomalos, Academic Advisor, Department of Nursing–Bloomington Division, Indiana University Bloomington, Room 401, Bloomington, IN 47405. *Telephone:* 812-855-2592. *Fax:* 812-855-6986. *E-mail:* dhrisoma@indiana.edu.

# Indiana University East

## School of Nursing
## Richmond, Indiana

***http://www.iue.edu/nursing/***

Founded in 1971

### DEGREE • BSN

**Nursing Program Faculty** 15 (7% with doctorates).

**Baccalaureate Enrollment** 201 **Women** 92.5% **Men** 7.5% **Minority** 5% **International** 1%

**Nursing Student Activities** Sigma Theta Tau, Student Nurses' Association.

**Nursing Student Resources** Academic advising; academic or career counseling; assistance for students with disabilities; bookstore; campus computer network; career placement assistance; computer lab; computer-assisted instruction; daycare for children of students; e-mail services; externships; interactive nursing skills videos; Internet; learning resource lab; library services; nursing audiovisuals; placement services for program completers; remedial services; resume preparation assistance; skills, simulation, or other laboratory; tutoring; unpaid internships.

**Library Facilities** 81,000 volumes (5,039 in health, 3,418 in nursing); 70 periodical subscriptions health-care related.

## BACCALAUREATE PROGRAMS

**Degree** BSN

**Available Programs** ADN to Baccalaureate; Generic Baccalaureate; RN Baccalaureate.
**Study Options** Full-time.
**Program Entrance Requirements** Minimum overall college GPA of 2.7, transcript of college record, CPR certification, high school biology, high school chemistry, 3 years high school math, 3 years high school science, high school transcript, immunizations, minimum high school GPA of 2.0, minimum high school rank 50%, minimum GPA in nursing prerequisites of 2.0, prerequisite course work. Transfer students are accepted. *Application deadline:* 3/1 (fall).
**Advanced Placement** Credit by examination available. Credit given for nursing courses completed elsewhere dependent upon specific evaluations.
**Contact** *Telephone:* 765-973-8353. *Fax:* 765-973-8220.

# Indiana University Kokomo

## Indiana University School of Nursing
## Kokomo, Indiana

Founded in 1945

### DEGREE • BSN

**Nursing Program Faculty** 14 (43% with doctorates).
**Baccalaureate Enrollment** 235 **Women** 95% **Men** 5% **Minority** 1% **International** 1% **Part-time** 32%
**Nursing Student Activities** Sigma Theta Tau, Student Nurses' Association.
**Nursing Student Resources** Academic advising; academic or career counseling; assistance for students with disabilities; bookstore; campus computer network; career placement assistance; computer lab; computer-assisted instruction; daycare for children of students; e-mail services; employment services for current students; externships; interactive nursing skills videos; Internet; learning resource lab; library services; nursing audiovisuals; paid internships; remedial services; resume preparation assistance; skills, simulation, or other laboratory; tutoring.
**Library Facilities** 138,653 volumes (2,881 in health, 1,513 in nursing); 75 periodical subscriptions health-care related.

### BACCALAUREATE PROGRAMS

**Degree** BSN
**Available Programs** Accelerated RN Baccalaureate; Generic Baccalaureate.
**Site Options** Peru, IN; Marion, IN; Logansport, IN.
**Study Options** Full-time.
**Program Entrance Requirements** Minimum overall college GPA of 2.5, transcript of college record, CPR certification, high school biology, high school chemistry, 4 years high school math, high school transcript, immunizations, minimum high school GPA of 2.0, minimum high school rank 50%, minimum GPA in nursing prerequisites of 2.7, prerequisite course work. Transfer students are accepted.
**Contact** *Telephone:* 765-455-9384. *Fax:* 765-455-9421.

### CONTINUING EDUCATION PROGRAM

**Contact** *Telephone:* 765-455-9384. *Fax:* 765-455-9421.

# Indiana University Northwest

## School of Nursing
## Gary, Indiana

*http://www.iun.edu/nursing*
Founded in 1959

### DEGREE • BSN

**Nursing Program Faculty** 25 (25% with doctorates).
**Baccalaureate Enrollment** 220 **Women** 87% **Men** 13% **Minority** 34% **Part-time** 10%
**Distance Learning Courses** Available.
**Nursing Student Activities** Sigma Theta Tau, Student Nurses' Association.
**Nursing Student Resources** Academic advising; academic or career counseling; assistance for students with disabilities; bookstore; campus computer network; career placement assistance; computer lab; computer-assisted instruction; e-mail services; externships; interactive nursing skills videos; Internet; learning resource lab; library services; nursing audiovisuals; placement services for program completers; remedial services; resume preparation assistance; skills, simulation, or other laboratory; tutoring.
**Library Facilities** 226,300 volumes (134,740 in health, 6,050 in nursing); 253 periodical subscriptions health-care related.

### BACCALAUREATE PROGRAMS

**Degree** BSN
**Available Programs** Accelerated Baccalaureate for Second Degree; Generic Baccalaureate; RN Baccalaureate.
**Study Options** Full-time.
**Online Degree Options** Yes.
**Program Entrance Requirements** Minimum overall college GPA of 2.7, transcript of college record, CPR certification, health exam, health insurance, immunizations, minimum GPA in nursing prerequisites of 2.7, prerequisite course work. Transfer students are accepted. *Application deadline:* 4/1 (fall), 1/1 (summer).
**Advanced Placement** Credit given for nursing courses completed elsewhere dependent upon specific evaluations.
**Expenses (2013–14)** *Tuition, state resident:* full-time $4650. *Tuition, nonresident:* full-time $13,000. *International tuition:* $13,000 full-time. *Required fees:* full-time $2200.
**Financial Aid** 75% of baccalaureate students in nursing programs received some form of financial aid in 2012–13.
**Contact** Ms. Anne Mitchell, Nursing Student Services Coordinator, School of Nursing, Indiana University Northwest, 3400 Broadway, Gary, IN 46408-1197. *Telephone:* 219-980-6611. *Fax:* 219-980-6578. *E-mail:* amitchel@iun.edu.

# Indiana University–Purdue University Fort Wayne

## Department of Nursing
## Fort Wayne, Indiana

*http://www.ipfw.edu/nursing*
Founded in 1917

### DEGREES • BS • MS

**Nursing Program Faculty** 53 (19% with doctorates).
**Baccalaureate Enrollment** 339 **Women** 86.3% **Men** 13.7% **Minority** 13.4% **International** 1% **Part-time** 31.3%
**Graduate Enrollment** 56 **Women** 95.5% **Men** 4.5% **Minority** 6% **Part-time** 97%
**Distance Learning Courses** Available.
**Nursing Student Activities** Sigma Theta Tau, nursing club.
**Nursing Student Resources** Academic advising; academic or career counseling; assistance for students with disabilities; bookstore; campus computer network; career placement assistance; computer lab; computer-assisted instruction; daycare for children of students; e-mail services; employment services for current students; housing assistance; interactive nursing skills videos; Internet; learning resource lab; library services; nursing audiovisuals; placement services for program completers; remedial services; resume preparation assistance; skills, simulation, or other laboratory; tutoring.
**Library Facilities** 369,101 volumes (1,100 in health, 500 in nursing); 27,840 periodical subscriptions (120 health-care related).

### BACCALAUREATE PROGRAMS

**Degree** BS
**Available Programs** Generic Baccalaureate; RN Baccalaureate.
**Study Options** Full-time and part-time.
**Program Entrance Requirements** Minimum overall college GPA of 2.5, transcript of college record, CPR certification, health exam, high school transcript, immunizations, minimum GPA in nursing prerequisites, professional liability insurance/malpractice insurance, prerequisite course work. Transfer students are accepted. *Application deadline:* 5/1 (fall), 12/1 (spring).
**Advanced Placement** Credit by examination available. Credit given for nursing courses completed elsewhere dependent upon specific evaluations.
**Expenses (2013–14)** *Tuition, state resident:* full-time $3117; part-time $260 per credit. *Tuition, nonresident:* full-time $7487; part-time $624 per credit. *International tuition:* $7487 full-time. *Room and board:* room only: $6120 per academic year. *Required fees:* full-time $461; part-time $230 per credit.
**Financial Aid** 60% of baccalaureate students in nursing programs received some form of financial aid in 2012–13.

Contact Ms. Joanne Bauman, Nursing Advisor, Department of Nursing, Indiana University–Purdue University Fort Wayne, 2101 East Coliseum Boulevard, Fort Wayne, IN 46805. *Telephone:* 260-481-6282. *Fax:* 260-481-6482. *E-mail:* baumanj@ipfw.edu.

## GRADUATE PROGRAMS

**Expenses (2013–14)** *Tuition, state resident:* part-time $325 per credit hour. *Tuition, nonresident:* part-time $325 per credit hour.
**Financial Aid** 52% of graduate students in nursing programs received some form of financial aid in 2012–13.
**Contact** Dr. Deb Poling, Director of Graduate Nursing Programs, Department of Nursing, Indiana University–Purdue University Fort Wayne, 2101 East Coliseum Boulevard, Fort Wayne, IN 46805. *Telephone:* 260-481-6276. *Fax:* 260-481-6276. *E-mail:* polingd@ipfw.edu.

### MASTER'S DEGREE PROGRAM

**Degree** MS
**Available Programs** Master's.
**Concentrations Available** Nursing administration; nursing education. *Nurse practitioner programs in:* adult health, primary care,women's health.
**Study Options** Part-time.
**Online Degree Options** Yes.
**Program Entrance Requirements** Computer literacy, minimum overall college GPA of 3.0, transcript of college record, CPR certification, immunizations, 3 letters of recommendation, nursing research course, physical assessment course, professional liability insurance/malpractice insurance, prerequisite course work, resume, statistics course. *Application deadline:* 6/30 (fall), 11/15 (spring), 4/1 (summer). *Application fee:* $40.
**Advanced Placement** Credit by examination available. Credit given for nursing courses completed elsewhere dependent upon specific evaluations.
**Degree Requirements** 46 total credit hours, thesis or project.

# Indiana University–Purdue University Indianapolis

**School of Nursing**
**Indianapolis, Indiana**

***http://www.nursing.iupui.edu/***
Founded in 1969

**DEGREES • BSN • MSN • PHD**
**Nursing Program Faculty** 182 (39% with doctorates).
**Baccalaureate Enrollment** 1,261 **Women** 88% **Men** 12% **Minority** 11% **International** 3% **Part-time** 20%
**Graduate Enrollment** 437 **Women** 93% **Men** 7% **Minority** 17% **International** 3% **Part-time** 86%
**Distance Learning Courses** Available.
**Nursing Student Activities** Sigma Theta Tau, Student Nurses' Association, nursing club.
**Nursing Student Resources** Academic advising; academic or career counseling; assistance for students with disabilities; bookstore; campus computer network; career placement assistance; computer lab; computer-assisted instruction; e-mail services; employment services for current students; externships; housing assistance; interactive nursing skills videos; Internet; learning resource lab; library services; nursing audiovisuals; other; paid internships; remedial services; resume preparation assistance; skills, simulation, or other laboratory; tutoring; unpaid internships.
**Library Facilities** 1.7 million volumes (318,211 in health, 8,258 in nursing); 1,951 periodical subscriptions health-care related.

## BACCALAUREATE PROGRAMS

**Degree** BSN
**Available Programs** ADN to Baccalaureate; Accelerated Baccalaureate for Second Degree; Generic Baccalaureate; RN Baccalaureate.
**Site Options** Columbus, IN; Bloomington, IN.
**Study Options** Full-time.
**Online Degree Options** Yes.
**Program Entrance Requirements** Minimum overall college GPA of 2.7, transcript of college record, CPR certification, health insurance, immunizations, minimum GPA in nursing prerequisites of 3.0, prerequisite course work. Transfer students are accepted. *Application deadline:* 3/15 (fall), 9/15 (spring).
**Advanced Placement** Credit by examination available.
**Expenses (2013–14)** *Tuition, state resident:* full-time $4664; part-time $258 per credit hour. *Tuition, nonresident:* full-time $12,990; part-time $952 per credit hour. *Room and board:* $8534; room only: $4042 per academic year. *Required fees:* full-time $1564; part-time $782 per term.
**Financial Aid** 75% of baccalaureate students in nursing programs received some form of financial aid in 2012–13.
**Contact** Dr. Susan Hendricks, PhD, Associate Dean for Undergraduate Programs, School of Nursing, Indiana University–Purdue University Indianapolis, 1111 Middle Drive, Indianapolis, IN 46202. *Telephone:* 317-274-2806. *Fax:* 317-274-2996. *E-mail:* nursing@iupui.edu.

## GRADUATE PROGRAMS

**Expenses (2013–14)** *Tuition, state resident:* full-time $8086; part-time $479 per credit hour. *Tuition, nonresident:* full-time $19,383; part-time $1421 per credit hour. *Room and board:* $8534; room only: $4042 per academic year. *Required fees:* full-time $2335; part-time $200 per credit; part-time $1006 per term.
**Financial Aid** 75% of graduate students in nursing programs received some form of financial aid in 2012–13. 9 fellowships with full tuition reimbursements available (averaging $7,039 per year), 7 teaching assistantships with full tuition reimbursements available (averaging $5,300 per year) were awarded; research assistantships with full tuition reimbursements available, Federal Work-Study, institutionally sponsored loans, scholarships, and tuition waivers (full) also available. Aid available to part-time students. *Financial aid application deadline:* 5/1.
**Contact** Dr. Patricia R. Ebright, PhD, Associate Dean for Graduate Programs, School of Nursing, Indiana University–Purdue University Indianapolis, 1111 Middle Drive, Indianapolis, IN 46202. *Telephone:* 317-274-3115. *Fax:* 317-274-2996. *E-mail:* nursing@iupui.edu.

### MASTER'S DEGREE PROGRAM

**Degree** MSN
**Available Programs** Master's; RN to Master's.
**Concentrations Available** Nursing administration; nursing education. *Clinical nurse specialist programs in:* acute care, adult health, critical care, gerontology, medical-surgical, oncology. *Nurse practitioner programs in:* acute care, adult health, family health, pediatric, psychiatric/mental health.
**Study Options** Full-time and part-time.
**Online Degree Options** Yes.
**Program Entrance Requirements** Clinical experience, computer literacy, minimum overall college GPA of 3.0, transcript of college record, CPR certification, written essay, immunizations, interview, 3 letters of recommendation, resume, statistics course. *Application deadline:* 9/15 (fall), 2/15 (spring). *Application fee:* $60.
**Advanced Placement** Credit given for nursing courses completed elsewhere dependent upon specific evaluations.
**Degree Requirements** 42 total credit hours, thesis or project.

### POST-MASTER'S PROGRAM

**Areas of Study** Nursing administration; nursing education; nursing informatics. *Clinical nurse specialist programs in:* acute care, adult health, critical care, gerontology, medical-surgical, oncology. *Nurse practitioner programs in:* acute care, adult health, family health, pediatric, psychiatric/mental health.

### DOCTORAL DEGREE PROGRAM

**Degree** PhD
**Available Programs** Doctorate; Post-Baccalaureate Doctorate.
**Areas of Study** Aging, bio-behavioral research, faculty preparation, family health, health policy, health promotion/disease prevention, health-care systems, human health and illness, information systems, nursing administration, nursing education, nursing policy, nursing research, nursing science, oncology.
**Program Entrance Requirements** Minimum overall college GPA of 3.0, interview by faculty committee, 3 letters of recommendation, statistics course, vita, writing sample, GRE General Test.
**Degree Requirements** 90 total credit hours, dissertation, oral exam, written exam, residency.

### POSTDOCTORAL PROGRAM

**Areas of Study** Adolescent health, cancer care, chronic illness, family health, health promotion/disease prevention, individualized study, nursing informatics, nursing research, nursing science.
**Postdoctoral Program Contact** Dr. Michael Weaver, PhD, Center for Academic Affairs, School of Nursing, Indiana University–Purdue University Indianapolis, 1111 Middle Drive, Indianapolis, IN 46202. *Telephone:* 317-274-2806. *Fax:* 317-274-2996. *E-mail:* nursing@iupui.edu.

## CONTINUING EDUCATION PROGRAM

**Contact** Ms. Lisa D. Wagnes, RN, Assistant Dean, Center for Professional Development and Lifelong Learning, School of Nursing, Indiana University–Purdue University Indianapolis, 1111 Middle Drive, Indianapolis, IN 46202. *Telephone:* 317-274-7779. *Fax:* 317-274-0012. *E-mail:* lwagnes@iu.edu.

# Indiana University South Bend

### College of Health Sciences
### South Bend, Indiana

***http://www.iusb.edu/nursing/***
Founded in 1922

**DEGREES • BSN • MSN**
**Nursing Program Faculty** 24 (30% with doctorates).
**Baccalaureate Enrollment** 205 **Women** 84% **Men** 16% **Minority** 11% **International** 2% **Part-time** 10%
**Graduate Enrollment** 47 **Women** 92% **Men** 8% **Minority** 20% **International** 8% **Part-time** 100%
**Distance Learning Courses** Available.
**Nursing Student Activities** Sigma Theta Tau, Student Nurses' Association.
**Nursing Student Resources** Academic advising; academic or career counseling; assistance for students with disabilities; bookstore; campus computer network; career placement assistance; computer lab; computer-assisted instruction; daycare for children of students; e-mail services; employment services for current students; externships; housing assistance; interactive nursing skills videos; Internet; learning resource lab; library services; nursing audiovisuals; placement services for program completers; resume preparation assistance; skills, simulation, or other laboratory; tutoring.
**Library Facilities** 329,139 volumes (4,300 in health, 2,300 in nursing); 145 periodical subscriptions health-care related.

## BACCALAUREATE PROGRAMS

**Degree** BSN
**Available Programs** Accelerated Baccalaureate for Second Degree; Generic Baccalaureate; RN Baccalaureate.
**Study Options** Full-time and part-time.
**Program Entrance Requirements** Minimum overall college GPA of 2.5, transcript of college record, CPR certification, written essay, health exam, high school biology, high school chemistry, high school transcript, immunizations, minimum high school GPA of 2.0, minimum high school rank 50%, minimum GPA in nursing prerequisites of 2.7, prerequisite course work. Transfer students are accepted. *Application deadline:* 3/1 (fall), 10/1 (spring), 2/1 (summer).
**Advanced Placement** Credit given for nursing courses completed elsewhere dependent upon specific evaluations.
**Expenses (2013–14)** *Tuition, state resident:* full-time $6227; part-time $208 per credit hour. *Tuition, nonresident:* full-time $17,190; part-time $573 per credit hour. *International tuition:* $17,190 full-time. *Room and board:* $6000 per academic year. *Required fees:* full-time $1665; part-time $125 per credit.
**Financial Aid** 65% of baccalaureate students in nursing programs received some form of financial aid in 2012–13.
**Contact** Office of Student Services, College of Health Sciences, Indiana University South Bend, 1700 Mishawaka Avenue, PO Box 7111, South Bend, IN 46634-7111. *Telephone:* 574-520-4571. *Fax:* 574-520-4461. *E-mail:* nursing@iusb.edu.

## GRADUATE PROGRAMS

**Expenses (2013–14)** *Tuition, state resident:* full-time $6030; part-time $335 per credit hour. *Tuition, nonresident:* full-time $17,586; part-time $977 per credit hour. *International tuition:* $23,448 full-time. *Required fees:* full-time $693; part-time $38 per credit.
**Financial Aid** 30% of graduate students in nursing programs received some form of financial aid in 2012–13.
**Contact** Dr. Sue Anderson, Director of Graduate Program in Nursing, College of Health Sciences, Indiana University South Bend, 1700 Mishawaka Avenue, PO Box 7111, South Bend, IN 46634-7111. *Telephone:* 574-520-4369. *Fax:* 574-520-4461. *E-mail:* sanderso@iusb.edu.

### MASTER'S DEGREE PROGRAM

**Degree** MSN
**Available Programs** Master's.
**Concentrations Available** *Nurse practitioner programs in:* family health.
**Study Options** Part-time.
**Program Entrance Requirements** Clinical experience, computer literacy, minimum overall college GPA of 3.0, transcript of college record, CPR certification, written essay, immunizations, 3 letters of recommendation, nursing research course, physical assessment course, statistics course. *Application deadline:* 4/1 (fall). *Application fee:* $40.
**Advanced Placement** Credit given for nursing courses completed elsewhere dependent upon specific evaluations.
**Degree Requirements** 42 total credit hours, thesis or project.

# Indiana University Southeast

### Division of Nursing
### New Albany, Indiana

***http://www.ius.edu/nursing/***
Founded in 1941

**DEGREE • BSN**
**Nursing Program Faculty** 23 (27% with doctorates).
**Baccalaureate Enrollment** 155 **Women** 91% **Men** 9% **Minority** 2% **International** 2%
**Distance Learning Courses** Available.
**Nursing Student Activities** Sigma Theta Tau, Student Nurses' Association.
**Nursing Student Resources** Academic advising; academic or career counseling; assistance for students with disabilities; bookstore; campus computer network; career placement assistance; computer lab; computer-assisted instruction; daycare for children of students; e-mail services; externships; housing assistance; interactive nursing skills videos; Internet; learning resource lab; library services; nursing audiovisuals; paid internships; remedial services; resume preparation assistance; skills, simulation, or other laboratory; tutoring.
**Library Facilities** 375,198 volumes (35 in health, 15 in nursing); 35 periodical subscriptions health-care related.

## BACCALAUREATE PROGRAMS

**Degree** BSN
**Available Programs** Generic Baccalaureate; RN Baccalaureate.
**Study Options** Full-time.
**Program Entrance Requirements** Transcript of college record, CPR certification, immunizations, minimum GPA in nursing prerequisites of 2.5, prerequisite course work. Transfer students are accepted.
**Advanced Placement** Credit given for nursing courses completed elsewhere dependent upon specific evaluations.
**Expenses (2013–14)** *Tuition, state resident:* part-time $204 per credit hour. *Tuition, nonresident:* part-time $573 per credit hour. *Room and board:* room only: $6185 per academic year.
**Financial Aid** 60% of baccalaureate students in nursing programs received some form of financial aid in 2012–13.
**Contact** Ms. Brenda Hackett, Nursing Advisor, Division of Nursing, Indiana University Southeast, 4201 Grant Line Road, Life Sciences Building, Room 276, New Albany, IN 47150-6405. *Telephone:* 812-941-2283. *Fax:* 812-941-2687. *E-mail:* bhackett@ius.edu.

# Indiana Wesleyan University

### School of Nursing
### Marion, Indiana

***http://www.indwes.edu/Academics/School-of-Nursing/***
Founded in 1920

**DEGREES • BSN • MSN**
**Nursing Program Faculty** 210 (21% with doctorates).
**Baccalaureate Enrollment** 1,581 **Women** 93% **Men** 7% **Minority** 16% **Part-time** 9%
**Graduate Enrollment** 427 **Women** 95% **Men** 5% **Minority** 13% **Part-time** 10%
**Distance Learning Courses** Available.
**Nursing Student Activities** Nursing Honor Society, Sigma Theta Tau, Student Nurses' Association, nursing club.
**Nursing Student Resources** Academic advising; academic or career counseling; assistance for students with disabilities; bookstore; campus computer network; career placement assistance; computer lab; computer-assisted instruction; e-mail services; housing assistance; interactive

nursing skills videos; Internet; learning resource lab; library services; nursing audiovisuals; remedial services; resume preparation assistance; skills, simulation, or other laboratory; tutoring.
**Library Facilities** 248,819 volumes (7,142 in health, 5,672 in nursing); 101,452 periodical subscriptions (160 health-care related).

## BACCALAUREATE PROGRAMS

**Degree** BSN
**Available Programs** Accelerated Baccalaureate for Second Degree; Generic Baccalaureate; RN Baccalaureate.
**Site Options** Lexington, KY; Merrillville, IN; Louisville, KY.
**Study Options** Full-time and part-time.
**Program Entrance Requirements** Minimum overall college GPA of 2.75, transcript of college record, CPR certification, written essay, health exam, health insurance, high school biology, high school chemistry, high school foreign language, 3 years high school math, 3 years high school science, high school transcript, immunizations, minimum high school GPA of 2.8, minimum GPA in nursing prerequisites of 2.75, prerequisite course work. Transfer students are accepted. *Application deadline:* 5/30 (fall), 12/1 (spring).
**Advanced Placement** Credit given for nursing courses completed elsewhere dependent upon specific evaluations.
**Contact** *Telephone:* 765-677-2268. *Fax:* 765-677-2284.

## GRADUATE PROGRAMS

**Contact** *Telephone:* 765-677-2045. *Fax:* 765-677-2380.

### MASTER'S DEGREE PROGRAM

**Degree** MSN
**Available Programs** Master's.
**Concentrations Available** Nursing administration; nursing education. *Nurse practitioner programs in:* family health.
**Site Options** Lexington, KY; Merrillville, IN; Louisville, KY.
**Study Options** Full-time and part-time.
**Online Degree Options** Yes.
**Program Entrance Requirements** Clinical experience, minimum overall college GPA of 3.0, transcript of college record, written essay, immunizations, interview, 3 letters of recommendation, nursing research course, physical assessment course, resume, statistics course.
**Advanced Placement** Credit given for nursing courses completed elsewhere dependent upon specific evaluations.
**Degree Requirements** 41 total credit hours, thesis or project.

### POST-MASTER'S PROGRAM

**Areas of Study** Nursing administration; nursing education. *Nurse practitioner programs in:* family health.

# Marian University

## School of Nursing
## Indianapolis, Indiana

*http://www.marian.edu/Nursing/Pages/default.aspx*
Founded in 1851

**DEGREE • BSN**
**Nursing Program Faculty** 35
**Baccalaureate Enrollment** 480 **Women** 95% **Men** 5% **Minority** 15% **International** 2% **Part-time** 10%
**Distance Learning Courses** Available.
**Nursing Student Activities** Nursing Honor Society, Sigma Theta Tau, Student Nurses' Association.
**Nursing Student Resources** Academic advising; academic or career counseling; assistance for students with disabilities; bookstore; campus computer network; career placement assistance; computer lab; computer-assisted instruction; e-mail services; employment services for current students; interactive nursing skills videos; Internet; learning resource lab; library services; nursing audiovisuals; remedial services; resume preparation assistance; skills, simulation, or other laboratory; tutoring; unpaid internships.
**Library Facilities** 130,000 volumes (3,250 in health, 2,000 in nursing); 337 periodical subscriptions (116 health-care related).

## BACCALAUREATE PROGRAMS

**Degree** BSN
**Available Programs** Accelerated Baccalaureate; Accelerated Baccalaureate for Second Degree; Accelerated RN Baccalaureate; Baccalaureate for Second Degree; Generic Baccalaureate; RN Baccalaureate.
**Site Options** Indianapolis, IN.
**Study Options** Full-time and part-time.
**Online Degree Options** Yes.
**Program Entrance Requirements** Minimum overall college GPA of 2.8, transcript of college record, CPR certification, health exam, health insurance, high school biology, high school chemistry, high school transcript, immunizations, minimum high school GPA of 2.3, minimum GPA in nursing prerequisites of 2.8, prerequisite course work. Transfer students are accepted. *Application deadline:* 7/15 (fall), 11/15 (winter), 12/15 (spring), 4/15 (summer). *Application fee:* $50.
**Expenses (2012–13)** *Tuition:* full-time $26,000; part-time $1200 per credit. *Required fees:* full-time $300; part-time $300 per term.
**Financial Aid** 97% of baccalaureate students in nursing programs received some form of financial aid in 2011–12.
**Contact** Ms. Marsha Schuler, Academic Advisor, School of Nursing, Marian University, 3200 Cold Spring Road, Indianapolis, IN 46222-1997. *Telephone:* 317-955-6157. *Fax:* 317-955-6135. *E-mail:* mschuler@marian.edu.

## CONTINUING EDUCATION PROGRAM

**Contact** Jodie Freeland, Assistant Dean, Associate Professor, School of Nursing, Marian University, 3200 Cold Spring Road, Indianapolis, IN 46222. *Telephone:* 317-955-6145. *Fax:* 317-955-6135. *E-mail:* freeland@marian.edu.

# Purdue University

## School of Nursing
## West Lafayette, Indiana

*http://www.nursing.purdue.edu/*
Founded in 1869

**DEGREES • BS • DNP • MS**
**Nursing Program Faculty** 60 (15% with doctorates).
**Baccalaureate Enrollment** 552 **Women** 94% **Men** 6% **Minority** 3% **International** .5% **Part-time** .06%
**Graduate Enrollment** 48 **Women** 96% **Men** 4% **Minority** 2% **Part-time** 50%
**Nursing Student Activities** Sigma Theta Tau, Student Nurses' Association.
**Nursing Student Resources** Academic advising; academic or career counseling; assistance for students with disabilities; bookstore; campus computer network; career placement assistance; computer lab; computer-assisted instruction; e-mail services; interactive nursing skills videos; Internet; learning resource lab; library services; nursing audiovisuals; remedial services; resume preparation assistance; skills, simulation, or other laboratory; tutoring.
**Library Facilities** 3.6 million volumes (200,000 in health, 10,000 in nursing); 1,000 periodical subscriptions health-care related.

## BACCALAUREATE PROGRAMS

**Degree** BS
**Available Programs** ADN to Baccalaureate; Accelerated Baccalaureate for Second Degree; Baccalaureate for Second Degree; Generic Baccalaureate; RN Baccalaureate.
**Site Options** Indianapolis, IN.
**Study Options** Full-time and part-time.
**Program Entrance Requirements** Transcript of college record, CPR certification, health exam, health insurance, high school biology, high school chemistry, high school foreign language, 3 years high school math, 3 years high school science, high school transcript, immunizations, letters of recommendation, minimum high school GPA of 3.0. Transfer students are accepted.
**Advanced Placement** Credit by examination available. Credit given for nursing courses completed elsewhere dependent upon specific evaluations.
**Contact** *Telephone:* 765-494-1776. *Fax:* 765-494-0544.

## GRADUATE PROGRAMS

**Contact** *Telephone:* 765-494-4015. *Fax:* 765-496-1800.

### MASTER'S DEGREE PROGRAM

**Degree** MS
**Available Programs** Master's.
**Concentrations Available** *Nurse practitioner programs in:* adult health, pediatric.
**Study Options** Full-time and part-time.

**Program Entrance Requirements** Clinical experience, computer literacy, minimum overall college GPA of 3.0, transcript of college record, CPR certification, written essay, interview, 3 letters of recommendation, professional liability insurance/malpractice insurance, prerequisite course work, resume, statistics course.
**Advanced Placement** Credit given for nursing courses completed elsewhere dependent upon specific evaluations.
**Degree Requirements** 46 total credit hours, thesis or project.

### POST-MASTER'S PROGRAM
**Areas of Study** *Nurse practitioner programs in:* adult health, pediatric.

### DOCTORAL DEGREE PROGRAM
**Degree** DNP
**Available Programs** Doctorate.
**Areas of Study** Advanced practice nursing, aging, biology of health and illness, clinical practice, critical care, ethics, gerontology, health policy, health promotion/disease prevention, health-care systems, illness and transition, individualized study, information systems, nursing administration, nursing education, nursing policy, nursing research, nursing science, oncology, urban health,women's health.
**Program Entrance Requirements** Clinical experience, minimum overall college GPA of 3.0, interview by faculty committee, interview, letters of recommendation, MSN or equivalent, statistics course, vita, writing sample.
**Degree Requirements** 83 total credit hours, oral exam, residency.

### CONTINUING EDUCATION PROGRAM
**Contact** *Telephone:* 765-494-4030. *Fax:* 765-494-6339.

## Purdue University Calumet
### School of Nursing
### Hammond, Indiana

*http://webs.purduecal.edu/nursing/*
Founded in 1951

**DEGREES • BS • MS**
**Nursing Program Faculty** 39 (33% with doctorates).
**Baccalaureate Enrollment** 621 **Women** 84.5% **Men** 15.5% **Minority** 16.7% **Part-time** 61.5%
**Graduate Enrollment** 127 **Women** 93% **Men** 7% **Minority** 23% **International** 3% **Part-time** 94%
**Distance Learning Courses** Available.
**Nursing Student Activities** Sigma Theta Tau, Student Nurses' Association, nursing club.
**Nursing Student Resources** Academic advising; academic or career counseling; assistance for students with disabilities; bookstore; campus computer network; career placement assistance; computer lab; computer-assisted instruction; daycare for children of students; e-mail services; employment services for current students; externships; housing assistance; interactive nursing skills videos; Internet; learning resource lab; library services; nursing audiovisuals; other; paid internships; placement services for program completers; remedial services; resume preparation assistance; skills, simulation, or other laboratory; tutoring; unpaid internships.
**Library Facilities** 287,564 volumes (7,900 in health, 1,140 in nursing); 6,688 periodical subscriptions (610 health-care related).

### BACCALAUREATE PROGRAMS
**Degree** BS
**Available Programs** Accelerated Baccalaureate for Second Degree; Accelerated RN Baccalaureate; Generic Baccalaureate; LPN to Baccalaureate.
**Study Options** Full-time and part-time.
**Online Degree Options** Yes.
**Program Entrance Requirements** Minimum overall college GPA of 2.5, transcript of college record, CPR certification, health exam, high school biology, high school chemistry, 3 years high school math, 4 years high school science, high school transcript, immunizations, minimum GPA in nursing prerequisites of 2.0, prerequisite course work. Transfer students are accepted. *Application deadline:* 2/1 (fall).
**Advanced Placement** Credit by examination available. Credit given for nursing courses completed elsewhere dependent upon specific evaluations.
**Contact** *Telephone:* 219-989-2859. *Fax:* 219-989-2848.

### GRADUATE PROGRAMS
**Contact** *Telephone:* 219-989-2815. *Fax:* 219-989-2848.

### MASTER'S DEGREE PROGRAM
**Degree** MS
**Available Programs** Master's.
**Concentrations Available** Nursing administration. *Clinical nurse specialist programs in:* adult health, critical care. *Nurse practitioner programs in:* family health.
**Study Options** Full-time and part-time.
**Online Degree Options** Yes.
**Program Entrance Requirements** Minimum overall college GPA of 3.0, transcript of college record, written essay, 3 letters of recommendation, physical assessment course, resume, statistics course. *Application deadline:* 2/15 (fall), 9/15 (spring), 2/15 (summer). *Application fee:* $55.
**Advanced Placement** Credit given for nursing courses completed elsewhere dependent upon specific evaluations.
**Degree Requirements** 45 total credit hours.

### POST-MASTER'S PROGRAM
**Areas of Study** Nursing education. *Clinical nurse specialist programs in:* adult health, critical care. *Nurse practitioner programs in:* family health.

## Purdue University North Central
### Department of Nursing
### Westville, Indiana

*https://www.pnc.edu/nu/*
Founded in 1967

**DEGREE • BS**
**Nursing Program Faculty** 34 (35% with doctorates).
**Baccalaureate Enrollment** 150 **Women** 97% **Men** 3% **Minority** 12% **Part-time** 87%
**Distance Learning Courses** Available.
**Nursing Student Activities** Nursing Honor Society, Student Nurses' Association.
**Nursing Student Resources** Academic advising; academic or career counseling; assistance for students with disabilities; bookstore; campus computer network; career placement assistance; computer lab; computer-assisted instruction; daycare for children of students; e-mail services; interactive nursing skills videos; Internet; learning resource lab; library services; nursing audiovisuals; placement services for program completers; resume preparation assistance; skills, simulation, or other laboratory; tutoring.
**Library Facilities** 87,848 volumes (1,100 in health, 560 in nursing); 42,367 periodical subscriptions (229 health-care related).

### BACCALAUREATE PROGRAMS
**Degree** BS
**Available Programs** ADN to Baccalaureate; Accelerated Baccalaureate; Accelerated Baccalaureate for Second Degree; Baccalaureate for Second Degree; LPN to Baccalaureate; RN Baccalaureate.
**Site Options** Valparaiso, IN.
**Study Options** Full-time and part-time.
**Program Entrance Requirements** Minimum overall college GPA of 2.5, transcript of college record, CPR certification, health exam, health insurance, high school biology, high school chemistry, 3 years high school math, 3 years high school science, high school transcript, immunizations, minimum high school GPA of 2.5, minimum high school rank 50%, minimum GPA in nursing prerequisites of 2.5, professional liability insurance/malpractice insurance, prerequisite course work. Transfer students are accepted. *Application deadline:* 1/16 (fall), 8/16 (spring).
**Advanced Placement** Credit by examination available. Credit given for nursing courses completed elsewhere dependent upon specific evaluations.
**Expenses (2012–13)** *Tuition, state resident:* part-time $215 per credit hour. *Tuition, nonresident:* part-time $539 per credit hour.
**Financial Aid** 44% of baccalaureate students in nursing programs received some form of financial aid in 2011–12.
**Contact** Ms. Nicole Hartford, Professional Academic Advisor for Nursing, Department of Nursing, Purdue University North Central, 1401 South U.S. Highway 421, Westville, IN 46391. *Telephone:* 219-785-5439. *Fax:* 219-785-5495. *E-mail:* nursing@pnc.edu.

# Saint Joseph's College
## St. Elizabeth School of Nursing
## Rensselaer, Indiana

*http://www.steson.org*
Founded in 1889

### DEGREE • BSN

**Nursing Program Faculty** 30 (.07% with doctorates).
**Baccalaureate Enrollment** 267 **Women** 96% **Men** 4% **Minority** 2% **International** 1% **Part-time** 2%
**Distance Learning Courses** Available.
**Nursing Student Activities** Student Nurses' Association.
**Nursing Student Resources** Academic advising; assistance for students with disabilities; campus computer network; computer lab; computer-assisted instruction; e-mail services; interactive nursing skills videos; Internet; learning resource lab; library services; nursing audiovisuals; remedial services; resume preparation assistance; skills, simulation, or other laboratory; tutoring.
**Library Facilities** 127,984 volumes (900 in health, 900 in nursing); 13,262 periodical subscriptions (50 health-care related).

### BACCALAUREATE PROGRAMS

**Degree** BSN
**Available Programs** Accelerated Baccalaureate for Second Degree; LPN to RN Baccalaureate; RN Baccalaureate.
**Site Options** Lafayette, IN.
**Study Options** Full-time and part-time.
**Program Entrance Requirements** Minimum overall college GPA of 2.0, transcript of college record, CPR certification, written essay, health exam, health insurance, high school biology, high school chemistry, 3 years high school math, 2 years high school science, high school transcript, immunizations, 3 letters of recommendation, minimum high school GPA of 2.0, minimum high school rank 51%. Transfer students are accepted. *Application deadline:* Applications may be processed on a rolling basis for some programs. *Application fee:* $25.
**Advanced Placement** Credit given for nursing courses completed elsewhere dependent upon specific evaluations.
**Expenses (2013–14)** *Tuition:* full-time $16,880; part-time $495 per credit hour. *Room and board:* $8440 per academic year. *Required fees:* full-time $800.
**Financial Aid** 98% of baccalaureate students in nursing programs received some form of financial aid in 2012–13. *Gift aid (need-based):* Federal Pell, FSEOG, state, private, college/university gift aid from institutional funds. *Loans:* Federal Direct (Subsidized and Unsubsidized Stafford PLUS), Perkins. *Work-study:* Federal Work-Study. *Financial aid application deadline (priority):* 3/1.
**Contact** Anita K. Reed, Coordinator of Admissions, St. Elizabeth School of Nursing, Saint Joseph's College, 1508 Tippecanoe Street, Lafayette, IN 47904. *Telephone:* 765-423-6285. *Fax:* 765-423-6383. *E-mail:* anita.reed@franciscanalliance.org.

# Saint Mary's College
## Department of Nursing
## Notre Dame, Indiana

*http://www3.saintmarys.edu/nursing*
Founded in 1844

### DEGREE • BS

**Nursing Program Faculty** 20 (25% with doctorates).
**Baccalaureate Enrollment** 258 **Women** 100% **Minority** 5%
**Distance Learning Courses** Available.
**Nursing Student Activities** Nursing Honor Society, Sigma Theta Tau, Student Nurses' Association.
**Nursing Student Resources** Academic advising; academic or career counseling; assistance for students with disabilities; bookstore; campus computer network; career placement assistance; computer lab; computer-assisted instruction; daycare for children of students; e-mail services; employment services for current students; externships; interactive nursing skills videos; Internet; learning resource lab; library services; nursing audiovisuals; paid internships; placement services for program completers; remedial services; resume preparation assistance; skills, simulation, or other laboratory; tutoring; unpaid internships.
**Library Facilities** 244,651 volumes (9,787 in health, 5,149 in nursing); 30,704 periodical subscriptions (70 health-care related).

### BACCALAUREATE PROGRAMS

**Degree** BS
**Available Programs** Generic Baccalaureate.
**Site Options** Goshen, IN; South Bend, IN.
**Study Options** Full-time.
**Program Entrance Requirements** Minimum overall college GPA of 3.0, transcript of college record, CPR certification, written essay, health exam, high school foreign language, 3 years high school math, 2 years high school science, high school transcript, immunizations, 2 letters of recommendation, minimum GPA in nursing prerequisites of 2.75. Transfer students are accepted. *Application deadline:* Applications may be processed on a rolling basis for some programs. *Application fee:* $30.
**Advanced Placement** Credit given for nursing courses completed elsewhere dependent upon specific evaluations.
**Expenses (2013–14)** *Tuition:* full-time $33,860; part-time $1340 per credit. *Room and board:* $10,600; room only: $6600 per academic year. *Required fees:* full-time $940.
**Financial Aid** 75% of baccalaureate students in nursing programs received some form of financial aid in 2012–13. *Gift aid (need-based):* Federal Pell, FSEOG, state, private, college/university gift aid from institutional funds. *Loans:* Federal Direct (Subsidized and Unsubsidized Stafford PLUS), Perkins. *Work-study:* Federal Work-Study, part-time campus jobs. *Financial aid application deadline:* 3/1(priority: 3/1).
**Contact** Mrs. Mona Bowe, Vice President for Enrollment Management, Department of Nursing, Saint Mary's College, 124 LeMans, Notre Dame, IN 46556. *Telephone:* 574-284-4587. *Fax:* 574-284-4716. *E-mail:* mbowe@saintmarys.edu.

# University of Evansville
## Department of Nursing
## Evansville, Indiana

*http://www.evansville.edu/majors/nursing/*
Founded in 1854

### DEGREE • BSN

**Nursing Program Faculty** 11 (28% with doctorates).
**Baccalaureate Enrollment** 188 **Women** 86% **Men** 14% **Minority** 4% **International** 1% **Part-time** 20%
**Distance Learning Courses** Available.
**Nursing Student Activities** Sigma Theta Tau, Student Nurses' Association.
**Nursing Student Resources** Academic advising; academic or career counseling; assistance for students with disabilities; bookstore; campus computer network; career placement assistance; computer lab; computer-assisted instruction; e-mail services; employment services for current students; externships; housing assistance; interactive nursing skills videos; Internet; learning resource lab; library services; nursing audiovisuals; paid internships; placement services for program completers; remedial services; resume preparation assistance; skills, simulation, or other laboratory; tutoring; unpaid internships.
**Library Facilities** 284,157 volumes (11,000 in nursing); 169 periodical subscriptions (155 health-care related).

### BACCALAUREATE PROGRAMS

**Degree** BSN
**Available Programs** Generic Baccalaureate; RN Baccalaureate.
**Site Options** Henderson, KY.
**Study Options** Full-time and part-time.
**Program Entrance Requirements** CPR certification, health exam, health insurance, high school chemistry, 3 years high school math, 2 years high school science, high school transcript, immunizations, minimum high school rank 67%, professional liability insurance/malpractice insurance. Transfer students are accepted. *Application deadline:* Applications may be processed on a rolling basis for some programs. *Application fee:* $35.
**Advanced Placement** Credit given for nursing courses completed elsewhere dependent upon specific evaluations.
**Expenses (2012–13)** *Tuition:* full-time $30,556; part-time $830 per credit hour. *International tuition:* $30,556 full-time. *Room and board:* $10,000 per academic year. *Required fees:* full-time $840; part-time $50 per term.
**Financial Aid** 100% of baccalaureate students in nursing programs received some form of financial aid in 2011–12.
**Contact** Dr. Amy M. Hall, Chair/Professor of Nursing, Department of Nursing, University of Evansville, 1800 Lincoln Avenue, Evansville, IN

47722. *Telephone:* 812-488-2414. *Fax:* 812-488-2717. *E-mail:* ah169@evansville.edu.

# University of Indianapolis

## School of Nursing
## Indianapolis, Indiana

***http://www.uindy.edu/***
Founded in 1902

**DEGREES • BSN • DNP • MSN**

**Nursing Program Faculty** 39 (50% with doctorates).
**Baccalaureate Enrollment** 475 **Women** 92.9% **Men** 7.1% **Minority** 14% **Part-time** 50%
**Graduate Enrollment** 297 **Women** 97.2% **Men** 2.8% **Minority** 15.5% **Part-time** 98%
**Distance Learning Courses** Available.
**Nursing Student Activities** Nursing Honor Society, Sigma Theta Tau, Student Nurses' Association.
**Nursing Student Resources** Academic advising; academic or career counseling; assistance for students with disabilities; bookstore; campus computer network; career placement assistance; computer lab; computer-assisted instruction; e-mail services; employment services for current students; externships; housing assistance; interactive nursing skills videos; Internet; learning resource lab; library services; nursing audiovisuals; other; paid internships; placement services for program completers; remedial services; resume preparation assistance; skills, simulation, or other laboratory; tutoring; unpaid internships.
**Library Facilities** 173,363 volumes (15,600 in health, 1,000 in nursing); 1,015 periodical subscriptions (600 health-care related).

### BACCALAUREATE PROGRAMS

**Degree** BSN
**Available Programs** ADN to Baccalaureate; Accelerated Baccalaureate for Second Degree; Generic Baccalaureate; RN Baccalaureate.
**Site Options** Indianapolis, IN.
**Study Options** Full-time and part-time.
**Online Degree Options** Yes.
**Program Entrance Requirements** Minimum overall college GPA of 2.82, transcript of college record, CPR certification, health exam, health insurance, high school biology, high school chemistry, 2 years high school math, 2 years high school science, high school transcript, immunizations, minimum GPA in nursing prerequisites of 2.0, prerequisite course work. Transfer students are accepted. *Application deadline:* 4/15 (fall), 10/15 (winter). *Application fee:* $25.
**Advanced Placement** Credit by examination available. Credit given for nursing courses completed elsewhere dependent upon specific evaluations.
**Expenses (2013–14)** *Tuition:* full-time $24,420. *Room and board:* $8790 per academic year. *Required fees:* full-time $300.
**Financial Aid** 98% of baccalaureate students in nursing programs received some form of financial aid in 2012–13.
**Contact** Mrs. Cheryl Conces, Undergraduate Program Director, School of Nursing, University of Indianapolis, 1400 East Hanna Avenue, Indianapolis, IN 46227-3697. *Telephone:* 317-788-3206. *Fax:* 317-788-6208. *E-mail:* cconces@uindy.edu.

### GRADUATE PROGRAMS

**Expenses (2013–14)** *Tuition:* part-time $652 per credit hour.
**Financial Aid** 90% of graduate students in nursing programs received some form of financial aid in 2012–13.
**Contact** Dr. Norma Hall, Director, Graduate Program, School of Nursing, University of Indianapolis, 1400 East Hanna Avenue, Indianapolis, IN 46227-3697. *Telephone:* 317-788-3206. *Fax:* 317-788-6208. *E-mail:* hallne@uindy.edu.

#### MASTER'S DEGREE PROGRAM

**Degree** MSN
**Available Programs** Accelerated Master's for Non-Nursing College Graduates; Master's.
**Concentrations Available** Nurse-midwifery; nursing administration; nursing education. *Nurse practitioner programs in:* adult health, family health, gerontology, neonatal health, primary care,women's health.
**Site Options** Indianapolis, IN.
**Study Options** Full-time and part-time.
**Online Degree Options** Yes.
**Program Entrance Requirements** Clinical experience, minimum overall college GPA of 3.0, transcript of college record, CPR certification, written essay, immunizations, interview, 3 letters of recommendation, nursing research course, professional liability insurance/malpractice insurance, prerequisite course work, resume, statistics course. *Application deadline:* 4/15 (fall). Applications may be processed on a rolling basis for some programs. *Application fee:* $60.
**Degree Requirements** 39 total credit hours, thesis or project, comprehensive exam.

#### POST-MASTER'S PROGRAM

**Areas of Study** Nurse-midwifery; nursing administration; nursing education. *Nurse practitioner programs in:* adult health, family health, gerontology, neonatal health, primary care,women's health.

#### DOCTORAL DEGREE PROGRAM

**Degree** DNP
**Available Programs** Doctorate.
**Areas of Study** Health-care systems.
**Online Degree Options** Yes (online only).
**Program Entrance Requirements** Clinical experience, minimum overall college GPA of 3.25, interview by faculty committee, 3 letters of recommendation, MSN or equivalent, statistics course, vita, writing sample. *Application deadline:* 4/15 (fall), 10/15 (winter). Applications may be processed on a rolling basis for some programs. *Application fee:* $60.
**Degree Requirements** 35 total credit hours, residency.

# University of Saint Francis

## Department of Nursing
## Fort Wayne, Indiana

***http://www.sf.edu/nursing***
Founded in 1890

**DEGREES • BSN • MSN**

**Nursing Program Faculty** 35 (5% with doctorates).
**Baccalaureate Enrollment** 279 **Women** 89% **Men** 11% **Minority** 10.7% **Part-time** 1.7%
**Graduate Enrollment** 102 **Women** 93% **Men** 7% **Minority** 5.8% **Part-time** 67.6%
**Distance Learning Courses** Available.
**Nursing Student Activities** Nursing Honor Society, Sigma Theta Tau, Student Nurses' Association.
**Nursing Student Resources** Academic advising; academic or career counseling; assistance for students with disabilities; bookstore; campus computer network; career placement assistance; computer lab; computer-assisted instruction; e-mail services; employment services for current students; externships; housing assistance; interactive nursing skills videos; Internet; learning resource lab; library services; nursing audiovisuals; paid internships; remedial services; resume preparation assistance; skills, simulation, or other laboratory; tutoring; unpaid internships.
**Library Facilities** 6,233 volumes in health, 3,376 volumes in nursing; 2,468 periodical subscriptions health-care related.

### BACCALAUREATE PROGRAMS

**Degree** BSN
**Available Programs** ADN to Baccalaureate; Generic Baccalaureate; RN Baccalaureate.
**Study Options** Full-time and part-time.
**Online Degree Options** Yes.
**Program Entrance Requirements** Minimum overall college GPA of 2.7, transcript of college record, CPR certification, health exam, high school biology, high school chemistry, 1 year of high school math, high school transcript, immunizations, minimum high school GPA of 2.7, minimum GPA in nursing prerequisites of 2.7, prerequisite course work. Transfer students are accepted. *Application deadline:* 7/31 (fall), 11/18 (spring). Applications may be processed on a rolling basis for some programs.
**Advanced Placement** Credit given for nursing courses completed elsewhere dependent upon specific evaluations.
**Expenses (2013–14)** *Tuition:* full-time $24,270; part-time $765 per credit hour. *International tuition:* $24,270 full-time. *Room and board:* $8312 per academic year. *Required fees:* full-time $910; part-time $22 per credit; part-time $125 per term.
**Financial Aid** 96% of baccalaureate students in nursing programs received some form of financial aid in 2012–13.

**Contact** Megan Winegarden, BSN Program Director, Department of Nursing, University of Saint Francis, 2701 Spring Street, Fort Wayne, IN 46808. *Telephone:* 260-399-7700 Ext. 8513. *Fax:* 260-399-8167. *E-mail:* mwinegarden@sf.edu.

## GRADUATE PROGRAMS

**Expenses (2013–14)** *Tuition:* part-time $805 per credit. *Required fees:* part-time $22 per credit; part-time $125 per term.

**Financial Aid** 97% of graduate students in nursing programs received some form of financial aid in 2012–13. Federal Work-Study, scholarships, tuition waivers (full and partial), and unspecified assistantships available.

**Contact** Wendy Clark, MSN Program Director, Department of Nursing, University of Saint Francis, 2701 Spring Street, Fort Wayne, IN 46808. *Telephone:* 260-399-7700 Ext. 8534. *Fax:* 260-399-8167. *E-mail:* wclark@sf.edu.

### MASTER'S DEGREE PROGRAM

**Degree** MSN
**Available Programs** Master's; Master's for Nurses with Non-Nursing Degrees.
**Concentrations Available** *Nurse practitioner programs in:* family health.
**Study Options** Full-time and part-time.
**Program Entrance Requirements** Computer literacy, minimum overall college GPA of 3.2, transcript of college record, CPR certification, written essay, immunizations, interview, 3 letters of recommendation, nursing research course, physical assessment course, resume, statistics course, GRE. *Application deadline:* 7/28 (fall), 4/14 (summer).
**Advanced Placement** Credit given for nursing courses completed elsewhere dependent upon specific evaluations.
**Degree Requirements** 48 total credit hours.

### POST-MASTER'S PROGRAM

**Areas of Study** *Nurse practitioner programs in:* family health.

# University of Southern Indiana

## College of Nursing and Health Professions
## Evansville, Indiana

***http://www.health.usi.edu/***
Founded in 1965

### DEGREES • BSN • DNP • MSN

**Nursing Program Faculty** 58 (68% with doctorates).
**Baccalaureate Enrollment** 413 **Women** 90% **Men** 10% **Minority** 5% **International** 1% **Part-time** 26%
**Graduate Enrollment** 457 **Women** 93% **Men** 7% **Minority** 8% **Part-time** 72%
**Distance Learning Courses** Available.
**Nursing Student Activities** Sigma Theta Tau, Student Nurses' Association.
**Nursing Student Resources** Academic advising; academic or career counseling; assistance for students with disabilities; bookstore; campus computer network; career placement assistance; computer lab; computer-assisted instruction; daycare for children of students; e-mail services; employment services for current students; housing assistance; interactive nursing skills videos; Internet; learning resource lab; library services; nursing audiovisuals; placement services for program completers; remedial services; resume preparation assistance; skills, simulation, or other laboratory; tutoring; unpaid internships.
**Library Facilities** 344,078 volumes (9,200 in health, 1,500 in nursing); 41,931 periodical subscriptions (2,000 health-care related).

## BACCALAUREATE PROGRAMS

**Degree** BSN
**Available Programs** Generic Baccalaureate; RN Baccalaureate.
**Study Options** Full-time.
**Online Degree Options** Yes.
**Program Entrance Requirements** Minimum overall college GPA of 3.0, transcript of college record, CPR certification, written essay, health exam, health insurance, high school transcript, immunizations, minimum GPA in nursing prerequisites of 2.0, professional liability insurance/malpractice insurance, prerequisite course work. Transfer students are accepted. *Application deadline:* 8/1 (fall).
**Advanced Placement** Credit given for nursing courses completed elsewhere dependent upon specific evaluations.
**Expenses (2013–14)** *Tuition, state resident:* full-time $6784; part-time $212 per credit hour. *Tuition, nonresident:* full-time $10,240; part-time $320 per credit hour. *International tuition:* $16,224 full-time. *Room and board:* $7680; room only: $4030 per academic year. *Required fees:* full-time $1780; part-time $55 per credit; part-time $890 per term.
**Financial Aid** 70% of baccalaureate students in nursing programs received some form of financial aid in 2012–13. *Gift aid (need-based):* Federal Pell, FSEOG, state, private, college/university gift aid from institutional funds, Federal Nursing. *Loans:* Federal Direct (Subsidized and Unsubsidized Stafford PLUS). *Work-study:* Federal Work-Study. *Financial aid application deadline:* 3/1.
**Contact** Dr. Sarah Stevens, Director of CNHP Advising Center, College of Nursing and Health Professions, University of Southern Indiana, 8600 University Boulevard, Evansville, IN 47712. *Telephone:* 812-461-5238. *Fax:* 812-465-7092. *E-mail:* sestevens@usi.edu.

## GRADUATE PROGRAMS

**Expenses (2013–14)** *Tuition, state resident:* full-time $7440; part-time $310 per credit hour. *Tuition, nonresident:* full-time $7440; part-time $310 per credit hour. *International tuition:* $14,640 full-time. *Room and board:* $7440; room only: $4030 per academic year. *Required fees:* full-time $3640; part-time $150 per credit; part-time $1350 per term.
**Financial Aid** 45% of graduate students in nursing programs received some form of financial aid in 2012–13. 1 research assistantship with partial tuition reimbursement available (averaging $3,000 per year) was awarded; Federal Work-Study, scholarships, tuition waivers (full and partial), and unspecified assistantships also available. *Financial aid application deadline:* 3/1.
**Contact** Dr. Mellisa Hall, Chair, College of Nursing and Health Professions, University of Southern Indiana, 8600 University Boulevard, Evansville, IN 47712. *Telephone:* 812-465-1168. *Fax:* 812-465-7092. *E-mail:* mhall@usi.edu.

### MASTER'S DEGREE PROGRAM

**Degree** MSN
**Available Programs** Master's.
**Concentrations Available** Nursing administration; nursing education. *Clinical nurse specialist programs in:* adult health. *Nurse practitioner programs in:* acute care, family health, psychiatric/mental health.
**Study Options** Full-time and part-time.
**Online Degree Options** Yes (online only).
**Program Entrance Requirements** Computer literacy, minimum overall college GPA of 3.0, transcript of college record, CPR certification, written essay, immunizations, 2 letters of recommendation, professional liability insurance/malpractice insurance, resume, statistics course. *Application deadline:* 2/15 (fall). *Application fee:* $25.
**Advanced Placement** Credit given for nursing courses completed elsewhere dependent upon specific evaluations.
**Degree Requirements** 42 total credit hours.

### POST-MASTER'S PROGRAM

**Areas of Study** Nursing administration; nursing education. *Clinical nurse specialist programs in:* adult health. *Nurse practitioner programs in:* acute care, family health, psychiatric/mental health.

### DOCTORAL DEGREE PROGRAM

**Degree** DNP
**Available Programs** Doctorate.
**Areas of Study** Clinical practice, nursing administration.
**Program Entrance Requirements** Clinical experience, minimum overall college GPA of 3.25, 3 letters of recommendation, MSN or equivalent, vita, writing sample. *Application deadline:* 1/15 (fall). *Application fee:* $25.
**Degree Requirements** 78 total credit hours.

## CONTINUING EDUCATION PROGRAM

**Contact** Peggy Graul, Coordinator of Continuing Education for Nursing and Health Professions, College of Nursing and Health Professions, University of Southern Indiana, 8600 University Boulevard, Evansville, IN 47712. *Telephone:* 812-465-1161. *Fax:* 812-465-7092. *E-mail:* pgraul@usi.edu.

# Valparaiso University
## College of Nursing
## Valparaiso, Indiana

*http://www.valpo.edu/nursing*
Founded in 1859

**DEGREES • BSN • MSN • MSN/MBA**

**Nursing Program Faculty** 13 (38% with doctorates).
**Baccalaureate Enrollment** 310 **Women** 92% **Men** 8% **Minority** 12% **International** 2% **Part-time** 6%
**Graduate Enrollment** 34 **Women** 91% **Men** 9% **Minority** 12% **Part-time** 59%
**Nursing Student Activities** Sigma Theta Tau, Student Nurses' Association.
**Nursing Student Resources** Academic advising; academic or career counseling; assistance for students with disabilities; bookstore; campus computer network; career placement assistance; computer lab; computer-assisted instruction; e-mail services; employment services for current students; externships; housing assistance; interactive nursing skills videos; Internet; learning resource lab; library services; nursing audiovisuals; placement services for program completers; remedial services; resume preparation assistance; skills, simulation, or other laboratory; tutoring; unpaid internships.
**Library Facilities** 580,732 volumes (9,500 in health, 995 in nursing); 43,700 periodical subscriptions (1,000 health-care related).

### BACCALAUREATE PROGRAMS

**Degree** BSN
**Available Programs** Accelerated Baccalaureate; Generic Baccalaureate; RN Baccalaureate.
**Study Options** Full-time and part-time.
**Program Entrance Requirements** Minimum overall college GPA of 3.0, transcript of college record, written essay, high school biology, high school chemistry, 2 years high school math, 4 years high school science, high school transcript, immunizations, minimum high school GPA of 2.0, minimum GPA in nursing prerequisites of 2.5. Transfer students are accepted.
**Advanced Placement** Credit by examination available. Credit given for nursing courses completed elsewhere dependent upon specific evaluations.
**Contact** *Telephone:* 219-464-5011. *Fax:* 219-464-6888.

### GRADUATE PROGRAMS

**Contact** *Telephone:* 219-464-5289. *Fax:* 219-464-5425.

#### MASTER'S DEGREE PROGRAM

**Degrees** MSN; MSN/MBA
**Available Programs** Master's; RN to Master's.
**Concentrations Available** *Clinical nurse specialist programs in:* adult health, gerontology,women's health.
**Study Options** Full-time and part-time.
**Program Entrance Requirements** Minimum overall college GPA of 3.0, transcript of college record, CPR certification, written essay, immunizations, 2 letters of recommendation, nursing research course, physical assessment course, statistics course.
**Advanced Placement** Credit given for nursing courses completed elsewhere dependent upon specific evaluations.
**Degree Requirements** 36 total credit hours, thesis or project.

#### POST-MASTER'S PROGRAM

**Areas of Study** *Nurse practitioner programs in:* family health.

### CONTINUING EDUCATION PROGRAM

**Contact** *Telephone:* 219-464-5291. *Fax:* 219-464-5425.

# Vincennes University
## Department of Nursing
## Vincennes, Indiana

Founded in 1801

**DEGREE • BSN**

### BACCALAUREATE PROGRAMS

**Degree** BSN
**Available Programs** RN Baccalaureate.
**Contact** *Telephone:* 812-888-8888.

# IOWA

# Allen College
## Program in Nursing
## Waterloo, Iowa

*http://www.allencollege.edu/*
Founded in 1989

**DEGREES • BSN • DNP • MSN**

**Nursing Program Faculty** 38 (34% with doctorates).
**Baccalaureate Enrollment** 334 **Women** 94% **Men** 6% **Minority** 96% **International** 1% **Part-time** 39%
**Graduate Enrollment** 178 **Women** 93% **Men** 7% **Minority** 97% **Part-time** 88%
**Distance Learning Courses** Available.
**Nursing Student Activities** Sigma Theta Tau, Student Nurses' Association, nursing club.
**Nursing Student Resources** Academic advising; academic or career counseling; campus computer network; career placement assistance; computer lab; computer-assisted instruction; e-mail services; externships; housing assistance; interactive nursing skills videos; Internet; library services; nursing audiovisuals; other; paid internships; placement services for program completers; resume preparation assistance; skills, simulation, or other laboratory; tutoring.
**Library Facilities** 3,300 volumes (4,900 in health, 4,900 in nursing); 214 periodical subscriptions (244 health-care related).

### BACCALAUREATE PROGRAMS

**Degree** BSN
**Available Programs** ADN to Baccalaureate; Accelerated Baccalaureate; Accelerated Baccalaureate for Second Degree; Accelerated RN Baccalaureate; Baccalaureate for Second Degree; Generic Baccalaureate; LPN to Baccalaureate; RN Baccalaureate.
**Study Options** Full-time and part-time.
**Online Degree Options** Yes.
**Program Entrance Requirements** Transcript of college record, CPR certification, health exam, immunizations, 1 letter of recommendation, minimum GPA in nursing prerequisites of 2.7, prerequisite course work. Transfer students are accepted. *Application deadline:* 2/1 (fall), 6/1 (spring), 6/1 (summer). Applications may be processed on a rolling basis for some programs. *Application fee:* $50.
**Advanced Placement** Credit given for nursing courses completed elsewhere dependent upon specific evaluations.
**Expenses (2013–14)** *Tuition:* full-time $16,771. *Room and board:* $7281; room only: $3641 per academic year. *Required fees:* full-time $2058.
**Financial Aid** 75% of baccalaureate students in nursing programs received some form of financial aid in 2012–13. *Gift aid (need-based):* Federal Pell, FSEOG, state, private, college/university gift aid from institutional funds, Federal Nursing, Scholarships for Disadvantaged Students (SDS). *Loans:* Federal Nursing Student Loans, Federal Direct (Subsidized and Unsubsidized Stafford PLUS), Perkins, state, college/university. *Work-study:* Federal Work-Study. *Financial aid application deadline:* Continuous.
**Contact** Ashlee Gilstrap, Student Services Education Secretary, Program in Nursing, Allen College, 1825 Logan Avenue, Waterloo, IA 50703. *Telephone:* 319-226-2014. *Fax:* 319-226-2010. *E-mail:* Admissions@AllenCollege.edu.

### GRADUATE PROGRAMS

**Expenses (2013–14)** *Tuition:* full-time $15,393. *Room and board:* $7281; room only: $3641 per academic year. *Required fees:* full-time $1146.
**Financial Aid** 82% of graduate students in nursing programs received some form of financial aid in 2012–13. Institutionally sponsored loans, scholarships, and traineeships available. Aid available to part-time students. *Financial aid application deadline:* 8/15.
**Contact** Ashlee Gilstrap, Student Services Education Secretary, Program in Nursing, Allen College, 1825 Logan Avenue, Waterloo, IA 50703.

*Telephone:* 319-226-2014. *Fax:* 319-226-2010. *E-mail:* Admissions@AllenCollege.edu.

### MASTER'S DEGREE PROGRAM

**Degree** MSN
**Available Programs** Master's; Master's for Nurses with Non-Nursing Degrees; RN to Master's.
**Concentrations Available** Nursing administration; nursing education. *Nurse practitioner programs in:* acute care, adult health, family health, gerontology, psychiatric/mental health.
**Study Options** Full-time and part-time.
**Online Degree Options** Yes.
**Program Entrance Requirements** Clinical experience, computer literacy, minimum overall college GPA of 3.0, transcript of college record, CPR certification, written essay, immunizations, interview, 3 letters of recommendation, nursing research course, professional liability insurance/malpractice insurance, prerequisite course work, resume, statistics course. *Application deadline:* 2/1 (fall), 9/1 (spring). Applications may be processed on a rolling basis for some programs. *Application fee:* $50.
**Advanced Placement** Credit given for nursing courses completed elsewhere dependent upon specific evaluations.
**Degree Requirements** 44 total credit hours, thesis or project.

### POST-MASTER'S PROGRAM

**Areas of Study** Nursing administration; nursing education. *Nurse practitioner programs in:* acute care, adult health, family health, gerontology, psychiatric/mental health.

### DOCTORAL DEGREE PROGRAM

**Degree** DNP
**Available Programs** Doctorate.
**Online Degree Options** Yes (online only).
**Program Entrance Requirements** Clinical experience, minimum overall college GPA of 3.25, interview by faculty committee, 3 letters of recommendation, MSN or equivalent, statistics course, vita, writing sample. *Application deadline:* Applications may be processed on a rolling basis for some programs. *Application fee:* $50.
**Degree Requirements** 33 total credit hours.

### POSTDOCTORAL PROGRAM

**Postdoctoral Program Contact** Dr. Diane Young, Department Chair, MSN Program, Program in Nursing, Allen College, 1825 Logan Avenue, Waterloo, IA 50703. *Telephone:* 319-226-2047. *Fax:* 319-226-2070. *E-mail:* youngdm@ihs.org.

### CONTINUING EDUCATION PROGRAM

**Contact** Dina Dowden, Continuing Education Coordinator, Program in Nursing, Allen College, 1825 Logan Avenue, Waterloo, IA 50703. *Telephone:* 319-226-2017. *Fax:* 319-226-2051. *E-mail:* Dina.Dowden@AllenCollege.edu.

# Briar Cliff University

## Department of Nursing
## Sioux City, Iowa

***http://www.briarcliff.edu/***
Founded in 1930

### DEGREES • BSN • DNP • MSN

**Nursing Program Faculty** 9 (33% with doctorates).
**Baccalaureate Enrollment** 125 **Women** 90% **Men** 10% **Minority** 5% **Part-time** 25%
**Graduate Enrollment** 50 **Women** 95% **Men** 5% **Minority** 5% **Part-time** 75%
**Distance Learning Courses** Available.
**Nursing Student Activities** Sigma Theta Tau, Student Nurses' Association, nursing club.
**Nursing Student Resources** Academic advising; academic or career counseling; assistance for students with disabilities; bookstore; campus computer network; career placement assistance; computer lab; computer-assisted instruction; e-mail services; employment services for current students; externships; interactive nursing skills videos; Internet; learning resource lab; library services; nursing audiovisuals; placement services for program completers; remedial services; resume preparation assistance; skills, simulation, or other laboratory; tutoring.
**Library Facilities** 82,007 volumes (7,954 in health, 266 in nursing); 151 periodical subscriptions (4,102 health-care related).

### BACCALAUREATE PROGRAMS

**Degree** BSN
**Available Programs** ADN to Baccalaureate; Generic Baccalaureate; LPN to Baccalaureate; RN Baccalaureate.
**Study Options** Full-time and part-time.
**Program Entrance Requirements** Minimum overall college GPA of 2.75, transcript of college record, CPR certification, written essay, health exam, high school foreign language, high school transcript, immunizations, minimum GPA in nursing prerequisites of 2.75, prerequisite course work. Transfer students are accepted. *Application deadline:* 8/15 (fall), 12/1 (winter), 12/1 (spring), 4/1 (summer). Applications may be processed on a rolling basis for some programs. *Application fee:* $25.
**Advanced Placement** Credit given for nursing courses completed elsewhere dependent upon specific evaluations.
**Expenses (2013–14)** *Tuition:* full-time $25,464; part-time $840 per credit hour. *International tuition:* $25,464 full-time. *Room and board:* $7760; room only: $3830 per academic year. *Required fees:* full-time $1296; part-time $28 per credit.
**Financial Aid** 99% of baccalaureate students in nursing programs received some form of financial aid in 2012–13.
**Contact** Dr. Richard A. Petersen, Department Chair and Associate Professor, Department of Nursing, Briar Cliff University, 3303 Rebecca Street, Sioux City, IA 51104. *Telephone:* 712-279-1662. *Fax:* 712-279-5299. *E-mail:* rick.petersen@briarcliff.edu.

### GRADUATE PROGRAMS

**Expenses (2013–14)** *Tuition:* part-time $540 per credit hour. *Required fees:* part-time $28 per credit.
**Financial Aid** 90% of graduate students in nursing programs received some form of financial aid in 2012–13.
**Contact** Dr. Richard A. Petersen, Department Chair and Associate Professor, Department of Nursing, Briar Cliff University, 3303 Rebecca Street, Sioux City, IA 51104. *Telephone:* 712-279-1662. *Fax:* 712-279-5299. *E-mail:* rick.petersen@briarcliff.edu.

### MASTER'S DEGREE PROGRAM

**Degree** MSN
**Available Programs** Master's.
**Concentrations Available** Nursing education.
**Study Options** Part-time.
**Online Degree Options** Yes (online only).
**Program Entrance Requirements** Clinical experience, computer literacy, minimum overall college GPA of 3.0, transcript of college record, CPR certification, written essay, immunizations, 2 letters of recommendation, nursing research course, physical assessment course, resume, statistics course. *Application deadline:* 7/15 (fall). Applications may be processed on a rolling basis for some programs. *Application fee:* $25.
**Advanced Placement** Credit given for nursing courses completed elsewhere dependent upon specific evaluations.
**Degree Requirements** 44 total credit hours, thesis or project, comprehensive exam.

### DOCTORAL DEGREE PROGRAM

**Degree** DNP
**Available Programs** Doctorate.
**Areas of Study** Advanced practice nursing, family health, gerontology.
**Online Degree Options** Yes (online only).
**Program Entrance Requirements** Clinical experience, minimum overall college GPA of 3.00, 2 letters of recommendation, statistics course, vita, writing sample. *Application deadline:* 7/15 (fall). *Application fee:* $25.
**Degree Requirements** 79 total credit hours, oral exam.

### CONTINUING EDUCATION PROGRAM

**Contact** Dr. Richard A. Petersen, Chair and Associate Professor, Department of Nursing, Briar Cliff University, 3303 Rebecca Street, Sioux City, IA 51104. *Telephone:* 712-279-1662. *Fax:* 712-279-5299. *E-mail:* rick.petersen@briarcliff.edu.

## Clarke University
### Department of Nursing and Health
### Dubuque, Iowa

*http://www.clarke.edu/*
Founded in 1843

**DEGREES • BS • MSN**

**Nursing Program Faculty** 18 (3% with doctorates).

**Baccalaureate Enrollment** 104 **Women** 92% **Men** 8% **Minority** 1% **International** 1% **Part-time** 9%

**Graduate Enrollment** 52 **Women** 99% **Men** 1% **Part-time** 35%

**Nursing Student Activities** Nursing Honor Society, Sigma Theta Tau, Student Nurses' Association.

**Nursing Student Resources** Academic advising; academic or career counseling; assistance for students with disabilities; bookstore; campus computer network; career placement assistance; computer lab; computer-assisted instruction; e-mail services; employment services for current students; externships; housing assistance; interactive nursing skills videos; Internet; learning resource lab; library services; nursing audiovisuals; paid internships; placement services for program completers; remedial services; resume preparation assistance; skills, simulation, or other laboratory; tutoring; unpaid internships.

**Library Facilities** 98,700 volumes (7,000 in health, 2,856 in nursing); 42,000 periodical subscriptions (124 health-care related).

#### BACCALAUREATE PROGRAMS

**Degree** BS

**Available Programs** Baccalaureate for Second Degree; Generic Baccalaureate; RN Baccalaureate.

**Site Options** Dubuque, IA.

**Study Options** Full-time and part-time.

**Program Entrance Requirements** Minimum overall college GPA of 2.75, transcript of college record, CPR certification, written essay, health exam, health insurance, high school chemistry, high school foreign language, high school math, high school transcript, immunizations, interview, 2 letters of recommendation, minimum high school GPA of 2.0, minimum GPA in nursing prerequisites of 1.67, professional liability insurance/malpractice insurance, prerequisite course work. Transfer students are accepted. *Application deadline:* Applications may be processed on a rolling basis for some programs.

**Advanced Placement** Credit given for nursing courses completed elsewhere dependent upon specific evaluations.

**Contact** *Telephone:* 563-588-8109. *Fax:* 563-588-8684.

#### GRADUATE PROGRAMS

**Contact** *Telephone:* 563-588-8109. *Fax:* 563-588-8684.

#### MASTER'S DEGREE PROGRAM

**Degree** MSN

**Available Programs** Master's.

**Concentrations Available** Nursing education. *Nurse practitioner programs in:* family health.

**Study Options** Full-time and part-time.

**Program Entrance Requirements** Computer literacy, minimum overall college GPA of 3.0, transcript of college record, CPR certification, written essay, immunizations, interview, 3 letters of recommendation, nursing research course, physical assessment course, prerequisite course work, resume, statistics course, GRE General Test or MAT. *Application deadline:* Applications may be processed on a rolling basis for some programs. *Application fee:* $35.

**Advanced Placement** Credit given for nursing courses completed elsewhere dependent upon specific evaluations.

**Degree Requirements** 37 total credit hours, thesis or project.

#### POST-MASTER'S PROGRAM

**Areas of Study** *Nurse practitioner programs in:* family health.

#### CONTINUING EDUCATION PROGRAM

**Contact** *Telephone:* 563-588-6378. *Fax:* 563-588-8684.

## Coe College
### Department of Nursing
### Cedar Rapids, Iowa

Founded in 1851

**DEGREE • BSN**

**Nursing Program Faculty** 7 (86% with doctorates).

**Baccalaureate Enrollment** 50 **Women** 85% **Men** 15% **Minority** 2% **International** 1%

**Nursing Student Activities** Student Nurses' Association.

**Nursing Student Resources** Academic advising; academic or career counseling; assistance for students with disabilities; bookstore; campus computer network; career placement assistance; computer lab; e-mail services; employment services for current students; housing assistance; Internet; learning resource lab; library services; nursing audiovisuals; remedial services; resume preparation assistance; skills, simulation, or other laboratory; tutoring; unpaid internships.

**Library Facilities** 301,894 volumes (2,929 in health, 492 in nursing); 36,879 periodical subscriptions (34 health-care related).

#### BACCALAUREATE PROGRAMS

**Degree** BSN

**Available Programs** Generic Baccalaureate.

**Study Options** Full-time and part-time.

**Program Entrance Requirements** Minimum overall college GPA of 2.7, transcript of college record, CPR certification, written essay, health exam, health insurance, high school chemistry, high school transcript, immunizations, minimum high school GPA of 2.0, minimum GPA in nursing prerequisites of 2.7, prerequisite course work. Transfer students are accepted. *Application deadline:* 12/1 (fall). Applications may be processed on a rolling basis for some programs. *Application fee:* $50.

**Advanced Placement** Credit given for nursing courses completed elsewhere dependent upon specific evaluations.

**Financial Aid** 100% of baccalaureate students in nursing programs received some form of financial aid in 2011–12.

**Contact** Ms. Julie Staker, Dean of Admission, Department of Nursing, Coe College, 1220 First Avenue NE, Cedar Rapids, IA 52402. *Telephone:* 319-399-8046. *Fax:* 319-399-8816. *E-mail:* jstaker@coe.edu.

## Dordt College
### Nursing Program
### Sioux Center, Iowa

Founded in 1955

**DEGREE • BSN**

**Nursing Program Faculty** 3

**Library Facilities** 185,000 volumes; 6,597 periodical subscriptions.

#### BACCALAUREATE PROGRAMS

**Degree** BSN

**Available Programs** Generic Baccalaureate.

**Contact** *Telephone:* 712-722-6000.

## Grand View University
### Division of Nursing
### Des Moines, Iowa

*http://www.grandview.edu*
Founded in 1896

**DEGREES • BSN • MS**

**Nursing Program Faculty** 18 (33% with doctorates).

**Baccalaureate Enrollment** 200 **Women** 90% **Men** 10% **Minority** 15% **Part-time** 5%

**Graduate Enrollment** 6 **Women** 83% **Men** 17% **Part-time** 100%

**Distance Learning Courses** Available.

**Nursing Student Activities** Sigma Theta Tau, Student Nurses' Association.

**Nursing Student Resources** Academic advising; academic or career counseling; assistance for students with disabilities; bookstore; campus computer network; career placement assistance; computer lab; computer-assisted instruction; e-mail services; employment services for current students; externships; housing assistance; interactive nursing skills videos;

Internet; learning resource lab; library services; nursing audiovisuals; placement services for program completers; remedial services; resume preparation assistance; skills, simulation, or other laboratory; tutoring; unpaid internships.
**Library Facilities** 135,448 volumes (5,672 in health, 4,061 in nursing); 27,077 periodical subscriptions (370 health-care related).

## BACCALAUREATE PROGRAMS

**Degree** BSN
**Available Programs** Generic Baccalaureate; RN Baccalaureate.
**Study Options** Full-time and part-time.
**Program Entrance Requirements** Minimum overall college GPA of 2.75, transcript of college record, CPR certification, health exam, health insurance, high school chemistry, high school transcript, immunizations, 3 letters of recommendation, minimum GPA in nursing prerequisites of 2.75, prerequisite course work. Transfer students are accepted. *Application deadline:* 2/1 (fall), 10/1 (spring). Applications may be processed on a rolling basis for some programs.
**Advanced Placement** Credit by examination available. Credit given for nursing courses completed elsewhere dependent upon specific evaluations.
**Contact** *Telephone:* 515-263-2859. *Fax:* 515-263-6077.

## GRADUATE PROGRAMS

**Contact** *Telephone:* 515-263-2859. *Fax:* 515-263-6077.

### MASTER'S DEGREE PROGRAM

**Degree** MS
**Available Programs** Master's.
**Concentrations Available** Clinical nurse leader.
**Study Options** Part-time.
**Program Entrance Requirements** Clinical experience, computer literacy, minimum overall college GPA of 3.0, transcript of college record, CPR certification, written essay, immunizations, interview, 3 letters of recommendation, nursing research course, physical assessment course, professional liability insurance/malpractice insurance, prerequisite course work, resume, statistics course. *Application deadline:* 7/1 (fall). Applications may be processed on a rolling basis for some programs.
**Degree Requirements** 40 total credit hours, thesis or project.

## CONTINUING EDUCATION PROGRAM

**Contact** *Telephone:* 515-263-2869. *Fax:* 515-263-6700.

# Iowa Wesleyan College

## Division of Nursing
## Mount Pleasant, Iowa

***http://www.iwc.edu/***
Founded in 1842

### DEGREE • BSN

**Nursing Program Faculty** 7 (29% with doctorates).
**Baccalaureate Enrollment** 80 **Women** 92% **Men** 8% **Minority** 7% **International** 1% **Part-time** 2%
**Distance Learning Courses** Available.
**Nursing Student Activities** Student Nurses' Association.
**Nursing Student Resources** Academic advising; academic or career counseling; assistance for students with disabilities; bookstore; campus computer network; career placement assistance; computer lab; computer-assisted instruction; e-mail services; employment services for current students; interactive nursing skills videos; Internet; learning resource lab; library services; nursing audiovisuals; remedial services; resume preparation assistance; skills, simulation, or other laboratory; tutoring; unpaid internships.
**Library Facilities** 84,778 volumes (500 in health, 300 in nursing); 44 periodical subscriptions (40 health-care related).

## BACCALAUREATE PROGRAMS

**Degree** BSN
**Available Programs** ADN to Baccalaureate; Baccalaureate for Second Degree; Generic Baccalaureate; LPN to Baccalaureate; LPN to RN Baccalaureate; RN Baccalaureate.
**Study Options** Full-time and part-time.
**Program Entrance Requirements** Minimum overall college GPA of 2.25, transcript of college record, CPR certification, health exam, health insurance, high school transcript, immunizations, interview, minimum high school GPA of 2.25, minimum high school rank 50%, minimum GPA in nursing prerequisites of 2.25, professional liability insurance/malpractice insurance, prerequisite course work. Transfer students are accepted. *Application deadline:* 8/1 (fall). Applications may be processed on a rolling basis for some programs.
**Expenses (2012–13)** *Tuition:* full-time $24,300; part-time $610 per credit hour. *Room and board:* $3790; room only: $1570 per academic year. *Required fees:* full-time $150; part-time $150 per term.
**Financial Aid** 98% of baccalaureate students in nursing programs received some form of financial aid in 2011–12. *Gift aid (need-based):* Federal Pell, FSEOG, state, private, college/university gift aid from institutional funds. *Loans:* Federal Direct (Subsidized and Unsubsidized Stafford PLUS), Perkins, alternative loans. *Work-study:* Federal Work-Study. *Financial aid application deadline (priority):* 4/1.
**Contact** Mr. Mark Petty, Dean for Admissions, Division of Nursing, Iowa Wesleyan College, 601 North Main Street, Mount Pleasant, IA 52641. *Telephone:* 800-582-2383 Ext. 6231. *Fax:* 319-385-6296. *E-mail:* mpetty@iwc.edu.

# Luther College

## Department of Nursing
## Decorah, Iowa

***http://www.nursing.luther.edu/***
Founded in 1861

### DEGREE • BA

**Nursing Program Faculty** 16 (3% with doctorates).
**Baccalaureate Enrollment** 130 **Women** 96% **Men** 4% **Minority** 3%
**Nursing Student Activities** Student Nurses' Association.
**Nursing Student Resources** Academic advising; academic or career counseling; assistance for students with disabilities; bookstore; campus computer network; career placement assistance; computer lab; computer-assisted instruction; e-mail services; employment services for current students; externships; Internet; learning resource lab; library services; nursing audiovisuals; placement services for program completers; remedial services; resume preparation assistance; skills, simulation, or other laboratory; tutoring; unpaid internships.
**Library Facilities** 335,949 volumes (4,324 in health, 3,337 in nursing); 38,495 periodical subscriptions (35 health-care related).

## BACCALAUREATE PROGRAMS

**Degree** BA
**Available Programs** Generic Baccalaureate.
**Site Options** Rochester, MN.
**Study Options** Full-time and part-time.
**Program Entrance Requirements** Minimum overall college GPA of 2.75, transcript of college record, CPR certification, health exam, health insurance, 3 years high school math, 2 years high school science, high school transcript, immunizations, minimum high school rank 50%, minimum GPA in nursing prerequisites of 2.75, professional liability insurance/malpractice insurance, prerequisite course work. Transfer students are accepted. *Application deadline:* Applications may be processed on a rolling basis for some programs.
**Advanced Placement** Credit given for nursing courses completed elsewhere dependent upon specific evaluations.
**Financial Aid** 100% of baccalaureate students in nursing programs received some form of financial aid in 2012–13. *Gift aid (need-based):* Federal Pell, FSEOG, state, private, college/university gift aid from institutional funds. *Loans:* Federal Direct (Subsidized and Unsubsidized Stafford PLUS), Perkins, college/university. *Work-study:* Federal Work-Study, part-time campus jobs. *Financial aid application deadline (priority):* 3/1.
**Contact** Ms. Tracy Elsbernd, Administrative Assistant, Department of Nursing, Luther College, 700 College Drive, Decorah, IA 52101. *Telephone:* 563-387-1057. *Fax:* 563-387-2149. *E-mail:* elsbtr01@luther.edu.

## CONTINUING EDUCATION PROGRAM

**Contact** Ms. Tracy Elsbernd, Administrative Assistant, Department of Nursing, Luther College, 700 College Drive, Decorah, IA 52101. *Telephone:* 563-387-1057. *Fax:* 563-387-2149. *E-mail:* elsbtr01@luther.edu.

***See display on next page and full description on page 478.***

## Mercy College of Health Sciences
### Division of Nursing
### Des Moines, Iowa

*http://www.mchs.edu/*
Founded in 1995

**DEGREE • BSN**

**Nursing Program Faculty** 22 (2% with doctorates).

**Baccalaureate Enrollment** 76 **Women** 98% **Men** 2% **Minority** 1% **Part-time** 98%

**Nursing Student Activities** Sigma Theta Tau, Student Nurses' Association.

**Nursing Student Resources** Academic advising; academic or career counseling; assistance for students with disabilities; campus computer network; career placement assistance; computer lab; computer-assisted instruction; daycare for children of students; e-mail services; employment services for current students; interactive nursing skills videos; Internet; learning resource lab; library services; nursing audiovisuals; placement services for program completers; skills, simulation, or other laboratory.

**BACCALAUREATE PROGRAMS**

**Degree** BSN

**Available Programs** ADN to Baccalaureate.

**Study Options** Full-time and part-time.

**Program Entrance Requirements** Minimum overall college GPA of 2.7, transcript of college record, CPR certification, health exam, high school biology, high school chemistry, high school transcript, immunizations, minimum GPA in nursing prerequisites of 2.7, prerequisite course work, RN licensure. Transfer students are accepted. *Application deadline:* Applications may be processed on a rolling basis for some programs. *Application fee:* $25.

**Advanced Placement** Credit given for nursing courses completed elsewhere dependent upon specific evaluations.

**Contact** *Telephone:* 515-643-3180. *Fax:* 515-643-6698.

## Morningside College
### Department of Nursing Education
### Sioux City, Iowa

*http://webs.morningside.edu/nursing/*
Founded in 1894

**DEGREE • BSN**

**Nursing Program Faculty** 16 (13% with doctorates).

**Baccalaureate Enrollment** 93 **Women** 89% **Men** 11% **Minority** 8% **Part-time** 2%

**Distance Learning Courses** Available.

**Nursing Student Activities** Sigma Theta Tau, Student Nurses' Association.

**Nursing Student Resources** Academic advising; academic or career counseling; assistance for students with disabilities; bookstore; campus computer network; computer lab; computer-assisted instruction; e-mail services; employment services for current students; externships; housing assistance; interactive nursing skills videos; Internet; learning resource lab; library services; nursing audiovisuals; remedial services; resume preparation assistance; skills, simulation, or other laboratory; tutoring; unpaid internships.

**Library Facilities** 49,359 volumes (1,086 in nursing); 165 periodical subscriptions (18 health-care related).

**BACCALAUREATE PROGRAMS**

**Degree** BSN

**Available Programs** Baccalaureate for Second Degree; Generic Baccalaureate; International Nurse to Baccalaureate; LPN to Baccalaureate; RN Baccalaureate.

**Study Options** Full-time and part-time.

**Online Degree Options** Yes.

**Program Entrance Requirements** Minimum overall college GPA of 2.75, transcript of college record, CPR certification, high school transcript, immunizations, interview, minimum GPA in nursing prerequisites of 2.75, prerequisite course work. Transfer students are accepted. *Application deadline:* 8/15 (fall).

**Advanced Placement** Credit given for nursing courses completed elsewhere dependent upon specific evaluations.

**Expenses (2013–14)** *Tuition:* full-time $24,720; part-time $455 per credit. *Room and board:* $7930 per academic year. *Required fees:* full-time $1270; part-time $245 per term.
**Financial Aid** 99% of baccalaureate students in nursing programs received some form of financial aid in 2012–13. *Gift aid (need-based):* Federal Pell, FSEOG, state, private, college/university gift aid from institutional funds. *Loans:* Federal Direct (Subsidized and Unsubsidized Stafford PLUS), Perkins, college/university, private loans. *Work-study:* Federal Work-Study, part-time campus jobs. *Financial aid application deadline (priority):* 3/1.
**Contact** Dr. Mary B. Kovarna, Professor and Chair, Department of Nursing Education, Morningside College, 1501 Morningside Avenue, Sioux City, IA 51106-1751. *Telephone:* 712-274-5156. *Fax:* 712-274-5101. *E-mail:* kovarna@morningside.edu.

# Mount Mercy University
## Department of Nursing
## Cedar Rapids, Iowa

*http://www.mtmercy.edu/*
Founded in 1928

**DEGREES • BSN • MSN**
**Nursing Program Faculty** 45 (9% with doctorates).
**Baccalaureate Enrollment** 257 **Women** 97% **Men** 3% **Minority** 3% **International** 2% **Part-time** 35%
**Graduate Enrollment** 41 **Women** 99% **Men** 1% **Minority** 1% **International** 1% **Part-time** 2%
**Nursing Student Activities** Sigma Theta Tau, Student Nurses' Association.
**Nursing Student Resources** Academic advising; academic or career counseling; assistance for students with disabilities; bookstore; campus computer network; career placement assistance; computer lab; computer-assisted instruction; e-mail services; employment services for current students; externships; housing assistance; interactive nursing skills videos; Internet; learning resource lab; library services; nursing audiovisuals; paid internships; placement services for program completers; remedial services; resume preparation assistance; skills, simulation, or other laboratory; tutoring; unpaid internships.
**Library Facilities** 130,508 volumes (5,400 in health, 1,475 in nursing); 3,511 periodical subscriptions (130 health-care related).

### BACCALAUREATE PROGRAMS

**Degree** BSN
**Available Programs** ADN to Baccalaureate; Accelerated RN Baccalaureate; Generic Baccalaureate.
**Study Options** Full-time and part-time.
**Program Entrance Requirements** Minimum overall college GPA of 2.7, transcript of college record, CPR certification, health exam, health insurance, high school chemistry, 2 years high school math, 2 years high school science, high school transcript, immunizations, minimum high school rank 75%, minimum GPA in nursing prerequisites of 2.7, prerequisite course work. Transfer students are accepted. *Application deadline:* 5/31 (fall), 10/1 (winter), 10/1 (spring), 4/1 (summer).
**Advanced Placement** Credit by examination available. Credit given for nursing courses completed elsewhere dependent upon specific evaluations.
**Expenses (2013–14)** *Tuition:* full-time $26,160; part-time $710 per credit hour. *International tuition:* $26,160 full-time. *Room and board:* $4200; room only: $2000 per academic year. *Required fees:* full-time $600.
**Financial Aid** 90% of baccalaureate students in nursing programs received some form of financial aid in 2012–13. *Gift aid (need-based):* Federal Pell, FSEOG, state, private, college/university gift aid from institutional funds. *Loans:* Federal Direct (Subsidized and Unsubsidized Stafford PLUS), Perkins, state, college/university. *Work-study:* Federal Work-Study, part-time campus jobs. *Financial aid application deadline (priority):* 3/1.
**Contact** Dr. Mary P. Tarbox, Professor and Chair, Department of Nursing, Mount Mercy University, 1330 Elmhurst Drive NE, Cedar Rapids, IA 52402. *Telephone:* 800-248-4504 Ext. 6460. *Fax:* 319-368-6479. *E-mail:* mtarbox@mtmercy.edu.

### GRADUATE PROGRAMS

**Expenses (2013–14)** *Tuition:* full-time $16,350; part-time $545 per credit hour. *Required fees:* full-time $415.
**Financial Aid** 50% of graduate students in nursing programs received some form of financial aid in 2012–13.
**Contact** Dr. Mary P. Tarbox, Chair, Department of Nursing, Mount Mercy University, 1330 Elmhurst Drive NE, Cedar Rapids, IA 52402. *Telephone:* 319-368-6471. *Fax:* 319-368-6479. *E-mail:* mtarbox@mtmercy.edu.

#### MASTER'S DEGREE PROGRAM

**Degree** MSN
**Available Programs** Master's.
**Concentrations Available** Health-care administration; nursing administration; nursing education. *Clinical nurse specialist programs in:* community health, public health.
**Study Options** Full-time and part-time.
**Program Entrance Requirements** Clinical experience, minimum overall college GPA of 3.0, transcript of college record, CPR certification, written essay, immunizations, 2 letters of recommendation, statistics course. *Application deadline:* Applications may be processed on a rolling basis for some programs.
**Advanced Placement** Credit given for nursing courses completed elsewhere dependent upon specific evaluations.
**Degree Requirements** 36 total credit hours, thesis or project.

### CONTINUING EDUCATION PROGRAM

**Contact** Dr. Mary P. Tarbox, Department Chair, Department of Nursing, Mount Mercy University, 1330 Elmhurst Drive NE, Cedar Rapids, IA 52402. *Telephone:* 319-368-6471. *Fax:* 319-368-6479. *E-mail:* mtarbox@mtmercy.edu.

# Northwestern College
## Nursing Program
## Orange City, Iowa

*http://www.nwciowa.edu/nursing*
Founded in 1882

**DEGREE • BSN**
**Nursing Program Faculty** 8 (12% with doctorates).
**Baccalaureate Enrollment** 58 **Women** 93% **Men** 7% **Part-time** 3%
**Nursing Student Activities** Nursing Honor Society, Sigma Theta Tau, Student Nurses' Association, nursing club.
**Nursing Student Resources** Academic advising; assistance for students with disabilities; bookstore; campus computer network; career placement assistance; computer lab; e-mail services; housing assistance; interactive nursing skills videos; Internet; learning resource lab; library services; nursing audiovisuals; placement services for program completers; remedial services; resume preparation assistance; skills, simulation, or other laboratory; tutoring.
**Library Facilities** 120,000 volumes; 840 periodical subscriptions.

### BACCALAUREATE PROGRAMS

**Degree** BSN
**Available Programs** Generic Baccalaureate.
**Study Options** Full-time.
**Program Entrance Requirements** Transcript of college record, CPR certification, written essay, health exam, immunizations, minimum GPA in nursing prerequisites of 2.7, prerequisite course work. Transfer students are accepted. *Application deadline:* 4/10 (spring). *Application fee:* $550.
**Advanced Placement** Credit given for nursing courses completed elsewhere dependent upon specific evaluations.
**Contact** *Telephone:* 712-707-7086.

# St. Ambrose University
## Program in Nursing (BSN)
## Davenport, Iowa

*http://www.sau.edu/*
Founded in 1882

**DEGREES • BSN • MSN**
**Nursing Program Faculty** 17 (35% with doctorates).
**Baccalaureate Enrollment** 266 **Women** 96% **Men** 4% **Minority** 7% **International** 2% **Part-time** 38%
**Graduate Enrollment** 14 **Women** 100% **Part-time** 100%

**Nursing Student Activities** Student Nurses' Association.
**Nursing Student Resources** Academic advising; academic or career counseling; assistance for students with disabilities; bookstore; campus computer network; career placement assistance; computer lab; e-mail services; employment services for current students; housing assistance; interactive nursing skills videos; Internet; learning resource lab; library services; nursing audiovisuals; resume preparation assistance; skills, simulation, or other laboratory; tutoring; unpaid internships.
**Library Facilities** 171,113 volumes (1,793 in health, 674 in nursing); 563,352 periodical subscriptions (157 health-care related).

## BACCALAUREATE PROGRAMS

**Degree** BSN
**Available Programs** Generic Baccalaureate; RN Baccalaureate.
**Study Options** Full-time and part-time.
**Program Entrance Requirements** Minimum overall college GPA of 3.0, transcript of college record, CPR certification, health exam, health insurance, high school biology, high school chemistry, high school foreign language, 3 years high school math, high school transcript, immunizations, minimum GPA in nursing prerequisites of 3.0, prerequisite course work. Transfer students are accepted. *Application deadline:* 4/1 (fall), 10/25 (winter), 11/30 (spring), 4/15 (summer). Applications may be processed on a rolling basis for some programs. *Application fee:* $25.
**Advanced Placement** Credit by examination available. Credit given for nursing courses completed elsewhere dependent upon specific evaluations.
**Contact** *Telephone:* 563-333-6076.

## GRADUATE PROGRAMS

**Contact** *Telephone:* 563-333-6069. *Fax:* 563-333-6063.

### MASTER'S DEGREE PROGRAM

**Degree** MSN
**Available Programs** Master's.
**Concentrations Available** Health-care administration; nursing administration.
**Study Options** Part-time.
**Program Entrance Requirements** Clinical experience, minimum overall college GPA of 3.0, transcript of college record, CPR certification, immunizations, 3 letters of recommendation, physical assessment course, resume, statistics course. *Application deadline:* 4/15 (fall). Applications may be processed on a rolling basis for some programs. *Application fee:* $25.
**Advanced Placement** Credit given for nursing courses completed elsewhere dependent upon specific evaluations.
**Degree Requirements** 37 total credit hours, thesis or project.

## CONTINUING EDUCATION PROGRAM

**Contact** *Telephone:* 563-333-6076. *Fax:* 563-333-6063.

# University of Dubuque

## School of Professional Programs
## Dubuque, Iowa

*http://www.dbq.edu*
Founded in 1852

## DEGREE • BSN

**Nursing Program Faculty** 8 (1% with doctorates).
**Baccalaureate Enrollment** 58 **Women** 86% **Men** 14% **Minority** 2%
**Nursing Student Activities** Student Nurses' Association.
**Nursing Student Resources** Academic advising; academic or career counseling; assistance for students with disabilities; bookstore; campus computer network; career placement assistance; computer lab; daycare for children of students; e-mail services; employment services for current students; interactive nursing skills videos; Internet; learning resource lab; library services; nursing audiovisuals; resume preparation assistance; skills, simulation, or other laboratory; tutoring; unpaid internships.
**Library Facilities** 183,336 volumes; 51,859 periodical subscriptions.

## BACCALAUREATE PROGRAMS

**Degree** BSN
**Available Programs** RN Baccalaureate.
**Study Options** Full-time.
**Program Entrance Requirements** Transcript of college record, CPR certification, health exam, health insurance, immunizations, 2 letters of recommendation, minimum GPA in nursing prerequisites of 2.75, professional liability insurance/malpractice insurance, prerequisite course work. Transfer students are accepted.
**Contact** *Telephone:* 563-589-3000.

# The University of Iowa

## College of Nursing
## Iowa City, Iowa

*http://www.nursing.uiowa.edu/*
Founded in 1847

## DEGREES • BSN • MSN • MSN/MBA • MSN/MPH • PHD

**Nursing Program Faculty** 67 (63% with doctorates).
**Baccalaureate Enrollment** 618 **Women** 93% **Men** 7% **Minority** 6% **Part-time** 25%
**Graduate Enrollment** 258 **Women** 89% **Men** 11% **Minority** 4% **International** 7% **Part-time** 50%
**Nursing Student Activities** Sigma Theta Tau, Student Nurses' Association.
**Nursing Student Resources** Academic advising; academic or career counseling; assistance for students with disabilities; campus computer network; career placement assistance; computer lab; computer-assisted instruction; e-mail services; employment services for current students; Internet; learning resource lab; nursing audiovisuals; placement services for program completers; resume preparation assistance; skills, simulation, or other laboratory; tutoring.
**Library Facilities** 5.3 million volumes (273,469 in health); 2,500 periodical subscriptions health-care related.

## BACCALAUREATE PROGRAMS

**Degree** BSN
**Available Programs** Generic Baccalaureate; RN Baccalaureate.
**Study Options** Full-time and part-time.
**Program Entrance Requirements** Minimum overall college GPA of 2.7, transcript of college record, CPR certification, written essay, health exam, health insurance, high school biology, high school chemistry, high school foreign language, 3 years high school math, 3 years high school science, high school transcript, immunizations, minimum GPA in nursing prerequisites of 2.7, professional liability insurance/malpractice insurance, prerequisite course work. Transfer students are accepted.
**Advanced Placement** Credit given for nursing courses completed elsewhere dependent upon specific evaluations.
**Contact** *Telephone:* 319-335-7016. *Fax:* 319-384-4423.

## GRADUATE PROGRAMS

**Contact** *Telephone:* 319-335-7021. *Fax:* 319-335-9990.

### MASTER'S DEGREE PROGRAM

**Degrees** MSN; MSN/MBA; MSN/MPH
**Available Programs** Accelerated RN to Master's; Master's; Master's for Nurses with Non-Nursing Degrees.
**Concentrations Available** Nurse anesthesia; nursing administration; nursing education; nursing informatics. *Clinical nurse specialist programs in:* adult health, community health, gerontology, occupational health, psychiatric/mental health. *Nurse practitioner programs in:* adult health, family health, gerontology, neonatal health, pediatric, psychiatric/mental health.
**Study Options** Full-time and part-time.
**Program Entrance Requirements** Computer literacy, minimum overall college GPA of 3.0, transcript of college record, written essay, immunizations, 3 letters of recommendation, nursing research course, physical assessment course, professional liability insurance/malpractice insurance, prerequisite course work, resume, statistics course.
**Advanced Placement** Credit given for nursing courses completed elsewhere dependent upon specific evaluations.
**Degree Requirements** 33 total credit hours, thesis or project.

### POST-MASTER'S PROGRAM

**Areas of Study** Nursing informatics. *Clinical nurse specialist programs in:* adult health, psychiatric/mental health. *Nurse practitioner programs in:* adult health, family health, gerontology, pediatric, psychiatric/mental health.

**DOCTORAL DEGREE PROGRAM**
**Degree** PhD
**Available Programs** Doctorate; Post-Baccalaureate Doctorate.
**Areas of Study** Aging, family health, gerontology, individualized study, information systems, nursing administration.
**Program Entrance Requirements** Minimum overall college GPA of 3.0, interview, 3 letters of recommendation, statistics course, vita, GRE General Test.
**Degree Requirements** 60 total credit hours, dissertation, oral exam, written exam, residency.

**POSTDOCTORAL PROGRAM**
**Areas of Study** Family health, nursing informatics, nursing interventions, outcomes.
**Postdoctoral Program Contact** *Telephone:* 319-335-7021. *Fax:* 319-335-9990.

### CONTINUING EDUCATION PROGRAM

**Contact** *Telephone:* 319-335-7075. *Fax:* 319-335-9990.

## Upper Iowa University

### RN-BSN Nursing Program
### Fayette, Iowa

*http://www.uiu.edu/nursing/*
Founded in 1857

**DEGREE • BSN**
**Nursing Program Faculty** 10
**Library Facilities** 74,813 volumes; 284 periodical subscriptions.

### BACCALAUREATE PROGRAMS

**Degree** BSN
**Available Programs** RN Baccalaureate.
**Site Options** Cedar Rapids, IA; West Des Moines, IA.
**Program Entrance Requirements** Minimum overall college GPA of 2.5, transcript of college record, CPR certification, health exam, high school transcript, RN licensure. Transfer students are accepted.
**Contact** *Telephone:* 563-425-5357.

# KANSAS

## Baker University

### School of Nursing
### Topeka, Kansas

*http://www.bakeru.edu/*
Founded in 1858

**DEGREE • BSN**
**Nursing Program Faculty** 16 (25% with doctorates).
**Baccalaureate Enrollment** 169 **Women** 90% **Men** 10% **Minority** 11% **Part-time** .2%
**Nursing Student Activities** Sigma Theta Tau, Student Nurses' Association.
**Nursing Student Resources** Academic advising; assistance for students with disabilities; campus computer network; computer lab; computer-assisted instruction; e-mail services; Internet; learning resource lab; library services; nursing audiovisuals; resume preparation assistance; skills, simulation, or other laboratory; tutoring.
**Library Facilities** 106,549 volumes (5,000 in health, 2,716 in nursing); 160 periodical subscriptions (414 health-care related).

### BACCALAUREATE PROGRAMS

**Degree** BSN
**Available Programs** Generic Baccalaureate; RN Baccalaureate.
**Study Options** Full-time and part-time.
**Program Entrance Requirements** Transcript of college record, CPR certification, written essay, health exam, health insurance, high school transcript, immunizations, interview, minimum GPA in nursing prerequisites of 2.7, prerequisite course work. Transfer students are accepted. *Application deadline:* 12/1 (fall), 8/1 (spring).
**Advanced Placement** Credit given for nursing courses completed elsewhere dependent upon specific evaluations.
**Expenses (2013–14)** *Tuition:* full-time $16,484. *International tuition:* $16,484 full-time.
**Financial Aid** 87% of baccalaureate students in nursing programs received some form of financial aid in 2012–13.
**Contact** Ms. Cara Bonfiglio, Student Affairs Specialist, School of Nursing, Baker University, 1500 SW 10th Street, Topeka, KS 66604-1353. *Telephone:* 785-354-5850. *Fax:* 785-354-5832. *E-mail:* cbonfig@stormontvail.org.

## Benedictine College

### Department of Nursing
### Atchison, Kansas

Founded in 1859

**DEGREE • BSN**
**Nursing Program Faculty** 8 (25% with doctorates).
**Baccalaureate Enrollment** 50 **Women** 96% **Men** 4% **Minority** 6% **International** 2%
**Nursing Student Activities** Student Nurses' Association.
**Nursing Student Resources** Academic advising; academic or career counseling; bookstore; campus computer network; career placement assistance; computer lab; e-mail services; employment services for current students; Internet; learning resource lab; library services; nursing audiovisuals; resume preparation assistance; skills, simulation, or other laboratory; tutoring.
**Library Facilities** 347,829 volumes; 27,467 periodical subscriptions.

### BACCALAUREATE PROGRAMS

**Degree** BSN
**Available Programs** Generic Baccalaureate.
**Study Options** Full-time.
**Program Entrance Requirements** Minimum overall college GPA of 2.75, CPR certification, written essay, health exam, health insurance, immunizations, 2 letters of recommendation, professional liability insurance/malpractice insurance, prerequisite course work. Transfer students are accepted. *Application deadline:* 1/15 (fall). *Application fee:* $40.
**Advanced Placement** Credit given for nursing courses completed elsewhere dependent upon specific evaluations.
**Expenses (2013–14)** *Tuition:* full-time $23,650; part-time $665 per credit hour. *International tuition:* $23,650 full-time. *Room and board:* $8175; room only: $6350 per academic year. *Required fees:* full-time $600.
**Financial Aid** 100% of baccalaureate students in nursing programs received some form of financial aid in 2012–13. *Gift aid (need-based):* Federal Pell, FSEOG, state, private, college/university gift aid from institutional funds. *Loans:* Perkins, alternative loans. *Work-study:* Federal Work-Study, part-time campus jobs. *Financial aid application deadline (priority):* 3/15.
**Contact** Lynne Connelly, Director of Nursing, Department of Nursing, Benedictine College, 1020 North 2nd Street, Atchison, KS 66002. *Telephone:* 913-360-7560. *E-mail:* lconnelly@benedictine.edu.

## Bethel College

### Department of Nursing
### North Newton, Kansas

*http://www.bethelks.edu/*
Founded in 1887

**DEGREE • BSN**
**Nursing Program Faculty** 8
**Baccalaureate Enrollment** 42 **Women** 75% **Men** 25% **Minority** 30% **International** 25% **Part-time** 1%
**Distance Learning Courses** Available.
**Nursing Student Activities** Nursing Honor Society, Sigma Theta Tau, Student Nurses' Association.
**Nursing Student Resources** Academic advising; academic or career counseling; assistance for students with disabilities; bookstore; campus computer network; computer lab; e-mail services; employment services for current students; housing assistance; Internet; learning resource lab; library services; nursing audiovisuals; resume preparation assistance; skills, simulation, or other laboratory; tutoring.

**Library Facilities** 5,690 volumes in health, 3,150 volumes in nursing; 445 periodical subscriptions health-care related.

### BACCALAUREATE PROGRAMS

**Degree** BSN
**Available Programs** Generic Baccalaureate; LPN to Baccalaureate; RN Baccalaureate.
**Study Options** Full-time and part-time.
**Online Degree Options** Yes.
**Program Entrance Requirements** Minimum overall college GPA of 3.0, transcript of college record, CPR certification, written essay, health exam, health insurance, high school transcript, immunizations, interview, 2 letters of recommendation, minimum high school GPA of 2.75, minimum GPA in nursing prerequisites of 2.0, prerequisite course work. Transfer students are accepted. *Application deadline:* 2/1 (fall).
**Advanced Placement** Credit given for nursing courses completed elsewhere dependent upon specific evaluations.
**Contact** *Telephone:* 316-283-5295 Ext. 377. *Fax:* 316-284-5286.

# Emporia State University

## Newman Division of Nursing
## Emporia, Kansas

***http://www.emporia.edu/nursing***
Founded in 1863

### DEGREE • BSN

**Nursing Program Faculty** 12 (17% with doctorates).
**Baccalaureate Enrollment** 125 **Women** 94% **Men** 6% **Minority** 20% **International** 2%
**Nursing Student Activities** Sigma Theta Tau, Student Nurses' Association.
**Nursing Student Resources** Academic advising; academic or career counseling; assistance for students with disabilities; bookstore; campus computer network; career placement assistance; computer lab; computer-assisted instruction; daycare for children of students; e-mail services; employment services for current students; housing assistance; interactive nursing skills videos; Internet; learning resource lab; library services; nursing audiovisuals; placement services for program completers; remedial services; resume preparation assistance; skills, simulation, or other laboratory; tutoring.
**Library Facilities** 799,061 volumes (53,197 in health, 2,200 in nursing); 27,318 periodical subscriptions (186 health-care related).

### BACCALAUREATE PROGRAMS

**Degree** BSN
**Available Programs** ADN to Baccalaureate; Generic Baccalaureate; LPN to Baccalaureate; RN Baccalaureate.
**Study Options** Full-time.
**Program Entrance Requirements** Transcript of college record, written essay, minimum GPA in nursing prerequisites of 2.5, prerequisite course work. Transfer students are accepted. *Application deadline:* 5/1 (fall). *Application fee:* $25.
**Advanced Placement** Credit given for nursing courses completed elsewhere dependent upon specific evaluations.
**Expenses (2012–13)** *Tuition, area resident:* full-time $4102; part-time $137 per credit hour. *Tuition, state resident:* full-time $6154; part-time $205 per credit hour. *Tuition, nonresident:* full-time $15,156; part-time $505 per credit hour. *International tuition:* $15,156 full-time. *Room and board:* $7133 per academic year. *Required fees:* full-time $1170; part-time $140 per credit.
**Financial Aid** 90% of baccalaureate students in nursing programs received some form of financial aid in 2011–12. *Gift aid (need-based):* Federal Pell, FSEOG, state, private, college/university gift aid from institutional funds, Jones Foundation Grants. *Loans:* Perkins, alternative loans, Alaska Loans. *Work-study:* Federal Work-Study, part-time campus jobs. *Financial aid application deadline (priority):* 3/15.
**Contact** Dr. Jean M. DeDonder, Interim Chair and Associate Professor, Newman Division of Nursing, Emporia State University, Newman Division of Nursing, 1127 Chestnut Street, Emporia, KS 66801. *Telephone:* 620-343-6800 Ext. 5640. *Fax:* 620-341-7871. *E-mail:* jdedonde@emporia.edu.

# Fort Hays State University

## Department of Nursing
## Hays, Kansas

***http://www.fhsu.edu/nursing/***
Founded in 1902

### DEGREES • BSN • MSN • MSN/ED D

**Nursing Program Faculty** 23 (13% with doctorates).
**Baccalaureate Enrollment** 235 **Women** 86% **Men** 14% **Minority** 12% **International** 1% **Part-time** 59%
**Graduate Enrollment** 108 **Women** 94% **Men** 6% **Minority** 13% **International** 1% **Part-time** 81%
**Distance Learning Courses** Available.
**Nursing Student Activities** Sigma Theta Tau, Student Nurses' Association, nursing club.
**Nursing Student Resources** Academic advising; academic or career counseling; assistance for students with disabilities; bookstore; campus computer network; career placement assistance; computer lab; computer-assisted instruction; daycare for children of students; e-mail services; employment services for current students; housing assistance; interactive nursing skills videos; Internet; learning resource lab; library services; nursing audiovisuals; paid internships; placement services for program completers; remedial services; resume preparation assistance; skills, simulation, or other laboratory; tutoring.
**Library Facilities** 12,338 volumes in health, 2,414 volumes in nursing; 243 periodical subscriptions health-care related.

### BACCALAUREATE PROGRAMS

**Degree** BSN
**Available Programs** Generic Baccalaureate; RN Baccalaureate.
**Study Options** Full-time and part-time.
**Online Degree Options** Yes.
**Program Entrance Requirements** Minimum overall college GPA of 2.75, transcript of college record, CPR certification, written essay, health exam, health insurance, high school transcript, immunizations, 2 letters of recommendation, minimum GPA in nursing prerequisites of 2.75, professional liability insurance/malpractice insurance, prerequisite course work, RN licensure. Transfer students are accepted. *Application deadline:* 3/1 (fall), 10/1 (spring).
**Advanced Placement** Credit by examination available. Credit given for nursing courses completed elsewhere dependent upon specific evaluations.
**Expenses (2013–14)** *Tuition, area resident:* full-time $2179; part-time $145 per credit hour. *Tuition, state resident:* full-time $3019; part-time $168 per credit hour. *Tuition, nonresident:* full-time $6411; part-time $394 per credit hour. *International tuition:* $6411 full-time. *Room and board:* $7660; room only: $4040 per academic year. *Required fees:* full-time $30.
**Financial Aid** 75% of baccalaureate students in nursing programs received some form of financial aid in 2012–13.
**Contact** Mrs. Carolyn Insley, Coordinator of BSN Program, Department of Nursing, Fort Hays State University, 600 Park Street, Stroup Hall, Room 147, Hays, KS 67601-4099. *Telephone:* 785-628-4514. *Fax:* 785-628-4080. *E-mail:* cinsley@fhsu.edu.

### GRADUATE PROGRAMS

**Expenses (2013–14)** *Tuition, area resident:* full-time $2408; part-time $201 per credit hour. *Tuition, state resident:* full-time $3412; part-time $251 per credit hour. *Tuition, nonresident:* full-time $6120; part-time $477 per credit hour. *International tuition:* $6120 full-time. *Room and board:* $7660; room only: $4040 per academic year. *Required fees:* full-time $35.
**Financial Aid** 56% of graduate students in nursing programs received some form of financial aid in 2012–13. 1 teaching assistantship (averaging $5,000 per year) was awarded; research assistantships.
**Contact** Mrs. Christine L. Hober, Associate Professor, Department of Nursing, Fort Hays State University, 600 Park Street, Stroup Hall, Room 127, Hays, KS 67601-4099. *Telephone:* 785-628-4511. *Fax:* 785-628-4080. *E-mail:* chober@fhsu.edu.

#### MASTER'S DEGREE PROGRAM

**Degrees** MSN; MSN/Ed D
**Available Programs** Master's.
**Concentrations Available** Nursing administration; nursing education. *Nurse practitioner programs in:* family health.
**Study Options** Full-time and part-time.

**Program Entrance Requirements** Clinical experience, computer literacy, minimum overall college GPA of 3.0, transcript of college record, CPR certification, written essay, immunizations, 2 letters of recommendation, physical assessment course, professional liability insurance/malpractice insurance, prerequisite course work, statistics course, GRE General Test or MAT. *Application deadline:* 2/1 (fall), 9/1 (spring), 2/1 (summer). *Application fee:* $35.
**Advanced Placement** Credit given for nursing courses completed elsewhere dependent upon specific evaluations.
**Degree Requirements** 51 total credit hours, thesis or project, comprehensive exam.

### POST-MASTER'S PROGRAM
**Areas of Study** Nursing administration; nursing education. *Nurse practitioner programs in:* family health.

## Kansas Wesleyan University
### Department of Nursing Education
### Salina, Kansas

***http://www.kwu.edu/academics/academic-departments/nursing***
Founded in 1886

### DEGREE • BSN
**Nursing Program Faculty** 8 (13% with doctorates).
**Baccalaureate Enrollment** 68 **Women** 91% **Men** 9% **Minority** 12% **International** 3% **Part-time** 2%
**Nursing Student Activities** Nursing club.
**Nursing Student Resources** Academic advising; academic or career counseling; assistance for students with disabilities; bookstore; campus computer network; career placement assistance; computer lab; computer-assisted instruction; e-mail services; employment services for current students; housing assistance; Internet; learning resource lab; library services; nursing audiovisuals; resume preparation assistance; skills, simulation, or other laboratory; tutoring.
**Library Facilities** 97,060 volumes (15,921 in health, 8,700 in nursing); 188 periodical subscriptions (1,123 health-care related).

### BACCALAUREATE PROGRAMS
**Degree** BSN
**Available Programs** ADN to Baccalaureate; Generic Baccalaureate; RN Baccalaureate.
**Study Options** Full-time and part-time.
**Program Entrance Requirements** Minimum overall college GPA of 2.6, transcript of college record, health exam, high school transcript, immunizations, minimum GPA in nursing prerequisites of 2.6, prerequisite course work. Transfer students are accepted. *Application deadline:* Applications may be processed on a rolling basis for some programs.
**Advanced Placement** Credit by examination available. Credit given for nursing courses completed elsewhere dependent upon specific evaluations.
**Contact** *Telephone:* 785-827-5541 Ext. 2311. *Fax:* 785-827-0927.

## MidAmerica Nazarene University
### Division of Nursing
### Olathe, Kansas

***http://www.mnu.edu/***
Founded in 1966

### DEGREES • BSN • MSN
**Nursing Program Faculty** 55 (52% with doctorates).
**Baccalaureate Enrollment** 393 **Women** 89% **Men** 11% **Minority** 31% **Part-time** 26%
**Graduate Enrollment** 92 **Women** 92% **Men** 8% **Minority** 34% **Part-time** 18%
**Distance Learning Courses** Available.
**Nursing Student Activities** Nursing Honor Society, Student Nurses' Association, nursing club.
**Nursing Student Resources** Academic advising; assistance for students with disabilities; bookstore; campus computer network; computer lab; e-mail services; interactive nursing skills videos; Internet; learning resource lab; library services; nursing audiovisuals; resume preparation assistance; skills, simulation, or other laboratory; tutoring; unpaid internships.
**Library Facilities** 106,268 volumes (1,903 in health, 547 in nursing); 275 periodical subscriptions (115 health-care related).

### BACCALAUREATE PROGRAMS
**Degree** BSN
**Available Programs** Accelerated Baccalaureate; Accelerated RN Baccalaureate; RN Baccalaureate.
**Site Options** Liberty, MO; North Kansas City, MO.
**Study Options** Full-time.
**Online Degree Options** Yes.
**Program Entrance Requirements** Minimum overall college GPA of 2.6, transcript of college record, CPR certification, health insurance, high school transcript, immunizations, 2 letters of recommendation, minimum GPA in nursing prerequisites of 3.6, prerequisite course work. Transfer students are accepted. *Application deadline:* 10/1 (fall), 2/1 (spring).
**Advanced Placement** Credit by examination available. Credit given for nursing courses completed elsewhere dependent upon specific evaluations.
**Expenses (2013–14)** *Tuition:* full-time $21,200; part-time $725 per credit hour. *Room and board:* $3625; room only: $1990 per academic year. *Required fees:* full-time $1025.
**Financial Aid** 80% of baccalaureate students in nursing programs received some form of financial aid in 2012–13.
**Contact** Dr. Susan G. Larson, Dean, School of Nursing and Health Science, Division of Nursing, MidAmerica Nazarene University, 2030 East College Way, Olathe, KS 66062-1899. *Telephone:* 913-971-3698. *Fax:* 913-971-3408. *E-mail:* slarson@mnu.edu.

### GRADUATE PROGRAMS
**Expenses (2013–14)** *Tuition:* full-time $14,580; part-time $405 per credit. *Required fees:* full-time $360.
**Financial Aid** 50% of graduate students in nursing programs received some form of financial aid in 2012–13.
**Contact** Dr. Karen D. Wiegman, Associate Dean, Graduate Studies in Nursing, Division of Nursing, MidAmerica Nazarene University, 2030 East College Way, Olathe, KS 66062-1899. *Telephone:* 913-971-3081. *E-mail:* kdwiegman@mnu.edu.

### MASTER'S DEGREE PROGRAM
**Degree** MSN
**Available Programs** Master's.
**Concentrations Available** Health-care administration; nursing education.
**Site Options** Liberty, MO; North Kansas City, MO.
**Study Options** Full-time and part-time.
**Online Degree Options** Yes.
**Program Entrance Requirements** Minimum overall college GPA of 3.0, transcript of college record, prerequisite course work, statistics course. *Application deadline:* Applications may be processed on a rolling basis for some programs.
**Advanced Placement** Credit by examination available. Credit given for nursing courses completed elsewhere dependent upon specific evaluations.
**Degree Requirements** 36 total credit hours, thesis or project.

## Newman University
### Division of Nursing
### Wichita, Kansas

***http://www.newmanu.edu/***
Founded in 1933

### DEGREES • BSN • MS
**Nursing Program Faculty** 18 (17% with doctorates).
**Baccalaureate Enrollment** 108 **Women** 89% **Men** 11% **Minority** 19% **International** 5% **Part-time** 3%
**Graduate Enrollment** 47 **Women** 46.8% **Men** 53.2% **Minority** .04%
**Distance Learning Courses** Available.
**Nursing Student Activities** Sigma Theta Tau, nursing club.
**Nursing Student Resources** Academic advising; academic or career counseling; assistance for students with disabilities; bookstore; campus computer network; computer lab; computer-assisted instruction; e-mail services; Internet; learning resource lab; library services; nursing audiovisuals; remedial services; resume preparation assistance; skills, simulation, or other laboratory; tutoring.

**Library Facilities** 72,849 volumes (1,528 in health, 938 in nursing); 99 periodical subscriptions (144 health-care related).

## BACCALAUREATE PROGRAMS

**Degree** BSN
**Available Programs** Generic Baccalaureate; LPN to Baccalaureate; RN Baccalaureate.
**Study Options** Full-time and part-time.
**Online Degree Options** Yes.
**Program Entrance Requirements** Minimum overall college GPA of 2.85, transcript of college record, CPR certification, written essay, health exam, health insurance, immunizations, interview, 2 letters of recommendation, minimum GPA in nursing prerequisites of 2.85, professional liability insurance/malpractice insurance, prerequisite course work. Transfer students are accepted. *Application deadline:* Applications may be processed on a rolling basis for some programs.
**Advanced Placement** Credit given for nursing courses completed elsewhere dependent upon specific evaluations.
**Expenses (2013–14)** *Tuition:* full-time $22,700; part-time $757 per credit hour. *International tuition:* $22,700 full-time. *Room and board:* $6666; room only: $4300 per academic year. *Required fees:* full-time $1500; part-time $750 per credit; part-time $375 per term.
**Financial Aid** 43% of baccalaureate students in nursing programs received some form of financial aid in 2012–13.
**Contact** Dr. Bernadette M. Fetterolf, RN, Associate Dean, School of Nursing and Allied Health, Division of Nursing, Newman University, 3100 McCormick Avenue, Wichita, KS 67213-2097. *Telephone:* 316-942-4291 Ext. 2244. *Fax:* 316-942-4483. *E-mail:* fetterolfb@newmanu.edu.

## GRADUATE PROGRAMS

**Expenses (2013–14)** *Tuition:* full-time $25,000; part-time $785 per credit hour. *International tuition:* $25,000 full-time. *Room and board:* $4000; room only: $2330 per academic year. *Required fees:* full-time $300.
**Financial Aid** 100% of graduate students in nursing programs received some form of financial aid in 2012–13. *Application deadline:* 8/15.
**Contact** Ms. Sharon Niemann, Director, Master of Science in Nurse Anesthesia Program, Division of Nursing, Newman University, 3100 McCormick Avenue, Wichita, KS 67213-2097. *Telephone:* 316-942-4291 Ext. 2272. *Fax:* 316-942-4483. *E-mail:* niemanns@newmanu.edu.

### MASTER'S DEGREE PROGRAM

**Degree** MS
**Available Programs** Master's.
**Concentrations Available** Nurse anesthesia.
**Program Entrance Requirements** Clinical experience, minimum overall college GPA of 3.45, transcript of college record, CPR certification, interview, 3 letters of recommendation, nursing research course, resume, statistics course, MAT. *Application deadline:* 11/15 (fall). *Application fee:* $25.
**Degree Requirements** 60 total credit hours, thesis or project.

# Pittsburg State University

**Department of Nursing**
**Pittsburg, Kansas**

***http://www.pittstate.edu/nurs***
Founded in 1903

## DEGREES • BSN • MSN

**Nursing Program Faculty** 18 (1% with doctorates).
**Baccalaureate Enrollment** 211 **Women** 90% **Men** 10% **Minority** 95% **International** 1%
**Graduate Enrollment** 46 **Women** 85% **Men** 15% **Minority** 100% **International** 1%
**Distance Learning Courses** Available.
**Nursing Student Activities** Nursing Honor Society, Sigma Theta Tau, Student Nurses' Association, nursing club.
**Nursing Student Resources** Academic advising; academic or career counseling; assistance for students with disabilities; bookstore; campus computer network; career placement assistance; computer lab; computer-assisted instruction; e-mail services; interactive nursing skills videos; Internet; learning resource lab; library services; nursing audiovisuals; remedial services; resume preparation assistance; skills, simulation, or other laboratory; tutoring; unpaid internships.
**Library Facilities** 712,681 volumes (45,044 in nursing); 35,360 periodical subscriptions.

## BACCALAUREATE PROGRAMS

**Degree** BSN
**Available Programs** Generic Baccalaureate; RN Baccalaureate.
**Study Options** Full-time.
**Online Degree Options** Yes.
**Program Entrance Requirements** Minimum overall college GPA of 2.5, transcript of college record, CPR certification, immunizations, 3 letters of recommendation, minimum GPA in nursing prerequisites of 2.5, professional liability insurance/malpractice insurance, prerequisite course work. Transfer students are accepted. *Application deadline:* 12/15 (fall). *Application fee:* $25.
**Advanced Placement** Credit by examination available. Credit given for nursing courses completed elsewhere dependent upon specific evaluations.
**Expenses (2013–14)** *Tuition, state resident:* full-time $2953; part-time $209 per credit hour. *Tuition, nonresident:* full-time $3313; part-time $279 per credit hour. *International tuition:* $15,786 full-time. *Room and board:* $6954 per academic year. *Required fees:* full-time $1000.
**Financial Aid** 95% of baccalaureate students in nursing programs received some form of financial aid in 2012–13.
**Contact** Dr. Barbara Ruth McClaskey, Coordinator of Bachelor of Science in Nursing Program, Department of Nursing, Pittsburg State University, Irene Ransom Bradley School of Nursing, 1701 South Broadway, Pittsburg, KS 66762. *Telephone:* 620-235-4437. *Fax:* 620-235-4449. *E-mail:* bmcclaskey@pittstate.edu.

## GRADUATE PROGRAMS

**Expenses (2013–14)** *Tuition, area resident:* part-time $279 per credit hour. *Tuition, state resident:* full-time $4966; part-time $279. *Tuition, nonresident:* full-time $7893; part-time $660 per credit hour. *International tuition:* $15,786 full-time. *Room and board:* $6734 per academic year.
**Financial Aid** 90% of graduate students in nursing programs received some form of financial aid in 2012–13.
**Contact** Dr. Mary Carol Pomatto, Master of Science Coordinator, Department of Nursing, Pittsburg State University, 1701 South Broadway, Pittsburg, KS 66762. *Telephone:* 620-235-4431. *Fax:* 620-235-4449. *E-mail:* mpomatto@pittstate.edu.

### MASTER'S DEGREE PROGRAM

**Degree** MSN
**Available Programs** Master's.
**Concentrations Available** Nursing administration; nursing education. *Nurse practitioner programs in:* family health.
**Study Options** Full-time and part-time.
**Program Entrance Requirements** Clinical experience, computer literacy, minimum overall college GPA of 3.0, transcript of college record, CPR certification, written essay, immunizations, 3 letters of recommendation, nursing research course, physical assessment course, professional liability insurance/malpractice insurance, prerequisite course work, resume, statistics course, GRE General Test. *Application deadline:* 3/15 (fall). *Application fee:* $50.
**Advanced Placement** Credit given for nursing courses completed elsewhere dependent upon specific evaluations.
**Degree Requirements** 47 total credit hours, thesis or project, comprehensive exam.

### POST-MASTER'S PROGRAM

**Areas of Study** Nursing administration; nursing education. *Nurse practitioner programs in:* family health.

## CONTINUING EDUCATION PROGRAM

**Contact** Dr. Kristy L. Frisbee, Coordinator of Continuing Nursing Education, Department of Nursing, Pittsburg State University, 1701 South Broadway, McPherson Hall, RM 121, Pittsburg, KS 66762. *Telephone:* 620-235-4434. *Fax:* 620-235-4449. *E-mail:* kfrisbee@pittstate.edu.

# Tabor College
## Department of Nursing
## Hillsboro, Kansas

***http://www.tabor.edu/***
Founded in 1908

**DEGREE • BSN**
**Nursing Program Faculty** 12
**Baccalaureate Enrollment** 71 **Women** 90% **Men** 10% **Minority** 10% **Part-time** 100%
**Distance Learning Courses** Available.
**Nursing Student Activities** Sigma Theta Tau.
**Nursing Student Resources** Academic advising; academic or career counseling; bookstore; campus computer network; computer lab; e-mail services; Internet; learning resource lab; library services; nursing audiovisuals; remedial services; resume preparation assistance; skills, simulation, or other laboratory; tutoring.
**Library Facilities** 77,456 volumes (240 in health, 140 in nursing); 151 periodical subscriptions (600 health-care related).

### BACCALAUREATE PROGRAMS
**Degree** BSN
**Available Programs** ADN to Baccalaureate; Accelerated RN Baccalaureate.
**Site Options** Wichita, KS; Colby, KS; Larned, KS.
**Study Options** Full-time and part-time.
**Online Degree Options** Yes (online only).
**Program Entrance Requirements** Minimum overall college GPA of 2.5, transcript of college record, RN licensure. Transfer students are accepted. *Application deadline:* 8/31 (fall), 12/31 (spring), 4/30 (summer). Applications may be processed on a rolling basis for some programs. *Application fee:* $30.
**Advanced Placement** Credit by examination available. Credit given for nursing courses completed elsewhere dependent upon specific evaluations.
**Contact** *Telephone:* 316-729-6333 Ext. 206. *Fax:* 316-773-5436.

# The University of Kansas
## School of Nursing
## Kansas City, Kansas

***http://www.nursing.kumc.edu***
Founded in 1866

**DEGREES • BSN • MS • MS/MHSA • MS/MPH • PHD**
**Nursing Program Faculty** 74 (58% with doctorates).
**Baccalaureate Enrollment** 260 **Women** 88% **Men** 12% **Minority** 11% **International** 1% **Part-time** 10%
**Graduate Enrollment** 411 **Women** 93% **Men** 7% **Minority** 16% **International** 1% **Part-time** 93%
**Distance Learning Courses** Available.
**Nursing Student Activities** Nursing Honor Society, Sigma Theta Tau, Student Nurses' Association, nursing club.
**Nursing Student Resources** Academic advising; academic or career counseling; assistance for students with disabilities; bookstore; campus computer network; computer lab; computer-assisted instruction; e-mail services; employment services for current students; interactive nursing skills videos; Internet; learning resource lab; library services; nursing audiovisuals; remedial services; resume preparation assistance; skills, simulation, or other laboratory.
**Library Facilities** 5.3 million volumes (180,000 in health, 5,050 in nursing); 6,500 periodical subscriptions health-care related.

### BACCALAUREATE PROGRAMS
**Degree** BSN
**Available Programs** ADN to Baccalaureate; Generic Baccalaureate; RN Baccalaureate.
**Study Options** Full-time and part-time.
**Program Entrance Requirements** Minimum overall college GPA of 2.5, transcript of college record, CPR certification, written essay, health exam, health insurance, immunizations, 3 letters of recommendation, minimum GPA in nursing prerequisites of 2.5, prerequisite course work. Transfer students are accepted. *Application deadline:* 10/15 (fall). *Application fee:* $60.
**Advanced Placement** Credit given for nursing courses completed elsewhere dependent upon specific evaluations.
**Contact** *Telephone:* 913-588-1619. *Fax:* 913-588-1615.

### GRADUATE PROGRAMS
**Contact** *Telephone:* 913-588-1619. *Fax:* 913-588-1615.

#### MASTER'S DEGREE PROGRAM
**Degrees** MS; MS/MHSA; MS/MPH
**Available Programs** Master's; RN to Master's.
**Concentrations Available** Health-care administration; nurse-midwifery; nursing administration; nursing informatics. *Clinical nurse specialist programs in:* adult health, gerontology. *Nurse practitioner programs in:* adult health, family health, gerontology, psychiatric/mental health.
**Site Options** Garden City, KS.
**Study Options** Full-time and part-time.
**Online Degree Options** Yes.
**Program Entrance Requirements** Clinical experience, minimum overall college GPA of 3.0, transcript of college record, CPR certification, immunizations, interview, 3 letters of recommendation, physical assessment course, resume, statistics course. *Application deadline:* 4/1 (fall), 9/1 (spring). *Application fee:* $60.
**Degree Requirements** 37 total credit hours, thesis or project, comprehensive exam.

#### POST-MASTER'S PROGRAM
**Areas of Study** Health-care administration; nurse-midwifery; nursing administration; nursing informatics. *Clinical nurse specialist programs in:* adult health, gerontology. *Nurse practitioner programs in:* adult health, family health, gerontology, psychiatric/mental health.

#### DOCTORAL DEGREE PROGRAM
**Degree** PhD
**Available Programs** Doctorate; Post-Baccalaureate Doctorate.
**Areas of Study** Nursing research.
**Online Degree Options** Yes.
**Program Entrance Requirements** Clinical experience, minimum overall college GPA of 3.5, interview by faculty committee, interview, 3 letters of recommendation, statistics course, vita, writing sample, GRE General Test. *Application deadline:* 12/1 (summer). *Application fee:* $60.
**Degree Requirements** 65 total credit hours, dissertation, oral exam, written exam, residency.

#### POSTDOCTORAL PROGRAM
**Areas of Study** Gerontology, nursing research, outcomes, self-care.
**Postdoctoral Program Contact***Telephone:* 913-588-1692.

### CONTINUING EDUCATION PROGRAM
**Contact** *Telephone:* 913-588-4488. *Fax:* 913-588-4486.

# University of Saint Mary
## Bachelor of Science in Nursing Program
## Leavenworth, Kansas

***http://www.stmary.edu/acad_nursing/default.asp***
Founded in 1923

**DEGREE • BSN**
**Nursing Program Faculty** 22 (9% with doctorates).
**Baccalaureate Enrollment** 168 **Women** 93% **Men** 7% **Minority** 12.5% **International** 3.5% **Part-time** 39%
**Distance Learning Courses** Available.
**Nursing Student Activities** Student Nurses' Association.
**Nursing Student Resources** Academic advising; academic or career counseling; bookstore; campus computer network; e-mail services; employment services for current students; Internet; learning resource lab; library services; nursing audiovisuals; placement services for program completers; resume preparation assistance; skills, simulation, or other laboratory; tutoring.
**Library Facilities** 119,625 volumes; 144 periodical subscriptions.

### BACCALAUREATE PROGRAMS
**Degree** BSN
**Available Programs** Generic Baccalaureate; RN Baccalaureate.
**Site Options** Overland Park, KS.
**Study Options** Full-time.

**Online Degree Options** Yes (online only).
**Program Entrance Requirements** Minimum overall college GPA of 2.5, transcript of college record, CPR certification, written essay, health exam, health insurance, immunizations, 2 letters of recommendation, minimum GPA in nursing prerequisites of 2.5, prerequisite course work. Transfer students are accepted. *Application deadline:* 3/1 (fall). Applications may be processed on a rolling basis for some programs.
**Contact** *Telephone:* 913-758-4381. *Fax:* 913-758-4356.

# Washburn University
## School of Nursing
## Topeka, Kansas

***http://www.washburn.edu/academics/college-schools/nursing/index.html***
Founded in 1865

**DEGREES • BSN • MSN**
**Nursing Program Faculty** 29 (24% with doctorates).
**Baccalaureate Enrollment** 315 **Women** 89% **Men** 11% **Minority** 10% **International** 1% **Part-time** 1%
**Graduate Enrollment** 51 **Women** 90% **Men** 10% **Minority** 1% **Part-time** 70%
**Nursing Student Activities** Sigma Theta Tau, Student Nurses' Association, nursing club.
**Nursing Student Resources** Academic advising; academic or career counseling; assistance for students with disabilities; bookstore; campus computer network; career placement assistance; computer lab; computer-assisted instruction; e-mail services; employment services for current students; interactive nursing skills videos; Internet; learning resource lab; library services; nursing audiovisuals; remedial services; resume preparation assistance; skills, simulation, or other laboratory; tutoring; unpaid internships.
**Library Facilities** 467,524 volumes (12,880 in health, 1,612 in nursing); 42,657 periodical subscriptions (84 health-care related).

### BACCALAUREATE PROGRAMS
**Degree** BSN
**Available Programs** ADN to Baccalaureate; Baccalaureate for Second Degree; Generic Baccalaureate; LPN to Baccalaureate; RN Baccalaureate.
**Study Options** Full-time.
**Program Entrance Requirements** Minimum overall college GPA of 2.7, transcript of college record, CPR certification, written essay, health exam, health insurance, immunizations, interview, 2 letters of recommendation, minimum GPA in nursing prerequisites of 2.0, professional liability insurance/malpractice insurance, prerequisite course work. Transfer students are accepted.
**Advanced Placement** Credit by examination available. Credit given for nursing courses completed elsewhere dependent upon specific evaluations.
**Contact** *Telephone:* 785-231-1032 Ext. 1525. *Fax:* 785-231-1032.

### GRADUATE PROGRAMS
**Contact** *Telephone:* 785-231-1010 Ext. 1533. *Fax:* 785-213-1032.

#### MASTER'S DEGREE PROGRAM
**Degree** MSN
**Available Programs** Master's.
**Concentrations Available** Nursing administration. *Nurse practitioner programs in:* adult health, family health.
**Study Options** Full-time and part-time.
**Program Entrance Requirements** Computer literacy, transcript of college record, CPR certification, written essay, immunizations, 2 letters of recommendation, nursing research course, physical assessment course, professional liability insurance/malpractice insurance, prerequisite course work, resume, statistics course. *Application deadline:* 3/15 (fall). *Application fee:* $35.
**Degree Requirements** 42 total credit hours, thesis or project.

#### POST-MASTER'S PROGRAM
**Areas of Study** Nursing education.

### CONTINUING EDUCATION PROGRAM
**Contact** *Telephone:* 785-231-1010 Ext. 1526. *Fax:* 785-231-1032.

# Wichita State University
## School of Nursing
## Wichita, Kansas

***http://www.wichita.edu/nurs***
Founded in 1895

**DEGREES • BSN • DNP**
**Nursing Program Faculty** 51 (25% with doctorates).
**Baccalaureate Enrollment** 251 **Women** 90% **Men** 10% **Minority** 21% **International** 4% **Part-time** 1%
**Graduate Enrollment** 150 **Women** 94% **Men** 6% **Minority** 6% **International** 1% **Part-time** 66%
**Distance Learning Courses** Available.
**Nursing Student Activities** Sigma Theta Tau, Student Nurses' Association.
**Nursing Student Resources** Academic advising; academic or career counseling; assistance for students with disabilities; bookstore; campus computer network; career placement assistance; computer lab; computer-assisted instruction; daycare for children of students; e-mail services; employment services for current students; housing assistance; interactive nursing skills videos; Internet; learning resource lab; library services; nursing audiovisuals; resume preparation assistance; skills, simulation, or other laboratory.
**Library Facilities** 1.9 million volumes (31,320 in health, 2,746 in nursing); 61,010 periodical subscriptions (406 health-care related).

### BACCALAUREATE PROGRAMS
**Degree** BSN
**Available Programs** ADN to Baccalaureate; Accelerated Baccalaureate; Accelerated Baccalaureate for Second Degree; Generic Baccalaureate; LPN to RN Baccalaureate; RN Baccalaureate.
**Site Options** Derby, KS.
**Study Options** Full-time.
**Online Degree Options** Yes.
**Program Entrance Requirements** Minimum overall college GPA of 2.75, transcript of college record, CPR certification, written essay, health exam, health insurance, immunizations, interview, minimum GPA in nursing prerequisites of 2.0, professional liability insurance/malpractice insurance, prerequisite course work. Transfer students are accepted. *Application deadline:* 2/1 (fall), 9/1 (spring).
**Advanced Placement** Credit given for nursing courses completed elsewhere dependent upon specific evaluations.
**Contact** *Telephone:* 316-978-5732. *Fax:* 316-978-3094.

### GRADUATE PROGRAMS
**Contact** *Telephone:* 316-978-3610. *Fax:* 316-978-3094.

#### MASTER'S DEGREE PROGRAM
**Program Entrance Requirements** *Application deadline:* Applications may be processed on a rolling basis for some programs. *Application fee:* $35.

#### DOCTORAL DEGREE PROGRAM
**Degree** DNP
**Available Programs** Doctorate; Post-Baccalaureate Doctorate.
**Areas of Study** Advanced practice nursing, clinical practice, critical care, faculty preparation, family health, health policy, health promotion/disease prevention, health-care systems, human health and illness, nursing administration, nursing education, nursing policy, nursing research, nursing science.
**Program Entrance Requirements** Clinical experience, minimum overall college GPA of 3.0, interview by faculty committee, interview, 2 letters of recommendation, statistics course, vita. *Application deadline:* 2/15 (fall), 10/15 (spring). *Application fee:* $35.
**Degree Requirements** 74 total credit hours, written exam, residency.

# KENTUCKY

## Bellarmine University

### Donna and Allan Lansing School of Nursing and Health Sciences
### Louisville, Kentucky

*http://www.bellarmine.edu/*
Founded in 1950

**DEGREES • BSN • DNP • MSN • MSN/MBA**

**Nursing Program Faculty** 85 (15% with doctorates).

**Baccalaureate Enrollment** 210 **Women** 88.8% **Men** 11.2% **Minority** 9.26% **International** .24% **Part-time** 18%

**Graduate Enrollment** 79 **Women** 92.8% **Men** 7.2% **Minority** 3.2% **Part-time** 89.6%

**Nursing Student Activities** Sigma Theta Tau, Student Nurses' Association.

**Nursing Student Resources** Academic advising; academic or career counseling; assistance for students with disabilities; bookstore; campus computer network; career placement assistance; computer lab; computer-assisted instruction; e-mail services; employment services for current students; externships; housing assistance; interactive nursing skills videos; Internet; learning resource lab; library services; nursing audiovisuals; paid internships; placement services for program completers; remedial services; resume preparation assistance; skills, simulation, or other laboratory; tutoring; unpaid internships.

**Library Facilities** 136,183 volumes (4,670 in health, 1,644 in nursing); 418 periodical subscriptions (93 health-care related).

#### BACCALAUREATE PROGRAMS

**Degree** BSN

**Available Programs** Accelerated Baccalaureate for Second Degree; Generic Baccalaureate; RN Baccalaureate.

**Study Options** Full-time and part-time.

**Program Entrance Requirements** Minimum overall college GPA of 2.5, transcript of college record, CPR certification, written essay, health exam, health insurance, high school biology, high school chemistry, 2 years high school math, 2 years high school science, high school transcript, immunizations, interview, minimum high school GPA of 2.75, minimum GPA in nursing prerequisites of 2.75, prerequisite course work. Transfer students are accepted. *Application deadline:* 8/15 (fall), 1/3 (winter), 1/3 (spring), 5/3 (summer). Applications may be processed on a rolling basis for some programs. *Application fee:* $25.

**Advanced Placement** Credit by examination available. Credit given for nursing courses completed elsewhere dependent upon specific evaluations.

**Financial Aid** 77% of baccalaureate students in nursing programs received some form of financial aid in 2011–12. *Gift aid (need-based):* Federal Pell, FSEOG, state, private, college/university gift aid from institutional funds. *Loans:* Federal Direct (Subsidized and Unsubsidized Stafford PLUS). *Work-study:* Federal Work-Study, part-time campus jobs. *Financial aid application deadline (priority):* 3/1.

**Contact** Dr. Beverley Holland, BSN Department Chairperson, Donna and Allan Lansing School of Nursing and Health Sciences, Bellarmine University, 2001 Newburg Road, Miles Hall, #202, Louisville, KY 40205-0671. *Telephone:* 502-452-8279. *Fax:* 502-452-8058. *E-mail:* bholland@bellarmine.edu.

#### GRADUATE PROGRAMS

**Financial Aid** 77% of graduate students in nursing programs received some form of financial aid in 2011–12. Career-related internships or fieldwork and scholarships available.

**Contact** Ms. Julie Armstrong-Binnix, Marketing/Recruiter, Donna and Allan Lansing School of Nursing and Health Sciences, Bellarmine University, 2001 Newburg Road, Miles Hall, #201, Louisville, KY 40205-0671. *Telephone:* 502-452-8364. *Fax:* 502-452-8058. *E-mail:* julieab@bellarmine.edu.

#### MASTER'S DEGREE PROGRAM

**Degrees** MSN; MSN/MBA

**Available Programs** Master's; Master's for Nurses with Non-Nursing Degrees; RN to Master's.

**Concentrations Available** Nursing administration; nursing education.

**Study Options** Part-time.

**Program Entrance Requirements** Minimum overall college GPA of 2.75, transcript of college record, professional liability insurance/malpractice insurance, GRE General Test. *Application deadline:* 8/20 (fall), 1/5 (winter), 1/5 (spring), 5/1 (summer). Applications may be processed on a rolling basis for some programs. *Application fee:* $25.

**Advanced Placement** Credit given for nursing courses completed elsewhere dependent upon specific evaluations.

**Degree Requirements** 38 total credit hours, thesis or project.

#### POST-MASTER'S PROGRAM

**Areas of Study** *Nurse practitioner programs in:* family health.

#### DOCTORAL DEGREE PROGRAM

**Degree** DNP

**Available Programs** Doctorate for Nurses with Non-Nursing Degrees.

**Areas of Study** Advanced practice nursing, family health.

**Program Entrance Requirements** Minimum overall college GPA of 3.5, interview by faculty committee, 3 letters of recommendation, MSN or equivalent, vita, GRE General Test. *Application deadline:* 8/15 (fall), 1/5 (spring), 5/3 (summer). *Application fee:* $25.

**Degree Requirements** Residency.

#### CONTINUING EDUCATION PROGRAM

**Contact** Ms. Linda Bailey, Director, Continuing Education, Donna and Allan Lansing School of Nursing and Health Sciences, Bellarmine University, 2001 Newburg Road, Continuing Education Office, Louisville, KY 40205-0671. *Telephone:* 502-452-8161. *Fax:* 502-452-8203. *E-mail:* lbailey@bellarmine.edu.

## Berea College

### Department of Nursing
### Berea, Kentucky

*http://www.berea.edu/nur/*
Founded in 1855

**DEGREE • BSN**

**Nursing Program Faculty** 9 (2% with doctorates).

**Baccalaureate Enrollment** 48 **Women** 90% **Men** 10% **Minority** 10% **International** 12.5%

**Nursing Student Activities** Student Nurses' Association.

**Nursing Student Resources** Academic advising; academic or career counseling; assistance for students with disabilities; bookstore; campus computer network; career placement assistance; computer lab; computer-assisted instruction; daycare for children of students; e-mail services; employment services for current students; externships; housing assistance; interactive nursing skills videos; Internet; learning resource lab; library services; nursing audiovisuals; paid internships; placement services for program completers; remedial services; resume preparation assistance; skills, simulation, or other laboratory; tutoring; unpaid internships.

**Library Facilities** 392,752 volumes; 1,438 periodical subscriptions.

#### BACCALAUREATE PROGRAMS

**Degree** BSN

**Available Programs** Generic Baccalaureate.

**Study Options** Full-time.

**Program Entrance Requirements** Minimum overall college GPA of 2.5, transcript of college record, CPR certification, written essay, high school transcript, immunizations, interview, 3 letters of recommendation, minimum high school GPA, minimum high school rank 15%, minimum GPA in nursing prerequisites of 2.5, prerequisite course work. Transfer students are accepted. *Application deadline:* Applications may be processed on a rolling basis for some programs.

**Advanced Placement** Credit given for nursing courses completed elsewhere dependent upon specific evaluations.

**Contact** *Telephone:* 859-985-3503.

## Eastern Kentucky University
### Department of Baccalaureate and Graduate Nursing
### Richmond, Kentucky

***http://www.bsn-gn.eku.edu/***
Founded in 1906

**DEGREES • BSN • MSN**

**Nursing Program Faculty** 42 (40% with doctorates).
**Baccalaureate Enrollment** 500
**Graduate Enrollment** 200
**Distance Learning Courses** Available.
**Nursing Student Activities** Sigma Theta Tau, Student Nurses' Association.
**Nursing Student Resources** Academic advising; academic or career counseling; assistance for students with disabilities; bookstore; campus computer network; computer lab; computer-assisted instruction; e-mail services; housing assistance; interactive nursing skills videos; Internet; learning resource lab; library services; nursing audiovisuals; skills, simulation, or other laboratory.
**Library Facilities** 799,496 volumes; 2,901 periodical subscriptions.

#### BACCALAUREATE PROGRAMS

**Degree** BSN
**Available Programs** Accelerated RN Baccalaureate; Baccalaureate for Second Degree; Generic Baccalaureate; RN Baccalaureate.
**Site Options** Hazard, KY; Corbin, KY; Danville, KY.
**Study Options** Full-time and part-time.
**Program Entrance Requirements** Minimum overall college GPA of 2.5, CPR certification, immunizations, professional liability insurance/malpractice insurance, prerequisite course work. Transfer students are accepted.
**Advanced Placement** Credit given for nursing courses completed elsewhere dependent upon specific evaluations.
**Contact** *Telephone:* 859-622-1827. *Fax:* 859-622-1972.

#### GRADUATE PROGRAMS

**Contact** *Telephone:* 859-622-1838. *Fax:* 859-622-1972.

**MASTER'S DEGREE PROGRAM**
**Degree** MSN
**Available Programs** Master's.
**Concentrations Available** Nursing education. *Clinical nurse specialist programs in:* public health. *Nurse practitioner programs in:* family health, psychiatric/mental health.
**Site Options** Hazard, KY; Corbin, KY; Danville, KY.
**Study Options** Full-time and part-time.
**Program Entrance Requirements** Minimum overall college GPA of 2.75, transcript of college record, written essay, 3 letters of recommendation, statistics course.
**Advanced Placement** Credit given for nursing courses completed elsewhere dependent upon specific evaluations.
**Degree Requirements** 48 total credit hours, thesis or project, comprehensive exam.

## Frontier Nursing University
### Nursing Degree Programs
### Hyden, Kentucky

Founded in 1939

**DEGREES • DNP • MSN**

#### GRADUATE PROGRAMS

**Contact** *Telephone:* 606-672-2312.

**MASTER'S DEGREE PROGRAM**
**Degree** MSN
**Available Programs** Accelerated AD/RN to Master's.

**DOCTORAL DEGREE PROGRAM**
**Degree** DNP
**Available Programs** Doctorate.

## Kentucky Christian University
### School of Nursing
### Grayson, Kentucky

***http://www.kcu.edu/yancey-nursing***
Founded in 1919

**DEGREE • BSN**

**Nursing Program Faculty** 6 (20% with doctorates).
**Baccalaureate Enrollment** 63 **Women** 90% **Men** 10% **Minority** 1% **International** 1%
**Nursing Student Activities** Student Nurses' Association.
**Nursing Student Resources** Academic advising; assistance for students with disabilities; bookstore; campus computer network; computer lab; e-mail services; housing assistance; interactive nursing skills videos; Internet; learning resource lab; library services; nursing audiovisuals; other; remedial services; skills, simulation, or other laboratory.
**Library Facilities** 204,752 volumes (400 in health, 300 in nursing); 190 periodical subscriptions (200 health-care related).

#### BACCALAUREATE PROGRAMS

**Degree** BSN
**Available Programs** Generic Baccalaureate.
**Study Options** Full-time.
**Program Entrance Requirements** Transcript of college record, written essay, health exam, health insurance, high school transcript, immunizations, minimum GPA in nursing prerequisites of 2.5, prerequisite course work. Transfer students are accepted.
**Contact** *Telephone:* 606-474-3255. *Fax:* 606-474-3342.

#### CONTINUING EDUCATION PROGRAM

**Contact** *Telephone:* 606-474-3271. *Fax:* 606-474-3342.

## Kentucky State University
### School of Nursing
### Frankfort, Kentucky

***http://www.kysu.edu/***
Founded in 1886

**DEGREE • BSN**

**Nursing Program Faculty** 18 (11% with doctorates).
**Baccalaureate Enrollment** 25
**Nursing Student Activities** Student Nurses' Association.
**Nursing Student Resources** Academic advising; academic or career counseling; assistance for students with disabilities; bookstore; campus computer network; career placement assistance; computer lab; computer-assisted instruction; e-mail services; externships; housing assistance; interactive nursing skills videos; Internet; learning resource lab; library services; nursing audiovisuals; other; placement services for program completers; remedial services; resume preparation assistance; skills, simulation, or other laboratory; tutoring.
**Library Facilities** 326,821 volumes; 785 periodical subscriptions.

#### BACCALAUREATE PROGRAMS

**Degree** BSN
**Available Programs** ADN to Baccalaureate.
**Program Entrance Requirements** Transfer students are accepted.
**Contact** *Telephone:* 502-597-6963. *Fax:* 502-597-5818.

## Midway College
### Program in Nursing (Baccalaureate)
### Midway, Kentucky

***http://www.midway.edu/academic-programs/nursing-science***
Founded in 1847

**DEGREE • BSN**

**Nursing Program Faculty** 3 (33% with doctorates).
**Baccalaureate Enrollment** 45 **Women** 99% **Men** 1% **Minority** 20% **Part-time** 50%
**Distance Learning Courses** Available.
**Nursing Student Activities** Student Nurses' Association.

**Nursing Student Resources** Academic advising; academic or career counseling; assistance for students with disabilities; bookstore; campus computer network; career placement assistance; computer lab; computer-assisted instruction; e-mail services; externships; interactive nursing skills videos; Internet; learning resource lab; library services; nursing audiovisuals; placement services for program completers; remedial services; resume preparation assistance; skills, simulation, or other laboratory; tutoring; unpaid internships.
**Library Facilities** 96,236 volumes (1,200 in health, 800 in nursing); 250 periodical subscriptions (102 health-care related).

## BACCALAUREATE PROGRAMS

**Degree** BSN
**Available Programs** ADN to Baccalaureate; Accelerated RN Baccalaureate; RN Baccalaureate.
**Study Options** Full-time and part-time.
**Program Entrance Requirements** Minimum overall college GPA of 2.5, CPR certification, health insurance, immunizations, interview, minimum GPA in nursing prerequisites of 2.5, prerequisite course work, RN licensure. Transfer students are accepted. *Application deadline:* 3/15 (fall), 3/15 (winter), 10/15 (spring), 3/15 (summer). Applications may be processed on a rolling basis for some programs. *Application fee:* $10.
**Advanced Placement** Credit given for nursing courses completed elsewhere dependent upon specific evaluations.
**Expenses (2013–14)** *Tuition:* part-time $530 per credit hour.
**Financial Aid** 100% of baccalaureate students in nursing programs received some form of financial aid in 2012–13.
**Contact** Dr. Barbara R. Kitchen, Dean, School of Health Sciences, Program in Nursing (Baccalaureate), Midway College, 512 East Stephens Street, Midway, KY 40347. *Telephone:* 859-846-5335. *Fax:* 859-846-5876. *E-mail:* bkitchen@midway.edu.

## CONTINUING EDUCATION PROGRAM

**Contact** Dr. Barbara R. Kitchen, Dean, School of Health Sciences, Program in Nursing (Baccalaureate), Midway College, 512 East Stephens Street, Midway, KY 40347. *Telephone:* 859-846-5335. *Fax:* 859-846-5876. *E-mail:* bkitchen@midway.edu.

# Morehead State University
### Department of Nursing
### Morehead, Kentucky

***http://www.moreheadstate.edu/nursing***
Founded in 1922

**DEGREE • BSN**
**Nursing Program Faculty** 51 (16% with doctorates).
**Baccalaureate Enrollment** 202 **Women** 92% **Men** 8% **Minority** 5% **Part-time** 23%
**Distance Learning Courses** Available.
**Nursing Student Activities** Student Nurses' Association.
**Nursing Student Resources** Academic advising; academic or career counseling; assistance for students with disabilities; bookstore; campus computer network; career placement assistance; computer lab; computer-assisted instruction; e-mail services; interactive nursing skills videos; Internet; learning resource lab; library services; nursing audiovisuals; remedial services; resume preparation assistance; skills, simulation, or other laboratory; tutoring.
**Library Facilities** 591,287 volumes (500,000 in health, 860 in nursing); 56,528 periodical subscriptions (286 health-care related).

## BACCALAUREATE PROGRAMS

**Degree** BSN
**Available Programs** ADN to Baccalaureate; Generic Baccalaureate; RN Baccalaureate.
**Site Options** Prestonsburg, KY; Mt. Sterling, KY; Ashland, KY.
**Study Options** Full-time.
**Online Degree Options** Yes.
**Program Entrance Requirements** Minimum overall college GPA of 2.0, transcript of college record, CPR certification, immunizations, minimum GPA in nursing prerequisites of 3.0, prerequisite course work. Transfer students are accepted. *Application deadline:* 3/15 (fall).
**Advanced Placement** Credit by examination available. Credit given for nursing courses completed elsewhere dependent upon specific evaluations.
**Expenses (2013–14)** *Tuition, state resident:* full-time $7498; part-time $320 per credit hour. *Tuition, nonresident:* full-time $18,746; part-time $800 per credit hour. *International tuition:* $18,746 full-time. *Room and board:* $6200; room only: $4040 per academic year. *Required fees:* full-time $325.
**Financial Aid** 80% of baccalaureate students in nursing programs received some form of financial aid in 2012–13. *Gift aid (need-based):* Federal Pell, FSEOG, state, private, college/university gift aid from institutional funds. *Loans:* Federal Direct (Subsidized and Unsubsidized Stafford PLUS), Perkins, college/university. *Work-study:* Federal Work-Study, part-time campus jobs. *Financial aid application deadline (priority):* 3/15.
**Contact** Ms. Carla June Aagaard, Academic Counseling Coordinator, Department of Nursing, Morehead State University, CHER 201A, Morehead, KY 40351. *Telephone:* 606-783-2641. *Fax:* 606-783-9123. *E-mail:* c.aagaard@moreheadstate.edu.

# Murray State University
### Program in Nursing
### Murray, Kentucky

***http://www.murraystate.edu/***
Founded in 1922

**DEGREES • BSN • MSN**
**Nursing Program Faculty** 16 (47% with doctorates).
**Baccalaureate Enrollment** 206 **Women** 94% **Men** 6% **Minority** 3%
**Graduate Enrollment** 48 **Women** 85% **Men** 15%
**Distance Learning Courses** Available.
**Nursing Student Activities** Sigma Theta Tau, Student Nurses' Association.
**Nursing Student Resources** Academic advising; academic or career counseling; assistance for students with disabilities; bookstore; campus computer network; career placement assistance; computer lab; computer-assisted instruction; daycare for children of students; e-mail services; employment services for current students; externships; housing assistance; interactive nursing skills videos; Internet; learning resource lab; library services; nursing audiovisuals; placement services for program completers; remedial services; resume preparation assistance; skills, simulation, or other laboratory; tutoring; unpaid internships.
**Library Facilities** 759,173 volumes (4,060 in health, 2,160 in nursing); 327,441 periodical subscriptions (124 health-care related).

## BACCALAUREATE PROGRAMS

**Degree** BSN
**Available Programs** Generic Baccalaureate; RN Baccalaureate.
**Site Options** Hopkinsville, KY; Paducah, KY; Madisonville, KY.
**Study Options** Full-time.
**Program Entrance Requirements** Transcript of college record, CPR certification, immunizations, minimum GPA in nursing prerequisites of 2.5, professional liability insurance/malpractice insurance, prerequisite course work. Transfer students are accepted. *Application deadline:* 5/1 (fall), 11/22 (spring).
**Advanced Placement** Credit by examination available. Credit given for nursing courses completed elsewhere dependent upon specific evaluations.
**Contact** *Telephone:* 270-809-2193. *Fax:* 270-809-6662.

## GRADUATE PROGRAMS

**Contact** *Telephone:* 270-809-6671. *Fax:* 270-809-6662.

### MASTER'S DEGREE PROGRAM

**Degree** MSN
**Available Programs** Master's.
**Concentrations Available** Nurse anesthesia. *Clinical nurse specialist programs in:* adult health, critical care, medical-surgical. *Nurse practitioner programs in:* family health.
**Site Options** Hopkinsville, KY; Paducah, KY; Madisonville, KY.
**Study Options** Full-time and part-time.
**Program Entrance Requirements** Clinical experience, minimum overall college GPA of 3.0, transcript of college record, CPR certification, immunizations, interview, 3 letters of recommendation, nursing research course, physical assessment course, professional liability insurance/malpractice insurance, prerequisite course work, statistics course, GRE General Test. *Application deadline:* 11/1 (fall).
**Advanced Placement** Credit given for nursing courses completed elsewhere dependent upon specific evaluations.
**Degree Requirements** 46 total credit hours.

**POST-MASTER'S PROGRAM**
**Areas of Study** Nurse anesthesia. *Clinical nurse specialist programs in:* adult health, critical care, medical-surgical. *Nurse practitioner programs in:* family health.

## CONTINUING EDUCATION PROGRAM

**Contact** *Telephone:* 270-809-6674. *Fax:* 270-809-6662.

# Northern Kentucky University

## Department of Nursing
## Highland Heights, Kentucky

***http://www.nku.edu/majors/nursing.html***
Founded in 1968

**DEGREES • BSN • DNP • MSN**
**Nursing Program Faculty** 100 (20% with doctorates).
**Baccalaureate Enrollment** 600 **Women** 93% **Men** 7% **Minority** 2% **International** 1% **Part-time** 50%
**Graduate Enrollment** 275 **Women** 95% **Men** 5% **Minority** 1% **Part-time** 90%
**Distance Learning Courses** Available.
**Nursing Student Activities** Sigma Theta Tau, Student Nurses' Association.
**Nursing Student Resources** Academic advising; academic or career counseling; assistance for students with disabilities; bookstore; campus computer network; career placement assistance; computer lab; computer-assisted instruction; daycare for children of students; e-mail services; employment services for current students; housing assistance; interactive nursing skills videos; Internet; learning resource lab; library services; nursing audiovisuals; resume preparation assistance; skills, simulation, or other laboratory; tutoring.
**Library Facilities** 888,132 volumes (6,380 in health, 3,500 in nursing); 46,140 periodical subscriptions (100 health-care related).

## BACCALAUREATE PROGRAMS

**Degree** BSN
**Available Programs** Accelerated Baccalaureate for Second Degree; Generic Baccalaureate; RN Baccalaureate.
**Study Options** Full-time.
**Program Entrance Requirements** Minimum overall college GPA of 2.5, transcript of college record, CPR certification, health exam, health insurance, high school biology, high school chemistry, 3 years high school math, high school transcript, immunizations, minimum GPA in nursing prerequisites of 3.0, prerequisite course work. Transfer students are accepted. *Application deadline:* 1/15 (fall), 8/15 (spring).
**Advanced Placement** Credit by examination available. Credit given for nursing courses completed elsewhere dependent upon specific evaluations.
**Expenses (2012–13)** *Tuition, state resident:* full-time $3936; part-time $328 per credit hour. *Tuition, nonresident:* full-time $7872; part-time $656 per credit hour. *Room and board:* $7600; room only: $4200 per academic year. *Required fees:* full-time $250; part-time $125 per term.
**Financial Aid** ***Gift aid (need-based):*** Federal Pell, FSEOG, state, private, college/university gift aid from institutional funds. *Loans:* Federal Direct (Subsidized and Unsubsidized Stafford PLUS), Perkins, college/university, private loans. *Work-study:* Federal Work-Study, part-time campus jobs. *Financial aid application deadline (priority):* 2/1.
**Contact** Dr. Carrie McCoy, Chair, Department of Nursing, Northern Kentucky University, Nunn Drive, AHC 303, Highland Heights, KY 41099. *Telephone:* 859-572-5248. *Fax:* 859-572-6098. *E-mail:* mccoy@nku.edu.

## GRADUATE PROGRAMS

**Expenses (2012–13)** *Tuition, state resident:* part-time $510 per credit hour. *Tuition, nonresident:* part-time $765 per credit hour. *Room and board:* $7600; room only: $4200 per academic year. *Required fees:* part-time $45 per term.
**Financial Aid** 10% of graduate students in nursing programs received some form of financial aid in 2011–12.
**Contact** Dr. Jayne Lancaster, Interim Chair of Advanced Nursing Studies, Department of Nursing, Northern Kentucky University, HC 206, Highland Heights, KY 41099. *Telephone:* 859-572-7966. *Fax:* 859-572-1934. *E-mail:* lancasterj1@nku.edu.

**MASTER'S DEGREE PROGRAM**
**Degree** MSN
**Available Programs** Master's.
**Concentrations Available** Nursing administration; nursing education; nursing informatics. *Nurse practitioner programs in:* acute care, adult health, family health, pediatric.
**Study Options** Full-time and part-time.
**Online Degree Options** Yes.
**Program Entrance Requirements** Clinical experience, minimum overall college GPA of 3.0, transcript of college record, CPR certification, immunizations, 1 letter of recommendation, nursing research course, physical assessment course, professional liability insurance/malpractice insurance, prerequisite course work, resume, statistics course. *Application deadline:* 2/15 (fall), 10/15 (spring).
**Advanced Placement** Credit by examination available. Credit given for nursing courses completed elsewhere dependent upon specific evaluations.
**Degree Requirements** 42 total credit hours, thesis or project.

**POST-MASTER'S PROGRAM**
**Areas of Study** Nursing administration; nursing education. *Nurse practitioner programs in:* acute care, adult health, family health, pediatric, psychiatric/mental health.

**DOCTORAL DEGREE PROGRAM**
**Degree** DNP
**Available Programs** Doctorate.
**Online Degree Options** Yes.
**Program Entrance Requirements** Minimum overall college GPA of 3.0, 3 letters of recommendation, MSN or equivalent, statistics course, vita, writing sample. *Application deadline:* 2/15 (fall), 10/15 (spring).
**Degree Requirements** 36 total credit hours, dissertation.

## CONTINUING EDUCATION PROGRAM

**Contact** Mary Gers, Director of Simulation and Technology, Department of Nursing, Northern Kentucky University, NKU, HC 303, Highland Heights, KY 41099. *Telephone:* 859-572-6322. *Fax:* 859-572-1934. *E-mail:* gersm@nku.edu.

# Spalding University

## School of Nursing
## Louisville, Kentucky

***http://www.spalding.edu/nursing***
Founded in 1814

**DEGREES • BSN • MSN**
**Nursing Program Faculty** 33 (18% with doctorates).
**Baccalaureate Enrollment** 170 **Women** 94% **Men** 6% **Minority** 10% **International** 6%
**Graduate Enrollment** 56 **Women** 99.5% **Men** .5% **Minority** 2% **International** 3.4% **Part-time** 50%
**Nursing Student Activities** Sigma Theta Tau, Student Nurses' Association.
**Nursing Student Resources** Academic advising; academic or career counseling; assistance for students with disabilities; bookstore; campus computer network; career placement assistance; computer lab; computer-assisted instruction; e-mail services; employment services for current students; externships; interactive nursing skills videos; Internet; learning resource lab; library services; nursing audiovisuals; remedial services; resume preparation assistance; skills, simulation, or other laboratory; tutoring; unpaid internships.
**Library Facilities** 101,988 volumes (2,875 in health, 1,125 in nursing); 102 periodical subscriptions (367 health-care related).

## BACCALAUREATE PROGRAMS

**Degree** BSN
**Available Programs** Accelerated Baccalaureate for Second Degree; Accelerated RN Baccalaureate; Generic Baccalaureate.
**Study Options** Full-time and part-time.
**Program Entrance Requirements** Minimum overall college GPA of 2.5, transcript of college record, CPR certification, health exam, health insurance, high school transcript, immunizations, minimum GPA in nursing prerequisites of 2.5, professional liability insurance/malpractice insurance, prerequisite course work. Transfer students are accepted.
**Advanced Placement** Credit given for nursing courses completed elsewhere dependent upon specific evaluations.
**Contact** *Telephone:* 502-585-7125. *Fax:* 502-588-7175.

## GRADUATE PROGRAMS

**Contact** *Telephone:* 502-585-9911 Ext. 2332. *Fax:* 502-588-7175.

**MASTER'S DEGREE PROGRAM**

**Degree** MSN
**Available Programs** Accelerated RN to Master's; Master's.
**Concentrations Available** Nursing administration; nursing education. *Nurse practitioner programs in:* adult health, family health, pediatric.
**Study Options** Full-time and part-time.
**Program Entrance Requirements** Computer literacy, minimum overall college GPA of 3.0, transcript of college record, CPR certification, written essay, immunizations, interview, 2 letters of recommendation, physical assessment course, professional liability insurance/malpractice insurance, prerequisite course work, resume, statistics course, GRE General Test.
**Advanced Placement** Credit by examination available. Credit given for nursing courses completed elsewhere dependent upon specific evaluations.
**Degree Requirements** 53 total credit hours, thesis or project.

**POST-MASTER'S PROGRAM**

**Areas of Study** Nursing administration; nursing education. *Nurse practitioner programs in:* adult health, family health, pediatric.

## CONTINUING EDUCATION PROGRAM

**Contact** *Telephone:* 502-585-9911 Ext. 2332. *Fax:* 502-588-7175.

# Thomas More College

### Program in Nursing
### Crestview Hills, Kentucky

***http://www.thomasmore.edu/***
Founded in 1921

**DEGREE • BSN**

**Nursing Program Faculty** 7 (29% with doctorates).
**Baccalaureate Enrollment** 100 **Women** 92% **Men** 8% **Minority** .03% **International** .01%
**Nursing Student Activities** Student Nurses' Association.
**Nursing Student Resources** Academic advising; academic or career counseling; assistance for students with disabilities; bookstore; campus computer network; career placement assistance; computer lab; computer-assisted instruction; e-mail services; employment services for current students; externships; interactive nursing skills videos; Internet; learning resource lab; library services; nursing audiovisuals; other; placement services for program completers; remedial services; resume preparation assistance; skills, simulation, or other laboratory; tutoring.
**Library Facilities** 113,904 volumes (350 in health, 200 in nursing); 421 periodical subscriptions (50 health-care related).

## BACCALAUREATE PROGRAMS

**Degree** BSN
**Available Programs** Generic Baccalaureate.
**Study Options** Full-time.
**Program Entrance Requirements** Transcript of college record, CPR certification, health exam, health insurance, high school transcript, immunizations, minimum GPA in nursing prerequisites of 2.75, professional liability insurance/malpractice insurance, prerequisite course work. Transfer students are accepted. *Application deadline:* 5/1 (fall). *Application fee:* $25.
**Advanced Placement** Credit given for nursing courses completed elsewhere dependent upon specific evaluations.
**Financial Aid** 90% of baccalaureate students in nursing programs received some form of financial aid in 2011–12. *Gift aid (need-based):* Federal Pell, FSEOG, state, private, college/university gift aid from institutional funds, Federal Nursing. *Loans:* Federal Nursing Student Loans, Federal Direct (Subsidized and Unsubsidized Stafford PLUS), Perkins, college/university. *Work-study:* Federal Work-Study, part-time campus jobs. *Financial aid application deadline (priority):* 3/15.
**Contact** Dr. Lisa Spangler Torok, Chair, Program in Nursing, Thomas More College, 333 Thomas More Parkway, Crestview Hills, KY 41017. *Telephone:* 859-344-3413. *Fax:* 859-344-3537. *E-mail:* lisa.spangler-torok@thomasmore.edu.

# Union College

### School of Nursing & Health Sciences
### Barbourville, Kentucky

Founded in 1879

**DEGREE • BSN**

**Library Facilities** 116,825 volumes; 16,223 periodical subscriptions.

## BACCALAUREATE PROGRAMS

**Degree** BSN
**Available Programs** Generic Baccalaureate.
**Study Options** Full-time and part-time.
**Contact** Dr. Lorene Putnam, Dean of Nursing and Health Sciences, School of Nursing & Health Sciences, Union College, 115 Health and Natural Sciences, Barbourville, KY 40906. *Telephone:* 606-546-1212. *E-mail:* lputnam@unionky.edu.

# University of Kentucky

### College of Nursing
### Lexington, Kentucky

***http://www.uknursing.uky.edu/***
Founded in 1865

**DEGREES • BSN • MSN • PHD**

**Nursing Program Faculty** 65 (54% with doctorates).
**Baccalaureate Enrollment** 260 **Women** 97% **Men** 3% **Minority** 6% **Part-time** 14%
**Graduate Enrollment** 221 **Women** 92% **Men** 8% **Minority** 9% **International** 5% **Part-time** 35%
**Nursing Student Activities** Sigma Theta Tau, Student Nurses' Association.
**Nursing Student Resources** Academic advising; academic or career counseling; assistance for students with disabilities; bookstore; campus computer network; career placement assistance; computer lab; computer-assisted instruction; e-mail services; interactive nursing skills videos; Internet; learning resource lab; library services; nursing audiovisuals; skills, simulation, or other laboratory.
**Library Facilities** 105,793 volumes in health; 3,347 periodical subscriptions health-care related.

## BACCALAUREATE PROGRAMS

**Degree** BSN
**Available Programs** Baccalaureate for Second Degree; Generic Baccalaureate; RN Baccalaureate.
**Study Options** Full-time and part-time.
**Program Entrance Requirements** Minimum overall college GPA of 2.5, transcript of college record, CPR certification, written essay, high school transcript, immunizations, minimum GPA in nursing prerequisites of 2.5, prerequisite course work. Transfer students are accepted.
**Advanced Placement** Credit by examination available. Credit given for nursing courses completed elsewhere dependent upon specific evaluations.
**Contact** *Telephone:* 859-323-5108. *Fax:* 859-323-1057.

## GRADUATE PROGRAMS

**Contact** *Telephone:* 859-323-5108. *Fax:* 859-323-1057.

**MASTER'S DEGREE PROGRAM**

**Degree** MSN
**Available Programs** Master's; RN to Master's.
**Concentrations Available** Nurse case management; nursing administration. *Clinical nurse specialist programs in:* acute care, adult health, community health, critical care, gerontology, medical-surgical, oncology, parent-child, pediatric, perinatal, psychiatric/mental health, public health,women's health. *Nurse practitioner programs in:* acute care, adult health, family health, gerontology, pediatric, psychiatric/mental health.
**Site Options** Morehead, KY.
**Study Options** Full-time and part-time.
**Program Entrance Requirements** Clinical experience, minimum overall college GPA of 2.75, transcript of college record, written essay, interview, 3 letters of recommendation, physical assessment course, statistics course.
**Advanced Placement** Credit given for nursing courses completed elsewhere dependent upon specific evaluations.

**Degree Requirements** 40 total credit hours, comprehensive exam.

### POST-MASTER'S PROGRAM

**Areas of Study** Nurse case management. *Nurse practitioner programs in:* acute care, adult health, family health, gerontology, pediatric, psychiatric/mental health.

### DOCTORAL DEGREE PROGRAM

**Degree** PhD
**Available Programs** Doctorate.
**Areas of Study** Nursing research.
**Program Entrance Requirements** Minimum overall college GPA of 3.3, interview, 3 letters of recommendation, MSN or equivalent, statistics course, writing sample, GRE General Test.
**Degree Requirements** 63 total credit hours, dissertation, oral exam, written exam, residency.

## CONTINUING EDUCATION PROGRAM

**Contact** *Telephone:* 859-323-3851. *Fax:* 859-323-1057.

# University of Louisville

## School of Nursing
## Louisville, Kentucky

***http://www.louisville.edu/nursing***
Founded in 1798

**DEGREES • BSN • MSN • PHD**
**Nursing Program Faculty** 72 (40% with doctorates).
**Baccalaureate Enrollment** 479 **Women** 89% **Men** 11% **Minority** 17% **International** 1% **Part-time** 18%
**Graduate Enrollment** 137 **Women** 89% **Men** 11% **Minority** 18% **International** 1% **Part-time** 48%
**Distance Learning Courses** Available.
**Nursing Student Activities** Sigma Theta Tau, Student Nurses' Association.
**Nursing Student Resources** Academic advising; academic or career counseling; assistance for students with disabilities; bookstore; campus computer network; career placement assistance; computer lab; computer-assisted instruction; e-mail services; employment services for current students; housing assistance; interactive nursing skills videos; Internet; learning resource lab; library services; nursing audiovisuals; skills, simulation, or other laboratory; tutoring.
**Library Facilities** 2.4 million volumes (253,595 in health, 2,806 in nursing); 4,329 periodical subscriptions health-care related.

## BACCALAUREATE PROGRAMS

**Degree** BSN
**Available Programs** Accelerated Baccalaureate for Second Degree; Generic Baccalaureate; RN Baccalaureate.
**Site Options** Owensboro, KY.
**Study Options** Full-time.
**Online Degree Options** Yes.
**Program Entrance Requirements** Minimum overall college GPA of 2.8, transcript of college record, CPR certification, written essay, health insurance, high school foreign language, 3 years high school math, 3 years high school science, high school transcript, immunizations, minimum high school GPA of 2.8, minimum GPA in nursing prerequisites of 2.8, professional liability insurance/malpractice insurance, prerequisite course work. Transfer students are accepted. *Application deadline:* 5/1 (fall), 9/15 (spring). *Application fee:* $40.
**Advanced Placement** Credit by examination available. Credit given for nursing courses completed elsewhere dependent upon specific evaluations.
**Expenses (2012–13)** *Tuition, state resident:* full-time $9466; part-time $395 per credit hour. *Tuition, nonresident:* full-time $22,950; part-time $957 per credit hour. *Room and board:* $5980; room only: $4520 per academic year. *Required fees:* full-time $1600.
**Financial Aid** 87% of baccalaureate students in nursing programs received some form of financial aid in 2011–12. *Gift aid (need-based):* Federal Pell, FSEOG, state, private, college/university gift aid from institutional funds. *Loans:* Federal Nursing Student Loans, Federal Direct (Subsidized and Unsubsidized Stafford PLUS), Perkins. *Work-study:* Federal Work-Study. *Financial aid application deadline (priority):* 3/15.
**Contact** Trish Hart, Director of Student Services, School of Nursing, University of Louisville, 555 South Floyd Street, Louisville, KY 40202. *Telephone:* 502-852-8298. *Fax:* 502-852-8783. *E-mail:* trish.hart@louisville.edu.

## GRADUATE PROGRAMS

**Expenses (2012–13)** *Tuition, state resident:* full-time $10,274; part-time $571 per credit hour. *Tuition, nonresident:* full-time $21,378; part-time $1188 per credit hour. *International tuition:* $21,378 full-time. *Room and board:* $5922 per academic year. *Required fees:* full-time $1600.
**Financial Aid** 87% of graduate students in nursing programs received some form of financial aid in 2011–12. 6 research assistantships with full tuition reimbursements available (averaging $20,000 per year), 6 teaching assistantships with full tuition reimbursements available (averaging $19,167 per year) were awarded; fellowships with full tuition reimbursements available, institutionally sponsored loans, scholarships, traineeships, and unspecified assistantships also available. Aid available to part-time students. *Financial aid application deadline:* 4/15.
**Contact** Dr. Rosalie Mainous, Associate Dean for Graduate Academic Affairs, School of Nursing, University of Louisville, 555 South Floyd Street, Louisville, KY 40292. *Telephone:* 502-852-8387. *Fax:* 502-852-8783. *E-mail:* rosalie.mainous@louisville.edu.

### MASTER'S DEGREE PROGRAM

**Degree** MSN
**Available Programs** Master's.
**Concentrations Available** Nursing education. *Nurse practitioner programs in:* acute care, adult health, family health, neonatal health, psychiatric/mental health,women's health.
**Study Options** Full-time and part-time.
**Program Entrance Requirements** Clinical experience, minimum overall college GPA of 3.0, transcript of college record, CPR certification, written essay, immunizations, 2 letters of recommendation, professional liability insurance/malpractice insurance, GRE General Test. *Application deadline:* 4/1 (fall), 10/1 (spring). *Application fee:* $50.
**Advanced Placement** Credit given for nursing courses completed elsewhere dependent upon specific evaluations.
**Degree Requirements** 45 total credit hours.

### POST-MASTER'S PROGRAM

**Areas of Study** *Nurse practitioner programs in:* acute care, adult health, family health, neonatal health, psychiatric/mental health,women's health.

### DOCTORAL DEGREE PROGRAM

**Degree** PhD
**Available Programs** Doctorate; Post-Baccalaureate Doctorate.
**Areas of Study** Faculty preparation, health policy, individualized study, nursing research, nursing science.
**Program Entrance Requirements** Minimum overall college GPA of 3.0, interview by faculty committee, 3 letters of recommendation, vita, writing sample, GRE General Test. *Application deadline:* 2/1 (fall). *Application fee:* $50.
**Degree Requirements** Dissertation, written exam.

### POSTDOCTORAL PROGRAM

**Postdoctoral Program Contact** Dr. Rosalie Mainous, Associate Dean for Graduate Academic Affairs, School of Nursing, University of Louisville, 555 South Floyd Street, Louisville, KY 40292. *Telephone:* 502-852-8387. *Fax:* 502-852-8783. *E-mail:* rosalie.mainous@louisville.edu.

## CONTINUING EDUCATION PROGRAM

**Contact** Dr. Deborah Thomas, Director, School of Nursing, University of Louisville, 555 South Floyd Street, K-3019, Louisville, KY 40292. *Telephone:* 502-852-8392. *Fax:* 502-852-8783. *E-mail:* dvthom01@louisville.edu.

# University of Pikeville

## RN to BSN Completion Program
## Pikeville, Kentucky

Founded in 1889

**DEGREE • BSN**
**Library Facilities** 82,945 volumes; 38,849 periodical subscriptions.

## BACCALAUREATE PROGRAMS

**Degree** BSN
**Available Programs** RN Baccalaureate.

**Contact** Mary Rado Simpson, Chair, Division of Nursing, RN to BSN Completion Program, University of Pikeville, 147 Sycamore Street, Pikeville, KY 41501. *Telephone:* 616-218-5750. *E-mail:* MarySimpson@upike.edu.

# Western Kentucky University

## School of Nursing
## Bowling Green, Kentucky

***http://www.wku.edu/nursing/***
Founded in 1906

### DEGREES • BSN • DNP • MSN

**Nursing Program Faculty** 50 (40% with doctorates).
**Baccalaureate Enrollment** 450 **Women** 92% **Men** 8% **Minority** 5% **International** 2% **Part-time** 30%
**Graduate Enrollment** 150 **Women** 96% **Men** 4% **Minority** 2% **International** 2% **Part-time** 75%
**Distance Learning Courses** Available.
**Nursing Student Activities** Nursing Honor Society, Sigma Theta Tau, Student Nurses' Association.
**Nursing Student Resources** Academic advising; academic or career counseling; assistance for students with disabilities; bookstore; campus computer network; career placement assistance; computer lab; computer-assisted instruction; e-mail services; employment services for current students; externships; housing assistance; interactive nursing skills videos; Internet; learning resource lab; library services; nursing audiovisuals; paid internships; placement services for program completers; remedial services; resume preparation assistance; skills, simulation, or other laboratory; tutoring; unpaid internships.
**Library Facilities** 1.9 million volumes (17,880 in health, 1,697 in nursing); 3,749 periodical subscriptions (217 health-care related).

### BACCALAUREATE PROGRAMS

**Degree** BSN
**Available Programs** ADN to Baccalaureate; Baccalaureate for Second Degree; Generic Baccalaureate; RN Baccalaureate.
**Study Options** Full-time.
**Program Entrance Requirements** Minimum overall college GPA of 2.75, transcript of college record, CPR certification, health exam, health insurance, high school transcript, immunizations, minimum GPA in nursing prerequisites of 3.0, professional liability insurance/malpractice insurance, prerequisite course work. Transfer students are accepted. *Application deadline:* 1/15 (fall), 7/15 (spring).
**Advanced Placement** Credit by examination available. Credit given for nursing courses completed elsewhere dependent upon specific evaluations.
**Expenses (2013–14)** *Tuition, state resident:* full-time $8472; part-time $353 per credit hour. *Tuition, nonresident:* full-time $21,000; part-time $875 per credit hour. *International tuition:* $21,000 full-time. *Required fees:* full-time $1000.
**Financial Aid** 50% of baccalaureate students in nursing programs received some form of financial aid in 2012–13.
**Contact** Dr. Sherry Lovan, Program Coordinator, School of Nursing, Western Kentucky University, School of Nursing, MCHC 2204, #11036, Bowling Green, KY 42101-3576. *Telephone:* 270-745-4379. *Fax:* 270-745-3392. *E-mail:* sherry.lovan@wku.edu.

### GRADUATE PROGRAMS

**Expenses (2013–14)** *Tuition, state resident:* part-time $467 per credit hour. *Tuition, nonresident:* part-time $583 per credit hour.
**Financial Aid** 75% of graduate students in nursing programs received some form of financial aid in 2012–13. Research assistantships with partial tuition reimbursements available, teaching assistantships with partial tuition reimbursements available, Federal Work-Study, institutionally sponsored loans, traineeships, tuition waivers (partial), and unspecified assistantships available. Aid available to part-time students. *Financial aid application deadline:* 4/1.
**Contact** Dr. Beverly C. Siegrist, Professor, School of Nursing, Western Kentucky University, School of Nursing, MCHC 3340, #11036, Bowling Green, KY 42101. *Telephone:* 270-745-3490. *Fax:* 270-745-3392. *E-mail:* beverly.siegrist@wku.edu.

#### MASTER'S DEGREE PROGRAM

**Degree** MSN
**Available Programs** Accelerated Master's for Nurses with Non-Nursing Degrees; Master's.
**Concentrations Available** Nursing administration; nursing education.
**Study Options** Full-time and part-time.
**Program Entrance Requirements** Clinical experience, computer literacy, minimum overall college GPA of 2.75, transcript of college record, CPR certification, written essay, immunizations, interview, 3 letters of recommendation, nursing research course, physical assessment course, professional liability insurance/malpractice insurance, statistics course, GRE General Test. *Application deadline:* Applications may be processed on a rolling basis for some programs.
**Advanced Placement** Credit given for nursing courses completed elsewhere dependent upon specific evaluations.
**Degree Requirements** 45 total credit hours, thesis or project, comprehensive exam.

#### DOCTORAL DEGREE PROGRAM

**Degree** DNP
**Available Programs** Doctorate; Post-Baccalaureate Doctorate.
**Areas of Study** Advanced practice nursing, nursing policy.
**Program Entrance Requirements** Clinical experience, minimum overall college GPA of 3.25, interview by faculty committee, statistics course, writing sample. *Application deadline:* Applications may be processed on a rolling basis for some programs. *Application fee:* $100.
**Degree Requirements** 76 total credit hours, written exam, residency.

### CONTINUING EDUCATION PROGRAM

**Contact** Ms. Kim Vickous, School of Nursing, Western Kentucky University, School of Nursing, MCHC 2220, #11036, Bowling Green, KY 42101-3576. *Telephone:* 270-745-3876. *Fax:* 270-745-3392. *E-mail:* kim.vickous@wku.edu.

# LOUISIANA

# Dillard University

## Division of Nursing
## New Orleans, Louisiana

***http://www.dillard.edu/index.php?option=com_content&view=article&id=106&Itemid=91***
Founded in 1869

### DEGREE • BSN

**Nursing Program Faculty** 13 (31% with doctorates).
**Baccalaureate Enrollment** 100 **Women** 98% **Men** 2% **Minority** 99% **International** 1%
**Nursing Student Activities** Nursing Honor Society, Sigma Theta Tau, Student Nurses' Association.
**Nursing Student Resources** Academic advising; academic or career counseling; assistance for students with disabilities; bookstore; campus computer network; career placement assistance; computer lab; computer-assisted instruction; e-mail services; externships; interactive nursing skills videos; Internet; learning resource lab; library services; nursing audiovisuals; paid internships; placement services for program completers; remedial services; resume preparation assistance; skills, simulation, or other laboratory; tutoring.
**Library Facilities** 105,286 volumes; 21 periodical subscriptions health-care related.

### BACCALAUREATE PROGRAMS

**Degree** BSN
**Available Programs** Generic Baccalaureate; LPN to Baccalaureate; LPN to RN Baccalaureate; RN Baccalaureate.
**Study Options** Full-time.
**Program Entrance Requirements** Minimum overall college GPA of 2.5, transcript of college record, CPR certification, health exam, health insurance, high school transcript, immunizations, minimum high school GPA of 2.5, minimum GPA in nursing prerequisites of 2.5, professional liability insurance/malpractice insurance, prerequisite course work. Transfer students are accepted. *Application deadline:* 3/1 (fall).
**Contact** *Telephone:* 504-816-4717. *Fax:* 504-816-4861.

### CONTINUING EDUCATION PROGRAM

**Contact** *Telephone:* 504-816-4717. *Fax:* 504-816-4861.

# Grambling State University
## School of Nursing
## Grambling, Louisiana

Founded in 1901

**DEGREES • BSN • MSN**
**Nursing Program Faculty** 23 (20% with doctorates).
**Baccalaureate Enrollment** 600 **Women** 85% **Men** 15% **Minority** 68% **International** 9% **Part-time** 5%
**Graduate Enrollment** 41 **Women** 86% **Men** 14% **Minority** 66% **International** 12%
**Distance Learning Courses** Available.
**Nursing Student Activities** Student Nurses' Association.
**Nursing Student Resources** Academic advising; academic or career counseling; assistance for students with disabilities; bookstore; campus computer network; career placement assistance; computer lab; computer-assisted instruction; e-mail services; employment services for current students; interactive nursing skills videos; Internet; learning resource lab; library services; nursing audiovisuals; skills, simulation, or other laboratory; tutoring.
**Library Facilities** 234,524 volumes (10,000 in health, 5,000 in nursing); 1.2 million periodical subscriptions (65 health-care related).

### BACCALAUREATE PROGRAMS

**Degree** BSN
**Available Programs** Generic Baccalaureate; LPN to RN Baccalaureate; RN Baccalaureate.
**Study Options** Full-time.
**Program Entrance Requirements** Transcript of college record, CPR certification, health exam, high school foreign language, 3 years high school math, 3 years high school science, high school transcript, immunizations, minimum high school GPA of 2.0, minimum GPA in nursing prerequisites of 2.75, professional liability insurance/malpractice insurance, prerequisite course work. Transfer students are accepted. *Application deadline:* 6/1 (fall), 12/1 (spring). *Application fee:* $20.
**Advanced Placement** Credit given for nursing courses completed elsewhere dependent upon specific evaluations.
**Contact** *Telephone:* 318-274-2528. *Fax:* 318-274-3491.

### GRADUATE PROGRAMS

**Contact** *Telephone:* 318-274-2897. *Fax:* 318-274-3491.

#### MASTER'S DEGREE PROGRAM

**Degree** MSN
**Available Programs** Master's.
**Concentrations Available** Nursing education. *Clinical nurse specialist programs in:* adult health, maternity-newborn, pediatric. *Nurse practitioner programs in:* family health, pediatric.
**Study Options** Full-time and part-time.
**Program Entrance Requirements** Clinical experience, minimum overall college GPA of 3.0, transcript of college record, CPR certification, immunizations, interview, 3 letters of recommendation, physical assessment course, professional liability insurance/malpractice insurance, prerequisite course work, statistics course, GRE. *Application deadline:* 6/1 (fall). *Application fee:* $20.
**Advanced Placement** Credit given for nursing courses completed elsewhere dependent upon specific evaluations.
**Degree Requirements** 49 total credit hours, thesis or project, comprehensive exam.

#### POST-MASTER'S PROGRAM

**Areas of Study** *Nurse practitioner programs in:* family health.

# Louisiana College
## Department of Nursing
## Pineville, Louisiana

*http://www.lacollege.edu/*
Founded in 1906

**DEGREE • BSN**
**Nursing Program Faculty** 6 (17% with doctorates).
**Baccalaureate Enrollment** 100
**Nursing Student Activities** Sigma Theta Tau, Student Nurses' Association.
**Nursing Student Resources** Academic advising; academic or career counseling; assistance for students with disabilities; bookstore; campus computer network; career placement assistance; computer lab; computer-assisted instruction; e-mail services; employment services for current students; externships; Internet; learning resource lab; library services; nursing audiovisuals; skills, simulation, or other laboratory; tutoring; unpaid internships.
**Library Facilities** 357,313 volumes (3,426 in health, 500 in nursing); 404 periodical subscriptions (142 health-care related).

### BACCALAUREATE PROGRAMS

**Degree** BSN
**Available Programs** Generic Baccalaureate.
**Study Options** Full-time.
**Program Entrance Requirements** Minimum overall college GPA of 2.6, transcript of college record, CPR certification, health exam, health insurance, immunizations, interview, minimum high school GPA of 2.0, minimum high school rank 50%, minimum GPA in nursing prerequisites of 2.6, professional liability insurance/malpractice insurance, prerequisite course work. Transfer students are accepted.
**Advanced Placement** Credit given for nursing courses completed elsewhere dependent upon specific evaluations.
**Contact** *Telephone:* 318-487-7127. *Fax:* 318-487-7488.

# Louisiana State University at Alexandria
## Nursing Program
## Alexandria, Louisiana

Founded in 1960

**DEGREE • BSN**
**Library Facilities** 166,340 volumes; 1,541 periodical subscriptions.

### BACCALAUREATE PROGRAMS

**Degree** BSN
**Available Programs** RN Baccalaureate.
**Program Entrance Requirements** Minimum overall college GPA of 2.5, RN licensure.
**Contact** *Telephone:* 318-473-6417.

# Louisiana State University Health Sciences Center
## School of Nursing
## New Orleans, Louisiana

*https://nursing.lsuhsc.edu/*
Founded in 1931

**DEGREES • BSN • DNP • MN**
**Nursing Program Faculty** 78 (25% with doctorates).
**Baccalaureate Enrollment** 739 **Women** 87% **Men** 13% **Minority** 21% **International** .13% **Part-time** 28%
**Graduate Enrollment** 278 **Women** 76% **Men** 24% **Minority** 21% **Part-time** 44%
**Nursing Student Activities** Nursing Honor Society, Sigma Theta Tau, Student Nurses' Association.
**Nursing Student Resources** Academic advising; academic or career counseling; assistance for students with disabilities; bookstore; campus computer network; computer lab; computer-assisted instruction; e-mail services; housing assistance; interactive nursing skills videos; Internet; learning resource lab; library services; nursing audiovisuals; skills, simulation, or other laboratory; tutoring.
**Library Facilities** 215,833 volumes in health, 9,490 volumes in nursing; 4,913 periodical subscriptions (5,389 health-care related).

### BACCALAUREATE PROGRAMS

**Degree** BSN
**Available Programs** Accelerated Baccalaureate for Second Degree; Generic Baccalaureate; RN Baccalaureate.
**Study Options** Full-time and part-time.
**Program Entrance Requirements** Minimum overall college GPA of 2.0, transcript of college record, written essay, interview, minimum GPA

in nursing prerequisites of 2.8, prerequisite course work. Transfer students are accepted. *Application deadline:* 1/15 (fall), 8/15 (spring). *Application fee:* $50.
**Expenses (2013–14)** *Tuition, state resident:* full-time $5275. *Tuition, nonresident:* full-time $10,053. *International tuition:* $10,053 full-time. *Room and board:* $4797 per academic year. *Required fees:* full-time $1013.
**Financial Aid** 79% of baccalaureate students in nursing programs received some form of financial aid in 2012–13.
**Contact** Dr. Catherine Lopez, Assistant Dean for Student Services, School of Nursing, Louisiana State University Health Sciences Center, 1900 Gravier Street, New Orleans, LA 70112. *Telephone:* 504-568-4180. *Fax:* 504-568-5853. *E-mail:* clopez@lsuhsc.edu.

## GRADUATE PROGRAMS

**Expenses (2013–14)** *Tuition, state resident:* full-time $6597. *Tuition, nonresident:* full-time $13,300. *International tuition:* $13,300 full-time. *Room and board:* $4797 per academic year. *Required fees:* full-time $954.
**Financial Aid** 66% of graduate students in nursing programs received some form of financial aid in 2012–13. Federal Work-Study, institutionally sponsored loans, scholarships, and traineeships available.
**Contact** Dr. Catherine Lopez, Assistant Dean for Student Services, School of Nursing, Louisiana State University Health Sciences Center, 1900 Gravier Street, New Orleans, LA 70112. *Telephone:* 504-568-4180. *Fax:* 504-568-5853. *E-mail:* clopez@lsuhsc.edu.

### MASTER'S DEGREE PROGRAM

**Degree** MN
**Available Programs** Master's.
**Concentrations Available** Nurse anesthesia; nursing administration; nursing education. *Clinical nurse specialist programs in:* adult health, community health, public health. *Nurse practitioner programs in:* family health, neonatal health.
**Study Options** Full-time and part-time.
**Program Entrance Requirements** Clinical experience, minimum overall college GPA of 3.0, transcript of college record, CPR certification, written essay, interview, 3 letters of recommendation, statistics course, GRE General Test, MAT. *Application deadline:* 2/1 (fall), 9/1 (spring), 1/15 (summer). *Application fee:* $100.
**Degree Requirements** 40 total credit hours.

### DOCTORAL DEGREE PROGRAM

**Degree** DNP
**Available Programs** Doctorate.
**Areas of Study** Advanced practice nursing, clinical practice, community health, gerontology, maternity-newborn, nursing administration.
**Program Entrance Requirements** Clinical experience, minimum overall college GPA of 3.5, interview, 3 letters of recommendation, MSN or equivalent, scholarly papers, vita, writing sample, GRE General Test. *Application deadline:* 2/1 (fall), 9/1 (spring). *Application fee:* $50.
**Degree Requirements** 54 total credit hours, dissertation, oral exam.

### POSTDOCTORAL PROGRAM

**Postdoctoral Program Contact** Dr. Anita Hufft, Associate Dean, School of Nursing, Louisiana State University Health Sciences Center, 1900 Gravier Street, New Orleans, LA 70112. *Telephone:* 504-568-4107. *Fax:* 504-568-5853. *E-mail:* ahufft@lsuhsc.edu.

## CONTINUING EDUCATION PROGRAM

**Contact** Ms. Kimberly Cheramie, RN, Coordinator of Continuing Nursing Education, School of Nursing, Louisiana State University Health Sciences Center, 1900 Gravier Street, New Orleans, LA 70112. *Telephone:* 504-568-4202. *E-mail:* kvanna@lsuhsc.edu.

# Loyola University New Orleans

**School of Nursing**
**New Orleans, Louisiana**

***http://www.css.loyno.edu/nursing***
Founded in 1912

**DEGREES • BSN • DNP • MSN**

**Nursing Program Faculty** 40 (100% with doctorates).
**Baccalaureate Enrollment** 25 **Women** 98% **Men** 2% **Minority** 22.7% **Part-time** 97.25%
**Graduate Enrollment** 490 **Women** 95% **Men** 5% **Minority** 36.5% **Part-time** 79.12%
**Distance Learning Courses** Available.
**Nursing Student Activities** Sigma Theta Tau.
**Nursing Student Resources** Academic advising; academic or career counseling; assistance for students with disabilities; bookstore; campus computer network; career placement assistance; computer lab; computer-assisted instruction; e-mail services; interactive nursing skills videos; Internet; learning resource lab; library services; nursing audiovisuals; skills, simulation, or other laboratory; tutoring.
**Library Facilities** 584,939 volumes (6,881 in health, 913 in nursing); 169,032 periodical subscriptions (6,716 health-care related).

## BACCALAUREATE PROGRAMS

**Degree** BSN
**Available Programs** RN Baccalaureate.
**Study Options** Full-time and part-time.
**Online Degree Options** Yes (online only).
**Program Entrance Requirements** Minimum overall college GPA of 2.5, transcript of college record, written essay, immunizations, minimum GPA in nursing prerequisites of 2.0, professional liability insurance/malpractice insurance, RN licensure. Transfer students are accepted. *Application deadline:* Applications may be processed on a rolling basis for some programs. *Application fee:* $40.
**Advanced Placement** Credit by examination available. Credit given for nursing courses completed elsewhere dependent upon specific evaluations.
**Expenses (2012–13)** *Tuition:* full-time $11,568; part-time $482 per credit hour. *Required fees:* full-time $1096; part-time $548 per term.
**Financial Aid** 96% of baccalaureate students in nursing programs received some form of financial aid in 2011–12. *Gift aid (need-based):* Federal Pell, FSEOG, private, college/university gift aid from institutional funds. *Loans:* Perkins. *Work-study:* Federal Work-Study. *Financial aid application deadline:* 6/1(priority: 2/15).
**Contact** Dr. Ann Cary, Director, RN-BSN Coordinator and Professor, School of Nursing, Loyola University New Orleans, 6363 St. Charles Avenue, Campus Box 45, New Orleans, LA 70118. *Telephone:* 504-865-2579. *Fax:* 504-865-3254. *E-mail:* ahcary@loyno.edu.

## GRADUATE PROGRAMS

**Financial Aid** 68% of graduate students in nursing programs received some form of financial aid in 2011–12. Traineeships and Incumbent Workers Training Program grants available. *Financial aid application deadline:* 5/1.
**Contact** Dr. Ann H. Cary, Director, School of Nursing, School of Nursing, Loyola University New Orleans, 6363 St. Charles Avenue, Campus Box 45, New Orleans, LA 70118. *Telephone:* 504-865-3142. *Fax:* 504-865-3254. *E-mail:* nursing@loyno.edu.

### MASTER'S DEGREE PROGRAM

**Degree** MSN
**Available Programs** Master's; Master's for Nurses with Non-Nursing Degrees; RN to Master's.
**Concentrations Available** Health-care administration; nurse case management. *Nurse practitioner programs in:* adult health, family health.
**Study Options** Full-time and part-time.
**Online Degree Options** Yes.
**Program Entrance Requirements** Clinical experience, minimum overall college GPA of 3.0, transcript of college record, CPR certification, written essay, immunizations, interview, 3 letters of recommendation, nursing research course, professional liability insurance/malpractice insurance, prerequisite course work, statistics course. *Application deadline:* Applications may be processed on a rolling basis for some programs.
**Advanced Placement** Credit given for nursing courses completed elsewhere dependent upon specific evaluations.
**Degree Requirements** 36 total credit hours, comprehensive exam.

### POST-MASTER'S PROGRAM

**Areas of Study** *Nurse practitioner programs in:* adult health, family health.

### DOCTORAL DEGREE PROGRAM

**Degree** DNP
**Available Programs** Doctorate; Post-Baccalaureate Doctorate.
**Areas of Study** Advanced practice nursing, clinical practice, faculty preparation, family health, nursing administration, nursing research.
**Online Degree Options** Yes (online only).

**Program Entrance Requirements** Clinical experience, minimum overall college GPA of 3.2, interview by faculty committee, interview, 3 letters of recommendation, MSN or equivalent, statistics course, writing sample. *Application deadline:* 11/1 (fall), 2/1 (spring). *Application fee:* $75.
**Degree Requirements** 39 total credit hours, dissertation, written exam, residency.

# McNeese State University

## College of Nursing
## Lake Charles, Louisiana

***http://www.mcneese.edu/***
Founded in 1939

### DEGREES • BSN • MSN

**Nursing Program Faculty** 59 (23% with doctorates).
**Baccalaureate Enrollment** 1,031 **Women** 83% **Men** 17% **Minority** 27% **International** 2% **Part-time** 11%
**Graduate Enrollment** 132 **Women** 78% **Men** 22% **Minority** 16% **Part-time** 88%
**Distance Learning Courses** Available.
**Nursing Student Activities** Sigma Theta Tau, Student Nurses' Association.
**Nursing Student Resources** Academic advising; academic or career counseling; assistance for students with disabilities; bookstore; campus computer network; career placement assistance; computer lab; computer-assisted instruction; daycare for children of students; e-mail services; employment services for current students; housing assistance; interactive nursing skills videos; Internet; learning resource lab; library services; nursing audiovisuals; placement services for program completers; resume preparation assistance; skills, simulation, or other laboratory; tutoring.
**Library Facilities** 41,000 volumes in health, 27,500 volumes in nursing; 120 periodical subscriptions health-care related.

### BACCALAUREATE PROGRAMS

**Degree** BSN
**Available Programs** ADN to Baccalaureate; Generic Baccalaureate; LPN to Baccalaureate; LPN to RN Baccalaureate.
**Study Options** Full-time and part-time.
**Program Entrance Requirements** Minimum overall college GPA of 2.7, transcript of college record, CPR certification, health exam, health insurance, high school transcript, immunizations, minimum high school GPA of 2.5, minimum GPA in nursing prerequisites of 2.7, prerequisite course work. Transfer students are accepted. *Application deadline:* 10/15 (fall), 3/10 (spring). *Application fee:* $30.
**Advanced Placement** Credit by examination available. Credit given for nursing courses completed elsewhere dependent upon specific evaluations.
**Expenses (2013–14)** *Tuition, state resident:* full-time $3681; part-time $1840 per semester. *Tuition, nonresident:* full-time $8763; part-time $4381 per semester. *International tuition:* $10,074 full-time. *Room and board:* $7274; room only: $4630 per academic year. *Required fees:* full-time $1320; part-time $54 per credit; part-time $660 per term.
**Financial Aid** 85% of baccalaureate students in nursing programs received some form of financial aid in 2012–13. *Gift aid (need-based):* Federal Pell, FSEOG, state. *Loans:* Federal Direct (Subsidized Stafford), Perkins. *Work-study:* Federal Work-Study, part-time campus jobs. *Financial aid application deadline (priority):* 5/1.
**Contact** Dr. Peggy L. Wolfe, Dean and Professor, College of Nursing, McNeese State University, PO Box 90415, Lake Charles, LA 70609-0415. *Telephone:* 337-475-5820. *Fax:* 337-475-5924. *E-mail:* pwolfe@mail.mcneese.edu.

### GRADUATE PROGRAMS

**Expenses (2013–14)** *Tuition, state resident:* full-time $5495; part-time $2748 per semester. *Tuition, nonresident:* full-time $15,576; part-time $7788 per semester. *International tuition:* $17,576 full-time. *Room and board:* $7274; room only: $4630 per academic year. *Required fees:* full-time $1264; part-time $59 per credit; part-time $632 per term.
**Financial Aid** 38% of graduate students in nursing programs received some form of financial aid in 2012–13. *Application deadline:* 5/1.
**Contact** Dr. Peggy Wolfe, Dean, College of Nursing, McNeese State University, PO Box 90415, Lake Charles, LA 70609-0415. *Telephone:* 337-475-5820. *Fax:* 337-475-5702. *E-mail:* pwolfe@mcneese.edu.

**MASTER'S DEGREE PROGRAM**
**Degree** MSN
**Available Programs** Master's.
**Concentrations Available** Nursing administration; nursing education. *Nurse practitioner programs in:* family health, psychiatric/mental health.
**Site Options** Lake Charles, LA; Baton Rouge, LA; Lafayette, LA.
**Study Options** Full-time and part-time.
**Online Degree Options** Yes (online only).
**Program Entrance Requirements** Minimum overall college GPA of 2.7, transcript of college record, written essay, immunizations, 2 letters of recommendation, physical assessment course, statistics course, GRE. *Application deadline:* 5/15 (fall), 11/1 (spring). *Application fee:* $20.
**Advanced Placement** Credit given for nursing courses completed elsewhere dependent upon specific evaluations.
**Degree Requirements** 46 total credit hours, thesis or project.

**POST-MASTER'S PROGRAM**
**Areas of Study** *Nurse practitioner programs in:* family health, psychiatric/mental health.

### CONTINUING EDUCATION PROGRAM

**Contact** Dr. Rhonda LeJeune Johnson, Continuing Education Coordinator, College of Nursing, McNeese State University, PO Box 90415, Lake Charles, LA 70609-0415. *Telephone:* 337-475-5929. *Fax:* 337-475-5924. *E-mail:* MSUconCE@mcneese.edu.

# Nicholls State University

## Department of Nursing
## Thibodaux, Louisiana

***http://www.nicholls.edu/nursing/***
Founded in 1948

### DEGREE • BSN

**Nursing Program Faculty** 19 (21% with doctorates).
**Library Facilities** 600,954 volumes; 11,149 periodical subscriptions.

### BACCALAUREATE PROGRAMS

**Degree** BSN
**Available Programs** Generic Baccalaureate; LPN to Baccalaureate; RN Baccalaureate.
**Program Entrance Requirements** Minimum overall college GPA of 2.75, transcript of college record, minimum GPA in nursing prerequisites of 2.0, prerequisite course work. Transfer students are accepted.
**Contact** *Telephone:* 985-448-4696. *Fax:* 985-448-4932.

### CONTINUING EDUCATION PROGRAM

**Contact** *Telephone:* 985-448-4696. *Fax:* 985-448-4932.

# Northwestern State University of Louisiana

## College of Nursing and Allied Health
## Shreveport, Louisiana

***http://www.nsula.edu/nursing***
Founded in 1884

### DEGREES • BSN • MSN

**Nursing Program Faculty** 54 (23% with doctorates).
**Baccalaureate Enrollment** 1,347 **Women** 85% **Men** 15% **Minority** 37% **Part-time** 35%
**Graduate Enrollment** 185 **Women** 92% **Men** 8% **Minority** 17% **International** 1% **Part-time** 92%
**Distance Learning Courses** Available.
**Nursing Student Activities** Sigma Theta Tau, Student Nurses' Association.
**Nursing Student Resources** Academic advising; academic or career counseling; assistance for students with disabilities; bookstore; campus computer network; computer lab; computer-assisted instruction; e-mail services; employment services for current students; interactive nursing skills videos; Internet; learning resource lab; library services; nursing audiovisuals; placement services for program completers; remedial services; skills, simulation, or other laboratory; tutoring.

**Library Facilities** 791,279 volumes (4,443 in health, 3,047 in nursing); 700 periodical subscriptions (1,360 health-care related).

## BACCALAUREATE PROGRAMS

**Degree** BSN
**Available Programs** ADN to Baccalaureate; Generic Baccalaureate; LPN to Baccalaureate; RN Baccalaureate.
**Site Options** Alexandria, LA; Ferriday, LA.
**Study Options** Full-time and part-time.
**Online Degree Options** Yes.
**Program Entrance Requirements** Minimum overall college GPA of 2.0, transcript of college record, CPR certification, health exam, health insurance, high school transcript, immunizations, minimum GPA in nursing prerequisites of 2.7, prerequisite course work. Transfer students are accepted. *Application deadline:* 5/15 (fall), 8/15 (spring). *Application fee:* $20.
**Advanced Placement** Credit by examination available. Credit given for nursing courses completed elsewhere dependent upon specific evaluations.
**Expenses (2012–13)** *Tuition, state resident:* full-time $3939; part-time $110 per credit hour. *Tuition, nonresident:* full-time $7183; part-time $600 per credit hour. *International tuition:* $7183 full-time. *Required fees:* full-time $1275; part-time $425 per term.
**Financial Aid** 80% of baccalaureate students in nursing programs received some form of financial aid in 2011–12. *Gift aid (need-based):* Federal Pell, state, private, college/university gift aid from institutional funds. *Loans:* Federal Nursing Student Loans, Federal Direct (Subsidized and Unsubsidized Stafford), Perkins, state, college/university, alternative loans. *Work-study:* Federal Work-Study, part-time campus jobs. *Financial aid application deadline (priority):* 5/1.
**Contact** Ms. Linda Copple, Coordinator, Baccalaureate Program, College of Nursing and Allied Health, Northwestern State University of Louisiana, 1800 Line Avenue, Shreveport, LA 71101. *Telephone:* 318-677-3100. *Fax:* 318-677-3127. *E-mail:* copplel@nsula.edu.

## GRADUATE PROGRAMS

**Expenses (2012–13)** *Tuition, state resident:* full-time $8508; part-time $260 per credit hour. *Tuition, nonresident:* full-time $22,557; part-time $650 per credit hour. *International tuition:* $22,557 full-time. *Required fees:* full-time $1275; part-time $425 per term.
**Financial Aid** 25% of graduate students in nursing programs received some form of financial aid in 2011–12. Career-related internships or fieldwork and Federal Work-Study available. Aid available to part-time students. *Financial aid application deadline:* 5/1.
**Contact** Dr. Dana Roe, Coordinator, Graduate Studies and Research in Nursing, College of Nursing and Allied Health, Northwestern State University of Louisiana, 1800 Line Avenue, Shreveport, LA 71101. *Telephone:* 318-677-3100. *Fax:* 318-677-3127. *E-mail:* roed@nsula.edu.

### MASTER'S DEGREE PROGRAM

**Degree** MSN
**Available Programs** Master's.
**Concentrations Available** Nursing administration; nursing education. *Clinical nurse specialist programs in:* adult health, critical care. *Nurse practitioner programs in:* acute care, family health, pediatric,women's health.
**Site Options** Alexandria, LA; Ferriday, LA.
**Study Options** Full-time and part-time.
**Program Entrance Requirements** Clinical experience, minimum overall college GPA of 3.0, transcript of college record, written essay, immunizations, 2 letters of recommendation, nursing research course, physical assessment course, professional liability insurance/malpractice insurance, prerequisite course work, statistics course, GRE General Test. *Application deadline:* 6/1 (fall). *Application fee:* $20.
**Advanced Placement** Credit given for nursing courses completed elsewhere dependent upon specific evaluations.
**Degree Requirements** 39 total credit hours, thesis or project, comprehensive exam.

### POST-MASTER'S PROGRAM

**Areas of Study** *Nurse practitioner programs in:* acute care, family health, pediatric,women's health.

## CONTINUING EDUCATION PROGRAM

**Contact** Ms. Heather Hayter, Lead Nurse Planner, College of Nursing and Allied Health, Northwestern State University of Louisiana, 1800 Line Avenue, Shreveport, LA 71101. *Telephone:* 318-677-3105. *Fax:* 318-677-3127. *E-mail:* hayterh@nsula.edu.

# Our Lady of Holy Cross College

**Division of Nursing**
**New Orleans, Louisiana**

*http://www.olhcc.edu/*
Founded in 1916

**DEGREE • BSN**

**Nursing Program Faculty** 16 (32% with doctorates).
**Baccalaureate Enrollment** 168 **Women** 90% **Men** 10% **Minority** 15% **Part-time** 11%
**Nursing Student Activities** Sigma Theta Tau, Student Nurses' Association, nursing club.
**Nursing Student Resources** Academic advising; academic or career counseling; assistance for students with disabilities; bookstore; campus computer network; career placement assistance; computer lab; computer-assisted instruction; e-mail services; interactive nursing skills videos; Internet; learning resource lab; library services; nursing audiovisuals; remedial services; resume preparation assistance; skills, simulation, or other laboratory; tutoring.
**Library Facilities** 83,631 volumes (5,000 in health, 3,100 in nursing); 1,002 periodical subscriptions (103 health-care related).

## BACCALAUREATE PROGRAMS

**Degree** BSN
**Available Programs** Generic Baccalaureate.
**Study Options** Full-time.
**Program Entrance Requirements** Minimum overall college GPA of 2.5, transcript of college record, CPR certification, written essay, health exam, health insurance, high school transcript, immunizations, 3 letters of recommendation, minimum high school GPA of 2.0, minimum GPA in nursing prerequisites of 2.5, professional liability insurance/malpractice insurance, prerequisite course work. Transfer students are accepted.
**Advanced Placement** Credit by examination available. Credit given for nursing courses completed elsewhere dependent upon specific evaluations.
**Contact** *Telephone:* 504-398-2215. *Fax:* 504-391-2421.

# Our Lady of the Lake College

**Division of Nursing**
**Baton Rouge, Louisiana**

*http://www.ollusa.edu/s/1190/start2012.aspx*
Founded in 1990

**DEGREES • BSN • MSN**

**Nursing Program Faculty** 38 (21% with doctorates).
**Baccalaureate Enrollment** 265 **Women** 85% **Men** 15% **Minority** 31% **Part-time** 19%
**Graduate Enrollment** 87 **Women** 45% **Men** 55% **Minority** 13%
**Distance Learning Courses** Available.
**Nursing Student Activities** Nursing Honor Society, Student Nurses' Association.
**Nursing Student Resources** Academic advising; academic or career counseling; assistance for students with disabilities; bookstore; campus computer network; career placement assistance; computer lab; computer-assisted instruction; e-mail services; employment services for current students; interactive nursing skills videos; Internet; learning resource lab; library services; nursing audiovisuals; paid internships; remedial services; resume preparation assistance; skills, simulation, or other laboratory; tutoring.
**Library Facilities** 10,000 volumes in health, 1,000 volumes in nursing; 215 periodical subscriptions (200 health-care related).

## BACCALAUREATE PROGRAMS

**Degree** BSN
**Available Programs** ADN to Baccalaureate; Accelerated Baccalaureate for Second Degree; Generic Baccalaureate; LPN to Baccalaureate; RN Baccalaureate.
**Study Options** Full-time.
**Online Degree Options** Yes.
**Program Entrance Requirements** Minimum overall college GPA of 2.0, transcript of college record, CPR certification, written essay, health exam, health insurance, immunizations, minimum GPA in nursing prerequisites of 2.75, professional liability insurance/malpractice insurance,

prerequisite course work. Transfer students are accepted. *Application deadline:* 1/15 (fall), 7/15 (spring). *Application fee:* $35.
**Advanced Placement** Credit given for nursing courses completed elsewhere dependent upon specific evaluations.
**Expenses (2012–13)** *Tuition:* full-time $12,614; part-time $394 per credit hour. *International tuition:* $12,614 full-time. *Required fees:* full-time $854; part-time $12 per credit; part-time $240 per term.
**Financial Aid** 94% of baccalaureate students in nursing programs received some form of financial aid in 2011–12.
**Contact** Dr. Phyllis LeBlanc, RN-BSN Program Director, Division of Nursing, Our Lady of the Lake College, 7500 Hennessy Boulevard, Baton Rouge, LA 70808. *Telephone:* 225-768-1793. *Fax:* 225-768-1760. *E-mail:* pleblanc@ololcollege.edu.

## GRADUATE PROGRAMS

**Expenses (2012–13)** *Tuition:* full-time $30,638; part-time $851 per credit hour. *International tuition:* $30,638 full-time. *Required fees:* full-time $1358; part-time $12 per credit; part-time $513 per term.
**Financial Aid** 97% of graduate students in nursing programs received some form of financial aid in 2011–12.
**Contact** Dr. Jennifer Beck, Dean, School of Nursing, Division of Nursing, Our Lady of the Lake College, 7500 Hennessy Boulevard, Baton Rouge, LA 70808. *Telephone:* 225-768-1779. *Fax:* 225-768-1760. *E-mail:* jbeck@ololcollege.edu.

### MASTER'S DEGREE PROGRAM

**Degree** MSN
**Available Programs** Master's.
**Concentrations Available** Nurse anesthesia; nursing administration; nursing education.
**Study Options** Full-time.
**Program Entrance Requirements** Clinical experience, minimum overall college GPA of 3.3, transcript of college record, interview, 3 letters of recommendation, nursing research course, physical assessment course, statistics course. *Application deadline:* 12/1 (fall), 7/15 (spring). *Application fee:* $35.
**Advanced Placement** Credit given for nursing courses completed elsewhere dependent upon specific evaluations.
**Degree Requirements** 80 total credit hours, thesis or project.

## CONTINUING EDUCATION PROGRAM

**Contact** Ms. Shantelle Steib-Dennis, Director of Continuing Education, Division of Nursing, Our Lady of the Lake College, 7434 Perkins Road, Baton Rouge, LA 70808. *Telephone:* 225-768-1708. *Fax:* 225-214-1940. *E-mail:* Shantelle.Steib-dennis@ololcollege.edu.

# Southeastern Louisiana University

### School of Nursing
### Hammond, Louisiana

***http://www.selu.edu/acad_research/depts/nurs***
Founded in 1925

## DEGREES • BS • DNP • MSN

**Nursing Program Faculty** 62 (29% with doctorates).
**Baccalaureate Enrollment** 1,481 **Women** 86% **Men** 14% **Minority** 31.9% **International** 1% **Part-time** 19.9%
**Graduate Enrollment** 138 **Women** 87.7% **Men** 12.3% **Minority** 14.5% **Part-time** 84.8%
**Distance Learning Courses** Available.
**Nursing Student Activities** Nursing Honor Society, Sigma Theta Tau, Student Nurses' Association.
**Nursing Student Resources** Academic advising; academic or career counseling; assistance for students with disabilities; bookstore; campus computer network; career placement assistance; computer lab; computer-assisted instruction; e-mail services; employment services for current students; interactive nursing skills videos; Internet; learning resource lab; library services; nursing audiovisuals; other; resume preparation assistance; skills, simulation, or other laboratory; tutoring.
**Library Facilities** 790,197 volumes (19,210 in health, 5,545 in nursing); 3,561 periodical subscriptions (6,893 health-care related).

## BACCALAUREATE PROGRAMS

**Degree** BS
**Available Programs** Accelerated Baccalaureate for Second Degree; Generic Baccalaureate; LPN to RN Baccalaureate; RN Baccalaureate.
**Site Options** Baton Rouge, LA.
**Study Options** Full-time and part-time.
**Online Degree Options** Yes.
**Program Entrance Requirements** Minimum overall college GPA of 2.0, CPR certification, health exam, high school biology, high school chemistry, 4 years high school math, 4 years high school science, high school transcript, immunizations, minimum high school GPA of 2.0, minimum GPA in nursing prerequisites of 3.0, prerequisite course work. Transfer students are accepted. *Application deadline:* 7/15 (fall), 12/1 (spring), 5/1 (summer). Applications may be processed on a rolling basis for some programs. *Application fee:* $20.
**Advanced Placement** Credit given for nursing courses completed elsewhere dependent upon specific evaluations.
**Expenses (2013–14)** *Tuition, state resident:* full-time $4362; part-time $238 per credit hour. *Tuition, nonresident:* full-time $16,381; part-time $739 per credit hour. *International tuition:* $16,381 full-time. *Room and board:* $7610; room only: $5290 per academic year. *Required fees:* full-time $1353.
**Financial Aid** 55% of baccalaureate students in nursing programs received some form of financial aid in 2012–13. *Gift aid (need-based):* Federal Pell, FSEOG, state, private, college/university gift aid from institutional funds. *Loans:* Federal Direct (Subsidized and Unsubsidized Stafford PLUS), Perkins, college/university. *Work-study:* Federal Work-Study, part-time campus jobs. *Financial aid application deadline (priority):* 5/1.
**Contact** Dr. Eileen Creel, Department Head, School of Nursing, Southeastern Louisiana University, SLU 10835, Hammond, LA 70402. *Telephone:* 985-549-2156. *Fax:* 985-549-2869. *E-mail:* nursing@selu.edu.

## GRADUATE PROGRAMS

**Expenses (2013–14)** *Tuition, state resident:* full-time $5047; part-time $348 per credit hour. *Tuition, nonresident:* full-time $17,066; part-time $1015 per credit hour. *International tuition:* $17,066 full-time. *Room and board:* $7610; room only: $5290 per academic year. *Required fees:* full-time $1213.
**Financial Aid** 51% of graduate students in nursing programs received some form of financial aid in 2012–13. Federal Work-Study, institutionally sponsored loans, scholarships, traineeships, and unspecified assistantships available. Aid available to part-time students. *Financial aid application deadline:* 5/1.
**Contact** Dr. Lorinda Sealey, Graduate Nursing Program Coordinator, School of Nursing, Southeastern Louisiana University, SLU 10448, Hammond, LA 70402. *Telephone:* 985-549-5045. *Fax:* 985-549-5087. *E-mail:* vjohnson@selu.edu.

### MASTER'S DEGREE PROGRAM

**Degree** MSN
**Available Programs** Master's.
**Concentrations Available** Nursing administration. *Nurse practitioner programs in:* family health, psychiatric/mental health.
**Site Options** Lake Charles, LA; Lafayette, LA.
**Study Options** Full-time and part-time.
**Online Degree Options** Yes.
**Program Entrance Requirements** Clinical experience, minimum overall college GPA of 2.7, transcript of college record, written essay, immunizations, letters of recommendation, physical assessment course, prerequisite course work, resume, statistics course, GRE (verbal and quantitative). *Application deadline:* 7/15 (fall), 12/1 (spring), 5/1 (summer). Applications may be processed on a rolling basis for some programs. *Application fee:* $20.
**Advanced Placement** Credit given for nursing courses completed elsewhere dependent upon specific evaluations.
**Degree Requirements** 39 total credit hours, thesis or project.

### POST-MASTER'S PROGRAM

**Areas of Study** *Nurse practitioner programs in:* family health, psychiatric/mental health.

### DOCTORAL DEGREE PROGRAM

**Degree** DNP
**Available Programs** Doctorate.
**Site Options** Lafayette, LA.
**Program Entrance Requirements** Minimum overall college GPA of 3.30, interview, 3 letters of recommendation, MSN or equivalent, vita. *Application deadline:* 7/15 (fall), 12/1 (spring), 5/1 (summer). Applica-

tions may be processed on a rolling basis for some programs. *Application fee:* $20.

**Degree Requirements** 39 total credit hours.

# Southern University and Agricultural and Mechanical College

## School of Nursing
## Baton Rouge, Louisiana

***http://www.subr.edu/***
Founded in 1880

**DEGREES • BSN • MSN • PHD**

**Nursing Program Faculty** 36 (3% with doctorates).

**Baccalaureate Enrollment** 1,020 **Women** 91% **Men** 9% **Minority** 96% **International** 1% **Part-time** 12%

**Nursing Student Activities** Nursing Honor Society, Student Nurses' Association, nursing club.

**Nursing Student Resources** Academic advising; academic or career counseling; assistance for students with disabilities; bookstore; campus computer network; computer lab; computer-assisted instruction; e-mail services; interactive nursing skills videos; Internet; learning resource lab; library services; nursing audiovisuals; resume preparation assistance; skills, simulation, or other laboratory; tutoring.

**Library Facilities** 880,098 volumes (4,220 in health, 716 in nursing); 8,882 periodical subscriptions (114 health-care related).

### BACCALAUREATE PROGRAMS

**Degree** BSN

**Available Programs** Generic Baccalaureate.

**Study Options** Full-time and part-time.

**Program Entrance Requirements** Minimum overall college GPA of 2.6, CPR certification, health exam, immunizations, minimum GPA in nursing prerequisites, prerequisite course work. Transfer students are accepted.

**Contact** *Telephone:* 225-771-3416. *Fax:* 225-771-2651.

### GRADUATE PROGRAMS

**Contact** *Telephone:* 225-771-2663. *Fax:* 225-771-3547.

#### MASTER'S DEGREE PROGRAM

**Degree** MSN

**Available Programs** Master's.

**Concentrations Available** Health-care administration; nursing education. *Clinical nurse specialist programs in:* family health. *Nurse practitioner programs in:* family health.

**Study Options** Full-time and part-time.

**Program Entrance Requirements** Minimum overall college GPA of 3.0, transcript of college record, 3 letters of recommendation, physical assessment course, statistics course, GRE General Test.

**Degree Requirements** 46 total credit hours, thesis or project, comprehensive exam.

#### POST-MASTER'S PROGRAM

**Areas of Study** *Nurse practitioner programs in:* family health.

#### DOCTORAL DEGREE PROGRAM

**Degree** PhD

**Areas of Study** Advanced practice nursing, nursing education, nursing research,women's health.

**Program Entrance Requirements** Clinical experience, minimum overall college GPA of 3.2, interview by faculty committee, 3 letters of recommendation, MSN or equivalent, scholarly papers, statistics course, vita, writing sample, GRE General Test.

**Degree Requirements** 60 total credit hours, dissertation, written exam.

# University of Louisiana at Lafayette

## College of Nursing
## Lafayette, Louisiana

***http://www.nursing.louisiana.edu/***
Founded in 1898

**DEGREES • BSN • MSN**

**Nursing Program Faculty** 47 (13% with doctorates).

**Baccalaureate Enrollment** 1,354 **Women** 83% **Men** 17% **Minority** 25% **Part-time** 10%

**Distance Learning Courses** Available.

**Nursing Student Activities** Nursing Honor Society, Sigma Theta Tau, Student Nurses' Association.

**Nursing Student Resources** Academic advising; academic or career counseling; assistance for students with disabilities; bookstore; campus computer network; career placement assistance; computer lab; computer-assisted instruction; daycare for children of students; e-mail services; employment services for current students; externships; housing assistance; interactive nursing skills videos; Internet; learning resource lab; library services; nursing audiovisuals; other; paid internships; placement services for program completers; remedial services; resume preparation assistance; skills, simulation, or other laboratory; tutoring; unpaid internships.

**Library Facilities** 1.1 million volumes (6,883 in health, 4,593 in nursing); 1,965 periodical subscriptions (184 health-care related).

### BACCALAUREATE PROGRAMS

**Degree** BSN

**Available Programs** ADN to Baccalaureate; Accelerated Baccalaureate for Second Degree; Generic Baccalaureate; LPN to Baccalaureate.

**Study Options** Full-time and part-time.

**Online Degree Options** Yes.

**Program Entrance Requirements** Minimum overall college GPA of 2.8, transcript of college record, CPR certification, health exam, health insurance, high school biology, high school chemistry, high school foreign language, 2 years high school math, 3 years high school science, high school transcript, immunizations, minimum high school GPA of 2.0, minimum high school rank 25%, minimum GPA in nursing prerequisites of 2.0, prerequisite course work. Transfer students are accepted. *Application deadline:* 4/1 (fall), 11/2 (spring).

**Advanced Placement** Credit by examination available. Credit given for nursing courses completed elsewhere dependent upon specific evaluations.

**Contact** *Telephone:* 337-482-5604. *Fax:* 337-482-5700.

### GRADUATE PROGRAMS

**Contact** *Telephone:* 337-482-5639. *Fax:* 337-482-5650.

#### MASTER'S DEGREE PROGRAM

**Degree** MSN

**Available Programs** Master's; RN to Master's.

**Concentrations Available** Health-care administration; nursing administration; nursing education. *Clinical nurse specialist programs in:* adult health, psychiatric/mental health. *Nurse practitioner programs in:* adult health, psychiatric/mental health.

**Site Options** Hammond, LA; Baton Rouge, LA; Lake Charles, LA.

**Study Options** Full-time and part-time.

**Online Degree Options** Yes (online only).

**Program Entrance Requirements** Minimum overall college GPA of 2.75, transcript of college record, immunizations, 3 letters of recommendation, physical assessment course, statistics course, GRE General Test. *Application deadline:* Applications may be processed on a rolling basis for some programs. *Application fee:* $25.

**Advanced Placement** Credit given for nursing courses completed elsewhere dependent upon specific evaluations.

**Degree Requirements** 38 total credit hours, thesis or project.

#### POST-MASTER'S PROGRAM

**Areas of Study** *Clinical nurse specialist programs in:* adult health, psychiatric/mental health. *Nurse practitioner programs in:* adult health, psychiatric/mental health.

### CONTINUING EDUCATION PROGRAM

**Contact** *Telephone:* 337-482-5648. *Fax:* 337-482-5053.

## University of Louisiana at Monroe
### Nursing
### Monroe, Louisiana

*http://www.ulm.edu/nursing*
Founded in 1931

**DEGREE • BS**

**Nursing Program Faculty** 29 (2% with doctorates).
**Baccalaureate Enrollment** 237 **Women** 85% **Men** 15% **Minority** 26% **International** 1% **Part-time** 20%
**Distance Learning Courses** Available.
**Nursing Student Activities** Sigma Theta Tau, Student Nurses' Association.
**Nursing Student Resources** Academic advising; academic or career counseling; assistance for students with disabilities; bookstore; campus computer network; computer lab; computer-assisted instruction; daycare for children of students; e-mail services; employment services for current students; interactive nursing skills videos; Internet; learning resource lab; library services; nursing audiovisuals; placement services for program completers; remedial services; resume preparation assistance; skills, simulation, or other laboratory; tutoring.
**Library Facilities** 629,606 volumes (20,924 in health, 3,000 in nursing); 95 periodical subscriptions (425 health-care related).

#### BACCALAUREATE PROGRAMS

**Degree** BS
**Available Programs** ADN to Baccalaureate; Generic Baccalaureate; LPN to Baccalaureate; RN Baccalaureate.
**Study Options** Full-time and part-time.
**Online Degree Options** Yes (online only).
**Program Entrance Requirements** Transcript of college record, CPR certification, health exam, health insurance, high school transcript, immunizations, minimum high school GPA of 2.0, minimum high school rank 50%, minimum GPA in nursing prerequisites of 2.8, professional liability insurance/malpractice insurance, prerequisite course work. Transfer students are accepted. *Application deadline:* 3/1 (fall), 9/1 (spring). *Application fee:* $50.
**Advanced Placement** Credit given for nursing courses completed elsewhere dependent upon specific evaluations.
**Contact** *Telephone:* 318-342-1640. *Fax:* 318-342-1567.

#### CONTINUING EDUCATION PROGRAM

**Contact** *Telephone:* 318-342-1640. *Fax:* 318-342-1567.

## University of Phoenix–Louisiana Campus
### College of Nursing
### Metairie, Louisiana

Founded in 1976

**DEGREE • BSN**

**Nursing Program Faculty** 2 (50% with doctorates).
**Baccalaureate Enrollment** 9
**Nursing Student Activities** Sigma Theta Tau.
**Nursing Student Resources** Academic advising; academic or career counseling; assistance for students with disabilities; bookstore; campus computer network; computer lab; computer-assisted instruction; e-mail services; interactive nursing skills videos; Internet; learning resource lab; library services; nursing audiovisuals; remedial services; tutoring.
**Library Facilities** 16,781 periodical subscriptions (1,300 health-care related).

#### BACCALAUREATE PROGRAMS

**Degree** BSN
**Available Programs** Accelerated Baccalaureate; LPN to Baccalaureate.
**Study Options** Full-time.
**Program Entrance Requirements** Transcript of college record, CPR certification, immunizations, 1 letter of recommendation, RN licensure. Transfer students are accepted. *Application deadline:* Applications may be processed on a rolling basis for some programs.
**Advanced Placement** Credit by examination available. Credit given for nursing courses completed elsewhere dependent upon specific evaluations.
**Contact** *Telephone:* 504-461-8852.

# MAINE

## Husson University
### School of Nursing
### Bangor, Maine

*http://www.husson.edu/*
Founded in 1898

**DEGREES • BSN • MSN**

**Nursing Program Faculty** 13 (15% with doctorates).
**Baccalaureate Enrollment** 291 **Women** 93% **Men** 7% **Minority** 4%
**Graduate Enrollment** 49 **Women** 92% **Men** 8% **Part-time** 26%
**Distance Learning Courses** Available.
**Nursing Student Activities** Sigma Theta Tau, Student Nurses' Association, nursing club.
**Nursing Student Resources** Academic advising; academic or career counseling; assistance for students with disabilities; bookstore; campus computer network; career placement assistance; computer lab; computer-assisted instruction; e-mail services; employment services for current students; externships; interactive nursing skills videos; Internet; learning resource lab; library services; nursing audiovisuals; remedial services; resume preparation assistance; skills, simulation, or other laboratory; tutoring; unpaid internships.
**Library Facilities** 119,501 volumes (3,450 in health, 1,100 in nursing); 114 periodical subscriptions (183 health-care related).

#### BACCALAUREATE PROGRAMS

**Degree** BSN
**Available Programs** Generic Baccalaureate.
**Study Options** Full-time and part-time.
**Program Entrance Requirements** Minimum overall college GPA of 3.0, transcript of college record, written essay, health exam, health insurance, high school biology, high school chemistry, 2 years high school math, 2 years high school science, high school transcript, immunizations, 2 letters of recommendation, minimum high school GPA of 3.0, minimum GPA in nursing prerequisites of 3.0, prerequisite course work. Transfer students are accepted. *Application deadline:* Applications may be processed on a rolling basis for some programs. *Application fee:* $25.
**Advanced Placement** Credit by examination available. Credit given for nursing courses completed elsewhere dependent upon specific evaluations.
**Contact** *Telephone:* 207-941-7058. *Fax:* 207-941-7198.

#### GRADUATE PROGRAMS

**Contact** *Telephone:* 207-941-7166. *Fax:* 207-941-7198.

**MASTER'S DEGREE PROGRAM**

**Degree** MSN
**Available Programs** Master's; Master's for Nurses with Non-Nursing Degrees.
**Concentrations Available** Nursing education. *Clinical nurse specialist programs in:* psychiatric/mental health. *Nurse practitioner programs in:* family health.
**Site Options** South Portland, ME; Presque Isle, ME.
**Study Options** Full-time and part-time.
**Program Entrance Requirements** Clinical experience, minimum overall college GPA of 3.0, transcript of college record, CPR certification, written essay, immunizations, interview, 3 letters of recommendation, physical assessment course, prerequisite course work, statistics course. *Application deadline:* Applications may be processed on a rolling basis for some programs. *Application fee:* $25.
**Advanced Placement** Credit by examination available. Credit given for nursing courses completed elsewhere dependent upon specific evaluations.
**Degree Requirements** 44 total credit hours, thesis or project.

**POST-MASTER'S PROGRAM**

**Areas of Study** Nursing education. *Clinical nurse specialist programs in:* psychiatric/mental health. *Nurse practitioner programs in:* family health, psychiatric/mental health.

## Saint Joseph's College of Maine

### Master of Science in Nursing Program
### Standish, Maine

Founded in 1912

**DEGREES • BSN • MSN • MSN/MHA**

**Nursing Program Faculty** 65 (8% with doctorates).
**Baccalaureate Enrollment** 558 **Women** 95% **Men** 5% **Minority** 1% **Part-time** 48%
**Graduate Enrollment** 343 **Women** 93% **Men** 7% **Minority** 3% **Part-time** 100%
**Distance Learning Courses** Available.
**Nursing Student Activities** Sigma Theta Tau, Student Nurses' Association.
**Nursing Student Resources** Academic advising; academic or career counseling; assistance for students with disabilities; bookstore; campus computer network; computer lab; computer-assisted instruction; e-mail services; interactive nursing skills videos; Internet; learning resource lab; library services; nursing audiovisuals; remedial services; resume preparation assistance; skills, simulation, or other laboratory; tutoring.
**Library Facilities** 85,000 volumes (4,114 in health, 409 in nursing); 45,141 periodical subscriptions (108 health-care related).

#### BACCALAUREATE PROGRAMS

**Degree** BSN
**Available Programs** Generic Baccalaureate; RN Baccalaureate.
**Study Options** Full-time and part-time.
**Program Entrance Requirements** Minimum overall college GPA of 2.0, transcript of college record, written essay, health exam, health insurance, high school biology, high school chemistry, 3 years high school math, 2 years high school science, high school transcript, immunizations, 1 letter of recommendation, minimum high school GPA of 2.0. *Application deadline:* 5/1 (spring). *Application fee:* $250.
**Advanced Placement** Credit given for nursing courses completed elsewhere dependent upon specific evaluations.
**Contact** *Telephone:* 207-893-7830. *Fax:* 207-892-7423.

#### GRADUATE PROGRAMS

**Contact** *Telephone:* 207-893-7956. *Fax:* 207-893-7520.

**MASTER'S DEGREE PROGRAM**
**Degrees** MSN; MSN/MHA
**Available Programs** Master's; Master's for Nurses with Non-Nursing Degrees; RN to Master's.
**Concentrations Available** Nursing administration; nursing education.
**Study Options** Full-time and part-time.
**Online Degree Options** Yes (online only).
**Program Entrance Requirements** Clinical experience, computer literacy, minimum overall college GPA of 3.0, transcript of college record, prerequisite course work, resume, MAT. *Application deadline:* Applications may be processed on a rolling basis for some programs.
**Advanced Placement** Credit given for nursing courses completed elsewhere dependent upon specific evaluations.
**Degree Requirements** 42 total credit hours, thesis or project.

#### CONTINUING EDUCATION PROGRAM

**Contact** *Telephone:* 207-893-7956. *Fax:* 207-893-7520.

## University of Maine

### School of Nursing
### Orono, Maine

Founded in 1865

**DEGREES • BSN • MSN**

**Nursing Program Faculty** 20 (40% with doctorates).
**Baccalaureate Enrollment** 407 **Women** 90% **Men** 10% **Minority** .4% **International** .1% **Part-time** .5%
**Graduate Enrollment** 27 **Women** 99% **Men** 1% **Part-time** 50%
**Distance Learning Courses** Available.
**Nursing Student Activities** Sigma Theta Tau, Student Nurses' Association.
**Nursing Student Resources** Academic advising; academic or career counseling; assistance for students with disabilities; bookstore; campus computer network; computer lab; daycare for children of students; e-mail services; employment services for current students; housing assistance; interactive nursing skills videos; Internet; learning resource lab; library services; nursing audiovisuals; skills, simulation, or other laboratory; tutoring.
**Library Facilities** 1.1 million volumes (20,600 in health, 2,100 in nursing); 16,988 periodical subscriptions (3,750 health-care related).

#### BACCALAUREATE PROGRAMS

**Degree** BSN
**Available Programs** Generic Baccalaureate; RN Baccalaureate.
**Site Options** Presque Isle, ME; Augusta, ME; Portland, ME.
**Study Options** Full-time and part-time.
**Program Entrance Requirements** Minimum overall college GPA of 2.75, transcript of college record, CPR certification, written essay, health exam, high school biology, high school chemistry, high school foreign language, 3 years high school math, 3 years high school science, high school transcript, immunizations, interview, minimum high school rank 30%. Transfer students are accepted.
**Advanced Placement** Credit by examination available. Credit given for nursing courses completed elsewhere dependent upon specific evaluations.
**Contact** *Telephone:* 207-581-2588. *Fax:* 207-581-2585.

#### GRADUATE PROGRAMS

**Contact** *Telephone:* 207-581-2605. *Fax:* 207-581-2585.

**MASTER'S DEGREE PROGRAM**
**Degree** MSN
**Available Programs** Master's; RN to Master's.
**Concentrations Available** Health-care administration; nursing education. *Nurse practitioner programs in:* family health.
**Study Options** Full-time and part-time.
**Program Entrance Requirements** Clinical experience, minimum overall college GPA of 3.0, transcript of college record, CPR certification, written essay, immunizations, interview, 3 letters of recommendation, nursing research course, physical assessment course, statistics course, GRE General Test.
**Advanced Placement** Credit given for nursing courses completed elsewhere dependent upon specific evaluations.
**Degree Requirements** 47 total credit hours, thesis or project.

## University of Maine at Fort Kent

### Department of Nursing
### Fort Kent, Maine

***http://www.umfk.edu/***
Founded in 1878

**DEGREE • BSN**

**Nursing Program Faculty** 6 (16% with doctorates).
**Baccalaureate Enrollment** 246 **Women** 90% **Men** 10% **Minority** 2% **International** 2% **Part-time** 63%
**Distance Learning Courses** Available.
**Nursing Student Activities** Nursing Honor Society, Student Nurses' Association, nursing club.
**Nursing Student Resources** Academic advising; academic or career counseling; assistance for students with disabilities; bookstore; campus computer network; career placement assistance; computer lab; computer-assisted instruction; e-mail services; employment services for current students; externships; housing assistance; interactive nursing skills videos; Internet; learning resource lab; library services; nursing audiovisuals; paid internships; placement services for program completers; remedial services; resume preparation assistance; skills, simulation, or other laboratory; tutoring; unpaid internships.
**Library Facilities** 205,000 volumes (3,386 in health, 2,425 in nursing); 44,000 periodical subscriptions (73 health-care related).

#### BACCALAUREATE PROGRAMS

**Degree** BSN
**Available Programs** Accelerated Baccalaureate; Generic Baccalaureate; RN Baccalaureate.
**Study Options** Full-time and part-time.
**Online Degree Options** Yes.
**Program Entrance Requirements** Minimum overall college GPA of 2.5, CPR certification, written essay, health exam, health insurance, high school chemistry, high school foreign language, high school math, high school transcript, immunizations, minimum GPA in nursing prerequisites

of 2.5, prerequisite course work. Transfer students are accepted. *Application deadline:* 8/15 (fall), 1/10 (spring). *Application fee:* $40.
**Advanced Placement** Credit given for nursing courses completed elsewhere dependent upon specific evaluations.
**Contact** *Telephone:* 207-834-8607. *Fax:* 207-834-7577.

# University of New England
## Department of Nursing
## Biddeford, Maine

***http://www.une.edu/chp/nursing/***
Founded in 1831

### DEGREE • BSN
**Nursing Program Faculty** 16 (26% with doctorates).
**Baccalaureate Enrollment** 133 **Women** 73% **Men** 27% **Minority** 3%
**Nursing Student Activities** Nursing Honor Society, Sigma Theta Tau, Student Nurses' Association, nursing club.
**Nursing Student Resources** Academic advising; academic or career counseling; assistance for students with disabilities; bookstore; campus computer network; career placement assistance; computer lab; computer-assisted instruction; e-mail services; employment services for current students; housing assistance; interactive nursing skills videos; Internet; learning resource lab; library services; nursing audiovisuals; placement services for program completers; remedial services; resume preparation assistance; skills, simulation, or other laboratory; tutoring; unpaid internships.
**Library Facilities** 235,776 volumes (10,000 in health, 5,500 in nursing); 67,970 periodical subscriptions (1,300 health-care related).

### BACCALAUREATE PROGRAMS
**Degree** BSN
**Available Programs** Accelerated RN Baccalaureate; Generic Baccalaureate; RN Baccalaureate.
**Study Options** Full-time and part-time.
**Program Entrance Requirements** Minimum overall college GPA of 3.0, transcript of college record, CPR certification, health exam, health insurance, high school biology, high school chemistry, 2 years high school math, 2 years high school science, high school transcript, immunizations, minimum high school GPA of 3.0, professional liability insurance/malpractice insurance. Transfer students are accepted. *Application deadline:* 2/15 (fall). *Application fee:* $100.
**Advanced Placement** Credit by examination available. Credit given for nursing courses completed elsewhere dependent upon specific evaluations.
**Contact** *Telephone:* 207-602-2297.

### CONTINUING EDUCATION PROGRAM
**Contact** *Telephone:* 207-602-2050. *Fax:* 207-602-5973.

# University of Southern Maine
## School of Nursing
## Portland, Maine

***http://www.usm.maine.edu/nursing***
Founded in 1878

### DEGREES • BS • DNP • MS • MS/MBA
**Nursing Program Faculty** 70 (22% with doctorates).
**Baccalaureate Enrollment** 397 **Women** 90% **Men** 10% **Minority** 11% **Part-time** 21%
**Graduate Enrollment** 102 **Women** 85% **Men** 15% **Minority** 5% **Part-time** 81%
**Distance Learning Courses** Available.
**Nursing Student Activities** Sigma Theta Tau, Student Nurses' Association.
**Nursing Student Resources** Academic advising; academic or career counseling; assistance for students with disabilities; bookstore; campus computer network; computer lab; computer-assisted instruction; e-mail services; interactive nursing skills videos; Internet; learning resource lab; library services; nursing audiovisuals; remedial services; resume preparation assistance; skills, simulation, or other laboratory; tutoring.
**Library Facilities** 469,292 volumes (18,042 in health, 622 in nursing); 1,177 periodical subscriptions (230 health-care related).

### BACCALAUREATE PROGRAMS
**Degree** BS
**Available Programs** ADN to Baccalaureate; Accelerated Baccalaureate for Second Degree; Generic Baccalaureate; RN Baccalaureate.
**Site Options** Lewiston, ME.
**Study Options** Full-time and part-time.
**Program Entrance Requirements** Minimum overall college GPA of 3.0, transcript of college record, written essay, high school biology, high school chemistry, 3 years high school math, 2 years high school science, high school transcript, immunizations, 2 letters of recommendation, minimum high school GPA of 3.0. Transfer students are accepted. *Application deadline:* 1/15 (fall). *Application fee:* $40.
**Advanced Placement** Credit by examination available. Credit given for nursing courses completed elsewhere dependent upon specific evaluations.
**Expenses (2013–14)** *Tuition, state resident:* full-time $7590; part-time $253 per credit. *Tuition, nonresident:* full-time $19,950; part-time $665 per credit. *International tuition:* $19,950 full-time. *Room and board:* $9820; room only: $4600 per academic year. *Required fees:* full-time $1330; part-time $28 per credit; part-time $245 per term.
**Financial Aid** 96% of baccalaureate students in nursing programs received some form of financial aid in 2012–13.
**Contact** Ms. Brenda D. Webster, Coordinator of Nursing Student Services, School of Nursing, University of Southern Maine, PO Box 9300, Portland, ME 04104-9300. *Telephone:* 207-780-4802. *Fax:* 207-780-4973. *E-mail:* bwebster@usm.maine.edu.

### GRADUATE PROGRAMS
**Expenses (2013–14)** *Tuition, state resident:* full-time $6840; part-time $380 per credit. *Tuition, nonresident:* full-time $18,468; part-time $1026 per credit. *International tuition:* $18,468 full-time. *Room and board:* $9820 per academic year. *Required fees:* full-time $867; part-time $28 per credit; part-time $363 per term.
**Financial Aid** 90% of graduate students in nursing programs received some form of financial aid in 2012–13. Research assistantships, teaching assistantships, career-related internships or fieldwork, Federal Work-Study, scholarships, traineeships, tuition waivers (full and partial), and unspecified assistantships available. Aid available to part-time students. *Financial aid application deadline:* 2/15.
**Contact** Ms. Brenda D. Webster, Coordinator of Nursing Student Services, School of Nursing, University of Southern Maine, PO Box 9300, Portland, ME 04104-9300. *Telephone:* 207-780-4802. *Fax:* 207-780-4973. *E-mail:* bwebster@usm.maine.edu.

#### MASTER'S DEGREE PROGRAM
**Degrees** MS; MS/MBA
**Available Programs** Master's; Master's for Non-Nursing College Graduates; Master's for Nurses with Non-Nursing Degrees; RN to Master's.
**Concentrations Available** Clinical nurse leader; nursing administration; nursing education. *Nurse practitioner programs in:* family health, psychiatric/mental health.
**Study Options** Full-time and part-time.
**Program Entrance Requirements** Minimum overall college GPA of 3.0, transcript of college record, written essay, 2 letters of recommendation, physical assessment course, prerequisite course work, statistics course, GRE General Test or MAT. *Application deadline:* 4/1 (fall), 10/1 (spring), 11/1 (summer). *Application fee:* $50.
**Advanced Placement** Credit given for nursing courses completed elsewhere dependent upon specific evaluations.
**Degree Requirements** 54 total credit hours.

#### POST-MASTER'S PROGRAM
**Areas of Study** *Nurse practitioner programs in:* family health, psychiatric/mental health.

#### DOCTORAL DEGREE PROGRAM
**Degree** DNP
**Available Programs** Doctorate.
**Areas of Study** Clinical practice, ethics, health policy, health-care systems, nursing policy.
**Program Entrance Requirements** Clinical experience, minimum overall college GPA of 3.25, interview by faculty committee, 3 letters of recommendation, MSN or equivalent, statistics course, vita, writing sample, GRE. *Application deadline:* 3/15 (fall). *Application fee:* $65.
**Degree Requirements** 43 total credit hours, residency.

## CONTINUING EDUCATION PROGRAM

**Contact** Professional and Continuing Education, School of Nursing, University of Southern Maine, USM Professional and Continuing Education, PO Box 9300, Portland, ME 04104-9300. *Telephone:* 207-780-5900. *E-mail:* pce@usm.maine.edu.

# MARYLAND

## Bowie State University

### Department of Nursing
### Bowie, Maryland

*http://www.bowiestate.edu/academics/departments/nursing*
Founded in 1865

**DEGREES • BSN • MSN**

**Nursing Program Faculty** 20 (35% with doctorates).

**Baccalaureate Enrollment** 225 **Women** 88% **Men** 12% **Minority** 93% **International** 5% **Part-time** 25%

**Graduate Enrollment** 43 **Women** 87% **Men** 13% **Minority** 93% **International** 47% **Part-time** 5%

**Distance Learning Courses** Available.

**Nursing Student Activities** Nursing Honor Society, Student Nurses' Association.

**Nursing Student Resources** Academic advising; academic or career counseling; assistance for students with disabilities; bookstore; campus computer network; computer lab; computer-assisted instruction; housing assistance; interactive nursing skills videos; Internet; library services; nursing audiovisuals; skills, simulation, or other laboratory; tutoring.

**Library Facilities** 287,586 volumes; 780 periodical subscriptions.

### BACCALAUREATE PROGRAMS

**Degree** BSN

**Available Programs** Accelerated Baccalaureate; Generic Baccalaureate; RN Baccalaureate.

**Study Options** Full-time.

**Program Entrance Requirements** Minimum overall college GPA of 2.75, transcript of college record, health exam, health insurance, high school biology, high school chemistry, 4 years high school math, 4 years high school science, high school transcript, immunizations, minimum high school GPA of 3.0, minimum GPA in nursing prerequisites of 2.75, prerequisite course work. Transfer students are accepted. *Application deadline:* 3/31 (fall).

**Advanced Placement** Credit given for nursing courses completed elsewhere dependent upon specific evaluations.

**Contact** *Telephone:* 301-860-3202. *Fax:* 301-860-3222.

### GRADUATE PROGRAMS

**Contact** *Telephone:* 301-860-3202. *Fax:* 301-860-3222.

#### MASTER'S DEGREE PROGRAM

**Degree** MSN

**Available Programs** Master's.

**Concentrations Available** Nursing education. *Nurse practitioner programs in:* family health.

**Study Options** Full-time and part-time.

**Program Entrance Requirements** Clinical experience, minimum overall college GPA of 2.5, CPR certification, written essay, immunizations, 3 letters of recommendation, physical assessment course, professional liability insurance/malpractice insurance, resume, statistics course. *Application deadline:* 11/30 (fall), 4/30 (spring). Applications may be processed on a rolling basis for some programs.

**Advanced Placement** Credit by examination available. Credit given for nursing courses completed elsewhere dependent upon specific evaluations.

**Degree Requirements** 45 total credit hours, comprehensive exam.

## Coppin State University

### Helene Fuld School of Nursing
### Baltimore, Maryland

*http://www.coppin.edu/nursing*
Founded in 1900

**DEGREES • BSN • MSN**

**Nursing Program Faculty** 45 (18% with doctorates).

**Baccalaureate Enrollment** 529 **Women** 91% **Men** 9% **Minority** 99% **International** 2% **Part-time** 33%

**Graduate Enrollment** 32 **Women** 94% **Men** 6% **Minority** 94% **Part-time** 22%

**Distance Learning Courses** Available.

**Nursing Student Activities** Nursing Honor Society, Sigma Theta Tau, Student Nurses' Association.

**Nursing Student Resources** Academic advising; academic or career counseling; assistance for students with disabilities; bookstore; campus computer network; career placement assistance; computer lab; computer-assisted instruction; e-mail services; externships; interactive nursing skills videos; Internet; learning resource lab; library services; nursing audiovisuals; other; placement services for program completers; remedial services; resume preparation assistance; skills, simulation, or other laboratory; tutoring; unpaid internships.

**Library Facilities** 134,983 volumes (1,339 in health, 1,298 in nursing); 665 periodical subscriptions (132 health-care related).

### BACCALAUREATE PROGRAMS

**Degree** BSN

**Available Programs** Accelerated RN Baccalaureate; Baccalaureate for Second Degree; Generic Baccalaureate; RN Baccalaureate.

**Site Options** Baltimore, MD.

**Study Options** Full-time and part-time.

**Program Entrance Requirements** Written essay, health exam, high school biology, high school chemistry, high school foreign language, 3 years high school math, 2 years high school science, high school transcript, immunizations, 3 letters of recommendation, minimum high school GPA of 2.5, minimum GPA in nursing prerequisites of 2.5. Transfer students are accepted.

**Contact** *Telephone:* 410-951-3988. *Fax:* 410-400-5978.

### GRADUATE PROGRAMS

**Contact** *Telephone:* 410-951-3988. *Fax:* 410-400-5978.

#### MASTER'S DEGREE PROGRAM

**Degree** MSN

**Available Programs** Master's.

**Concentrations Available** *Nurse practitioner programs in:* family health.

**Site Options** Baltimore, MD.

**Study Options** Full-time and part-time.

**Program Entrance Requirements** Clinical experience, computer literacy, minimum overall college GPA of 3.0, transcript of college record, CPR certification, written essay, immunizations, interview, 3 letters of recommendation, nursing research course, physical assessment course, statistics course.

**Advanced Placement** Credit given for nursing courses completed elsewhere dependent upon specific evaluations.

**Degree Requirements** 48 total credit hours, thesis or project, comprehensive exam.

#### POST-MASTER'S PROGRAM

**Areas of Study** *Nurse practitioner programs in:* family health.

## Frostburg State University

### Nursing Department
### Frostburg, Maryland

Founded in 1898

**DEGREE • BSN**

**Library Facilities** 345,691 volumes; 3,899 periodical subscriptions.

### BACCALAUREATE PROGRAMS

**Degree** BSN

**Available Programs** RN Baccalaureate.

**Study Options** Part-time.
**Online Degree Options** Yes (online only).
**Program Entrance Requirements** Prerequisite course work, RN licensure. *Application deadline:* 4/1 (summer).
**Contact** Roxanne Weighley, Nursing Department, Nursing Department, Frostburg State University, 101 Braddock Road, Frostburg, MD 21532-2303. *Telephone:* 301-687-4141. *E-mail:* rmweighley@frostburg.edu.

# The Johns Hopkins University
## School of Nursing
## Baltimore, Maryland

*http://www.nursing.jhu.edu*
Founded in 1876

**DEGREES • BS • DNP • MSN • MSN/MBA • MSN/MPH • MSN/PHD • PHD**

**Nursing Program Faculty** 222 (32% with doctorates).
**Baccalaureate Enrollment** 497 **Women** 90.5% **Men** 9.5% **Minority** 27.2% **International** .7% **Part-time** 19.3%
**Graduate Enrollment** 205 **Women** 94.1% **Men** 5.9% **Minority** 23.9% **International** 3.9% **Part-time** 42.9%
**Distance Learning Courses** Available.
**Nursing Student Activities** Nursing Honor Society, Sigma Theta Tau, Student Nurses' Association, nursing club.
**Nursing Student Resources** Academic advising; academic or career counseling; assistance for students with disabilities; bookstore; campus computer network; career placement assistance; computer lab; computer-assisted instruction; e-mail services; employment services for current students; housing assistance; Internet; learning resource lab; library services; nursing audiovisuals; other; resume preparation assistance; skills, simulation, or other laboratory; tutoring.
**Library Facilities** 3.7 million volumes; 171,000 periodical subscriptions.

### BACCALAUREATE PROGRAMS

**Degree** BS
**Available Programs** Accelerated Baccalaureate; Accelerated Baccalaureate for Second Degree.
**Study Options** Full-time and part-time.
**Program Entrance Requirements** Minimum overall college GPA of 3.0, transcript of college record, CPR certification, written essay, health exam, health insurance, immunizations, interview, 3 letters of recommendation, minimum GPA in nursing prerequisites of 3.0, prerequisite course work. Transfer students are accepted. *Application deadline:* 1/15 (fall), 11/15 (summer). *Application fee:* $75.
**Advanced Placement** Credit by examination available. Credit given for nursing courses completed elsewhere dependent upon specific evaluations.
**Financial Aid** 85% of baccalaureate students in nursing programs received some form of financial aid in 2012–13. *Gift aid (need-based):* Federal Pell, FSEOG, state, private, college/university gift aid from institutional funds. *Loans:* Federal Direct (Subsidized and Unsubsidized Stafford PLUS), Perkins, college/university. *Work-study:* Federal Work-Study. *Financial aid application deadline:* 3/1.
**Contact** Office of Admissions and Student Services, School of Nursing, The Johns Hopkins University, 525 North Wolfe Street, Baltimore, MD 21205-2110. *Telephone:* 410-955-7548. *Fax:* 410-614-7086. *E-mail:* jhuson@jhu.edu.

### GRADUATE PROGRAMS

**Financial Aid** 80% of graduate students in nursing programs received some form of financial aid in 2012–13. 6 fellowships with partial tuition reimbursements available (averaging $23,272 per year) were awarded; research assistantships with full tuition reimbursements available, teaching assistantships with full tuition reimbursements available, career-related internships or fieldwork, Federal Work-Study, scholarships, traineeships, and tuition waivers (partial) also available. Aid available to part-time students. *Financial aid application deadline:* 3/1.
**Contact** Office of Admissions and Student Services, School of Nursing, The Johns Hopkins University, 525 North Wolfe Street, Baltimore, MD 21205-2110. *Telephone:* 410-955-7548. *Fax:* 410-614-7086. *E-mail:* jhuson@jhu.edu.

#### MASTER'S DEGREE PROGRAM

**Degrees** MSN; MSN/MBA; MSN/MPH; MSN/PhD
**Available Programs** Master's.
**Concentrations Available** Health-care administration; nurse case management; nurse-midwifery; nursing administration. *Clinical nurse specialist programs in:* acute care, adult health, gerontology, pediatric. *Nurse practitioner programs in:* acute care, adult health, family health, gerontology, pediatric, primary care.
**Study Options** Full-time and part-time.
**Online Degree Options** Yes.
**Program Entrance Requirements** Clinical experience, computer literacy, minimum overall college GPA of 3.0, transcript of college record, CPR certification, written essay, immunizations, interview, 3 letters of recommendation, nursing research course, physical assessment course, prerequisite course work, resume, statistics course. *Application deadline:* Applications may be processed on a rolling basis for some programs. *Application fee:* $75.
**Advanced Placement** Credit by examination available. Credit given for nursing courses completed elsewhere dependent upon specific evaluations.
**Degree Requirements** 36 total credit hours, thesis or project.

#### POST-MASTER'S PROGRAM

**Areas of Study** Nursing education. *Nurse practitioner programs in:* acute care, adult health, family health, gerontology, pediatric, primary care.

#### DOCTORAL DEGREE PROGRAM

**Degree** DNP
**Available Programs** Doctorate.
**Areas of Study** Advanced practice nursing, clinical practice, community health, critical care, family health, forensic nursing, gerontology, health policy, health promotion/disease prevention, health-care systems, human health and illness, illness and transition, individualized study, information systems, maternity-newborn, neuro-behavior, nurse case management, nursing administration, nursing education, nursing policy, nursing research, nursing science, oncology, urban health,women's health.
**Program Entrance Requirements** Minimum overall college GPA of 3.0, clinical experience, interview, 3 letters of recommendation, MSN or equivalent, statistics course, vita, writing sample. *Application deadline:* 1/1 (summer). *Application fee:* $100.
**Degree Requirements** 42 total credit hours, Capstone project.

**Degree** PhD
**Available Programs** Doctorate.
**Areas of Study** Addiction/substance abuse, advanced practice nursing, aging, bio-behavioral research, biology of health and illness, clinical practice, community health, critical care, family health, forensic nursing, gerontology, health policy, health promotion/disease prevention, health-care systems, human health and illness, illness and transition, individualized study, information systems, nurse case management, nursing research, nursing science, oncology, urban health,women's health.
**Program Entrance Requirements** Clinical experience, minimum overall college GPA of 3.0, interview, 3 letters of recommendation, MSN or equivalent, scholarly papers, statistics course, vita, writing sample, GRE (for PhD). *Application fee:* $100.
**Degree Requirements** Dissertation, oral exam, written exam.

#### POSTDOCTORAL PROGRAM

**Areas of Study** Health promotion/disease prevention, individualized study, vulnerable population.
**Postdoctoral Program Contact** Office of Admissions and Student Services, School of Nursing, The Johns Hopkins University, 525 North Wolfe Street, Baltimore, MD 21205-2110. *Telephone:* 410-955-7548. *Fax:* 410-614-7086. *E-mail:* jhuson@jhu.edu.

### CONTINUING EDUCATION PROGRAM

**Contact** David Newton, Executive Director, Professional Programs, School of Nursing, The Johns Hopkins University, 525 North Wolfe Street, Baltimore, MD 21205-2110. *Telephone:* 410-502-3335. *Fax:* 443-769-1232. *E-mail:* son-professionalprgm@jhu.edu.

***See display on next page and full description on page 476.***

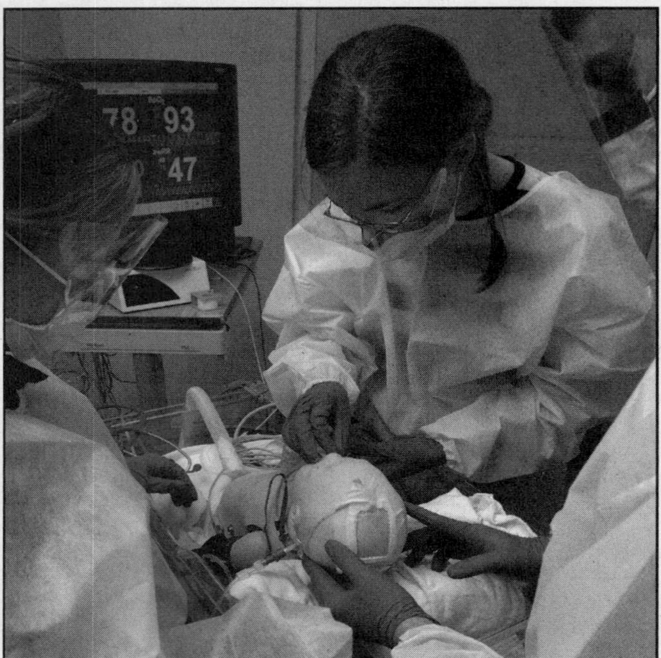



# Notre Dame of Maryland University

## Department of Nursing
## Baltimore, Maryland

***http://www.ndm.edu/academics/departments-and-programs/nursing/***
Founded in 1873

**DEGREE • BS**
**Nursing Program Faculty** 5 (60% with doctorates).
**Nursing Student Resources** Library services.
**Library Facilities** 999,295 volumes; 42,427 periodical subscriptions.

### BACCALAUREATE PROGRAMS

**Degree** BS
**Available Programs** Accelerated RN Baccalaureate; RN Baccalaureate.
**Site Options** Frederick, MD; Aberdeen, MD.
**Study Options** Full-time and part-time.
**Program Entrance Requirements** Minimum overall college GPA of 2.5, transcript of college record, interview, minimum GPA in nursing prerequisites of 2.0, prerequisite course work, RN licensure. Transfer students are accepted.
**Advanced Placement** Credit by examination available. Credit given for nursing courses completed elsewhere dependent upon specific evaluations.
**Contact** *Telephone:* 410-532-5500.

# Salisbury University

## Nursing DNP Program
## Salisbury, Maryland

***http://www.salisbury.edu/nursing***
Founded in 1925

**DEGREES • BS • DNP • MS**
**Nursing Program Faculty** 53 (85% with doctorates).
**Baccalaureate Enrollment** 570 **Women** 92% **Men** 8% **Minority** 23% **International** .5% **Part-time** 4%
**Graduate Enrollment** 50 **Women** 94% **Men** 6% **Minority** 16% **Part-time** 62%
**Distance Learning Courses** Available.
**Nursing Student Activities** Nursing Honor Society, Sigma Theta Tau, Student Nurses' Association.
**Nursing Student Resources** Academic advising; academic or career counseling; assistance for students with disabilities; bookstore; campus computer network; career placement assistance; computer lab; computer-assisted instruction; e-mail services; employment services for current students; externships; housing assistance; interactive nursing skills videos; Internet; learning resource lab; library services; nursing audiovisuals; paid internships; placement services for program completers; remedial services; resume preparation assistance; skills, simulation, or other laboratory; tutoring; unpaid internships.
**Library Facilities** 287,318 volumes (8,945 in health, 1,380 in nursing); 942 periodical subscriptions (75 health-care related).

### BACCALAUREATE PROGRAMS

**Degree** BS
**Available Programs** ADN to Baccalaureate; Accelerated Baccalaureate for Second Degree; Generic Baccalaureate; RN Baccalaureate.
**Study Options** Full-time and part-time.
**Program Entrance Requirements** Minimum overall college GPA of 3.0, transcript of college record, CPR certification, health exam, high school biology, high school chemistry, 2 years high school math, high school transcript, immunizations, minimum GPA in nursing prerequisites of 3.0, prerequisite course work. Transfer students are accepted. *Application deadline:* 2/1 (winter). *Application fee:* $45.
**Expenses (2012–13)** *Tuition, state resident:* full-time $5576. *Tuition, nonresident:* full-time $13,922. *Room and board:* $10,500; room only: $6350 per academic year. *Required fees:* full-time $2124.
**Financial Aid** 75% of baccalaureate students in nursing programs received some form of financial aid in 2011–12. *Gift aid (need-based):* Federal Pell, FSEOG, state, private, college/university gift aid from institutional funds. *Loans:* Federal Direct (Subsidized and Unsubsidized

Stafford PLUS), Perkins. *Work-study:* Federal Work-Study. *Financial aid application deadline:* 12/31(priority: 3/1).
**Contact** Dr. Lisa A. Seldomridge, Chair and Professor, Department of Nursing, Nursing DNP Program, Salisbury University, 1101 Camden Avenue, Salisbury, MD 21801. *Telephone:* 410-543-6413. *Fax:* 410-548-3313. *E-mail:* laseldomridge@salisbury.edu.

## GRADUATE PROGRAMS

**Expenses (2012–13)** *Tuition, state resident:* part-time $584 per credit. *Tuition, nonresident:* part-time $742 per credit. *Required fees:* part-time $77 per credit.
**Financial Aid** Career-related internships or fieldwork, institutionally sponsored loans, scholarships, and unspecified assistantships available.
**Contact** Dr. Mary T. Parsons, Director, Graduate and Second Degree Programs, Nursing DNP Program, Salisbury University, 1101 Camden Avenue, Salisbury, MD 21801. *Telephone:* 410-543-6416. *Fax:* 410-548-3313. *E-mail:* mtparsons@salisbury.edu.

### MASTER'S DEGREE PROGRAM

**Degree** MS
**Available Programs** Master's; RN to Master's.
**Concentrations Available** Health-care administration; nursing education. *Nurse practitioner programs in:* family health.
**Study Options** Full-time and part-time.
**Program Entrance Requirements** Minimum overall college GPA of 3.0, transcript of college record, CPR certification, written essay, immunizations, interview, 2 letters of recommendation, nursing research course, physical assessment course, professional liability insurance/malpractice insurance, prerequisite course work, resume, statistics course. *Application deadline:* Applications may be processed on a rolling basis for some programs. *Application fee:* $45.
**Advanced Placement** Credit given for nursing courses completed elsewhere dependent upon specific evaluations.
**Degree Requirements** 45 total credit hours, thesis or project.

### POST-MASTER'S PROGRAM

**Areas of Study** Health-care administration; nursing education. *Nurse practitioner programs in:* family health.

### DOCTORAL DEGREE PROGRAM

**Degree** DNP
**Available Programs** Doctorate.
**Areas of Study** Advanced practice nursing, biology of health and illness, clinical practice, community health, family health, gerontology, health policy, health promotion/disease prevention, health-care systems, individualized study, information systems, nursing policy,women's health.
**Program Entrance Requirements** Clinical experience, minimum overall college GPA of 3.5, interview, 3 letters of recommendation, MSN or equivalent, statistics course, vita, writing sample. *Application deadline:* 5/1 (fall). Applications may be processed on a rolling basis for some programs. *Application fee:* $45.
**Degree Requirements** 38 total credit hours, dissertation.

# Stevenson University

## Nursing Division
## Stevenson, Maryland

***http://www.stevenson.edu***
Founded in 1952

**DEGREES • BS • MS**

**Nursing Program Faculty** 50 (30% with doctorates).
**Baccalaureate Enrollment** 700 **Women** 94% **Men** 6% **Minority** 25% **Part-time** 52%
**Graduate Enrollment** 150 **Women** 95% **Men** 5% **Minority** 30% **Part-time** 100%
**Distance Learning Courses** Available.
**Nursing Student Activities** Sigma Theta Tau, Student Nurses' Association, nursing club.
**Nursing Student Resources** Academic advising; academic or career counseling; assistance for students with disabilities; bookstore; campus computer network; career placement assistance; computer lab; computer-assisted instruction; e-mail services; employment services for current students; externships; interactive nursing skills videos; Internet; learning resource lab; library services; nursing audiovisuals; placement services for program completers; remedial services; resume preparation assistance; skills, simulation, or other laboratory; tutoring.

**Library Facilities** 81,802 volumes (3,301 in health, 776 in nursing); 1,058 periodical subscriptions (635 health-care related).

## BACCALAUREATE PROGRAMS

**Degree** BS
**Available Programs** ADN to Baccalaureate; Accelerated RN Baccalaureate; Baccalaureate for Second Degree; Generic Baccalaureate; RN Baccalaureate.
**Site Options** Eastern shore, MD; southern state, MD; Baltimore, MD.
**Study Options** Full-time and part-time.
**Online Degree Options** Yes (online only).
**Program Entrance Requirements** Minimum overall college GPA of 3.0, transcript of college record, written essay, health exam, health insurance, high school biology, high school chemistry, 2 years high school math, high school transcript, immunizations, interview, minimum high school GPA of 3.0, minimum GPA in nursing prerequisites of 3.0. Transfer students are accepted. *Application deadline:* 2/1 (spring).
**Advanced Placement** Credit by examination available. Credit given for nursing courses completed elsewhere dependent upon specific evaluations.
**Expenses (2012–13)** *Tuition:* full-time $23,562; part-time $596 per credit. *Room and board:* $11,888; room only: $7888 per academic year. *Required fees:* full-time $1748.
**Financial Aid** 85% of baccalaureate students in nursing programs received some form of financial aid in 2011–12.
**Contact** Dr. Denise Seigart, Associate Dean for Nursing Education, Nursing Division, Stevenson University, 1525 Greenspring Valley Road, Stevenson, MD 21153-0641. *Telephone:* 443-334-2821. *Fax:* 443-334-2148. *E-mail:* dseigart@stevenson.edu.

## GRADUATE PROGRAMS

**Expenses (2012–13)** *Tuition:* part-time $560 per credit.
**Financial Aid** 20% of graduate students in nursing programs received some form of financial aid in 2011–12.
**Contact** Dr. Judith Feustle, Associate Dean, GPS Nursing, Nursing Division, Stevenson University, Garrison Hall, 100 Campus Circle, Owings MIlls, MD 21117. *Telephone:* 443-352-4292. *Fax:* 443-394-0538. *E-mail:* jfeustle@stevenson.edu.

### MASTER'S DEGREE PROGRAM

**Degree** MS
**Available Programs** Accelerated Master's; Accelerated RN to Master's; RN to Master's.
**Concentrations Available** Health-care administration; nursing administration; nursing education.
**Site Options** Eastern shore, MD; southern state, MD; Baltimore, MD.
**Study Options** Part-time.
**Online Degree Options** Yes (online only).
**Program Entrance Requirements** Computer literacy, minimum overall college GPA of 3.0, transcript of college record, immunizations, letters of recommendation, nursing research course.
**Advanced Placement** Credit given for nursing courses completed elsewhere dependent upon specific evaluations.
**Degree Requirements** 36 total credit hours, thesis or project.

# Towson University

## Department of Nursing
## Towson, Maryland

***http://www.towson.edu/nursing***
Founded in 1866

**DEGREES • BS • MS**

**Nursing Program Faculty** 80 (15% with doctorates).
**Baccalaureate Enrollment** 345 **Women** 87% **Men** 13% **Minority** 30% **International** 1% **Part-time** 3%
**Graduate Enrollment** 106 **Women** 95% **Men** 5% **Minority** 23% **International** 1% **Part-time** 60%
**Distance Learning Courses** Available.
**Nursing Student Activities** Sigma Theta Tau, Student Nurses' Association.
**Nursing Student Resources** Academic advising; academic or career counseling; assistance for students with disabilities; bookstore; campus computer network; career placement assistance; computer lab; computer-assisted instruction; daycare for children of students; e-mail services; housing assistance; interactive nursing skills videos; Internet; learning resource lab; library services; nursing audiovisuals; remedial services;

resume preparation assistance; skills, simulation, or other laboratory; tutoring.
**Library Facilities** 719,299 volumes (16,457 in health, 1,460 in nursing); 36,657 periodical subscriptions (721 health-care related).

## BACCALAUREATE PROGRAMS

**Degree** BS
**Available Programs** Generic Baccalaureate; RN Baccalaureate.
**Site Options** Hagerstown, MD.
**Study Options** Full-time and part-time.
**Program Entrance Requirements** Minimum overall college GPA of 3.0, transcript of college record, CPR certification, health exam, health insurance, immunizations, prerequisite course work. Transfer students are accepted. *Application deadline:* 1/15 (fall), 8/15 (spring). *Application fee:* $50.
**Advanced Placement** Credit given for nursing courses completed elsewhere dependent upon specific evaluations.
**Expenses (2013–14)** *Tuition, state resident:* full-time $5830; part-time $253 per credit. *Tuition, nonresident:* full-time $17,508; part-time $733 per credit. *International tuition:* $17,508 full-time. *Room and board:* $10,662 per academic year. *Required fees:* full-time $2512; part-time $105 per credit.
**Financial Aid** *Gift aid (need-based):* Federal Pell, FSEOG, state, private, college/university gift aid from institutional funds. *Loans:* Federal Direct (Subsidized and Unsubsidized Stafford PLUS), Perkins. *Work-study:* Federal Work-Study. *Financial aid application deadline (priority):* 2/15.
**Contact** Ms. Brook R. Necker, Admissions and Retention Coordinator, Department of Nursing, Towson University, 8000 York Road, Towson, MD 21252-0001. *Telephone:* 410-704-4170. *E-mail:* bnecker@towson.edu.

## GRADUATE PROGRAMS

**Expenses (2013–14)** *Tuition, state resident:* part-time $365 per credit. *Tuition, nonresident:* part-time $751 per credit. *Required fees:* part-time $105 per credit.
**Financial Aid** 15% of graduate students in nursing programs received some form of financial aid in 2012–13.
**Contact** Dr. Kathleen Ogle, Graduate Program Director, Department of Nursing, Towson University, 8000 York Road, Towson, MD 21252-0001. *Telephone:* 410-704-4389. *Fax:* 410-704-4325. *E-mail:* kogle@towson.edu.

### MASTER'S DEGREE PROGRAM

**Degree** MS
**Available Programs** Master's.
**Concentrations Available** Health-care administration; nursing education.
**Site Options** Hagerstown, MD.
**Study Options** Full-time and part-time.
**Program Entrance Requirements** Minimum overall college GPA of 3.0, transcript of college record, written essay, nursing research course, physical assessment course, resume, statistics course. *Application deadline:* 8/1 (fall), 12/1 (spring), 5/1 (summer). Applications may be processed on a rolling basis for some programs. *Application fee:* $50.
**Advanced Placement** Credit given for nursing courses completed elsewhere dependent upon specific evaluations.
**Degree Requirements** 36 total credit hours.

### POST-MASTER'S PROGRAM

**Areas of Study** Health-care administration; nursing education.

# University of Maryland, Baltimore

## Master's Program in Nursing
## Baltimore, Maryland

*http://www.nursing.umaryland.edu/*
Founded in 1807

**DEGREES • BSN • DNP • MS • MSN/MBA • MSN/MPH • PHD**

**Nursing Program Faculty** 146 (66% with doctorates).
**Baccalaureate Enrollment** 641 **Women** 85% **Men** 15% **Minority** 41.19% **International** 3.9% **Part-time** 25.59%
**Graduate Enrollment** 1,102 **Women** 89% **Men** 11% **Minority** 34.75% **International** 2.54% **Part-time** 65.06%
**Distance Learning Courses** Available.
**Nursing Student Activities** Nursing Honor Society, Sigma Theta Tau, Student Nurses' Association.
**Nursing Student Resources** Academic advising; academic or career counseling; assistance for students with disabilities; bookstore; campus computer network; career placement assistance; computer lab; computer-assisted instruction; e-mail services; interactive nursing skills videos; Internet; learning resource lab; library services; nursing audiovisuals; remedial services; skills, simulation, or other laboratory; tutoring.
**Library Facilities** 360,000 volumes in health, 60 volumes in nursing; 2,400 periodical subscriptions health-care related.

## BACCALAUREATE PROGRAMS

**Degree** BSN
**Available Programs** Generic Baccalaureate; RN Baccalaureate.
**Site Options** Baltimore-Shady Grove, MD.
**Study Options** Full-time and part-time.
**Online Degree Options** Yes.
**Program Entrance Requirements** Minimum overall college GPA of 3.0, transcript of college record, CPR certification, written essay, health exam, health insurance, immunizations, 2 letters of recommendation, minimum GPA in nursing prerequisites of 3.0, prerequisite course work. Transfer students are accepted. *Application deadline:* 2/1 (fall), 9/1 (spring). *Application fee:* $50.
**Advanced Placement** Credit by examination available.
**Financial Aid** 61% of baccalaureate students in nursing programs received some form of financial aid in 2012–13.
**Contact** Mr. Kevin Nies, Associate Director of Admissions, Master's Program in Nursing, University of Maryland, Baltimore, 655 West Lombard Street, Room 102G, Baltimore, MD 21201. *Telephone:* 410-706-1281. *Fax:* 410-706-7238. *E-mail:* nies@son.umaryland.edu.

## GRADUATE PROGRAMS

**Expenses (2013–14)** *Tuition, state resident:* full-time $10,476; part-time $604 per credit. *Tuition, nonresident:* full-time $19,332; part-time $1116 per credit. *Required fees:* full-time $1672.
**Financial Aid** 53% of graduate students in nursing programs received some form of financial aid in 2012–13. Fellowships, research assistantships, teaching assistantships, career-related internships or fieldwork and traineeships available. Aid available to part-time students. *Financial aid application deadline:* 2/15.
**Contact** Ms. Marchelle Payne-Gassaway, Director of Admissions, Master's Program in Nursing, University of Maryland, Baltimore, 655 West Lombard Street, Room 102, Baltimore, MD 21201-1579. *Telephone:* 410-706-1281. *Fax:* 410-706-2326. *E-mail:* gassaway@son.umaryland.edu.

### MASTER'S DEGREE PROGRAM

**Degrees** MS; MSN/MBA; MSN/MPH
**Available Programs** Accelerated Master's for Non-Nursing College Graduates; Master's; RN to Master's.
**Concentrations Available** Clinical nurse leader; nursing informatics. *Clinical nurse specialist programs in:* community health, public health.
**Site Options** Baltimore-Shady Grove, MD.
**Study Options** Full-time and part-time.
**Online Degree Options** Yes.
**Program Entrance Requirements** Computer literacy, minimum overall college GPA of 3.0, transcript of college record, CPR certification, written essay, immunizations, interview, 2 letters of recommendation, nursing research course, physical assessment course, professional liability insurance/malpractice insurance, prerequisite course work, resume, statistics course. *Application deadline:* 2/1 (fall), 9/1 (spring). *Application fee:* $50.
**Advanced Placement** Credit given for nursing courses completed elsewhere dependent upon specific evaluations.
**Degree Requirements** 36 total credit hours, thesis or project.

### POST-MASTER'S PROGRAM

**Areas of Study** Nursing informatics. *Clinical nurse specialist programs in:* community health, public health.

### DOCTORAL DEGREE PROGRAM

**Degree** DNP
**Available Programs** Doctorate; Post-Baccalaureate Doctorate.
**Areas of Study** Addiction/substance abuse, advanced practice nursing, aging, bio-behavioral research, biology of health and illness, clinical practice, clinical research, community health, critical care, ethics, faculty preparation, family health, gerontology, health policy, health promotion/disease prevention, health-care systems, human health and

illness, illness and transition, individualized study, information systems, maternity-newborn, neuro-behavior, nurse case management, nursing administration, nursing education, nursing policy, nursing research, nursing science, oncology, palliative care, urban health,women's health.

**Program Entrance Requirements** Clinical experience, minimum overall college GPA of 3.0, interview by faculty committee, interview, 3 letters of recommendation, MSN or equivalent, vita, writing sample. *Application deadline:* 2/1 (fall). *Application fee:* $50.

**Degree Requirements** 36 total credit hours, oral exam, written exam.

**Degree** PhD

**Available Programs** Doctorate, Post-Baccalaureate Doctorate.

**Areas of Study** Addiction/substance abuse, aging, bio-behavioral research, biology of health and illness, critical care, faculty preparation, gerontology, health promotion/disease prevention, illness and transition, individualized study, information systems, neuro-behavior, nursing administration, nursing education, nursing research, nursing science, oncology.

**Program Entrance Requirements** Minimum overall college GPA of 3.5, interview, interview by faculty committee, 3 letters of recommendation, MSN or equivalent, statistics course, vita. *Application deadline:* 2/15 (fall). *Application fee:* $50.

**Degree Requirements** 60 total credit hours, dissertation, oral exam, residency, written exam.

### CONTINUING EDUCATION PROGRAM

**Contact** Sonia Smith, Program Coordinator, Master's Program in Nursing, University of Maryland, Baltimore, 655 West Lombard Street, Room 311G, Baltimore, MD 21201-1579. *Telephone:* 410-706-3768. *E-mail:* Ssmith@son.umaryland.edu.

## Washington Adventist University

### Nursing Department
### Takoma Park, Maryland

*http://www.wau.edu/*

Founded in 1904

**DEGREE • BS**

**Nursing Program Faculty** 8 (14% with doctorates).

**Baccalaureate Enrollment** 240 **Women** 90% **Men** 10% **Minority** 75% **International** 1% **Part-time** 10%

**Nursing Student Activities** Student Nurses' Association, nursing club.

**Nursing Student Resources** Academic advising; academic or career counseling; bookstore; campus computer network; computer lab; e-mail services; externships; interactive nursing skills videos; Internet; learning resource lab; library services; nursing audiovisuals; remedial services; skills, simulation, or other laboratory; tutoring; unpaid internships.

### BACCALAUREATE PROGRAMS

**Degree** BS

**Available Programs** Accelerated RN Baccalaureate; Generic Baccalaureate.

**Study Options** Full-time.

**Program Entrance Requirements** Minimum overall college GPA of 2.75, transcript of college record, CPR certification, written essay, health exam, immunizations, interview, 2 letters of recommendation, minimum GPA in nursing prerequisites of 2.75, prerequisite course work. Transfer students are accepted.

**Advanced Placement** Credit given for nursing courses completed elsewhere dependent upon specific evaluations.

**Contact** *Telephone:* 301-891-4144. *Fax:* 301-891-4191.

# MASSACHUSETTS

## American International College

### Division of Nursing
### Springfield, Massachusetts

*http://www.aic.edu/academics/hs/nursing*

Founded in 1885

**DEGREES • BSN • MSN**

**Nursing Program Faculty** 16 (13% with doctorates).

**Baccalaureate Enrollment** 372 **Women** 87% **Men** 13% **Minority** 29% **Part-time** 8%

**Graduate Enrollment** 23 **Women** 91% **Men** 9% **Minority** 17% **Part-time** 48%

**Distance Learning Courses** Available.

**Nursing Student Activities** Nursing Honor Society, Sigma Theta Tau, Student Nurses' Association.

**Nursing Student Resources** Academic advising; academic or career counseling; assistance for students with disabilities; bookstore; campus computer network; career placement assistance; computer lab; e-mail services; employment services for current students; externships; housing assistance; interactive nursing skills videos; Internet; learning resource lab; library services; nursing audiovisuals; other; placement services for program completers; remedial services; resume preparation assistance; skills, simulation, or other laboratory; tutoring; unpaid internships.

**Library Facilities** 70,741 volumes (2,125 in health, 226 in nursing); 7,211 periodical subscriptions (67 health-care related).

### BACCALAUREATE PROGRAMS

**Degree** BSN

**Available Programs** ADN to Baccalaureate; Generic Baccalaureate; RN Baccalaureate.

**Study Options** Full-time and part-time.

**Program Entrance Requirements** Minimum overall college GPA of 2.5, transcript of college record, health exam, health insurance, high school biology, high school chemistry, 3 years high school math, 2 years high school science, high school transcript, immunizations, minimum high school GPA of 2.5, minimum GPA in nursing prerequisites of 2.5, professional liability insurance/malpractice insurance, prerequisite course work. Transfer students are accepted. *Application deadline:* 2/15 (fall). Applications may be processed on a rolling basis for some programs. *Application fee:* $25.

**Advanced Placement** Credit by examination available. Credit given for nursing courses completed elsewhere dependent upon specific evaluations.

**Expenses (2013–14)** *Tuition:* full-time $30,040; part-time $620 per credit. *International tuition:* $30,040 full-time. *Room and board:* $12,150; room only: $6270 per academic year. *Required fees:* full-time $1500; part-time $750 per term.

**Financial Aid** 99% of baccalaureate students in nursing programs received some form of financial aid in 2012–13. *Gift aid (need-based):* Federal Pell, FSEOG, state, private, college/university gift aid from institutional funds. *Loans:* Federal Direct (Subsidized and Unsubsidized Stafford PLUS), Perkins. *Work-study:* Federal Work-Study, part-time campus jobs. *Financial aid application deadline (priority):* 5/1.

**Contact** Ms. Janelle Holmboe, Admission Services, Division of Nursing, American International College, 1000 State Street, Springfield, MA 01109. *Telephone:* 413-205-3201. *Fax:* 413-205-3275. *E-mail:* janelle.holmboe@aic.edu.

### GRADUATE PROGRAMS

**Expenses (2013–14)** *Tuition:* part-time $549 per credit. *Room and board:* $12,150; room only: $6270 per academic year.

**Financial Aid** 50% of graduate students in nursing programs received some form of financial aid in 2012–13.

**Contact** Ms. Janelle Holmboe, Dean of Admissions, Division of Nursing, American International College, 1000 State Street, Springfield, MA 01109. *Telephone:* 413-205-3275. *Fax:* 413-205-3201. *E-mail:* janelle.holmboe@aic.edu.

**MASTER'S DEGREE PROGRAM**

**Degree** MSN

**Available Programs** Master's.

**Concentrations Available** Nursing administration; nursing education.

**Study Options** Full-time and part-time.

**Online Degree Options** Yes (online only).

**Program Entrance Requirements** Clinical experience, minimum overall college GPA of 3.0, transcript of college record, CPR certification, immunizations, interview, 2 letters of recommendation, professional liability insurance/malpractice insurance, prerequisite course work, resume. *Application deadline:* Applications may be processed on a rolling basis for some programs. *Application fee:* $50.

**Advanced Placement** Credit given for nursing courses completed elsewhere dependent upon specific evaluations.

**Degree Requirements** 36 total credit hours, thesis or project.

# Anna Maria College
## Department of Nursing
## Paxton, Massachusetts

*http://www.annamaria.edu/*

Founded in 1946

### DEGREE • BSN

**Nursing Program Faculty** 6 (16% with doctorates).

**Baccalaureate Enrollment** 32 **Women** 94% **Men** 6% **Minority** 6% **Part-time** 100%

**Nursing Student Activities** Sigma Theta Tau.

**Nursing Student Resources** Academic advising; academic or career counseling; assistance for students with disabilities; bookstore; campus computer network; career placement assistance; computer lab; e-mail services; employment services for current students; Internet; learning resource lab; library services; nursing audiovisuals; placement services for program completers; remedial services; resume preparation assistance; skills, simulation, or other laboratory; tutoring; unpaid internships.

**Library Facilities** 3,000 volumes in health, 400 volumes in nursing; 22 periodical subscriptions health-care related.

### BACCALAUREATE PROGRAMS

**Degree** BSN

**Available Programs** ADN to Baccalaureate; RN Baccalaureate.

**Study Options** Part-time.

**Program Entrance Requirements** Minimum overall college GPA of 2.5, transcript of college record, interview, 1 letter of recommendation, minimum high school GPA of 2.5, minimum GPA in nursing prerequisites of 2.5, RN licensure. Transfer students are accepted. *Application deadline:* Applications may be processed on a rolling basis for some programs. *Application fee:* $40.

**Advanced Placement** Credit by examination available. Credit given for nursing courses completed elsewhere dependent upon specific evaluations.

**Contact** *Telephone:* 508-829-3316 Ext. 316. *Fax:* 508-849-3343 Ext. 371.

### CONTINUING EDUCATION PROGRAM

**Contact** *Telephone:* 508-849-3316 Ext. 316. *Fax:* 508-849-3343 Ext. 371.

# Becker College
## Nursing Programs
## Worcester, Massachusetts

Founded in 1784

### DEGREE • BSN

**Library Facilities** 75,000 volumes; 400 periodical subscriptions.

### BACCALAUREATE PROGRAMS

**Degree** BSN

**Available Programs** Generic Baccalaureate; RN Baccalaureate.

**Contact** Linda Esper, Director and Professor of Nursing, Nursing Programs, Becker College, 61 Sever Street, Worcester, MA 01609. *Telephone:* 508-373-9727. *Fax:* 508-849-5385. *E-mail:* linda.esper@becker.edu.

# Boston College
## William F. Connell School of Nursing
## Chestnut Hill, Massachusetts

*http://www.bc.edu/nursing*

Founded in 1863

### DEGREES • BS • MS • MS/MA • MS/MBA • MSN/PHD • PHD

**Nursing Program Faculty** 122 (35% with doctorates).

**Baccalaureate Enrollment** 385 **Women** 96% **Men** 4% **Minority** 27% **International** 1%

**Graduate Enrollment** 280 **Women** 91% **Men** 9% **Minority** 16% **International** 3% **Part-time** 28%

**Nursing Student Activities** Nursing Honor Society, Sigma Theta Tau, Student Nurses' Association.

**Nursing Student Resources** Academic advising; academic or career counseling; assistance for students with disabilities; bookstore; campus computer network; career placement assistance; computer lab; computer-assisted instruction; e-mail services; employment services for current students; externships; housing assistance; interactive nursing skills videos; Internet; learning resource lab; library services; nursing audiovisuals; other; placement services for program completers; remedial services; resume preparation assistance; skills, simulation, or other laboratory; tutoring; unpaid internships.

**Library Facilities** 2.8 million volumes (65,000 in health, 20,000 in nursing); 271,513 periodical subscriptions (5,395 health-care related).

### BACCALAUREATE PROGRAMS

**Degree** BS

**Available Programs** Generic Baccalaureate.

**Study Options** Full-time.

**Program Entrance Requirements** Transcript of college record, written essay, health exam, health insurance, high school biology, high school chemistry, high school foreign language, 4 years high school math, 3 years high school science, high school transcript, immunizations, 2 letters of recommendation. Transfer students are accepted. *Application deadline:* 1/1 (fall), 11/1 (winter). *Application fee:* $70.

**Advanced Placement** Credit given for nursing courses completed elsewhere dependent upon specific evaluations.

**Expenses (2013–14)** *Tuition:* full-time $44,870. *Room and board:* $6442; room only: $3985 per academic year. *Required fees:* full-time $3975.

**Financial Aid** 76% of baccalaureate students in nursing programs received some form of financial aid in 2012–13.

**Contact** Ms. Christine Murphy, Undergraduate Program Assistant, William F. Connell School of Nursing, Boston College, 140 Commonwealth Avenue, Cushing Hall 202D, Chestnut Hill, MA 02467-3812. *Telephone:* 617-552-4925. *Fax:* 617-552-0745. *E-mail:* christine.murphy.1@bc.edu.

### GRADUATE PROGRAMS

**Expenses (2013–14)** *Tuition:* full-time $27,696. *Room and board:* $6442; room only: $3985 per academic year. *Required fees:* full-time $3274.

**Financial Aid** 76% of graduate students in nursing programs received some form of financial aid in 2012–13. 5 fellowships with full tuition reimbursements available (averaging $22,000 per year), 12 teaching assistantships (averaging $7,000 per year) were awarded; research assistantships, Federal Work-Study, scholarships, tuition waivers (partial), and unspecified assistantships also available. Aid available to part-time students. *Financial aid application deadline:* 3/1.

**Contact** Ms. Marybeth Crowley, Graduate Programs Office, William F. Connell School of Nursing, Boston College, 140 Commonwealth Avenue, Cushing Hall, Chestnut Hill, MA 02467-3812. *Telephone:* 617-552-4928. *Fax:* 617-552-2121. *E-mail:* csongrad@bc.edu.

#### MASTER'S DEGREE PROGRAM

**Degrees** MS; MS/MA; MS/MBA; MSN/PhD

**Available Programs** Accelerated Master's; Accelerated Master's for Non-Nursing College Graduates; Master's; RN to Master's.

**Concentrations Available** Nurse anesthesia. *Clinical nurse specialist programs in:* adult health, community health, gerontology, pediatric. *Nurse practitioner programs in:* adult health, family health, gerontology, pediatric, psychiatric/mental health,women's health.

**Study Options** Full-time and part-time.

**Program Entrance Requirements** Minimum overall college GPA of 3.0, transcript of college record, written essay, 2 letters of recommen-

dation, statistics course. *Application deadline:* 4/30 (fall), 9/15 (spring). *Application fee:* $40.
**Advanced Placement** Credit given for nursing courses completed elsewhere dependent upon specific evaluations.
**Degree Requirements** 45 total credit hours, comprehensive exam.

### POST-MASTER'S PROGRAM
**Areas of Study** Nurse anesthesia; nursing education. *Nurse practitioner programs in:* adult health, family health, gerontology, pediatric, psychiatric/mental health,women's health.

### DOCTORAL DEGREE PROGRAM
**Degree** PhD
**Available Programs** Doctorate; Post-Baccalaureate Doctorate.
**Areas of Study** Addiction/substance abuse, advanced practice nursing, aging, bio-behavioral research, biology of health and illness, clinical practice, community health, ethics, family health, forensic nursing, gerontology, health promotion/disease prevention, human health and illness, illness and transition, individualized study, maternity-newborn, neurobehavior, nurse case management, nursing research, nursing science, oncology, urban health,women's health.
**Program Entrance Requirements** Minimum overall college GPA of 3.5, interview by faculty committee, interview, 3 letters of recommendation, MSN or equivalent, statistics course, vita, writing sample, GRE General Test. *Application deadline:* 1/15 (fall). *Application fee:* $40.
**Degree Requirements** 46 total credit hours, dissertation, oral exam, written exam.

### CONTINUING EDUCATION PROGRAM
**Contact** Dr. Jean Weyman, Assistant Dean, Continuing Education, William F. Connell School of Nursing, Boston College, 140 Commonwealth Avenue, Service Building, 211F, Chestnut Hill, MA 02467-3812. *Telephone:* 617-552-4256. *Fax:* 617-552-0745. *E-mail:* jean.weyman@bc.edu.

# Curry College
## Division of Nursing
## Milton, Massachusetts

***http://www.curry.edu/***
Founded in 1879

### DEGREES • BS • MSN
**Nursing Program Faculty** 48 (33% with doctorates).
**Baccalaureate Enrollment** 611 **Women** 92% **Men** 8% **Minority** 15% **Part-time** 48%
**Graduate Enrollment** 31 **Women** 97% **Men** 3% **Minority** 20% **Part-time** 100%
**Nursing Student Activities** Sigma Theta Tau, Student Nurses' Association.
**Nursing Student Resources** Academic advising; academic or career counseling; assistance for students with disabilities; bookstore; campus computer network; career placement assistance; computer lab; computer-assisted instruction; daycare for children of students; e-mail services; employment services for current students; housing assistance; interactive nursing skills videos; Internet; learning resource lab; library services; nursing audiovisuals; placement services for program completers; remedial services; resume preparation assistance; skills, simulation, or other laboratory; tutoring.
**Library Facilities** 154,100 volumes (5,867 in health, 4,589 in nursing); 47,600 periodical subscriptions (162 health-care related).

### BACCALAUREATE PROGRAMS
**Degree** BS
**Available Programs** Accelerated Baccalaureate for Second Degree; Generic Baccalaureate; RN Baccalaureate; RPN to Baccalaureate.
**Site Options** Boston, MA; Plymouth, MA.
**Study Options** Full-time.
**Program Entrance Requirements** Written essay, health exam, health insurance, high school biology, high school chemistry, high school foreign language, 4 years high school math, 4 years high school science, high school transcript, immunizations, 1 letter of recommendation, minimum high school GPA of 2.75, minimum GPA in nursing prerequisites of 3.0. Transfer students are accepted. *Application deadline:* 4/1 (fall). Applications may be processed on a rolling basis for some programs. *Application fee:* $50.
**Advanced Placement** Credit by examination available. Credit given for nursing courses completed elsewhere dependent upon specific evaluations.
**Contact** *Telephone:* 800-669-0686. *Fax:* 617-333-2114.

### GRADUATE PROGRAMS
**Contact** *Telephone:* 617-333-2243. *Fax:* 617-333-6680.

### MASTER'S DEGREE PROGRAM
**Degree** MSN
**Available Programs** Master's; RN to Master's.
**Concentrations Available** Clinical nurse leader.
**Site Options** Boston, MA.
**Program Entrance Requirements** Minimum overall college GPA of 3.0, transcript of college record, written essay, immunizations, 2 letters of recommendation, nursing research course, physical assessment course, resume, statistics course. *Application deadline:* Applications may be processed on a rolling basis for some programs. *Application fee:* $50.
**Degree Requirements** 37 total credit hours, thesis or project.

# Elms College
## Division of Nursing
## Chicopee, Massachusetts

***http://www.elms.edu/***
Founded in 1928

### DEGREES • BS • MSN
**Nursing Program Faculty** 13 (46% with doctorates).
**Baccalaureate Enrollment** 200 **Women** 87% **Men** 13% **Minority** 11% **Part-time** 35%
**Graduate Enrollment** 42 **Women** 97% **Men** 3% **Minority** 5% **Part-time** 50%
**Nursing Student Activities** Nursing Honor Society, Sigma Theta Tau, Student Nurses' Association.
**Nursing Student Resources** Academic advising; academic or career counseling; assistance for students with disabilities; bookstore; campus computer network; career placement assistance; computer lab; computer-assisted instruction; e-mail services; employment services for current students; externships; interactive nursing skills videos; Internet; learning resource lab; library services; nursing audiovisuals; resume preparation assistance; skills, simulation, or other laboratory; tutoring.
**Library Facilities** 3,832 volumes in health, 3,000 volumes in nursing; 130 periodical subscriptions health-care related.

### BACCALAUREATE PROGRAMS
**Degree** BS
**Available Programs** Generic Baccalaureate; RN Baccalaureate.
**Study Options** Full-time and part-time.
**Program Entrance Requirements** Minimum overall college GPA of 2.5, transcript of college record, CPR certification, written essay, health exam, health insurance, high school biology, high school chemistry, high school transcript, immunizations, interview, 2 letters of recommendation, minimum high school GPA of 3.3, minimum high school rank 25%, minimum GPA in nursing prerequisites of 2.5, professional liability insurance/malpractice insurance. Transfer students are accepted. *Application deadline:* Applications may be processed on a rolling basis for some programs. *Application fee:* $30.
**Advanced Placement** Credit given for nursing courses completed elsewhere dependent upon specific evaluations.
**Contact** *Telephone:* 413-265-2237. *Fax:* 413-265-2335.

### GRADUATE PROGRAMS
**Contact** *Telephone:* 413-265-2455.

### MASTER'S DEGREE PROGRAM
**Degree** MSN
**Available Programs** Master's; RN to Master's.
**Concentrations Available** Nursing administration; nursing education.
**Study Options** Full-time and part-time.
**Program Entrance Requirements** Minimum overall college GPA of 3.0, transcript of college record, CPR certification, written essay, immunizations, interview, 2 letters of recommendation, professional liability insurance/malpractice insurance, resume. *Application deadline:* Applica-

tions may be processed on a rolling basis for some programs. *Application fee:* $30.
**Degree Requirements** 36 total credit hours, thesis or project.

# Emmanuel College
## Department of Nursing
## Boston, Massachusetts

***http://www.emmanuel.edu/graduate-studies-nursing/academics/nursing-bsn-msn.html***
Founded in 1919

### DEGREES • BS • MS

**Nursing Program Faculty** 19 (27% with doctorates).
**Baccalaureate Enrollment** 146 **Women** 93% **Men** 7% **Minority** 20% **Part-time** 97%
**Graduate Enrollment** 47 **Women** 92% **Men** 8% **Minority** 27% **Part-time** 88%
**Distance Learning Courses** Available.
**Nursing Student Activities** Sigma Theta Tau.
**Nursing Student Resources** Academic advising; academic or career counseling; assistance for students with disabilities; bookstore; campus computer network; computer lab; computer-assisted instruction; e-mail services; interactive nursing skills videos; Internet; library services; nursing audiovisuals; resume preparation assistance; skills, simulation, or other laboratory; tutoring.
**Library Facilities** 150,000 volumes (3,680 in health, 3,130 in nursing); 2,100 periodical subscriptions (7,625 health-care related).

### BACCALAUREATE PROGRAMS

**Degree** BS
**Available Programs** RN Baccalaureate.
**Site Options** Boston, MA.
**Study Options** Full-time and part-time.
**Program Entrance Requirements** Transcript of college record, written essay, interview, 2 letters of recommendation, RN licensure. Transfer students are accepted. *Application deadline:* Applications may be processed on a rolling basis for some programs.
**Advanced Placement** Credit by examination available. Credit given for nursing courses completed elsewhere dependent upon specific evaluations.
**Expenses (2013–14)** *Tuition:* part-time $1816 per course. *International tuition:* $10,896 full-time.
**Financial Aid** 43% of baccalaureate students in nursing programs received some form of financial aid in 2012–13. *Gift aid (need-based):* Federal Pell, FSEOG, state, private, college/university gift aid from institutional funds. *Loans:* Federal Direct (Subsidized and Unsubsidized Stafford PLUS), Perkins, state. *Work-study:* Federal Work-Study, part-time campus jobs. *Financial aid application deadline (priority):* 2/15.
**Contact** Dr. Mary Diane Arathuzik, RN, Chair and Associate Professor, Department of Nursing, Emmanuel College, Department of Nursing, 400 The Fenway, Boston, MA 02115. *Telephone:* 617-735-9845. *Fax:* 617-507-0434. *E-mail:* arathuzi@emmanuel.edu.

### GRADUATE PROGRAMS

**Financial Aid** 32% of graduate students in nursing programs received some form of financial aid in 2012–13.
**Contact** Dr. Mary Diane Arathuzik, RN, Chair and Associate Professor of Nursing, Department of Nursing, Emmanuel College, Department of Nursing, 400 The Fenway, Boston, MA 02115. *Telephone:* 617-735-9845. *Fax:* 617-507-0434. *E-mail:* arathuzi@emmanuel.edu.

### MASTER'S DEGREE PROGRAM

**Degree** MS
**Available Programs** Master's.
**Concentrations Available** Nursing administration; nursing education.
**Site Options** Boston, MA.
**Study Options** Full-time and part-time.
**Program Entrance Requirements** Clinical experience, minimum overall college GPA of 3.0, transcript of college record, written essay, 2 letters of recommendation, resume. *Application deadline:* 4/30 (fall).
**Advanced Placement** Credit given for nursing courses completed elsewhere dependent upon specific evaluations.
**Degree Requirements** 36 total credit hours, comprehensive exam.

***See display below and full description on page 474.***

# Endicott College

## Major in Nursing
## Beverly, Massachusetts

*http://www.endicott.edu/*
Founded in 1939

**DEGREES • BS • MSN**

**Nursing Program Faculty** 27 (25% with doctorates).

**Baccalaureate Enrollment** 170 **Women** 95% **Men** 5% **Minority** 2% **Part-time** 20%

**Graduate Enrollment** 25 **Women** 97% **Men** 3% **Minority** 1%

**Distance Learning Courses** Available.

**Nursing Student Activities** Nursing Honor Society, Sigma Theta Tau, Student Nurses' Association.

**Nursing Student Resources** Academic advising; academic or career counseling; assistance for students with disabilities; bookstore; campus computer network; career placement assistance; computer lab; computer-assisted instruction; e-mail services; externships; interactive nursing skills videos; Internet; learning resource lab; library services; nursing audiovisuals; resume preparation assistance; skills, simulation, or other laboratory; tutoring; unpaid internships.

**Library Facilities** 120,000 volumes (2,828 in health, 624 in nursing); 82,037 periodical subscriptions (55 health-care related).

### BACCALAUREATE PROGRAMS

**Degree** BS

**Available Programs** Generic Baccalaureate; RN Baccalaureate.

**Site Options** Beverly, MA.

**Study Options** Full-time.

**Program Entrance Requirements** Minimum overall college GPA of 2.5, transcript of college record, written essay, health exam, health insurance, high school biology, high school chemistry, 3 years high school math, 2 years high school science, high school transcript, immunizations, 1 letter of recommendation, minimum high school GPA of 2.5, minimum high school rank 50%, minimum GPA in nursing prerequisites of 2.5. Transfer students are accepted.

**Advanced Placement** Credit given for nursing courses completed elsewhere dependent upon specific evaluations.

**Financial Aid** 88% of baccalaureate students in nursing programs received some form of financial aid in 2011–12.

**Contact** Mr. Thomas J. Redman, Vice President for Admissions and Financial Aid, Major in Nursing, Endicott College, 376 Hale Street, Beverly, MA 01915. *Telephone:* 978-232-2005. *Fax:* 978-232-2500. *E-mail:* admissio@endicott.edu.

### GRADUATE PROGRAMS

**Contact** Dr. Kelly L. Fisher, Dean, School of Nursing, Major in Nursing, Endicott College, 375 Hale Street, Beverly, MA 01915. *E-mail:* kfisher@endicott.edu.

#### MASTER'S DEGREE PROGRAM

**Degree** MSN

**Available Programs** Master's.

**Concentrations Available** Nursing administration; nursing education.

**Site Options** Beverly, MA.

**Study Options** Full-time and part-time.

**Program Entrance Requirements** Clinical experience, transcript of college record, written essay, letters of recommendation, statistics course.

**Advanced Placement** Credit given for nursing courses completed elsewhere dependent upon specific evaluations.

**Degree Requirements** 33 total credit hours, thesis or project.

### CONTINUING EDUCATION PROGRAM

**Contact** Dr. Kelly Fisher, Dean, School of Nursing, Major in Nursing, Endicott College, 376 Hale Street, Beverly, MA 01915. *Telephone:* 978-232-2328. *Fax:* 978-232-3100. *E-mail:* kfisher@endicott.edu.

# Fitchburg State University

## Department of Nursing
## Fitchburg, Massachusetts

*http://www.fitchburgstate.edu/academics/academic-departments/department-homepage-nursing/*
Founded in 1894

**DEGREES • BS • MS**

**Nursing Program Faculty** 16 (31% with doctorates).

**Baccalaureate Enrollment** 435 **Women** 93% **Men** 7% **Minority** 8% **Part-time** 29%

**Graduate Enrollment** 21 **Women** 100% **International** .05% **Part-time** 100%

**Distance Learning Courses** Available.

**Nursing Student Activities** Sigma Theta Tau, Student Nurses' Association.

**Nursing Student Resources** Academic advising; academic or career counseling; assistance for students with disabilities; bookstore; campus computer network; career placement assistance; computer lab; computer-assisted instruction; e-mail services; employment services for current students; housing assistance; interactive nursing skills videos; Internet; learning resource lab; library services; nursing audiovisuals; remedial services; resume preparation assistance; skills, simulation, or other laboratory; tutoring; unpaid internships.

**Library Facilities** 222,517 volumes (10,753 in health, 9,949 in nursing); 3,050 periodical subscriptions (5,444 health-care related).

### BACCALAUREATE PROGRAMS

**Degree** BS

**Available Programs** Accelerated LPN to Baccalaureate; Generic Baccalaureate; RN Baccalaureate.

**Study Options** Full-time.

**Online Degree Options** Yes.

**Program Entrance Requirements** Transcript of college record, written essay, health insurance, high school biology, high school chemistry, high school foreign language, 3 years high school math, 3 years high school science, high school transcript, immunizations, minimum high school GPA of 3.0, minimum GPA in nursing prerequisites of 2.5. Transfer students are accepted. *Application deadline:* 1/1 (fall). Applications may be processed on a rolling basis for some programs. *Application fee:* $25.

**Expenses (2013–14)** *Tuition, state resident:* full-time $970; part-time $40 per credit. *Tuition, nonresident:* full-time $7050; part-time $294 per credit. *Room and board:* $8830; room only: $5780 per academic year. *Required fees:* part-time $334 per credit; part-time $4008 per term.

**Financial Aid** 76% of baccalaureate students in nursing programs received some form of financial aid in 2012–13.

**Contact** Mr. Michael L. Gantt, Interim Director of Admissions, Department of Nursing, Fitchburg State University, 160 Pearl Street, Fitchburg, MA 01420-2697. *Telephone:* 978-665-3144. *Fax:* 978-665-4540. *E-mail:* admissions@fitchburgstate.edu.

### GRADUATE PROGRAMS

**Expenses (2013–14)** *Tuition, state resident:* part-time $218 per credit. *Tuition, nonresident:* part-time $218 per credit. *Required fees:* part-time $161 per credit.

**Financial Aid** 11% of graduate students in nursing programs received some form of financial aid in 2012–13.

**Contact** Dr. Robert Dumas, Chairperson, Forensic Nursing Program, Department of Nursing, Fitchburg State University, 160 Pearl Street, Fitchburg, MA 01420-2697. *Telephone:* 978-665-3026. *Fax:* 978-665-4501. *E-mail:* rdumas@fitchburgstate.edu.

#### MASTER'S DEGREE PROGRAM

**Degree** MS

**Available Programs** Master's.

**Concentrations Available** *Clinical nurse specialist programs in:* forensic nursing.

**Study Options** Part-time.

**Online Degree Options** Yes (online only).

**Program Entrance Requirements** Clinical experience, computer literacy, minimum overall college GPA of 2.8, transcript of college record, written essay, immunizations, 3 letters of recommendation, nursing research course, physical assessment course, prerequisite course work, resume, statistics course. *Application deadline:* Applications may be processed on a rolling basis for some programs. *Application fee:* $25.

**Degree Requirements** 36 total credit hours, thesis or project.

**POST-MASTER'S PROGRAM**
**Areas of Study** *Clinical nurse specialist programs in:* forensic nursing.

# Framingham State University

## Department of Nursing
## Framingham, Massachusetts

***http://www.framingham.edu/nursing***
Founded in 1839

**DEGREES • BS • MSN**
**Nursing Program Faculty** 8 (75% with doctorates).
**Baccalaureate Enrollment** 74 **Women** 85% **Men** 15% **Minority** 33% **International** 2% **Part-time** 90%
**Graduate Enrollment** 58 **Women** 98% **Men** 2% **Minority** 3% **International** 1% **Part-time** 100%
**Nursing Student Activities** Sigma Theta Tau.
**Nursing Student Resources** Academic advising; academic or career counseling; assistance for students with disabilities; bookstore; campus computer network; career placement assistance; computer lab; computer-assisted instruction; daycare for children of students; e-mail services; employment services for current students; housing assistance; interactive nursing skills videos; Internet; learning resource lab; library services; nursing audiovisuals; placement services for program completers; remedial services; resume preparation assistance; skills, simulation, or other laboratory; tutoring.
**Library Facilities** 216,902 volumes (5,338 in health, 5,338 in nursing); 163 periodical subscriptions (1,200 health-care related).

### BACCALAUREATE PROGRAMS

**Degree** BS
**Available Programs** ADN to Baccalaureate.
**Study Options** Full-time and part-time.
**Program Entrance Requirements** Minimum overall college GPA of 3.0, transcript of college record, written essay, RN licensure. Transfer students are accepted. *Application deadline:* Applications may be processed on a rolling basis for some programs. *Application fee:* $50.
**Advanced Placement** Credit by examination available. Credit given for nursing courses completed elsewhere dependent upon specific evaluations.
**Contact** *Telephone:* 508-626-4713. *Fax:* 508-626-4746.

### GRADUATE PROGRAMS

**Contact** *Telephone:* 508-626-4713. *Fax:* 508-626-4746.

**MASTER'S DEGREE PROGRAM**
**Degree** MSN
**Available Programs** Master's.
**Concentrations Available** Nursing administration; nursing education.
**Study Options** Part-time.
**Program Entrance Requirements** Minimum overall college GPA of 3.0, transcript of college record, written essay, interview, 3 letters of recommendation, nursing research course, resume, statistics course. *Application deadline:* 6/1 (fall). Applications may be processed on a rolling basis for some programs. *Application fee:* $50.
**Degree Requirements** 36 total credit hours, thesis or project.

### CONTINUING EDUCATION PROGRAM

**Contact** *Telephone:* 508-626-4713. *Fax:* 508-626-4746.

# Labouré College

## Bachelor of Science in Nursing Program
## Boston, Massachusetts

Founded in 1971

**DEGREE • BSN**
**Library Facilities** 10,975 volumes; 155 periodical subscriptions.

### BACCALAUREATE PROGRAMS

**Degree** BSN
**Available Programs** Generic Baccalaureate.
**Contact** Admissions Office, Bachelor of Science in Nursing Program, Labouré College, 303 Adams Street, Milton, MA 02186. *Telephone:* 617-202-3149.

# MCPHS University

## School of Nursing
## Boston, Massachusetts

***http://www.mcphs.edu/***
Founded in 1823

**DEGREE • BSN**
**Nursing Program Faculty** 16 (44% with doctorates).
**Baccalaureate Enrollment** 358 **Women** 66.3% **Men** 33.7% **Minority** 35% **International** 3%
**Distance Learning Courses** Available.
**Nursing Student Activities** Nursing Honor Society, Sigma Theta Tau, Student Nurses' Association, nursing club.
**Nursing Student Resources** Academic advising; academic or career counseling; assistance for students with disabilities; bookstore; campus computer network; career placement assistance; computer lab; computer-assisted instruction; e-mail services; employment services for current students; housing assistance; interactive nursing skills videos; Internet; learning resource lab; library services; nursing audiovisuals; remedial services; resume preparation assistance; skills, simulation, or other laboratory; tutoring.
**Library Facilities** 17,400 volumes in health, 1,200 volumes in nursing; 10,000 periodical subscriptions health-care related.

### BACCALAUREATE PROGRAMS

**Degree** BSN
**Available Programs** Accelerated Baccalaureate; Accelerated Baccalaureate for Second Degree.
**Site Options** Manchester , NH; Worcester , MA.
**Study Options** Full-time.
**Program Entrance Requirements** Minimum overall college GPA of 2.5, written essay, high school biology, high school chemistry, 3 years high school math, 2 years high school science, high school transcript, 2 letters of recommendation, prerequisite course work. Transfer students are accepted. *Application deadline:* 2/1 (fall), 10/1 (spring). *Application fee:* $70.
**Contact** *Telephone:* 800-225-5506.

### CONTINUING EDUCATION PROGRAM

**Contact** *Telephone:* 617-735-1080.

# MGH Institute of Health Professions

## School of Nursing
## Boston, Massachusetts

***http://www.mghihp.edu/academics/nursing/***
Founded in 1977

**DEGREES • BSN • DNP • MS**
**Nursing Program Faculty** 62 (55% with doctorates).
**Baccalaureate Enrollment** 160 **Women** 86% **Men** 14% **Minority** 19% **International** 1%
**Graduate Enrollment** 401 **Women** 88% **Men** 12% **Minority** 18% **International** 1% **Part-time** 18%
**Distance Learning Courses** Available.
**Nursing Student Activities** Nursing Honor Society, Sigma Theta Tau, Student Nurses' Association, nursing club.
**Nursing Student Resources** Academic advising; academic or career counseling; assistance for students with disabilities; bookstore; campus computer network; career placement assistance; computer lab; computer-assisted instruction; daycare for children of students; e-mail services; employment services for current students; interactive nursing skills videos; Internet; learning resource lab; library services; nursing audiovisuals; remedial services; resume preparation assistance; skills, simulation, or other laboratory; tutoring.
**Library Facilities** 11,858 volumes in health, 11,081 volumes in nursing; 1,389 periodical subscriptions health-care related.

## BACCALAUREATE PROGRAMS

**Degree** BSN
**Available Programs** Accelerated Baccalaureate.
**Site Options** Boston, MA.
**Study Options** Full-time.
**Program Entrance Requirements** Transcript of college record, written essay, health insurance, immunizations, 3 letters of recommendation, minimum GPA in nursing prerequisites of 3.0, prerequisite course work. Transfer students are accepted. *Application deadline:* 7/1 (spring), 11/1 (summer). *Application fee:* $100.
**Advanced Placement** Credit by examination available. Credit given for nursing courses completed elsewhere dependent upon specific evaluations.
**Expenses (2013–14)** *Tuition:* full-time $59,000. *International tuition:* $59,000 full-time. *Required fees:* full-time $2095.
**Financial Aid** 81% of baccalaureate students in nursing programs received some form of financial aid in 2012–13.
**Contact** Admissions, School of Nursing, MGH Institute of Health Professions, 36 1st Avenue, Boston, MA 02129. *Telephone:* 617-726-3140. *Fax:* 617-726-8010. *E-mail:* admissions@mghihp.edu.

## GRADUATE PROGRAMS

**Expenses (2013–14)** *Tuition:* full-time $17,267. *International tuition:* $17,267 full-time. *Required fees:* full-time $1800.
**Financial Aid** 81% of graduate students in nursing programs received some form of financial aid in 2012–13. 4 research assistantships (averaging $1,200 per year), 17 teaching assistantships (averaging $1,200 per year) were awarded; career-related internships or fieldwork, scholarships, traineeships, and unspecified assistantships also available. Aid available to part-time students. *Financial aid application deadline:* 4/1.
**Contact** Office of Admissions, School of Nursing, MGH Institute of Health Professions, PO Box 6357, Boston, MA 02114. *Telephone:* 617-726-3140. *Fax:* 617-726-8010. *E-mail:* admissions@mghihp.edu.

### MASTER'S DEGREE PROGRAM

**Degree** MS
**Available Programs** Master's; Master's for Non-Nursing College Graduates; Master's for Nurses with Non-Nursing Degrees; RN to Master's.
**Concentrations Available** Clinical nurse leader; health-care administration; nursing administration; nursing education. *Nurse practitioner programs in:* acute care, adult health, family health, gerontology, pediatric, primary care, psychiatric/mental health,women's health.
**Site Options** Boston, MA.
**Study Options** Full-time and part-time.
**Program Entrance Requirements** Minimum overall college GPA of 3.0, transcript of college record, CPR certification, written essay, immunizations, 3 letters of recommendation, professional liability insurance/malpractice insurance, prerequisite course work, resume, statistics course, GRE General Test. *Application deadline:* 1/10 (fall). *Application fee:* $100.
**Advanced Placement** Credit by examination available. Credit given for nursing courses completed elsewhere dependent upon specific evaluations.
**Degree Requirements** 93 total credit hours, thesis or project.

### POST-MASTER'S PROGRAM

**Areas of Study** Clinical nurse leader; health-care administration. *Nurse practitioner programs in:* acute care, adult health, gerontology, pediatric, primary care, psychiatric/mental health,women's health.

### DOCTORAL DEGREE PROGRAM

**Degree** DNP
**Available Programs** Doctorate; Doctorate for Nurses with Non-Nursing Degrees.
**Areas of Study** Nursing administration.
**Site Options** Boston, MA.
**Program Entrance Requirements** Minimum overall college GPA of 3.0, interview by faculty committee, 3 letters of recommendation, MSN or equivalent, vita. *Application deadline:* 6/1 (fall). Applications may be processed on a rolling basis for some programs. *Application fee:* $100.
**Degree Requirements** 43 total credit hours, residency.

# Northeastern University
## School of Nursing
## Boston, Massachusetts

***http://www.northeastern.edu/bouve/nursing/index.html***
Founded in 1898

**DEGREES • BSN • DNP • MS**
**Distance Learning Courses** Available.
**Library Facilities** 1.5 million volumes; 128,027 periodical subscriptions.

## BACCALAUREATE PROGRAMS

**Degree** BSN
**Available Programs** Generic Baccalaureate.
**Program Entrance Requirements** *Application deadline:* 1/15 (fall).
**Contact** Undergraduate Admissions, School of Nursing, Northeastern University, 360 Huntington Avenue, 200 Kerr Hall, Boston, MA 02115. *Telephone:* 617-373-2200. *Fax:* 617-373-8780. *E-mail:* admissions@neu.edu.

## GRADUATE PROGRAMS

**Financial Aid** Fellowships, research assistantships, teaching assistantships, career-related internships or fieldwork, institutionally sponsored loans, scholarships, traineeships, tuition waivers (full and partial), and unspecified assistantships available.
**Contact** Bouve Grad, School of Nursing, Northeastern University, 360 Huntington Avenue, 123 Behrakis Health Sciences Building, Boston, MA 02115. *Telephone:* 617-373-3501. *E-mail:* bouvegrad@neu.edu.

### MASTER'S DEGREE PROGRAM

**Degree** MS
**Available Programs** Master's.
**Program Entrance Requirements** GRE General Test.

### DOCTORAL DEGREE PROGRAM

**Degree** DNP
**Available Programs** Post-Baccalaureate Doctorate.

## CONTINUING EDUCATION PROGRAM

**Contact** Bouve College of Health Sciences, School of Nursing, Northeastern University, 360 Huntington Avenue, 123 Behrakis Health Sciences Building, Boston, MA 02115. *Telephone:* 617-373-2708. *E-mail:* bouvegrad@neu.edu.

# Regis College
## School of Nursing, Science and Health Professions
## Weston, Massachusetts

***http://www.regiscollege.edu/grad***
Founded in 1927

**DEGREES • BSN • DNP • MSN**
**Nursing Program Faculty** 36 (75% with doctorates).
**Baccalaureate Enrollment** 78
**Graduate Enrollment** 600 **Women** 90% **Men** 10%
**Nursing Student Activities** Sigma Theta Tau, Student Nurses' Association, nursing club.
**Nursing Student Resources** Academic advising; academic or career counseling; assistance for students with disabilities; bookstore; campus computer network; computer lab; e-mail services; Internet; learning resource lab; library services; nursing audiovisuals; resume preparation assistance; skills, simulation, or other laboratory; tutoring.
**Library Facilities** 134,706 volumes (6,300 in health, 4,700 in nursing); 397 periodical subscriptions (228 health-care related).

## BACCALAUREATE PROGRAMS

**Degree** BSN
**Available Programs** ADN to Baccalaureate; Accelerated Baccalaureate; Accelerated Baccalaureate for Second Degree; Accelerated RN Baccalaureate; Baccalaureate for Second Degree; Generic Baccalaureate; RN Baccalaureate.
**Site Options** Medford, MA; Brighton, MA; Boston, MA.
**Study Options** Full-time.

**Program Entrance Requirements** Written essay, health exam, health insurance, high school foreign language, 3 years high school math, 2 years high school science, high school transcript, immunizations, 2 letters of recommendation, minimum high school GPA of 3.0, minimum high school rank 40%, minimum GPA in nursing prerequisites. Transfer students are accepted. *Application deadline:* Applications may be processed on a rolling basis for some programs. *Application fee:* $50.
**Advanced Placement** Credit by examination available. Credit given for nursing courses completed elsewhere dependent upon specific evaluations.
**Expenses (2012–13)** *Tuition:* full-time $33,000; part-time $660 per credit. *Room and board:* $11,000 per academic year.
**Financial Aid** 85% of baccalaureate students in nursing programs received some form of financial aid in 2011–12.
**Contact** Dr. Antionette Hays, Dean, School of Nursing and Health Professions, School of Nursing, Science and Health Professions, Regis College, 235 Wellesley Street, Weston, MA 02493. *Telephone:* 781-768-7090. *Fax:* 781-768-7071. *E-mail:* antoinette.hays@regiscollege.edu.

## GRADUATE PROGRAMS

**Expenses (2012–13)** *Tuition:* full-time $33,000; part-time $915 per credit. *International tuition:* $33,000 full-time. *Room and board:* $11,000 per academic year.
**Financial Aid** 52% of graduate students in nursing programs received some form of financial aid in 2011–12. Research assistantships, Federal Work-Study, scholarships, traineeships, and unspecified assistantships available. Aid available to part-time students.
**Contact** Ms. Claudia C. Pouravelis, Director of Graduate Admission, School of Nursing, Science and Health Professions, Regis College, 235 Wellesley Street, Weston, MA 02493. *Telephone:* 781-768-7058. *Fax:* 781-768-7071. *E-mail:* claudia.pouravelis@regiscollege.edu.

### MASTER'S DEGREE PROGRAM

**Degree** MSN
**Available Programs** Accelerated AD/RN to Master's; Accelerated Master's; Accelerated Master's for Non-Nursing College Graduates; Accelerated Master's for Nurses with Non-Nursing Degrees; Accelerated RN to Master's; Master's; Master's for Non-Nursing College Graduates; Master's for Nurses with Non-Nursing Degrees; RN to Master's.
**Concentrations Available** Clinical nurse leader; health-care administration; nurse case management; nursing administration; nursing education; nursing informatics. *Clinical nurse specialist programs in:* acute care. *Nurse practitioner programs in:* adult health, family health, pediatric, primary care, psychiatric/mental health,women's health.
**Site Options** Medford, MA; Brighton, MA; Boston, MA.
**Study Options** Full-time and part-time.
**Program Entrance Requirements** Computer literacy, minimum overall college GPA of 3.0, transcript of college record, CPR certification, written essay, immunizations, interview, 3 letters of recommendation, physical assessment course, professional liability insurance/malpractice insurance, prerequisite course work, resume, statistics course, GRE General Test or MAT. *Application deadline:* Applications may be processed on a rolling basis for some programs. *Application fee:* $50.
**Advanced Placement** Credit by examination available. Credit given for nursing courses completed elsewhere dependent upon specific evaluations.
**Degree Requirements** 44 total credit hours, thesis or project.

### POST-MASTER'S PROGRAM

**Areas of Study** Clinical nurse leader; health-care administration; nurse case management; nursing administration; nursing education. *Nurse practitioner programs in:* adult health, family health, pediatric, primary care, psychiatric/mental health,women's health.

### DOCTORAL DEGREE PROGRAM

**Degree** DNP
**Available Programs** Doctorate; Post-Baccalaureate Doctorate.
**Areas of Study** Gerontology, health policy, nursing administration, nursing education, nursing policy.
**Program Entrance Requirements** Clinical experience, minimum overall college GPA of 3.5, interview by faculty committee, interview, 2 letters of recommendation, MSN or equivalent, statistics course, vita, writing sample, MAT or GRE if GPA from master's lower than 3.5. *Application deadline:* Applications may be processed on a rolling basis for some programs. *Application fee:* $75.
**Degree Requirements** 50 total credit hours.

## CONTINUING EDUCATION PROGRAM

**Contact** Dr. Claudia Pouravelis, Associate Dean of Graduate Affairs, School of Nursing, Science and Health Professions, Regis College, 235 Wellesley Street, Weston, MA 02493. *Telephone:* 781-768-7058. *Fax:* 781-768-7089. *E-mail:* claudia.pouravelis@regiscollege.edu.

# Salem State University

**Program in Nursing**
**Salem, Massachusetts**

*http://www.salemstate.edu/*
Founded in 1854

**DEGREES • BSN • MSN • MSN/MBA**
**Nursing Program Faculty** 100 (25% with doctorates).
**Distance Learning Courses** Available.
**Nursing Student Activities** Nursing Honor Society, Sigma Theta Tau, Student Nurses' Association.
**Nursing Student Resources** Academic advising; academic or career counseling; assistance for students with disabilities; bookstore; campus computer network; career placement assistance; computer lab; computer-assisted instruction; daycare for children of students; e-mail services; employment services for current students; externships; housing assistance; interactive nursing skills videos; Internet; learning resource lab; library services; nursing audiovisuals; paid internships; remedial services; resume preparation assistance; skills, simulation, or other laboratory; tutoring.
**Library Facilities** 264,085 volumes (2,000 in health, 1,600 in nursing); 76,948 periodical subscriptions (50 health-care related).

## BACCALAUREATE PROGRAMS

**Degree** BSN
**Available Programs** ADN to Baccalaureate; Accelerated Baccalaureate for Second Degree; Generic Baccalaureate; International Nurse to Baccalaureate; LPN to Baccalaureate; LPN to RN Baccalaureate.
**Site Options** Haverhill, MA.
**Study Options** Full-time.
**Program Entrance Requirements** Minimum overall college GPA of 3.5, transcript of college record, CPR certification, health exam, health insurance, high school biology, high school chemistry, 3 years high school math, 2 years high school science, high school transcript, immunizations, interview, minimum high school GPA of 3.5, professional liability insurance/malpractice insurance. Transfer students are accepted. *Application deadline:* 2/1 (fall), 10/1 (spring), 4/1 (summer). Applications may be processed on a rolling basis for some programs. *Application fee:* $40.
**Advanced Placement** Credit by examination available. Credit given for nursing courses completed elsewhere dependent upon specific evaluations.
**Contact** *Telephone:* 978-542-6200.

## GRADUATE PROGRAMS

**Contact** *Telephone:* 978-542-7018. *Fax:* 978-542-2016.

### MASTER'S DEGREE PROGRAM

**Degrees** MSN; MSN/MBA
**Available Programs** Accelerated Master's for Non-Nursing College Graduates; Master's; Master's for Nurses with Non-Nursing Degrees.
**Concentrations Available** Clinical nurse leader; nursing administration; nursing education. *Clinical nurse specialist programs in:* community health, public health, rehabilitation. *Nurse practitioner programs in:* women's health.
**Study Options** Full-time and part-time.
**Program Entrance Requirements** Clinical experience, computer literacy, minimum overall college GPA of 3.0, transcript of college record, CPR certification, written essay, immunizations, interview, 3 letters of recommendation, professional liability insurance/malpractice insurance, resume, statistics course, GRE or MAT. *Application deadline:* 3/1 (fall), 10/1 (winter), 10/1 (spring), 3/1 (summer). Applications may be processed on a rolling basis for some programs. *Application fee:* $50.
**Advanced Placement** Credit given for nursing courses completed elsewhere dependent upon specific evaluations.
**Degree Requirements** 39 total credit hours, thesis or project.

## CONTINUING EDUCATION PROGRAM

**Contact** *Telephone:* 978-542-6805. *Fax:* 978-542-2016.

# Simmons College
## School of Nursing and Health Sciences
## Boston, Massachusetts

*http://www.simmons.edu/snhs/*
Founded in 1899

**DEGREES • BS • DNP • MS**
**Nursing Program Faculty** 138 (19% with doctorates).
**Baccalaureate Enrollment** 509 **Women** 100% **Minority** 20% **International** 1% **Part-time** 17%
**Graduate Enrollment** 273 **Women** 96% **Men** 4% **Minority** 19% **Part-time** 76%
**Distance Learning Courses** Available.
**Nursing Student Activities** Nursing Honor Society, Sigma Theta Tau, Student Nurses' Association, nursing club.
**Nursing Student Resources** Academic advising; academic or career counseling; assistance for students with disabilities; bookstore; campus computer network; career placement assistance; computer lab; computer-assisted instruction; e-mail services; employment services for current students; housing assistance; interactive nursing skills videos; Internet; learning resource lab; library services; nursing audiovisuals; placement services for program completers; remedial services; resume preparation assistance; skills, simulation, or other laboratory; tutoring; unpaid internships.
**Library Facilities** 277,169 volumes (3,103 in health, 2,226 in nursing); 59,134 periodical subscriptions (562 health-care related).

### BACCALAUREATE PROGRAMS

**Degree** BS
**Available Programs** ADN to Baccalaureate; Accelerated Baccalaureate; Accelerated Baccalaureate for Second Degree; Baccalaureate for Second Degree; Generic Baccalaureate; LPN to Baccalaureate; RN Baccalaureate.
**Site Options** Weymouth (South Shore Hospital), MA.
**Study Options** Full-time and part-time.
**Program Entrance Requirements** Transcript of college record, written essay, health exam, health insurance, high school biology, high school chemistry, high school foreign language, 4 years high school math, 3 years high school science, high school transcript, immunizations, 2 letters of recommendation, minimum GPA in nursing prerequisites of 3.0, prerequisite course work. Transfer students are accepted. *Application deadline:* 2/1 (fall), 11/1 (spring). *Application fee:* $55.
**Advanced Placement** Credit given for nursing courses completed elsewhere dependent upon specific evaluations.
**Expenses (2013–14)** *Tuition:* full-time $37,690; part-time $1178 per credit. *Room and board:* $13,400 per academic year. *Required fees:* full-time $1030.
**Financial Aid** 88% of baccalaureate students in nursing programs received some form of financial aid in 2012–13. *Gift aid (need-based):* Federal Pell, FSEOG, state, private, college/university gift aid from institutional funds. *Loans:* Federal Direct (Subsidized and Unsubsidized Stafford PLUS), Perkins, college/university. *Work-study:* Federal Work-Study. *Financial aid application deadline (priority):* 2/15.
**Contact** Ellen Johnson, Director of Undergraduate Admission, School of Nursing and Health Sciences, Simmons College, 300 The Fenway, Boston, MA 02115. *Telephone:* 617-521-2515. *Fax:* 617-521-3190. *E-mail:* ugadm@simmons.edu.

### GRADUATE PROGRAMS

**Expenses (2013–14)** *Tuition:* part-time $1198 per credit. *Room and board:* $15,000 per academic year.
**Financial Aid** 78% of graduate students in nursing programs received some form of financial aid in 2012–13.
**Contact** Ms. Carmen Fortin, Assistant Dean, Director of Admission, School of Nursing and Health Sciences, Simmons College, 300 The Fenway, Boston, MA 02115. *Telephone:* 617-521-2605. *Fax:* 617-521-3137. *E-mail:* carmen.fortin@simmons.edu.

#### MASTER'S DEGREE PROGRAM

**Degree** MS
**Available Programs** Accelerated Master's; Accelerated Master's for Non-Nursing College Graduates; Master's; RN to Master's.
**Concentrations Available** Nursing administration. *Nurse practitioner programs in:* family health, primary care.
**Site Options** Weymouth (South Shore Hospital), MA; Boston (Longwood Medical Area), MA.
**Study Options** Part-time.
**Online Degree Options** Yes.
**Program Entrance Requirements** Clinical experience, computer literacy, minimum overall college GPA of 3.0, transcript of college record, written essay, 3 letters of recommendation, physical assessment course, prerequisite course work, resume, statistics course. *Application deadline:* 2/5 (fall), 1/10 (summer). *Application fee:* $50.
**Degree Requirements** 48 total credit hours.

#### DOCTORAL DEGREE PROGRAM

**Degree** DNP
**Available Programs** Doctorate.
**Areas of Study** Clinical nurse leader.
**Program Entrance Requirements** Clinical experience, minimum overall college GPA of 3.0, 3 letters of recommendation, MSN or equivalent, statistics course, vita, writing sample. *Application deadline:* 6/1 (fall), 10/1 (spring). *Application fee:* $50.
**Degree Requirements** 36 total credit hours.

# University of Massachusetts Amherst
## School of Nursing
## Amherst, Massachusetts

*http://www.umass.edu/nursing*
Founded in 1863

**DEGREES • BS • MS • PHD**
**Nursing Program Faculty** 65 (40% with doctorates).
**Baccalaureate Enrollment** 441 **Women** 90% **Men** 10% **Minority** 19% **International** 3% **Part-time** 1%
**Graduate Enrollment** 234 **Women** 91% **Men** 9% **Minority** 13% **International** 1% **Part-time** 79%
**Distance Learning Courses** Available.
**Nursing Student Activities** Sigma Theta Tau, Student Nurses' Association.
**Nursing Student Resources** Academic advising; academic or career counseling; bookstore; campus computer network; career placement assistance; computer lab; computer-assisted instruction; e-mail services; employment services for current students; housing assistance; interactive nursing skills videos; Internet; learning resource lab; library services; nursing audiovisuals; resume preparation assistance; skills, simulation, or other laboratory; tutoring; unpaid internships.
**Library Facilities** 363,696 volumes in health, 41,844 volumes in nursing; 4,088 periodical subscriptions health-care related.

### BACCALAUREATE PROGRAMS

**Degree** BS
**Available Programs** Accelerated Baccalaureate for Second Degree; Accelerated RN Baccalaureate; Generic Baccalaureate.
**Study Options** Full-time.
**Online Degree Options** Yes.
**Program Entrance Requirements** Minimum overall college GPA of 3.0, transcript of college record, CPR certification, written essay, health exam, health insurance, high school foreign language, 3 years high school math, 3 years high school science, high school transcript, immunizations, 1 letter of recommendation, minimum high school GPA of 3.5, minimum GPA in nursing prerequisites of 2.5, professional liability insurance/malpractice insurance, prerequisite course work. *Application deadline:* 1/15 (fall). *Application fee:* $70.
**Advanced Placement** Credit given for nursing courses completed elsewhere dependent upon specific evaluations.
**Financial Aid** 86% of baccalaureate students in nursing programs received some form of financial aid in 2011–12.
**Contact** Ms. Elizabeth Theroux, Academic Secretary, Undergraduate Nursing Education, School of Nursing, University of Massachusetts Amherst, 024 Skinner Hall, 651 North Pleasant Street, Amherst, MA 01003-9304. *Telephone:* 413-545-5096. *Fax:* 413-577-2550. *E-mail:* etheroux@acad.umass.edu.

### GRADUATE PROGRAMS

**Financial Aid** 38% of graduate students in nursing programs received some form of financial aid in 2011–12. Fellowships with full and partial tuition reimbursements available, research assistantships with full and partial tuition reimbursements available, teaching assistantships with full and partial tuition reimbursements available, career-related internships or fieldwork, Federal Work-Study, scholarships, traineeships, tuition

waivers (full and partial), and unspecified assistantships available. Aid available to part-time students. *Financial aid application deadline:* 2/1.
**Contact** Ms. Karen Ayotte, Academic Services Graduate Program Assistant, School of Nursing, University of Massachusetts Amherst, 125 Skinner Hall, 651 North Pleasant Street, Amherst, MA 01003-9299. *Telephone:* 413-545-1302. *Fax:* 413-577-2550. *E-mail:* kayotte@nursing.umass.edu.

### MASTER'S DEGREE PROGRAM

**Degree** MS
**Available Programs** Master's.
**Concentrations Available** Clinical nurse leader.
**Study Options** Full-time and part-time.
**Online Degree Options** Yes (online only).
**Program Entrance Requirements** Minimum overall college GPA of 3.0, transcript of college record, CPR certification, written essay, immunizations, 2 letters of recommendation, physical assessment course, professional liability insurance/malpractice insurance, prerequisite course work, statistics course. *Application deadline:* 12/15 (fall). Applications may be processed on a rolling basis for some programs. *Application fee:* $65.
**Advanced Placement** Credit given for nursing courses completed elsewhere dependent upon specific evaluations.
**Degree Requirements** 37 total credit hours.

### DOCTORAL DEGREE PROGRAM

**Degree** PhD
**Available Programs** Doctorate; Post-Baccalaureate Doctorate.
**Areas of Study** Faculty preparation, health promotion/disease prevention, health-care systems, individualized study, nursing education, nursing research, nursing science.
**Program Entrance Requirements** Minimum overall college GPA of 3.2, interview, 2 letters of recommendation, MSN or equivalent, scholarly papers, statistics course, vita, writing sample. *Application deadline:* 12/15 (fall). Applications may be processed on a rolling basis for some programs. *Application fee:* $65.
**Degree Requirements** 57 total credit hours, dissertation, oral exam, written exam, residency.

### CONTINUING EDUCATION PROGRAM

**Contact** Ms. Karen Ayotte, Academic Services Graduate Program Assistant, School of Nursing, University of Massachusetts Amherst, 104 Skinner Hall, 651 North Pleasant Street, Amherst, MA 01003-9299. *Telephone:* 413-545-1302. *Fax:* 413-577-2550. *E-mail:* kayotte@nursing.umass.edu.

# University of Massachusetts Boston

## College of Nursing and Health Sciences
## Boston, Massachusetts

***http://www.umb.edu***
Founded in 1964

### DEGREES • BS • DNP • MS • PHD

**Nursing Program Faculty** 152 (30% with doctorates).
**Baccalaureate Enrollment** 1,325 **Women** 86% **Men** 14% **Minority** 40% **International** .4% **Part-time** 50%
**Graduate Enrollment** 209 **Women** 92.4% **Men** 7.6% **Minority** 20% **International** 2% **Part-time** 70%
**Distance Learning Courses** Available.
**Nursing Student Activities** Nursing Honor Society, Sigma Theta Tau, Student Nurses' Association.
**Nursing Student Resources** Academic advising; academic or career counseling; assistance for students with disabilities; bookstore; campus computer network; career placement assistance; computer lab; computer-assisted instruction; daycare for children of students; e-mail services; employment services for current students; housing assistance; interactive nursing skills videos; Internet; learning resource lab; library services; nursing audiovisuals; other; paid internships; remedial services; resume preparation assistance; skills, simulation, or other laboratory; tutoring.
**Library Facilities** 600,000 volumes (3,700 in health, 603 in nursing); 75,000 periodical subscriptions (4,815 health-care related).

### BACCALAUREATE PROGRAMS

**Degree** BS
**Available Programs** Accelerated Baccalaureate for Second Degree; Generic Baccalaureate; RN Baccalaureate.
**Site Options** West Barnstable, MA.
**Study Options** Full-time.
**Online Degree Options** Yes.
**Program Entrance Requirements** Minimum overall college GPA of 3.0, transcript of college record, written essay, health insurance, 3 years high school math, high school transcript, immunizations, 2 letters of recommendation, minimum high school GPA of 3.0, minimum GPA in nursing prerequisites of 2.7, minimum GPA in nursing prerequisites of 2.7, TEAS test. Transfer students are accepted. *Application deadline:* 2/1 (fall), 11/1 (spring). *Application fee:* $60.
**Advanced Placement** Credit given for nursing courses completed elsewhere dependent upon specific evaluations.
**Expenses (2013–14)** *Tuition, state resident:* full-time $14,278; part-time $72 per credit. *Tuition, nonresident:* full-time $29,742; part-time $407 per credit. *International tuition:* $29,742 full-time. *Required fees:* full-time $800; part-time $400 per term.
**Financial Aid** 70% of baccalaureate students in nursing programs received some form of financial aid in 2012–13.
**Contact** Mr. Jon Hutton, Director of Enrollment Information Services, College of Nursing and Health Sciences, University of Massachusetts Boston, 100 Morrissey Boulevard, Boston, MA 02125. *Telephone:* 617-287-6000. *Fax:* 617-287-5999. *E-mail:* enrollment.information@umb.edu.

### GRADUATE PROGRAMS

**Expenses (2013–14)** *Tuition, state resident:* full-time $16,480; part-time $108 per credit. *Tuition, nonresident:* full-time $29,756; part-time $407 per credit. *International tuition:* $29,756 full-time. *Required fees:* full-time $1200; part-time $600 per term.
**Financial Aid** 35% of graduate students in nursing programs received some form of financial aid in 2012–13. 3 research assistantships with full tuition reimbursements available (averaging $13,000 per year), 13 teaching assistantships with full tuition reimbursements available (averaging $13,000 per year) were awarded; career-related internships or fieldwork, Federal Work-Study, and unspecified assistantships also available. Aid available to part-time students. *Financial aid application deadline:* 3/1.
**Contact** Mr. Jon Hutton, Director of Enrollment Information Services, College of Nursing and Health Sciences, University of Massachusetts Boston, 100 Morrissey Boulevard, Boston, MA 02125. *Telephone:* 617-287-6000. *Fax:* 617-287-6040. *E-mail:* enrollment.information@umb.edu.

### MASTER'S DEGREE PROGRAM

**Degree** MS
**Available Programs** Master's.
**Concentrations Available** *Clinical nurse specialist programs in:* acute care, adult health, critical care, gerontology. *Nurse practitioner programs in:* acute care, adult health, family health, gerontology.
**Study Options** Full-time and part-time.
**Program Entrance Requirements** Clinical experience, minimum overall college GPA of 3.0, transcript of college record, written essay, immunizations, 3 letters of recommendation, physical assessment course, statistics course. *Application deadline:* 3/15 (fall), 10/15 (spring). *Application fee:* $60.
**Advanced Placement** Credit given for nursing courses completed elsewhere dependent upon specific evaluations.
**Degree Requirements** 48 total credit hours, thesis or project.

### POST-MASTER'S PROGRAM

**Areas of Study** Nursing education. *Clinical nurse specialist programs in:* acute care, adult health, critical care, gerontology. *Nurse practitioner programs in:* acute care, adult health, family health, gerontology.

### DOCTORAL DEGREE PROGRAM

**Degree** DNP
**Available Programs** Doctorate.
**Areas of Study** Advanced practice nursing.
**Online Degree Options** Yes (online only).
**Program Entrance Requirements** Minimum overall college GPA of 3.2, clinical experience, 3 letters of recommendation, MSN or equivalent, statistics course, vita, writing sample. *Application deadline:* 5/1 (fall), 12/1 (winter). *Application fee:* $60.
**Degree Requirements** 39 total credit hours, Capstone project, residency.

**Degree** PhD
**Available Programs** Doctorate; Post-Baccalaureate Doctorate.

**Areas of Study** Health policy, health promotion/disease prevention.
**Program Entrance Requirements** Clinical experience, minimum overall college GPA of 3.3, interview by faculty committee, interview, 3 letters of recommendation, MSN or equivalent, statistics course, vita, writing sample, GRE General Test. *Application deadline:* 2/15 (fall). Applications may be processed on a rolling basis for some programs. *Application fee:* $100.
**Degree Requirements** 60 total credit hours, dissertation, oral exam, written exam, residency.

### POSTDOCTORAL PROGRAM
**Areas of Study** Cancer care, nursing research.
**Postdoctoral Program Contact** Dr. Suzanne G. Leveille, PhD Program Director, College of Nursing and Health Sciences, University of Massachusetts Boston, College of Nursing and Health Sciences, 100 Morrissey Boulevard, Boston, MA 02125. *Telephone:* 617-287-7279. *E-mail:* suzanne.leveille@umb.edu.

### CONTINUING EDUCATION PROGRAM
**Contact** Ms. Wanda Willard, Director of Credit Programs, College of Nursing and Health Sciences, University of Massachusetts Boston, 100 Morrissey Boulevard, Wheatley Building, 2nd Floor, Boston, MA 02125-3393. *Telephone:* 617-287-7874. *Fax:* 617-287-7922. *E-mail:* wanda.willard@umb.edu.

## University of Massachusetts Dartmouth
**College of Nursing**
**North Dartmouth, Massachusetts**

*http://www.umassd.edu/nursing*
Founded in 1895

**DEGREES • BSN • MS • PHD**
**Nursing Program Faculty** 52 (33% with doctorates).
**Nursing Student Activities** Sigma Theta Tau, Student Nurses' Association, nursing club.
**Nursing Student Resources** Academic advising; academic or career counseling; assistance for students with disabilities; bookstore; campus computer network; career placement assistance; computer lab; computer-assisted instruction; daycare for children of students; e-mail services; employment services for current students; externships; housing assistance; interactive nursing skills videos; Internet; learning resource lab; library services; nursing audiovisuals; placement services for program completers; resume preparation assistance; skills, simulation, or other laboratory; tutoring; unpaid internships.
**Library Facilities** 438,887 volumes; 2,017 periodical subscriptions.

### BACCALAUREATE PROGRAMS
**Degree** BSN
**Available Programs** Generic Baccalaureate; RN Baccalaureate.
**Site Options** Fall River, MA.
**Study Options** Full-time and part-time.
**Program Entrance Requirements** Transcript of college record, CPR certification, written essay, health exam, health insurance, high school biology, high school chemistry, high school foreign language, 3 years high school math, 3 years high school science, high school transcript, immunizations, letters of recommendation, minimum high school GPA of 3.0, minimum high school rank 66%, professional liability insurance/malpractice insurance. Transfer students are accepted.
**Advanced Placement** Credit by examination available. Credit given for nursing courses completed elsewhere dependent upon specific evaluations.
**Contact** *Telephone:* 508-999-8605. *Fax:* 508-999-8755.

### GRADUATE PROGRAMS
**Contact** *Telephone:* 508-999-8251.

### MASTER'S DEGREE PROGRAM
**Degree** MS
**Available Programs** Master's.
**Concentrations Available** *Clinical nurse specialist programs in:* adult health, community health. *Nurse practitioner programs in:* adult health.
**Study Options** Full-time and part-time.
**Program Entrance Requirements** Clinical experience, computer literacy, minimum overall college GPA of 3.0, transcript of college record, CPR certification, written essay, immunizations, interview, 3 letters of recommendation, nursing research course, physical assessment course, professional liability insurance/malpractice insurance, statistics course.
**Advanced Placement** Credit given for nursing courses completed elsewhere dependent upon specific evaluations.
**Degree Requirements** 39 total credit hours, thesis or project.

### POST-MASTER'S PROGRAM
**Areas of Study** *Nurse practitioner programs in:* adult health.

### DOCTORAL DEGREE PROGRAM
**Degree** PhD
**Available Programs** Doctorate.
**Areas of Study** Nursing education.
**Program Entrance Requirements** Clinical experience, minimum overall college GPA of 3.3, 3 letters of recommendation, MSN or equivalent, statistics course, vita, writing sample, GRE (for PHD).
**Degree Requirements** 52 total credit hours.

### CONTINUING EDUCATION PROGRAM
**Contact** *Telephone:* 508-999-8591.

## University of Massachusetts Lowell
**School of Nursing**
**Lowell, Massachusetts**

*http://www.uml.edu/SHE/Nursing/default.aspx*
Founded in 1894

**DEGREES • BS • DNP • MS • PHD**
**Nursing Program Faculty** 50 (42% with doctorates).
**Baccalaureate Enrollment** 500 **Women** 90% **Men** 10% **Minority** 27% **Part-time** 14%
**Graduate Enrollment** 133 **Women** 95% **Men** 5% **Minority** 5% **International** .1% **Part-time** 72%
**Distance Learning Courses** Available.
**Nursing Student Activities** Nursing Honor Society, Sigma Theta Tau, Student Nurses' Association, nursing club.
**Nursing Student Resources** Academic advising; academic or career counseling; assistance for students with disabilities; bookstore; campus computer network; career placement assistance; computer lab; computer-assisted instruction; e-mail services; employment services for current students; housing assistance; interactive nursing skills videos; Internet; learning resource lab; library services; nursing audiovisuals; other; placement services for program completers; resume preparation assistance; skills, simulation, or other laboratory; tutoring.
**Library Facilities** 298,756 volumes (29,100 in health, 4,465 in nursing); 45,105 periodical subscriptions (350 health-care related).

### BACCALAUREATE PROGRAMS
**Degree** BS
**Available Programs** Generic Baccalaureate; RN Baccalaureate.
**Study Options** Full-time.
**Program Entrance Requirements** Minimum overall college GPA of 2.7, transcript of college record, CPR certification, health exam, health insurance, high school chemistry, high school foreign language, 3 years high school math, 3 years high school science, high school transcript, immunizations, minimum high school GPA of 3.25, minimum GPA in nursing prerequisites of 2.7, professional liability insurance/malpractice insurance. Transfer students are accepted. *Application deadline:* 11/1 (fall), 1/1 (winter). Applications may be processed on a rolling basis for some programs. *Application fee:* $50.
**Advanced Placement** Credit by examination available.
**Expenses (2013–14)** *Tuition, state resident:* full-time $11,847. *Tuition, nonresident:* full-time $24,896. *Room and board:* $10,282 per academic year.
**Financial Aid** 68% of baccalaureate students in nursing programs received some form of financial aid in 2012–13.
**Contact** Office of Undergraduate Admissions, School of Nursing, University of Massachusetts Lowell, 883 Broadway Street, Suite 110, Lowell, MA 01854-3931. *Telephone:* 978-934-3931. *E-mail:* admissions@uml.edu.

## GRADUATE PROGRAMS

**Expenses (2013–14)** *Tuition, area resident:* part-time $535 per credit hour. *Tuition, state resident:* full-time $11,228; part-time $535 per credit hour. *Tuition, nonresident:* full-time $20,773.
**Financial Aid** 50% of graduate students in nursing programs received some form of financial aid in 2012–13. 37 fellowships with tuition reimbursements available, 10 teaching assistantships with full tuition reimbursements available were awarded; research assistantships with full tuition reimbursements available, career-related internships or fieldwork, Federal Work-Study, institutionally sponsored loans, scholarships, and traineeships also available. Aid available to part-time students. *Financial aid application deadline:* 4/1.
**Contact** Dr. Barbara Mawn, PhD and Graduate Program Director, School of Nursing, University of Massachusetts Lowell, 113 Wilder Street, Suite 200, Lowell, MA 01854-5126. *Telephone:* 978-934-4845. *Fax:* 978-934-2015. *E-mail:* barbara_mawn@uml.edu.

### MASTER'S DEGREE PROGRAM

**Degree** MS
**Available Programs** Accelerated Master's; Accelerated RN to Master's; Master's.
**Concentrations Available** *Clinical nurse specialist programs in:* family health, psychiatric/mental health. *Nurse practitioner programs in:* family health, gerontology, psychiatric/mental health.
**Study Options** Full-time and part-time.
**Program Entrance Requirements** Computer literacy, minimum overall college GPA of 3.0, transcript of college record, CPR certification, written essay, immunizations, interview, 3 letters of recommendation, statistics course, GRE General Test. *Application deadline:* Applications may be processed on a rolling basis for some programs. *Application fee:* $50.
**Advanced Placement** Credit given for nursing courses completed elsewhere dependent upon specific evaluations.
**Degree Requirements** 42 total credit hours, thesis or project.

### POST-MASTER'S PROGRAM

**Areas of Study** *Clinical nurse specialist programs in:* psychiatric/mental health.

### DOCTORAL DEGREE PROGRAM

**Degree** DNP
**Available Programs** Doctorate.
**Areas of Study** Advanced practice nursing.
**Program Entrance Requirements** Minimum overall college GPA of 3.0, interview, interview by faculty committee, letters of recommendation, MSN or equivalent, statistics course, vita. *Application deadline:* 11/1 (fall), 4/1 (spring). Applications may be processed on a rolling basis for some programs. *Application fee:* $50.
**Degree Requirements** 33 total credit hours, scholarly project.

**Degree** PhD
**Available Programs** Doctorate.
**Areas of Study** Health promotion/disease prevention.
**Online Degree Options** Yes (hybrid module, online and weekends).
**Program Entrance Requirements** Minimum overall college GPA of 3.4, interview by faculty committee, interview, 3 letters of recommendation, MSN or equivalent, scholarly papers, statistics course, writing sample, GRE General Test. *Application deadline:* Applications may be processed on a rolling basis for some programs.
**Degree Requirements** 48 total credit hours, dissertation, oral exam, 2 qualifying papers (one in theory, one in methods), written exam.

# University of Massachusetts Worcester

## Graduate School of Nursing
## Worcester, Massachusetts

***http://www.umassmed.edu/gsn/***
Founded in 1962

### DEGREES • MS • PHD

**Nursing Program Faculty** 51 (40% with doctorates).
**Graduate Enrollment** 174 **Women** 87% **Men** 13% **Minority** 23% **International** 1% **Part-time** 4%
**Distance Learning Courses** Available.
**Nursing Student Activities** Sigma Theta Tau, Student Nurses' Association.
**Nursing Student Resources** Academic advising; academic or career counseling; assistance for students with disabilities; bookstore; campus computer network; computer lab; computer-assisted instruction; e-mail services; interactive nursing skills videos; Internet; learning resource lab; library services; nursing audiovisuals; skills, simulation, or other laboratory; unpaid internships.
**Library Facilities** 207,500 volumes in health, 1,173 volumes in nursing; 5,400 periodical subscriptions health-care related.

## GRADUATE PROGRAMS

**Contact** *Telephone:* 508-856-5756. *Fax:* 508-856-5756.

### MASTER'S DEGREE PROGRAM

**Degree** MS
**Available Programs** Accelerated Master's for Non-Nursing College Graduates; Master's.
**Concentrations Available** Nursing education. *Nurse practitioner programs in:* acute care, family health, gerontology, primary care.
**Site Options** Shrewsbury, MA; Worcester, MA.
**Study Options** Full-time and part-time.
**Program Entrance Requirements** Clinical experience, computer literacy, minimum overall college GPA of 3.0, transcript of college record, CPR certification, written essay, immunizations, interview, 3 letters of recommendation, physical assessment course, prerequisite course work, resume, statistics course, GRE General Test. *Application deadline:* 3/15 (fall). Applications may be processed on a rolling basis for some programs.
**Advanced Placement** Credit given for nursing courses completed elsewhere dependent upon specific evaluations.
**Degree Requirements** 42 total credit hours.

### POST-MASTER'S PROGRAM

**Areas of Study** Nursing education. *Nurse practitioner programs in:* acute care, gerontology, primary care.

### DOCTORAL DEGREE PROGRAM

**Degree** PhD
**Available Programs** Doctorate.
**Areas of Study** Advanced practice nursing, bio-behavioral research, clinical practice, critical care, family health, health promotion/disease prevention, human health and illness, illness and transition, nursing research, nursing science, oncology.
**Site Options** Worcester, MA.
**Program Entrance Requirements** Minimum overall college GPA of 3.0, interview by faculty committee, interview, 3 letters of recommendation, MSN or equivalent, scholarly papers, statistics course, vita, writing sample, GRE General Test. *Application deadline:* 3/15 (fall). Applications may be processed on a rolling basis for some programs.
**Degree Requirements** 57 total credit hours, dissertation, oral exam, written exam.

## CONTINUING EDUCATION PROGRAM

**Contact** *Telephone:* 508-856-3488. *Fax:* 508-856-6552.

# Worcester State University

## Department of Nursing
## Worcester, Massachusetts

***http://www.worcester.edu/***
Founded in 1874

### DEGREES • BS • MS

**Nursing Program Faculty** 45 (40% with doctorates).
**Baccalaureate Enrollment** 354 **Women** 90% **Men** 10% **Minority** 10%
**Graduate Enrollment** 81 **Women** 70% **Men** 30% **Minority** 30% **Part-time** 100%
**Nursing Student Activities** Nursing Honor Society, Sigma Theta Tau, Student Nurses' Association, nursing club.
**Nursing Student Resources** Academic advising; academic or career counseling; assistance for students with disabilities; bookstore; campus computer network; career placement assistance; computer lab; computer-assisted instruction; e-mail services; employment services for current students; externships; housing assistance; interactive nursing skills videos; Internet; learning resource lab; library services; nursing audiovisuals; paid internships; remedial services; resume preparation assistance; skills, simulation, or other laboratory; tutoring; unpaid internships.

**Library Facilities** 204,971 volumes (5,400 in health, 500 in nursing); 496 periodical subscriptions (385 health-care related).

### BACCALAUREATE PROGRAMS

**Degree** BS
**Available Programs** ADN to Baccalaureate; Generic Baccalaureate; LPN to RN Baccalaureate.
**Site Options** Worcester, MA.
**Study Options** Full-time.
**Program Entrance Requirements** Transcript of college record, high school foreign language, 3 years high school math, 3 years high school science, high school transcript, minimum high school GPA of 3.2. *Application deadline:* 1/15 (fall). Applications may be processed on a rolling basis for some programs. *Application fee:* $40.
**Advanced Placement** Credit by examination available.
**Expenses (2013–14)** *Tuition, state resident:* full-time $970; part-time $40 per credit. *Tuition, nonresident:* full-time $7050; part-time $294 per credit. *Room and board:* $10,530; room only: $7210 per academic year. *Required fees:* part-time $299 per credit; part-time $3594 per term.
**Financial Aid** 76% of baccalaureate students in nursing programs received some form of financial aid in 2012–13.
**Contact** Mr. Joseph Dicarlo, Director, Admissions, Department of Nursing, Worcester State University, 486 Chandler Street, Worcester, MA 01602. *Telephone:* 508-929-8040. *Fax:* 508-929-8183. *E-mail:* Joseph.Dicarlo@worcester.edu.

### GRADUATE PROGRAMS

**Expenses (2013–14)** *Tuition, state resident:* part-time $150 per credit. *Tuition, nonresident:* part-time $150 per credit. *Required fees:* part-time $115 per credit.
**Financial Aid** 35% of graduate students in nursing programs received some form of financial aid in 2012–13.
**Contact** Dr. Stephanie Chalupka, Associate Dean for Nursing, Department of Nursing, Worcester State University, 486 Chandler Street, Worcester, MA 01602. *Telephone:* 508-929-8129. *Fax:* 508-929-8168. *E-mail:* schalupka@worcester.edu.

#### MASTER'S DEGREE PROGRAM

**Degree** MS
**Available Programs** Master's; Master's for Nurses with Non-Nursing Degrees; RN to Master's.
**Concentrations Available** Nursing education. *Clinical nurse specialist programs in:* community health, public health.
**Study Options** Full-time and part-time.
**Program Entrance Requirements** Clinical experience, computer literacy, minimum overall college GPA of 3.0, transcript of college record, CPR certification, written essay, immunizations, 2 letters of recommendation, nursing research course, professional liability insurance/malpractice insurance, prerequisite course work, resume, statistics course. *Application deadline:* 4/1 (fall), 11/1 (winter). Applications may be processed on a rolling basis for some programs. *Application fee:* $40.
**Degree Requirements** 42 total credit hours, thesis or project.

#### POST-MASTER'S PROGRAM

**Areas of Study** Nursing education.

### CONTINUING EDUCATION PROGRAM

**Contact** Ms. Gina Fleury, RN, Continuing Education Coordinator, Department of Nursing, Worcester State University, 486 Chandler Street, Worcester, MA 01602. *Telephone:* 508-929-8683. *E-mail:* gfleury@worcester.edu.

# MICHIGAN

## Andrews University
**Department of Nursing**
**Berrien Springs, Michigan**

Founded in 1874

**DEGREES • BS • MS**
**Nursing Program Faculty** 11 (50% with doctorates).
**Baccalaureate Enrollment** 106
**Graduate Enrollment** 10
**Nursing Student Activities** Nursing Honor Society, Sigma Theta Tau, Student Nurses' Association.
**Nursing Student Resources** Academic advising; academic or career counseling; assistance for students with disabilities; bookstore; campus computer network; career placement assistance; computer lab; computer-assisted instruction; daycare for children of students; e-mail services; employment services for current students; externships; housing assistance; interactive nursing skills videos; Internet; learning resource lab; library services; nursing audiovisuals; paid internships; placement services for program completers; remedial services; resume preparation assistance; skills, simulation, or other laboratory; tutoring; unpaid internships.
**Library Facilities** 678,734 volumes (77,000 in health, 500 in nursing); 94,000 periodical subscriptions (700 health-care related).

### BACCALAUREATE PROGRAMS

**Degree** BS
**Available Programs** ADN to Baccalaureate; Generic Baccalaureate.
**Study Options** Full-time.
**Program Entrance Requirements** Minimum overall college GPA of 2.5, transcript of college record, health exam, high school transcript, immunizations, minimum GPA in nursing prerequisites of 2.5. Transfer students are accepted.
**Contact** *Telephone:* 269-471-3192. *Fax:* 269-471-3454.

### GRADUATE PROGRAMS

**Contact** *Telephone:* 269-471-3337. *Fax:* 269-471-3454.

#### MASTER'S DEGREE PROGRAM

**Degree** MS
**Available Programs** Master's.
**Concentrations Available** Nursing education.
**Study Options** Part-time.
**Program Entrance Requirements** Minimum overall college GPA of 3.0, transcript of college record, CPR certification, immunizations, 3 letters of recommendation, GRE.
**Degree Requirements** 38 total credit hours, thesis or project.

#### POST-MASTER'S PROGRAM

**Areas of Study** Nursing education.

## Calvin College
**Department of Nursing**
**Grand Rapids, Michigan**

*http://www.calvin.edu/academic/nursing*
Founded in 1876

**DEGREE • BSN**
**Nursing Program Faculty** 20 (20% with doctorates).
**Baccalaureate Enrollment** 120 **Women** 95% **Men** 5% **Minority** 10% **International** 10%
**Nursing Student Activities** Sigma Theta Tau, Student Nurses' Association, nursing club.
**Nursing Student Resources** Academic advising; academic or career counseling; assistance for students with disabilities; bookstore; campus computer network; career placement assistance; computer lab; computer-assisted instruction; e-mail services; employment services for current students; externships; housing assistance; interactive nursing skills videos; Internet; learning resource lab; library services; nursing audiovisuals; paid internships; placement services for program completers; remedial services; resume preparation assistance; skills, simulation, or other laboratory; tutoring.
**Library Facilities** 1.3 million volumes; 37,307 periodical subscriptions.

### BACCALAUREATE PROGRAMS

**Degree** BSN
**Available Programs** Generic Baccalaureate.
**Site Options** Grand Rapids, MI.
**Study Options** Full-time.
**Program Entrance Requirements** Minimum overall college GPA of 2.5, transcript of college record, CPR certification, health exam, health insurance, immunizations, 2 letters of recommendation, minimum GPA in nursing prerequisites of 2.5, professional liability insurance/malpractice insurance, prerequisite course work. Transfer students are accepted.

**Contact** *Telephone:* 616-526-6268. *Fax:* 616-526-8567.

# Davenport University
## Division of Nursing
## Grand Rapids, Michigan

Founded in 1866

**DEGREE • BSN**

**Nursing Program Faculty** 40

**Baccalaureate Enrollment** 215 **Women** 94% **Men** 6% **Minority** 30% **Part-time** 17%

**Distance Learning Courses** Available.

**Nursing Student Activities** Student Nurses' Association.

**Nursing Student Resources** Academic advising; academic or career counseling; assistance for students with disabilities; bookstore; campus computer network; career placement assistance; computer lab; computer-assisted instruction; e-mail services; employment services for current students; externships; housing assistance; interactive nursing skills videos; Internet; learning resource lab; library services; nursing audiovisuals; placement services for program completers; remedial services; resume preparation assistance; skills, simulation, or other laboratory; tutoring.

**Library Facilities** 74,714 volumes (100 in health, 50 in nursing); 219 periodical subscriptions (20 health-care related).

### BACCALAUREATE PROGRAMS

**Degree** BSN

**Available Programs** ADN to Baccalaureate; Generic Baccalaureate; RN Baccalaureate.

**Site Options** Midland, MI; Warren, MI.

**Study Options** Full-time and part-time.

**Online Degree Options** Yes.

**Program Entrance Requirements** Minimum overall college GPA of 3.5, transcript of college record, CPR certification, written essay, health exam, health insurance, high school biology, high school chemistry, 2 years high school math, 3 years high school science, high school transcript, immunizations, 2 letters of recommendation, minimum high school GPA of 3.5, minimum GPA in nursing prerequisites. Transfer students are accepted. *Application deadline:* 1/31 (fall).

**Advanced Placement** Credit by examination available. Credit given for nursing courses completed elsewhere dependent upon specific evaluations.

**Contact** *Telephone:* 616-451-3511. *Fax:* 616-732-1145.

# Davenport University
## Bachelor of Science in Nursing Program
## Kalamazoo, Michigan

Founded in 1977

**DEGREE • BSN**

### BACCALAUREATE PROGRAMS

**Degree** BSN

**Available Programs** Generic Baccalaureate; RN Baccalaureate.

**Contact** *Telephone:* 616-871-3977. *Fax:* 616-554-5225.

# Eastern Michigan University
## School of Nursing
## Ypsilanti, Michigan

*http://www.emich.edu/nursing*

Founded in 1849

**DEGREES • BSN • MSN • PHD**

**Nursing Program Faculty** 76 (25% with doctorates).

**Baccalaureate Enrollment** 592 **Women** 85% **Men** 15% **Minority** 24% **International** 1% **Part-time** 55%

**Graduate Enrollment** 28 **Women** 82% **Men** 18% **Minority** 43% **Part-time** 89%

**Distance Learning Courses** Available.

**Nursing Student Activities** Sigma Theta Tau, Student Nurses' Association.

**Nursing Student Resources** Academic advising; academic or career counseling; assistance for students with disabilities; bookstore; campus computer network; career placement assistance; computer lab; computer-assisted instruction; daycare for children of students; e-mail services; employment services for current students; housing assistance; interactive nursing skills videos; Internet; learning resource lab; library services; nursing audiovisuals; placement services for program completers; remedial services; resume preparation assistance; skills, simulation, or other laboratory; tutoring.

**Library Facilities** 1 million volumes (10,000 in health, 4,966 in nursing); 28,120 periodical subscriptions (8,851 health-care related).

### BACCALAUREATE PROGRAMS

**Degree** BSN

**Available Programs** ADN to Baccalaureate; Baccalaureate for Second Degree; Generic Baccalaureate; RN Baccalaureate.

**Site Options** Livonia, MI; Monroe, MI; Jackson, MI; Brighton, MI; Detroit, MI.

**Study Options** Full-time and part-time.

**Online Degree Options** Yes.

**Program Entrance Requirements** Transcript of college record, CPR certification, health exam, health insurance, immunizations, minimum GPA in nursing prerequisites of 3.0, prerequisite course work, RN licensure. Transfer students are accepted. *Application deadline:* 5/15 (fall). *Application fee:* $30.

**Advanced Placement** Credit by examination available. Credit given for nursing courses completed elsewhere dependent upon specific evaluations.

**Expenses (2013–14)** *Tuition, area resident:* full-time $6391; part-time $266 per credit hour. *Tuition, state resident:* full-time $6391; part-time $266. *Tuition, nonresident:* full-time $18,827; part-time $784 per credit hour. *International tuition:* $18,827 full-time. *Room and board:* $8481; room only: $3900 per academic year. *Required fees:* full-time $2857; part-time $119 per credit; part-time $50 per term.

**Financial Aid** 79% of baccalaureate students in nursing programs received some form of financial aid in 2012–13.

**Contact** Ms. Nancy Higgins, BSN Program Coordinator, School of Nursing, Eastern Michigan University, 323 Marshall Building, Ypsilanti, MI 48197. *Telephone:* 734-487-2334. *Fax:* 734-487-6946. *E-mail:* nancy.higgins@emich.edu.

### GRADUATE PROGRAMS

**Expenses (2013–14)** *Tuition, area resident:* full-time $11,180; part-time $466 per credit hour. *Tuition, state resident:* full-time $11,180; part-time $466. *Tuition, nonresident:* full-time $22,039; part-time $918 per credit hour. *Room and board:* $8481; room only: $3900 per academic year. *Required fees:* full-time $3200; part-time $133 per credit; part-time $50 per term.

**Financial Aid** 37% of graduate students in nursing programs received some form of financial aid in 2012–13.

**Contact** Dr. Laurie Blondy, Graduate Programs Coordinator, School of Nursing, Eastern Michigan University, 311 Marshall Building, Ypsilanti, MI 48197. *Telephone:* 734-487-3275. *Fax:* 734-487-6946. *E-mail:* lblondy@emich.edu.

#### MASTER'S DEGREE PROGRAM

**Degree** MSN

**Available Programs** Master's; Master's for Nurses with Non-Nursing Degrees.

**Concentrations Available** *Clinical nurse specialist programs in:* adult health. *Nurse practitioner programs in:* adult health, primary care.

**Site Options** Livonia, MI; Monroe, MI.

**Study Options** Part-time.

**Program Entrance Requirements** Clinical experience, minimum overall college GPA of 3.0, transcript of college record, CPR certification, written essay, immunizations, 2 letters of recommendation, physical assessment course, statistics course. *Application deadline:* 3/1 (fall).

**Advanced Placement** Credit by examination available. Credit given for nursing courses completed elsewhere dependent upon specific evaluations.

**Degree Requirements** 44 total credit hours, thesis or project.

#### DOCTORAL DEGREE PROGRAM

**Degree** PhD

**Available Programs** Doctorate.

**Areas of Study** Faculty preparation, nursing education.

**Program Entrance Requirements** Clinical experience, interview by faculty committee, 3 letters of recommendation, MSN or equivalent, statistics course, vita, writing sample. *Application deadline:* 2/1 (fall).

**Degree Requirements** 60 total credit hours, dissertation, oral exam, written exam.

# Ferris State University

## School of Nursing
## Big Rapids, Michigan

*http://www.ferris.edu/*
Founded in 1884

### DEGREES • BSN • MSN • MSN/MBA

**Nursing Program Faculty** 24 (20% with doctorates).

**Baccalaureate Enrollment** 643 **Women** 89% **Men** 11% **Minority** 8% **Part-time** 79%

**Graduate Enrollment** 108 **Women** 89% **Men** 11% **Minority** .5% **Part-time** 100%

**Distance Learning Courses** Available.

**Nursing Student Activities** Sigma Theta Tau, Student Nurses' Association, nursing club.

**Nursing Student Resources** Academic advising; academic or career counseling; assistance for students with disabilities; bookstore; campus computer network; career placement assistance; computer lab; computer-assisted instruction; daycare for children of students; e-mail services; employment services for current students; housing assistance; interactive nursing skills videos; Internet; library services; nursing audiovisuals; resume preparation assistance; skills, simulation, or other laboratory; tutoring.

**Library Facilities** 273,210 volumes (12,177 in health, 785 in nursing); 74,452 periodical subscriptions (515 health-care related).

### BACCALAUREATE PROGRAMS

**Degree** BSN

**Available Programs** Accelerated Baccalaureate for Second Degree; Accelerated RN Baccalaureate; Baccalaureate for Second Degree; RN Baccalaureate.

**Site Options** Greenville, MI; Traverse City, MI; Grand Rapids, MI.

**Study Options** Full-time.

**Online Degree Options** Yes.

**Program Entrance Requirements** Minimum overall college GPA of 2.7, transcript of college record, CPR certification, health insurance, immunizations, minimum GPA in nursing prerequisites of 2.7, prerequisite course work. Transfer students are accepted. *Application deadline:* 4/15 (spring).

**Advanced Placement** Credit by examination available. Credit given for nursing courses completed elsewhere dependent upon specific evaluations.

**Expenses (2013–14)** *Tuition, state resident:* full-time $15,330; part-time $365 per credit hour. *Tuition, nonresident:* full-time $23,016; part-time $548 per credit hour. *International tuition:* $24,612 full-time. *Room and board:* $8910; room only: $7470 per academic year. *Required fees:* full-time $1810; part-time $1000 per term.

**Financial Aid** 85% of baccalaureate students in nursing programs received some form of financial aid in 2012–13. *Gift aid (need-based):* Federal Pell, FSEOG, state, private, college/university gift aid from institutional funds. *Loans:* Federal Nursing Student Loans, Federal Direct (Subsidized and Unsubsidized Stafford PLUS), Perkins, college/university, alternative loans. *Work-study:* Federal Work-Study, part-time campus jobs. *Financial aid application deadline (priority):* 2/15.

**Contact** Dr. Susan J. Owens, Interim Chair, School of Nursing, School of Nursing, Ferris State University, 200 Ferris Drive, VFS 400-A, Big Rapids, MI 49307. *Telephone:* 231-591-2267. *Fax:* 231-591-2325. *E-mail:* owenss3@ferris.edu.

### GRADUATE PROGRAMS

**Expenses (2013–14)** *Tuition, state resident:* part-time $497 per credit hour. *Tuition, nonresident:* part-time $746 per credit hour.

**Financial Aid** 20% of graduate students in nursing programs received some form of financial aid in 2012–13.

**Contact** Dr. Susan Owens, MSN Program Coordinator, School of Nursing, Ferris State University, 200 Ferris Drive, VFS 300-A, Big Rapids, MI 49307. *Telephone:* 231-591-2290. *Fax:* 231-591-2325. *E-mail:* owenss3@ferris.edu.

#### MASTER'S DEGREE PROGRAM

**Degrees** MSN; MSN/MBA

**Available Programs** Accelerated AD/RN to Master's; Accelerated RN to Master's; Master's; RN to Master's.

**Concentrations Available** Nursing administration; nursing education; nursing informatics.

**Study Options** Full-time and part-time.

**Online Degree Options** Yes (online only).

**Program Entrance Requirements** Clinical experience, minimum overall college GPA of 3.0, transcript of college record, written essay, immunizations, 3 letters of recommendation, resume. *Application deadline:* 8/1 (fall), 12/1 (winter), 12/2 (spring).

**Advanced Placement** Credit given for nursing courses completed elsewhere dependent upon specific evaluations.

**Degree Requirements** 37 total credit hours, thesis or project, comprehensive exam.

# Finlandia University

## College of Professional Studies
## Hancock, Michigan

*http://www.finlandia.edu/*
Founded in 1896

### DEGREE • BSN

**Nursing Program Faculty** 12 (25% with doctorates).

**Baccalaureate Enrollment** 75 **Women** 87% **Men** 13% **Minority** 3% **Part-time** 2%

**Distance Learning Courses** Available.

**Nursing Student Activities** Student Nurses' Association, nursing club.

**Nursing Student Resources** Academic advising; academic or career counseling; assistance for students with disabilities; bookstore; campus computer network; career placement assistance; computer lab; computer-assisted instruction; e-mail services; externships; interactive nursing skills videos; Internet; learning resource lab; library services; nursing audiovisuals; placement services for program completers; remedial services; resume preparation assistance; skills, simulation, or other laboratory; tutoring.

**Library Facilities** 68,803 volumes (4,601 in health, 2,316 in nursing); 997 periodical subscriptions (97 health-care related).

### BACCALAUREATE PROGRAMS

**Degree** BSN

**Available Programs** Generic Baccalaureate; RN Baccalaureate.

**Study Options** Full-time.

**Online Degree Options** Yes.

**Program Entrance Requirements** Minimum overall college GPA of 2.5, transcript of college record, CPR certification, health exam, health insurance, high school biology, high school chemistry, 1 year of high school math, 2 years high school science, high school transcript, immunizations, minimum high school GPA of 2.5, minimum GPA in nursing prerequisites of 2.7, prerequisite course work. Transfer students are accepted. *Application deadline:* Applications may be processed on a rolling basis for some programs.

**Advanced Placement** Credit given for nursing courses completed elsewhere dependent upon specific evaluations.

**Expenses (2013–14)** *Tuition:* full-time $19,980; part-time $665 per credit hour. *International tuition:* $19,980 full-time. *Room and board:* $7210 per academic year. *Required fees:* full-time $400; part-time $200 per term.

**Financial Aid** 98% of baccalaureate students in nursing programs received some form of financial aid in 2012–13. *Gift aid (need-based):* Federal Pell, FSEOG, state, private, college/university gift aid from institutional funds. *Loans:* Federal Direct (Subsidized and Unsubsidized Stafford PLUS), private loans. *Work-study:* Federal Work-Study. *Financial aid application deadline (priority):* 3/1.

**Contact** Julie Jennerjohn, Admissions Office, College of Professional Studies, Finlandia University, 601 Quincy Street, Hancock, MI 49930. *Telephone:* 906-487-7352. *E-mail:* julie.jennerjohn@finlandia.edu.

# Grand Valley State University

## Kirkhof College of Nursing
## Allendale, Michigan

***http://www.gvsu.edu/kcon***
Founded in 1960

**DEGREES • BSN • DNP • MSN**

**Nursing Program Faculty** 78 (46% with doctorates).
**Baccalaureate Enrollment** 293 **Women** 87% **Men** 13% **Minority** 7% **Part-time** 7%
**Graduate Enrollment** 84 **Women** 87% **Men** 13% **Minority** 1% **Part-time** 13%
**Distance Learning Courses** Available.
**Nursing Student Activities** Sigma Theta Tau, Student Nurses' Association.
**Nursing Student Resources** Academic advising; academic or career counseling; assistance for students with disabilities; bookstore; campus computer network; career placement assistance; computer lab; computer-assisted instruction; daycare for children of students; e-mail services; employment services for current students; housing assistance; interactive nursing skills videos; Internet; learning resource lab; library services; nursing audiovisuals; remedial services; resume preparation assistance; skills, simulation, or other laboratory; tutoring.
**Library Facilities** 18,430 volumes in health, 1,354 volumes in nursing; 4,575 periodical subscriptions health-care related.

### BACCALAUREATE PROGRAMS

**Degree** BSN
**Available Programs** ADN to Baccalaureate; Accelerated Baccalaureate for Second Degree; Generic Baccalaureate; RN Baccalaureate.
**Site Options** Grand Rapids, MI.
**Study Options** Full-time and part-time.
**Program Entrance Requirements** Minimum overall college GPA of 3.0, transcript of college record, CPR certification, health exam, immunizations, interview, minimum GPA in nursing prerequisites of 3.0, prerequisite course work. Transfer students are accepted. *Application deadline:* 1/31 (fall), 8/31 (winter).
**Advanced Placement** Credit given for nursing courses completed elsewhere dependent upon specific evaluations.
**Expenses (2013–14)** *Tuition, state resident:* full-time $10,454; part-time $435 per credit hour. *Tuition, nonresident:* full-time $15,114; part-time $629 per credit hour. *Room and board:* $8080; room only: $6340 per academic year. *Required fees:* part-time $25 per credit.
**Financial Aid** 78% of baccalaureate students in nursing programs received some form of financial aid in 2012–13. *Gift aid (need-based):* Federal Pell, FSEOG, state, private, college/university gift aid from institutional funds. *Loans:* Federal Nursing Student Loans, Federal Direct (Subsidized and Unsubsidized Stafford PLUS), Perkins. *Work-study:* Federal Work-Study, part-time campus jobs. *Financial aid application deadline (priority):* 3/1.
**Contact** Ms. Kristin Norton, Director of Student Services, Kirkhof College of Nursing, Grand Valley State University, Cook-DeVos Center for Health Sciences, 301 Michigan Street NE, Room 322, Grand Rapids, MI 49503-3314. *Telephone:* 616-331-5637. *Fax:* 616-331-2510. *E-mail:* nortonkr@gvsu.edu.

### GRADUATE PROGRAMS

**Expenses (2013–14)** *Tuition, state resident:* part-time $591 per credit. *Tuition, nonresident:* part-time $781 per credit. *Room and board:* $8080; room only: $6340 per academic year.
**Financial Aid** 83% of graduate students in nursing programs received some form of financial aid in 2012–13. 32 fellowships (averaging $9,233 per year), 28 research assistantships with full and partial tuition reimbursements available (averaging $8,000 per year) were awarded; career-related internships or fieldwork, Federal Work-Study, institutionally sponsored loans, and traineeships also available. *Financial aid application deadline:* 2/15.
**Contact** Ms. Linda Buck, Student Services Coordinator, Kirkhof College of Nursing, Grand Valley State University, Cook-DeVos Center for Health Sciences, 301 Michigan Street NE, Room 318, Grand Rapids, MI 49503-3314. *Telephone:* 616-331-5785. *Fax:* 616-331-2510. *E-mail:* buckli@gvsu.edu.

#### MASTER'S DEGREE PROGRAM

**Degree** MSN
**Available Programs** Master's.
**Concentrations Available** Clinical nurse leader.
**Site Options** Grand Rapids, MI.
**Study Options** Full-time and part-time.
**Program Entrance Requirements** Minimum overall college GPA of 3.0, transcript of college record, CPR certification, written essay, immunizations, interview, resume, GRE. *Application deadline:* 2/1 (fall). *Application fee:* $30.
**Advanced Placement** Credit given for nursing courses completed elsewhere dependent upon specific evaluations.
**Degree Requirements** 41 total credit hours, thesis or project.

#### DOCTORAL DEGREE PROGRAM

**Degree** DNP
**Available Programs** Post-Baccalaureate Doctorate.
**Areas of Study** Advanced practice nursing, nursing administration.
**Site Options** Grand Rapids, MI.
**Program Entrance Requirements** Minimum overall college GPA of 3.0, interview by faculty committee, vita, writing sample. *Application deadline:* 2/1 (fall). *Application fee:* $30.
**Degree Requirements** 79–93 total credit hours, dissertation.

### CONTINUING EDUCATION PROGRAM

**Contact** Ms. Tamara Mohr, Academic Community Liaison, Kirkhof College of Nursing, Grand Valley State University, Cook-DeVos Center for Health Sciences, 301 Michigan Street NE, Room 310, Grand Rapids, MI 49503-3314. *Telephone:* 616-331-5763. *Fax:* 616-331-2510. *E-mail:* mohrt@gvsu.edu.

# Hope College

## Department of Nursing
## Holland, Michigan

Founded in 1866

**DEGREE • BSN**

**Nursing Program Faculty** 13 (30% with doctorates).
**Baccalaureate Enrollment** 135 **Women** 90% **Men** 10% **Minority** 10%
**Nursing Student Activities** Sigma Theta Tau, Student Nurses' Association.
**Nursing Student Resources** Academic advising; academic or career counseling; assistance for students with disabilities; bookstore; campus computer network; career placement assistance; computer lab; computer-assisted instruction; e-mail services; employment services for current students; externships; housing assistance; interactive nursing skills videos; Internet; learning resource lab; library services; nursing audiovisuals; remedial services; resume preparation assistance; skills, simulation, or other laboratory; tutoring; unpaid internships.
**Library Facilities** 368,860 volumes; 7,329 periodical subscriptions.

### BACCALAUREATE PROGRAMS

**Degree** BSN
**Available Programs** Generic Baccalaureate.
**Study Options** Full-time and part-time.
**Program Entrance Requirements** Minimum overall college GPA of 3.0, transcript of college record, written essay, 2 letters of recommendation. Transfer students are accepted. *Application deadline:* 10/1 (fall), 2/1 (winter).
**Financial Aid** ***Gift aid (need-based):*** Federal Pell, FSEOG, state, private, college/university gift aid from institutional funds. *Loans:* Federal Direct (Subsidized and Unsubsidized Stafford PLUS), Perkins. *Work-study:* Federal Work-Study, part-time campus jobs. *Financial aid application deadline (priority):* 3/1.
**Contact** Nursing Contact, Department of Nursing, Hope College, 35 East 12th Street, Holland, MI 49422-9000. *Telephone:* 616-395-7420. *Fax:* 616-395-7163. *E-mail:* nursing@hope.edu.

# Lake Superior State University

## Department of Nursing
## Sault Sainte Marie, Michigan

***http://www.lssu.edu/nursing/***
Founded in 1946

**DEGREE • BSN**

**Nursing Program Faculty** 20 (15% with doctorates).

**Baccalaureate Enrollment** 115 **Women** 90% **Men** 10% **Minority** 10% **International** 3%
**Distance Learning Courses** Available.
**Nursing Student Activities** Nursing Honor Society, Student Nurses' Association, nursing club.
**Nursing Student Resources** Academic advising; academic or career counseling; assistance for students with disabilities; bookstore; campus computer network; career placement assistance; computer lab; computer-assisted instruction; daycare for children of students; e-mail services; employment services for current students; interactive nursing skills videos; Internet; learning resource lab; library services; nursing audiovisuals; placement services for program completers; remedial services; resume preparation assistance; skills, simulation, or other laboratory; tutoring.
**Library Facilities** 200,449 volumes (5,246 in health, 942 in nursing); 850 periodical subscriptions (1,196 health-care related).

## BACCALAUREATE PROGRAMS

**Degree** BSN
**Available Programs** ADN to Baccalaureate; Generic Baccalaureate; LPN to Baccalaureate; LPN to RN Baccalaureate; RN Baccalaureate; RPN to Baccalaureate.
**Site Options** Escanaba, MI; Petoskey, MI.
**Study Options** Full-time and part-time.
**Program Entrance Requirements** Minimum overall college GPA of 2.5, transcript of college record, CPR certification, health exam, health insurance, high school biology, high school chemistry, high school transcript, immunizations, 1 letter of recommendation, minimum high school GPA of 2.0, minimum GPA in nursing prerequisites of 2.5, professional liability insurance/malpractice insurance, prerequisite course work. Transfer students are accepted. *Application deadline:* 2/1 (fall), 10/1 (spring).
**Advanced Placement** Credit given for nursing courses completed elsewhere dependent upon specific evaluations.
**Contact** *Telephone:* 906-635-2446. *Fax:* 906-635-2266.

# Madonna University

### College of Nursing and Health
### Livonia, Michigan

*http://www.madonna.edu/*
Founded in 1947

**DEGREES • BSN • DNP • MSN • MSN/MBA**
**Nursing Program Faculty** 71 (26% with doctorates).
**Baccalaureate Enrollment** 405 **Women** 87% **Men** 13% **Minority** 17% **International** 2% **Part-time** 32%
**Graduate Enrollment** 251 **Women** 88% **Men** 12% **Minority** 22% **International** 12% **Part-time** 98%
**Distance Learning Courses** Available.
**Nursing Student Activities** Sigma Theta Tau, Student Nurses' Association.
**Nursing Student Resources** Academic advising; academic or career counseling; assistance for students with disabilities; bookstore; campus computer network; career placement assistance; computer lab; computer-assisted instruction; e-mail services; employment services for current students; interactive nursing skills videos; Internet; learning resource lab; library services; nursing audiovisuals; remedial services; resume preparation assistance; skills, simulation, or other laboratory; tutoring.
**Library Facilities** 191,242 volumes (3,632 in health); 415 periodical subscriptions (2,778 health-care related).

## BACCALAUREATE PROGRAMS

**Degree** BSN
**Available Programs** ADN to Baccalaureate; Generic Baccalaureate; LPN to Baccalaureate; RN Baccalaureate.
**Study Options** Full-time and part-time.
**Program Entrance Requirements** Minimum overall college GPA of 3.0, transcript of college record, CPR certification, written essay, health exam, high school biology, high school chemistry, 1 year of high school math, high school transcript, immunizations, minimum high school GPA of 3.0, minimum GPA in nursing prerequisites of 3.0, professional liability insurance/malpractice insurance. Transfer students are accepted. *Application deadline:* 1/31 (fall), 7/31 (winter).
**Advanced Placement** Credit by examination available. Credit given for nursing courses completed elsewhere dependent upon specific evaluations.
**Expenses (2013–14)** *Tuition:* full-time $15,000; part-time $600 per credit hour. *International tuition:* $18,750 full-time. *Room and board:* room only: $5718 per academic year. *Required fees:* full-time $410.
**Financial Aid** 75% of baccalaureate students in nursing programs received some form of financial aid in 2012–13.
**Contact** Ms. Lauren Stemberger, Pre-Nursing Admissions Officer, College of Nursing and Health, Madonna University, 36600 Schoolcraft Road, Livonia, MI 48150-1173. *Telephone:* 734-432-5346. *E-mail:* lstemberger@madonna.edu.

## GRADUATE PROGRAMS

**Expenses (2013–14)** *Tuition:* full-time $10,980; part-time $610 per credit hour. *International tuition:* $13,725 full-time. *Required fees:* full-time $470.
**Financial Aid** 35% of graduate students in nursing programs received some form of financial aid in 2012–13.
**Contact** Mr. Sandro Faber-Bermudez, Admissions Officer, Graduate Nursing program, College of Nursing and Health, Madonna University, 36600 Schoolcraft Road, Livonia, MI 48150-1173. *Telephone:* 734-432-5407. *Fax:* 734-432-5463. *E-mail:* sfaber-bermudez@madonna.edu.

### MASTER'S DEGREE PROGRAM

**Degrees** MSN; MSN/MBA
**Available Programs** Master's.
**Concentrations Available** Nursing administration. *Nurse practitioner programs in:* acute care, primary care.
**Study Options** Full-time and part-time.
**Program Entrance Requirements** Clinical experience, computer literacy, minimum overall college GPA of 3.0, transcript of college record, written essay, interview, 2 letters of recommendation, nursing research course, physical assessment course, prerequisite course work, resume, statistics course. *Application deadline:* 2/1 (fall), 9/30 (winter), 2/1 (spring), 2/1 (summer). *Application fee:* $25.
**Degree Requirements** 48 total credit hours.

### POST-MASTER'S PROGRAM

**Areas of Study** Nursing administration. *Nurse practitioner programs in:* acute care, primary care.

### DOCTORAL DEGREE PROGRAM

**Degree** DNP
**Available Programs** Doctorate.
**Areas of Study** Advanced practice nursing, individualized study, nursing administration.
**Program Entrance Requirements** Clinical experience, minimum overall college GPA of 3.0, interview by faculty committee, interview, 3 letters of recommendation, MSN or equivalent, scholarly papers, vita, writing sample. *Application deadline:* 3/1 (fall). *Application fee:* $25.
**Degree Requirements** 38 total credit hours, oral exam, written exam, residency.

## CONTINUING EDUCATION PROGRAM

**Contact** Dr. Susan Hasenau, Coordinator of Nursing Continuing Education, College of Nursing and Health, Madonna University, 36600 Schoolcraft Road, Livonia, MI 48150-1173. *Telephone:* 734-432-5863. *Fax:* 734-432-5463. *E-mail:* shasenau@madonna.edu.

# Michigan State University

### College of Nursing
### East Lansing, Michigan

*http://www.nursing.msu.edu/*
Founded in 1855

**DEGREES • BSN • DNP • MSN • PHD**
**Nursing Program Faculty** 88 (42% with doctorates).
**Baccalaureate Enrollment** 336 **Women** 87.5% **Men** 12.5% **Minority** 9.7% **International** .3% **Part-time** 10.4%
**Graduate Enrollment** 196 **Women** 90.8% **Men** 9.2% **Minority** 7.2% **International** 1% **Part-time** 54.1%
**Distance Learning Courses** Available.
**Nursing Student Activities** Sigma Theta Tau, Student Nurses' Association.
**Nursing Student Resources** Academic advising; academic or career counseling; assistance for students with disabilities; bookstore; campus computer network; career placement assistance; computer lab; computer-assisted instruction; daycare for children of students; e-mail services;

employment services for current students; externships; housing assistance; interactive nursing skills videos; Internet; learning resource lab; library services; nursing audiovisuals; placement services for program completers; remedial services; resume preparation assistance; skills, simulation, or other laboratory; tutoring.
**Library Facilities** 6.7 million volumes (311,091 in health, 8,579 in nursing); 172,144 periodical subscriptions (8,451 health-care related).

## BACCALAUREATE PROGRAMS

**Degree** BSN
**Available Programs** Accelerated Baccalaureate for Second Degree; Generic Baccalaureate; RN Baccalaureate.
**Study Options** Full-time.
**Online Degree Options** Yes.
**Program Entrance Requirements** Minimum overall college GPA of 2.75, transcript of college record, written essay, 2 letters of recommendation, minimum GPA in nursing prerequisites of 2.0, prerequisite course work. Transfer students are accepted. *Application deadline:* 3/1 (fall), 10/1 (spring), 12/15 (summer).
**Advanced Placement** Credit given for nursing courses completed elsewhere dependent upon specific evaluations.
**Financial Aid** 79% of baccalaureate students in nursing programs received some form of financial aid in 2012–13.
**Contact** Office of Student Support Services, College of Nursing, Michigan State University, Bott Building for Nursing Education & Research, 1355 Bogue Street, Room C120, East Lansing, MI 48824. *Telephone:* 517-353-4827. *Fax:* 517-432-8251. *E-mail:* nurse@hc.msu.edu.

## GRADUATE PROGRAMS

**Financial Aid** 85% of graduate students in nursing programs received some form of financial aid in 2012–13. 1 research assistantship with tuition reimbursement available (averaging $6,110 per year), 2 teaching assistantships with tuition reimbursements available (averaging $7,076 per year) were awarded.
**Contact** Ms. Nikki O'Brien, Program Advisor, College of Nursing, Michigan State University, Bott Building for Nursing Education and Research, 1355 Bogue Street, Room C120, East Lansing, MI 48824. *Telephone:* 517-353-4827. *Fax:* 517-432-8251. *E-mail:* obrienni@msu.edu.

### MASTER'S DEGREE PROGRAM

**Degree** MSN
**Available Programs** Master's.
**Concentrations Available** Nurse anesthesia. *Clinical nurse specialist programs in:* adult health. *Nurse practitioner programs in:* adult health, family health, gerontology.
**Study Options** Full-time and part-time.
**Online Degree Options** Yes.
**Program Entrance Requirements** Clinical experience, minimum overall college GPA of 3.0, transcript of college record, CPR certification, written essay, immunizations, interview, 3 letters of recommendation, prerequisite course work, resume, statistics course. *Application deadline:* 2/1 (fall), 3/15 (spring). Applications may be processed on a rolling basis for some programs.
**Advanced Placement** Credit given for nursing courses completed elsewhere dependent upon specific evaluations.
**Degree Requirements** Thesis or project.

### POST-MASTER'S PROGRAM

**Areas of Study** *Clinical nurse specialist programs in:* adult health. *Nurse practitioner programs in:* adult health, family health, gerontology.

### DOCTORAL DEGREE PROGRAM

**Degree** PhD
**Available Programs** Doctorate.
**Areas of Study** Advanced practice nursing.
**Program Entrance Requirements** Minimum overall college GPA of 3.0, clinical experience, interview by faculty committee, MSN or equivalent, statistics course, vita, writing sample. *Application deadline:* 5/2 (spring).
**Degree Requirements** 36 total credit hours, scholarly/synthesis project, oral presentation of project.

**Degree** PhD
**Available Programs** Doctorate; Post-Baccalaureate Doctorate.
**Areas of Study** Family health, gerontology, health promotion/disease prevention, human health and illness, individualized study, maternity-newborn, nursing research, oncology,women's health.
**Program Entrance Requirements** Minimum overall college GPA of 3.0, interview by faculty committee, interview, 3 letters of recommendation, statistics course, vita, writing sample. *Application deadline:* 12/1 (fall). Applications may be processed on a rolling basis for some programs.
**Degree Requirements** 72 total credit hours, dissertation, written exam, residency.

## CONTINUING EDUCATION PROGRAM

**Contact** Kathy Forrest, Instructor and Coordinator Professional Programs, College of Nursing, Michigan State University, Life Sciences Building, 1355 Bogue Street, Room A112, East Lansing, MI 48824. *Telephone:* 517-432-0393. *Fax:* 517-432-8131. *E-mail:* kathy.forrest@hc.msu.edu.

# Northern Michigan University

## College of Nursing and Allied Health Science
## Marquette, Michigan

*http://www.nmu.edu/nursing/*
Founded in 1899

### DEGREES • BSN • MSN

**Nursing Program Faculty** 16 (69% with doctorates).
**Baccalaureate Enrollment** 221 **Women** 81% **Men** 19% **Minority** 4% **Part-time** 7%
**Graduate Enrollment** 16 **Women** 81% **Men** 19% **Part-time** 100%
**Distance Learning Courses** Available.
**Nursing Student Activities** Sigma Theta Tau, Student Nurses' Association.
**Nursing Student Resources** Academic advising; academic or career counseling; assistance for students with disabilities; bookstore; campus computer network; career placement assistance; computer lab; computer-assisted instruction; e-mail services; employment services for current students; housing assistance; interactive nursing skills videos; Internet; learning resource lab; library services; nursing audiovisuals; other; paid internships; remedial services; resume preparation assistance; skills, simulation, or other laboratory; tutoring.
**Library Facilities** 32,879 volumes in health, 2,733 volumes in nursing; 5,000 periodical subscriptions health-care related.

## BACCALAUREATE PROGRAMS

**Degree** BSN
**Available Programs** Accelerated Baccalaureate; Generic Baccalaureate; LPN to Baccalaureate; RN Baccalaureate.
**Study Options** Full-time.
**Program Entrance Requirements** Minimum overall college GPA of 2.75, transcript of college record, CPR certification, health exam, high school transcript, immunizations, minimum GPA in nursing prerequisites of 2.0, prerequisite course work. Transfer students are accepted. *Application deadline:* 2/1 (fall), 10/1 (winter).
**Advanced Placement** Credit by examination available. Credit given for nursing courses completed elsewhere dependent upon specific evaluations.
**Contact** *Telephone:* 906-227-2834. *Fax:* 906-227-1658.

## GRADUATE PROGRAMS

**Contact** *Telephone:* 906-227-2488. *Fax:* 906-227-1658.

### MASTER'S DEGREE PROGRAM

**Degree** MSN
**Available Programs** Master's.
**Concentrations Available** *Nurse practitioner programs in:* family health.
**Study Options** Part-time.
**Program Entrance Requirements** Clinical experience, computer literacy, minimum overall college GPA of 3.0, transcript of college record, CPR certification, written essay, immunizations, 2 letters of recommendation, physical assessment course, professional liability insurance/malpractice insurance, GRE General Test. *Application deadline:* 2/1 (fall).
**Advanced Placement** Credit given for nursing courses completed elsewhere dependent upon specific evaluations.
**Degree Requirements** 45 total credit hours, thesis or project, comprehensive exam.

### POST-MASTER'S PROGRAM

**Areas of Study** *Nurse practitioner programs in:* family health.

## CONTINUING EDUCATION PROGRAM

**Contact** *Telephone:* 906-227-2044. *Fax:* 906-227-2928.

# Oakland University

## School of Nursing
## Rochester, Michigan

*http://www.oakland.edu/*
Founded in 1957

**DEGREES • BSN • MSN**

**Nursing Program Faculty** 44 (50% with doctorates).
**Baccalaureate Enrollment** 462 **Women** 89% **Men** 11% **Minority** 12% **Part-time** 29%
**Graduate Enrollment** 123 **Women** 79% **Men** 21% **Minority** 11% **International** 1% **Part-time** 35%
**Nursing Student Activities** Nursing Honor Society, Sigma Theta Tau, Student Nurses' Association.
**Nursing Student Resources** Academic advising; academic or career counseling; assistance for students with disabilities; bookstore; campus computer network; career placement assistance; computer lab; computer-assisted instruction; e-mail services; employment services for current students; externships; housing assistance; interactive nursing skills videos; Internet; learning resource lab; library services; nursing audiovisuals; paid internships; placement services for program completers; remedial services; resume preparation assistance; skills, simulation, or other laboratory; tutoring; unpaid internships.
**Library Facilities** 826,421 volumes (12,652 in health, 2,780 in nursing); 20,610 periodical subscriptions (375 health-care related).

## BACCALAUREATE PROGRAMS

**Degree** BSN
**Available Programs** Generic Baccalaureate; RN Baccalaureate.
**Site Options** Royal Oak, MI.
**Study Options** Full-time and part-time.
**Program Entrance Requirements** Minimum overall college GPA of 3.0, transcript of college record, CPR certification, health exam, high school biology, high school chemistry, 2 years high school math, 1 year of high school science, high school transcript, immunizations, minimum high school GPA of 3.0, minimum GPA in nursing prerequisites of 3.0, professional liability insurance/malpractice insurance, prerequisite course work. Transfer students are accepted.
**Advanced Placement** Credit given for nursing courses completed elsewhere dependent upon specific evaluations.
**Contact** *Telephone:* 248-370-4065. *Fax:* 248-370-4279.

## GRADUATE PROGRAMS

**Contact** *Telephone:* 248-370-4082. *Fax:* 248-370-2996.

### MASTER'S DEGREE PROGRAM

**Degree** MSN
**Available Programs** Master's.
**Concentrations Available** Nurse anesthesia; nursing education. *Nurse practitioner programs in:* adult health, family health, gerontology.
**Site Options** Royal Oak, MI.
**Study Options** Full-time and part-time.
**Program Entrance Requirements** Clinical experience, minimum overall college GPA of 3.0, transcript of college record, CPR certification, written essay, immunizations, interview, 2 letters of recommendation, professional liability insurance/malpractice insurance, prerequisite course work, GRE General Test.
**Advanced Placement** Credit given for nursing courses completed elsewhere dependent upon specific evaluations.
**Degree Requirements** 45 total credit hours, thesis or project.

### POST-MASTER'S PROGRAM

**Areas of Study** Nurse anesthesia; nursing education. *Nurse practitioner programs in:* adult health, family health, gerontology.

## CONTINUING EDUCATION PROGRAM

**Contact** *Telephone:* 248-370-4013. *Fax:* 248-370-4279.

# The Robert B. Miller College

## School of Nursing
## Battle Creek, Michigan

**DEGREE • BSN**

## BACCALAUREATE PROGRAMS

**Degree** BSN
**Available Programs** RN Baccalaureate.
**Study Options** Full-time and part-time.
**Program Entrance Requirements** Minimum overall college GPA of 2.5, RN licensure.
**Contact** Nursing Program, School of Nursing, The Robert B. Miller College, 450 North Avenue, Battle Creek, MI 49017-3397. *Telephone:* 269-660-8021. *Fax:* 269-565-2180. *E-mail:* info@millercollege.edu.

# Rochester College

## School of Nursing
## Rochester Hills, Michigan

*http://www.rc.edu*
Founded in 1959

**DEGREE • BSN**

**Baccalaureate Enrollment** 42
**Distance Learning Courses** Available.
**Nursing Student Resources** Academic advising; academic or career counseling; assistance for students with disabilities; bookstore; campus computer network; career placement assistance; computer lab; computer-assisted instruction; e-mail services; externships; housing assistance; interactive nursing skills videos; Internet; learning resource lab; library services; nursing audiovisuals; remedial services; resume preparation assistance; skills, simulation, or other laboratory; tutoring; unpaid internships.
**Library Facilities** 55,000 volumes; 200 periodical subscriptions.

## BACCALAUREATE PROGRAMS

**Degree** BSN
**Available Programs** Generic Baccalaureate; RN Baccalaureate.
**Study Options** Full-time.
**Program Entrance Requirements** Minimum overall college GPA of 3.0, transcript of college record, written essay, interview, minimum GPA in nursing prerequisites of 3.0, prerequisite course work. Transfer students are accepted. *Application deadline:* 6/1 (fall).
**Expenses (2012–13)** *Tuition:* full-time $8000; part-time $500 per credit. *Room and board:* $8000 per academic year. *Required fees:* full-time $300.
**Financial Aid** 75% of baccalaureate students in nursing programs received some form of financial aid in 2011–12. *Gift aid (need-based):* Federal Pell, FSEOG, state, private, college/university gift aid from institutional funds. *Loans:* Federal Direct (Subsidized and Unsubsidized Stafford PLUS), Perkins. *Work-study:* Federal Work-Study, part-time campus jobs. *Financial aid application deadline:* Continuous.
**Contact** Mrs. Jaime M. Sinutko, Director of Nursing, School of Nursing, Rochester College, 800 West Avon Road, Rochester Hills, MI 48085. *Telephone:* 248-218-2283. *E-mail:* jsinutko@rc.edu.

# Saginaw Valley State University

## College of Health and Human Services
## University Center, Michigan

*http://www.svsu.edu/collegeofhealthhumanservices*
Founded in 1963

**DEGREES • BSN • DNP • MSN**

**Nursing Program Faculty** 18 (50% with doctorates).
**Baccalaureate Enrollment** 384 **Women** 80% **Men** 20%
**Graduate Enrollment** 95 **Women** 92% **Men** 8% **Part-time** 100%
**Nursing Student Activities** Sigma Theta Tau, Student Nurses' Association.
**Nursing Student Resources** Academic advising; academic or career counseling; assistance for students with disabilities; bookstore; campus computer network; career placement assistance; computer lab; computer-assisted instruction; e-mail services; employment services for current stu-

dents; externships; interactive nursing skills videos; Internet; learning resource lab; library services; nursing audiovisuals; remedial services; resume preparation assistance; skills, simulation, or other laboratory; tutoring.
**Library Facilities** 364,160 volumes; 48,336 periodical subscriptions.

## BACCALAUREATE PROGRAMS

**Degree** BSN
**Available Programs** ADN to Baccalaureate; Accelerated Baccalaureate for Second Degree; Baccalaureate for Second Degree; Generic Baccalaureate; RN Baccalaureate.
**Study Options** Full-time and part-time.
**Program Entrance Requirements** Minimum overall college GPA of 2.5, transcript of college record, CPR certification, health exam, immunizations, interview, minimum GPA in nursing prerequisites of 2.5, professional liability insurance/malpractice insurance, prerequisite course work. Transfer students are accepted. *Application deadline:* 4/15 (fall), 10/15 (winter).
**Advanced Placement** Credit by examination available. Credit given for nursing courses completed elsewhere dependent upon specific evaluations.
**Expenses (2012–13)** *Tuition, state resident:* full-time $6145. *Tuition, nonresident:* full-time $14,900. *Required fees:* full-time $200.
**Financial Aid** ***Gift aid (need-based):*** Federal Pell, FSEOG, state, private, college/university gift aid from institutional funds. *Loans:* Federal Direct (Subsidized and Unsubsidized Stafford PLUS), CitiAssist Loans, Chase Select loans, Charter One TruFit Student Loans. *Work-study:* Federal Work-Study, part-time campus jobs. *Financial aid application deadline (priority):* 2/14.
**Contact** Dr. Sally Decker, Nursing Department Chair, College of Health and Human Services, Saginaw Valley State University, 7400 Bay Road, H 226, University Center, MI 48710-0001. *Telephone:* 989-964-4098. *Fax:* 989-964-4925. *E-mail:* decker@svsu.edu.

## GRADUATE PROGRAMS

**Expenses (2012–13)** *Tuition, state resident:* full-time $7420. *Tuition, nonresident:* full-time $14,165. *Required fees:* full-time $800.
**Financial Aid** Federal Work-Study and scholarships available.
**Contact** Dr. Karen Brown-Fackler, MSN Coordinator, College of Health and Human Services, Saginaw Valley State University, 7400 Bay Road, H 219, University Center, MI 48710-0001. *Telephone:* 989-964-2185. *Fax:* 989-964-4925. *E-mail:* kmbrown4@svsu.edu.

### MASTER'S DEGREE PROGRAM

**Degree** MSN
**Available Programs** Accelerated AD/RN to Master's; Master's; RN to Master's.
**Concentrations Available** Clinical nurse leader; nursing administration; nursing education. *Clinical nurse specialist programs in:* family health. *Nurse practitioner programs in:* family health.
**Site Options** Gaylord, MI.
**Study Options** Part-time.
**Program Entrance Requirements** Clinical experience, minimum overall college GPA of 3.0, transcript of college record, CPR certification, written essay, immunizations, interview, 3 letters of recommendation, professional liability insurance/malpractice insurance, resume, statistics course, GRE. *Application deadline:* Applications may be processed on a rolling basis for some programs.
**Advanced Placement** Credit given for nursing courses completed elsewhere dependent upon specific evaluations.
**Degree Requirements** 39 total credit hours, thesis or project.

### POST-MASTER'S PROGRAM

**Areas of Study** Nursing administration; nursing education.

### DOCTORAL DEGREE PROGRAM

**Degree** DNP
**Available Programs** Doctorate.
**Program Entrance Requirements** Interview, letters of recommendation, vita. *Application deadline:* Applications may be processed on a rolling basis for some programs.

## CONTINUING EDUCATION PROGRAM

**Contact** CE Coordinator, College of Health and Human Services, Saginaw Valley State University, 7400 Bay Road, University Center, MI 48710-0001. *Telephone:* 989-964-4595. *Fax:* 989-964-4925.

# Siena Heights University

## Nursing Program
## Adrian, Michigan

*http://www.sienaheights.edu/*
Founded in 1919

### DEGREE • BSN

**Nursing Program Faculty** 7 (10% with doctorates).
**Baccalaureate Enrollment** 80 **Women** 87% **Men** 13% **Minority** 5% **International** 5% **Part-time** 48%
**Distance Learning Courses** Available.
**Nursing Student Activities** Student Nurses' Association.
**Nursing Student Resources** Academic advising; academic or career counseling; bookstore; campus computer network; career placement assistance; computer lab; computer-assisted instruction; e-mail services; interactive nursing skills videos; Internet; learning resource lab; library services; nursing audiovisuals; skills, simulation, or other laboratory; tutoring.
**Library Facilities** 200 volumes in health, 80 volumes in nursing; 150 periodical subscriptions health-care related.

## BACCALAUREATE PROGRAMS

**Degree** BSN
**Available Programs** Generic Baccalaureate; RN Baccalaureate.
**Site Options** Monroe, MI.
**Study Options** Full-time.
**Program Entrance Requirements** Minimum overall college GPA of 3.0, transcript of college record, CPR certification, written essay, health exam, health insurance, high school transcript, immunizations, interview, minimum GPA in nursing prerequisites of 3.0, professional liability insurance/malpractice insurance, prerequisite course work. Transfer students are accepted. *Application deadline:* 10/1 (fall).
**Expenses (2013–14)** *Tuition:* full-time $21,250; part-time $440 per credit hour. *International tuition:* $23,450 full-time. *Room and board:* $8710; room only: $4200 per academic year. *Required fees:* full-time $1120; part-time $260 per term.
**Financial Aid** 90% of baccalaureate students in nursing programs received some form of financial aid in 2012–13.
**Contact** Mrs. Trudy Mohre, Director of Admissions, Nursing Program, Siena Heights University, 1247 East Siena Heights Drive, Adrian, MI 49221. *Telephone:* 517-264-7180. *E-mail:* tmohre@sienaheighs.edu.

# Spring Arbor University

## Program in Nursing
## Spring Arbor, Michigan

*http://www.arbor.edu/bsn*
Founded in 1873

### DEGREES • BSN • MSN • MSN/MBA

**Nursing Program Faculty** 19 (26% with doctorates).
**Baccalaureate Enrollment** 217 **Women** 89% **Men** 11% **Minority** 7%
**Graduate Enrollment** 80 **Women** 92% **Men** 8% **Minority** 5%
**Distance Learning Courses** Available.
**Nursing Student Resources** Academic advising; academic or career counseling; assistance for students with disabilities; bookstore; campus computer network; career placement assistance; computer lab; computer-assisted instruction; e-mail services; Internet; library services; nursing audiovisuals; other; tutoring.
**Library Facilities** 115,987 volumes (1,000 in health, 350 in nursing); 523 periodical subscriptions (52 health-care related).

## BACCALAUREATE PROGRAMS

**Degree** BSN
**Available Programs** ADN to Baccalaureate.
**Site Options** Battle Creek, MI; Gaylord, MI; Jackson, MI; Flint, MI; Traverse City, MI; Southfield, MI; Grand Rapids, MI; Lambertville, MI; Lansing, MI; Kalamazoo, MI.
**Program Entrance Requirements** Minimum overall college GPA of 2.5, transcript of college record, written essay, high school biology, high school chemistry, 1 year of high school math, 2 years high school science, high school transcript, minimum GPA in nursing prerequisites of 2.5, RN licensure. Transfer students are accepted. *Application deadline:* Applications may be processed on a rolling basis for some programs.

**Financial Aid** 85% of baccalaureate students in nursing programs received some form of financial aid in 2012–13. *Gift aid (need-based):* Federal Pell, FSEOG, private, college/university gift aid from institutional funds. *Loans:* Federal Direct (Subsidized and Unsubsidized Stafford PLUS), Perkins. *Work-study:* Federal Work-Study. *Financial aid application deadline (priority):* 3/1.
**Contact** Mr. Alvin V. Kauffman, Director of Nursing, Program in Nursing, Spring Arbor University, 106 East Main Street, Suite #3, Spring Arbor, MI 49283-9799. *Telephone:* 517-750-6579. *Fax:* 517-750-6602. *E-mail:* alvin.kauffman@arbor.edu.

### GRADUATE PROGRAMS

**Financial Aid** 67% of graduate students in nursing programs received some form of financial aid in 2012–13.
**Contact** Mr. Dale Glinz, Lead Recruitment Specialist, Program in Nursing, Spring Arbor University, 106 East Main Street, Station 30, Spring Arbor, MI 49283. *Telephone:* 800-968-0011 Ext. 1703. *Fax:* 517-750-6799. *E-mail:* dglinz@arbor.edu.

#### MASTER'S DEGREE PROGRAM

**Degrees** MSN; MSN/MBA
**Available Programs** Master's.
**Concentrations Available** Nursing education. *Nurse practitioner programs in:* adult health, gerontology.
**Study Options** Full-time.
**Online Degree Options** Yes (online only).
**Program Entrance Requirements** Minimum overall college GPA of 3.0, transcript of college record, written essay, interview, 2 letters of recommendation, nursing research course, prerequisite course work, statistics course. *Application deadline:* 7/1 (fall), 1/5 (spring). *Application fee:* $30.
**Degree Requirements** 54 total credit hours, thesis or project.

## University of Detroit Mercy
### McAuley School of Nursing
### Detroit, Michigan

*http://www.udmercy.edu/healthprof/nursing/*
Founded in 1877

**DEGREES • BSN • MSN**
**Nursing Program Faculty** 80
**Baccalaureate Enrollment** 933 **Women** 88% **Men** 12% **Minority** 24% **International** 6% **Part-time** 46%
**Graduate Enrollment** 132 **Women** 95% **Men** 5% **Minority** 27% **International** 2% **Part-time** 96%
**Distance Learning Courses** Available.
**Nursing Student Activities** Sigma Theta Tau, Student Nurses' Association.
**Nursing Student Resources** Academic advising; academic or career counseling; bookstore; campus computer network; career placement assistance; computer lab; computer-assisted instruction; e-mail services; Internet; learning resource lab; library services; nursing audiovisuals; other; paid internships; placement services for program completers; remedial services; resume preparation assistance; skills, simulation, or other laboratory; tutoring.
**Library Facilities** 32,330 volumes in health, 3,404 volumes in nursing; 2,670 periodical subscriptions health-care related.

### BACCALAUREATE PROGRAMS

**Degree** BSN
**Available Programs** Accelerated Baccalaureate for Second Degree; Generic Baccalaureate; RN Baccalaureate.
**Site Options** Dearborn, MI; Grand Rapids, MI; Wayne, MI.
**Study Options** Full-time and part-time.
**Program Entrance Requirements** Minimum overall college GPA of 2.5, transcript of college record, CPR certification, health exam, health insurance, high school biology, high school chemistry, 2 years high school math, 2 years high school science, high school transcript, immunizations, minimum high school GPA of 2.5, minimum GPA in nursing prerequisites of 2.5, prerequisite course work. Transfer students are accepted.
**Advanced Placement** Credit given for nursing courses completed elsewhere dependent upon specific evaluations.
**Contact** *Telephone:* 313-993-1245. *Fax:* 313-993-3325.

### GRADUATE PROGRAMS

**Contact** *Telephone:* 313-993-6423. *Fax:* 313-993-6175.

#### MASTER'S DEGREE PROGRAM

**Degree** MSN
**Available Programs** Accelerated AD/RN to Master's; Master's; Master's for Nurses with Non-Nursing Degrees.
**Concentrations Available** Nursing administration; nursing education. *Nurse practitioner programs in:* family health.
**Study Options** Full-time and part-time.
**Program Entrance Requirements** Clinical experience, minimum overall college GPA of 3.0, transcript of college record, CPR certification, immunizations, interview, 3 letters of recommendation, resume.
**Degree Requirements** 50 total credit hours.

#### POST-MASTER'S PROGRAM

**Areas of Study** Nursing administration; nursing education. *Nurse practitioner programs in:* family health.

## University of Michigan
### School of Nursing
### Ann Arbor, Michigan

*http://www.nursing.umich.edu/*
Founded in 1817

**DEGREES • BSN • MS • MSN/MBA • MSN/MPH • PHD**
**Nursing Program Faculty** 130 (66% with doctorates).
**Baccalaureate Enrollment** 618 **Women** 90% **Men** 10% **Minority** 20% **International** 3% **Part-time** 13%
**Graduate Enrollment** 240 **Women** 95% **Men** 5% **Minority** 30% **International** 11% **Part-time** 40%
**Distance Learning Courses** Available.
**Nursing Student Activities** Nursing Honor Society, Sigma Theta Tau, Student Nurses' Association, nursing club.
**Nursing Student Resources** Academic advising; academic or career counseling; assistance for students with disabilities; bookstore; campus computer network; career placement assistance; computer lab; computer-assisted instruction; daycare for children of students; e-mail services; employment services for current students; externships; housing assistance; interactive nursing skills videos; Internet; learning resource lab; library services; nursing audiovisuals; paid internships; placement services for program completers; remedial services; resume preparation assistance; skills, simulation, or other laboratory; tutoring; unpaid internships.
**Library Facilities** 11.5 million volumes (1.2 million in nursing); 134,359 periodical subscriptions.

### BACCALAUREATE PROGRAMS

**Degree** BSN
**Available Programs** Accelerated Baccalaureate for Second Degree; Generic Baccalaureate; RN Baccalaureate.
**Site Options** Kalamazoo, MI; Traverse City, MI.
**Study Options** Full-time and part-time.
**Program Entrance Requirements** Minimum overall college GPA of 3.0, transcript of college record, written essay, high school chemistry, 2 years high school math, 2 years high school science, high school transcript, minimum high school GPA of 3.0, prerequisite course work. Transfer students are accepted. *Application deadline:* 2/1 (fall). Applications may be processed on a rolling basis for some programs. *Application fee:* $80.
**Advanced Placement** Credit given for nursing courses completed elsewhere dependent upon specific evaluations.
**Contact** *Telephone:* 734-647-1443. *Fax:* 734-936-0740.

### GRADUATE PROGRAMS

**Contact** *Telephone:* 734-764-7188. *Fax:* 734-647-1419.

#### MASTER'S DEGREE PROGRAM

**Degrees** MS; MSN/MBA; MSN/MPH
**Available Programs** Accelerated RN to Master's; Master's; RN to Master's.
**Concentrations Available** Health-care administration; nurse-midwifery; nursing administration; nursing informatics. *Clinical nurse specialist programs in:* community health, gerontology, home health care, medical-surgical, occupational health, psychiatric/mental health. *Nurse*

*practitioner programs in:* acute care, adult health, family health, gerontology, pediatric, primary care, psychiatric/mental health.
**Study Options** Full-time and part-time.
**Program Entrance Requirements** Computer literacy, minimum overall college GPA of 3.0, transcript of college record, written essay, interview, 3 letters of recommendation, resume. *Application deadline:* 2/1 (fall). Applications may be processed on a rolling basis for some programs. *Application fee:* $80.
**Advanced Placement** Credit given for nursing courses completed elsewhere dependent upon specific evaluations.
**Degree Requirements** 37 total credit hours, thesis or project.

### POST-MASTER'S PROGRAM

**Areas of Study** Health-care administration; nurse-midwifery; nursing administration; nursing informatics. *Clinical nurse specialist programs in:* community health, gerontology, home health care, medical-surgical, occupational health, psychiatric/mental health,women's health. *Nurse practitioner programs in:* acute care, adult health, family health, gerontology, pediatric, primary care, psychiatric/mental health,women's health.

### DOCTORAL DEGREE PROGRAM

**Degree** PhD
**Available Programs** Doctorate; Post-Baccalaureate Doctorate.
**Areas of Study** Advanced practice nursing, aging, bio-behavioral research, biology of health and illness, community health, critical care, ethics, family health, gerontology, health policy, health promotion/disease prevention, health-care systems, individualized study, information systems, neuro-behavior, nursing administration, nursing policy, nursing research, nursing science,women's health.
**Program Entrance Requirements** Minimum overall college GPA of 3.0, interview, 3 letters of recommendation, scholarly papers, vita, writing sample. *Application deadline:* 12/11 (fall). *Application fee:* $80.
**Degree Requirements** 50 total credit hours, dissertation, oral exam, written exam, residency.

### POSTDOCTORAL PROGRAM

**Areas of Study** Addiction/substance abuse, aging, chronic illness, community health, family health, gerontology, health promotion/disease prevention, individualized study, information systems, neuro-behavior, nursing interventions, nursing research, nursing science, vulnerable population,women's health.
**Postdoctoral Program Contact***Telephone:* 734-764-9454. *Fax:* 734-763-6668.

## University of Michigan–Flint

**Department of Nursing**
**Flint, Michigan**

***http://www.umflint.edu/nursing***
Founded in 1956

### DEGREES • BSN • DNP • MSN

**Nursing Program Faculty** 103 (19% with doctorates).
**Baccalaureate Enrollment** 904 **Women** 84.96% **Men** 15.04% **Minority** 17.04% **International** 1% **Part-time** 74.56%
**Graduate Enrollment** 252 **Women** 81.35% **Men** 18.65% **Minority** 17.06% **International** 1.59% **Part-time** 46.43%
**Distance Learning Courses** Available.
**Nursing Student Activities** Nursing Honor Society, Sigma Theta Tau, Student Nurses' Association, nursing club.
**Nursing Student Resources** Academic advising; academic or career counseling; assistance for students with disabilities; bookstore; campus computer network; career placement assistance; computer lab; computer-assisted instruction; daycare for children of students; e-mail services; employment services for current students; externships; housing assistance; interactive nursing skills videos; Internet; library services; nursing audiovisuals; remedial services; resume preparation assistance; skills, simulation, or other laboratory; tutoring.
**Library Facilities** 353,617 volumes (16,552 in health, 1,709 in nursing); 559 periodical subscriptions (204 health-care related).

### BACCALAUREATE PROGRAMS

**Degree** BSN
**Available Programs** Accelerated Baccalaureate for Second Degree; RN Baccalaureate; RPN to Baccalaureate.
**Site Options** Flint, MI; Lansing, MI; Detroit, MI; Alpena Community College/Alpena, MI.
**Study Options** Full-time.
**Online Degree Options** Yes.
**Program Entrance Requirements** Minimum overall college GPA of 3.0, transcript of college record, CPR certification, written essay, health exam, health insurance, immunizations, 2 letters of recommendation, minimum high school GPA of 3.0, minimum GPA in nursing prerequisites of 3.0, prerequisite course work. Transfer students are accepted. *Application deadline:* 1/10 (fall), 9/1 (winter). *Application fee:* $30.
**Advanced Placement** Credit by examination available. Credit given for nursing courses completed elsewhere dependent upon specific evaluations.
**Expenses (2013–14)** *Tuition, state resident:* full-time $10,584. *Tuition, nonresident:* full-time $21,156. *International tuition:* $21,156 full-time. *Room and board:* $7703 per academic year. *Required fees:* full-time $548.
**Financial Aid** 75% of baccalaureate students in nursing programs received some form of financial aid in 2012–13.
**Contact** Ms. Laura Martin, Senior Secretary, Department of Nursing, University of Michigan–Flint, 303 East Kearsley Street, 2102 William S. White, Flint, MI 48502-1950. *Telephone:* 810-762-3420. *Fax:* 810-766-6851. *E-mail:* lmart@umflint.edu.

### GRADUATE PROGRAMS

**Expenses (2013–14)** *Tuition, state resident:* full-time $7984. *Tuition, nonresident:* full-time $11,968. *International tuition:* $11,968 full-time. *Room and board:* $7703 per academic year. *Required fees:* full-time $418.
**Financial Aid** 65% of graduate students in nursing programs received some form of financial aid in 2012–13.
**Contact** Ms. Laura Martin, Senior Secretary, Department of Nursing, University of Michigan–Flint, 303 East Kearsley Street, 2102 William S. White, Flint, MI 48502-1950. *Telephone:* 810-762-3420. *Fax:* 810-766-6851. *E-mail:* lmartin@umflint.edu.

### MASTER'S DEGREE PROGRAM

**Degree** MSN
**Available Programs** Accelerated RN to Master's; RN to Master's.
**Concentrations Available** Nurse anesthesia. *Nurse practitioner programs in:* adult health.
**Site Options** Flint, MI.
**Study Options** Full-time.
**Online Degree Options** Yes.
**Program Entrance Requirements** Minimum overall college GPA of 3.2, transcript of college record, written essay, 3 letters of recommendation, resume, statistics course. *Application deadline:* 8/1 (fall), 10/1 (winter). *Application fee:* $55.
**Advanced Placement** Credit by examination available. Credit given for nursing courses completed elsewhere dependent upon specific evaluations.
**Degree Requirements** 43 total credit hours.

### DOCTORAL DEGREE PROGRAM

**Degree** DNP
**Available Programs** Doctorate.
**Areas of Study** Advanced practice nursing, family health, gerontology.
**Site Options** Flint, MI.
**Online Degree Options** Yes (online only).
**Program Entrance Requirements** Clinical experience, minimum overall college GPA of 3.2, interview, 3 letters of recommendation, statistics course, vita, writing sample. *Application deadline:* 3/1 (fall). *Application fee:* $55.
**Degree Requirements** 37 total credit hours.

## Wayne State University

**College of Nursing**
**Detroit, Michigan**

***http://www.nursing.wayne.edu/***
Founded in 1868

### DEGREES • BSN • DNP • MSN

**Nursing Program Faculty** 92 (51% with doctorates).
**Baccalaureate Enrollment** 249 **Women** 77% **Men** 23% **Minority** 21% **International** 1% **Part-time** 12%
**Graduate Enrollment** 420 **Women** 92% **Men** 8% **Minority** 27% **International** 6% **Part-time** 67%
**Distance Learning Courses** Available.

**Nursing Student Activities** Nursing Honor Society, Sigma Theta Tau, Student Nurses' Association, nursing club.

**Nursing Student Resources** Academic advising; academic or career counseling; assistance for students with disabilities; bookstore; campus computer network; career placement assistance; computer lab; computer-assisted instruction; e-mail services; employment services for current students; interactive nursing skills videos; Internet; learning resource lab; library services; nursing audiovisuals; placement services for program completers; resume preparation assistance; skills, simulation, or other laboratory; tutoring.

**Library Facilities** 3.4 million volumes (156,000 in health, 6,600 in nursing); 71,737 periodical subscriptions (5,000 health-care related).

## BACCALAUREATE PROGRAMS

**Degree** BSN
**Available Programs** Accelerated Baccalaureate for Second Degree; Generic Baccalaureate.
**Study Options** Full-time and part-time.
**Program Entrance Requirements** Minimum overall college GPA of 2.0, transcript of college record, interview, minimum GPA in nursing prerequisites of 2.5, prerequisite course work. Transfer students are accepted. *Application deadline:* 3/31 (fall). *Application fee:* $50.
**Expenses (2013–14)** *Tuition, state resident:* full-time $19,739; part-time $617 per credit hour. *Tuition, nonresident:* full-time $35,718; part-time $1116 per credit hour. *International tuition:* $35,718 full-time. *Room and board:* $9269 per academic year. *Required fees:* full-time $1372.
**Financial Aid** 86% of baccalaureate students in nursing programs received some form of financial aid in 2012–13.
**Contact** Office of Student Affairs, College of Nursing, Wayne State University, 5557 Cass Avenue, Detroit, MI 48202. *Telephone:* 313-577-4082. *Fax:* 313-577-6949.

## GRADUATE PROGRAMS

**Expenses (2013–14)** *Tuition, state resident:* full-time $24,190; part-time $1007 per credit hour. *Tuition, nonresident:* full-time $39,490; part-time $1645 per credit hour. *International tuition:* $39,490 full-time. *Room and board:* $8989 per academic year. *Required fees:* full-time $1446.
**Financial Aid** 68% of graduate students in nursing programs received some form of financial aid in 2012–13. 1 fellowship with tuition reimbursement available (averaging $16,000 per year), 1 research assistantship with tuition reimbursement available (averaging $17,391 per year), 5 teaching assistantships with tuition reimbursements available (averaging $27,572 per year) were awarded; Federal Work-Study, institutionally sponsored loans, scholarships, traineeships, and unspecified assistantships also available. Aid available to part-time students.
**Contact** Office of Student Affairs, College of Nursing, Wayne State University, 5557 Cass Avenue, Detroit, MI 48202. *Telephone:* 313-577-4082. *Fax:* 313-577-6949.

### MASTER'S DEGREE PROGRAM

**Degree** MSN
**Available Programs** Master's.
**Concentrations Available** Nurse-midwifery. *Clinical nurse specialist programs in:* acute care, community health, critical care, psychiatric/mental health. *Nurse practitioner programs in:* acute care, gerontology, neonatal health, pediatric, primary care, psychiatric/mental health,women's health.
**Study Options** Full-time and part-time.
**Program Entrance Requirements** Minimum overall college GPA of 3.0, transcript of college record, written essay, 3 letters of recommendation, resume. *Application deadline:* 7/1 (fall), 11/1 (winter), 4/1 (spring), 4/1 (summer).
**Advanced Placement** Credit given for nursing courses completed elsewhere dependent upon specific evaluations.
**Degree Requirements** 47 total credit hours.

### POST-MASTER'S PROGRAM

**Areas of Study** Nurse-midwifery; nursing education. *Clinical nurse specialist programs in:* psychiatric/mental health. *Nurse practitioner programs in:* acute care, gerontology, pediatric, primary care, psychiatric/mental health,women's health.

### DOCTORAL DEGREE PROGRAM

**Degree** DNP
**Available Programs** Doctorate; Post-Baccalaureate Doctorate.
**Areas of Study** Advanced practice nursing, clinical practice.
**Program Entrance Requirements** Clinical experience, minimum overall college GPA of 3.0, interview by faculty committee, interview, 2 letters of recommendation, vita, writing sample, GRE General Test (for PhD applicants). *Application deadline:* 1/15 (fall). Applications may be processed on a rolling basis for some programs. *Application fee:* $50.
**Degree Requirements** 90 total credit hours, written exam, residency.

### POSTDOCTORAL PROGRAM

**Postdoctoral Program Contact** Mr. Dennis Ross, Academic Services Officer, College of Nursing, Wayne State University, 5557 Cass Avenue, Detroit, MI 48202. *Telephone:* 313-577-4082. *Fax:* 313-577-6949. *E-mail:* nursinginfo@wayne.edu.

# Western Michigan University

**College of Health and Human Services**
**Kalamazoo, Michigan**

Founded in 1903

**DEGREES • BSN • MSN**

**Nursing Program Faculty** 38 (26% with doctorates).
**Baccalaureate Enrollment** 383 **Women** 85% **Men** 15% **Minority** 11% **International** 1% **Part-time** 21%
**Graduate Enrollment** 7 **Women** 85% **Men** 15% **Minority** 15% **Part-time** 100%
**Nursing Student Activities** Sigma Theta Tau, Student Nurses' Association.
**Nursing Student Resources** Academic advising; academic or career counseling; assistance for students with disabilities; bookstore; campus computer network; career placement assistance; computer lab; computer-assisted instruction; daycare for children of students; e-mail services; employment services for current students; externships; housing assistance; interactive nursing skills videos; Internet; learning resource lab; library services; nursing audiovisuals; placement services for program completers; remedial services; resume preparation assistance; skills, simulation, or other laboratory.
**Library Facilities** 2 million volumes (766 in nursing); 67,458 periodical subscriptions (362 health-care related).

## BACCALAUREATE PROGRAMS

**Degree** BSN
**Available Programs** ADN to Baccalaureate; Generic Baccalaureate.
**Site Options** St. Joseph, MI.
**Study Options** Full-time and part-time.
**Program Entrance Requirements** Minimum overall college GPA of 3.0, transcript of college record, CPR certification, high school biology, high school chemistry, 3 years high school math, 3 years high school science, high school transcript, immunizations, minimum high school GPA of 3.0, minimum GPA in nursing prerequisites of 3.0, prerequisite course work. Transfer students are accepted. *Application deadline:* Applications may be processed on a rolling basis for some programs. *Application fee:* $35.
**Advanced Placement** Credit given for nursing courses completed elsewhere dependent upon specific evaluations.
**Contact** *Telephone:* 269-387-8150. *Fax:* 269-387-8170.

## GRADUATE PROGRAMS

**Contact** *Telephone:* 269-387-8162.

### MASTER'S DEGREE PROGRAM

**Degree** MSN
**Available Programs** Master's.
**Concentrations Available** Nursing administration; nursing education.
**Site Options** St. Joseph, MI.
**Study Options** Part-time.
**Program Entrance Requirements** Minimum overall college GPA of 3.4, transcript of college record, interview, 3 letters of recommendation, resume. *Application deadline:* Applications may be processed on a rolling basis for some programs. *Application fee:* $40.
**Degree Requirements** 36 total credit hours, thesis or project, comprehensive exam.

## CONTINUING EDUCATION PROGRAM

**Contact** *Telephone:* 269-387-8150.

# MINNESOTA

## Augsburg College

### Program in Nursing
### Minneapolis, Minnesota

***http://www.augsburg.edu/nursing***
Founded in 1869

**DEGREES • BS • MA**

**Nursing Program Faculty** 9 (50% with doctorates).
**Baccalaureate Enrollment** 169 **Women** 83% **Men** 17% **Part-time** 89%
**Graduate Enrollment** 42 **Women** 100% **Minority** 2% **Part-time** 90%
**Nursing Student Resources** Academic advising; academic or career counseling; assistance for students with disabilities; bookstore; campus computer network; computer lab; computer-assisted instruction; e-mail services; Internet; library services; tutoring.
**Library Facilities** 146,433 volumes (1,550 in health, 200 in nursing); 754 periodical subscriptions (70 health-care related).

#### BACCALAUREATE PROGRAMS

**Degree** BS
**Available Programs** ADN to Baccalaureate.
**Site Options** Rochester, MN; Saint Paul, MN.
**Study Options** Full-time and part-time.
**Program Entrance Requirements** Minimum overall college GPA of 2.5, transcript of college record, CPR certification, written essay, high school transcript, immunizations, letters of recommendation, prerequisite course work, RN licensure. Transfer students are accepted.
**Contact** *Telephone:* 612-330-1101. *Fax:* 612-330-1784.

#### GRADUATE PROGRAMS

**Contact** *Telephone:* 612-330-1101. *Fax:* 612-330-1784.

**MASTER'S DEGREE PROGRAM**
**Degree** MA
**Available Programs** Master's.
**Concentrations Available** *Clinical nurse specialist programs in:* community health.
**Site Options** Rochester, MN; Saint Paul, MN.
**Study Options** Full-time and part-time.
**Program Entrance Requirements** Computer literacy, minimum overall college GPA of 3.0, transcript of college record, written essay, immunizations, 3 letters of recommendation, prerequisite course work, statistics course.
**Advanced Placement** Credit given for nursing courses completed elsewhere dependent upon specific evaluations.
**Degree Requirements** 48 total credit hours, thesis or project.

## Bemidji State University

### Department of Nursing
### Bemidji, Minnesota

***http://www.bemidjistate.edu/academics/departments/nursing/***
Founded in 1919

**DEGREE • BS**

**Nursing Program Faculty** 5 (60% with doctorates).
**Baccalaureate Enrollment** 62 **Women** 95% **Men** 5% **Minority** 3% **Part-time** 68%
**Distance Learning Courses** Available.
**Nursing Student Resources** Academic advising; academic or career counseling; assistance for students with disabilities; bookstore; campus computer network; career placement assistance; computer lab; computer-assisted instruction; daycare for children of students; e-mail services; employment services for current students; housing assistance; Internet; library services; nursing audiovisuals; remedial services; tutoring.
**Library Facilities** 9,000 volumes in health, 1,000 volumes in nursing; 300 periodical subscriptions health-care related.

#### BACCALAUREATE PROGRAMS

**Degree** BS
**Available Programs** Generic Baccalaureate; RN Baccalaureate.
**Study Options** Full-time and part-time.
**Program Entrance Requirements** Minimum overall college GPA, transcript of college record, immunizations, professional liability insurance/malpractice insurance, RN licensure. Transfer students are accepted.
**Contact** *Telephone:* 218-755-3892. *Fax:* 218-755-4402.

#### CONTINUING EDUCATION PROGRAM

**Contact** *Telephone:* 218-755-3892. *Fax:* 218-755-4402.

## Bethel University

### Department of Nursing
### St. Paul, Minnesota

***http://cas.bethel.edu/academics/departments/nursing/***
Founded in 1871

**DEGREES • BSN • MA**

**Nursing Program Faculty** 36 (40% with doctorates).
**Baccalaureate Enrollment** 283 **Women** 93.6% **Men** 6.4% **Minority** 11%
**Graduate Enrollment** 66 **Women** 97% **Men** 3% **Minority** 9.1%
**Distance Learning Courses** Available.
**Nursing Student Activities** Sigma Theta Tau, nursing club.
**Nursing Student Resources** Academic advising; academic or career counseling; assistance for students with disabilities; bookstore; campus computer network; career placement assistance; computer lab; computer-assisted instruction; daycare for children of students; e-mail services; employment services for current students; interactive nursing skills videos; Internet; learning resource lab; library services; nursing audiovisuals; paid internships; placement services for program completers; remedial services; resume preparation assistance; skills, simulation, or other laboratory; tutoring.
**Library Facilities** 198,836 volumes (4,900 in nursing); 44,016 periodical subscriptions (1,006 health-care related).

#### BACCALAUREATE PROGRAMS

**Degree** BSN
**Available Programs** Generic Baccalaureate; RN Baccalaureate.
**Site Options** Brooklyn Park, MN.
**Study Options** Full-time and part-time.
**Program Entrance Requirements** Minimum overall college GPA of 2.5, transcript of college record, CPR certification, written essay, health exam, health insurance, high school transcript, immunizations, interview, 2 letters of recommendation, minimum GPA in nursing prerequisites of 2.5, professional liability insurance/malpractice insurance, prerequisite course work. Transfer students are accepted. *Application deadline:* 9/15 (fall).
**Advanced Placement** Credit given for nursing courses completed elsewhere dependent upon specific evaluations.
**Contact** *Telephone:* 651-638-6455. *Fax:* 651-635-1965.

#### GRADUATE PROGRAMS

**Contact** *Telephone:* 651-635-8080. *Fax:* 651-635-1965.

**MASTER'S DEGREE PROGRAM**
**Degree** MA
**Available Programs** Master's.
**Concentrations Available** Nursing administration; nursing education.
**Study Options** Full-time and part-time.
**Program Entrance Requirements** Clinical experience, computer literacy, minimum overall college GPA of 3.0, transcript of college record, written essay, immunizations, interview, 3 letters of recommendation, professional liability insurance/malpractice insurance, resume, statistics course, MAT. *Application deadline:* Applications may be processed on a rolling basis for some programs. *Application fee:* $25.
**Advanced Placement** Credit given for nursing courses completed elsewhere dependent upon specific evaluations.
**Degree Requirements** 43 total credit hours, thesis or project.

## Capella University
### Nursing Programs
### Minneapolis, Minnesota

Founded in 1993

**DEGREES • BSN • DNP • MSN**

#### BACCALAUREATE PROGRAMS

**Degree** BSN
**Available Programs** RN Baccalaureate.
**Program Entrance Requirements** RN licensure. *Application fee:* $50.
**Contact** Nursing Program, Nursing Programs, Capella University, 225 South 6th Street, 9th Floor, Minneapolis, MN 55402. *Telephone:* 866-283-7921. *Fax:* 612-337-5396.

#### GRADUATE PROGRAMS

**Contact** Nursing Program, Nursing Programs, Capella University, 225 South 6th Street, 9th Floor, Minneapolis, MN 55402. *Telephone:* 866-283-7921. *Fax:* 612-337-5396.

**MASTER'S DEGREE PROGRAM**
**Degree** MSN
**Available Programs** Accelerated RN to Master's; Master's.
**Concentrations Available** Nursing administration; nursing education. *Clinical nurse specialist programs in:* gerontology.
**Program Entrance Requirements** Minimum overall college GPA of 3.0. *Application fee:* $50.

**DOCTORAL DEGREE PROGRAM**
**Degree** DNP
**Available Programs** Doctorate.
**Areas of Study** Nursing administration.
**Program Entrance Requirements** Minimum overall college GPA of 3.0. *Application fee:* $50.

## College of Saint Benedict
### Department of Nursing
### Saint Joseph, Minnesota

*http://www.csbsju.edu/nursing/*
Founded in 1887

**DEGREE • BS**
**Nursing Program Faculty** 17 (50% with doctorates).
**Baccalaureate Enrollment** 162 **Women** 90% **Men** 10% **Minority** 8% **International** 1% **Part-time** 1%
**Nursing Student Activities** Nursing Honor Society, Sigma Theta Tau, Student Nurses' Association, nursing club.
**Nursing Student Resources** Academic advising; academic or career counseling; assistance for students with disabilities; bookstore; campus computer network; career placement assistance; computer lab; computer-assisted instruction; e-mail services; employment services for current students; interactive nursing skills videos; Internet; learning resource lab; library services; nursing audiovisuals; paid internships; placement services for program completers; remedial services; resume preparation assistance; skills, simulation, or other laboratory; tutoring; unpaid internships.
**Library Facilities** 647,908 volumes (7,300 in health, 700 in nursing); 43,129 periodical subscriptions (335 health-care related).

#### BACCALAUREATE PROGRAMS

**Degree** BS
**Available Programs** Generic Baccalaureate.
**Study Options** Full-time.
**Program Entrance Requirements** Transcript of college record, CPR certification, health exam, health insurance, immunizations, minimum GPA in nursing prerequisites of 2.75, professional liability insurance/malpractice insurance, prerequisite course work. *Application deadline:* 5/1 (fall).
**Advanced Placement** Credit given for nursing courses completed elsewhere dependent upon specific evaluations.
**Expenses (2013–14)** *Tuition:* full-time $37,926; part-time $350 per credit. *International tuition:* $37,926 full-time. *Room and board:* $9644 per academic year. *Required fees:* full-time $700.
**Financial Aid** 96% of baccalaureate students in nursing programs received some form of financial aid in 2012–13.
**Contact** Dr. Carie Ann Braun, Professor and Chair, Department of Nursing, College of Saint Benedict, 37 College Avenue South, St. Joseph, MN 56374. *Telephone:* 320-363-5223. *Fax:* 320-363-6099. *E-mail:* cbraun@csbsju.edu.

## The College of St. Scholastica
### Department of Nursing
### Duluth, Minnesota

*http://www.css.edu*
Founded in 1912

**DEGREES • BS • DNP • MA**
**Nursing Program Faculty** 36 (44% with doctorates).
**Baccalaureate Enrollment** 621 **Women** 88% **Men** 12% **Minority** 19% **International** 1% **Part-time** 39%
**Graduate Enrollment** 181 **Women** 91% **Men** 9% **Minority** 11% **International** 1% **Part-time** 57%
**Distance Learning Courses** Available.
**Nursing Student Activities** Sigma Theta Tau, Student Nurses' Association.
**Nursing Student Resources** Academic advising; academic or career counseling; assistance for students with disabilities; bookstore; campus computer network; career placement assistance; computer lab; computer-assisted instruction; e-mail services; Internet; learning resource lab; library services; nursing audiovisuals; paid internships; placement services for program completers; resume preparation assistance; skills, simulation, or other laboratory; tutoring; unpaid internships.
**Library Facilities** 124,652 volumes (7,280 in health, 1,150 in nursing); 54,961 periodical subscriptions (291 health-care related).

#### BACCALAUREATE PROGRAMS

**Degree** BS
**Available Programs** ADN to Baccalaureate; Accelerated Baccalaureate for Second Degree; Generic Baccalaureate.
**Site Options** St. Cloud, MN; Duluth, MN.
**Study Options** Full-time.
**Online Degree Options** Yes.
**Program Entrance Requirements** Minimum overall college GPA of 3.0, transcript of college record, CPR certification, health exam, health insurance, high school transcript, immunizations, minimum GPA in nursing prerequisites of 2.0, prerequisite course work. Transfer students are accepted. *Application deadline:* 9/20 (fall).
**Expenses (2013–14)** *Tuition:* full-time $30,208; part-time $943 per credit. *Room and board:* $8040; room only: $4088 per academic year. *Required fees:* full-time $320; part-time $160 per term.
**Financial Aid** 98% of baccalaureate students in nursing programs received some form of financial aid in 2012–13. *Gift aid (need-based):* Federal Pell, FSEOG, state, private, college/university gift aid from institutional funds. *Loans:* Federal Nursing Student Loans, Federal Direct (Subsidized and Unsubsidized Stafford PLUS), Perkins, state, private loans. *Work-study:* Federal Work-Study, part-time campus jobs. *Financial aid application deadline (priority):* 3/1.
**Contact** Ms. Paula Byrne, Chair, Department of Traditional Undergraduate Nursing, Department of Nursing, The College of St. Scholastica, 1200 Kenwood Avenue, Duluth, MN 55811. *Telephone:* 218-723-6020. *Fax:* 218-733-2221. *E-mail:* pbyrne@css.edu.

#### GRADUATE PROGRAMS

**Expenses (2013–14)** *Tuition:* part-time $740 per credit. *Room and board:* $8040; room only: $4088 per academic year.
**Financial Aid** 90% of graduate students in nursing programs received some form of financial aid in 2012–13. Scholarships and traineeships available. Aid available to part-time students.
**Contact** Dr. Sally Fauchald, Chair, Graduate Nursing Department, Department of Nursing, The College of St. Scholastica, 1200 Kenwood Avenue, Duluth, MN 55811. *Telephone:* 218-723-6590. *Fax:* 218-733-2221. *E-mail:* sfauchal@css.edu.

**MASTER'S DEGREE PROGRAM**
**Degree** MA
**Available Programs** Master's.
**Concentrations Available** *Nurse practitioner programs in:* adult health, family health, gerontology, psychiatric/mental health.
**Site Options** St. Cloud, MN; Duluth, MN.

**Study Options** Full-time and part-time.
**Program Entrance Requirements** Clinical experience, computer literacy, minimum overall college GPA of 3.0, transcript of college record, CPR certification, written essay, immunizations, interview, 3 letters of recommendation, nursing research course, physical assessment course, professional liability insurance/malpractice insurance, resume, statistics course, GRE General Test. *Application deadline:* 3/1 (spring). *Application fee:* $50.
**Advanced Placement** Credit given for nursing courses completed elsewhere dependent upon specific evaluations.
**Degree Requirements** 47 total credit hours, thesis or project.

### POST-MASTER'S PROGRAM
**Areas of Study** Nursing informatics. *Nurse practitioner programs in:* adult health, family health, gerontology, psychiatric/mental health.

### DOCTORAL DEGREE PROGRAM
**Degree** DNP
**Available Programs** Doctorate; Post-Baccalaureate Doctorate.
**Areas of Study** Advanced practice nursing, gerontology, health policy, nursing education, nursing policy.
**Site Options** St. Cloud, MN; Duluth, MN.
**Program Entrance Requirements** Clinical experience, minimum overall college GPA of 3.0, interview by faculty committee, 3 letters of recommendation, MSN or equivalent, vita, writing sample. *Application deadline:* 3/1 (spring). *Application fee:* $50.
**Degree Requirements** 30 total credit hours, dissertation.

### POSTDOCTORAL PROGRAM
**Postdoctoral Program Contact** Dr. Carleen A. Maynard, Chair, Graduate Nursing Department, Department of Nursing, The College of St. Scholastica, 1200 Kenwood Avenue, Duluth, MN 55811. *Telephone:* 218-723-6452. *Fax:* 218-733-2295. *E-mail:* cmaynard@css.edu.

# Concordia College
## Department of Nursing
## Moorhead, Minnesota

*http://www.cord.edu/Academics/Nursing/index.php*
Founded in 1891

**DEGREES • BA • MS**
**Nursing Program Faculty** 6 (33% with doctorates).
**Baccalaureate Enrollment** 75
**Graduate Enrollment** 2 **Women** 100%
**Nursing Student Activities** Sigma Theta Tau, Student Nurses' Association.
**Nursing Student Resources** Academic advising; academic or career counseling; assistance for students with disabilities; bookstore; campus computer network; career placement assistance; computer lab; computer-assisted instruction; e-mail services; employment services for current students; externships; housing assistance; interactive nursing skills videos; Internet; learning resource lab; library services; nursing audiovisuals; paid internships; placement services for program completers; remedial services; resume preparation assistance; skills, simulation, or other laboratory; tutoring; unpaid internships.
**Library Facilities** 346,744 volumes (2,135 in health, 837 in nursing); 4,342 periodical subscriptions (81 health-care related).

### BACCALAUREATE PROGRAMS
**Degree** BA
**Available Programs** Accelerated Baccalaureate for Second Degree; Generic Baccalaureate.
**Study Options** Full-time.
**Program Entrance Requirements** Minimum overall college GPA of 2.9, transcript of college record, CPR certification, health exam, health insurance, immunizations, interview, 2 letters of recommendation, minimum GPA in nursing prerequisites of 2.7, professional liability insurance/malpractice insurance, prerequisite course work. Transfer students are accepted.
**Advanced Placement** Credit by examination available. Credit given for nursing courses completed elsewhere dependent upon specific evaluations.
**Contact** *Telephone:* 218-299-3879. *Fax:* 218-299-4309.

### GRADUATE PROGRAMS
**Contact** *Telephone:* 218-299-3879. *Fax:* 218-299-4309.

### MASTER'S DEGREE PROGRAM
**Degree** MS
**Available Programs** Master's.
**Concentrations Available** Nursing education.
**Study Options** Full-time and part-time.
**Program Entrance Requirements** Computer literacy, minimum overall college GPA of 3.0, transcript of college record, written essay, interview, 3 letters of recommendation.
**Advanced Placement** Credit given for nursing courses completed elsewhere dependent upon specific evaluations.
**Degree Requirements** 36 total credit hours, thesis or project, comprehensive exam.

# Crown College
## Nursing Department
## St. Bonifacius, Minnesota

*http://www.crown.edu/*
Founded in 1916

**DEGREE • BSN**
**Nursing Program Faculty** 6
**Baccalaureate Enrollment** 20 **Women** 100% **International** 10%
**Distance Learning Courses** Available.
**Nursing Student Activities** Student Nurses' Association.
**Nursing Student Resources** Academic advising; academic or career counseling; assistance for students with disabilities; bookstore; campus computer network; computer lab; computer-assisted instruction; e-mail services; employment services for current students; housing assistance; interactive nursing skills videos; Internet; learning resource lab; library services; nursing audiovisuals; remedial services; resume preparation assistance; skills, simulation, or other laboratory; tutoring; unpaid internships.
**Library Facilities** 148,561 volumes; 29,308 periodical subscriptions.

### BACCALAUREATE PROGRAMS
**Degree** BSN
**Available Programs** Generic Baccalaureate.
**Site Options** Owatonna, MN.
**Study Options** Full-time.
**Program Entrance Requirements** CPR certification, written essay, health exam, immunizations, 2 letters of recommendation, minimum high school GPA, minimum GPA in nursing prerequisites of 2.5, prerequisite course work. Transfer students are accepted. *Application deadline:* 2/1 (spring).
**Contact** *Telephone:* 952-446-4482.

# Globe University–Woodbury
## Bachelor of Science in Nursing
## Woodbury, Minnesota

*http://www.globeuniversity.edu/*
Founded in 1885

**DEGREE • BS**
**Nursing Program Faculty** 16
**Baccalaureate Enrollment** 135
**Nursing Student Activities** Student Nurses' Association.
**Nursing Student Resources** Academic advising; academic or career counseling; assistance for students with disabilities; bookstore; campus computer network; career placement assistance; computer lab; computer-assisted instruction; e-mail services; employment services for current students; interactive nursing skills videos; Internet; learning resource lab; library services; nursing audiovisuals; placement services for program completers; remedial services; resume preparation assistance; skills, simulation, or other laboratory; tutoring; unpaid internships.
**Library Facilities** 8,069 volumes; 63,753 periodical subscriptions.

### BACCALAUREATE PROGRAMS
**Degree** BS
**Available Programs** Generic Baccalaureate.
**Study Options** Full-time and part-time.
**Program Entrance Requirements** Minimum overall college GPA of 2.75, transcript of college record, CPR certification, written essay, health exam, high school biology, high school chemistry, 2 years high school

science, high school transcript, immunizations, interview, 2 letters of recommendation, minimum high school GPA of 2.75, minimum high school rank 60%, minimum GPA in nursing prerequisites of 2.75, prerequisite course work. Transfer students are accepted. *Application deadline:* Applications may be processed on a rolling basis for some programs. *Application fee:* $50.
**Advanced Placement** Credit given for nursing courses completed elsewhere dependent upon specific evaluations.
**Contact** *Telephone:* 612-798-3762.

# Gustavus Adolphus College
## Department of Nursing
## St. Peter, Minnesota

*http://www.gustavus.edu/*
Founded in 1862

**DEGREE • BA**

**Nursing Program Faculty** 9 (20% with doctorates).
**Baccalaureate Enrollment** 76 **Women** 92% **Men** 8% **Minority** 8% **International** 4%
**Nursing Student Activities** Sigma Theta Tau, Student Nurses' Association.
**Nursing Student Resources** Academic advising; academic or career counseling; assistance for students with disabilities; bookstore; campus computer network; career placement assistance; computer lab; computer-assisted instruction; e-mail services; employment services for current students; housing assistance; interactive nursing skills videos; Internet; learning resource lab; library services; nursing audiovisuals; paid internships; remedial services; resume preparation assistance; skills, simulation, or other laboratory; tutoring; unpaid internships.
**Library Facilities** 357,186 volumes; 23,619 periodical subscriptions.

### BACCALAUREATE PROGRAMS

**Degree** BA
**Available Programs** Generic Baccalaureate.
**Study Options** Full-time.
**Program Entrance Requirements** Minimum overall college GPA of 2.7, transcript of college record, written essay, high school transcript, immunizations, interview, minimum GPA in nursing prerequisites, prerequisite course work. Transfer students are accepted.
**Contact** *Telephone:* 507-933-6126. *Fax:* 507-933-6153.

# Herzing University
## Nursing Program
## Minneapolis, Minnesota

Founded in 1961

**DEGREE • BSN**

### BACCALAUREATE PROGRAMS

**Degree** BSN
**Available Programs** Generic Baccalaureate.
**Contact** Nursing Information, Nursing Program, Herzing University, 5700 West Broadway, Crystal, MN 55428. *Telephone:* 763-535-3000. *Fax:* 763-535-9205. *E-mail:* mpl-info@herzing.edu.

# Metropolitan State University
## College of Health, Community and Professional Studies
## St. Paul, Minnesota

*http://www.metrostate.edu/msweb/explore/chcps/departments/nursing/*
Founded in 1971

**DEGREES • BSN • DNP • MSN**

**Nursing Program Faculty** 16 (62% with doctorates).
**Baccalaureate Enrollment** 270 **Women** 90% **Men** 10% **Minority** 28% **International** 5% **Part-time** 50%
**Graduate Enrollment** 45 **Women** 95% **Men** 5% **Minority** 10% **International** 2% **Part-time** 20%
**Distance Learning Courses** Available.
**Nursing Student Activities** Student Nurses' Association.
**Nursing Student Resources** Academic advising; academic or career counseling; assistance for students with disabilities; bookstore; campus computer network; computer lab; computer-assisted instruction; e-mail services; interactive nursing skills videos; Internet; learning resource lab; library services; nursing audiovisuals; remedial services; skills, simulation, or other laboratory.

### BACCALAUREATE PROGRAMS

**Degree** BSN
**Available Programs** Generic Baccalaureate; RN Baccalaureate.
**Site Options** Minneapolis, MN.
**Study Options** Full-time.
**Program Entrance Requirements** Transcript of college record, immunizations, minimum GPA in nursing prerequisites of 2.75, prerequisite course work. Transfer students are accepted. *Application deadline:* 2/1 (fall). *Application fee:* $20.
**Advanced Placement** Credit given for nursing courses completed elsewhere dependent upon specific evaluations.
**Expenses (2013–14)** *Tuition, state resident:* part-time $286 per credit. *Tuition, nonresident:* part-time $286 per credit.
**Financial Aid** 10% of baccalaureate students in nursing programs received some form of financial aid in 2012–13. *Gift aid (need-based):* Federal Pell, FSEOG, state, private, college/university gift aid from institutional funds. *Loans:* Federal Direct (Subsidized and Unsubsidized Stafford PLUS), state. *Work-study:* Federal Work-Study, part-time campus jobs. *Financial aid application deadline (priority):* 6/1.
**Contact** Sandi Gerick, Director of Advising, College of Health, Community and Professional Studies, Metropolitan State University, 700 East Seventh Street, St. Paul, MN 55106-5000. *Telephone:* 651-793-1379. *Fax:* 651-793-1382. *E-mail:* sandi.gerick@metrostate.edu.

### GRADUATE PROGRAMS

**Expenses (2013–14)** *Tuition, state resident:* part-time $447 per credit. *Tuition, nonresident:* part-time $447 per credit.
**Financial Aid** 10% of graduate students in nursing programs received some form of financial aid in 2012–13. Fellowships, career-related internships or fieldwork, Federal Work-Study, institutionally sponsored loans, and traineeships available.
**Contact** Ms. Lynn Iverson-Eyestone, Academic Advisor, College of Health, Community and Professional Studies, Metropolitan State University, 700 East Seventh Street, St. Paul, MN 55106-5000. *Telephone:* 651-793-1356. *Fax:* 651-793-1382. *E-mail:* lynn.iversoneyestone@metropolitanstate.edu.

#### MASTER'S DEGREE PROGRAM

**Degree** MSN
**Available Programs** Master's for Nurses with Non-Nursing Degrees; RN to Master's.
**Concentrations Available** Nursing administration; nursing education.
**Study Options** Full-time and part-time.
**Online Degree Options** Yes.
**Program Entrance Requirements** Computer literacy, minimum overall college GPA of 3.0, transcript of college record, written essay, immunizations, interview, 2 letters of recommendation, statistics course, GRE General Test. *Application deadline:* 1/31 (fall). *Application fee:* $20.
**Advanced Placement** Credit given for nursing courses completed elsewhere dependent upon specific evaluations.
**Degree Requirements** 41 total credit hours, thesis or project.

#### POST-MASTER'S PROGRAM

**Areas of Study** Nursing administration; nursing education.

#### DOCTORAL DEGREE PROGRAM

**Degree** DNP
**Available Programs** Doctorate.
**Areas of Study** Advanced practice nursing.
**Program Entrance Requirements** Minimum overall college GPA of 3.0, 3 letters of recommendation, writing sample. *Application deadline:* 1/15 (fall). *Application fee:* $40.
**Degree Requirements** Oral exam, written exam.

# Minnesota Intercollegiate Nursing Consortium

## Minnesota Intercollegiate Nursing Consortium
## Northfield, Minnesota

***http://www.stolaf.edu/depts/nursing/***

**DEGREE • BA**

**Nursing Program Faculty** 11 (45% with doctorates).
**Baccalaureate Enrollment** 95 **Women** 86% **Men** 14% **Minority** 11% **International** 1%
**Nursing Student Activities** Sigma Theta Tau, Student Nurses' Association.
**Nursing Student Resources** Academic advising; academic or career counseling; assistance for students with disabilities; bookstore; campus computer network; career placement assistance; computer lab; computer-assisted instruction; e-mail services; employment services for current students; externships; interactive nursing skills videos; Internet; learning resource lab; library services; nursing audiovisuals; paid internships; remedial services; resume preparation assistance; skills, simulation, or other laboratory; tutoring; unpaid internships.

### BACCALAUREATE PROGRAMS

**Degree** BA
**Available Programs** Generic Baccalaureate.
**Site Options** St. Peter, MN; Northfield, MN.
**Study Options** Full-time.
**Program Entrance Requirements** Minimum overall college GPA of 2.85, transcript of college record, CPR certification, written essay, health exam, health insurance, immunizations, interview, minimum GPA in nursing prerequisites of 2.7, prerequisite course work. Transfer students are accepted. *Application deadline:* 11/15 (fall).
**Advanced Placement** Credit given for nursing courses completed elsewhere dependent upon specific evaluations.
**Contact** *Telephone:* 507-786-3265. *Fax:* 507-786-3733.

# Minnesota State University Mankato

## School of Nursing
## Mankato, Minnesota

***http://www.mnsu.edu/nursing/***
Founded in 1868

**DEGREES • BS • DNP • MSN • MSN/MS**

**Nursing Program Faculty** 48 (21% with doctorates).
**Baccalaureate Enrollment** 292 **Women** 90% **Men** 10% **Minority** 9% **International** 1% **Part-time** 1%
**Graduate Enrollment** 60 **Women** 96% **Men** 4% **Part-time** 48%
**Distance Learning Courses** Available.
**Nursing Student Activities** Nursing Honor Society, Sigma Theta Tau, Student Nurses' Association.
**Nursing Student Resources** Academic advising; academic or career counseling; assistance for students with disabilities; bookstore; campus computer network; career placement assistance; computer lab; computer-assisted instruction; daycare for children of students; e-mail services; employment services for current students; Internet; learning resource lab; library services; nursing audiovisuals; paid internships; placement services for program completers; resume preparation assistance; skills, simulation, or other laboratory; tutoring.
**Library Facilities** 1.2 million volumes (35,852 in health, 1,500 in nursing); 20,000 periodical subscriptions (156 health-care related).

### BACCALAUREATE PROGRAMS

**Degree** BS
**Available Programs** Accelerated Baccalaureate for Second Degree; Generic Baccalaureate; RN Baccalaureate.
**Study Options** Full-time and part-time.
**Program Entrance Requirements** Minimum overall college GPA of 2.5, transcript of college record, health exam, health insurance, minimum GPA in nursing prerequisites of 2.0, prerequisite course work. Transfer students are accepted.
**Advanced Placement** Credit by examination available. Credit given for nursing courses completed elsewhere dependent upon specific evaluations.
**Contact** *Telephone:* 507-389-6828. *Fax:* 507-389-6516.

### GRADUATE PROGRAMS

**Contact** *Telephone:* 507-389-1317. *Fax:* 507-389-6516.

#### MASTER'S DEGREE PROGRAM

**Degrees** MSN; MSN/MS
**Available Programs** Accelerated RN to Master's; Master's; Master's for Nurses with Non-Nursing Degrees; RN to Master's.
**Concentrations Available** Nursing education. *Clinical nurse specialist programs in:* adult health, family health, pediatric. *Nurse practitioner programs in:* family health.
**Study Options** Full-time and part-time.
**Program Entrance Requirements** Clinical experience, computer literacy, minimum overall college GPA of 3.0, transcript of college record, CPR certification, written essay, immunizations, 3 letters of recommendation, nursing research course, professional liability insurance/malpractice insurance, prerequisite course work, resume, statistics course.
**Advanced Placement** Credit given for nursing courses completed elsewhere dependent upon specific evaluations.
**Degree Requirements** 53 total credit hours, thesis or project.

#### POST-MASTER'S PROGRAM

**Areas of Study** Nursing education. *Clinical nurse specialist programs in:* family health. *Nurse practitioner programs in:* family health.

#### DOCTORAL DEGREE PROGRAM

**Degree** DNP
**Available Programs** Doctorate.
**Degree Requirements** 36 total credit hours.

### CONTINUING EDUCATION PROGRAM

**Contact** *Telephone:* 507-389-5194. *Fax:* 507-389-6516.

# Minnesota State University Moorhead

## School of Nursing and Healthcare Leadership
## Moorhead, Minnesota

***http://www.mnstate.edu/snhl/***
Founded in 1885

**DEGREES • BSN • MS**

**Nursing Program Faculty** 11 (36% with doctorates).
**Baccalaureate Enrollment** 212 **Women** 95% **Men** 5% **Minority** 3% **Part-time** 12%
**Graduate Enrollment** 43 **Women** 97% **Men** 3% **Minority** 6% **Part-time** 90%
**Distance Learning Courses** Available.
**Nursing Student Activities** Sigma Theta Tau, Student Nurses' Association.
**Nursing Student Resources** Academic advising; academic or career counseling; assistance for students with disabilities; bookstore; campus computer network; career placement assistance; computer lab; computer-assisted instruction; daycare for children of students; e-mail services; employment services for current students; Internet; library services; nursing audiovisuals; placement services for program completers; remedial services; resume preparation assistance; tutoring; unpaid internships.
**Library Facilities** 600,891 volumes (5,560 in health, 824 in nursing); 8,585 periodical subscriptions (50 health-care related).

### BACCALAUREATE PROGRAMS

**Degree** BSN
**Available Programs** ADN to Baccalaureate; RN Baccalaureate.
**Online Degree Options** Yes (online only).
**Program Entrance Requirements** CPR certification, written essay, high school transcript, immunizations, 2 letters of recommendation, RN licensure. Transfer students are accepted. *Application deadline:* 3/15 (fall), 10/1 (spring).
**Contact** *Telephone:* 218-477-2695. *Fax:* 218-477-5990.

### GRADUATE PROGRAMS

**Contact** *Telephone:* 218-477-2695. *Fax:* 218-477-5990.

**MASTER'S DEGREE PROGRAM**

**Degree** MS

**Available Programs** Master's.

**Concentrations Available** Nursing education. *Clinical nurse specialist programs in:* adult health, gerontology.

**Study Options** Full-time and part-time.

**Online Degree Options** Yes (online only).

**Program Entrance Requirements** Computer literacy, minimum overall college GPA of 3.0, transcript of college record, written essay, interview, 3 letters of recommendation, resume, statistics course. *Application deadline:* Applications may be processed on a rolling basis for some programs.

**Advanced Placement** Credit given for nursing courses completed elsewhere dependent upon specific evaluations.

**Degree Requirements** 45 total credit hours, thesis or project.

# St. Catherine University

## Department of Nursing
## St. Paul, Minnesota

***http://www.stkate.edu/academic/nursing/***

Founded in 1905

**DEGREES • BS • DNP • MS**

**Nursing Program Faculty** 74 (39% with doctorates).

**Baccalaureate Enrollment** 290 **Women** 99% **Men** 1% **Minority** 34% **International** .3% **Part-time** 37%

**Graduate Enrollment** 132 **Women** 98% **Men** 2% **Minority** 17% **International** .7% **Part-time** 9%

**Distance Learning Courses** Available.

**Nursing Student Activities** Nursing Honor Society, Sigma Theta Tau, Student Nurses' Association.

**Nursing Student Resources** Academic advising; academic or career counseling; assistance for students with disabilities; bookstore; campus computer network; career placement assistance; computer lab; computer-assisted instruction; daycare for children of students; e-mail services; employment services for current students; housing assistance; interactive nursing skills videos; Internet; learning resource lab; library services; nursing audiovisuals; paid internships; remedial services; resume preparation assistance; skills, simulation, or other laboratory; tutoring; unpaid internships.

**Library Facilities** 9,644 volumes in health, 1,121 volumes in nursing; 6,034 periodical subscriptions health-care related.

### BACCALAUREATE PROGRAMS

**Degree** BS

**Available Programs** ADN to Baccalaureate; Baccalaureate for Second Degree; Generic Baccalaureate; RN Baccalaureate.

**Site Options** Burnsville, MN; St. Louis Park, MN; Minneapolis, MN.

**Study Options** Full-time.

**Program Entrance Requirements** Minimum overall college GPA of 2.75, transcript of college record, CPR certification, written essay, health insurance, immunizations, 2 letters of recommendation, minimum GPA in nursing prerequisites of 2.75, prerequisite course work. Transfer students are accepted. *Application deadline:* 10/1 (fall).

**Expenses (2013–14)** *Tuition:* full-time $34,464; part-time $1077 per credit. *International tuition:* $34,464 full-time. *Room and board:* $6800; room only: $3092 per academic year. *Required fees:* part-time $550 per term.

**Financial Aid** 72% of baccalaureate students in nursing programs received some form of financial aid in 2012–13. *Gift aid (need-based):* Federal Pell, FSEOG, state, private, college/university gift aid from institutional funds. *Loans:* Federal Nursing Student Loans, Federal Direct (Subsidized and Unsubsidized Stafford PLUS), Perkins, state, alternative loans. *Work-study:* Federal Work-Study, part-time campus jobs. *Financial aid application deadline (priority):* 4/15.

**Contact** Dr. Susan Ellen Campbell, Assistant Dean Undergraduate Nursing, Department of Nursing, St. Catherine University, 2004 Randolph Avenue, St. Paul, MN 55105. *Telephone:* 651-690-7733. *Fax:* 651-690-6941. *E-mail:* secampbell@stkate.edu.

### GRADUATE PROGRAMS

**Expenses (2013–14)** *Tuition:* part-time $876 per credit. *Room and board:* $5540; room only: $1832 per academic year. *Required fees:* part-time $30 per term.

**Financial Aid** 52% of graduate students in nursing programs received some form of financial aid in 2012–13.

**Contact** Dr. Suzan Ulrich, Assistant Dean for Graduate Nursing, Department of Nursing, St. Catherine University, 2004 Randolph Avenue, #4250, St. Paul, MN 55105. *Telephone:* 651-690-6580. *Fax:* 651-690-6941. *E-mail:* sculrich@stkate.edu.

**MASTER'S DEGREE PROGRAM**

**Degree** MS

**Available Programs** Master's; Master's for Nurses with Non-Nursing Degrees.

**Concentrations Available** Nursing education. *Nurse practitioner programs in:* adult health, gerontology, pediatric.

**Study Options** Full-time and part-time.

**Program Entrance Requirements** Clinical experience, minimum overall college GPA of 3.0, transcript of college record, CPR certification, written essay, immunizations, interview, 3 letters of recommendation, professional liability insurance/malpractice insurance, resume, statistics course. *Application deadline:* 12/15 (fall).

**Advanced Placement** Credit given for nursing courses completed elsewhere dependent upon specific evaluations.

**Degree Requirements** 39 total credit hours, thesis or project.

**POST-MASTER'S PROGRAM**

**Areas of Study** Nursing education. *Nurse practitioner programs in:* adult health, gerontology, pediatric.

**DOCTORAL DEGREE PROGRAM**

**Degree** DNP

**Available Programs** Doctorate.

**Areas of Study** Advanced practice nursing, health policy, health-care systems.

**Program Entrance Requirements** Minimum overall college GPA of 3.0, interview by faculty committee, interview, 3 letters of recommendation, MSN or equivalent, statistics course, vita, writing sample. *Application deadline:* 1/15 (winter).

**Degree Requirements** 33 total credit hours, dissertation.

# St. Cloud State University

## Department of Nursing Science
## St. Cloud, Minnesota

Founded in 1869

**DEGREE • BS**

**Nursing Program Faculty** 12 (25% with doctorates).

**Baccalaureate Enrollment** 111

**Nursing Student Activities** Nursing club.

**Nursing Student Resources** Academic advising; academic or career counseling; assistance for students with disabilities; bookstore; campus computer network; career placement assistance; computer lab; computer-assisted instruction; daycare for children of students; e-mail services; interactive nursing skills videos; Internet; learning resource lab; library services; nursing audiovisuals; remedial services; resume preparation assistance; skills, simulation, or other laboratory; tutoring; unpaid internships.

**Library Facilities** 947,787 volumes (18,000 in health, 750 in nursing); 955 periodical subscriptions (100 health-care related).

### BACCALAUREATE PROGRAMS

**Degree** BS

**Available Programs** Generic Baccalaureate.

**Study Options** Full-time.

**Program Entrance Requirements** Minimum overall college GPA of 2.75, transcript of college record, CPR certification, health exam, immunizations, 2 letters of recommendation, minimum GPA in nursing prerequisites of 2.75, prerequisite course work.

**Contact** *Telephone:* 320-308-1749.

## Saint Mary's University of Minnesota
### B.S. in Nursing
### Winona, Minnesota

Founded in 1912

**DEGREE • BS**

**Library Facilities** 209,807 volumes; 40,015 periodical subscriptions.

#### BACCALAUREATE PROGRAMS

**Degree** BS

**Available Programs** RN Baccalaureate.

**Program Entrance Requirements** Transcript of college record, written essay, interview, letters of recommendation, RN licensure. *Application fee:* $25.

**Contact** Admissions Office, B.S. in Nursing, Saint Mary's University of Minnesota, 2500 Park Avenue, Minneapolis, MN 55404. *Telephone:* 612-728-5100. *E-mail:* tc-admission@smumn.edu.

## St. Olaf College
### Department of Nursing
### Northfield, Minnesota

*http://www.stolaf.edu/depts/nursing/*

Founded in 1874

**DEGREE • BA**

**Nursing Program Faculty** 5 (40% with doctorates).

**Baccalaureate Enrollment** 46 **Women** 80% **Men** 20% **Minority** 13% **International** 4%

**Nursing Student Activities** Sigma Theta Tau, Student Nurses' Association.

**Nursing Student Resources** Academic advising; academic or career counseling; assistance for students with disabilities; bookstore; campus computer network; career placement assistance; computer lab; computer-assisted instruction; e-mail services; employment services for current students; externships; interactive nursing skills videos; Internet; learning resource lab; library services; nursing audiovisuals; paid internships; placement services for program completers; remedial services; resume preparation assistance; skills, simulation, or other laboratory; tutoring; unpaid internships.

**Library Facilities** 742,064 volumes; 53,758 periodical subscriptions.

#### BACCALAUREATE PROGRAMS

**Degree** BA

**Available Programs** Generic Baccalaureate.

**Site Options** St. Peter, MN.

**Study Options** Full-time.

**Program Entrance Requirements** Minimum overall college GPA of 2.85, transcript of college record, CPR certification, written essay, health exam, health insurance, immunizations, interview, minimum GPA in nursing prerequisites of 2.7, prerequisite course work. Transfer students are accepted. *Application deadline:* 11/15 (fall).

**Advanced Placement** Credit given for nursing courses completed elsewhere dependent upon specific evaluations.

**Expenses (2012–13)** *Tuition:* full-time $48,650. *Room and board:* $9090; room only: $4260 per academic year. *Required fees:* full-time $1475.

**Financial Aid** 43% of baccalaureate students in nursing programs received some form of financial aid in 2011–12. *Gift aid (need-based):* Federal Pell, FSEOG, state, private, college/university gift aid from institutional funds. *Loans:* Federal Nursing Student Loans, Federal Direct (Subsidized and Unsubsidized Stafford PLUS), Perkins, state, college/university. *Work-study:* Federal Work-Study, part-time campus jobs. *Financial aid application deadline:* 3/1(priority: 2/1).

**Contact** Dr. Diana Odland Neal, Chair, Department of Nursing, St. Olaf College, 1520 St. Olaf Avenue, Northfield, MN 55057-1098. *Telephone:* 507-786-3349. *Fax:* 507-786-3733. *E-mail:* neal@stolaf.edu.

## University of Minnesota, Twin Cities Campus
### School of Nursing
### Minneapolis, Minnesota

*http://www.nursing.umn.edu/*

Founded in 1851

**DEGREES • BSN • DNP • PHD**

**Nursing Program Faculty** 85 (90% with doctorates).

**Baccalaureate Enrollment** 392 **Women** 87% **Men** 13% **Minority** 20% **Part-time** 8%

**Graduate Enrollment** 512 **Women** 88% **Men** 12% **Minority** 13% **International** 5% **Part-time** 44%

**Distance Learning Courses** Available.

**Nursing Student Activities** Nursing Honor Society, Sigma Theta Tau, Student Nurses' Association, nursing club.

**Nursing Student Resources** Academic advising; academic or career counseling; assistance for students with disabilities; bookstore; campus computer network; computer lab; computer-assisted instruction; daycare for children of students; e-mail services; employment services for current students; housing assistance; Internet; learning resource lab; library services; skills, simulation, or other laboratory.

**Library Facilities** 5.7 million volumes (4,000 in health, 1,500 in nursing); 45,000 periodical subscriptions (4,800 health-care related).

#### BACCALAUREATE PROGRAMS

**Degree** BSN

**Available Programs** Generic Baccalaureate.

**Site Options** Rochester, MN.

**Study Options** Full-time.

**Program Entrance Requirements** Minimum overall college GPA of 2.8, transcript of college record, CPR certification, written essay, health exam, health insurance, immunizations, minimum GPA in nursing prerequisites of 2.8, prerequisite course work. Transfer students are accepted. *Application deadline:* 2/1 (fall). *Application fee:* $60.

**Expenses (2012–13)** *Tuition, state resident:* full-time $12,100; part-time $6030 per semester. *Tuition, nonresident:* full-time $17,300; part-time $8655 per semester. *International tuition:* $17,300 full-time. *Room and board:* $12,000; room only: $9000 per academic year. *Required fees:* full-time $1456.

**Financial Aid** 73% of baccalaureate students in nursing programs received some form of financial aid in 2011–12. *Gift aid (need-based):* Federal Pell, FSEOG, state, private, college/university gift aid from institutional funds, Federal Nursing, ROTC Scholarships, Academic Merit scholarships. *Loans:* Federal Nursing Student Loans, Federal Direct (Subsidized and Unsubsidized Stafford PLUS), Perkins, state, college/university, Health Professions Student Loans (HPSL). *Work-study:* Federal Work-Study, part-time campus jobs. *Financial aid application deadline (priority):* 3/1.

**Contact** Office of Student Services, School of Nursing, University of Minnesota, Twin Cities Campus, 5-160 Weaver-Densford Hall, 308 Harvard Street SE, Minneapolis, MN 55455-0213. *Telephone:* 612-625-7980. *Fax:* 612-625-7727. *E-mail:* sonstudentinfo@umn.edu.

#### GRADUATE PROGRAMS

**Expenses (2012–13)** *Tuition, state resident:* full-time $22,000; part-time $11,000 per semester. *Tuition, nonresident:* full-time $22,000; part-time $11,000 per semester. *International tuition:* $22,000 full-time. *Room and board:* $12,000; room only: $9000 per academic year. *Required fees:* full-time $6550; part-time $3070 per term.

**Financial Aid** Fellowships, research assistantships, teaching assistantships, career-related internships or fieldwork and traineeships available.

**Contact** Office of Student Services, School of Nursing, University of Minnesota, Twin Cities Campus, 5-160 Weaver-Densford Hall, 308 Harvard Street SE, Minneapolis, MN 55455-0213. *Telephone:* 612-625-7980. *Fax:* 612-625-7727. *E-mail:* sonstudentinfo@umn.edu.

**MASTER'S DEGREE PROGRAM**

**Program Entrance Requirements** GRE General Test.

**DOCTORAL DEGREE PROGRAM**

**Degree** DNP

**Available Programs** Doctorate, Doctorate for Nurses with Non-Nursing Degrees, Post-Baccalaureate Doctorate.

**Areas of Study** Advanced practice nursing, community health, gerontology, information systems, maternity-newborn,women's health.

**Program Entrance Requirements** Minimum overall college GPA of 3.0, interview, interview by faculty committee, 2 letters of recommendation, writing sample, vita. *Application deadline:* 3/1 (fall). Applications may be processed on a rolling basis for some programs. *Application fee:* $60.
**Degree Requirements** 30-60 total credit hours, project and thesis presentation.

**Degree** PhD
**Available Programs** Doctorate; Doctorate for Nurses with Non-Nursing Degrees; Post-Baccalaureate Doctorate.
**Program Entrance Requirements** Minimum overall college GPA of 3.0, interview by faculty committee, interview, 2 letters of recommendation, vita, writing sample, GRE General Test. *Application deadline:* 3/1 (fall). Applications may be processed on a rolling basis for some programs. *Application fee:* $60.
**Degree Requirements** 60 total credit hours, dissertation, oral exam, written exam.

### CONTINUING EDUCATION PROGRAM

**Contact** Office of Student Services, School of Nursing, University of Minnesota, Twin Cities Campus, 5-160 Weaver-Densford Hall, 308 Harvard Street SE, Minneapolis, MN 55455-0213. *Telephone:* 612-625-7980. *Fax:* 612-625-7727. *E-mail:* sonstudentinfo@umn.edu.

## Walden University

### Nursing Programs
### Minneapolis, Minnesota

***http://www.waldenu.edu/Colleges-and-Schools/College-of-Health-Sciences/School-of-Nursing.htm***
Founded in 1970

**DEGREES • BSN • DNP • MSN**
**Nursing Program Faculty** 213 (100% with doctorates).
**Baccalaureate Enrollment** 1,048 **Women** 93% **Men** 7% **Minority** 27% **International** 2% **Part-time** 81%
**Graduate Enrollment** 6,501 **Women** 92% **Men** 8% **Minority** 35% **International** 2% **Part-time** 23%
**Distance Learning Courses** Available.
**Nursing Student Activities** Nursing Honor Society.
**Nursing Student Resources** Academic advising; academic or career counseling; assistance for students with disabilities; bookstore; campus computer network; career placement assistance; e-mail services; library services; nursing audiovisuals; placement services for program completers; remedial services; resume preparation assistance; tutoring.
**Library Facilities** 2.9 million volumes; 56,087 periodical subscriptions (6,689 health-care related).

### BACCALAUREATE PROGRAMS

**Degree** BSN
**Available Programs** RN Baccalaureate.
**Study Options** Full-time and part-time.
**Online Degree Options** Yes (online only).
**Program Entrance Requirements** Transcript of college record, high school transcript, prerequisite course work, RN licensure. Transfer students are accepted. *Application deadline:* Applications may be processed on a rolling basis for some programs. *Application fee:* $50.
**Expenses (2012–13)** *Tuition:* full-time $10,440; part-time $290 per credit. *International tuition:* $10,440 full-time. *Required fees:* full-time $285; part-time $95 per term.
**Contact** Dr. Karen Ouzts, Program Director, Nursing Programs, Walden University, 100 Washington Avenue South, Suite 900, Minneapolis, MN 55401. *Telephone:* 720-383-1356. *E-mail:* karen.ouzts@waldenu.edu.

### GRADUATE PROGRAMS

**Expenses (2012–13)** *Tuition:* part-time $395 per credit.
**Contact** Dr. Vincent Hall, Program Director, Nursing Programs, Walden University, 100 Washington Avenue South, Suite 900, Minneapolis, MN 55401. *E-mail:* vincent.hall@waldenu.edu.

#### MASTER'S DEGREE PROGRAM

**Degree** MSN
**Available Programs** Master's; RN to Master's.
**Concentrations Available** Nursing administration; nursing education; nursing informatics. *Nurse practitioner programs in:* family health, gerontology.
**Study Options** Full-time and part-time.
**Online Degree Options** Yes (online only).
**Program Entrance Requirements** Minimum overall college GPA of 2.5, transcript of college record. *Application deadline:* Applications may be processed on a rolling basis for some programs. *Application fee:* $50.
**Degree Requirements** 56 total credit hours, thesis or project.

#### POST-MASTER'S PROGRAM

**Areas of Study** Nursing administration; nursing education; nursing informatics.

#### DOCTORAL DEGREE PROGRAM

**Degree** DNP
**Available Programs** Doctorate.
**Online Degree Options** Yes (online only).
**Program Entrance Requirements** Minimum overall college GPA of 3.0, MSN or equivalent. *Application deadline:* Applications may be processed on a rolling basis for some programs. *Application fee:* $50.
**Degree Requirements** 53 total credit hours.

## Winona State University

### College of Nursing and Health Sciences
### Winona, Minnesota

***http://www.winona.edu/nursing/***
Founded in 1858

**DEGREES • BS • DNP • MS**
**Nursing Program Faculty** 39 (46% with doctorates).
**Baccalaureate Enrollment** 400 **Women** 94% **Men** 6% **Minority** 3% **International** 2% **Part-time** 13%
**Graduate Enrollment** 110 **Women** 89% **Men** 11% **Minority** 5% **International** 1% **Part-time** 65%
**Distance Learning Courses** Available.
**Nursing Student Activities** Sigma Theta Tau, Student Nurses' Association, nursing club.
**Nursing Student Resources** Academic advising; academic or career counseling; assistance for students with disabilities; bookstore; campus computer network; career placement assistance; computer lab; computer-assisted instruction; daycare for children of students; e-mail services; employment services for current students; externships; housing assistance; Internet; learning resource lab; library services; nursing audiovisuals; paid internships; placement services for program completers; remedial services; resume preparation assistance; skills, simulation, or other laboratory; tutoring.
**Library Facilities** 320,353 volumes (6,132 in health, 3,920 in nursing); 36,660 periodical subscriptions (413 health-care related).

### BACCALAUREATE PROGRAMS

**Degree** BS
**Available Programs** Generic Baccalaureate; RN Baccalaureate.
**Site Options** Rochester, MN.
**Study Options** Full-time and part-time.
**Program Entrance Requirements** Minimum overall college GPA of 3.0, transcript of college record, CPR certification, health exam, health insurance, immunizations, minimum GPA in nursing prerequisites of 3.3, professional liability insurance/malpractice insurance, prerequisite course work. Transfer students are accepted. *Application deadline:* 11/1 (fall), 1/31 (spring).
**Contact** *Telephone:* 507-457-5120. *Fax:* 507-457-5550.

### GRADUATE PROGRAMS

**Contact** *Telephone:* 507-285-7135. *Fax:* 507-292-5127.

#### MASTER'S DEGREE PROGRAM

**Degree** MS
**Available Programs** Master's; Master's for Nurses with Non-Nursing Degrees; RN to Master's.
**Concentrations Available** Nursing administration; nursing education. *Clinical nurse specialist programs in:* adult health. *Nurse practitioner programs in:* adult health, family health.
**Site Options** Rochester, MN.
**Study Options** Full-time and part-time.
**Program Entrance Requirements** Clinical experience, computer literacy, minimum overall college GPA of 3.0, transcript of college record, CPR certification, written essay, immunizations, interview, 3 letters of recommendation, nursing research course, physical assessment course,

professional liability insurance/malpractice insurance, statistics course, GRE (if GPA less than 3.0). *Application deadline:* 12/1 (fall). *Application fee:* $20.
**Advanced Placement** Credit given for nursing courses completed elsewhere dependent upon specific evaluations.
**Degree Requirements** 43 total credit hours, thesis or project.

**POST-MASTER'S PROGRAM**
**Areas of Study** Nursing administration; nursing education. *Clinical nurse specialist programs in:* adult health. *Nurse practitioner programs in:* adult health, family health.

**DOCTORAL DEGREE PROGRAM**
**Degree** DNP
**Available Programs** Doctorate.
**Areas of Study** Advanced practice nursing, faculty preparation, nursing administration.
**Site Options** Rochester, MN.
**Online Degree Options** Yes (online only).
**Program Entrance Requirements** Clinical experience, minimum overall college GPA of 3.0, 2 letters of recommendation, MSN or equivalent, statistics course, vita, writing sample. *Application deadline:* 3/15 (spring). *Application fee:* $20.
**Degree Requirements** 36 total credit hours, oral exam.

# MISSISSIPPI

## Alcorn State University
### School of Nursing
### Natchez, Mississippi

*http://www.alcorn.edu/nursing/*
Founded in 1871

**DEGREES • BSN • MSN**
**Nursing Program Faculty** 21 (29% with doctorates).
**Baccalaureate Enrollment** 63 **Women** 88.8% **Men** 11.2% **Minority** 42.8% **Part-time** 7.9%
**Graduate Enrollment** 53 **Women** 89.3% **Men** 10.7% **Minority** 35.7% **Part-time** 78.6%
**Distance Learning Courses** Available.
**Nursing Student Activities** Nursing Honor Society, Sigma Theta Tau, Student Nurses' Association.
**Nursing Student Resources** Academic advising; campus computer network; computer lab; housing assistance; learning resource lab; library services; nursing audiovisuals; paid internships; skills, simulation, or other laboratory.
**Library Facilities** 390,419 volumes (2,082 in health, 1,385 in nursing); 82,054 periodical subscriptions (30 health-care related).

### BACCALAUREATE PROGRAMS
**Degree** BSN
**Available Programs** Generic Baccalaureate; LPN to RN Baccalaureate; RN Baccalaureate.
**Study Options** Full-time.
**Online Degree Options** Yes.
**Program Entrance Requirements** Minimum overall college GPA of 2.5, transcript of college record, health exam, immunizations, minimum high school GPA of 2.5, professional liability insurance/malpractice insurance, prerequisite course work. Transfer students are accepted. *Application deadline:* 12/19 (fall).
**Contact** *Telephone:* 601-304-4305. *Fax:* 601-304-4398.

### GRADUATE PROGRAMS
**Contact** *Telephone:* 601-304-4303. *Fax:* 601-304-4398.

**MASTER'S DEGREE PROGRAM**
**Degree** MSN
**Available Programs** Master's.
**Concentrations Available** Nursing education. *Nurse practitioner programs in:* family health.
**Study Options** Full-time and part-time.
**Online Degree Options** Yes.
**Program Entrance Requirements** Computer literacy, minimum overall college GPA of 3.0, transcript of college record, written essay, 2 letters of recommendation, statistics course. *Application deadline:* 7/15 (fall). *Application fee:* $10.
**Advanced Placement** Credit given for nursing courses completed elsewhere dependent upon specific evaluations.
**Degree Requirements** 43 total credit hours, thesis or project.

**POST-MASTER'S PROGRAM**
**Areas of Study** Nursing education. *Nurse practitioner programs in:* family health.

## Delta State University
### School of Nursing
### Cleveland, Mississippi

*http://nursing.deltastate.edu/*
Founded in 1924

**DEGREES • BSN • DNP • MSN**
**Nursing Program Faculty** 17 (53% with doctorates).
**Baccalaureate Enrollment** 95 **Women** 81% **Men** 19% **Minority** 19% **Part-time** 17%
**Graduate Enrollment** 38 **Women** 89% **Men** 11% **Minority** 26% **Part-time** 26%
**Distance Learning Courses** Available.
**Nursing Student Activities** Sigma Theta Tau, Student Nurses' Association.
**Nursing Student Resources** Academic advising; academic or career counseling; assistance for students with disabilities; bookstore; campus computer network; career placement assistance; computer lab; computer-assisted instruction; daycare for children of students; e-mail services; externships; housing assistance; interactive nursing skills videos; Internet; learning resource lab; library services; nursing audiovisuals; other; remedial services; resume preparation assistance; skills, simulation, or other laboratory; tutoring.
**Library Facilities** 445,626 volumes (5,000 in health, 1,000 in nursing); 24,101 periodical subscriptions (120 health-care related).

### BACCALAUREATE PROGRAMS
**Degree** BSN
**Available Programs** ADN to Baccalaureate; Generic Baccalaureate.
**Study Options** Full-time and part-time.
**Program Entrance Requirements** Transcript of college record, CPR certification, health exam, health insurance, immunizations, 3 letters of recommendation, minimum GPA in nursing prerequisites of 2.5, professional liability insurance/malpractice insurance, prerequisite course work. Transfer students are accepted. *Application deadline:* 3/1 (fall).
**Advanced Placement** Credit given for nursing courses completed elsewhere dependent upon specific evaluations.
**Expenses (2013–14)** *Tuition, state resident:* full-time $6012; part-time $251 per credit hour. *Tuition, nonresident:* full-time $6012. *International tuition:* $6012 full-time. *Room and board:* $6803; room only: $4095 per academic year. *Required fees:* full-time $1470; part-time $61 per credit; part-time $735 per term.
**Financial Aid** 95% of baccalaureate students in nursing programs received some form of financial aid in 2012–13.
**Contact** Dr. Vicki L. Bingham, Chair of Academic Programs, School of Nursing, Delta State University, PO Box 3343, Cleveland, MS 38733. *Telephone:* 662-846-4255. *Fax:* 662-846-4267. *E-mail:* vbingham@deltastate.edu.

### GRADUATE PROGRAMS
**Expenses (2013–14)** *Tuition, state resident:* full-time $6012; part-time $334 per credit hour. *Tuition, nonresident:* full-time $6012; part-time $334 per credit hour. *International tuition:* $6012 full-time. *Room and board:* $6803; room only: $4095 per academic year. *Required fees:* full-time $723; part-time $30 per credit; part-time $361 per term.
**Financial Aid** 70% of graduate students in nursing programs received some form of financial aid in 2012–13. Research assistantships, career-related internships or fieldwork, Federal Work-Study, and institutionally sponsored loans available. *Financial aid application deadline:* 6/1.
**Contact** Dr. Vicki L. Bingham, Chair of Academic Programs, School of Nursing, Delta State University, PO Box 3343, Cleveland, MS 38733. *Telephone:* 662-846-4255. *Fax:* 662-846-4267. *E-mail:* vbingham@deltastate.edu.

**MASTER'S DEGREE PROGRAM**
**Degree** MSN
**Available Programs** Master's; Master's for Nurses with Non-Nursing Degrees.
**Concentrations Available** Nursing administration; nursing education. *Nurse practitioner programs in:* family health, gerontology, psychiatric/mental health.
**Study Options** Full-time and part-time.
**Online Degree Options** Yes (online only).
**Program Entrance Requirements** Clinical experience, computer literacy, minimum overall college GPA of 3.0, transcript of college record, CPR certification, written essay, immunizations, interview, 3 letters of recommendation, nursing research course, physical assessment course, professional liability insurance/malpractice insurance, prerequisite course work, resume, statistics course, GRE General Test. *Application deadline:* 2/1 (fall).
**Advanced Placement** Credit given for nursing courses completed elsewhere dependent upon specific evaluations.
**Degree Requirements** 44 total credit hours, thesis or project, comprehensive exam.

**POST-MASTER'S PROGRAM**
**Areas of Study** Nursing administration; nursing education. *Nurse practitioner programs in:* family health, gerontology, psychiatric/mental health.

**DOCTORAL DEGREE PROGRAM**
**Degree** DNP
**Available Programs** Doctorate; Post-Baccalaureate Doctorate.
**Areas of Study** Advanced practice nursing, family health.
**Online Degree Options** Yes (online only).
**Program Entrance Requirements** Clinical experience, minimum overall college GPA of 3.2, interview, 3 letters of recommendation, statistics course, vita, writing sample. *Application deadline:* 4/1 (fall).
**Degree Requirements** 31–95 total credit hours.

# Mississippi College
## School of Nursing
## Clinton, Mississippi

***http://www.mc.edu/***
Founded in 1826

### DEGREE • BSN
**Nursing Program Faculty** 20 (20% with doctorates).
**Baccalaureate Enrollment** 141 **Women** 80% **Men** 20% **Minority** 35% **International** 3% **Part-time** 7%
**Distance Learning Courses** Available.
**Nursing Student Activities** Sigma Theta Tau, Student Nurses' Association, nursing club.
**Nursing Student Resources** Academic advising; academic or career counseling; assistance for students with disabilities; bookstore; campus computer network; career placement assistance; computer lab; computer-assisted instruction; e-mail services; employment services for current students; externships; housing assistance; interactive nursing skills videos; Internet; learning resource lab; library services; nursing audiovisuals; paid internships; placement services for program completers; remedial services; resume preparation assistance; skills, simulation, or other laboratory; tutoring; unpaid internships.
**Library Facilities** 247,916 volumes (43,000 in health, 8,000 in nursing); 79,074 periodical subscriptions (290 health-care related).

### BACCALAUREATE PROGRAMS
**Degree** BSN
**Available Programs** Generic Baccalaureate; RN Baccalaureate.
**Study Options** Full-time and part-time.
**Program Entrance Requirements** Minimum overall college GPA of 2.5, transcript of college record, CPR certification, health exam, high school biology, high school chemistry, high school transcript, immunizations, 2 letters of recommendation, minimum GPA in nursing prerequisites of 2.5, professional liability insurance/malpractice insurance, prerequisite course work. Transfer students are accepted. *Application deadline:* 2/1 (fall), 9/1 (spring), 4/1 (summer).
**Advanced Placement** Credit given for nursing courses completed elsewhere dependent upon specific evaluations.
**Expenses (2013–14)** *Tuition:* full-time $14,120; part-time $442 per credit hour. *International tuition:* $14,120 full-time. *Room and board:* $8100 per academic year. *Required fees:* full-time $680; part-time $173 per term.
**Financial Aid** 95% of baccalaureate students in nursing programs received some form of financial aid in 2012–13.
**Contact** Dr. Mary Jean Padgett, Dean, School of Nursing, Mississippi College, Box 4037, 200 South Capitol Street, Clinton, MS 39058. *Telephone:* 601-925-3278. *Fax:* 601-925-3379. *E-mail:* padgett@mc.edu.

# Mississippi University for Women
## College of Nursing and Speech Language Pathology
## Columbus, Mississippi

***http://www.muw.edu/nursing***
Founded in 1884

### DEGREES • BSN • DNP • MSN
**Nursing Program Faculty** 43 (35% with doctorates).
**Baccalaureate Enrollment** 500 **Women** 80% **Men** 20% **Minority** 30% **International** 1% **Part-time** 1%
**Graduate Enrollment** 41 **Women** 90% **Men** 10% **Minority** 15% **Part-time** 1%
**Distance Learning Courses** Available.
**Nursing Student Activities** Sigma Theta Tau, Student Nurses' Association.
**Nursing Student Resources** Academic advising; academic or career counseling; assistance for students with disabilities; bookstore; campus computer network; career placement assistance; computer lab; computer-assisted instruction; daycare for children of students; e-mail services; employment services for current students; externships; housing assistance; interactive nursing skills videos; Internet; learning resource lab; library services; nursing audiovisuals; paid internships; placement services for program completers; remedial services; resume preparation assistance; skills, simulation, or other laboratory; tutoring; unpaid internships.
**Library Facilities** 31,682 volumes (27,520 in health, 23,600 in nursing); 4,347 periodical subscriptions (240 health-care related).

### BACCALAUREATE PROGRAMS
**Degree** BSN
**Available Programs** ADN to Baccalaureate; Generic Baccalaureate.
**Site Options** Tupelo, MS.
**Study Options** Full-time.
**Online Degree Options** Yes.
**Program Entrance Requirements** Minimum overall college GPA of 2.75, transcript of college record, CPR certification, health exam, health insurance, immunizations, minimum GPA in nursing prerequisites of 2.75, professional liability insurance/malpractice insurance, prerequisite course work. Transfer students are accepted. *Application deadline:* 1/15 (fall).
**Advanced Placement** Credit given for nursing courses completed elsewhere dependent upon specific evaluations.
**Expenses (2013–14)** *Tuition, state resident:* full-time $5640; part-time $235 per credit hour. *Tuition, nonresident:* full-time $7680; part-time $640 per credit hour. *Room and board:* $3200; room only: $1800 per academic year. *Required fees:* full-time $500.
**Financial Aid** 90% of baccalaureate students in nursing programs received some form of financial aid in 2012–13.
**Contact** Dr. Tammie McCoy, Baccalaureate Nursing Department Chair, College of Nursing and Speech Language Pathology, Mississippi University for Women, 1100 College Street, MUW-910, Columbus, MS 39701-5800. *Telephone:* 662-329-7301. *Fax:* 662-329-8559. *E-mail:* tmmccoy@muw.edu.

### GRADUATE PROGRAMS
**Expenses (2013–14)** *Tuition, state resident:* full-time $5640; part-time $313 per credit hour. *Tuition, nonresident:* full-time $7680; part-time $640 per credit hour. *Room and board:* $3200; room only: $1800 per academic year. *Required fees:* full-time $1000.
**Financial Aid** 80% of graduate students in nursing programs received some form of financial aid in 2012–13. Fellowships, Federal Work-Study, institutionally sponsored loans, and traineeships available. *Financial aid application deadline:* 4/1.
**Contact** Dr. Johnnie Sue Wijewardane, Graduate Nursing Program Department Chair, College of Nursing and Speech Language Pathology, Mississippi University for Women, 1100 College Street, MUW-910,

Columbus, MS 39701-5800. *Telephone:* 662-329-7323. *Fax:* 662-329-7372. *E-mail:* jswijewardane@muw.edu.

**MASTER'S DEGREE PROGRAM**
**Degree** MSN
**Available Programs** Master's.
**Concentrations Available** *Nurse practitioner programs in:* family health, gerontology, pediatric, psychiatric/mental health.
**Study Options** Full-time.
**Program Entrance Requirements** Clinical experience, computer literacy, minimum overall college GPA of 3.0, transcript of college record, CPR certification, written essay, immunizations, interview, 3 letters of recommendation, nursing research course, physical assessment course, professional liability insurance/malpractice insurance, prerequisite course work, resume, statistics course, GRE General Test. *Application deadline:* 4/1 (fall). *Application fee:* $25.
**Advanced Placement** Credit given for nursing courses completed elsewhere dependent upon specific evaluations.
**Degree Requirements** 39 total credit hours, thesis or project, comprehensive exam.

**POST-MASTER'S PROGRAM**
**Areas of Study** *Nurse practitioner programs in:* family health, gerontology, pediatric, psychiatric/mental health.

**DOCTORAL DEGREE PROGRAM**
**Degree** DNP
**Available Programs** Doctorate; Post-Baccalaureate Doctorate.
**Areas of Study** Advanced practice nursing.
**Program Entrance Requirements** Clinical experience, minimum overall college GPA of 3.0, interview, letters of recommendation, MSN or equivalent, statistics course, vita, writing sample. *Application deadline:* 6/1 (fall).
**Degree Requirements** 44 total credit hours, dissertation, oral exam, written exam, residency.

# University of Mississippi Medical Center

## School of Nursing
## Jackson, Mississippi

*http://www.umc.edu/son/*
Founded in 1955

**DEGREES • BSN • DNP • MSN**
**Nursing Program Faculty** 72 (60% with doctorates).
**Baccalaureate Enrollment** 373 **Women** 86.5% **Men** 13.5% **Minority** 18.8% **Part-time** 9%
**Graduate Enrollment** 330 **Women** 91% **Men** 9% **Minority** 15% **Part-time** 41%
**Distance Learning Courses** Available.
**Nursing Student Activities** Nursing Honor Society, Sigma Theta Tau, Student Nurses' Association, nursing club.
**Nursing Student Resources** Academic advising; academic or career counseling; assistance for students with disabilities; bookstore; campus computer network; career placement assistance; computer lab; computer-assisted instruction; e-mail services; employment services for current students; externships; interactive nursing skills videos; Internet; learning resource lab; library services; nursing audiovisuals; remedial services; skills, simulation, or other laboratory; tutoring; unpaid internships.
**Library Facilities** 310,016 volumes (72,557 in health, 8,170 in nursing); 2,732 periodical subscriptions (4,180 health-care related).

**BACCALAUREATE PROGRAMS**
**Degree** BSN
**Available Programs** ADN to Baccalaureate; Accelerated Baccalaureate for Second Degree; Generic Baccalaureate.
**Site Options** Oxford, MS.
**Study Options** Full-time and part-time.
**Program Entrance Requirements** Minimum overall college GPA of 2.5, transcript of college record, CPR certification, health exam, health insurance, immunizations, minimum GPA in nursing prerequisites of 2.5, professional liability insurance/malpractice insurance, prerequisite course work. Transfer students are accepted. *Application deadline:* 1/15 (spring). *Application fee:* $25.
**Advanced Placement** Credit given for nursing courses completed elsewhere dependent upon specific evaluations.
**Expenses (2013–14)** *Tuition, state resident:* full-time $6660; part-time $278 per contact hour. *Tuition, nonresident:* full-time $10,968; part-time $457 per contact hour. *Required fees:* full-time $1500.
**Financial Aid** 78% of baccalaureate students in nursing programs received some form of financial aid in 2012–13.
**Contact** Dr. Patricia A. Waltman, Associate Dean for Academic Affairs, School of Nursing, University of Mississippi Medical Center, 2500 North State Street, Jackson, MS 39216-4505. *Telephone:* 601-984-6211. *Fax:* 601-815-9309. *E-mail:* pwaltman@son.umsmed.edu.

**GRADUATE PROGRAMS**
**Expenses (2013–14)** *Tuition, state resident:* full-time $9990; part-time $370 per contact hour. *Required fees:* full-time $1500.
**Financial Aid** 80% of graduate students in nursing programs received some form of financial aid in 2012–13. Institutionally sponsored loans and scholarships available. Aid available to part-time students. *Financial aid application deadline:* 4/1.
**Contact** Dr. Marcia Rachel, Associate Dean for Graduate Studies, School of Nursing, University of Mississippi Medical Center, 2500 North State Street, Jackson, MS 39216-4505. *Telephone:* 601-984-6228. *Fax:* 601-815-4067. *E-mail:* mrachel@umc.edu.

**MASTER'S DEGREE PROGRAM**
**Degree** MSN
**Available Programs** Master's; RN to Master's.
**Concentrations Available** Nursing administration; nursing education. *Nurse practitioner programs in:* acute care, family health, gerontology, psychiatric/mental health.
**Study Options** Full-time and part-time.
**Program Entrance Requirements** Computer literacy, minimum overall college GPA of 3.0, transcript of college record, CPR certification, immunizations, 3 letters of recommendation, professional liability insurance/malpractice insurance, resume, statistics course, GRE. *Application deadline:* 10/15 (fall), 2/15 (winter), 3/31 (spring). Applications may be processed on a rolling basis for some programs. *Application fee:* $25.
**Advanced Placement** Credit given for nursing courses completed elsewhere dependent upon specific evaluations.
**Degree Requirements** 46 total credit hours, comprehensive exam.

**POST-MASTER'S PROGRAM**
**Areas of Study** Nursing administration; nursing education. *Nurse practitioner programs in:* acute care, family health, gerontology, psychiatric/mental health.

**DOCTORAL DEGREE PROGRAM**
**Degree** DNP
**Available Programs** Doctorate; Post-Baccalaureate Doctorate.
**Areas of Study** Advanced practice nursing, nursing administration.
**Program Entrance Requirements** Minimum overall college GPA of 3.0, interview by faculty committee, interview, letters of recommendation, MSN or equivalent, statistics course, vita, GRE. *Application deadline:* 5/1 (fall). *Application fee:* $25.
**Degree Requirements** 60 total credit hours, dissertation, oral exam, written exam, residency.

**CONTINUING EDUCATION PROGRAM**
**Contact** Dr. Renee Williams, Director of Continuing Education, School of Nursing, University of Mississippi Medical Center, 2500 North State Street, Jackson, MS 39216-4505. *Telephone:* 601-984-6227. *Fax:* 601-984-6214. *E-mail:* rwilliams@son.umsmed.edu.

# University of Southern Mississippi

## School of Nursing
## Hattiesburg, Mississippi

*http://www.usm.edu/nursing/*
Founded in 1910

**DEGREES • BSN • MSN • PHD**
**Nursing Program Faculty** 57 (49% with doctorates).
**Baccalaureate Enrollment** 416 **Women** 81% **Men** 19% **Minority** 19% **Part-time** 2%
**Graduate Enrollment** 143 **Women** 84% **Men** 16% **Minority** 24% **Part-time** 25%
**Distance Learning Courses** Available.

**Nursing Student Activities** Nursing Honor Society, Sigma Theta Tau, Student Nurses' Association.
**Nursing Student Resources** Academic advising; academic or career counseling; assistance for students with disabilities; bookstore; campus computer network; career placement assistance; computer lab; computer-assisted instruction; e-mail services; externships; housing assistance; interactive nursing skills videos; Internet; learning resource lab; library services; nursing audiovisuals; remedial services; resume preparation assistance; skills, simulation, or other laboratory; tutoring.
**Library Facilities** 1.2 million volumes; 33,307 periodical subscriptions (170 health-care related).

## BACCALAUREATE PROGRAMS

**Degree** BSN
**Available Programs** ADN to Baccalaureate; Generic Baccalaureate.
**Site Options** Meridian, MS; Long Beach, MS.
**Study Options** Full-time and part-time.
**Online Degree Options** Yes.
**Program Entrance Requirements** Minimum overall college GPA of 2.5, transcript of college record, CPR certification, written essay, health exam, health insurance, high school transcript, immunizations, minimum GPA in nursing prerequisites of 2.5, professional liability insurance/malpractice insurance, prerequisite course work. Transfer students are accepted. *Application deadline:* 2/1 (fall), 9/1 (spring).
**Expenses (2012–13)** *Tuition, state resident:* full-time $6336; part-time $244 per credit. *Tuition, nonresident:* full-time $8112; part-time $576 per credit. *International tuition:* $8112 full-time. *Room and board:* $8388; room only: $5618 per academic year. *Required fees:* full-time $800; part-time $75 per credit.
**Financial Aid** 85% of baccalaureate students in nursing programs received some form of financial aid in 2011–12. *Gift aid (need-based):* Federal Pell, FSEOG, state, private, college/university gift aid from institutional funds. *Loans:* Federal Direct (Subsidized and Unsubsidized Stafford PLUS). *Work-study:* Federal Work-Study. *Financial aid application deadline (priority):* 3/15.
**Contact** Cindy Sheffield, Assistant to the Dean for Academic/Advisement Records, School of Nursing, University of Southern Mississippi, 118 College Drive, Box 5095, Hattiesburg, MS 39406-5095. *Telephone:* 601-266-5454. *Fax:* 601-266-5711. *E-mail:* cynthia.sheffield@usm.edu.

## GRADUATE PROGRAMS

**Expenses (2012–13)** *Tuition, state resident:* full-time $5834; part-time $325 per credit. *Tuition, nonresident:* full-time $13,790; part-time $767 per credit. *International tuition:* $13,790 full-time. *Required fees:* full-time $300; part-time $50 per credit.
**Financial Aid** 85% of graduate students in nursing programs received some form of financial aid in 2011–12. 14 research assistantships with full tuition reimbursements available (averaging $12,577 per year), teaching assistantships (averaging $12,000 per year) were awarded; Federal Work-Study, institutionally sponsored loans, scholarships, traineeships, and unspecified assistantships also available. *Financial aid application deadline:* 3/15.
**Contact** Ms. Cynthia Sheffield, Assistant to the Dean for Academic/Advisement Records, School of Nursing, University of Southern Mississippi, 118 College Drive, Box 5095, Hattiesburg, MS 39406-5095. *Telephone:* 601-266-5454. *Fax:* 601-266-5711. *E-mail:* Cynthia.Sheffield@usm.edu.

### MASTER'S DEGREE PROGRAM

**Degree** MSN
**Available Programs** Master's; RN to Master's.
**Concentrations Available** Nursing administration. *Nurse practitioner programs in:* family health, gerontology, psychiatric/mental health.
**Site Options** Meridian, MS; Long Beach, MS.
**Study Options** Full-time and part-time.
**Program Entrance Requirements** Minimum overall college GPA of 3.0, transcript of college record, CPR certification, immunizations, 3 letters of recommendation, professional liability insurance/malpractice insurance, statistics course, GRE General Test. *Application deadline:* 2/1 (fall), 9/1 (spring).
**Degree Requirements** 45 total credit hours, thesis or project, comprehensive exam.

### POST-MASTER'S PROGRAM

**Areas of Study** Nursing administration. *Nurse practitioner programs in:* family health, gerontology, psychiatric/mental health.

### DOCTORAL DEGREE PROGRAM

**Degree** PhD
**Available Programs** Doctorate; Post-Baccalaureate Doctorate.
**Program Entrance Requirements** Clinical experience, minimum overall college GPA of 3.5, interview by faculty committee, 3 letters of recommendation, MSN or equivalent, statistics course, vita, writing sample, GRE General Test. *Application deadline:* 2/1 (fall).
**Degree Requirements** 72 total credit hours, dissertation, written exam.

# William Carey University
## School of Nursing
## Hattiesburg, Mississippi

*http://www.wmcarey.edu/*
Founded in 1906

**DEGREES • BSN • MSN • PHD**

**Nursing Program Faculty** 25 (40% with doctorates).
**Baccalaureate Enrollment** 214 **Women** 85% **Men** 15% **Minority** 36% **International** .5% **Part-time** 26%
**Graduate Enrollment** 91 **Women** 89% **Men** 11% **Minority** 41% **Part-time** 45%
**Distance Learning Courses** Available.
**Nursing Student Activities** Sigma Theta Tau, Student Nurses' Association.
**Nursing Student Resources** Academic advising; academic or career counseling; assistance for students with disabilities; bookstore; campus computer network; computer lab; computer-assisted instruction; e-mail services; interactive nursing skills videos; Internet; learning resource lab; library services; nursing audiovisuals; resume preparation assistance; skills, simulation, or other laboratory; tutoring.
**Library Facilities** 450 volumes in health, 450 volumes in nursing; 50 periodical subscriptions health-care related.

## BACCALAUREATE PROGRAMS

**Degree** BSN
**Available Programs** ADN to Baccalaureate; Generic Baccalaureate.
**Site Options** Biloxi, MS; New Orleans, LA.
**Study Options** Full-time and part-time.
**Program Entrance Requirements** Minimum overall college GPA of 2.75, transcript of college record, CPR certification, health exam, high school transcript, immunizations, minimum GPA in nursing prerequisites, professional liability insurance/malpractice insurance, prerequisite course work. Transfer students are accepted. *Application deadline:* 2/22 (fall), 8/10 (spring). *Application fee:* $40.
**Advanced Placement** Credit given for nursing courses completed elsewhere dependent upon specific evaluations.
**Expenses (2012–13)** *Tuition:* part-time $335 per contact hour. *Room and board:* room only: $1800 per academic year. *Required fees:* part-time $250 per term.
**Financial Aid** 90% of baccalaureate students in nursing programs received some form of financial aid in 2011–12.
**Contact** Dr. Janet K. Williams, Dean, School of Nursing, William Carey University, 498 Tuscan Avenue, Box 8, Hattiesburg, MS 39401. *Telephone:* 601-318-6478. *Fax:* 601-318-6446. *E-mail:* jwilliams@wmcarey.edu.

## GRADUATE PROGRAMS

**Expenses (2012–13)** *Tuition:* part-time $310 per contact hour. *International tuition:* $310 full-time. *Required fees:* full-time $1000; part-time $50 per credit.
**Financial Aid** 50% of graduate students in nursing programs received some form of financial aid in 2011–12.
**Contact** Dr. Marilyn McLeod Cooksey, Associate Dean of Graduate Studies, School of Nursing, William Carey University, 498 Tuscan Avenue, Hattiesburg, MS 39401. *Telephone:* 601-318-6478. *E-mail:* mcooksey@wmcarey.edu.

### MASTER'S DEGREE PROGRAM

**Degree** MSN
**Available Programs** Master's.
**Concentrations Available** Nursing education.
**Site Options** Biloxi, MS.
**Study Options** Full-time and part-time.
**Program Entrance Requirements** Computer literacy, minimum overall college GPA of 3.0, transcript of college record, CPR certification, written essay, immunizations, 2 letters of recommendation, nursing

research course, professional liability insurance/malpractice insurance, prerequisite course work, resume. *Application deadline:* 8/15 (fall), 2/15 (spring). Applications may be processed on a rolling basis for some programs. *Application fee:* $30.
**Advanced Placement** Credit given for nursing courses completed elsewhere dependent upon specific evaluations.
**Degree Requirements** 35 total credit hours, thesis or project.

**DOCTORAL DEGREE PROGRAM**
**Degree** PhD
**Available Programs** Doctorate.
**Areas of Study** Nursing education.
**Program Entrance Requirements** Minimum overall college GPA of 3.5, 3 letters of recommendation, MSN or equivalent, statistics course, vita, writing sample. *Application deadline:* 6/22 (fall). Applications may be processed on a rolling basis for some programs. *Application fee:* $390.
**Degree Requirements** 56 total credit hours, dissertation, written exam.

# MISSOURI

## Avila University
### School of Nursing
### Kansas City, Missouri

***http://www.avila.edu/nursing***
Founded in 1916

**DEGREE • BSN**
**Nursing Program Faculty** 17 (12% with doctorates).
**Baccalaureate Enrollment** 106 **Women** 87% **Men** 13% **Minority** 20% **Part-time** .02%
**Nursing Student Activities** Student Nurses' Association.
**Nursing Student Resources** Academic advising; academic or career counseling; assistance for students with disabilities; bookstore; campus computer network; career placement assistance; computer lab; computer-assisted instruction; e-mail services; employment services for current students; externships; interactive nursing skills videos; Internet; learning resource lab; library services; nursing audiovisuals; remedial services; resume preparation assistance; skills, simulation, or other laboratory; tutoring.
**Library Facilities** 80,845 volumes (463 in health, 439 in nursing); 22,464 periodical subscriptions (60 health-care related).

**BACCALAUREATE PROGRAMS**
**Degree** BSN
**Available Programs** Generic Baccalaureate.
**Study Options** Full-time.
**Program Entrance Requirements** Minimum overall college GPA of 2.7, transcript of college record, CPR certification, written essay, health insurance, immunizations, interview, minimum GPA in nursing prerequisites of 2.0, prerequisite course work. Transfer students are accepted. *Application deadline:* 1/10 (fall). *Application fee:* $45.
**Advanced Placement** Credit given for nursing courses completed elsewhere dependent upon specific evaluations.
**Expenses (2013–14)** *Tuition:* full-time $24,750; part-time $630 per credit. *Room and board:* $7500 per academic year. *Required fees:* full-time $1460; part-time $36 per credit.
**Financial Aid** 99% of baccalaureate students in nursing programs received some form of financial aid in 2012–13.
**Contact** Office of Admissions, School of Nursing, Avila University, 11901 Wornall Road, Kansas City, MO 64145-1698. *Telephone:* 816-501-2400. *Fax:* 816-501-2453. *E-mail:* admissions@avila.edu.

## Central Methodist University
### College of Liberal Arts and Sciences
### Fayette, Missouri

***http://www.centralmethodist.edu/***
Founded in 1854

**DEGREES • BSN • MSN**
**Nursing Program Faculty** 30 (26% with doctorates).
**Baccalaureate Enrollment** 325 **Women** 92% **Men** 8% **Minority** 11% **International** 1%
**Graduate Enrollment** 33 **Women** 96% **Men** 4% **Minority** 7%
**Distance Learning Courses** Available.
**Nursing Student Activities** Sigma Theta Tau, Student Nurses' Association.
**Nursing Student Resources** Academic advising; academic or career counseling; assistance for students with disabilities; bookstore; campus computer network; computer lab; computer-assisted instruction; e-mail services; interactive nursing skills videos; Internet; learning resource lab; library services; nursing audiovisuals; resume preparation assistance; skills, simulation, or other laboratory; tutoring.
**Library Facilities** 97,793 volumes; 316 periodical subscriptions.

**BACCALAUREATE PROGRAMS**
**Degree** BSN
**Available Programs** ADN to Baccalaureate; Accelerated Baccalaureate for Second Degree; Generic Baccalaureate.
**Site Options** Columbia, MO; St. Louis, MO; Rolla, MO.
**Study Options** Full-time.
**Online Degree Options** Yes.
**Program Entrance Requirements** Minimum overall college GPA, transcript of college record, CPR certification, written essay, health insurance, high school transcript, immunizations, minimum GPA in nursing prerequisites, prerequisite course work. Transfer students are accepted. *Application deadline:* 4/1 (fall), 1/1 (spring). Applications may be processed on a rolling basis for some programs.
**Advanced Placement** Credit by examination available. Credit given for nursing courses completed elsewhere dependent upon specific evaluations.
**Expenses (2013–14)** *Tuition:* full-time $10,295; part-time $190 per credit hour. *International tuition:* $10,295 full-time. *Room and board:* $3520; room only: $3250 per academic year. *Required fees:* full-time $1380.
**Financial Aid** 95% of baccalaureate students in nursing programs received some form of financial aid in 2012–13.
**Contact** Prof. Megan Hess, Chair, Division of Health Professions. *Telephone:* 660-248-6359. *E-mail:* mhess@centralmethodist.edu.

**GRADUATE PROGRAMS**
**Expenses (2013–14)** *Tuition:* part-time $360 per credit hour.
**Financial Aid** 90% of graduate students in nursing programs received some form of financial aid in 2012–13.
**Contact** Stephanie Brink, Associate Dean of Online Programming, College of Liberal Arts and Sciences, Central Methodist University, 411 Central Methodist Square, Fayette, MO 65248. *Telephone:* 660-248-6639. *Fax:* 660-248-6243. *E-mail:* sbrink@centralmethodist.edu.

**MASTER'S DEGREE PROGRAM**
**Degree** MSN
**Available Programs** Master's.
**Concentrations Available** Clinical nurse leader; nursing education.
**Study Options** Full-time and part-time.
**Online Degree Options** Yes (online only).
**Program Entrance Requirements** Clinical experience, computer literacy, minimum overall college GPA of 3.0, transcript of college record, CPR certification, written essay, immunizations, nursing research course, professional liability insurance/malpractice insurance, prerequisite course work, statistics course. *Application deadline:* Applications may be processed on a rolling basis for some programs.
**Advanced Placement** Credit given for nursing courses completed elsewhere dependent upon specific evaluations.
**Degree Requirements** 34 total credit hours, thesis or project.

## Chamberlain College of Nursing
### Chamberlain College of Nursing
### St. Louis, Missouri

***http://www.chamberlain.edu/***
Founded in 1889

**DEGREE • BSN**
**Nursing Program Faculty** 80 (21% with doctorates).
**Distance Learning Courses** Available.
**Nursing Student Activities** Student Nurses' Association.
**Nursing Student Resources** Academic advising; academic or career counseling; assistance for students with disabilities; bookstore; campus

computer network; career placement assistance; computer lab; computer-assisted instruction; e-mail services; employment services for current students; housing assistance; Internet; learning resource lab; library services; nursing audiovisuals; placement services for program completers; skills, simulation, or other laboratory; tutoring.
**Library Facilities** 3,287 volumes in health, 957 volumes in nursing; 182 periodical subscriptions health-care related.

### BACCALAUREATE PROGRAMS

**Degree** BSN
**Available Programs** ADN to Baccalaureate; Accelerated RN Baccalaureate; Generic Baccalaureate; LPN to RN Baccalaureate; RN Baccalaureate.
**Site Options** Columbus, OH; Phoenix, AZ; Addison, IL.
**Study Options** Full-time.
**Online Degree Options** Yes (online only).
**Program Entrance Requirements** Minimum overall college GPA of 2.75, transcript of college record, written essay, health exam, health insurance, high school biology, high school chemistry, 3 years high school math, 3 years high school science, high school transcript, immunizations, interview, minimum high school GPA of 2.75, minimum high school rank 33%. Transfer students are accepted.
**Advanced Placement** Credit by examination available. Credit given for nursing courses completed elsewhere dependent upon specific evaluations.
**Contact** *Telephone:* 800-942-4310 Ext. 1. *Fax:* 314-768-3044.

## College of the Ozarks
### Armstrong McDonald School of Nursing
### Point Lookout, Missouri

***http://www.cofo.edu/***
Founded in 1906

### DEGREE • BSN
**Nursing Program Faculty** 9 (22% with doctorates).
**Baccalaureate Enrollment** 59 **Women** 78% **Men** 22% **Minority** 6.8% **International** 3.4%
**Nursing Student Activities** Nursing club.
**Nursing Student Resources** Academic advising; academic or career counseling; assistance for students with disabilities; bookstore; campus computer network; career placement assistance; computer lab; computer-assisted instruction; daycare for children of students; e-mail services; employment services for current students; externships; housing assistance; interactive nursing skills videos; Internet; learning resource lab; library services; nursing audiovisuals; paid internships; placement services for program completers; remedial services; resume preparation assistance; skills, simulation, or other laboratory; tutoring; unpaid internships.
**Library Facilities** 265,081 volumes (1,225 in health, 861 in nursing); 470 periodical subscriptions (68 health-care related).

### BACCALAUREATE PROGRAMS

**Degree** BSN
**Available Programs** Generic Baccalaureate.
**Study Options** Full-time and part-time.
**Program Entrance Requirements** Minimum overall college GPA of 2.5, transcript of college record, health exam, 2 years high school math, high school transcript, immunizations, interview, 2 letters of recommendation, minimum high school GPA of 3.0, minimum high school rank 51%, minimum GPA in nursing prerequisites of 2.5, professional liability insurance/malpractice insurance, prerequisite course work. Transfer students are accepted. *Application deadline:* 10/1 (fall), 3/1 (spring).
**Expenses (2013–14)** *Room and board:* $5900; room only: $2900 per academic year.
**Financial Aid** 100% of baccalaureate students in nursing programs received some form of financial aid in 2012–13. *Gift aid (need-based):* Federal Pell, FSEOG, state, private, college/university gift aid from institutional funds. *Work-study:* Federal Work-Study, part-time campus jobs. *Financial aid application deadline (priority):* 2/15.
**Contact** Mrs. Deborah J. Lyon, Office Manager, Armstrong McDonald School of Nursing, College of the Ozarks, PO Box 17, Point Lookout, MO 65726. *Telephone:* 417-690-2421. *Fax:* 417-690-2422. *E-mail:* dlyon@cofo.edu.

## Cox College
### Department of Nursing
### Springfield, Missouri

Founded in 1994

### DEGREES • BSN • MSN
**Nursing Program Faculty** 61 (10% with doctorates).
**Baccalaureate Enrollment** 240 **Women** 87% **Men** 13% **Minority** 5% **Part-time** 80%
**Graduate Enrollment** 83 **Women** 92% **Men** 8%
**Distance Learning Courses** Available.
**Nursing Student Activities** Nursing Honor Society, Student Nurses' Association, nursing club.
**Nursing Student Resources** Academic advising; academic or career counseling; assistance for students with disabilities; bookstore; campus computer network; career placement assistance; computer lab; computer-assisted instruction; daycare for children of students; e-mail services; employment services for current students; externships; housing assistance; interactive nursing skills videos; Internet; learning resource lab; library services; nursing audiovisuals; placement services for program completers; remedial services; resume preparation assistance; skills, simulation, or other laboratory; tutoring.
**Library Facilities** 29,750 volumes (5,500 in health, 1,900 in nursing); 249 periodical subscriptions (250 health-care related).

### BACCALAUREATE PROGRAMS

**Degree** BSN
**Available Programs** ADN to Baccalaureate; Accelerated Baccalaureate; Accelerated Baccalaureate for Second Degree; Baccalaureate for Second Degree; Generic Baccalaureate; LPN to Baccalaureate; LPN to RN Baccalaureate; RN Baccalaureate.
**Site Options** Springfield, MO.
**Study Options** Full-time.
**Online Degree Options** Yes (online only).
**Program Entrance Requirements** Minimum overall college GPA of 3.0, transcript of college record, CPR certification, high school transcript, immunizations, interview, minimum high school GPA of 3.0, minimum GPA in nursing prerequisites of 3.0, professional liability insurance/malpractice insurance, prerequisite course work, RN licensure. Transfer students are accepted. *Application deadline:* 1/15 (fall), 8/15 (spring). *Application fee:* $45.
**Advanced Placement** Credit given for nursing courses completed elsewhere dependent upon specific evaluations.
**Contact** *Telephone:* 417-269-3401. *Fax:* 417-269-3586.

### GRADUATE PROGRAMS

**Contact** *Telephone:* 417-269-3401.

#### MASTER'S DEGREE PROGRAM
**Degree** MSN
**Available Programs** Master's; RN to Master's.
**Concentrations Available** Clinical nurse leader; nursing education. *Clinical nurse specialist programs in:* family health.
**Site Options** Springfield, MO.
**Study Options** Full-time and part-time.
**Online Degree Options** Yes (online only).
**Program Entrance Requirements** Clinical experience, computer literacy, minimum overall college GPA of 3.0, transcript of college record, CPR certification, written essay, immunizations, interview, letters of recommendation, resume. *Application deadline:* 3/1 (fall). *Application fee:* $45.
**Degree Requirements** 42 total credit hours, thesis or project.

### CONTINUING EDUCATION PROGRAM

**Contact** *Telephone:* 417-269-5062.

## Culver-Stockton College
### Blessing–Rieman College of Nursing
### Canton, Missouri

***http://www.culver.edu/***

***See description of programs under Blessing–Rieman College of Nursing (Quincy, Illinois).***

# Goldfarb School of Nursing at Barnes-Jewish College

## Goldfarb School of Nursing at Barnes-Jewish College
## St. Louis, Missouri

Founded in 1902

### DEGREES • BSN • MSN • PHD

**Nursing Program Faculty** 51 (45% with doctorates).
**Baccalaureate Enrollment** 658 **Women** 91% **Men** 9% **Minority** 12%
**Graduate Enrollment** 166 **Women** 88% **Men** 12% **Minority** 18% **International** .6% **Part-time** 50%
**Distance Learning Courses** Available.
**Nursing Student Activities** Nursing Honor Society, Sigma Theta Tau, Student Nurses' Association, nursing club.
**Nursing Student Resources** Academic advising; academic or career counseling; assistance for students with disabilities; bookstore; campus computer network; career placement assistance; computer lab; computer-assisted instruction; e-mail services; employment services for current students; externships; housing assistance; interactive nursing skills videos; Internet; learning resource lab; library services; nursing audiovisuals; placement services for program completers; remedial services; resume preparation assistance; skills, simulation, or other laboratory; tutoring.
**Library Facilities** 1,125 volumes (13,000 in health, 8,200 in nursing); 47 periodical subscriptions (250 health-care related).

### BACCALAUREATE PROGRAMS

**Degree** BSN
**Available Programs** ADN to Baccalaureate; Accelerated Baccalaureate; Accelerated Baccalaureate for Second Degree; Generic Baccalaureate; RN Baccalaureate.
**Site Options** Town and Country, MO.
**Study Options** Full-time.
**Program Entrance Requirements** Minimum overall college GPA of 3.0, transcript of college record, CPR certification, health exam, high school biology, high school transcript, immunizations, minimum high school GPA of 3.0, minimum GPA in nursing prerequisites of 3.0, prerequisite course work. Transfer students are accepted. *Application deadline:* 8/15 (fall), 12/15 (spring), 4/1 (summer). Applications may be processed on a rolling basis for some programs. *Application fee:* $50.
**Advanced Placement** Credit by examination available. Credit given for nursing courses completed elsewhere dependent upon specific evaluations.
**Expenses (2013–14)** *Tuition:* full-time $25,768; part-time $633 per credit hour. *Required fees:* full-time $1565.
**Financial Aid** 95% of baccalaureate students in nursing programs received some form of financial aid in 2012–13.
**Contact** Karen Sartorius, Enrollment Coordinator, Goldfarb School of Nursing at Barnes-Jewish College, 4483 Duncan, MS #90-36-697, St. Louis, MO 63110-1091. *Telephone:* 314-454-7057. *Fax:* 314-362-9250. *E-mail:* ksartorius@bjc.org.

### GRADUATE PROGRAMS

**Expenses (2013–14)** *Tuition:* full-time $16,755; part-time $685 per credit hour. *Required fees:* full-time $295.
**Financial Aid** 80% of graduate students in nursing programs received some form of financial aid in 2012–13.
**Contact** Dr. Gretchen Drinkard, Associate Dean/Graduate Programs, Goldfarb School of Nursing at Barnes-Jewish College, 4483 Duncan, MS #90-36-697, St. Louis, MO 63110-1091. *Telephone:* 314-454-7540. *Fax:* 314-362-9222. *E-mail:* gdrinkard@bjc.org.

#### MASTER'S DEGREE PROGRAM

**Degree** MSN
**Available Programs** Master's.
**Concentrations Available** Health-care administration; nurse anesthesia; nursing administration; nursing education. *Nurse practitioner programs in:* acute care, adult health.
**Study Options** Full-time and part-time.
**Program Entrance Requirements** Clinical experience, computer literacy, minimum overall college GPA of 3.0, transcript of college record, CPR certification, immunizations, 2 letters of recommendation, nursing research course, physical assessment course, resume, statistics course. *Application deadline:* 8/20 (fall), 12/15 (spring), 4/15 (summer). Applications may be processed on a rolling basis for some programs. *Application fee:* $50.
**Advanced Placement** Credit given for nursing courses completed elsewhere dependent upon specific evaluations.
**Degree Requirements** 34 total credit hours, thesis or project.

#### POST-MASTER'S PROGRAM

**Areas of Study** Health-care administration; nursing administration; nursing education. *Nurse practitioner programs in:* acute care, adult health.

#### DOCTORAL DEGREE PROGRAM

**Degree** PhD
**Available Programs** Doctorate.
**Areas of Study** Clinical practice, nursing administration, nursing education.
**Program Entrance Requirements** Minimum overall college GPA of 3.0, interview by faculty committee, interview, 3 letters of recommendation, MSN or equivalent, statistics course, vita, writing sample. *Application deadline:* 7/15 (fall). Applications may be processed on a rolling basis for some programs. *Application fee:* $50.
**Degree Requirements** 111 total credit hours, dissertation, oral exam, written exam, residency.

# Graceland University

## School of Nursing
## Independence, Missouri

*http://www.graceland.edu/nursing*
Founded in 1895

### DEGREES • BSN • DNP • MSN

**Nursing Program Faculty** 21 (57% with doctorates).
**Baccalaureate Enrollment** 122 **Women** 89% **Men** 11% **Minority** 5% **Part-time** 5%
**Graduate Enrollment** 493 **Women** 91% **Men** 9% **Minority** 2% **Part-time** 50%
**Distance Learning Courses** Available.
**Nursing Student Activities** Nursing Honor Society, Sigma Theta Tau, Student Nurses' Association, nursing club.
**Nursing Student Resources** Academic advising; academic or career counseling; assistance for students with disabilities; bookstore; campus computer network; computer lab; computer-assisted instruction; e-mail services; housing assistance; interactive nursing skills videos; Internet; learning resource lab; library services; nursing audiovisuals; resume preparation assistance; skills, simulation, or other laboratory; tutoring.
**Library Facilities** 143,989 volumes (4,195 in health, 2,234 in nursing); 903 periodical subscriptions (561 health-care related).

### BACCALAUREATE PROGRAMS

**Degree** BSN
**Available Programs** ADN to Baccalaureate; Accelerated Baccalaureate; Generic Baccalaureate; RN Baccalaureate.
**Site Options** Independence, MO.
**Study Options** Full-time and part-time.
**Program Entrance Requirements** Minimum overall college GPA of 2.75, transcript of college record, written essay, health exam, high school chemistry, high school transcript, immunizations, interview, 2 letters of recommendation, minimum high school GPA of 2.75, minimum GPA in nursing prerequisites of 2.0, prerequisite course work. Transfer students are accepted. *Application deadline:* 11/30 (fall). *Application fee:* $50.
**Advanced Placement** Credit given for nursing courses completed elsewhere dependent upon specific evaluations.
**Expenses (2013–14)** *Tuition:* full-time $23,180; part-time $725 per credit hour. *International tuition:* $23,180 full-time. *Required fees:* full-time $1795; part-time $897 per term.
**Financial Aid** 90% of baccalaureate students in nursing programs received some form of financial aid in 2012–13. *Gift aid (need-based):* Federal Pell, FSEOG, state, private, college/university gift aid from institutional funds. *Loans:* Federal Direct (Subsidized and Unsubsidized Stafford PLUS), Perkins, state, college/university. *Work-study:* Federal Work-Study, part-time campus jobs. *Financial aid application deadline:* Continuous.
**Contact** Ms. Laurie Hale, Admissions Counselor, School of Nursing, Graceland University, 1401 West Truman Road, Independence, MO 64050-3434. *Telephone:* 800-423-4675. *Fax:* 816-833-2990. *E-mail:* lhale@graceland.edu.

## GRADUATE PROGRAMS

**Expenses (2013–14)** *Tuition:* part-time $650 per credit hour.

**Financial Aid** 80% of graduate students in nursing programs received some form of financial aid in 2012–13.

**Contact** Ms. Jill Whitworth, Program Consultant, School of Nursing, Graceland University, 1401 West Truman Road, Independence, MO 64050-3434. *Telephone:* 816-423-4712. *Fax:* 816-833-2990. *E-mail:* jwhitwor@graceland.edu.

### MASTER'S DEGREE PROGRAM

**Degree** MSN

**Available Programs** Master's; RN to Master's.

**Concentrations Available** Nursing education. *Nurse practitioner programs in:* family health.

**Site Options** Independence, MO.

**Study Options** Full-time and part-time.

**Online Degree Options** Yes (online only).

**Program Entrance Requirements** Clinical experience, minimum overall college GPA of 3.0, transcript of college record, written essay, 3 letters of recommendation, nursing research course, physical assessment course, prerequisite course work, statistics course. *Application deadline:* 6/1 (fall), 10/1 (winter), 2/1 (spring). *Application fee:* $50.

**Advanced Placement** Credit given for nursing courses completed elsewhere dependent upon specific evaluations.

**Degree Requirements** 47 total credit hours, thesis or project, comprehensive exam.

### POST-MASTER'S PROGRAM

**Areas of Study** Nursing education. *Nurse practitioner programs in:* family health.

### DOCTORAL DEGREE PROGRAM

**Degree** DNP

**Available Programs** Doctorate.

**Areas of Study** Advanced practice nursing, family health, health policy, health promotion/disease prevention, health-care systems, human health and illness, nursing policy, nursing science.

**Site Options** Independence, MO.

**Online Degree Options** Yes (online only).

**Program Entrance Requirements** Minimum overall college GPA of 3.2, 3 letters of recommendation, MSN or equivalent, writing sample. *Application deadline:* 5/15 (fall). *Application fee:* $50.

**Degree Requirements** 31 total credit hours, dissertation, residency.

# Lincoln University

### Department of Nursing
### Jefferson City, Missouri

***http://www.lincolnu.edu/web/dept.-of-nursing-science/nursing-science***

Founded in 1866

**DEGREE • BSN**

**Distance Learning Courses** Available.

**Nursing Student Resources** Academic advising; academic or career counseling; assistance for students with disabilities; bookstore; campus computer network; computer lab; e-mail services; Internet; library services; remedial services; tutoring.

**Library Facilities** 328,418 volumes; 334 periodical subscriptions.

## BACCALAUREATE PROGRAMS

**Degree** BSN

**Available Programs** RN Baccalaureate.

**Contact** Dr. Connie Hamacher, Department Head of Nursing Science, Department of Nursing, Lincoln University, 820 Chestnut, Elliff Hall, Room 100, Jefferson City, MO 65101. *Telephone:* 573-681-5421. *E-mail:* nursing@lincolnu.edu.

# Maryville University of Saint Louis

### Nursing Program, School of Health Professions
### St. Louis, Missouri

***http://www.maryville.edu/academics-hp-nursing.htm***

Founded in 1872

**DEGREES • BSN • DNP • MSN**

**Nursing Program Faculty** 65 (4% with doctorates).

**Baccalaureate Enrollment** 463 **Women** 95% **Men** 5% **Minority** 10% **International** 1% **Part-time** 45%

**Graduate Enrollment** 116 **Women** 92% **Men** 8% **Minority** 14% **Part-time** 79%

**Nursing Student Activities** Sigma Theta Tau, Student Nurses' Association.

**Nursing Student Resources** Academic advising; academic or career counseling; assistance for students with disabilities; bookstore; campus computer network; career placement assistance; computer lab; computer-assisted instruction; e-mail services; externships; interactive nursing skills videos; Internet; learning resource lab; library services; nursing audiovisuals; paid internships; remedial services; resume preparation assistance; skills, simulation, or other laboratory; tutoring.

**Library Facilities** 108,733 volumes (8,680 in health, 1,464 in nursing); 85,674 periodical subscriptions (4,315 health-care related).

## BACCALAUREATE PROGRAMS

**Degree** BSN

**Available Programs** Accelerated Baccalaureate; Accelerated RN Baccalaureate; Generic Baccalaureate; LPN to Baccalaureate; RN Baccalaureate.

**Study Options** Full-time and part-time.

**Program Entrance Requirements** Minimum overall college GPA of 2.75, transcript of college record, health exam, high school transcript, immunizations, minimum high school GPA of 2.75, minimum GPA in nursing prerequisites of 2.75. Transfer students are accepted. *Application deadline:* 12/15 (fall). Applications may be processed on a rolling basis for some programs.

**Advanced Placement** Credit given for nursing courses completed elsewhere dependent upon specific evaluations.

**Contact** *Telephone:* 314-529-9453. *Fax:* 314-529-9495.

## GRADUATE PROGRAMS

**Contact** *Telephone:* 314-529-9453. *Fax:* 314-529-9495.

### MASTER'S DEGREE PROGRAM

**Degree** MSN

**Available Programs** Accelerated RN to Master's; Master's; RN to Master's.

**Concentrations Available** Nursing education. *Nurse practitioner programs in:* adult health, family health.

**Study Options** Full-time and part-time.

**Program Entrance Requirements** Minimum overall college GPA of 3.0, transcript of college record, written essay, 3 letters of recommendation, resume, statistics course. *Application deadline:* Applications may be processed on a rolling basis for some programs.

**Advanced Placement** Credit by examination available. Credit given for nursing courses completed elsewhere dependent upon specific evaluations.

**Degree Requirements** 42 total credit hours, thesis or project.

### DOCTORAL DEGREE PROGRAM

**Degree** DNP

**Available Programs** Doctorate.

**Areas of Study** Advanced practice nursing, ethics, health policy, nursing research.

**Program Entrance Requirements** Minimum overall college GPA of 3.5, 3 letters of recommendation, MSN or equivalent, vita, writing sample. *Application deadline:* Applications may be processed on a rolling basis for some programs.

**Degree Requirements** 30 total credit hours.

# Missouri Southern State University

## Department of Nursing
## Joplin, Missouri

*http://www.mssu.edu*
Founded in 1937

**DEGREES • BSN • MSN**
**Nursing Program Faculty** 10 (10% with doctorates).
**Baccalaureate Enrollment** 107 **Women** 79.44% **Men** 20.56% **Minority** 12.15%
**Graduate Enrollment** 49 **Women** 96% **Men** 4% **Minority** 8% **Part-time** 31%
**Distance Learning Courses** Available.
**Nursing Student Activities** Nursing Honor Society, Student Nurses' Association.
**Nursing Student Resources** Academic advising; academic or career counseling; assistance for students with disabilities; bookstore; campus computer network; career placement assistance; computer lab; computer-assisted instruction; daycare for children of students; e-mail services; employment services for current students; housing assistance; interactive nursing skills videos; Internet; learning resource lab; library services; nursing audiovisuals; remedial services; resume preparation assistance; skills, simulation, or other laboratory; tutoring.
**Library Facilities** 4,872 volumes in health, 4,470 volumes in nursing; 4,412 periodical subscriptions health-care related.

### BACCALAUREATE PROGRAMS

**Degree** BSN
**Available Programs** ADN to Baccalaureate; Baccalaureate for Second Degree; Generic Baccalaureate; LPN to Baccalaureate; RN Baccalaureate.
**Study Options** Full-time.
**Program Entrance Requirements** Transcript of college record, CPR certification, health exam, health insurance, immunizations, minimum GPA in nursing prerequisites of 2.5, professional liability insurance/malpractice insurance, prerequisite course work, RN licensure. Transfer students are accepted. *Application deadline:* 1/31 (fall). *Application fee:* $50.
**Advanced Placement** Credit by examination available. Credit given for nursing courses completed elsewhere dependent upon specific evaluations.
**Contact** *Telephone:* 417-625-9322. *Fax:* 417-625-3186.

### GRADUATE PROGRAMS

**Contact** *Telephone:* 417-625-9322. *Fax:* 417-625-3186.

#### MASTER'S DEGREE PROGRAM

**Degree** MSN
**Available Programs** Master's.
**Concentrations Available** Nursing education. *Clinical nurse specialist programs in:* family health.
**Study Options** Full-time and part-time.
**Program Entrance Requirements** Minimum overall college GPA of 3.0, transcript of college record, resume. *Application deadline:* 12/1 (fall). *Application fee:* $35.
**Degree Requirements** 42 total credit hours.

# Missouri State University

## Department of Nursing
## Springfield, Missouri

*http://www.missouristate.edu/nursing*
Founded in 1905

**DEGREES • BSN • DNP • MSN**
**Nursing Program Faculty** 14 (36% with doctorates).
**Baccalaureate Enrollment** 210 **Women** 90% **Men** 10% **Minority** 4% **International** 1% **Part-time** 25%
**Graduate Enrollment** 51 **Women** 97% **Men** 3% **Minority** 2% **Part-time** 40%
**Distance Learning Courses** Available.
**Nursing Student Activities** Sigma Theta Tau, Student Nurses' Association.
**Nursing Student Resources** Academic advising; academic or career counseling; assistance for students with disabilities; bookstore; campus computer network; career placement assistance; computer lab; computer-assisted instruction; daycare for children of students; e-mail services; employment services for current students; externships; housing assistance; interactive nursing skills videos; Internet; learning resource lab; library services; nursing audiovisuals; paid internships; placement services for program completers; remedial services; resume preparation assistance; skills, simulation, or other laboratory; tutoring; unpaid internships.
**Library Facilities** 10,500 volumes in health, 3,516 volumes in nursing; 370 periodical subscriptions health-care related.

### BACCALAUREATE PROGRAMS

**Degree** BSN
**Available Programs** ADN to Baccalaureate; Accelerated RN Baccalaureate; Generic Baccalaureate; LPN to Baccalaureate; RN Baccalaureate.
**Study Options** Full-time.
**Online Degree Options** Yes.
**Program Entrance Requirements** Minimum overall college GPA of 2.75, transcript of college record, CPR certification, written essay, health insurance, immunizations, prerequisite course work. Transfer students are accepted. *Application deadline:* 1/31 (summer). *Application fee:* $50.
**Advanced Placement** Credit given for nursing courses completed elsewhere dependent upon specific evaluations.
**Expenses (2012–13)** *Tuition, state resident:* full-time $6264; part-time $200 per credit hour. *Tuition, nonresident:* full-time $12,610; part-time $412 per credit hour. *International tuition:* $12,610 full-time. *Room and board:* $7204; room only: $5768 per academic year. *Required fees:* full-time $1228.
**Financial Aid** 65% of baccalaureate students in nursing programs received some form of financial aid in 2011–12.
**Contact** Dr. Kathryn L. Hope, Head, Department of Nursing, Department of Nursing, Missouri State University, 901 South National Avenue, Springfield, MO 65897. *Telephone:* 417-836-5310. *Fax:* 417-836-5484. *E-mail:* kathrynhope@missouristate.edu.

### GRADUATE PROGRAMS

**Expenses (2012–13)** *Tuition, state resident:* full-time $4356; part-time $242 per credit hour. *Tuition, nonresident:* full-time $8712; part-time $484 per credit hour. *International tuition:* $8712 full-time. *Room and board:* $7204; room only: $5768 per academic year. *Required fees:* full-time $778.
**Financial Aid** 25% of graduate students in nursing programs received some form of financial aid in 2011–12. Federal Work-Study, institutionally sponsored loans, scholarships, and unspecified assistantships available. *Financial aid application deadline:* 3/31.
**Contact** Dr. Kathryn L. Hope, Head, Department of Nursing, Department of Nursing, Missouri State University, 901 South National Avenue, Springfield, MO 65897. *Telephone:* 417-836-5310. *Fax:* 417-836-5484. *E-mail:* kathrynhope@missouristate.edu.

#### MASTER'S DEGREE PROGRAM

**Degree** MSN
**Available Programs** Accelerated AD/RN to Master's; Master's; RN to Master's.
**Concentrations Available** Nursing education. *Nurse practitioner programs in:* family health.
**Study Options** Full-time and part-time.
**Online Degree Options** Yes (online only).
**Program Entrance Requirements** Computer literacy, minimum overall college GPA of 3.0, transcript of college record, CPR certification, written essay, immunizations, interview, nursing research course, physical assessment course, professional liability insurance/malpractice insurance, prerequisite course work, statistics course, GRE General Test. *Application deadline:* 2/15 (fall). *Application fee:* $50.
**Advanced Placement** Credit given for nursing courses completed elsewhere dependent upon specific evaluations.
**Degree Requirements** 51 total credit hours, thesis or project, comprehensive exam.

#### POST-MASTER'S PROGRAM

**Areas of Study** Nursing education. *Nurse practitioner programs in:* family health.

#### DOCTORAL DEGREE PROGRAM

**Degree** DNP
**Available Programs** Doctorate; Post-Baccalaureate Doctorate.
**Areas of Study** Advanced practice nursing, health-care systems.

**Online Degree Options** Yes.
**Program Entrance Requirements** Clinical experience, minimum overall college GPA of 3.25, interview by faculty committee, interview, statistics course, vita, writing sample. *Application deadline:* 12/1 (summer). *Application fee:* $50.
**Degree Requirements** 29 total credit hours, oral exam.

### CONTINUING EDUCATION PROGRAM

**Contact** Virginia Cordova, Program Coordinator, Department of Nursing, Missouri State University, 901 South National Avenue, Department of Continuing Education, Springfield, MO 65897. *Telephone:* 417-836-6660. *Fax:* 417-836-7674. *E-mail:* virginiacordova@missouristate.edu.

## Missouri Western State University

### Department of Nursing
### St. Joseph, Missouri

***http://www.missouriwestern.edu/nursing***
Founded in 1915

**DEGREES • BSN • MSN**
**Nursing Program Faculty** 35 (23% with doctorates).
**Baccalaureate Enrollment** 200 **Women** 86% **Men** 14% **Minority** 4% **Part-time** 7%
**Graduate Enrollment** 17 **Women** 100% **Part-time** 100%
**Distance Learning Courses** Available.
**Nursing Student Activities** Sigma Theta Tau, Student Nurses' Association.
**Nursing Student Resources** Academic advising; academic or career counseling; assistance for students with disabilities; bookstore; campus computer network; career placement assistance; computer lab; computer-assisted instruction; e-mail services; employment services for current students; interactive nursing skills videos; Internet; learning resource lab; library services; nursing audiovisuals; placement services for program completers; remedial services; resume preparation assistance; skills, simulation, or other laboratory; tutoring; unpaid internships.
**Library Facilities** 224,131 volumes; 3,214 periodical subscriptions (29 health-care related).

### BACCALAUREATE PROGRAMS

**Degree** BSN
**Available Programs** ADN to Baccalaureate; Generic Baccalaureate.
**Site Options** Kansas City, MO.
**Study Options** Full-time.
**Program Entrance Requirements** Minimum overall college GPA of 2.7, transcript of college record, CPR certification, written essay, health insurance, high school transcript, immunizations, minimum GPA in nursing prerequisites of 2.7, prerequisite course work. Transfer students are accepted. *Application deadline:* 1/15 (fall), 7/31 (spring). *Application fee:* $45.
**Advanced Placement** Credit by examination available. Credit given for nursing courses completed elsewhere dependent upon specific evaluations.
**Expenses (2012–13)** *Tuition, state resident:* part-time $189 per credit. *Tuition, nonresident:* part-time $372 per credit. *Room and board:* $9036 per academic year.
**Financial Aid** 88% of baccalaureate students in nursing programs received some form of financial aid in 2011–12. *Gift aid (need-based):* Federal Pell, FSEOG, state, private, college/university gift aid from institutional funds. *Loans:* Federal Direct (Subsidized and Unsubsidized Stafford PLUS), Perkins. *Work-study:* Federal Work-Study, part-time campus jobs. *Financial aid application deadline:* Continuous.
**Contact** Rebecca Boettcher, Admissions/Advisement Counselor, Department of Nursing, Missouri Western State University, 4525 Downs Drive, Murphy Hall 309, St. Joseph, MO 64507. *Telephone:* 816-271-4415. *Fax:* 816-271-5849. *E-mail:* rboettcher@missouriwestern.edu.

### GRADUATE PROGRAMS

**Expenses (2012–13)** *Tuition, state resident:* part-time $281 per credit hour. *Tuition, nonresident:* part-time $540 per credit hour.
**Financial Aid** 78% of graduate students in nursing programs received some form of financial aid in 2011–12.
**Contact** Dr. Kathleen E. O'Connor, Associate Professor and Chairperson, Department of Nursing, Missouri Western State University, 4525 Downs Drive, St. Joseph, MO 64507. *Telephone:* 816-271-4415. *Fax:* 816-271-5849. *E-mail:* koconnor5@missouriwestern.edu.

**MASTER'S DEGREE PROGRAM**
**Degree** MSN
**Available Programs** Master's.
**Concentrations Available** Health-care administration.
**Study Options** Part-time.
**Program Entrance Requirements** Minimum overall college GPA of 2.75, transcript of college record, written essay, interview, nursing research course, prerequisite course work, statistics course. *Application deadline:* 7/15 (fall), 10/15 (spring). *Application fee:* $30.
**Degree Requirements** 36 total credit hours, thesis or project.

### CONTINUING EDUCATION PROGRAM

**Contact** Rebecca Boettcher, Admissions/Advisement Counselor, Department of Nursing, Missouri Western State University, 4525 Downs Drive, Murphy Hall 309, St. Joseph, MO 64507. *Telephone:* 816-271-4415. *Fax:* 816-271-5849. *E-mail:* rboettcher@missouriwestern.edu.

## Research College of Nursing

### College of Nursing
### Kansas City, Missouri

***http://www.researchcollege.edu/***
Founded in 1980

**DEGREES • BSN • MSN**
**Nursing Program Faculty** 37 (16% with doctorates).
**Baccalaureate Enrollment** 345 **Women** 92% **Men** 8% **Minority** 7%
**Graduate Enrollment** 124 **Women** 95% **Men** 5% **Minority** 13% **Part-time** 90%
**Distance Learning Courses** Available.
**Nursing Student Activities** Sigma Theta Tau, Student Nurses' Association.
**Nursing Student Resources** Academic advising; academic or career counseling; bookstore; campus computer network; career placement assistance; computer lab; computer-assisted instruction; daycare for children of students; e-mail services; housing assistance; Internet; learning resource lab; library services; resume preparation assistance; skills, simulation, or other laboratory; tutoring.
**Library Facilities** 150,000 volumes; 675 periodical subscriptions.

### BACCALAUREATE PROGRAMS

**Degree** BSN
**Available Programs** Accelerated Baccalaureate; Accelerated Baccalaureate for Second Degree; Baccalaureate for Second Degree; Generic Baccalaureate.
**Study Options** Full-time.
**Program Entrance Requirements** Transcript of college record, high school chemistry, 3 years high school math, 2 years high school science, high school transcript, minimum high school rank 50%, minimum GPA in nursing prerequisites of 2.7. Transfer students are accepted. *Application deadline:* 2/15 (spring). *Application fee:* $45.
**Advanced Placement** Credit given for nursing courses completed elsewhere dependent upon specific evaluations.
**Expenses (2013–14)** *Tuition:* full-time $30,550; part-time $1020 per credit hour. *Room and board:* $7500; room only: $4000 per academic year. *Required fees:* full-time $730; part-time $300 per term.
**Financial Aid** 90% of baccalaureate students in nursing programs received some form of financial aid in 2012–13.
**Contact** Ms. Leslie Ann Mendenhall, Director of Transfer and Graduate Admissions, College of Nursing, Research College of Nursing, 2525 East Meyer Boulevard, Kansas City, MO 64132-1199. *Telephone:* 816-995-2820. *Fax:* 816-995-2813. *E-mail:* leslie.mendenhall@researchcollege.edu.

### GRADUATE PROGRAMS

**Expenses (2013–14)** *Tuition:* part-time $465 per credit hour. *Required fees:* part-time $25 per credit.
**Financial Aid** 15% of graduate students in nursing programs received some form of financial aid in 2012–13.
**Contact** Ms. Leslie Ann Mendenhall, Director of Transfer and Graduate Admissions, College of Nursing, Research College of Nursing, 2525 East Meyer Boulevard, Kansas City, MO 64132-1199. *Telephone:* 816-995-2820. *Fax:* 816-995-2813. *E-mail:* leslie.mendenhall@researchcollege.edu.

**MASTER'S DEGREE PROGRAM**
**Degree** MSN
**Available Programs** Master's; RN to Master's.
**Concentrations Available** Clinical nurse leader; nursing administration; nursing education. *Nurse practitioner programs in:* adult health, family health.
**Study Options** Part-time.
**Online Degree Options** Yes.
**Program Entrance Requirements** Minimum overall college GPA of 3.0, transcript of college record, written essay, interview, 3 letters of recommendation, physical assessment course, resume, statistics course. *Application deadline:* 3/1 (fall). *Application fee:* $60.
**Advanced Placement** Credit given for nursing courses completed elsewhere dependent upon specific evaluations.
**Degree Requirements** 45 total credit hours, thesis or project.

**POST-MASTER'S PROGRAM**
**Areas of Study** Clinical nurse leader; nursing administration; nursing education. *Nurse practitioner programs in:* adult health, family health.

## Saint Louis University
### School of Nursing
### St. Louis, Missouri

***http://www.nursing.slu.edu***
Founded in 1818

**DEGREES • BSN • DNP • MSN • PHD**
**Nursing Program Faculty** 54 (63% with doctorates).
**Baccalaureate Enrollment** 581 **Women** 91% **Men** 9% **Minority** 14% **International** 1% **Part-time** 11%
**Graduate Enrollment** 511 **Women** 91% **Men** 9% **Minority** 15% **Part-time** 70%
**Distance Learning Courses** Available.
**Nursing Student Activities** Sigma Theta Tau, Student Nurses' Association.
**Nursing Student Resources** Academic advising; academic or career counseling; assistance for students with disabilities; bookstore; campus computer network; career placement assistance; computer lab; e-mail services; employment services for current students; housing assistance; interactive nursing skills videos; Internet; library services; nursing audiovisuals; remedial services; resume preparation assistance; skills, simulation, or other laboratory; tutoring; unpaid internships.
**Library Facilities** 1.9 million volumes (275,000 in health, 4,800 in nursing); 7,735 periodical subscriptions (8,429 health-care related).

**BACCALAUREATE PROGRAMS**
**Degree** BSN
**Available Programs** Accelerated Baccalaureate; Accelerated Baccalaureate for Second Degree; Generic Baccalaureate; RN Baccalaureate.
**Site Options** St. Louis, MO.
**Study Options** Full-time and part-time.
**Online Degree Options** Yes.
**Program Entrance Requirements** Minimum overall college GPA of 3.4, transcript of college record, health exam, high school biology, high school chemistry, high school transcript, immunizations, minimum high school GPA of 3.2. Transfer students are accepted. *Application deadline:* 12/1 (fall).
**Advanced Placement** Credit by examination available. Credit given for nursing courses completed elsewhere dependent upon specific evaluations.
**Expenses (2013–14)** *Tuition:* full-time $36,090; part-time $1260 per credit hour. *International tuition:* $36,090 full-time. *Room and board:* $9868 per academic year. *Required fees:* full-time $636; part-time $30 per credit; part-time $163 per term.
**Financial Aid** 97% of baccalaureate students in nursing programs received some form of financial aid in 2012–13.
**Contact** Mr. Scott Ragsdale, Recruitment Specialist, School of Nursing, Saint Louis University, 3525 Caroline Street, St. Louis, MO 63104. *Telephone:* 314-977-8995. *Fax:* 314-977-8949. *E-mail:* sragsda2@slu.edu.

**GRADUATE PROGRAMS**
**Expenses (2013–14)** *Tuition:* part-time $1010 per credit hour. *Required fees:* part-time $30 per credit; part-time $128 per term.
**Financial Aid** 50% of graduate students in nursing programs received some form of financial aid in 2012–13. 2 research assistantships (averaging $10,250 per year), 5 teaching assistantships with full tuition reimbursements available (averaging $11,000 per year) were awarded; Federal Work-Study, scholarships, traineeships, tuition waivers, and unspecified assistantships also available. Aid available to part-time students. *Financial aid application deadline:* 6/1.
**Contact** Dr. Mary Lee Barron, Advanced Nursing Practice Program Director, School of Nursing, Saint Louis University, 3525 Caroline Street, St. Louis, MO 63104. *Telephone:* 314-977-8978. *Fax:* 314-977-8949. *E-mail:* barronml@slu.edu.

**MASTER'S DEGREE PROGRAM**
**Degree** MSN
**Available Programs** Accelerated Master's for Non-Nursing College Graduates; Master's; Master's for Nurses with Non-Nursing Degrees.
**Concentrations Available** Nursing education. *Nurse practitioner programs in:* acute care, adult health, family health, gerontology, pediatric, primary care, psychiatric/mental health.
**Site Options** St. Louis, MO.
**Study Options** Full-time and part-time.
**Online Degree Options** Yes (online only).
**Program Entrance Requirements** Minimum overall college GPA of 3.2, transcript of college record, CPR certification, immunizations, 3 letters of recommendation, resume. *Application deadline:* 4/1 (fall), 9/1 (spring). *Application fee:* $55.
**Advanced Placement** Credit given for nursing courses completed elsewhere dependent upon specific evaluations.
**Degree Requirements** 39 total credit hours, comprehensive exam.

**POST-MASTER'S PROGRAM**
**Areas of Study** Nursing education. *Nurse practitioner programs in:* acute care, adult health, family health, gerontology, pediatric, primary care, psychiatric/mental health.

**DOCTORAL DEGREE PROGRAM**
**Degree** DNP
**Available Programs** Doctorate.
**Areas of Study** Advanced practice nursing.
**Online Degree Options** Yes (online only).
**Program Entrance Requirements** Minimum overall college GPA of 3.25, 3 letters of recommendation, MSN or equivalent, statistics course, vita, writing sample. *Application deadline:* 3/15 (fall). Applications may be processed on a rolling basis for some programs. *Application fee:* $40.
**Degree Requirements** 28 total credit hours, dissertation.

**Degree** PhD
**Available Programs** Doctorate.
**Areas of Study** Nursing research.
**Site Options** St. Louis, MO.
**Program Entrance Requirements** Minimum overall college GPA of 3.25, 3 letters of recommendation, MSN or equivalent, statistics course, vita, writing sample, GRE General Test. *Application deadline:* 6/1 (fall), 11/1 (spring). Applications may be processed on a rolling basis for some programs. *Application fee:* $55.
**Degree Requirements** 69 total credit hours, dissertation, oral exam, written exam, residency.

**CONTINUING EDUCATION PROGRAM**
**Contact** Mrs. Cathi Slinkard, Continuing Education Director, School of Nursing, Saint Louis University, 3525 Caroline Street, St. Louis, MO 63104. *Telephone:* 314-977-1909. *Fax:* 314-977-8949. *E-mail:* cslinkar@slu.edu.

## Saint Luke's College of Health Sciences
### Nursing College
### Kansas City, Missouri

***http://www.saintlukescollege.edu/***
Founded in 1903

**DEGREE • BSN**
**Nursing Program Faculty** 17 (18% with doctorates).
**Baccalaureate Enrollment** 115 **Women** 95% **Men** 5% **Minority** 10% **International** 1% **Part-time** 12%
**Nursing Student Activities** Student Nurses' Association.
**Nursing Student Resources** Academic advising; assistance for students with disabilities; bookstore; campus computer network; career placement

assistance; computer lab; computer-assisted instruction; e-mail services; employment services for current students; interactive nursing skills videos; Internet; learning resource lab; library services; nursing audiovisuals; paid internships; skills, simulation, or other laboratory; tutoring.

### BACCALAUREATE PROGRAMS

**Degree** BSN
**Available Programs** Generic Baccalaureate.
**Site Options** Kansas City, MO.
**Study Options** Full-time and part-time.
**Program Entrance Requirements** Transcript of college record, CPR certification, written essay, health exam, health insurance, high school transcript, immunizations, interview, 3 letters of recommendation, minimum GPA in nursing prerequisites of 2.7, prerequisite course work. Transfer students are accepted.
**Advanced Placement** Credit given for nursing courses completed elsewhere dependent upon specific evaluations.
**Contact** *Telephone:* 816-932-2367.

## Southeast Missouri State University

### Department of Nursing
### Cape Girardeau, Missouri

***http://www.semo.edu/nursing***
Founded in 1873

### DEGREES • BSN • MSN

**Nursing Program Faculty** 27 (35% with doctorates).
**Baccalaureate Enrollment** 202 **Women** 95% **Men** 5% **Minority** 2% **International** 1% **Part-time** 5%
**Graduate Enrollment** 18 **Women** 99% **Men** 1% **Minority** 1%
**Distance Learning Courses** Available.
**Nursing Student Activities** Sigma Theta Tau, Student Nurses' Association.
**Nursing Student Resources** Academic advising; academic or career counseling; assistance for students with disabilities; bookstore; campus computer network; career placement assistance; computer lab; computer-assisted instruction; e-mail services; employment services for current students; externships; housing assistance; Internet; learning resource lab; library services; nursing audiovisuals; remedial services; resume preparation assistance; skills, simulation, or other laboratory; tutoring.
**Library Facilities** 439,445 volumes (450,750 in health, 16,145 in nursing); 71,045 periodical subscriptions (75 health-care related).

### BACCALAUREATE PROGRAMS

**Degree** BSN
**Available Programs** Generic Baccalaureate; RN Baccalaureate.
**Study Options** Full-time.
**Online Degree Options** Yes.
**Program Entrance Requirements** Minimum overall college GPA of 2.8, transcript of college record, CPR certification, health exam, health insurance, immunizations, minimum GPA in nursing prerequisites of 2.8, professional liability insurance/malpractice insurance, prerequisite course work. Transfer students are accepted. *Application deadline:* 3/1 (fall), 10/1 (spring).
**Advanced Placement** Credit given for nursing courses completed elsewhere dependent upon specific evaluations.
**Expenses (2013–14)** *Tuition, state resident:* full-time $5814; part-time $194 per credit hour. *Tuition, nonresident:* full-time $11,049; part-time $368 per credit hour. *International tuition:* $11,049 full-time. *Room and board:* $8540; room only: $5850 per academic year. *Required fees:* full-time $1836; part-time $61 per credit; part-time $918 per term.
**Financial Aid** 65% of baccalaureate students in nursing programs received some form of financial aid in 2012–13.
**Contact** Dr. Ann Sprengel, Chairperson of Student Affairs Committee, Department of Nursing, Southeast Missouri State University, One University Plaza, Mail Stop 8300, Cape Girardeau, MO 63701-4799. *Telephone:* 573-651-2956. *Fax:* 573-651-2142. *E-mail:* asprengel@semo.edu.

### GRADUATE PROGRAMS

**Expenses (2013–14)** *Tuition, state resident:* full-time $3735; part-time $249 per credit hour. *Tuition, nonresident:* full-time $6987; part-time $466 per credit hour. *International tuition:* $6987 full-time. *Required fees:* full-time $468; part-time $31 per credit; part-time $234 per term.
**Financial Aid** 50% of graduate students in nursing programs received some form of financial aid in 2012–13. 4 teaching assistantships with full tuition reimbursements available (averaging $7,900 per year) were awarded; career-related internships or fieldwork, Federal Work-Study, scholarships, traineeships, tuition waivers (full), and unspecified assistantships also available. *Financial aid application deadline:* 6/30.
**Contact** Dr. Elaine Jackson, Director, Graduate Studies, Department of Nursing, Southeast Missouri State University, One University Plaza, Mail Stop 8300, Cape Girardeau, MO 63701-4799. *Telephone:* 573-651-2871. *Fax:* 573-651-2142. *E-mail:* ejackson@semo.edu.

#### MASTER'S DEGREE PROGRAM

**Degree** MSN
**Available Programs** Master's.
**Concentrations Available** Nursing education. *Nurse practitioner programs in:* family health.
**Site Options** Sikeston, MO; Poplar Bluff, MO; Kennett, MO.
**Study Options** Full-time.
**Program Entrance Requirements** Clinical experience, minimum overall college GPA of 3.25, transcript of college record, CPR certification, written essay, immunizations, 2 letters of recommendation, physical assessment course, professional liability insurance/malpractice insurance, prerequisite course work, resume, statistics course. *Application deadline:* Applications may be processed on a rolling basis for some programs.
**Degree Requirements** 45 total credit hours, comprehensive exam.

#### POST-MASTER'S PROGRAM

**Areas of Study** *Nurse practitioner programs in:* family health.

## Southwest Baptist University

### College of Nursing
### Bolivar, Missouri

***http://www.sbuniv.edu/collegeofnursing***
Founded in 1878

### DEGREES • BSN • MSN

**Nursing Program Faculty** 12 (25% with doctorates).
**Baccalaureate Enrollment** 143 **Women** 87.5% **Men** 12.5% **Minority** 2.1% **Part-time** 82.5%
**Graduate Enrollment** 31 **Women** 96.8% **Men** 3.2% **Part-time** 74.1%
**Distance Learning Courses** Available.
**Nursing Student Activities** Nursing Honor Society, Student Nurses' Association.
**Nursing Student Resources** Academic advising; bookstore; campus computer network; computer lab; computer-assisted instruction; e-mail services; interactive nursing skills videos; Internet; learning resource lab; library services; nursing audiovisuals; skills, simulation, or other laboratory.
**Library Facilities** 301,745 volumes (4,042 in health, 3,602 in nursing); 323,485 periodical subscriptions (41,500 health-care related).

### BACCALAUREATE PROGRAMS

**Degree** BSN
**Available Programs** RN Baccalaureate.
**Site Options** Springfield, MO.
**Study Options** Full-time and part-time.
**Program Entrance Requirements** Minimum overall college GPA of 2.5, transcript of college record, CPR certification, high school transcript, immunizations, letters of recommendation, minimum GPA in nursing prerequisites of 2.5, professional liability insurance/malpractice insurance, prerequisite course work, RN licensure. Transfer students are accepted. *Application deadline:* 8/15 (fall), 1/1 (winter), 1/15 (spring), 6/1 (summer). Applications may be processed on a rolling basis for some programs.
**Advanced Placement** Credit given for nursing courses completed elsewhere dependent upon specific evaluations.
**Expenses (2012–13)** *Tuition:* full-time $7440; part-time $310 per credit hour. *International tuition:* $7440 full-time. *Room and board:* $6350; room only: $3150 per academic year. *Required fees:* full-time $910; part-time $600 per credit.
**Financial Aid** 70% of baccalaureate students in nursing programs received some form of financial aid in 2011–12.
**Contact** Ms. Dana Hunt, Director, BSN Program, College of Nursing, Southwest Baptist University, 4431 South Fremont Avenue, Springfield,

MO 65804. *Telephone:* 417-820-5060. *Fax:* 417-887-4847. *E-mail:* dhunt@sbuniv.edu.

## GRADUATE PROGRAMS

**Expenses (2012–13)** *Tuition:* full-time $9600; part-time $400 per credit hour. *International tuition:* $9600 full-time. *Required fees:* full-time $1820.

**Financial Aid** 60% of graduate students in nursing programs received some form of financial aid in 2011–12.

**Contact** Dr. Martha Cheryl Baker, Dean, College of Nursing, Southwest Baptist University, 4431 South Fremont Avenue, Springfield, MO 65804. *Telephone:* 417-820-5058. *Fax:* 417-887-4847. *E-mail:* mbaker@sbuniv.edu.

### MASTER'S DEGREE PROGRAM

**Degree** MSN

**Available Programs** Master's.

**Concentrations Available** Nursing administration; nursing education.

**Site Options** Springfield, MO.

**Study Options** Full-time and part-time.

**Online Degree Options** Yes.

**Program Entrance Requirements** Computer literacy, minimum overall college GPA of 3.0, transcript of college record, CPR certification, written essay, immunizations, letters of recommendation, nursing research course, physical assessment course, professional liability insurance/malpractice insurance, statistics course. *Application deadline:* 7/15 (fall), 1/1 (spring). Applications may be processed on a rolling basis for some programs. *Application fee:* $30.

**Advanced Placement** Credit given for nursing courses completed elsewhere dependent upon specific evaluations.

**Degree Requirements** 36 total credit hours, thesis or project, comprehensive exam.

# Truman State University

## Program in Nursing
## Kirksville, Missouri

***http://nursing.truman.edu/***
Founded in 1867

### DEGREE • BSN

**Nursing Program Faculty** 11 (18% with doctorates).

**Baccalaureate Enrollment** 172 **Women** 94% **Men** 6% **Minority** 5% **International** 5% **Part-time** 1%

**Nursing Student Activities** Nursing Honor Society, Sigma Theta Tau, Student Nurses' Association, nursing club.

**Nursing Student Resources** Academic advising; academic or career counseling; assistance for students with disabilities; bookstore; campus computer network; career placement assistance; computer lab; computer-assisted instruction; e-mail services; employment services for current students; externships; interactive nursing skills videos; Internet; learning resource lab; library services; nursing audiovisuals; paid internships; remedial services; resume preparation assistance; skills, simulation, or other laboratory; tutoring; unpaid internships.

**Library Facilities** 512,535 volumes (6,923 in health, 1,654 in nursing); 3,315 periodical subscriptions (900 health-care related).

## BACCALAUREATE PROGRAMS

**Degree** BSN

**Available Programs** Generic Baccalaureate.

**Study Options** Full-time.

**Program Entrance Requirements** Minimum overall college GPA of 2.75, transcript of college record, written essay, high school biology, high school chemistry, high school foreign language, 3 years high school math, 3 years high school science, high school transcript, immunizations, minimum high school GPA of 3.3, minimum GPA in nursing prerequisites of 3.0. Transfer students are accepted.

**Contact** *Telephone:* 660-785-4557. *Fax:* 660-785-7424.

# University of Central Missouri

## Department of Nursing
## Warrensburg, Missouri

***http://www.ucmo.edu/nursing***
Founded in 1871

### DEGREES • BS • MS

**Nursing Program Faculty** 18 (39% with doctorates).
**Baccalaureate Enrollment** 153 **Women** 95% **Men** 5% **Minority** 7% **International** 1%
**Graduate Enrollment** 152 **Women** 95% **Men** 5% **Minority** 8% **Part-time** 99%
**Distance Learning Courses** Available.
**Nursing Student Activities** Nursing club.
**Nursing Student Resources** Academic advising; academic or career counseling; assistance for students with disabilities; bookstore; campus computer network; career placement assistance; computer lab; computer-assisted instruction; daycare for children of students; e-mail services; employment services for current students; externships; housing assistance; interactive nursing skills videos; Internet; learning resource lab; library services; nursing audiovisuals; placement services for program completers; remedial services; resume preparation assistance; skills, simulation, or other laboratory; tutoring.
**Library Facilities** 1.3 million volumes (17,000 in health, 1,000 in nursing); 835 periodical subscriptions (300 health-care related).

## BACCALAUREATE PROGRAMS

**Degree** BS
**Available Programs** ADN to Baccalaureate; Generic Baccalaureate; RN Baccalaureate.
**Site Options** Lee's Summit, MO; Warrensburg, MO.
**Study Options** Full-time.
**Online Degree Options** Yes.
**Program Entrance Requirements** Minimum overall college GPA of 2.75, minimum GPA in nursing prerequisites of 2.0, prerequisite course work. Transfer students are accepted. *Application deadline:* 1/1 (fall), 7/1 (spring). *Application fee:* $45.
**Advanced Placement** Credit by examination available. Credit given for nursing courses completed elsewhere dependent upon specific evaluations.
**Expenses (2013–14)** *Tuition, state resident:* full-time $7265; part-time $242 per credit hour. *Tuition, nonresident:* full-time $13,656; part-time $455 per credit hour. *International tuition:* $13,656 full-time. *Room and board:* $6173; room only: $4888 per academic year. *Required fees:* full-time $400.
**Financial Aid** 89% of baccalaureate students in nursing programs received some form of financial aid in 2012–13.
**Contact** Dr. Julie Ann Clawson, Chair, Department of Nursing, University of Central Missouri, 600 South College, UHC 106A, Warrensburg, MO 64093. *Telephone:* 660-543-4775. *Fax:* 660-543-8304. *E-mail:* clawson@ucmo.edu.

## GRADUATE PROGRAMS

**Expenses (2013–14)** *Tuition, state resident:* full-time $3663; part-time $305 per credit hour. *Tuition, nonresident:* full-time $6978; part-time $582 per credit hour. *International tuition:* $6978 full-time. *Room and board:* $6173; room only: $4888 per academic year.
**Financial Aid** 70% of graduate students in nursing programs received some form of financial aid in 2012–13.
**Contact** Dr. Joseph Vaughn, Dean, Department of Nursing, University of Central Missouri, Graduate Studies, WDE 1800, Warrensburg, MO 64093. *Telephone:* 660-543-4621. *E-mail:* vaughn@ucmo.edu.

### MASTER'S DEGREE PROGRAM

**Degree** MS
**Available Programs** Master's.
**Concentrations Available** Nursing education. *Nurse practitioner programs in:* family health.
**Site Options** Lee's Summit, MO; Warrensburg, MO.
**Study Options** Part-time.
**Online Degree Options** Yes (online only).
**Program Entrance Requirements** Clinical experience, minimum overall college GPA of 3.0, transcript of college record, CPR certification, immunizations, professional liability insurance/malpractice insurance. *Application deadline:* 2/15 (fall), 9/15 (spring), 2/15 (summer). Applications may be processed on a rolling basis for some programs.

**Advanced Placement** Credit given for nursing courses completed elsewhere dependent upon specific evaluations.
**Degree Requirements** 32 total credit hours, thesis or project.

# University of Missouri
## Sinclair School of Nursing
## Columbia, Missouri

*http://www.nursing.missouri.edu/*
Founded in 1839

**DEGREES • BSN • MSN • MSN/PHD • PHD**
**Baccalaureate Enrollment** 380 **Women** 90% **Men** 10% **Minority** 6% **International** 3% **Part-time** 31%
**Graduate Enrollment** 200 **Women** 95% **Men** 5% **Minority** 8% **International** 2% **Part-time** 77%
**Distance Learning Courses** Available.
**Nursing Student Activities** Nursing Honor Society, Sigma Theta Tau, Student Nurses' Association, nursing club.
**Nursing Student Resources** Academic advising; academic or career counseling; assistance for students with disabilities; bookstore; campus computer network; career placement assistance; computer lab; computer-assisted instruction; daycare for children of students; e-mail services; employment services for current students; externships; housing assistance; interactive nursing skills videos; Internet; learning resource lab; library services; nursing audiovisuals; paid internships; remedial services; resume preparation assistance; skills, simulation, or other laboratory; tutoring; unpaid internships.
**Library Facilities** 2.7 million volumes (114,580 in health, 6,416 in nursing).

### BACCALAUREATE PROGRAMS
**Degree** BSN
**Available Programs** ADN to Baccalaureate; Accelerated Baccalaureate; Accelerated Baccalaureate for Second Degree; Generic Baccalaureate; RN Baccalaureate.
**Study Options** Full-time and part-time.
**Online Degree Options** Yes.
**Program Entrance Requirements** Minimum overall college GPA of 2.5, transcript of college record, CPR certification, high school biology, high school chemistry, 4 years high school math, 3 years high school science, high school transcript, immunizations, interview, minimum GPA in nursing prerequisites of 2.5, prerequisite course work. Transfer students are accepted.
**Advanced Placement** Credit by examination available. Credit given for nursing courses completed elsewhere dependent upon specific evaluations.
**Contact** *Telephone:* 573-882-0277. *Fax:* 573-884-4544.

### GRADUATE PROGRAMS
**Contact** *Telephone:* 573-882-0277.

#### MASTER'S DEGREE PROGRAM
**Degrees** MSN; MSN/PhD
**Available Programs** Master's.
**Concentrations Available** Nursing administration; nursing education. *Clinical nurse specialist programs in:* acute care, adult health, cardiovascular, community health, critical care, home health care, maternity-newborn, oncology, palliative care, pediatric, public health, rehabilitation, school health,women's health. *Nurse practitioner programs in:* family health, gerontology, pediatric, primary care, psychiatric/mental health.
**Study Options** Full-time and part-time.
**Online Degree Options** Yes (online only).
**Program Entrance Requirements** Computer literacy, minimum overall college GPA of 3.0, transcript of college record, CPR certification, immunizations, interview, 2 letters of recommendation, nursing research course, prerequisite course work, statistics course, GRE General Test.
**Advanced Placement** Credit given for nursing courses completed elsewhere dependent upon specific evaluations.
**Degree Requirements** 43 total credit hours, comprehensive exam.

#### POST-MASTER'S PROGRAM
**Areas of Study** Nursing administration; nursing education. *Clinical nurse specialist programs in:* acute care, adult health, cardiovascular, community health, critical care, home health care, maternity-newborn, oncology, palliative care, pediatric, public health, rehabilitation, school health,women's health. *Nurse practitioner programs in:* family health, gerontology, pediatric, primary care, psychiatric/mental health.

#### DOCTORAL DEGREE PROGRAM
**Degree** PhD
**Available Programs** Doctorate; Post-Baccalaureate Doctorate.
**Areas of Study** Aging, family health, gerontology, health promotion/disease prevention, health-care systems, human health and illness, nursing research, oncology,women's health.
**Program Entrance Requirements** Minimum overall college GPA of 3.5, interview by faculty committee, 3 letters of recommendation, vita, writing sample.
**Degree Requirements** 72 total credit hours, dissertation, oral exam, written exam, residency.

### CONTINUING EDUCATION PROGRAM
**Contact** *Telephone:* 573-882-0215. *Fax:* 573-884-4544.

# University of Missouri–Kansas City
## School of Nursing and Health Studies
## Kansas City, Missouri

*http://www.umkc.edu/nursing*
Founded in 1929

**DEGREES • BSN • DNP • MSN • PHD**
**Nursing Program Faculty** 99 (44% with doctorates).
**Baccalaureate Enrollment** 597 **Women** 86% **Men** 14% **Minority** 25% **Part-time** 41%
**Graduate Enrollment** 444 **Women** 91% **Men** 9% **Minority** 10% **Part-time** 82%
**Distance Learning Courses** Available.
**Nursing Student Activities** Sigma Theta Tau, Student Nurses' Association.
**Nursing Student Resources** Academic advising; academic or career counseling; assistance for students with disabilities; bookstore; campus computer network; career placement assistance; computer lab; computer-assisted instruction; e-mail services; employment services for current students; housing assistance; interactive nursing skills videos; Internet; learning resource lab; library services; nursing audiovisuals; other; placement services for program completers; remedial services; resume preparation assistance; skills, simulation, or other laboratory; tutoring.
**Library Facilities** 1.5 million volumes (118,853 in health, 1 in nursing); 53,976 periodical subscriptions (32,569 health-care related).

### BACCALAUREATE PROGRAMS
**Degree** BSN
**Available Programs** Accelerated Baccalaureate; Generic Baccalaureate; RN Baccalaureate.
**Study Options** Full-time.
**Online Degree Options** Yes (online only).
**Program Entrance Requirements** Minimum overall college GPA of 2.75, transcript of college record, written essay, high school foreign language, 4 years high school math, 4 years high school science, high school transcript, 1 letter of recommendation, minimum GPA in nursing prerequisites of 2.75, prerequisite course work. Transfer students are accepted. *Application deadline:* 1/31 (fall). *Application fee:* $25.
**Expenses (2013–14)** *Tuition, state resident:* full-time $6662; part-time $270 per credit hour. *Tuition, nonresident:* full-time $16,680; part-time $695 per credit hour. *International tuition:* $16,680 full-time. *Room and board:* $9284; room only: $8007 per academic year. *Required fees:* full-time $1320; part-time $55 per credit.
**Financial Aid** 85% of baccalaureate students in nursing programs received some form of financial aid in 2012–13. *Gift aid (need-based):* Federal Pell, FSEOG, state, private, college/university gift aid from institutional funds, United Negro College Fund, Federal Nursing. *Loans:* Federal Nursing Student Loans, Federal Direct (Subsidized and Unsubsidized Stafford PLUS), Perkins, state, college/university. *Work-study:* Federal Work-Study. *Financial aid application deadline (priority):* 3/1.
**Contact** Mrs. Judy A. Jellison, Director, Nursing Student Services, School of Nursing and Health Studies, University of Missouri–Kansas City, 2464 Charlotte Street, Kansas City, MO 64108. *Telephone:* 816-235-1740. *Fax:* 816-235-6593. *E-mail:* jellisonj@umkc.edu.

## GRADUATE PROGRAMS

**Expenses (2013–14)** *Tuition, state resident:* full-time $6073; part-time $337 per credit hour. *Tuition, nonresident:* full-time $15,680; part-time $1209 per credit hour. *International tuition:* $15,680 full-time. *Required fees:* full-time $241; part-time $14 per credit.

**Financial Aid** 72% of graduate students in nursing programs received some form of financial aid in 2012–13. 12 teaching assistantships with partial tuition reimbursements available (averaging $9,125 per year) were awarded; fellowships, research assistantships, career-related internships or fieldwork, Federal Work-Study, institutionally sponsored loans, and tuition waivers (full and partial) also available. Aid available to part-time students. *Financial aid application deadline:* 3/1.

**Contact** Mrs. Judy A. Jellison, Director, Nursing Student Services, School of Nursing and Health Studies, University of Missouri–Kansas City, 2464 Charlotte Street, Kansas City, MO 64108. *Telephone:* 816-235-1740. *Fax:* 816-235-6593. *E-mail:* jellisonj@umkc.edu.

### MASTER'S DEGREE PROGRAM

**Degree** MSN

**Available Programs** Master's.

**Concentrations Available** Nursing education. *Nurse practitioner programs in:* neonatal health, psychiatric/mental health.

**Site Options** St. Joseph, MO; Joplin, MO.

**Study Options** Full-time and part-time.

**Program Entrance Requirements** Clinical experience, computer literacy, minimum overall college GPA of 3.2, transcript of college record, written essay, 3 letters of recommendation, physical assessment course, prerequisite course work, resume, statistics course. *Application deadline:* 12/1 (fall), 12/1 (summer). *Application fee:* $25.

**Degree Requirements** 43 total credit hours.

### POST-MASTER'S PROGRAM

**Areas of Study** Nursing education. *Nurse practitioner programs in:* neonatal health, psychiatric/mental health.

### DOCTORAL DEGREE PROGRAM

**Degree** DNP

**Available Programs** Doctorate, Post-Baccalaureate Doctorate.

**Areas of Study** Adult gerontology, family health, nurse anesthesia, pediatric, women's health.

**Program Entrance Requirements** Vary by program. *Application deadline:* Varies by program.

**Degree Requirements** 73-74 total credit hours, depending on program chosen.

**Degree** DNP (MS to DNP)

**Available Programs** Doctorate; Post-Baccalaureate Doctorate.

**Areas of Study** Advanced practice nursing, adult gerontology, family nurse, pediatric, women's health.

**Program Entrance Requirements** Minimum overall college GPA of 3.5, interview by faculty committee, interview, 3 letters of recommendation, MSN or equivalent, vita, writing sample, GRE. *Application deadline:* 12/1 (fall), 2/1 (summer). *Application fee:* $25.

**Degree** Requirements 31-55 total credit hours, dissertation, oral exam, written exam, residency.

**Degree** PhD

**Available Programs** Doctorate; Post-Baccalaureate Doctorate.

**Areas of Study** Biology of health and illness, individualized study, nursing education.

**Program Entrance Requirements** Minimum overall college GPA of 3.5, interview by faculty committee, interview, 3 letters of recommendation, MSN or equivalent, vita, writing sample, GRE. *Application deadline:* 2/1 (fall). *Application fee:* $25.

**Degree Requirements** 61 total credit hours, dissertation, oral exam, written exam, residency.

## CONTINUING EDUCATION PROGRAM

**Contact** Jodi M. Baker, Continuing Education Coordinator, School of Nursing and Health Studies, University of Missouri–Kansas City, 2464 Charlotte Street, Kansas City, MO 64108. *Telephone:* 816-235-6463. *Fax:* 816-235-1701. *E-mail:* bakerjm@umkc.edu.

# University of Missouri–St. Louis

**College of Nursing**
**St. Louis, Missouri**

*http://www.umsl.edu/divisions/nursing/*
Founded in 1963

**DEGREES • BSN • DNP • MSN**

**Nursing Program Faculty** 90 (31% with doctorates).

**Baccalaureate Enrollment** 955 **Women** 87% **Men** 13% **Minority** 26% **Part-time** 38%

**Graduate Enrollment** 227 **Women** 96% **Men** 4% **Minority** 18% **Part-time** 100%

**Distance Learning Courses** Available.

**Nursing Student Activities** Nursing Honor Society, Sigma Theta Tau, Student Nurses' Association.

**Nursing Student Resources** Academic advising; academic or career counseling; assistance for students with disabilities; bookstore; campus computer network; career placement assistance; computer lab; computer-assisted instruction; daycare for children of students; e-mail services; employment services for current students; externships; interactive nursing skills videos; Internet; learning resource lab; library services; nursing audiovisuals; resume preparation assistance; skills, simulation, or other laboratory; tutoring; unpaid internships.

**Library Facilities** 1.3 million volumes (89,479 in health, 18,229 in nursing); 2,631 periodical subscriptions (7,683 health-care related).

## BACCALAUREATE PROGRAMS

**Degree** BSN

**Available Programs** Accelerated Baccalaureate; Baccalaureate for Second Degree; Generic Baccalaureate; RN Baccalaureate.

**Site Options** Bridgeton, MO; Creve Coeur, MO; St. Louis, MO; St. Charles, MO.

**Study Options** Full-time and part-time.

**Online Degree Options** Yes.

**Program Entrance Requirements** Minimum overall college GPA of 2.5, transcript of college record, CPR certification, health exam, 4 years high school math, 3 years high school science, high school transcript, immunizations, minimum high school GPA of 2.5, minimum GPA in nursing prerequisites, professional liability insurance/malpractice insurance. Transfer students are accepted. *Application deadline:* 2/1 (fall), 10/1 (spring). *Application fee:* $35.

**Advanced Placement** Credit given for nursing courses completed elsewhere dependent upon specific evaluations.

**Expenses (2013–14)** *Tuition, state resident:* full-time $9474; part-time $316 per credit hour. *Tuition, nonresident:* full-time $24,429; part-time $814 per credit hour. *International tuition:* $24,429 full-time. *Room and board:* $8830; room only: $3630 per academic year.

**Financial Aid** 77% of baccalaureate students in nursing programs received some form of financial aid in 2012–13. *Gift aid (need-based):* Federal Pell, FSEOG, state, private, college/university gift aid from institutional funds, United Negro College Fund, Federal Nursing, TEACH Grants. *Loans:* Federal Nursing Student Loans, Federal Direct (Subsidized and Unsubsidized Stafford PLUS), Perkins, state. *Work-study:* Federal Work-Study. *Financial aid application deadline (priority):* 3/1.

**Contact** Dr. Sandra J. Lindquist, Associate Dean for the Undergraduate Program, College of Nursing, University of Missouri–St. Louis, One University Boulevard, 233 Nursing Administration Building, St. Louis, MO 63121-4499. *Telephone:* 314-516-6066. *Fax:* 314-516-7519. *E-mail:* sandy_lindquist@umsl.edu.

## GRADUATE PROGRAMS

**Expenses (2013–14)** *Tuition, state resident:* full-time $9818; part-time $409 per credit hour. *Tuition, nonresident:* full-time $24,204; part-time $1009 per credit hour. *International tuition:* $24,204 full-time. *Room and board:* $8830; room only: $5200 per academic year.

**Financial Aid** 56% of graduate students in nursing programs received some form of financial aid in 2012–13. *Application deadline:* 4/1.

**Contact** Dr. Nancy Magnuson, Acting Associate Dean for Advanced Nursing Education, College of Nursing, University of Missouri–St. Louis, One University Boulevard, Nursing Administration Building, St. Louis, MO 63121-4499. *Telephone:* 314-516-6066. *Fax:* 314-516-7519. *E-mail:* magnusonn@umsl.edu.

### MASTER'S DEGREE PROGRAM

**Degree** MSN

**Available Programs** Master's.

**Concentrations Available** Nursing education. *Nurse practitioner programs in:* adult health, family health, neonatal health, pediatric,women's health.
**Site Options** Park Hills, MO; Town & Country, MO; St. Charles, MO.
**Study Options** Full-time and part-time.
**Online Degree Options** Yes.
**Program Entrance Requirements** Clinical experience, minimum overall college GPA of 3.0, transcript of college record, CPR certification, immunizations, 2 letters of recommendation, physical assessment course, statistics course. *Application deadline:* 2/15 (fall), 10/1 (spring). *Application fee:* $35.
**Advanced Placement** Credit given for nursing courses completed elsewhere dependent upon specific evaluations.
**Degree Requirements** 43 total credit hours.

**POST-MASTER'S PROGRAM**
**Areas of Study** *Nurse practitioner programs in:* adult health, family health, pediatric,women's health.

**DOCTORAL DEGREE PROGRAM**
**Degree** DNP
**Available Programs** Doctorate.
**Areas of Study** Advanced practice nursing.
**Program Entrance Requirements** Minimum overall college GPA of 3.0, interview, 2 letters of recommendation, MSN or equivalent, statistics course, writing sample, GRE. *Application deadline:* 4/1 (fall). *Application fee:* $35.
**Degree Requirements** 30 total credit hours, dissertation.

### CONTINUING EDUCATION PROGRAM

**Contact** Vanessa Loyd, Director of Continuing Education and Outreach, College of Nursing, University of Missouri–St. Louis, One University Boulevard, St. Louis, MO 63121-4400. *Telephone:* 314-516-6066. *Fax:* 314-516-6730. *E-mail:* loydv@umsl.edu.

## Webster University
**Department of Nursing**
**St. Louis, Missouri**

*http://www.webster.edu/arts-and-sciences/departments/nursing/*
Founded in 1915

**DEGREES • BSN • MSN**
**Nursing Program Faculty** 12 (72% with doctorates).
**Baccalaureate Enrollment** 150 **Women** 93% **Men** 7% **Minority** 14% **International** 1% **Part-time** 90%
**Graduate Enrollment** 75 **Women** 90% **Men** 10% **Minority** 20% **International** 10% **Part-time** 100%
**Nursing Student Activities** Nursing Honor Society, Sigma Theta Tau.
**Nursing Student Resources** Academic advising; academic or career counseling; assistance for students with disabilities; bookstore; campus computer network; career placement assistance; computer lab; e-mail services; employment services for current students; Internet; learning resource lab; library services; nursing audiovisuals; placement services for program completers; remedial services; resume preparation assistance; skills, simulation, or other laboratory; tutoring.
**Library Facilities** 280,051 volumes (7,030 in health, 3,114 in nursing); 1,622 periodical subscriptions (108 health-care related).

### BACCALAUREATE PROGRAMS

**Degree** BSN
**Available Programs** ADN to Baccalaureate; RN Baccalaureate.
**Site Options** Kansas City, MO.
**Program Entrance Requirements** Minimum overall college GPA of 2.5, transcript of college record, immunizations, interview, prerequisite course work, RN licensure. Transfer students are accepted.
**Contact** *Telephone:* 314-968-7483. *Fax:* 314-963-6101.

### GRADUATE PROGRAMS

**Contact** *Telephone:* 314-968-7483. *Fax:* 314-963-6101.

**MASTER'S DEGREE PROGRAM**
**Degree** MSN
**Available Programs** Master's; RN to Master's.
**Concentrations Available** Nursing administration; nursing education. *Clinical nurse specialist programs in:* family health.
**Site Options** Kansas City, MO.
**Study Options** Part-time.
**Program Entrance Requirements** Clinical experience, computer literacy, minimum overall college GPA of 3.0, transcript of college record, written essay, immunizations, interview, 3 letters of recommendation, nursing research course, physical assessment course, resume, statistics course.
**Advanced Placement** Credit given for nursing courses completed elsewhere dependent upon specific evaluations.
**Degree Requirements** 36 total credit hours, thesis or project.

## William Jewell College
**Department of Nursing**
**Liberty, Missouri**

*http://www.jewell.edu/*
Founded in 1849

**DEGREE • BS**
**Nursing Program Faculty** 36 (25% with doctorates).
**Baccalaureate Enrollment** 150 **Women** 89% **Men** 11% **Minority** 3% **International** 1%
**Nursing Student Activities** Nursing Honor Society, Sigma Theta Tau, Student Nurses' Association.
**Nursing Student Resources** Academic advising; academic or career counseling; assistance for students with disabilities; bookstore; campus computer network; career placement assistance; computer lab; computer-assisted instruction; e-mail services; employment services for current students; externships; housing assistance; interactive nursing skills videos; Internet; learning resource lab; library services; nursing audiovisuals; paid internships; placement services for program completers; resume preparation assistance; skills, simulation, or other laboratory; tutoring; unpaid internships.
**Library Facilities** 143,567 volumes (4,000 in health, 1,000 in nursing); 83,352 periodical subscriptions (250 health-care related).

### BACCALAUREATE PROGRAMS

**Degree** BS
**Available Programs** Accelerated Baccalaureate; Generic Baccalaureate.
**Study Options** Full-time.
**Program Entrance Requirements** Minimum overall college GPA of 2.7, transcript of college record, CPR certification, written essay, health insurance, high school foreign language, high school transcript, immunizations, interview, 2 letters of recommendation, minimum high school GPA of 3.0, minimum GPA in nursing prerequisites of 2.7, professional liability insurance/malpractice insurance, prerequisite course work. Transfer students are accepted. *Application deadline:* 6/1 (spring), 8/1 (summer). *Application fee:* $25.
**Advanced Placement** Credit given for nursing courses completed elsewhere dependent upon specific evaluations.
**Contact** *Telephone:* 816-415-5072. *Fax:* 816-415-5024.

# MONTANA

## Carroll College
**Department of Nursing**
**Helena, Montana**

*http://www.carroll.edu/*
Founded in 1909

**DEGREE • BS**
**Nursing Program Faculty** 18 (5% with doctorates).
**Baccalaureate Enrollment** 119 **Women** 88% **Men** 12% **Minority** 2% **Part-time** 3%
**Nursing Student Activities** Nursing Honor Society, Sigma Theta Tau, Student Nurses' Association, nursing club.
**Nursing Student Resources** Academic advising; academic or career counseling; assistance for students with disabilities; bookstore; campus computer network; career placement assistance; computer lab; computer-assisted instruction; e-mail services; employment services for current students; externships; housing assistance; interactive nursing skills videos;

Internet; learning resource lab; library services; nursing audiovisuals; paid internships; placement services for program completers; remedial services; resume preparation assistance; skills, simulation, or other laboratory; tutoring; unpaid internships.
**Library Facilities** 320,000 volumes (1,000 in health, 150 in nursing); 35,980 periodical subscriptions (9,000 health-care related).

## BACCALAUREATE PROGRAMS

**Degree** BS
**Available Programs** Generic Baccalaureate.
**Study Options** Full-time.
**Program Entrance Requirements** Minimum overall college GPA of 2.75, transcript of college record, health insurance, high school transcript, immunizations, minimum GPA in nursing prerequisites of 2.75, preadmission exam, prerequisite course work. Transfer students are accepted. *Application deadline:* 3/1 (spring).
**Expenses (2013–14)** *Tuition:* full-time $27,304; part-time $1138 per credit. *International tuition:* $27,304 full-time. *Room and board:* $8304; room only: $4420 per academic year. *Required fees:* full-time $915; part-time $457 per term.
**Financial Aid** 95% of baccalaureate students in nursing programs received some form of financial aid in 2012–13.
**Contact** Ms. Cynthia Thornquist, Director of Admissions and Enrollment, Department of Nursing, Carroll College, 1601 North Benton Avenue, Helena, MT 59625. *Telephone:* 406-447-4384. *Fax:* 406-447-4533. *E-mail:* cthornqu@carroll.edu.

# Montana State University

### College of Nursing
### Bozeman, Montana

***http://www.montana.edu/nursing***
Founded in 1893

**DEGREES • BSN • DNP • MN**
**Nursing Program Faculty** 103 (20% with doctorates).
**Baccalaureate Enrollment** 902 **Women** 85.6% **Men** 14.4% **Minority** 10.1% **Part-time** 16%
**Graduate Enrollment** 82 **Women** 84.1% **Men** 15.9% **Minority** 13.4% **Part-time** 34.1%
**Distance Learning Courses** Available.
**Nursing Student Activities** Sigma Theta Tau, Student Nurses' Association.
**Nursing Student Resources** Academic advising; academic or career counseling; assistance for students with disabilities; bookstore; campus computer network; career placement assistance; computer lab; computer-assisted instruction; daycare for children of students; e-mail services; employment services for current students; housing assistance; Internet; library services; nursing audiovisuals; paid internships; placement services for program completers; remedial services; resume preparation assistance; skills, simulation, or other laboratory; tutoring; unpaid internships.
**Library Facilities** 868,041 volumes (80,389 in health, 11,535 in nursing); 15,615 periodical subscriptions (1,690 health-care related).

## BACCALAUREATE PROGRAMS

**Degree** BSN
**Available Programs** Accelerated Baccalaureate for Second Degree; Baccalaureate for Second Degree; Generic Baccalaureate; LPN to Baccalaureate.
**Site Options** Billings, MT; Great Falls, MT; Missoula, MT.
**Study Options** Full-time and part-time.
**Program Entrance Requirements** Minimum overall college GPA of 2.75, transcript of college record, CPR certification, health insurance, high school transcript, immunizations, minimum high school GPA of 2.5, minimum high school rank 50%, minimum GPA in nursing prerequisites of 2.75, prerequisite course work. Transfer students are accepted. *Application deadline:* 8/1 (fall), 1/1 (spring), 5/1 (summer). Applications may be processed on a rolling basis for some programs. *Application fee:* $30.
**Advanced Placement** Credit by examination available. Credit given for nursing courses completed elsewhere dependent upon specific evaluations.
**Expenses (2013–14)** *Tuition, state resident:* full-time $6705; part-time $326 per credit. *Tuition, nonresident:* full-time $20,062; part-time $882 per credit. *Room and board:* $8070 per academic year. *Required fees:* full-time $986.
**Financial Aid** 70% of baccalaureate students in nursing programs received some form of financial aid in 2012–13.
**Contact** Ms. Debbie McCray, Undergraduate Student Services Coordinator, College of Nursing, Montana State University, 111 Sherrick Hall, PO Box 173560, Bozeman, MT 59717-3560. *Telephone:* 406-994-2660. *Fax:* 406-994-6020. *E-mail:* dmccray@montana.edu.

## GRADUATE PROGRAMS

**Expenses (2013–14)** *Tuition, state resident:* full-time $6033. *Tuition, nonresident:* full-time $16,051. *Room and board:* $8070 per academic year.
**Financial Aid** 70% of graduate students in nursing programs received some form of financial aid in 2012–13. 8 teaching assistantships with partial tuition reimbursements available (averaging $7,050 per year) were awarded; scholarships, traineeships, and tuition waivers (partial) also available. *Financial aid application deadline:* 3/1.
**Contact** Ms. Lynn Taylor, Graduate Program Assistant, College of Nursing, Montana State University, 122 Sherrick Hall, PO Box 173560, Bozeman, MT 59717-3560. *Telephone:* 406-994-3500. *Fax:* 406-994-6020. *E-mail:* lynnt@montana.edu.

### MASTER'S DEGREE PROGRAM

**Degree** MN
**Available Programs** Master's.
**Concentrations Available** Clinical nurse leader.
**Site Options** Billings, MT; Great Falls, MT; Missoula, MT.
**Study Options** Full-time and part-time.
**Program Entrance Requirements** Computer literacy, minimum overall college GPA of 3.0, transcript of college record, CPR certification, written essay, immunizations, interview, 3 letters of recommendation, nursing research course, physical assessment course, prerequisite course work, statistics course, GRE General Test. *Application deadline:* 2/15 (fall). *Application fee:* $60.
**Advanced Placement** Credit given for nursing courses completed elsewhere dependent upon specific evaluations.
**Degree Requirements** 35 total credit hours, thesis or project, comprehensive exam.

### POST-MASTER'S PROGRAM

**Areas of Study** Nursing education.

### DOCTORAL DEGREE PROGRAM

**Degree** DNP
**Available Programs** Doctorate; Post-Baccalaureate Doctorate.
**Areas of Study** Advanced practice nursing.
**Site Options** Billings, MT; Great Falls, MT; Missoula, MT.
**Program Entrance Requirements** Minimum overall college GPA of 3.0, interview by faculty committee, 3 letters of recommendation, statistics course, vita, writing sample. *Application deadline:* 2/15 (fall). *Application fee:* $60.
**Degree Requirements** 65 total credit hours.

# Montana State University–Northern

### College of Nursing
### Havre, Montana

***http://www.msun.edu/academics/nursing***
Founded in 1929

**DEGREE • BSN**
**Nursing Program Faculty** 12 (8% with doctorates).
**Baccalaureate Enrollment** 53 **Women** 96% **Men** 4% **Part-time** 92%
**Distance Learning Courses** Available.
**Nursing Student Activities** Nursing club.
**Nursing Student Resources** Academic advising; academic or career counseling; assistance for students with disabilities; bookstore; campus computer network; career placement assistance; computer lab; computer-assisted instruction; e-mail services; employment services for current students; housing assistance; interactive nursing skills videos; Internet; learning resource lab; library services; nursing audiovisuals; remedial services; resume preparation assistance; skills, simulation, or other laboratory; tutoring.
**Library Facilities** 2,600 volumes in health, 1,300 volumes in nursing; 40 periodical subscriptions health-care related.

## BACCALAUREATE PROGRAMS

**Degree** BSN

**Available Programs** ADN to Baccalaureate; RN Baccalaureate.

**Site Options** Great Falls, MT; Lewistown, MT.

**Study Options** Full-time and part-time.

**Online Degree Options** Yes (online only).

**Program Entrance Requirements** Minimum overall college GPA of 2.25, transcript of college record, CPR certification, health exam, health insurance, immunizations, professional liability insurance/malpractice insurance, prerequisite course work, RN licensure. Transfer students are accepted. *Application deadline:* 8/1 (fall), 1/10 (winter), 5/2 (summer). Applications may be processed on a rolling basis for some programs. *Application fee:* $30.

**Advanced Placement** Credit given for nursing courses completed elsewhere dependent upon specific evaluations.

**Contact** *Telephone:* 406-265-4196 Ext. 4196. *Fax:* 406-265-3772.

# Salish Kootenai College

### Nursing Department
### Pablo, Montana

Founded in 1977

**DEGREE • BS**

**Nursing Program Faculty** 7

**Nursing Student Activities** Nursing club.

**Nursing Student Resources** Academic advising; academic or career counseling; bookstore; computer lab; daycare for children of students; employment services for current students; Internet; library services.

**Library Facilities** 24,000 volumes; 200 periodical subscriptions.

## BACCALAUREATE PROGRAMS

**Degree** BS

**Available Programs** RN Baccalaureate.

**Study Options** Full-time and part-time.

**Program Entrance Requirements** Transcript of college record, CPR certification, health exam, health insurance, high school biology, high school chemistry, 2 years high school math, 2 years high school science, high school transcript, immunizations, minimum high school GPA of 2.5, professional liability insurance/malpractice insurance, prerequisite course work, RN licensure.

**Contact** *Telephone:* 406-275-4800.

# University of Great Falls

### B.S. in Nursing Degree Completion Program
### Great Falls, Montana

Founded in 1932

**DEGREE • BSN**

## BACCALAUREATE PROGRAMS

**Degree** BSN

**Available Programs** RN Baccalaureate.

**Study Options** Part-time.

**Program Entrance Requirements** Transcript of college record, prerequisite course work. *Application deadline:* 4/5 (fall).

**Expenses (2012–13)** *Tuition:* part-time $453 per credit hour.

**Contact** Nicole Brandt, RN to BSN Admission Liaison, B.S. in Nursing Degree Completion Program, University of Great Falls, 1301 20th Street South, Great Falls, MT 59405. *Telephone:* 406-791-5234. *E-mail:* rn2bsn@ugf.edu.

# NEBRASKA

# Bryan College of Health Sciences

### School of Nursing
### Lincoln, Nebraska

*http://www.bryanhealth.com/collegeofhealthsciences*

**DEGREES • BSN • MS**

**Nursing Program Faculty** 30 (10% with doctorates).

**Baccalaureate Enrollment** 470 **Women** 90.2% **Men** 9.8% **Minority** 8.1% **Part-time** 52.77%

**Graduate Enrollment** 64 **Women** 67.2% **Men** 32.8% **Minority** 15.6% **Part-time** 29.69%

**Distance Learning Courses** Available.

**Nursing Student Activities** Sigma Theta Tau, Student Nurses' Association.

**Nursing Student Resources** Academic advising; academic or career counseling; assistance for students with disabilities; bookstore; campus computer network; career placement assistance; computer lab; computer-assisted instruction; e-mail services; employment services for current students; housing assistance; interactive nursing skills videos; Internet; learning resource lab; library services; nursing audiovisuals; remedial services; resume preparation assistance; skills, simulation, or other laboratory; tutoring.

**Library Facilities** 6,000 volumes in health, 5,000 volumes in nursing; 26,000 periodical subscriptions health-care related.

## BACCALAUREATE PROGRAMS

**Degree** BSN

**Available Programs** Generic Baccalaureate; RN Baccalaureate.

**Study Options** Full-time.

**Program Entrance Requirements** Minimum overall college GPA of 2.0, transcript of college record, CPR certification, written essay, health insurance, high school chemistry, high school foreign language, 3 years high school math, 3 years high school science, high school transcript, immunizations, interview, 3 letters of recommendation, minimum high school GPA of 2.75, minimum GPA in nursing prerequisites of 2.5, professional liability insurance/malpractice insurance. Transfer students are accepted. *Application deadline:* 1/15 (fall), 6/1 (spring). *Application fee:* $50.

**Advanced Placement** Credit given for nursing courses completed elsewhere dependent upon specific evaluations.

**Expenses (2013–14)** *Tuition:* full-time $15,680; part-time $7840 per semester. *Required fees:* full-time $768; part-time $24 per credit.

**Financial Aid** 64% of baccalaureate students in nursing programs received some form of financial aid in 2012–13.

**Contact** Kelli Backman, Director of Enrollment, School of Nursing, Bryan College of Health Sciences, 5035 Everett Street, Lincoln, NE 68505. *Telephone:* 402-481-8698. *Fax:* 402-481-8421. *E-mail:* kelli.backman@bryanhealth.org.

## GRADUATE PROGRAMS

**Expenses (2013–14)** *Tuition:* full-time $25,916. *Required fees:* full-time $585.

**Financial Aid** 93% of graduate students in nursing programs received some form of financial aid in 2012–13.

**Contact** Dr. Sharon Hadenfeldt, RN, Dean of Graduate Studies, School of Nursing, Bryan College of Health Sciences, 5035 Everett Street, Lincoln, NE 68506. *Telephone:* 402-481-8606. *Fax:* 402-481-8404. *E-mail:* sharon.hadenfeldt@bryanhealth.org.

### MASTER'S DEGREE PROGRAM

**Degree** MS

**Available Programs** Master's.

**Concentrations Available** Nurse anesthesia; nursing education.

**Study Options** Full-time.

**Program Entrance Requirements** Clinical experience, computer literacy, minimum overall college GPA of 3.0, transcript of college record, CPR certification, written essay, immunizations, interview, 4 letters of recommendation, prerequisite course work, resume. *Application deadline:* 5/30 (fall), 10/31 (spring), 5/30 (summer). *Application fee:* $75.

**Degree Requirements** 71 total credit hours, thesis or project.

# Clarkson College
## Master of Science in Nursing Program
## Omaha, Nebraska

*http://www.clarksoncollege.edu/academics/nursing/*
Founded in 1888

**DEGREES • BSN • MSN**

**Nursing Program Faculty** 42 (6% with doctorates).

**Baccalaureate Enrollment** 500 **Women** 90% **Men** 10% **Minority** 10% **Part-time** 15%

**Graduate Enrollment** 200 **Women** 90% **Men** 10% **Minority** 10% **Part-time** 50%

**Distance Learning Courses** Available.

**Nursing Student Activities** Sigma Theta Tau, Student Nurses' Association.

**Nursing Student Resources** Academic advising; academic or career counseling; assistance for students with disabilities; bookstore; campus computer network; career placement assistance; computer lab; computer-assisted instruction; daycare for children of students; e-mail services; employment services for current students; interactive nursing skills videos; Internet; learning resource lab; library services; nursing audiovisuals; placement services for program completers; resume preparation assistance; skills, simulation, or other laboratory; tutoring.

**Library Facilities** 8,807 volumes (7,500 in health, 2,200 in nursing); 262 periodical subscriptions (600 health-care related).

### BACCALAUREATE PROGRAMS

**Degree** BSN

**Available Programs** ADN to Baccalaureate; Accelerated RN Baccalaureate; Baccalaureate for Second Degree; Generic Baccalaureate; LPN to Baccalaureate; LPN to RN Baccalaureate; RN Baccalaureate.

**Study Options** Full-time and part-time.

**Online Degree Options** Yes.

**Program Entrance Requirements** Minimum overall college GPA of 2.5, transcript of college record, CPR certification, written essay, health exam, health insurance, 2 years high school math, 2 years high school science, high school transcript, immunizations, minimum high school GPA of 2.5, minimum high school rank 50%. Transfer students are accepted. *Application fee:* $35.

**Advanced Placement** Credit given for nursing courses completed elsewhere dependent upon specific evaluations.

**Contact** *Telephone:* 402-552-3100. *Fax:* 402-552-6057.

### GRADUATE PROGRAMS

**Contact** *Telephone:* 800-647-5500. *Fax:* 402-552-6057.

#### MASTER'S DEGREE PROGRAM

**Degree** MSN

**Available Programs** Master's; RN to Master's.

**Concentrations Available** Health-care administration; nurse anesthesia; nursing administration; nursing education. *Nurse practitioner programs in:* adult health, family health.

**Study Options** Full-time and part-time.

**Online Degree Options** Yes (online only).

**Program Entrance Requirements** Clinical experience, minimum overall college GPA of 3.0, transcript of college record, written essay, 2 letters of recommendation, resume. *Application deadline:* 7/1 (fall), 11/15 (spring), 4/1 (summer). *Application fee:* $35.

**Advanced Placement** Credit given for nursing courses completed elsewhere dependent upon specific evaluations.

**Degree Requirements** 46 total credit hours, thesis or project.

#### POST-MASTER'S PROGRAM

**Areas of Study** Health-care administration; nurse anesthesia; nursing administration; nursing education. *Nurse practitioner programs in:* adult health, family health.

### CONTINUING EDUCATION PROGRAM

**Contact** *Telephone:* 402-552-3100. *Fax:* 402-552-6057.

# College of Saint Mary
## Division of Health Care Professions
## Omaha, Nebraska

Founded in 1923

**DEGREES • BSN • MSN**

**Nursing Program Faculty** 18 (6% with doctorates).

**Baccalaureate Enrollment** 45 **Women** 100% **Minority** 10% **Part-time** 65%

**Graduate Enrollment** 20 **Women** 100% **Minority** 5% **Part-time** 50%

**Distance Learning Courses** Available.

**Nursing Student Activities** Nursing Honor Society, Sigma Theta Tau, Student Nurses' Association, nursing club.

**Nursing Student Resources** Academic advising; academic or career counseling; assistance for students with disabilities; bookstore; campus computer network; career placement assistance; computer lab; computer-assisted instruction; daycare for children of students; e-mail services; employment services for current students; housing assistance; interactive nursing skills videos; Internet; learning resource lab; library services; nursing audiovisuals; other; placement services for program completers; remedial services; resume preparation assistance; skills, simulation, or other laboratory; tutoring; unpaid internships.

**Library Facilities** 88,503 volumes (30 in health, 30 in nursing); 178 periodical subscriptions (100 health-care related).

### BACCALAUREATE PROGRAMS

**Degree** BSN

**Available Programs** ADN to Baccalaureate; Generic Baccalaureate; LPN to Baccalaureate.

**Study Options** Full-time and part-time.

**Program Entrance Requirements** Minimum overall college GPA of 2.75, transcript of college record, CPR certification, health exam, health insurance, high school biology, high school chemistry, high school foreign language, high school transcript, immunizations, minimum high school GPA of 3.0, minimum GPA in nursing prerequisites of 2.75. Transfer students are accepted.

**Financial Aid** 90% of baccalaureate students in nursing programs received some form of financial aid in 2012–13.

**Contact** Ms. Christi Glesmann, Undergraduate Nursing Program Director, Division of Health Care Professions, College of Saint Mary, 7000 Mercy Road, Omaha, NE 68106. *Telephone:* 402-399-2400. *E-mail:* cglesmann@csm.edu.

### GRADUATE PROGRAMS

**Financial Aid** 100% of graduate students in nursing programs received some form of financial aid in 2012–13.

**Contact** Dr. Kari Wade, Graduate Nursing Program Director, Division of Health Care Professions, College of Saint Mary, 7000 Mercy Road, Omaha, NE 68106. *Telephone:* 402-399-2400. *E-mail:* kwade@csm.edu.

#### MASTER'S DEGREE PROGRAM

**Degree** MSN

**Available Programs** Master's.

**Concentrations Available** Nursing education.

**Study Options** Full-time and part-time.

**Program Entrance Requirements** Computer literacy, minimum overall college GPA of 3.0, transcript of college record, CPR certification, immunizations, prerequisite course work. *Application deadline:* Applications may be processed on a rolling basis for some programs.

**Degree Requirements** Thesis or project.

# Creighton University
## School of Nursing
## Omaha, Nebraska

*http://www.creighton.edu/nursing/*
Founded in 1878

**DEGREES • BSN • DNP • MSN**

**Nursing Program Faculty** 54 (46% with doctorates).

**Baccalaureate Enrollment** 548 **Women** 90.7% **Men** 9.3% **Minority** 20.4% **International** .3% **Part-time** 3.2%

**Graduate Enrollment** 165 **Women** 95.8% **Men** 4.2% **Minority** 7.9% **Part-time** 54.5%

**Distance Learning Courses** Available.

**Nursing Student Activities** Nursing Honor Society, Sigma Theta Tau, Student Nurses' Association.
**Nursing Student Resources** Academic advising; academic or career counseling; assistance for students with disabilities; bookstore; campus computer network; career placement assistance; computer lab; computer-assisted instruction; daycare for children of students; e-mail services; employment services for current students; Internet; learning resource lab; library services; nursing audiovisuals; remedial services; resume preparation assistance; skills, simulation, or other laboratory; tutoring; unpaid internships.
**Library Facilities** 722,682 volumes (184,619 in health, 3,861 in nursing); 59,602 periodical subscriptions (10,376 health-care related).

### BACCALAUREATE PROGRAMS

**Degree** BSN
**Available Programs** Accelerated Baccalaureate for Second Degree; Generic Baccalaureate; RN Baccalaureate.
**Site Options** Hastings, NE.
**Study Options** Full-time and part-time.
**Online Degree Options** Yes.
**Program Entrance Requirements** Minimum overall college GPA of 2.0, transcript of college record, written essay, health exam, health insurance, high school chemistry, 3 years high school math, 2 years high school science, high school transcript, immunizations, 1 letter of recommendation, minimum high school GPA of 3.0, minimum high school rank 50%. Transfer students are accepted. *Application deadline:* Applications may be processed on a rolling basis for some programs. *Application fee:* $50.
**Advanced Placement** Credit given for nursing courses completed elsewhere dependent upon specific evaluations.
**Contact** *Telephone:* 402-280-2067. *Fax:* 402-280-2045.

### GRADUATE PROGRAMS

**Contact** *Telephone:* 402-280-2067. *Fax:* 402-280-2045.

#### MASTER'S DEGREE PROGRAM

**Degree** MSN
**Available Programs** Master's.
**Concentrations Available** Clinical nurse leader; nursing administration; nursing education. *Clinical nurse specialist programs in:* adult health, cardiovascular, family health, gerontology, maternity-newborn, oncology, pediatric. *Nurse practitioner programs in:* acute care, adult health, family health, gerontology, neonatal health, oncology, pediatric, psychiatric/mental health.
**Site Options** Hastings, NE.
**Study Options** Full-time and part-time.
**Program Entrance Requirements** Clinical experience, minimum overall college GPA of 3.0, transcript of college record, CPR certification, written essay, immunizations, 3 letters of recommendation, physical assessment course, prerequisite course work, resume, statistics course. *Application deadline:* Applications may be processed on a rolling basis for some programs. *Application fee:* $50.
**Advanced Placement** Credit given for nursing courses completed elsewhere dependent upon specific evaluations.
**Degree Requirements** 36 total credit hours, thesis or project.

#### POST-MASTER'S PROGRAM

**Areas of Study** Clinical nurse leader; nursing administration; nursing education. *Clinical nurse specialist programs in:* adult health, cardiovascular, family health, gerontology, maternity-newborn, oncology, pediatric. *Nurse practitioner programs in:* acute care, adult health, family health, gerontology, neonatal health, oncology, pediatric, psychiatric/mental health.

#### DOCTORAL DEGREE PROGRAM

**Degree** DNP
**Available Programs** Doctorate; Post-Baccalaureate Doctorate.
**Areas of Study** Advanced practice nursing, clinical practice, critical care, family health, gerontology, health promotion/disease prevention, maternity-newborn, neuro-behavior, nursing administration, nursing education, oncology.
**Site Options** Hastings, NE.
**Program Entrance Requirements** Clinical experience, minimum overall college GPA of 3.0, 3 letters of recommendation, statistics course, vita. *Application deadline:* Applications may be processed on a rolling basis for some programs. *Application fee:* $50.
**Degree Requirements** 32 total credit hours, residency.

## Midland University
### Department of Nursing
### Fremont, Nebraska

***http://www.midlandu.edu/***
Founded in 1883

**DEGREE • BSN**
**Nursing Program Faculty** 12 (25% with doctorates).
**Baccalaureate Enrollment** 130 **Women** 93% **Men** 7% **Minority** 4% **International** 3% **Part-time** 9%
**Distance Learning Courses** Available.
**Nursing Student Activities** Sigma Theta Tau, Student Nurses' Association.
**Nursing Student Resources** Academic advising; academic or career counseling; assistance for students with disabilities; bookstore; campus computer network; career placement assistance; computer lab; computer-assisted instruction; e-mail services; employment services for current students; housing assistance; interactive nursing skills videos; Internet; learning resource lab; library services; nursing audiovisuals; paid internships; placement services for program completers; remedial services; resume preparation assistance; skills, simulation, or other laboratory; tutoring; unpaid internships.
**Library Facilities** 110,000 volumes (4,700 in health, 2,000 in nursing); 900 periodical subscriptions (550 health-care related).

### BACCALAUREATE PROGRAMS

**Degree** BSN
**Available Programs** ADN to Baccalaureate; Generic Baccalaureate; LPN to RN Baccalaureate; RN Baccalaureate.
**Site Options** Columbus, NE.
**Study Options** Full-time and part-time.
**Program Entrance Requirements** Minimum overall college GPA of 2.5, transcript of college record, CPR certification, written essay, health exam, high school transcript, immunizations, interview, 2 letters of recommendation, minimum GPA in nursing prerequisites of 2.5, prerequisite course work. Transfer students are accepted. *Application deadline:* 3/1 (spring). Applications may be processed on a rolling basis for some programs.
**Advanced Placement** Credit given for nursing courses completed elsewhere dependent upon specific evaluations.
**Contact** *Telephone:* 402-941-6505. *Fax:* 402-941-6513.

## Nebraska Methodist College
### Department of Nursing
### Omaha, Nebraska

***http://www.methodistcollege.edu/***
Founded in 1891

**DEGREES • BSN • MSN**
**Nursing Program Faculty** 35 (31% with doctorates).
**Baccalaureate Enrollment** 550 **Women** 93% **Men** 7% **Minority** 11% **International** 1% **Part-time** 44%
**Graduate Enrollment** 121 **Women** 97% **Men** 3% **Minority** 2% **Part-time** 32%
**Distance Learning Courses** Available.
**Nursing Student Activities** Nursing Honor Society, Sigma Theta Tau, Student Nurses' Association.
**Nursing Student Resources** Academic advising; academic or career counseling; assistance for students with disabilities; bookstore; campus computer network; career placement assistance; computer lab; computer-assisted instruction; e-mail services; employment services for current students; interactive nursing skills videos; Internet; learning resource lab; library services; nursing audiovisuals; remedial services; resume preparation assistance; skills, simulation, or other laboratory; tutoring.
**Library Facilities** 10,300 volumes (8,000 in health, 4,500 in nursing); 640 periodical subscriptions (13,600 health-care related).

### BACCALAUREATE PROGRAMS

**Degree** BSN
**Available Programs** Accelerated Baccalaureate for Second Degree; Accelerated RN Baccalaureate; Generic Baccalaureate; LPN to Baccalaureate; LPN to RN Baccalaureate; RN Baccalaureate.
**Study Options** Full-time and part-time.

**Program Entrance Requirements** Minimum overall college GPA of 2.5, transcript of college record, written essay, high school biology, high school chemistry, 2 years high school math, 2 years high school science, high school transcript, interview, minimum high school GPA of 2.5, minimum GPA in nursing prerequisites of 2.5. Transfer students are accepted. *Application deadline:* Applications may be processed on a rolling basis for some programs. *Application fee:* $25.
**Advanced Placement** Credit given for nursing courses completed elsewhere dependent upon specific evaluations.
**Expenses (2013–14)** *Tuition:* full-time $15,240; part-time $508 per credit hour. *International tuition:* $15,240 full-time. *Room and board:* room only: $7032 per academic year. *Required fees:* full-time $630; part-time $20 per credit; part-time $75 per term.
**Financial Aid** 96% of baccalaureate students in nursing programs received some form of financial aid in 2012–13. *Gift aid (need-based):* Federal Pell, FSEOG, state, private, college/university gift aid from institutional funds, Federal Nursing. *Loans:* Federal Nursing Student Loans, Federal Direct (Subsidized and Unsubsidized Stafford PLUS), Perkins, college/university, private loans. *Work-study:* Federal Work-Study. *Financial aid application deadline (priority):* 4/1.
**Contact** Sara Hanson, Director, Enrollment Services, Department of Nursing, Nebraska Methodist College, 720 North 87th Street, Omaha, NE 68114-2852. *Telephone:* 402-354-7200. *Fax:* 402-354-7020. *E-mail:* admissions@methodistcollege.edu.

## GRADUATE PROGRAMS

**Expenses (2013–14)** *Tuition:* full-time $11,898; part-time $661 per credit hour. *International tuition:* $11,898 full-time. *Room and board:* room only: $7032 per academic year. *Required fees:* full-time $360; part-time $20 per credit.
**Financial Aid** 82% of graduate students in nursing programs received some form of financial aid in 2012–13.
**Contact** Sara Hanson, Director, Enrollment Services, Department of Nursing, Nebraska Methodist College, 720 North 87th Street, Omaha, NE 68114-2852. *Telephone:* 402-354-7200. *Fax:* 402-354-7020. *E-mail:* admissions@methodistcollege.edu.

### MASTER'S DEGREE PROGRAM

**Degree** MSN
**Available Programs** Master's; Master's for Nurses with Non-Nursing Degrees; RN to Master's.
**Concentrations Available** Nursing administration; nursing education.
**Study Options** Full-time and part-time.
**Online Degree Options** Yes (online only).
**Program Entrance Requirements** Computer literacy, minimum overall college GPA of 3.0, transcript of college record, CPR certification, written essay, immunizations, interview, 2 letters of recommendation, nursing research course, physical assessment course, prerequisite course work, resume, statistics course. *Application deadline:* Applications may be processed on a rolling basis for some programs. *Application fee:* $25.
**Advanced Placement** Credit given for nursing courses completed elsewhere dependent upon specific evaluations.
**Degree Requirements** 36 total credit hours, thesis or project.

### POST-MASTER'S PROGRAM

**Areas of Study** Nursing administration; nursing education.

## CONTINUING EDUCATION PROGRAM

**Contact** Phyllis Zimmermann, Director, Continuing Education, Department of Nursing, Nebraska Methodist College, 720 North 87th Street, Omaha, NE 68114-2852. *Telephone:* 402-354-7109. *Fax:* 402-354-7055. *E-mail:* phyllis.zimmermann@methodistcollege.edu.

# Nebraska Wesleyan University

## Department of Nursing
## Lincoln, Nebraska

*http://www.nebrwesleyan.edu/*
Founded in 1887

### DEGREES • BSN • MSN

**Nursing Program Faculty** 15 (50% with doctorates).
**Baccalaureate Enrollment** 87 **Women** 92% **Men** 8% **Minority** 7% **International** 11% **Part-time** 40%
**Graduate Enrollment** 54 **Women** 96% **Men** 4% **Minority** 12% **International** 2% **Part-time** 50%
**Distance Learning Courses** Available.
**Nursing Student Activities** Sigma Theta Tau.
**Nursing Student Resources** Academic advising; academic or career counseling; assistance for students with disabilities; bookstore; campus computer network; career placement assistance; computer lab; e-mail services; Internet; library services; nursing audiovisuals; resume preparation assistance; unpaid internships.
**Library Facilities** 225,771 volumes (5,000 in health, 3,700 in nursing); 1,551 periodical subscriptions (470 health-care related).

## BACCALAUREATE PROGRAMS

**Degree** BSN
**Available Programs** ADN to Baccalaureate; Accelerated RN Baccalaureate; International Nurse to Baccalaureate; RN Baccalaureate.
**Site Options** Omaha, NE.
**Study Options** Full-time and part-time.
**Program Entrance Requirements** Transfer students are accepted. *Application deadline:* Applications may be processed on a rolling basis for some programs. *Application fee:* $100.
**Advanced Placement** Credit by examination available. Credit given for nursing courses completed elsewhere dependent upon specific evaluations.
**Contact** *Telephone:* 800-541-3818 Ext. 2330. *Fax:* 402-465-2479.

## GRADUATE PROGRAMS

**Contact** *Telephone:* 402-465-2336. *Fax:* 402-465-2179.

### MASTER'S DEGREE PROGRAM

**Degree** MSN
**Available Programs** Accelerated AD/RN to Master's; Accelerated Master's; Accelerated RN to Master's; Master's; RN to Master's.
**Concentrations Available** Nursing administration; nursing education.
**Site Options** Omaha, NE.
**Study Options** Full-time and part-time.
**Program Entrance Requirements** Clinical experience, computer literacy, minimum overall college GPA of 3.0, transcript of college record, written essay, immunizations, 2 letters of recommendation, nursing research course, resume, statistics course. *Application deadline:* 8/1 (fall), 12/10 (spring). Applications may be processed on a rolling basis for some programs. *Application fee:* $100.
**Advanced Placement** Credit by examination available. Credit given for nursing courses completed elsewhere dependent upon specific evaluations.
**Degree Requirements** 40 total credit hours, thesis or project, comprehensive exam.

### POST-MASTER'S PROGRAM

**Areas of Study** Nursing administration; nursing education.

# Union College

## Division of Health Sciences
## Lincoln, Nebraska

*http://www.ucollege.edu/*
Founded in 1891

### DEGREE • BSN

**Nursing Program Faculty** 15
**Baccalaureate Enrollment** 110 **Women** 82% **Men** 18% **Minority** 10% **International** 5.2% **Part-time** 12.7%
**Nursing Student Activities** Sigma Theta Tau, nursing club.
**Nursing Student Resources** Academic advising; academic or career counseling; assistance for students with disabilities; bookstore; campus computer network; career placement assistance; computer lab; computer-assisted instruction; e-mail services; employment services for current students; externships; housing assistance; interactive nursing skills videos; Internet; learning resource lab; library services; nursing audiovisuals; placement services for program completers; remedial services; resume preparation assistance; skills, simulation, or other laboratory; tutoring; unpaid internships.
**Library Facilities** 176,653 volumes (450 in health, 350 in nursing); 32,990 periodical subscriptions (100 health-care related).

## BACCALAUREATE PROGRAMS

**Degree** BSN
**Available Programs** ADN to Baccalaureate; Generic Baccalaureate; LPN to Baccalaureate.
**Study Options** Full-time and part-time.

**Program Entrance Requirements** Minimum overall college GPA of 2.75, transcript of college record, CPR certification, written essay, health exam, health insurance, high school transcript, immunizations, interview, 2 letters of recommendation, professional liability insurance/malpractice insurance, prerequisite course work. Transfer students are accepted. *Application deadline:* 3/1 (fall), 10/1 (spring). *Application fee:* $250.
**Advanced Placement** Credit given for nursing courses completed elsewhere dependent upon specific evaluations.
**Expenses (2013–14)** *Room and board:* $3260 per academic year.
**Financial Aid** 83% of baccalaureate students in nursing programs received some form of financial aid in 2012–13.
**Contact** Mrs. Angela Heam, Program Development and Enrollment Counselor, Division of Health Sciences, Union College, 3800 South 48th Street, Lincoln, NE 68506. *Telephone:* 402-486-2674. *Fax:* 402-486-2582. *E-mail:* anheam@ucollege.edu.

# University of Nebraska Medical Center
## College of Nursing
## Omaha, Nebraska

***http://www.unmc.edu/nursing/***
Founded in 1869

**DEGREES • BSN • MSN • PHD**
**Nursing Program Faculty** 112 (60% with doctorates).
**Baccalaureate Enrollment** 600
**Graduate Enrollment** 300
**Nursing Student Activities** Nursing Honor Society, Sigma Theta Tau, Student Nurses' Association, nursing club.
**Nursing Student Resources** Academic advising; academic or career counseling; assistance for students with disabilities; bookstore; campus computer network; career placement assistance; computer lab; computer-assisted instruction; daycare for children of students; e-mail services; employment services for current students; externships; housing assistance; interactive nursing skills videos; Internet; learning resource lab; library services; nursing audiovisuals; other; paid internships; placement services for program completers; remedial services; resume preparation assistance; skills, simulation, or other laboratory; tutoring.
**Library Facilities** 251,347 volumes (240,000 in health, 3,500 in nursing); 7,603 periodical subscriptions (2,200 health-care related).

### BACCALAUREATE PROGRAMS
**Degree** BSN
**Available Programs** ADN to Baccalaureate; Accelerated Baccalaureate; Accelerated Baccalaureate for Second Degree; Accelerated RN Baccalaureate; Baccalaureate for Second Degree; Generic Baccalaureate; International Nurse to Baccalaureate; LPN to Baccalaureate; LPN to RN Baccalaureate; RN Baccalaureate; RPN to Baccalaureate.
**Study Options** Full-time.
**Program Entrance Requirements** Minimum overall college GPA of 2.5, transcript of college record, CPR certification, health insurance, high school transcript, immunizations, 2 letters of recommendation, prerequisite course work. Transfer students are accepted.
**Advanced Placement** Credit by examination available. Credit given for nursing courses completed elsewhere dependent upon specific evaluations.
**Contact** *Telephone:* 402-559-5184.

### GRADUATE PROGRAMS
**Contact** *Telephone:* 402-559-5184.

#### MASTER'S DEGREE PROGRAM
**Degree** MSN
**Available Programs** Master's; Master's for Non-Nursing College Graduates; RN to Master's.
**Concentrations Available** Health-care administration; nurse case management; nursing administration; nursing education; nursing informatics. *Clinical nurse specialist programs in:* acute care, adult health, cardiovascular, community health, critical care, family health, gerontology, maternity-newborn, medical-surgical, oncology, parent-child, pediatric, perinatal, psychiatric/mental health, public health,women's health. *Nurse practitioner programs in:* acute care, adult health, community health, family health, gerontology, neonatal health, oncology, pediatric, primary care, psychiatric/mental health,women's health.
**Study Options** Full-time and part-time.
**Program Entrance Requirements** Computer literacy, minimum overall college GPA of 3.0, transcript of college record, CPR certification, immunizations, interview, 3 letters of recommendation, nursing research course, statistics course.
**Advanced Placement** Credit given for nursing courses completed elsewhere dependent upon specific evaluations.
**Degree Requirements** 45 total credit hours.

#### POST-MASTER'S PROGRAM
**Areas of Study** Health-care administration; nurse case management; nursing administration; nursing education; nursing informatics. *Clinical nurse specialist programs in:* acute care, adult health, cardiovascular, community health, critical care, family health, gerontology, maternity-newborn, medical-surgical, oncology, parent-child, pediatric, perinatal, psychiatric/mental health, public health,women's health. *Nurse practitioner programs in:* acute care, adult health, community health, family health, gerontology, neonatal health, oncology, pediatric, primary care, psychiatric/mental health,women's health.

#### DOCTORAL DEGREE PROGRAM
**Degree** PhD
**Available Programs** Doctorate; Doctorate for Nurses with Non-Nursing Degrees; Post-Baccalaureate Doctorate.
**Areas of Study** Advanced practice nursing, aging, bio-behavioral research, biology of health and illness, clinical practice, community health, critical care, faculty preparation, family health, gerontology, health policy, health promotion/disease prevention, health-care systems, human health and illness, illness and transition, individualized study, information systems, maternity-newborn, neuro-behavior, nurse case management, nursing administration, nursing policy, nursing research, nursing science, oncology,women's health.
**Program Entrance Requirements** Minimum overall college GPA of 3.2, interview by faculty committee, interview, 3 letters of recommendation, scholarly papers, statistics course, vita, writing sample.
**Degree Requirements** Dissertation, oral exam, written exam.

#### POSTDOCTORAL PROGRAM
**Postdoctoral Program Contact***Telephone:* 402-559-7457. *Fax:* 410-706-0945.

### CONTINUING EDUCATION PROGRAM
**Contact** *Telephone:* 402-559-7487.

# NEVADA

# Great Basin College
## BSN Program
## Elko, Nevada

***http://www.gbcnv.edu/programs/show.cgi?BS-NUR***
Founded in 1967

**DEGREE • BSN**
**Nursing Program Faculty** 6 (33% with doctorates).
**Baccalaureate Enrollment** 38 **Women** 95% **Men** 5% **Minority** 35%
**Distance Learning Courses** Available.
**Nursing Student Activities** Nursing club.
**Nursing Student Resources** Academic advising; academic or career counseling; assistance for students with disabilities; bookstore; campus computer network; computer lab; computer-assisted instruction; daycare for children of students; e-mail services; employment services for current students; Internet; learning resource lab; library services; nursing audiovisuals; resume preparation assistance; skills, simulation, or other laboratory.
**Library Facilities** 113,341 volumes; 142 periodical subscriptions.

### BACCALAUREATE PROGRAMS
**Degree** BSN
**Available Programs** ADN to Baccalaureate; RN Baccalaureate.
**Online Degree Options** Yes.
**Program Entrance Requirements** CPR certification, written essay, health exam, health insurance, immunizations, 3 letters of recommendation, minimum GPA in nursing prerequisites of 3.0, prerequisite course work, RN licensure.
**Contact** *Telephone:* 775-738-8493.

# Nevada State College at Henderson

## Nursing Program
## Henderson, Nevada

*http://www.nsc.nevada.edu/83.asp*
Founded in 2002

### DEGREE • BSN

**Nursing Program Faculty** 31 (16% with doctorates).
**Baccalaureate Enrollment** 312 **Women** 86% **Men** 14% **Minority** 34% **Part-time** 66%
**Distance Learning Courses** Available.
**Nursing Student Activities** Sigma Theta Tau, Student Nurses' Association.
**Nursing Student Resources** Academic advising; academic or career counseling; assistance for students with disabilities; bookstore; campus computer network; computer lab; computer-assisted instruction; e-mail services; interactive nursing skills videos; Internet; learning resource lab; library services; nursing audiovisuals; skills, simulation, or other laboratory; tutoring.
**Library Facilities** 16,016 volumes (1,075 in health, 647 in nursing); 47 periodical subscriptions (4,981 health-care related).

### BACCALAUREATE PROGRAMS

**Degree** BSN
**Available Programs** Accelerated Baccalaureate for Second Degree; Generic Baccalaureate; RN Baccalaureate.
**Study Options** Full-time and part-time.
**Online Degree Options** Yes.
**Program Entrance Requirements** Minimum overall college GPA of 2.5, transcript of college record, CPR certification, health exam, health insurance, high school transcript, immunizations, minimum GPA in nursing prerequisites of 3.25, prerequisite course work. Transfer students are accepted. *Application deadline:* 3/15 (fall), 9/15 (spring).
**Advanced Placement** Credit given for nursing courses completed elsewhere dependent upon specific evaluations.
**Contact** *Telephone:* 702-992-2638. *Fax:* 702-992-2058.

# Roseman University of Health Sciences

## College of Nursing
## Henderson, Nevada

*http://www.roseman.edu/*
Founded in 2000

### DEGREE • BSN

**Nursing Program Faculty** 52 (25% with doctorates).
**Baccalaureate Enrollment** 205 **Women** 78% **Men** 22% **Minority** 57%
**Distance Learning Courses** Available.
**Nursing Student Activities** Nursing Honor Society, Student Nurses' Association.
**Nursing Student Resources** Academic advising; academic or career counseling; assistance for students with disabilities; campus computer network; career placement assistance; computer lab; computer-assisted instruction; e-mail services; interactive nursing skills videos; Internet; learning resource lab; library services; nursing audiovisuals; remedial services; resume preparation assistance; skills, simulation, or other laboratory; unpaid internships.

### BACCALAUREATE PROGRAMS

**Degree** BSN
**Available Programs** Accelerated Baccalaureate; Accelerated Baccalaureate for Second Degree; Generic Baccalaureate.
**Site Options** South Jordan, UT; Las Vegas, NV.
**Study Options** Full-time.
**Program Entrance Requirements** Transcript of college record, written essay, health exam, health insurance, immunizations, interview, minimum GPA in nursing prerequisites of 2.75, prerequisite course work. Transfer students are accepted. *Application deadline:* 5/1 (fall), 10/1 (spring). Applications may be processed on a rolling basis for some programs. *Application fee:* $100.
**Advanced Placement** Credit given for nursing courses completed elsewhere dependent upon specific evaluations.
**Financial Aid** 90% of baccalaureate students in nursing programs received some form of financial aid in 2012–13.
**Contact** Mr. Erik D. Dillon, Recruitment, Admissions, and Enrollment Coordinator, College of Nursing, Roseman University of Health Sciences, 11 Sunset Way, Henderson, NV 89014. *Telephone:* 702-968-2075. *Fax:* 702-968-2097. *E-mail:* edillon@roseman.edu.

# Touro University

## School of Nursing
## Henderson, Nevada

### DEGREES • BSN • DNP • MSN

**Nursing Program Faculty** 10 (60% with doctorates).
**Baccalaureate Enrollment** 31 **Women** 77.5% **Men** 22.5% **Minority** 41.9%
**Graduate Enrollment** 6 **Women** 83% **Men** 17% **Minority** 70% **Part-time** 100%
**Distance Learning Courses** Available.
**Nursing Student Activities** Sigma Theta Tau, Student Nurses' Association.
**Nursing Student Resources** Academic advising; assistance for students with disabilities; bookstore; campus computer network; computer lab; computer-assisted instruction; e-mail services; interactive nursing skills videos; Internet; learning resource lab; library services; nursing audiovisuals; remedial services; skills, simulation, or other laboratory; tutoring.
**Library Facilities** 86 volumes in health; 6,002 periodical subscriptions health-care related.

### BACCALAUREATE PROGRAMS

**Degree** BSN
**Available Programs** ADN to Baccalaureate; Generic Baccalaureate; RN Baccalaureate.
**Study Options** Full-time.
**Online Degree Options** Yes.
**Program Entrance Requirements** Minimum overall college GPA of 3.0, transcript of college record, CPR certification, health exam, health insurance, immunizations, minimum GPA in nursing prerequisites of 3.0, prerequisite course work, RN licensure. Transfer students are accepted. *Application deadline:* 7/30 (fall), 12/31 (spring). Applications may be processed on a rolling basis for some programs. *Application fee:* $50.
**Advanced Placement** Credit given for nursing courses completed elsewhere dependent upon specific evaluations.
**Expenses (2012–13)** *Tuition, area resident:* full-time $18,240. *Required fees:* full-time $1600.
**Financial Aid** 90% of baccalaureate students in nursing programs received some form of financial aid in 2011–12.
**Contact** Oscar Espinoza-Parra, Director of Admissions, School of Nursing, Touro University, 874 American Pacific Drive, Henderson, NV 89014. *Telephone:* 702-777-1751. *Fax:* 702-777-1752. *E-mail:* oscar.parra@tun.touro.edu.

### GRADUATE PROGRAMS

**Expenses (2012–13)** *Tuition, state resident:* part-time $600 per credit.
**Financial Aid** 90% of graduate students in nursing programs received some form of financial aid in 2011–12.
**Contact** Dr. Douglas Turner, Graduate Coordinator, School of Nursing, Touro University, 874 American Pacific Drive, Henderson, NV 89014. *Telephone:* 702-777-3997. *Fax:* 702-777-1752. *E-mail:* douglas.turner@tun.touro.edu.

#### MASTER'S DEGREE PROGRAM

**Degree** MSN
**Available Programs** Master's.
**Concentrations Available** Nursing education.
**Study Options** Full-time and part-time.
**Online Degree Options** Yes (online only).
**Program Entrance Requirements** Clinical experience, computer literacy, minimum overall college GPA of 3.0, transcript of college record, CPR certification, 2 letters of recommendation, statistics course. *Application deadline:* Applications may be processed on a rolling basis for some programs. *Application fee:* $50.

**Advanced Placement** Credit given for nursing courses completed elsewhere dependent upon specific evaluations.
**Degree Requirements** 36 total credit hours, thesis or project, comprehensive exam.

**DOCTORAL DEGREE PROGRAM**
**Degree** DNP
**Available Programs** Doctorate.
**Areas of Study** Individualized study.
**Online Degree Options** Yes (online only).
**Program Entrance Requirements** Clinical experience, minimum overall college GPA of 3.0, 3 letters of recommendation, MSN or equivalent, statistics course, vita, writing sample. *Application deadline:* Applications may be processed on a rolling basis for some programs. *Application fee:* $50.
**Degree Requirements** 39 total credit hours, oral exam, residency.

# University of Nevada, Las Vegas
## School of Nursing
## Las Vegas, Nevada

***http://www.unlv.edu/nursing***
Founded in 1957

**DEGREES • BSN • DNP • MSN • PHD**
**Nursing Program Faculty** 35 (54% with doctorates).
**Baccalaureate Enrollment** 181 **Women** 82% **Men** 18% **Minority** 53%
**Graduate Enrollment** 129 **Women** 85% **Men** 15% **Minority** 15% **Part-time** 58%
**Distance Learning Courses** Available.
**Nursing Student Activities** Nursing Honor Society, Sigma Theta Tau, Student Nurses' Association.
**Nursing Student Resources** Academic advising; academic or career counseling; assistance for students with disabilities; bookstore; campus computer network; career placement assistance; computer lab; computer-assisted instruction; e-mail services; employment services for current students; housing assistance; interactive nursing skills videos; Internet; learning resource lab; library services; nursing audiovisuals; remedial services; resume preparation assistance; skills, simulation, or other laboratory; tutoring.
**Library Facilities** 35,800 volumes in health, 12,000 volumes in nursing; 305 periodical subscriptions health-care related.

### BACCALAUREATE PROGRAMS
**Degree** BSN
**Available Programs** Accelerated Baccalaureate; Generic Baccalaureate.
**Study Options** Full-time.
**Program Entrance Requirements** Minimum overall college GPA of 3.0, transcript of college record, CPR certification, health exam, health insurance, high school transcript, immunizations, minimum GPA in nursing prerequisites of 3.0, prerequisite course work. Transfer students are accepted. *Application deadline:* Applications may be processed on a rolling basis for some programs.
**Advanced Placement** Credit by examination available. Credit given for nursing courses completed elsewhere dependent upon specific evaluations.
**Expenses (2013–14)** *Tuition, state resident:* full-time $9950; part-time $383 per credit. *Tuition, nonresident:* full-time $23,860. *International tuition:* $25,838 full-time. *Room and board:* $5262; room only: $2940 per academic year. *Required fees:* part-time $380 per term.
**Financial Aid** 67% of baccalaureate students in nursing programs received some form of financial aid in 2012–13. *Gift aid (need-based):* Federal Pell, FSEOG, state, private, college/university gift aid from institutional funds. *Loans:* Federal Nursing Student Loans, Federal Direct (Subsidized and Unsubsidized Stafford PLUS), Perkins, state, college/university. *Work-study:* Federal Work-Study, part-time campus jobs. *Financial aid application deadline (priority):* 2/1.
**Contact** Ms. Cheryl Perna, Undergraduate Coordinator, School of Nursing, University of Nevada, Las Vegas, 4505 Maryland Parkway, Las Vegas, NV 89154-3018. *Telephone:* 702-895-0167. *Fax:* 702-895-4807. *E-mail:* cheryl.perna@unlv.edu.

### GRADUATE PROGRAMS
**Expenses (2013–14)** *Tuition, state resident:* full-time $10,672; part-time $524 per credit. *Tuition, nonresident:* full-time $21,094; part-time $1103 per credit. *International tuition:* $28,044 full-time. *Room and board:* $5262; room only: $2940 per academic year. *Required fees:* full-time $1240; part-time $620 per term.
**Financial Aid** 40% of graduate students in nursing programs received some form of financial aid in 2012–13. 4 teaching assistantships with partial tuition reimbursements available (averaging $11,500 per year) were awarded; institutionally sponsored loans, scholarships, and unspecified assistantships also available. *Financial aid application deadline:* 3/1.
**Contact** Dr. Michelle Giddings, Coordinator, MSN Program, School of Nursing, University of Nevada, Las Vegas, 4505 Maryland Parkway, Box 453018, Las Vegas, NV 89154-3018. *Telephone:* 702-895-3404. *Fax:* 702-895-4807. *E-mail:* michelle.giddings@unlv.edu.

**MASTER'S DEGREE PROGRAM**
**Degree** MSN
**Available Programs** Master's.
**Concentrations Available** Nursing education. *Nurse practitioner programs in:* family health.
**Study Options** Full-time and part-time.
**Online Degree Options** Yes (online only).
**Program Entrance Requirements** Clinical experience, minimum overall college GPA of 3.0, transcript of college record, CPR certification, written essay, immunizations, interview, 2 letters of recommendation, nursing research course, professional liability insurance/malpractice insurance, prerequisite course work, resume, statistics course. *Application deadline:* 2/1 (fall), 2/1 (spring). *Application fee:* $60.
**Advanced Placement** Credit given for nursing courses completed elsewhere dependent upon specific evaluations.
**Degree Requirements** 46 total credit hours, thesis or project.

**POST-MASTER'S PROGRAM**
**Areas of Study** Nursing education. *Nurse practitioner programs in:* family health.

**DOCTORAL DEGREE PROGRAM**
**Degree** DNP
**Available Programs** Doctorate.
**Areas of Study** Advanced practice nursing, nursing administration.
**Online Degree Options** Yes (online only).
**Program Entrance Requirements** Minimum overall college GPA of 3.5, clinical experience, interview by faculty committee, 3 letters of recommendation, MSN or equivalent, vita. *Application deadline:* Applications are processed on a rolling basis. *Application fee:* $60.
**Degree Requirements** 39 total credit hours, DNP scholarly project, residency.

**Degree** PhD
**Available Programs** Doctorate.
**Areas of Study** Human health and illness, nursing education.
**Online Degree Options** Yes (online only).
**Program Entrance Requirements** Clinical experience, minimum overall college GPA of 3.5, interview by faculty committee, 2 letters of recommendation, MSN or equivalent, scholarly papers, statistics course, vita, writing sample, GRE General Test. *Application deadline:* 2/1 (fall). *Application fee:* $60.
**Degree Requirements** 62 total credit hours, dissertation, oral exam, written exam.

### CONTINUING EDUCATION PROGRAM
**Contact** Ms. Jill Racicot, Continuing Education Coordinator Assistant, School of Nursing, University of Nevada, Las Vegas, 4505 Maryland Parkway, Las Vegas, NV 89154-3018. *Telephone:* 702-895-5920. *Fax:* 702-895-4807. *E-mail:* Jill.Racicot@unlv.edu.

# University of Nevada, Reno
## Orvis School of Nursing
## Reno, Nevada

***http://www.unr.edu/nursing***
Founded in 1874

**DEGREES • BSN • DNP • MSN • MSN/MPH**
**Nursing Program Faculty** 30 (45% with doctorates).
**Baccalaureate Enrollment** 144 **Women** 60% **Men** 40% **Minority** 16%
**International** 5%

**Graduate Enrollment** 67 **Women** 90% **Men** 10% **Minority** 1% **Part-time** 75%
**Distance Learning Courses** Available.
**Nursing Student Activities** Nursing Honor Society, Sigma Theta Tau, Student Nurses' Association.
**Nursing Student Resources** Academic advising; academic or career counseling; assistance for students with disabilities; bookstore; campus computer network; career placement assistance; computer lab; computer-assisted instruction; e-mail services; housing assistance; Internet; learning resource lab; library services; nursing audiovisuals; resume preparation assistance; skills, simulation, or other laboratory; tutoring.
**Library Facilities** 1.2 million volumes (5,000 in health, 3,000 in nursing); 25,360 periodical subscriptions (172 health-care related). .

## BACCALAUREATE PROGRAMS

**Degree** BSN
**Available Programs** ADN to Baccalaureate; Accelerated Baccalaureate; Baccalaureate for Second Degree; Generic Baccalaureate; RN Baccalaureate.
**Site Options** Reno , NV.
**Study Options** Full-time.
**Program Entrance Requirements** Transcript of college record, CPR certification, health exam, health insurance, immunizations, interview, minimum GPA in nursing prerequisites of 3.0, professional liability insurance/malpractice insurance, prerequisite course work. Transfer students are accepted. *Application deadline:* 2/15 (fall), 9/7 (spring).
**Advanced Placement** Credit given for nursing courses completed elsewhere dependent upon specific evaluations.
**Expenses (2013–14)** *Tuition, state resident:* full-time $33,600. *Tuition, nonresident:* full-time $47,100. *Room and board:* $9000; room only: $5000 per academic year. *Required fees:* full-time $500.
**Financial Aid** 60% of baccalaureate students in nursing programs received some form of financial aid in 2012–13.
**Contact** Kimberly Diane Baxter, Associate Director of Undergraduate Programs, Orvis School of Nursing, University of Nevada, Reno, Mail Stop 0134, Reno, NV 89557. *Telephone:* 775-682-7145. *Fax:* 775-784-4262. *E-mail:* kimbaxter@unr.edu.

## GRADUATE PROGRAMS

**Expenses (2013–14)** *Tuition, area resident:* part-time $504 per credit.
**Financial Aid** 30% of graduate students in nursing programs received some form of financial aid in 2012–13. Research assistantships with partial tuition reimbursements available, teaching assistantships with partial tuition reimbursements available, Federal Work-Study, institutionally sponsored loans, scholarships, and unspecified assistantships available. *Financial aid application deadline:* 3/1.
**Contact** Dr. Stephanie DeBoor, Coordinator, Graduate Program, Orvis School of Nursing, University of Nevada, Reno, Pennington Health Sciences Building, Reno, NV 89557-0134. *Telephone:* 775-682-7156. *Fax:* 775-784-4262. *E-mail:* deboors2@unr.edu.

### MASTER'S DEGREE PROGRAM

**Degrees** MSN; MSN/MPH
**Available Programs** Master's.
**Concentrations Available** Clinical nurse leader; nursing education. *Nurse practitioner programs in:* acute care, family health.
**Site Options** Reno, NV.
**Study Options** Full-time and part-time.
**Program Entrance Requirements** Clinical experience, computer literacy, minimum overall college GPA of 3.0, transcript of college record, CPR certification, written essay, immunizations, 3 letters of recommendation, physical assessment course, professional liability insurance/malpractice insurance, prerequisite course work, resume, statistics course. *Application deadline:* 3/1 (fall), 10/1 (spring). *Application fee:* $60.
**Advanced Placement** Credit given for nursing courses completed elsewhere dependent upon specific evaluations.
**Degree Requirements** 37 total credit hours, thesis or project, comprehensive exam.

### POST-MASTER'S PROGRAM

**Areas of Study** Clinical nurse leader; nursing education. *Nurse practitioner programs in:* acute care, family health.

### DOCTORAL DEGREE PROGRAM

**Degree** DNP
**Available Programs** Doctorate.
**Areas of Study** Advanced practice nursing, nursing administration.
**Online Degree Options** Yes (online only).
**Program Entrance Requirements** Clinical experience, minimum overall college GPA of 3.5, 2 letters of recommendation, MSN or equivalent, vita, writing sample. *Application deadline:* 3/15 (fall).
**Degree Requirements** 39 total credit hours, written exam, residency.

# NEW HAMPSHIRE

## Colby-Sawyer College
**Department of Nursing**
**New London, New Hampshire**

***http://www.colby-sawyer.edu/nursing/index.html***
Founded in 1837

**DEGREE • BSN**
**Nursing Program Faculty** 14 (.14% with doctorates).
**Baccalaureate Enrollment** 169 **Women** 93% **Men** 7% **Minority** 4% **International** 1% **Part-time** 1%
**Nursing Student Activities** Nursing Honor Society, Student Nurses' Association.
**Nursing Student Resources** Academic advising; academic or career counseling; assistance for students with disabilities; bookstore; campus computer network; career placement assistance; computer lab; computer-assisted instruction; e-mail services; employment services for current students; housing assistance; interactive nursing skills videos; Internet; learning resource lab; library services; nursing audiovisuals; remedial services; resume preparation assistance; skills, simulation, or other laboratory; tutoring; unpaid internships.
**Library Facilities** 93,696 volumes (12,050 in health, 760 in nursing); 27,072 periodical subscriptions (135 health-care related).

### BACCALAUREATE PROGRAMS

**Degree** BSN
**Available Programs** Generic Baccalaureate.
**Study Options** Full-time and part-time.
**Program Entrance Requirements** Minimum overall college GPA of 2.7, transcript of college record, CPR certification, written essay, health exam, health insurance, high school biology, high school chemistry, high school foreign language, 3 years high school math, 3 years high school science, high school transcript, immunizations, 2 letters of recommendation, minimum high school GPA of 2.75, minimum GPA in nursing prerequisites of 2.7, prerequisite course work. Transfer students are accepted. *Application deadline:* Applications may be processed on a rolling basis for some programs.
**Advanced Placement** Credit by examination available. Credit given for nursing courses completed elsewhere dependent upon specific evaluations.
**Contact** *Telephone:* 603-526-3795. *Fax:* 603-526-3159.

## Franklin Pierce University
**Master of Science in Nursing**
**Rindge, New Hampshire**

***http://www.franklinpierce.edu/***
Founded in 1962

**DEGREES • BS • MSN**
**Nursing Program Faculty** 4 (50% with doctorates).
**Baccalaureate Enrollment** 110 **Women** 97% **Men** 3% **Minority** 3% **Part-time** 100%
**Graduate Enrollment** 24 **Women** 96% **Men** 4% **Minority** 8% **Part-time** 100%
**Distance Learning Courses** Available.
**Nursing Student Resources** Academic advising; assistance for students with disabilities; bookstore; campus computer network; computer lab; library services.
**Library Facilities** 200 periodical subscriptions health-care related.

### BACCALAUREATE PROGRAMS

**Degree** BS
**Available Programs** ADN to Baccalaureate; RN Baccalaureate.
**Site Options** Concord, NH; Lebanon, NH; Portsmouth, NH.

**Study Options** Part-time.
**Program Entrance Requirements** RN licensure. Transfer students are accepted. *Application deadline:* Applications may be processed on a rolling basis for some programs.
**Advanced Placement** Credit by examination available.
**Contact** *Telephone:* 603-433-2000 Ext. 2000. *Fax:* 603-899-1067 Ext. 1067.

## GRADUATE PROGRAMS

**Contact** *Telephone:* 603-322-2000. *Fax:* 603-899-1067.

### MASTER'S DEGREE PROGRAM

**Degree** MSN
**Available Programs** Master's; Master's for Nurses with Non-Nursing Degrees; RN to Master's.
**Concentrations Available** Nursing administration; nursing education.
**Site Options** Concord, NH; Lebanon, NH; Portsmouth, NH.
**Study Options** Part-time.
**Program Entrance Requirements** Computer literacy, minimum overall college GPA of 2.8, transcript of college record, written essay, interview, 3 letters of recommendation, resume, statistics course. *Application deadline:* Applications may be processed on a rolling basis for some programs.
**Degree Requirements** 34 total credit hours, thesis or project.

# Rivier University

## Division of Nursing
## Nashua, New Hampshire

***http://www.rivier.edu/***
Founded in 1933

**DEGREES • BS • MS**

**Nursing Program Faculty** 28
**Baccalaureate Enrollment** 710 **Women** 94% **Men** 6% **Minority** 10% **Part-time** 45%
**Graduate Enrollment** 136 **Women** 95% **Men** 5% **Minority** 7% **Part-time** 89%
**Distance Learning Courses** Available.
**Nursing Student Activities** Nursing Honor Society, Sigma Theta Tau, Student Nurses' Association.
**Nursing Student Resources** Academic advising; academic or career counseling; assistance for students with disabilities; bookstore; campus computer network; career placement assistance; computer lab; computer-assisted instruction; e-mail services; employment services for current students; externships; housing assistance; interactive nursing skills videos; Internet; learning resource lab; library services; nursing audiovisuals; other; remedial services; resume preparation assistance; skills, simulation, or other laboratory; tutoring.
**Library Facilities** 177,535 volumes (3,777 in health, 1,170 in nursing); 317 periodical subscriptions (4,000 health-care related).

## BACCALAUREATE PROGRAMS

**Degree** BS
**Available Programs** ADN to Baccalaureate; Generic Baccalaureate; LPN to Baccalaureate; LPN to RN Baccalaureate; RN Baccalaureate.
**Site Options** Manchester, NH.
**Study Options** Full-time and part-time.
**Online Degree Options** Yes.
**Program Entrance Requirements** Minimum overall college GPA, transcript of college record, written essay, health exam, health insurance, high school biology, high school chemistry, high school foreign language, 3 years high school math, 2 years high school science, high school transcript, immunizations, 2 letters of recommendation, minimum high school GPA, minimum high school rank, prerequisite course work. Transfer students are accepted. *Application deadline:* Applications may be processed on a rolling basis for some programs. *Application fee:* $25.
**Advanced Placement** Credit by examination available. Credit given for nursing courses completed elsewhere dependent upon specific evaluations.
**Expenses (2013–14)** *Tuition:* full-time $27,480. *Room and board:* $10,570; room only: $5720 per academic year.
**Contact** Ms. Valerie Leclair, Director of Undergraduate Admissions, Division of Nursing, Rivier University, 420 South Main Street, Nashua, NH 03060-5086. *Telephone:* 603-897-8515. *Fax:* 603-897-8808. *E-mail:* vleclair@rivier.edu.

## GRADUATE PROGRAMS

**Expenses (2013–14)** *Tuition:* full-time $29,000. *International tuition:* $29,000 full-time. *Required fees:* full-time $75.
**Financial Aid** 42% of graduate students in nursing programs received some form of financial aid in 2012–13. Available to part-time students. *Application deadline:* 2/1.
**Contact** Pamela A. Slawinowski, Assistant to Program Director, Division of Nursing, Rivier University, 420 South Main Street, Nashua, NH 03060-5086. *Telephone:* 603-897-8528. *Fax:* 603-897-8884. *E-mail:* pslawinowski@rivier.edu.

### MASTER'S DEGREE PROGRAM

**Degree** MS
**Available Programs** Master's; Master's for Nurses with Non-Nursing Degrees; RN to Master's.
**Concentrations Available** Nursing education. *Nurse practitioner programs in:* family health, psychiatric/mental health.
**Study Options** Full-time and part-time.
**Program Entrance Requirements** Clinical experience, minimum overall college GPA of 3.0, transcript of college record, written essay, immunizations, interview, 2 letters of recommendation, resume, statistics course, GRE, MAT. *Application deadline:* Applications may be processed on a rolling basis for some programs. *Application fee:* $25.
**Advanced Placement** Credit by examination available. Credit given for nursing courses completed elsewhere dependent upon specific evaluations.
**Degree Requirements** 43 total credit hours, thesis or project.

### POST-MASTER'S PROGRAM

**Areas of Study** Nursing education. *Nurse practitioner programs in:* family health, psychiatric/mental health.

# Saint Anselm College

## Department of Nursing
## Manchester, New Hampshire

***http://www.anselm.edu/Academics/Majors-and-Departments/Nursing.htm***
Founded in 1889

**DEGREE • BSN**

**Nursing Program Faculty** 21 (33% with doctorates).
**Baccalaureate Enrollment** 331 **Women** 97% **Men** 3%
**Nursing Student Activities** Sigma Theta Tau, Student Nurses' Association, nursing club.
**Nursing Student Resources** Academic advising; academic or career counseling; assistance for students with disabilities; bookstore; campus computer network; career placement assistance; computer lab; computer-assisted instruction; e-mail services; employment services for current students; externships; housing assistance; interactive nursing skills videos; Internet; learning resource lab; library services; nursing audiovisuals; resume preparation assistance; skills, simulation, or other laboratory; tutoring.
**Library Facilities** 222,000 volumes (6,346 in health); 1,900 periodical subscriptions (4,575 health-care related).

## BACCALAUREATE PROGRAMS

**Degree** BSN
**Available Programs** RN Baccalaureate.
**Study Options** Full-time and part-time.
**Program Entrance Requirements** Transcript of college record, written essay, health exam, health insurance, high school biology, high school chemistry, high school foreign language, 3 years high school math, 3 years high school science, high school transcript, immunizations, 2 letters of recommendation. Transfer students are accepted. *Application deadline:* 11/15 (fall). *Application fee:* $50.
**Advanced Placement** Credit by examination available. Credit given for nursing courses completed elsewhere dependent upon specific evaluations.
**Expenses (2013–14)** *Tuition:* full-time $34,084. *Room and board:* $12,690 per academic year. *Required fees:* full-time $1550.
**Financial Aid** 97% of baccalaureate students in nursing programs received some form of financial aid in 2012–13. *Gift aid (need-based):* Federal Pell, FSEOG, state, private, college/university gift aid from institutional funds. *Loans:* Federal Direct (Subsidized and Unsubsidized Stafford PLUS), Perkins. *Work-study:* Federal Work-Study, part-time campus jobs. *Financial aid application deadline:* 3/15(priority: 3/15).

**Contact** Mr. Eric Nichols, Director of Admission, Department of Nursing, Saint Anselm College, 100 Saint Anselm Drive, Manchester, NH 03102-1310. *Telephone:* 603-641-7500. *Fax:* 603-641-7550. *E-mail:* enichols@anselm.edu.

### CONTINUING EDUCATION PROGRAM

**Contact** Sharon George, Dean of Nursing, Department of Nursing, Saint Anselm College, 100 Saint Anselm Drive, #1745, Manchester, NH 03102-1310. *Telephone:* 603-641-7084. *Fax:* 603-641-7089. *E-mail:* sgeorge@anselm.edu.

## University of New Hampshire
### Department of Nursing
### Durham, New Hampshire

***http://www.chhs.unh.edu/nursing***
Founded in 1866

**DEGREES • BS • MS**
**Nursing Program Faculty** 13 (75% with doctorates).
**Baccalaureate Enrollment** 268 **Women** 91% **Men** 9% **Minority** 1%
**Graduate Enrollment** 54 **Women** 95% **Men** 5% **Minority** 1%
**Nursing Student Activities** Nursing Honor Society, Sigma Theta Tau, Student Nurses' Association.
**Nursing Student Resources** Academic advising; academic or career counseling; assistance for students with disabilities; bookstore; campus computer network; computer lab; computer-assisted instruction; daycare for children of students; e-mail services; housing assistance; interactive nursing skills videos; Internet; learning resource lab; nursing audiovisuals; paid internships; resume preparation assistance; skills, simulation, or other laboratory; tutoring.
**Library Facilities** 1.8 million volumes; 58,875 periodical subscriptions.

### BACCALAUREATE PROGRAMS

**Degree** BS
**Available Programs** Generic Baccalaureate; RN Baccalaureate.
**Study Options** Full-time and part-time.
**Program Entrance Requirements** High school transcript, prerequisite course work. Transfer students are accepted.
**Contact** *Telephone:* 603-862-4715. *Fax:* 603-862-4771.

### GRADUATE PROGRAMS

**Contact** *Telephone:* 603-862-2285. *Fax:* 603-862-4771.

**MASTER'S DEGREE PROGRAM**
**Degree** MS
**Available Programs** Master's; Master's for Nurses with Non-Nursing Degrees.
**Concentrations Available** *Clinical nurse specialist programs in:* adult health. *Nurse practitioner programs in:* adult health, family health.
**Program Entrance Requirements** GRE General Test or MAT.
**Degree Requirements** 45 total credit hours, thesis or project, comprehensive exam.

**POST-MASTER'S PROGRAM**
**Areas of Study** *Clinical nurse specialist programs in:* adult health. *Nurse practitioner programs in:* adult health, family health.

# NEW JERSEY

## Bloomfield College
### Division of Nursing
### Bloomfield, New Jersey

***http://www.bloomfield.edu/***
Founded in 1868

**DEGREE • BS**
**Nursing Program Faculty** 15 (40% with doctorates).
**Baccalaureate Enrollment** 160 **Women** 89% **Men** 11% **Minority** 67%
**International** 3% **Part-time** 23%
**Distance Learning Courses** Available.
**Nursing Student Activities** Nursing Honor Society, Sigma Theta Tau, Student Nurses' Association, nursing club.
**Nursing Student Resources** Academic advising; academic or career counseling; assistance for students with disabilities; bookstore; campus computer network; career placement assistance; computer lab; computer-assisted instruction; e-mail services; employment services for current students; interactive nursing skills videos; Internet; learning resource lab; library services; nursing audiovisuals; other; placement services for program completers; resume preparation assistance; skills, simulation, or other laboratory; tutoring; unpaid internships.
**Library Facilities** 64,000 volumes (2,000 in health, 2,000 in nursing); 460 periodical subscriptions (44 health-care related).

### BACCALAUREATE PROGRAMS

**Degree** BS
**Available Programs** Generic Baccalaureate; RN Baccalaureate.
**Study Options** Full-time and part-time.
**Program Entrance Requirements** Transcript of college record, CPR certification, health exam, immunizations, minimum GPA in nursing prerequisites of 2.5, prerequisite course work. Transfer students are accepted. *Application deadline:* 5/1 (fall). *Application fee:* $40.
**Advanced Placement** Credit given for nursing courses completed elsewhere dependent upon specific evaluations.
**Expenses (2013–14)** *Tuition:* full-time $24,680; part-time $3085 per course. *International tuition:* $24,680 full-time. *Room and board:* $10,900; room only: $5450 per academic year. *Required fees:* full-time $1200; part-time $150 per credit.
**Financial Aid** 92% of baccalaureate students in nursing programs received some form of financial aid in 2012–13. *Gift aid (need-based):* Federal Pell, FSEOG, state, private, college/university gift aid from institutional funds. *Loans:* Federal Direct (Subsidized and Unsubsidized Stafford PLUS). *Work-study:* Federal Work-Study, part-time campus jobs. *Financial aid application deadline:* 6/1(priority: 3/15).
**Contact** Dr. Neddie Serra, Chair, Division of Nursing, Bloomfield College, Bloomfield, NJ 07003. *Telephone:* 973-748-9000 Ext. 1120. *Fax:* 973-743-3998. *E-mail:* neddie_serra@bloomfield.edu.

## Caldwell College
### Nursing Programs
### Caldwell, New Jersey

***http://www.caldwell.edu/***
Founded in 1939

**DEGREE • BSN**
**Nursing Program Faculty** 13 (24% with doctorates).
**Baccalaureate Enrollment** 150
**Distance Learning Courses** Available.
**Nursing Student Activities** Student Nurses' Association, nursing club.
**Nursing Student Resources** Academic advising; academic or career counseling; assistance for students with disabilities; bookstore; campus computer network; computer lab; computer-assisted instruction; e-mail services; employment services for current students; housing assistance; Internet; learning resource lab; library services; nursing audiovisuals; paid internships; remedial services; skills, simulation, or other laboratory; tutoring.
**Library Facilities** 151,293 volumes (4,794 in health, 97 in nursing); 422 periodical subscriptions (5,215 health-care related).

### BACCALAUREATE PROGRAMS

**Degree** BSN
**Available Programs** Accelerated Baccalaureate; Baccalaureate for Second Degree; Generic Baccalaureate; RN Baccalaureate.
**Study Options** Full-time and part-time.
**Online Degree Options** Yes.
**Program Entrance Requirements** Minimum overall college GPA of 2.75, transcript of college record, CPR certification, written essay, health exam, health insurance, high school biology, high school chemistry, high school foreign language, 4 years high school math, 3 years high school science, high school transcript, immunizations, 2 letters of recommendation, minimum high school GPA of 2.75, minimum GPA in nursing prerequisites of 2.75, professional liability insurance/malpractice insurance, prerequisite course work. Transfer students are accepted. *Application deadline:* Applications may be processed on a rolling basis for some programs. *Application fee:* $40.
**Advanced Placement** Credit by examination available.

**Contact** Ms. Michelle Perez, Academic Advisor, Nursing Programs, Caldwell College, 120 Bloomfield Avenue, Caldwell, NJ 07006. *Telephone:* 973-618-3339. *E-mail:* miperez@caldwell.edu.

# The College of New Jersey

## School of Nursing, Health and Exercise Science
## Ewing, New Jersey

***http://www.nursing.pages.tcnj.edu/***
Founded in 1855

**DEGREES • BSN • MSN**
**Nursing Program Faculty** 16 (38% with doctorates).
**Baccalaureate Enrollment** 286 **Women** 90% **Men** 10% **Minority** 38% **Part-time** 3%
**Graduate Enrollment** 25 **Women** 88% **Men** 12% **Minority** 24% **Part-time** 88%
**Nursing Student Activities** Sigma Theta Tau, Student Nurses' Association.
**Nursing Student Resources** Academic advising; academic or career counseling; assistance for students with disabilities; bookstore; campus computer network; career placement assistance; computer lab; computer-assisted instruction; daycare for children of students; e-mail services; employment services for current students; externships; interactive nursing skills videos; Internet; learning resource lab; library services; nursing audiovisuals; paid internships; resume preparation assistance; skills, simulation, or other laboratory; tutoring; unpaid internships.
**Library Facilities** 694,144 volumes (30,000 in health, 18,800 in nursing); 73,733 periodical subscriptions (228 health-care related).

### BACCALAUREATE PROGRAMS

**Degree** BSN
**Available Programs** Generic Baccalaureate; RN Baccalaureate.
**Study Options** Full-time and part-time.
**Program Entrance Requirements** Written essay, health exam, high school transcript, immunizations. Transfer students are accepted. *Application deadline:* 1/15 (fall), 11/15 (spring). *Application fee:* $75.
**Advanced Placement** Credit by examination available. Credit given for nursing courses completed elsewhere dependent upon specific evaluations.
**Expenses (2012–13)** *Tuition, state resident:* full-time $10,102; part-time $358 per credit hour. *Tuition, nonresident:* full-time $20,254; part-time $717 per credit hour. *International tuition:* $20,254 full-time. *Room and board:* $10,998; room only: $8006 per academic year. *Required fees:* full-time $4600; part-time $170 per credit.
**Financial Aid** 80% of baccalaureate students in nursing programs received some form of financial aid in 2011–12. *Gift aid (need-based):* Federal Pell, FSEOG, state, private, college/university gift aid from institutional funds, Federal Nursing. *Loans:* Federal Nursing Student Loans, Federal Direct (Subsidized and Unsubsidized Stafford PLUS), Perkins. *Work-study:* Federal Work-Study. *Financial aid application deadline (priority):* 3/1.
**Contact** Antonino Scarpati, Assistant Dean for Student Services, School of Nursing, Health and Exercise Science, The College of New Jersey, PO Box 7718, 2000 Pennington Road, Ewing, NJ 08628-0718. *Telephone:* 609-771-2669. *Fax:* 609-637-5159. *E-mail:* roger@tcnj.edu.

### GRADUATE PROGRAMS

**Expenses (2012–13)** *Tuition, state resident:* full-time $11,616; part-time $645 per credit hour. *Tuition, nonresident:* full-time $18,321; part-time $1018 per credit hour. *International tuition:* $18,321 full-time. *Required fees:* full-time $3206; part-time $159 per credit.
**Financial Aid** 48% of graduate students in nursing programs received some form of financial aid in 2011–12. Tuition waivers (partial) and unspecified assistantships available. *Financial aid application deadline:* 5/1.
**Contact** Dr. Claire Lindberg, Chair, Division of Advanced Nursing Education and Practice, School of Nursing, Health and Exercise Science, The College of New Jersey, PO Box 7718, 2000 Pennington Road, Ewing, NJ 08628-0718. *Telephone:* 609-771-2591. *Fax:* 609-637-5159. *E-mail:* lindberg@tcnj.edu.

#### MASTER'S DEGREE PROGRAM

**Degree** MSN
**Available Programs** Master's; Master's for Nurses with Non-Nursing Degrees; RN to Master's.
**Concentrations Available** Clinical nurse leader. *Clinical nurse specialist programs in:* adult health. *Nurse practitioner programs in:* adult health, family health, neonatal health, school health.
**Study Options** Full-time and part-time.
**Program Entrance Requirements** Computer literacy, minimum overall college GPA of 3.0, transcript of college record, written essay, immunizations, interview, 3 letters of recommendation, physical assessment course, statistics course, GRE General Test. *Application deadline:* 2/1 (fall), 2/1 (summer). *Application fee:* $75.
**Advanced Placement** Credit given for nursing courses completed elsewhere dependent upon specific evaluations.
**Degree Requirements** 47 total credit hours, comprehensive exam.

#### POST-MASTER'S PROGRAM

**Areas of Study** Nursing administration. *Clinical nurse specialist programs in:* adult health. *Nurse practitioner programs in:* adult health, family health, neonatal health.

# College of Saint Elizabeth

## Department of Nursing
## Morristown, New Jersey

***http://www.cse.edu/academics/academic-programs/health-wellness/nursing/***
Founded in 1899

**DEGREE • BSN**
**Nursing Program Faculty** 13 (25% with doctorates).
**Baccalaureate Enrollment** 231 **Women** 95% **Men** 5% **Minority** 48% **Part-time** 99%
**Nursing Student Activities** Nursing Honor Society, Sigma Theta Tau, nursing club.
**Nursing Student Resources** Academic advising; academic or career counseling; assistance for students with disabilities; bookstore; campus computer network; career placement assistance; computer lab; computer-assisted instruction; e-mail services; employment services for current students; interactive nursing skills videos; Internet; learning resource lab; library services; nursing audiovisuals; other; remedial services; resume preparation assistance; skills, simulation, or other laboratory; tutoring.
**Library Facilities** 119,438 volumes (4,246 in health, 702 in nursing); 1,048 periodical subscriptions (194 health-care related).

### BACCALAUREATE PROGRAMS

**Degree** BSN
**Available Programs** ADN to Baccalaureate; Accelerated RN Baccalaureate; International Nurse to Baccalaureate; RN Baccalaureate.
**Site Options** Randolph, NJ; Elizabeth , NJ; Hoboken, NJ.
**Study Options** Part-time.
**Program Entrance Requirements** Minimum overall college GPA of 2.0, transcript of college record, CPR certification, health exam, immunizations, prerequisite course work, RN licensure. Transfer students are accepted.
**Advanced Placement** Credit by examination available. Credit given for nursing courses completed elsewhere dependent upon specific evaluations.
**Contact** *Telephone:* 973-290-4056. *Fax:* 973-290-4177.

### CONTINUING EDUCATION PROGRAM

**Contact** *Telephone:* 973-290-4073. *Fax:* 973-290-4177.

# Fairleigh Dickinson University, Metropolitan Campus

## Henry P. Becton School of Nursing and Allied Health
## Teaneck, New Jersey

***http://www.fduinfo.com/depts/ucnah.php***
Founded in 1942

**DEGREES • BSN • DNP • MSN**
**Nursing Program Faculty** 20 (60% with doctorates).
**Baccalaureate Enrollment** 381 **Women** 88% **Men** 12% **Minority** 55% **International** 6% **Part-time** 26%

**Graduate Enrollment** 483 **Women** 88% **Men** 12% **Minority** 66% **International** 3% **Part-time** 95%
**Distance Learning Courses** Available.
**Nursing Student Activities** Nursing Honor Society, Sigma Theta Tau, Student Nurses' Association.
**Nursing Student Resources** Academic advising; academic or career counseling; assistance for students with disabilities; bookstore; campus computer network; career placement assistance; computer lab; computer-assisted instruction; e-mail services; employment services for current students; externships; housing assistance; interactive nursing skills videos; Internet; learning resource lab; library services; nursing audiovisuals; other; placement services for program completers; remedial services; resume preparation assistance; skills, simulation, or other laboratory; tutoring; unpaid internships.
**Library Facilities** 155,753 volumes (2,336 in health, 2,336 in nursing); 1,526 periodical subscriptions health-care related.

## BACCALAUREATE PROGRAMS

**Degree** BSN
**Available Programs** Accelerated Baccalaureate for Second Degree; Generic Baccalaureate; RN Baccalaureate.
**Site Options** Morristown, NJ; Summit, NJ; Teaneck, NJ.
**Study Options** Full-time.
**Program Entrance Requirements** Minimum overall college GPA of 3.0, transcript of college record, CPR certification, health exam, health insurance, high school biology, high school chemistry, 2 years high school math, 2 years high school science, high school transcript, immunizations, 2 letters of recommendation, professional liability insurance/malpractice insurance. Transfer students are accepted. *Application deadline:* Applications may be processed on a rolling basis for some programs.
**Advanced Placement** Credit given for nursing courses completed elsewhere dependent upon specific evaluations.
**Expenses (2013–14)** *Tuition:* full-time $33,920; part-time $925 per credit. *Room and board:* $12,742; room only: $8586 per academic year. *Required fees:* full-time $958; part-time $16 per credit; part-time $600 per term.
**Financial Aid** 94% of baccalaureate students in nursing programs received some form of financial aid in 2012–13.
**Contact** Ms. Sylvia Cabassa, Associate Director, Undergraduate Nursing, Henry P. Becton School of Nursing and Allied Health, Fairleigh Dickinson University, Metropolitan Campus, 1000 River Road, H-DH4-02, Teaneck, NJ 07666-1914. *Telephone:* 201-692-2880. *Fax:* 201-692-2388. *E-mail:* scabassa@fdu.edu.

## GRADUATE PROGRAMS

**Expenses (2013–14)** *Tuition:* full-time $20,754; part-time $1153 per credit. *Room and board:* $12,742; room only: $8586 per academic year. *Required fees:* full-time $958; part-time $16 per credit; part-time $600 per term.
**Financial Aid** 91% of graduate students in nursing programs received some form of financial aid in 2012–13.
**Contact** Dr. Elizabeth S. Parietti, Associate Director of Graduate Programs, Henry P. Becton School of Nursing and Allied Health, Fairleigh Dickinson University, Metropolitan Campus, 1000 River Road, H-DH4-02, Teaneck, NJ 07666-1914. *Telephone:* 201-692-2881. *Fax:* 201-692-2388. *E-mail:* parietti@fdu.edu.

### MASTER'S DEGREE PROGRAM

**Degree** MSN
**Available Programs** Accelerated RN to Master's; Master's; RN to Master's.
**Concentrations Available** Nursing administration; nursing education; nursing informatics. *Nurse practitioner programs in:* adult health, family health, gerontology, psychiatric/mental health.
**Site Options** Morristown, NJ; Summit, NJ; Teaneck, NJ.
**Study Options** Full-time and part-time.
**Online Degree Options** Yes.
**Program Entrance Requirements** Clinical experience, minimum overall college GPA of 3.0, transcript of college record, CPR certification, immunizations, 2 letters of recommendation, nursing research course, physical assessment course, professional liability insurance/malpractice insurance, resume, statistics course. *Application deadline:* Applications may be processed on a rolling basis for some programs. *Application fee:* $40.
**Advanced Placement** Credit given for nursing courses completed elsewhere dependent upon specific evaluations.
**Degree Requirements** 31 total credit hours, thesis or project.

### POST-MASTER'S PROGRAM

**Areas of Study** Nursing administration; nursing education; nursing informatics. *Nurse practitioner programs in:* adult health, family health, gerontology, psychiatric/mental health.

### DOCTORAL DEGREE PROGRAM

**Degree** DNP
**Available Programs** Doctorate.
**Areas of Study** Advanced practice nursing, clinical practice, health policy, health-care systems, human health and illness, information systems, nursing administration, nursing policy, nursing research, nursing science.
**Program Entrance Requirements** Clinical experience, minimum overall college GPA of 3.5, interview by faculty committee, interview, 3 letters of recommendation, MSN or equivalent, vita, writing sample. *Application deadline:* Applications may be processed on a rolling basis for some programs.
**Degree Requirements** 36 total credit hours, dissertation, oral exam, residency.

## CONTINUING EDUCATION PROGRAM

**Contact** Mrs. Marian L. Rutherford, RN, Administrator for Clinical Affairs, Henry P. Becton School of Nursing and Allied Health, Fairleigh Dickinson University, Metropolitan Campus, 1000 River Road, H-DH4-02, Teaneck, NJ 07666-1914. *Telephone:* 201-692-2520. *Fax:* 201-692-2388. *E-mail:* marian@fdu.edu.

# Felician College

## Division of Nursing and Health Management
## Lodi, New Jersey

***http://www.felician.edu/***
Founded in 1942

**DEGREES • BSN • MA/MSM • MSN**
**Nursing Program Faculty** 25 (32% with doctorates).
**Baccalaureate Enrollment** 512 **Women** 92% **Men** 8% **Minority** 32% **International** 2% **Part-time** 20%
**Graduate Enrollment** 93 **Women** 89% **Men** 11% **Minority** 33% **Part-time** 88%
**Distance Learning Courses** Available.
**Nursing Student Activities** Nursing Honor Society, Sigma Theta Tau, Student Nurses' Association.
**Nursing Student Resources** Academic advising; academic or career counseling; assistance for students with disabilities; bookstore; campus computer network; career placement assistance; computer lab; computer-assisted instruction; daycare for children of students; e-mail services; interactive nursing skills videos; Internet; learning resource lab; library services; nursing audiovisuals; placement services for program completers; remedial services; resume preparation assistance; skills, simulation, or other laboratory; tutoring.
**Library Facilities** 158,728 volumes (12,519 in health, 12,519 in nursing); 22,575 periodical subscriptions (21 health-care related).

## BACCALAUREATE PROGRAMS

**Degree** BSN
**Available Programs** Accelerated Baccalaureate for Second Degree; Generic Baccalaureate.
**Site Options** East Orange, NJ; Long Branch, NJ; Edison, NJ.
**Study Options** Full-time and part-time.
**Program Entrance Requirements** Minimum overall college GPA of 3.0, transcript of college record, written essay, health exam, health insurance, high school biology, high school chemistry, 2 years high school math, 2 years high school science, high school transcript, immunizations, minimum high school GPA of 3.0, minimum GPA in nursing prerequisites of 2.8, professional liability insurance/malpractice insurance. Transfer students are accepted. *Application deadline:* 8/15 (fall), 1/10 (spring). Applications may be processed on a rolling basis for some programs. *Application fee:* $30.
**Advanced Placement** Credit by examination available. Credit given for nursing courses completed elsewhere dependent upon specific evaluations.
**Contact** *Telephone:* 201-559-6131. *Fax:* 201-559-6138.

## GRADUATE PROGRAMS

**Contact** *Telephone:* 201-559-6077. *Fax:* 201-559-6138.

### MASTER'S DEGREE PROGRAM

**Degrees** MA/MSM; MSN
**Available Programs** Accelerated RN to Master's; Master's.
**Concentrations Available** Nursing administration; nursing education. *Nurse practitioner programs in:* adult health, family health.
**Study Options** Full-time and part-time.
**Online Degree Options** Yes.
**Program Entrance Requirements** Clinical experience, computer literacy, minimum overall college GPA of 3.0, transcript of college record, CPR certification, written essay, immunizations, 2 letters of recommendation, nursing research course, physical assessment course, professional liability insurance/malpractice insurance, prerequisite course work, statistics course. *Application deadline:* Applications may be processed on a rolling basis for some programs. *Application fee:* $40.
**Advanced Placement** Credit given for nursing courses completed elsewhere dependent upon specific evaluations.
**Degree Requirements** 46 total credit hours, thesis or project.

### POST-MASTER'S PROGRAM

**Areas of Study** Nursing administration; nursing education. *Nurse practitioner programs in:* adult health, family health.

# Georgian Court University

## The Georgian Court-Meridian Health School of Nursing
## Lakewood, New Jersey

Founded in 1908

**DEGREE • BSN**

**Library Facilities** 187,772 volumes; 51,048 periodical subscriptions.

### BACCALAUREATE PROGRAMS

**Degree** BSN
**Available Programs** Generic Baccalaureate.
**Contact** Dr. Theresa Wurmser, Chair, The Georgian Court-Meridian Health School of Nursing, Georgian Court University, 900 Lakewood Avenue, Lakewood, NJ 08701. *Telephone:* 732-987-2760. *E-mail:* wurmsert@georgian.edu.

# Kean University

## Department of Nursing
## Union, New Jersey

*http://www.kean.edu/KU/School-of-Nursing*
Founded in 1855

**DEGREES • BSN • MSN • MSN/MPA**

**Nursing Program Faculty** 31 (32% with doctorates).
**Baccalaureate Enrollment** 313 **Women** 93% **Men** 7% **Minority** 45% **International** 35% **Part-time** 90%
**Graduate Enrollment** 102 **Women** 93% **Men** 7% **Minority** 40% **International** 20% **Part-time** 95%
**Nursing Student Activities** Nursing Honor Society, Sigma Theta Tau, nursing club.
**Nursing Student Resources** Academic advising; academic or career counseling; assistance for students with disabilities; bookstore; campus computer network; career placement assistance; computer lab; computer-assisted instruction; daycare for children of students; e-mail services; employment services for current students; housing assistance; interactive nursing skills videos; Internet; learning resource lab; library services; nursing audiovisuals; placement services for program completers; remedial services; resume preparation assistance; tutoring.
**Library Facilities** 224,487 volumes; 47,721 periodical subscriptions.

### BACCALAUREATE PROGRAMS

**Degree** BSN
**Available Programs** ADN to Baccalaureate; RN Baccalaureate.
**Site Options** Branchburg, NJ; Toms River, NJ.
**Study Options** Full-time and part-time.
**Program Entrance Requirements** Minimum overall college GPA of 2.0, written essay, 2 letters of recommendation, prerequisite course work, RN licensure. Transfer students are accepted. *Application deadline:* Applications may be processed on a rolling basis for some programs.
**Advanced Placement** Credit by examination available. Credit given for nursing courses completed elsewhere dependent upon specific evaluations.
**Contact** *Telephone:* 908-737-3390. *Fax:* 908-737-3393.

### GRADUATE PROGRAMS

**Contact** *Telephone:* 908-737-3390. *Fax:* 908-737-3393.

### MASTER'S DEGREE PROGRAM

**Degrees** MSN; MSN/MPA
**Available Programs** Accelerated Master's for Nurses with Non-Nursing Degrees; Master's; Master's for Nurses with Non-Nursing Degrees.
**Concentrations Available** Health-care administration; nursing administration. *Clinical nurse specialist programs in:* community health, school health.
**Site Options** Toms River, NJ.
**Study Options** Full-time and part-time.
**Program Entrance Requirements** Clinical experience, computer literacy, minimum overall college GPA of 3.0, transcript of college record, written essay, immunizations, interview, 2 letters of recommendation, nursing research course, physical assessment course, professional liability insurance/malpractice insurance, statistics course.
**Advanced Placement** Credit given for nursing courses completed elsewhere dependent upon specific evaluations.
**Degree Requirements** 36 total credit hours, thesis or project.

# Monmouth University

## Marjorie K. Unterberg School of Nursing
## West Long Branch, New Jersey

*http://www.monmouth.edu/*
Founded in 1933

**DEGREES • BSN • MSN**

**Nursing Program Faculty** 17 (67% with doctorates).
**Baccalaureate Enrollment** 71 **Women** 93% **Men** 7% **Minority** 23% **Part-time** 98%
**Graduate Enrollment** 245 **Women** 97% **Men** 3% **Minority** 25% **International** .08% **Part-time** 92%
**Distance Learning Courses** Available.
**Nursing Student Activities** Sigma Theta Tau, Student Nurses' Association.
**Nursing Student Resources** Academic advising; academic or career counseling; assistance for students with disabilities; bookstore; campus computer network; career placement assistance; computer lab; computer-assisted instruction; e-mail services; employment services for current students; interactive nursing skills videos; Internet; learning resource lab; library services; nursing audiovisuals; paid internships; remedial services; resume preparation assistance; skills, simulation, or other laboratory; tutoring.
**Library Facilities** 286,000 volumes (250,000 in health, 25,000 in nursing); 43,200 periodical subscriptions (98 health-care related).

### BACCALAUREATE PROGRAMS

**Degree** BSN
**Available Programs** ADN to Baccalaureate; RN Baccalaureate.
**Site Options** Red Bank, NJ; Freehold, NJ.
**Study Options** Full-time and part-time.
**Program Entrance Requirements** Transcript of college record, health exam, immunizations, 2 letters of recommendation, minimum GPA in nursing prerequisites of 2.0, professional liability insurance/malpractice insurance, prerequisite course work, RN licensure. Transfer students are accepted. *Application deadline:* 7/15 (fall), 11/15 (spring), 5/1 (summer). Applications may be processed on a rolling basis for some programs. *Application fee:* $50.
**Advanced Placement** Credit by examination available. Credit given for nursing courses completed elsewhere dependent upon specific evaluations.
**Contact** *Telephone:* 732-571-3443. *Fax:* 732-263-5131.

### GRADUATE PROGRAMS

**Contact** *Telephone:* 732-571-3443. *Fax:* 732-263-5131.

### MASTER'S DEGREE PROGRAM

**Degree** MSN
**Available Programs** Master's; Master's for Nurses with Non-Nursing Degrees; RN to Master's.

**Concentrations Available** Nursing administration; nursing education. *Clinical nurse specialist programs in:* forensic nursing, school health. *Nurse practitioner programs in:* adult health, family health, psychiatric/mental health.
**Site Options** Edison, NJ.
**Study Options** Full-time and part-time.
**Program Entrance Requirements** Minimum overall college GPA of 2.75, transcript of college record, immunizations, 2 letters of recommendation, professional liability insurance/malpractice insurance. *Application deadline:* 7/15 (fall), 11/15 (spring), 5/1 (summer). Applications may be processed on a rolling basis for some programs. *Application fee:* $50.
**Advanced Placement** Credit by examination available. Credit given for nursing courses completed elsewhere dependent upon specific evaluations.
**Degree Requirements** 42 total credit hours.

### POST-MASTER'S PROGRAM
**Areas of Study** Nursing administration; nursing education. *Clinical nurse specialist programs in:* forensic nursing, school health. *Nurse practitioner programs in:* adult health, family health, psychiatric/mental health.

### CONTINUING EDUCATION PROGRAM
**Contact** *Telephone:* 732-571-3694. *Fax:* 732-263-5131.

## New Jersey City University
**Department of Nursing**
**Jersey City, New Jersey**

***https://www.njcu.edu/nursing/***
Founded in 1927

**DEGREE • BSN**
**Nursing Program Faculty** 10 (70% with doctorates).
**Baccalaureate Enrollment** 125 **Women** 85% **Men** 15% **Minority** 75% **International** 15% **Part-time** 40%
**Nursing Student Activities** Nursing Honor Society, Sigma Theta Tau, Student Nurses' Association.
**Nursing Student Resources** Academic advising; academic or career counseling; assistance for students with disabilities; bookstore; campus computer network; computer lab; computer-assisted instruction; daycare for children of students; e-mail services; interactive nursing skills videos; Internet; learning resource lab; library services; nursing audiovisuals; remedial services; skills, simulation, or other laboratory.
**Library Facilities** 319,360 volumes; 25,214 periodical subscriptions.

### BACCALAUREATE PROGRAMS
**Degree** BSN
**Available Programs** Accelerated Baccalaureate for Second Degree; RN Baccalaureate.
**Site Options** Wall Township, NJ; East Orange, NJ.
**Study Options** Full-time.
**Program Entrance Requirements** Minimum overall college GPA of 3.0, transcript of college record, CPR certification, written essay, health exam, immunizations, 2 letters of recommendation, professional liability insurance/malpractice insurance, prerequisite course work, RN licensure. Transfer students are accepted. *Application deadline:* 5/15 (fall), 3/15 (summer). *Application fee:* $35.
**Advanced Placement** Credit by examination available. Credit given for nursing courses completed elsewhere dependent upon specific evaluations.
**Contact** *Telephone:* 201-200-2511. *Fax:* 201-200-3222.

## Ramapo College of New Jersey
**Master of Science in Nursing Program**
**Mahwah, New Jersey**

***http://ww2.ramapo.edu/nursing/***
Founded in 1969

**DEGREES • BSN • MSN**
**Nursing Program Faculty** 29 (20% with doctorates).
**Baccalaureate Enrollment** 435 **Women** 90% **Men** 10% **Minority** 35% **International** 7% **Part-time** 15%
**Graduate Enrollment** 41 **Women** 95% **Men** 5% **Minority** 17% **Part-time** 90%
**Distance Learning Courses** Available.
**Nursing Student Activities** Nursing Honor Society, Student Nurses' Association.
**Nursing Student Resources** Academic advising; academic or career counseling; assistance for students with disabilities; bookstore; campus computer network; career placement assistance; computer lab; computer-assisted instruction; e-mail services; employment services for current students; externships; housing assistance; interactive nursing skills videos; Internet; learning resource lab; library services; nursing audiovisuals; placement services for program completers; remedial services; resume preparation assistance; skills, simulation, or other laboratory; tutoring; unpaid internships.
**Library Facilities** 3,500 volumes in nursing; 200 periodical subscriptions health-care related.

### BACCALAUREATE PROGRAMS
**Degree** BSN
**Available Programs** Generic Baccalaureate; RN Baccalaureate.
**Site Options** Englewood, NJ.
**Study Options** Full-time.
**Online Degree Options** Yes.
**Program Entrance Requirements** CPR certification, health exam, 3 years high school science, immunizations, minimum high school GPA of 2.5, minimum high school rank 20%, professional liability insurance/malpractice insurance. Transfer students are accepted. *Application deadline:* 3/1 (fall), 3/1 (spring). Applications may be processed on a rolling basis for some programs. *Application fee:* $60.
**Advanced Placement** Credit given for nursing courses completed elsewhere dependent upon specific evaluations.
**Contact** *Telephone:* 201-684-7737. *Fax:* 201-684-7934.

### GRADUATE PROGRAMS
**Contact** *Telephone:* 201-684-7737. *Fax:* 201-684-7934.

### MASTER'S DEGREE PROGRAM
**Degree** MSN
**Available Programs** Master's.
**Concentrations Available** Nursing education.
**Study Options** Full-time and part-time.
**Online Degree Options** Yes (online only).
**Program Entrance Requirements** Clinical experience, computer literacy, minimum overall college GPA of 3.0, transcript of college record, CPR certification, 2 letters of recommendation, nursing research course, professional liability insurance/malpractice insurance, statistics course. *Application deadline:* Applications may be processed on a rolling basis for some programs. *Application fee:* $60.
**Advanced Placement** Credit given for nursing courses completed elsewhere dependent upon specific evaluations.
**Degree Requirements** 32 total credit hours.

### POST-MASTER'S PROGRAM
**Areas of Study** Nursing education.

### CONTINUING EDUCATION PROGRAM
**Contact** *Telephone:* 201-684-7206. *Fax:* 201-684-7954.

## The Richard Stockton College of New Jersey
**Program in Nursing**
**Galloway, New Jersey**

***http://www.stockton.edu***
Founded in 1969

**DEGREES • BSN • MSN**
**Nursing Program Faculty** 6 (66% with doctorates).
**Baccalaureate Enrollment** 69 **Women** 98% **Men** 2% **Minority** 10% **Part-time** 80%
**Graduate Enrollment** 20 **Women** 90% **Men** 10% **Minority** 15% **Part-time** 95%
**Nursing Student Activities** Sigma Theta Tau.
**Nursing Student Resources** Academic advising; academic or career counseling; assistance for students with disabilities; bookstore; campus computer network; computer lab; computer-assisted instruction; daycare

for children of students; e-mail services; housing assistance; Internet; learning resource lab; library services; nursing audiovisuals; resume preparation assistance; skills, simulation, or other laboratory; tutoring.
**Library Facilities** 308,800 volumes (9,761 in health, 1,258 in nursing); 47,250 periodical subscriptions (83 health-care related).

### BACCALAUREATE PROGRAMS

**Degree** BSN
**Available Programs** RN Baccalaureate.
**Study Options** Full-time and part-time.
**Program Entrance Requirements** Transfer students are accepted.
**Advanced Placement** Credit given for nursing courses completed elsewhere dependent upon specific evaluations.
**Contact** *Telephone:* 609-652-4837.

### GRADUATE PROGRAMS

**Contact** *Telephone:* 609-652-4501.

**MASTER'S DEGREE PROGRAM**
**Degree** MSN
**Concentrations Available** *Nurse practitioner programs in:* adult health.
**Study Options** Full-time and part-time.
**Program Entrance Requirements** Clinical experience, computer literacy, minimum overall college GPA of 3.0, transcript of college record, CPR certification, written essay, immunizations, 2 letters of recommendation, nursing research course, physical assessment course, professional liability insurance/malpractice insurance, statistics course.
**Advanced Placement** Credit given for nursing courses completed elsewhere dependent upon specific evaluations.
**Degree Requirements** 42 total credit hours, thesis or project.

## Rowan University
### RN to BSN Program
### Glassboro, New Jersey

Founded in 1923

**DEGREE • BSN**
**Library Facilities** 438,135 volumes; 50,883 periodical subscriptions.

### BACCALAUREATE PROGRAMS

**Degree** BSN
**Available Programs** RN Baccalaureate.
**Study Options** Part-time.
**Program Entrance Requirements** Minimum overall college GPA of 2.75, transcript of college record, prerequisite course work, RN licensure. *Application fee:* $65.
**Contact** Admissions, RN to BSN Program, Rowan University, 201 Mullica Hill Road, Glassboro, NJ 08028. *Telephone:* 856-256-5435. *E-mail:* cgceenrollement@rowan.edu.

## Rutgers, The State University of New Jersey, Camden
### Rutgers School of Nursing–Camden
### Camden, New Jersey

*http://www.nursing.camden.rutgers.edu/*
Founded in 1927

**DEGREE • BS**
**Nursing Program Faculty** 42 (79% with doctorates).
**Baccalaureate Enrollment** 431 **Women** 81% **Men** 19% **Minority** 38% **International** 5% **Part-time** 33%
**Distance Learning Courses** Available.
**Nursing Student Activities** Sigma Theta Tau, Student Nurses' Association.
**Nursing Student Resources** Academic advising; academic or career counseling; assistance for students with disabilities; bookstore; campus computer network; career placement assistance; computer lab; computer-assisted instruction; e-mail services; employment services for current students; externships; housing assistance; interactive nursing skills videos; Internet; learning resource lab; library services; nursing audiovisuals; remedial services; resume preparation assistance; skills, simulation, or other laboratory; tutoring.
**Library Facilities** 729,987 volumes; 15,013 periodical subscriptions.

### BACCALAUREATE PROGRAMS

**Degree** BS
**Available Programs** Accelerated RN Baccalaureate; Generic Baccalaureate; RN Baccalaureate.
**Site Options** Mercer, NJ; Atlantic City, NJ.
**Study Options** Full-time.
**Program Entrance Requirements** Written essay, health insurance, high school biology, high school chemistry, 2 years high school math, high school transcript, minimum high school GPA of 3.0. Transfer students are accepted. *Application deadline:* 3/15 (summer). *Application fee:* $65.
**Expenses (2013–14)** *Tuition, state resident:* full-time $13,499; part-time $345 per credit. *Tuition, nonresident:* full-time $27,523; part-time $803 per credit. *International tuition:* $39,101 full-time. *Room and board:* $11,578 per academic year. *Required fees:* full-time $3435.
**Financial Aid** ***Gift aid (need-based):*** Federal Pell, FSEOG, state, private, college/university gift aid from institutional funds, Federal Nursing. *Loans:* Federal Nursing Student Loans, Federal Direct (Subsidized and Unsubsidized Stafford PLUS), Perkins, state, college/university, alternative loans. *Work-study:* Federal Work-Study, part-time campus jobs. *Financial aid application deadline (priority):* 3/15.
**Contact** Mahirym Holguin, Administrative Assistant, Rutgers School of Nursing–Camden, Rutgers, The State University of New Jersey, Camden, 311 North Fifth Street, Armitage Hall, Room 407, Camden, NJ 08102. *Telephone:* 856-225-6226. *Fax:* 856-225-6250. *E-mail:* nursecam@camden.rutgers.edu.

### GRADUATE PROGRAMS

**Contact** Dr. Claudia Beckman, Associate Dean, Graduate and Professional Programs and Associate Professor, Rutgers School of Nursing–Camden, Rutgers, The State University of New Jersey, Camden, 419 Cooper Street, Room 202, Camden, NJ 08102. *Telephone:* 856-225-6226. *Fax:* 856-225-6250. *E-mail:* cbeckman@camden.rutgers.edu.

## Rutgers, The State University of New Jersey, Newark
### Rutgers School of Nursing
### Newark, New Jersey

*http://sn.rutgers.edu/*
Founded in 1956

**DEGREES • BSN • DNP • MSN • MSN/MPH**
**Nursing Program Faculty** 234 (30% with doctorates).
**Baccalaureate Enrollment** 340 **Women** 85% **Men** 15% **Minority** 48%
**Graduate Enrollment** 976 **Women** 80% **Men** 20% **Minority** 30% **Part-time** 80%
**Distance Learning Courses** Available.
**Nursing Student Activities** Nursing Honor Society, Sigma Theta Tau, Student Nurses' Association.
**Nursing Student Resources** Academic advising; academic or career counseling; assistance for students with disabilities; bookstore; campus computer network; computer lab; computer-assisted instruction; daycare for children of students; e-mail services; housing assistance; interactive nursing skills videos; Internet; learning resource lab; library services; nursing audiovisuals; remedial services; resume preparation assistance; skills, simulation, or other laboratory; tutoring.
**Library Facilities** 249,841 volumes (92,000 in health, 3,300 in nursing); 4,784 periodical subscriptions (4,500 health-care related).

### BACCALAUREATE PROGRAMS

**Degree** BSN
**Available Programs** Accelerated Baccalaureate for Second Degree; RN Baccalaureate.
**Site Options** Stratford, NJ.
**Study Options** Full-time.
**Program Entrance Requirements** Minimum overall college GPA of 3.3, transcript of college record, CPR certification, written essay, health exam, health insurance, immunizations, 2 letters of recommendation, minimum GPA in nursing prerequisites of 2.75, prerequisite course work. *Application deadline:* 3/15 (fall), 7/15 (spring), 3/15 (summer). *Application fee:* $45.
**Advanced Placement** Credit given for nursing courses completed elsewhere dependent upon specific evaluations.

**Financial Aid** 82% of baccalaureate students in nursing programs received some form of financial aid in 2012–13.
**Contact** Ms. Angie Pichardo, Admissions Coordinator, Rutgers School of Nursing, Rutgers, The State University of New Jersey, Newark, 65 Bergen Street, Newark, NJ 07101. *Telephone:* 973-972-5336. *E-mail:* picharan@umdnj.edu.

## GRADUATE PROGRAMS

**Financial Aid** 32% of graduate students in nursing programs received some form of financial aid in 2012–13. Teaching assistantships, institutionally sponsored loans and scholarships available. Aid available to part-time students. *Financial aid application deadline:* 5/1.
**Contact** Ms. Angie Pichardo, Admissions Coordinator, Rutgers School of Nursing, Rutgers, The State University of New Jersey, Newark, 65 Bergen Street, Newark, NJ 07101. *Telephone:* 973-972-5336. *E-mail:* picharan@umdnj.edu.

### MASTER'S DEGREE PROGRAM

**Degrees** MSN; MSN/MPH
**Available Programs** Master's; Master's for Nurses with Non-Nursing Degrees; RN to Master's.
**Concentrations Available** Clinical nurse leader; nurse anesthesia; nurse-midwifery; nursing education; nursing informatics. *Nurse practitioner programs in:* acute care, adult health, family health, gerontology, psychiatric/mental health,women's health.
**Site Options** Somers Point, NJ; Stratford, NJ; Voorhees, NJ.
**Study Options** Full-time and part-time.
**Online Degree Options** Yes.
**Program Entrance Requirements** Clinical experience, minimum overall college GPA of 3.0, transcript of college record, CPR certification, 2 letters of recommendation, physical assessment course, prerequisite course work, resume, statistics course, GRE. *Application deadline:* 3/15 (fall). *Application fee:* $50.
**Advanced Placement** Credit given for nursing courses completed elsewhere dependent upon specific evaluations.
**Degree Requirements** 40 total credit hours.

### POST-MASTER'S PROGRAM

**Areas of Study** Clinical nurse leader; nurse-midwifery; nursing informatics. *Nurse practitioner programs in:* acute care, adult health, family health, gerontology, psychiatric/mental health,women's health.

### DOCTORAL DEGREE PROGRAM

**Degree** DNP
**Available Programs** Doctorate; Doctorate for Nurses with Non-Nursing Degrees; Post-Baccalaureate Doctorate.
**Areas of Study** Clinical practice, nursing administration.
**Site Options** Stratford, NJ.
**Program Entrance Requirements** Clinical experience, minimum overall college GPA of 3.0, interview by faculty committee, interview, 2 letters of recommendation, MSN or equivalent, statistics course, vita, writing sample. *Application deadline:* 6/1 (fall), 12/9 (spring). Applications may be processed on a rolling basis for some programs. *Application fee:* $50.
**Degree Requirements** 32 total credit hours, dissertation.

## CONTINUING EDUCATION PROGRAM

**Contact** Dr. Donna Cill, Assistant Dean and Director of the Center for Lifelong Learning, Rutgers School of Nursing, Rutgers, The State University of New Jersey, Newark, 65 Bergen Street, Room 1132-A, Newark, NJ 07101-1709. *Telephone:* 973-972-9793. Fax: 973-972-7904. *E-mail:* donna.cill@rutgers.edu.

# Saint Peter's University

## Nursing Program
## Jersey City, New Jersey

***http://www.saintpeters.edu/***
Founded in 1872

## DEGREES • BSN • MSN

**Nursing Program Faculty** 15 (73% with doctorates).
**Baccalaureate Enrollment** 161 **Women** 85% **Men** 15% **Minority** 40%
**Graduate Enrollment** 55 **Women** 99% **Men** 1% **Minority** 45%
**Distance Learning Courses** Available.
**Nursing Student Activities** Nursing Honor Society, Sigma Theta Tau, Student Nurses' Association.
**Nursing Student Resources** Academic advising; academic or career counseling; assistance for students with disabilities; bookstore; campus computer network; career placement assistance; computer lab; computer-assisted instruction; e-mail services; externships; interactive nursing skills videos; Internet; learning resource lab; library services; nursing audiovisuals; remedial services; resume preparation assistance; skills, simulation, or other laboratory; tutoring.
**Library Facilities** 7,200 volumes in health; 1,586 periodical subscriptions health-care related.

## BACCALAUREATE PROGRAMS

**Degree** BSN
**Available Programs** ADN to Baccalaureate; Generic Baccalaureate; RN Baccalaureate.
**Site Options** Englewood Cliffs, NJ.
**Study Options** Full-time.
**Program Entrance Requirements** Minimum overall college GPA of 2.7, transcript of college record, written essay, high school biology, high school chemistry, high school foreign language, 3 years high school math, 3 years high school science, high school transcript, immunizations, 2 letters of recommendation, minimum high school GPA of 3.0. Transfer students are accepted. *Application deadline:* Applications may be processed on a rolling basis for some programs.
**Contact** *Telephone:* 201-761-7113. *Fax:* 201-761-7105.

## GRADUATE PROGRAMS

**Contact** *Telephone:* 201-761-6272. *Fax:* 201-761-6271.

### MASTER'S DEGREE PROGRAM

**Degree** MSN
**Available Programs** Master's; Master's for Nurses with Non-Nursing Degrees.
**Concentrations Available** Nurse case management; nursing administration. *Nurse practitioner programs in:* adult health.
**Site Options** Englewood Cliffs, NJ.
**Study Options** Part-time.
**Program Entrance Requirements** Clinical experience, minimum overall college GPA of 3.0, transcript of college record, written essay, immunizations, 3 letters of recommendation, nursing research course, physical assessment course, professional liability insurance/malpractice insurance, statistics course. *Application deadline:* 8/25 (fall), 10/24 (winter), 12/15 (spring), 5/5 (summer). *Application fee:* $40.
**Degree Requirements** 39 total credit hours, thesis or project.

### POST-MASTER'S PROGRAM

**Areas of Study** *Nurse practitioner programs in:* adult health.

# Seton Hall University

## College of Nursing
## South Orange, New Jersey

***http://www.shu.edu/academics/nursing/***
Founded in 1856

## DEGREES • BSN • DNP • MSN • MSN/MA • MSN/MBA

**Nursing Program Faculty** 43 (65% with doctorates).
**Baccalaureate Enrollment** 962 **Women** 86% **Men** 14% **Minority** 43% **International** 1% **Part-time** 10%
**Graduate Enrollment** 255 **Women** 89% **Men** 11% **Minority** 17% **Part-time** 74%
**Distance Learning Courses** Available.
**Nursing Student Activities** Nursing Honor Society, Sigma Theta Tau, Student Nurses' Association.
**Nursing Student Resources** Academic advising; academic or career counseling; assistance for students with disabilities; bookstore; campus computer network; career placement assistance; computer lab; computer-assisted instruction; e-mail services; employment services for current students; externships; housing assistance; interactive nursing skills videos; Internet; learning resource lab; library services; nursing audiovisuals; paid internships; placement services for program completers; remedial services; resume preparation assistance; skills, simulation, or other laboratory; tutoring; unpaid internships.
**Library Facilities** 506,042 volumes; 1,475 periodical subscriptions.

## BACCALAUREATE PROGRAMS

**Degree** BSN
**Available Programs** ADN to Baccalaureate; Accelerated Baccalaureate for Second Degree; Accelerated RN Baccalaureate; Baccalaureate for Second Degree; Generic Baccalaureate; International Nurse to Baccalaureate; RN Baccalaureate.
**Site Options** Brick/Toms River, NJ; Lakewood, NJ; Camden, NJ.
**Study Options** Full-time and part-time.
**Program Entrance Requirements** Minimum overall college GPA of 3.0, transcript of college record, CPR certification, written essay, health exam, high school biology, high school chemistry, high school foreign language, 3 years high school math, 2 years high school science, high school transcript, immunizations, minimum high school GPA of 3.0, professional liability insurance/malpractice insurance. Transfer students are accepted. *Application deadline:* Applications may be processed on a rolling basis for some programs.
**Expenses (2013–14)** *Tuition:* full-time $33,740; part-time $1028 per credit. *Room and board:* $10,500; room only: $8500 per academic year.
**Financial Aid** 75% of baccalaureate students in nursing programs received some form of financial aid in 2012–13.
**Contact** Ms. Kristyn Kent-Wuillermin, Director of Strategic Alliances, Marketing, and Enrollment, College of Nursing, Seton Hall University, 400 South Orange Avenue, South Orange, NJ 07079-2697. *Telephone:* 973-761-9291. *Fax:* 973-761-9607. *E-mail:* kristyn.kent@shu.edu.

## GRADUATE PROGRAMS

**Expenses (2013–14)** *Tuition:* part-time $1066 per credit.
**Financial Aid** 31% of graduate students in nursing programs received some form of financial aid in 2012–13. Institutionally sponsored loans, scholarships, traineeships, tuition waivers (partial), and unspecified assistantships available. Aid available to part-time students.
**Contact** Ms. Kristyn Kent-Wuillermin, Director of Strategic Alliances, Marketing, and Enrollment, College of Nursing, Seton Hall University, 400 South Orange Avenue, South Orange, NJ 07079-2697. *Telephone:* 973-761-9291. *Fax:* 973-761-9607. *E-mail:* kristyn.kent@shu.edu.

### MASTER'S DEGREE PROGRAM

**Degrees** MSN; MSN/MA; MSN/MBA
**Available Programs** Accelerated Master's for Non-Nursing College Graduates; Accelerated Master's for Nurses with Non-Nursing Degrees; Accelerated RN to Master's; Master's; Master's for Non-Nursing College Graduates; Master's for Nurses with Non-Nursing Degrees; RN to Master's.
**Concentrations Available** Clinical nurse leader; health-care administration; nurse case management; nursing administration; nursing education. *Nurse practitioner programs in:* acute care, adult health, gerontology, pediatric, primary care, school health.
**Study Options** Full-time and part-time.
**Online Degree Options** Yes (online only).
**Program Entrance Requirements** Clinical experience, computer literacy, minimum overall college GPA of 3.0, transcript of college record, CPR certification, written essay, immunizations, interview, 2 letters of recommendation, nursing research course, physical assessment course, professional liability insurance/malpractice insurance, prerequisite course work, resume, statistics course. *Application deadline:* 4/15 (fall), 11/1 (spring). Applications may be processed on a rolling basis for some programs. *Application fee:* $75.
**Degree Requirements** 45 total credit hours, thesis or project.

### POST-MASTER'S PROGRAM

**Areas of Study** Health-care administration; nurse case management; nursing administration; nursing education. *Nurse practitioner programs in:* acute care, adult health, gerontology, pediatric, primary care, school health.

### DOCTORAL DEGREE PROGRAM

**Degree** DNP
**Available Programs** Doctorate; Post-Baccalaureate Doctorate.
**Areas of Study** Advanced practice nursing, aging, clinical practice, clinical research, faculty preparation, gerontology, health policy, health promotion/disease prevention, health-care systems, illness and transition, individualized study, nursing administration, nursing policy, nursing research, nursing science.
**Online Degree Options** Yes.
**Program Entrance Requirements** Clinical experience, minimum overall college GPA of 3.0, interview by faculty committee, interview, 2 letters of recommendation, MSN or equivalent, scholarly papers, statistics course, vita, writing sample, GRE (waived for students with GPA of 3.5 or higher).
**Degree Requirements** 31 total credit hours, dissertation, residency.

# Thomas Edison State College
## W. Cary Edwards School of Nursing
## Trenton, New Jersey

*http://www.tesc.edu/nursing*
Nursing program founded in 1983

### DEGREES • ACCELERATED 2ND DEGREE BSN • RN-BSN • RN-BSN/MSN • BSN-MSN

**Nursing Student Resources** Students in the W. Cary Edwards School of Nursing have the opportunity to earn degrees through traditional and non-traditional methods, which take into consideration the individual needs and interests of each student. All post-licensure nursing courses are designed and delivered online. Students in these courses communicate with fellow students and mentors, who guide students in the course and grade assignments and exams in an asynchronous environment, which allows for a flexible learning schedule. Students may earn credit toward a degree by demonstrating college-level knowledge through testing and assessment of prior learning; by transfer credit for courses taken through other regionally accredited institutions; through the College's *e*-Pack® courses; and for licenses, certificates, and courses taken at work or through military training, if approved and recommended for academic credit.
**W. Cary Edwards School of Nursing Mentors** The School utilizes mentors, who are off-site nurse educators from a variety of nursing education and service settings to develop, implement, and evaluate the program. All mentors have a minimum of a master's degree in nursing, with approximately 76% prepared at the doctoral level and many tenured at their home institution. With its courses offered by distance learning, the School has the opportunity to draw nurse educators from across the country, resulting in a diverse and experienced group of online nurse mentors. The W. Cary Edwards School of Nursing programs are accredited by the Accreditation Commission for Education in Nursing (ACEN), formerly the National League for Nursing Accrediting Commission (NLNAC), 3343 Peachtree Road, N.E., Suite 850, Atlanta, GA 30326, (404) 975-5000, http://www.acenursing.org and the Commission on Collegiate Nursing Education (CCNE), One Dupont Circle, N.W., Suite 530, Washington, D.C. 20036-1120, (202) 887-6791, http://www.aacn.nche.edu/accreditation. The W. Cary Edwards School of Nursing programs at Thomas Edison State College are approved by the New Jersey Board of Nursing., P.O. Box 45010, Newark, NJ 07101, (973) 504-6430, www.state.nj.us/lps/ca/medical/nursing.htm.

### BACHELOR'S AND MASTER'S DEGREE PROGRAMS

**Degrees** Accelerated 2nd Degree BSN • RN-BSN • RN-BSN/MSN • MSN
**Master's degree has three specialties: Nurse Educator, Nursing Informatics** and **Nursing Administration**
**ACCELERATED 2$^{ND}$ DEGREE BSN PROGRAM** A one-year baccalaureate program designed for adults who already possess a bachelor's degree (non-nursing) completed prior to admission and who are interested in becoming registered nurses. The program includes 60 credits of professional nursing completed both online and onground at Thomas Edison State College in Trenton, NJ. The Accelerated 2$^{nd}$ Degree BSN Program prepares graduates for the National Council Licensure Examination for Registered Nurses (NCLEX-RN). Due to the rigorous nature of this full-time program, outside employment is not recommended.
**RN-BSN/MSN DEGREE PROGRAMS** The online RN-BSN/MSN degree programs are designed for experienced registered nurses (RNs) who want an alternative to campus-based instruction. Three options are offered: BSN (Bachelor of Science in Nursing), BSN/MSN (Bachelor of Science in Nursing and Master of Science in Nursing), and MSN (Master of Science in Nursing). Three nursing specialties are offered in the MSN degree: Nurse Educator, Nursing Informatics, and Nursing Administration.
**Study Options** Self-paced RN-BSN and RN-BSN/MSN programs; online nursing courses offered quarterly; multiple options for credit earning; no time limit for RN-BSN and RN-BSN/MSN degree completion; no residency requirement with maximum flexibility in transfer credit.
**CERTIFICATE PROGRAMS** Three 12–18 credit graduate nursing certificate programs—Nurse Educator; Nursing Informatics; and Nursing Administration—are available to RNs with a master's degree in another area of nursing specialty.

PROGRAM ENTRANCE REQUIREMENTS

**Accelerated 2nd Degree BSN Program**, admission requirements include a bachelor's degree from a regionally accredited college or university completed prior to admission with an earned cumulative GPA of 3.0 or higher, all science prerequisites completed within five years prior to admission, a grade of B or better in all prerequisite science and math courses, completed general education and nursing prerequisites prior to admission, a criminal background check, drug screen, health and immunization verification, malpractice and health insurance, and CPR certification.

**RN-BSN** and **RN-BSN/MSN,** admission is open and rolling. RNs can enroll any day of the year. In addition to the documentation of their current RN license valid in the United States, all applicants must submit a completed online application with $75 fee, and have official transcripts of all completed course work sent to the Office of the Registrar (undergraduate students) or Office of Admissions for graduate students. Up to 80 credits may be accepted from a community college, and up to 60 credits, will be awarded to diploma graduates based on current licensure. There is no age restriction on credits transferred in to meet general education requirements or lower-division nursing requirements. Any upper-division nursing credits accepted for transfer must be from an accredited baccalaureate or higher degree nursing program, and newer than 10 years at the application date.

All credits used in the nursing requirement must have a grade equivalent of C or better. All previously completed graduate credits transferred in to meet MSN degree and graduate certificate requirements must be newer than seven years at the application date, have a grade equivalent of B or better, and be from a **regionally accredited college or university or recognized foreign institution**. For more information on acceptance of foreign credit go to: http://www.tesc.edu/nursing/MSN-Admission-Requirements.cfm. Applicants to the BSN/MSN (BSNM) program will be enrolled in the MSN degree on certification for graduation from the BSN degree. Up to 9 graduate credits required in the BSN degree may be applied to the MSN degree requirements.

**Expenses (2013–14)** *Accelerated 2nd Degree BSN Program Tuition,* $32,600. *RN-BSN Tuition, state resident:* $395 per credit. RN-BSN *Tuition, nonresident:* $476 per credit; $599 for the *MSN degree and Graduate Nursing Certificate Programs*.

**Financial Aid** 10% of the RNs in the undergraduate nursing program and 4% in the graduate nursing program received some form of financial aid in 2012–2013.

**Contact** Thomas Edison State College, 101 W. State St., Trenton, NJ 08608-1176. *Telephone*: 888-442-8372. *E-mail*: nursinginfo@tesc.edu.

# William Paterson University of New Jersey

## Department of Nursing
## Wayne, New Jersey

***http://www.wpunj.edu/***

Founded in 1855

### DEGREES • BSN • DNP • MSN

**Nursing Program Faculty** 55 (33% with doctorates).

**Baccalaureate Enrollment** 412 **Women** 81% **Men** 19% **Minority** 55%

**Graduate Enrollment** 80 **Women** 95% **Men** 5% **Minority** 57% **International** 5% **Part-time** 70%

**Distance Learning Courses** Available.

**Nursing Student Activities** Sigma Theta Tau, Student Nurses' Association.

**Nursing Student Resources** Academic advising; academic or career counseling; assistance for students with disabilities; bookstore; campus computer network; career placement assistance; computer lab; computer-assisted instruction; daycare for children of students; e-mail services; employment services for current students; housing assistance; interactive nursing skills videos; Internet; learning resource lab; library services; nursing audiovisuals; placement services for program completers; remedial services; resume preparation assistance; skills, simulation, or other laboratory; tutoring.

**Library Facilities** 338,573 volumes (15,000 in health, 12,700 in nursing); 6,569 periodical subscriptions (150 health-care related).

### BACCALAUREATE PROGRAMS

**Degree** BSN

**Available Programs** ADN to Baccalaureate; Accelerated Baccalaureate for Second Degree; Generic Baccalaureate; LPN to Baccalaureate; RN Baccalaureate.

**Study Options** Full-time.

**Program Entrance Requirements** Minimum overall college GPA of 2.5, transcript of college record, CPR certification, health exam, health insurance, high school biology, high school chemistry, 1 year of high school math, 2 years high school science, high school transcript, immunizations, minimum high school GPA of 3.25, professional liability insurance/malpractice insurance, prerequisite course work. Transfer students are accepted. *Application deadline:* 5/1 (fall). Applications may be processed on a rolling basis for some programs. *Application fee:* $50.

**Expenses (2013–14)** *Tuition, state resident:* full-time $7421; part-time $237 per credit. *Tuition, nonresident:* full-time $14,961; part-time $485 per credit. *International tuition:* $14,961 full-time. *Room and board:* $8130; room only: $6180 per academic year. *Required fees:* full-time $3297; part-time $290 per term.

**Financial Aid** 67% of baccalaureate students in nursing programs received some form of financial aid in 2012–13.

**Contact** Dr. Nadine Aktan, Chairperson, Department of Nursing, William Paterson University of New Jersey, 300 Pompton Road, W106, Wayne, NJ 07470. *Telephone:* 973-720-2527. *Fax:* 973-720-2668. *E-mail:* aktann@wpunj.edu.

### GRADUATE PROGRAMS

**Expenses (2013–14)** *Tuition, state resident:* part-time $512 per credit. *Tuition, nonresident:* full-time $12,284. *International tuition:* $12,284 full-time. *Required fees:* full-time $3417; part-time $200 per credit.

**Financial Aid** 15% of graduate students in nursing programs received some form of financial aid in 2012–13. Research assistantships with tuition reimbursements available, unspecified assistantships available. *Financial aid application deadline:* 4/1.

**Contact** Dr. Kem Louie, Director, Graduate Program, Department of Nursing, William Paterson University of New Jersey, 300 Pompton Road, W240, Wayne, NJ 07470. *Telephone:* 973-720-3511. *Fax:* 973-720-3517. *E-mail:* louiek@wpunj.edu.

#### MASTER'S DEGREE PROGRAM

**Degree** MSN

**Available Programs** Master's; Master's for Nurses with Non-Nursing Degrees.

**Concentrations Available** Nursing administration; nursing education. *Clinical nurse specialist programs in:* community health. *Nurse practitioner programs in:* adult health, family health.

**Site Options** Paramus, NJ; Englewood, NJ.

**Study Options** Full-time and part-time.

**Program Entrance Requirements** Computer literacy, minimum overall college GPA of 3.0, transcript of college record, CPR certification, written essay, 2 letters of recommendation, nursing research course, physical assessment course, professional liability insurance/malpractice insurance, resume, statistics course, GRE General Test. *Application deadline:* Applications may be processed on a rolling basis for some programs. *Application fee:* $50.

**Advanced Placement** Credit given for nursing courses completed elsewhere dependent upon specific evaluations.

**Degree Requirements** 42 total credit hours, thesis or project.

#### POST-MASTER'S PROGRAM

**Areas of Study** *Clinical nurse specialist programs in:* school health. *Nurse practitioner programs in:* adult health, family health.

#### DOCTORAL DEGREE PROGRAM

**Degree** DNP

**Available Programs** Doctorate.

**Areas of Study** Advanced practice nursing, clinical practice, health-care systems, individualized study.

**Program Entrance Requirements** Clinical experience, minimum overall college GPA of 3.3, interview by faculty committee, letters of recommendation, MSN or equivalent, statistics course, vita, writing sample. *Application deadline:* 4/15 (fall). *Application fee:* $75.

**Degree Requirements** 42 total credit hours.

# NEW MEXICO

## Eastern New Mexico University

### Department of Allied Health–Nursing
### Portales, New Mexico

***https://www.enmu.edu/***
Founded in 1934

**DEGREE • BSN**

**Nursing Program Faculty** 7 (1% with doctorates).
**Baccalaureate Enrollment** 243 **Women** 90% **Men** 10% **Minority** 45% **International** 5% **Part-time** 95%
**Distance Learning Courses** Available.
**Nursing Student Activities** Nursing Honor Society.
**Nursing Student Resources** Academic advising; academic or career counseling; assistance for students with disabilities; bookstore; campus computer network; career placement assistance; computer lab; computer-assisted instruction; e-mail services; housing assistance; Internet; library services; other; resume preparation assistance; tutoring.
**Library Facilities** 8 million volumes (100 in health, 50 in nursing); 62,670 periodical subscriptions (15 health-care related).

#### BACCALAUREATE PROGRAMS

**Degree** BSN
**Available Programs** ADN to Baccalaureate.
**Study Options** Full-time and part-time.
**Online Degree Options** Yes (online only).
**Program Entrance Requirements** Minimum overall college GPA of 2.0, transcript of college record, CPR certification, immunizations, interview, 3 letters of recommendation, minimum GPA in nursing prerequisites of 2.0, professional liability insurance/malpractice insurance, prerequisite course work, RN licensure. Transfer students are accepted. *Application deadline:* 8/20 (fall), 1/4 (winter), 1/20 (spring), 6/1 (summer).
**Advanced Placement** Credit given for nursing courses completed elsewhere dependent upon specific evaluations.
**Expenses (2013–14)** *Tuition, state resident:* full-time $2073; part-time $187 per credit hour. *Tuition, nonresident:* full-time $4829; part-time $402 per credit hour. *International tuition:* $4829 full-time. *Room and board:* $6238; room only: $3018 per academic year. *Required fees:* part-time $186 per credit; part-time $25 per term.
**Financial Aid** 10% of baccalaureate students in nursing programs received some form of financial aid in 2012–13.
**Contact** Dr. Leslie Paternoster, Nursing Program Director, Department of Allied Health–Nursing, Eastern New Mexico University, 1500 South Avenue K, Station 12, Portales, NM 88130. *Telephone:* 575-562-2773. *Fax:* 575-562-2293. *E-mail:* leslie.paternoster@enmu.edu.

## New Mexico Highlands University

### Department of Nursing
### Las Vegas, New Mexico

***http://www.nmhu.edu/nursing***
Founded in 1893

**DEGREE • BSN**

**Nursing Program Faculty** 3 (75% with doctorates).
**Baccalaureate Enrollment** 51 **Women** 90% **Men** 10% **Minority** 67% **Part-time** 80%
**Distance Learning Courses** Available.
**Nursing Student Resources** Academic advising; academic or career counseling; assistance for students with disabilities; bookstore; campus computer network; career placement assistance; e-mail services; housing assistance; Internet; library services; nursing audiovisuals; placement services for program completers; resume preparation assistance; tutoring.
**Library Facilities** 500 volumes in nursing.

#### BACCALAUREATE PROGRAMS

**Degree** BSN
**Available Programs** RN Baccalaureate.
**Online Degree Options** Yes (online only).
**Program Entrance Requirements** Minimum overall college GPA of 2.5, minimum GPA in nursing prerequisites of 2.0, RN licensure. *Application deadline:* 6/15 (fall).
**Advanced Placement** Credit given for nursing courses completed elsewhere dependent upon specific evaluations.
**Expenses (2012–13)** *Tuition, state resident:* full-time $3504; part-time $146 per credit hour. *Tuition, nonresident:* full-time $5671; part-time $236 per credit hour. *International tuition:* $7231 full-time. *Room and board:* $7160; room only: $3990 per academic year. *Required fees:* full-time $20.
**Financial Aid** 3% of baccalaureate students in nursing programs received some form of financial aid in 2011–12. *Gift aid (need-based):* Federal Pell, FSEOG, state, private, college/university gift aid from institutional funds. *Loans:* Federal Direct (Subsidized and Unsubsidized Stafford PLUS), Perkins. *Work-study:* Federal Work-Study, part-time campus jobs. *Financial aid application deadline:* Continuous.
**Contact** Ms. Susan M. Martin, Recruiter/Advisor Coordinator, RN-BSN Program, Department of Nursing, New Mexico Highlands University, Box 9000, Las Vegas, NM 87701. *Telephone:* 505-426-2116. *Fax:* 505-426-2109. *E-mail:* smmartin@nmhu.edu.

## New Mexico State University

### School of Nursing
### Las Cruces, New Mexico

***http://www.nmsu.edu/~nursing***
Founded in 1888

**DEGREES • BSN • MSN • PHD**

**Nursing Program Faculty** 35 (37% with doctorates).
**Baccalaureate Enrollment** 171 **Women** 84% **Men** 16% **Minority** 49% **International** 1% **Part-time** 15%
**Graduate Enrollment** 116 **Women** 88% **Men** 12% **Minority** 24% **International** 1% **Part-time** 25%
**Distance Learning Courses** Available.
**Nursing Student Activities** Sigma Theta Tau, Student Nurses' Association.
**Nursing Student Resources** Academic advising; academic or career counseling; assistance for students with disabilities; bookstore; campus computer network; computer lab; computer-assisted instruction; daycare for children of students; e-mail services; housing assistance; interactive nursing skills videos; Internet; learning resource lab; library services; nursing audiovisuals; paid internships; remedial services; skills, simulation, or other laboratory; tutoring.
**Library Facilities** 1.8 million volumes (33,000 in health, 17,500 in nursing); 61,113 periodical subscriptions (620 health-care related).

#### BACCALAUREATE PROGRAMS

**Degree** BSN
**Available Programs** Generic Baccalaureate; RN Baccalaureate.
**Site Options** Carlsbad, NM; Alamagordo, NM; Grants, NM.
**Study Options** Full-time.
**Online Degree Options** Yes.
**Program Entrance Requirements** Minimum overall college GPA of 3.0, transcript of college record, CPR certification, health insurance, immunizations, minimum GPA in nursing prerequisites of 3.0, prerequisite course work. Transfer students are accepted.
**Advanced Placement** Credit given for nursing courses completed elsewhere dependent upon specific evaluations.
**Contact** *Telephone:* 575-646-2164. *Fax:* 505-646-6166.

#### GRADUATE PROGRAMS

**Contact** *Telephone:* 505-646-8170. *Fax:* 505-646-2167.

**MASTER'S DEGREE PROGRAM**

**Degree** MSN
**Available Programs** Master's; Master's for Nurses with Non-Nursing Degrees.
**Concentrations Available** Nursing administration.
**Study Options** Full-time and part-time.
**Online Degree Options** Yes (online only).
**Program Entrance Requirements** Minimum overall college GPA of 3.0, transcript of college record, CPR certification, written essay, immunizations, 3 letters of recommendation, resume, statistics course, NCLEX exam.
**Advanced Placement** Credit given for nursing courses completed elsewhere dependent upon specific evaluations.
**Degree Requirements** 38 total credit hours, comprehensive exam.

**DOCTORAL DEGREE PROGRAM**
**Degree** PhD
**Available Programs** Doctorate.
**Areas of Study** Nursing research.
**Online Degree Options** Yes (online only).
**Program Entrance Requirements** Minimum overall college GPA of 3.0, interview by faculty committee, 3 letters of recommendation, MSN or equivalent, statistics course, vita, writing sample, NCLEX exam.
**Degree Requirements** 60 total credit hours, dissertation, oral exam, written exam.

## CONTINUING EDUCATION PROGRAM

**Contact** *Telephone:* 505-646-3812. *Fax:* 505-646-2167.

# Northern New Mexico College

## College of Nursing and Health Sciences
## Española, New Mexico

Founded in 1909

**DEGREE • BSN**
**Library Facilities** 18,065 volumes; 222 periodical subscriptions.

## BACCALAUREATE PROGRAMS

**Degree** BSN
**Available Programs** RN Baccalaureate.
**Program Entrance Requirements** RN licensure.
**Contact** Director, RN to BSN Program, College of Nursing and Health Sciences, Northern New Mexico College, 921 North Paseo de Oate, Espanola, NM 87532. *Telephone:* 505-747-2278. *E-mail:* nklebanoff@nnmc.edu.

# University of New Mexico

## College of Nursing
## Albuquerque, New Mexico

***http://nursing.unm.edu/***
Founded in 1889

**DEGREES • BSN • DNP • MSN • PHD**
**Nursing Program Faculty** 64 (56% with doctorates).
**Baccalaureate Enrollment** 258 **Women** 85% **Men** 15% **Minority** 55% **Part-time** 41%
**Graduate Enrollment** 159 **Women** 87% **Men** 13% **Minority** 34% **Part-time** 55%
**Distance Learning Courses** Available.
**Nursing Student Activities** Sigma Theta Tau, Student Nurses' Association.
**Nursing Student Resources** Academic advising; academic or career counseling; assistance for students with disabilities; bookstore; campus computer network; career placement assistance; computer lab; computer-assisted instruction; daycare for children of students; e-mail services; housing assistance; interactive nursing skills videos; Internet; learning resource lab; library services; nursing audiovisuals; remedial services; skills, simulation, or other laboratory.
**Library Facilities** 4.3 million volumes (92,207 in health, 158 in nursing); 71,932 periodical subscriptions (2,344 health-care related).

## BACCALAUREATE PROGRAMS

**Degree** BSN
**Available Programs** Generic Baccalaureate; RN Baccalaureate.
**Study Options** Full-time.
**Program Entrance Requirements** Minimum overall college GPA of 3.0, transcript of college record, written essay, 2 letters of recommendation, minimum GPA in nursing prerequisites of 3.0, prerequisite course work. Transfer students are accepted. *Application deadline:* 2/15 (fall), 9/15 (spring). *Application fee:* $60.
**Advanced Placement** Credit given for nursing courses completed elsewhere dependent upon specific evaluations.
**Expenses (2013–14)** *Tuition, state resident:* part-time $470 per credit hour. *Tuition, nonresident:* part-time $1047 per credit hour. *Required fees:* part-time $386 per term.
**Financial Aid** 70% of baccalaureate students in nursing programs received some form of financial aid in 2012–13. *Gift aid (need-based):* Federal Pell, FSEOG, state, private, college/university gift aid from institutional funds, United Negro College Fund, Federal Nursing. *Loans:* Federal Nursing Student Loans, Federal Direct (Subsidized and Unsubsidized Stafford PLUS), Perkins, state, college/university. *Work-study:* Federal Work-Study, part-time campus jobs. *Financial aid application deadline (priority):* 3/1.
**Contact** Ms. Ann Marie Oechsler, Director of Student Services, College of Nursing, University of New Mexico, 1 University of New Mexico, MSC09 5350, Albuquerque, NM 87131-0001. *Telephone:* 505-272-4223. *Fax:* 505-272-3970. *E-mail:* aoechsler@salud.unm.edu.

## GRADUATE PROGRAMS

**Expenses (2013–14)** *Tuition, state resident:* part-time $551 per credit hour. *Tuition, nonresident:* part-time $1137 per credit hour. *Required fees:* part-time $500 per term.
**Financial Aid** 47% of graduate students in nursing programs received some form of financial aid in 2012–13. 10 fellowships (averaging $24,000 per year), 4 research assistantships with partial tuition reimbursements available (averaging $10,083 per year), 10 teaching assistantships with partial tuition reimbursements available (averaging $10,083 per year) were awarded; institutionally sponsored loans, scholarships, and unspecified assistantships also available. Aid available to part-time students. *Financial aid application deadline:* 3/1.
**Contact** Ms. Nissane Capps, Senior Academic Advisor, College of Nursing, University of New Mexico, UNM College of Nursing, MSC09 5350, 1 University of New Mexico, Albuquerque, NM 87131-0001. *Telephone:* 505-272-4223. *Fax:* 505-272-3970. *E-mail:* ncapps@salud.unm.edu.

**MASTER'S DEGREE PROGRAM**
**Degree** MSN
**Available Programs** Master's.
**Concentrations Available** Nurse-midwifery; nursing administration; nursing education. *Nurse practitioner programs in:* acute care, family health, pediatric.
**Study Options** Full-time and part-time.
**Online Degree Options** Yes (online only).
**Program Entrance Requirements** Clinical experience, minimum overall college GPA of 3.0, transcript of college record, interview, 3 letters of recommendation, resume. *Application deadline:* 2/15 (fall), 10/15 (spring). *Application fee:* $60.
**Advanced Placement** Credit given for nursing courses completed elsewhere dependent upon specific evaluations.
**Degree Requirements** 32 total credit hours, thesis or project, comprehensive exam.

**POST-MASTER'S PROGRAM**
**Areas of Study** Nurse-midwifery; nursing administration; nursing education. *Nurse practitioner programs in:* acute care, family health, pediatric.

**DOCTORAL DEGREE PROGRAM**
**Degree** DNP
**Available Programs** Doctorate.
**Areas of Study** Nursing administration.
**Online Degree Options** Yes.
**Program Entrance Requirements** Minimum overall college GPA of 3.0, clinical experience, interview by faculty committee, 3 letters of recommendation, MSN or equivalent, scholarly papers, vita, writing sample. *Application deadline:* 12/1 (summer). *Application fee:* $60.
**Degree Requirements** 69 total credit hours, written exam.

**Degree** PhD
**Available Programs** Doctorate.
**Areas of Study** Health policy, nursing research.
**Online Degree Options** Yes.
**Program Entrance Requirements** Clinical experience, minimum overall college GPA of 3.0, interview by faculty committee, 3 letters of recommendation, MSN or equivalent, vita, writing sample. *Application deadline:* 2/15 (summer). *Application fee:* $60.
**Degree Requirements** 69 total credit hours, dissertation.

## University of Phoenix–New Mexico Campus
### College of Nursing
### Albuquerque, New Mexico

**DEGREES • BSN • MSN • MSN/ED D**
**Nursing Program Faculty** 18 (13% with doctorates).
**Baccalaureate Enrollment** 24 **Women** 100% **Minority** 33.3%
**Graduate Enrollment** 14 **Women** 100% **Minority** 21.43%
**Nursing Student Activities** Sigma Theta Tau.
**Nursing Student Resources** Academic advising; academic or career counseling; assistance for students with disabilities; bookstore; campus computer network; computer lab; computer-assisted instruction; e-mail services; interactive nursing skills videos; Internet; learning resource lab; library services; nursing audiovisuals; remedial services; skills, simulation, or other laboratory; tutoring.
**Library Facilities** 16,781 periodical subscriptions (1,300 health-care related).

**BACCALAUREATE PROGRAMS**

**Degree** BSN
**Available Programs** Accelerated Baccalaureate.
**Site Options** Santa Fe, NM; Santa Teresa, NM.
**Study Options** Full-time.
**Program Entrance Requirements** Transcript of college record, CPR certification, immunizations, 1 letter of recommendation, RN licensure. Transfer students are accepted.
**Advanced Placement** Credit by examination available. Credit given for nursing courses completed elsewhere dependent upon specific evaluations.
**Contact** *Telephone:* 505-821-4800.

**GRADUATE PROGRAMS**

**Contact** *Telephone:* 505-821-4800.

**MASTER'S DEGREE PROGRAM**
**Degrees** MSN; MSN/Ed D
**Available Programs** Master's.
**Concentrations Available** Nursing administration; nursing education.
**Site Options** Santa Fe, NM; Santa Teresa, NM.
**Study Options** Full-time.
**Online Degree Options** Yes.
**Program Entrance Requirements** Clinical experience, computer literacy, minimum overall college GPA of 2.5, transcript of college record. *Application deadline:* Applications may be processed on a rolling basis for some programs. *Application fee:* $45.
**Advanced Placement** Credit given for nursing courses completed elsewhere dependent upon specific evaluations.
**Degree Requirements** 39 total credit hours, thesis or project.

## Western New Mexico University
### Nursing Department
### Silver City, New Mexico

Founded in 1893

**DEGREE • BNSC**
**Nursing Program Faculty** 16 (8% with doctorates).
**Baccalaureate Enrollment** 85 **Women** 91% **Men** 9% **Minority** 39% **Part-time** 88%
**Distance Learning Courses** Available.
**Nursing Student Activities** Student Nurses' Association, nursing club.
**Nursing Student Resources** Academic advising; academic or career counseling; assistance for students with disabilities; bookstore; campus computer network; career placement assistance; computer lab; computer-assisted instruction; daycare for children of students; e-mail services; housing assistance; interactive nursing skills videos; Internet; learning resource lab; library services; nursing audiovisuals; placement services for program completers; remedial services; resume preparation assistance; skills, simulation, or other laboratory; tutoring.
**Library Facilities** 245,146 volumes (4,980 in health, 4,900 in nursing); 236 periodical subscriptions (14 health-care related).

**BACCALAUREATE PROGRAMS**

**Degree** BNSc
**Available Programs** RN Baccalaureate.
**Site Options** Deming , NM.
**Study Options** Full-time and part-time.
**Online Degree Options** Yes (online only).
**Program Entrance Requirements** Minimum overall college GPA of 2.5, transcript of college record, CPR certification, immunizations, minimum high school GPA, prerequisite course work, RN licensure. Transfer students are accepted. *Application deadline:* 7/15 (fall), 7/15 (winter), 11/15 (spring), 4/15 (summer). Applications may be processed on a rolling basis for some programs. *Application fee:* $30.
**Advanced Placement** Credit given for nursing courses completed elsewhere dependent upon specific evaluations.
**Financial Aid** 40% of baccalaureate students in nursing programs received some form of financial aid in 2012–13.
**Contact** Ms. Kim Woodard, BSN Advisor, Nursing Department, Western New Mexico University, PO Box 680, Silver City, NM 88062. *Telephone:* 575-538-6976. *Fax:* 575-538-6961. *E-mail:* kim.woodard@wnmu.edu.

# NEW YORK

## Adelphi University
### College of Nursing and Public Health
### Garden City, New York

***http://www.adelphi.edu/***
Founded in 1896

**DEGREES • BS • MS • MS/MBA • PHD**
**Nursing Program Faculty** 183 (15% with doctorates).
**Baccalaureate Enrollment** 1,063 **Women** 87.1% **Men** 12.9% **Minority** 53% **International** .6% **Part-time** 5.8%
**Graduate Enrollment** 152 **Women** 86.8% **Men** 13.2% **Minority** 63% **Part-time** 98%
**Distance Learning Courses** Available.
**Nursing Student Activities** Nursing Honor Society, Sigma Theta Tau, Student Nurses' Association, nursing club.
**Nursing Student Resources** Academic advising; academic or career counseling; assistance for students with disabilities; bookstore; campus computer network; career placement assistance; computer lab; computer-assisted instruction; daycare for children of students; e-mail services; employment services for current students; externships; housing assistance; interactive nursing skills videos; Internet; learning resource lab; library services; nursing audiovisuals; paid internships; placement services for program completers; remedial services; resume preparation assistance; skills, simulation, or other laboratory; tutoring; unpaid internships.
**Library Facilities** 605,791 volumes (29,918 in health, 2,666 in nursing); 77,060 periodical subscriptions (364 health-care related).

**BACCALAUREATE PROGRAMS**

**Degree** BS
**Available Programs** Accelerated Baccalaureate for Second Degree; Generic Baccalaureate; RN Baccalaureate.
**Site Options** Sayville, NY; Poughkeepsie, NY; Manhattan, NY.
**Study Options** Full-time.
**Program Entrance Requirements** Minimum overall college GPA of 3.0, transcript of college record, written essay, health exam, high school foreign language, 3 years high school math, 3 years high school science, high school transcript, immunizations, interview, 2 letters of recommendation, minimum high school GPA of 3.0, minimum GPA in nursing prerequisites of 2.7. Transfer students are accepted. *Application deadline:* Applications may be processed on a rolling basis for some programs. *Application fee:* $40.
**Advanced Placement** Credit given for nursing courses completed elsewhere dependent upon specific evaluations.
**Expenses (2013–14)** *Tuition:* full-time $29,550; part-time $920 per credit hour. *International tuition:* $29,550 full-time. *Room and board:* $11,800; room only: $8760 per academic year. *Required fees:* full-time $3530; part-time $1410 per term.
**Financial Aid** 90% of baccalaureate students in nursing programs received some form of financial aid in 2012–13. *Gift aid (need-based):*

Federal Pell, FSEOG, state, private, college/university gift aid from institutional funds, United Negro College Fund, endowed and restricted scholarships and grants. *Loans:* Federal Nursing Student Loans, Federal Direct (Subsidized and Unsubsidized Stafford PLUS), Perkins, New York HELP Program, private loans. *Work-study:* Federal Work-Study, part-time campus jobs. *Financial aid application deadline (priority):* 3/1.

**Contact** Mrs. Christine Murphy, Director of Admissions, College of Nursing and Public Health, Adelphi University, One South Avenue, Levermore Hall, Garden City, NY 11530. *Telephone:* 516-877-3050. *E-mail:* murphy2@adelphi.edu.

## GRADUATE PROGRAMS

**Expenses (2013–14)** *Tuition:* part-time $1005 per credit hour. *International tuition:* $1005 full-time. *Required fees:* full-time $660; part-time $330 per term.

**Financial Aid** 50% of graduate students in nursing programs received some form of financial aid in 2012–13. 8 research assistantships (averaging $5,370 per year) were awarded; career-related internships or fieldwork, unspecified assistantships, and achievement awards also available. Aid available to part-time students. *Financial aid application deadline:* 2/15.

**Contact** Mrs. Christine Murphy, Director of Admissions, College of Nursing and Public Health, Adelphi University, One South Avenue, Levermore Hall, Garden City, NY 11530. *Telephone:* 516-877-3050. *Fax:* 516-877-3039. *E-mail:* murphy2@adelphi.edu.

### MASTER'S DEGREE PROGRAM

**Degrees** MS; MS/MBA

**Available Programs** Master's.

**Concentrations Available** Health-care administration; nursing administration; nursing education; nursing informatics. *Nurse practitioner programs in:* adult health.

**Study Options** Full-time and part-time.

**Program Entrance Requirements** Clinical experience, computer literacy, minimum overall college GPA of 3.0, transcript of college record, CPR certification, written essay, immunizations, interview, 2 letters of recommendation, nursing research course, professional liability insurance/malpractice insurance, resume, statistics course. *Application deadline:* 3/1 (fall). Applications may be processed on a rolling basis for some programs. *Application fee:* $50.

**Advanced Placement** Credit given for nursing courses completed elsewhere dependent upon specific evaluations.

**Degree Requirements** 42 total credit hours, thesis or project, comprehensive exam.

### POST-MASTER'S PROGRAM

**Areas of Study** Health-care administration; nursing administration; nursing education; nursing informatics. *Clinical nurse specialist programs in:* public health. *Nurse practitioner programs in:* adult health.

### DOCTORAL DEGREE PROGRAM

**Degree** PhD

**Available Programs** Doctorate.

**Areas of Study** Faculty preparation, health-care systems, nursing administration, nursing education, nursing policy, nursing research, nursing science.

**Program Entrance Requirements** Minimum overall college GPA of 3.5, interview by faculty committee, interview, 3 letters of recommendation, MSN or equivalent, statistics course, vita, writing sample, GRE. *Application deadline:* 2/15 (fall). *Application fee:* $50.

**Degree Requirements** 54 total credit hours, dissertation, oral exam, written exam.

## CONTINUING EDUCATION PROGRAM

**Contact** Mrs. Karen Pappas, Director of Continuing Education, College of Nursing and Public Health, Adelphi University, One South Avenue, Garden City, NY 11530. *Telephone:* 516-877-4554. *E-mail:* pappas@adelphi.edu.

***See display below and full description on page 468.***

# Binghamton University, State University of New York

## Decker School of Nursing
## Vestal, New York

*http://www.binghamton.edu/dson/*
Founded in 1946

**DEGREES • BS • DNP • MS • PHD**

**Nursing Program Faculty** 58 (40% with doctorates).
**Baccalaureate Enrollment** 354
**Graduate Enrollment** 191
**Distance Learning Courses** Available.
**Nursing Student Activities** Sigma Theta Tau, Student Nurses' Association.
**Nursing Student Resources** Academic advising; assistance for students with disabilities; campus computer network; computer lab; e-mail services; Internet; learning resource lab; library services; skills, simulation, or other laboratory.
**Library Facilities** 2.5 million volumes (7,000 in health); 87,696 periodical subscriptions (9,300 health-care related).

### BACCALAUREATE PROGRAMS

**Degree** BS
**Available Programs** Accelerated RN Baccalaureate; Generic Baccalaureate.
**Study Options** Full-time and part-time.
**Program Entrance Requirements** Minimum overall college GPA of 2.7, transcript of college record, CPR certification, written essay, health exam, high school biology, high school chemistry, high school foreign language, 3 years high school math, 2 years high school science, high school transcript, 2 letters of recommendation, minimum high school GPA of 3.0, prerequisite course work. Transfer students are accepted. *Application deadline:* Applications may be processed on a rolling basis for some programs. *Application fee:* $50.
**Advanced Placement** Credit by examination available. Credit given for nursing courses completed elsewhere dependent upon specific evaluations.
**Contact** *Telephone:* 607-777-4954. *Fax:* 607-777-4440.

### GRADUATE PROGRAMS

**Contact** *Telephone:* 607-777-4614. *Fax:* 607-777-4440.

#### MASTER'S DEGREE PROGRAM

**Degree** MS
**Available Programs** Master's.
**Concentrations Available** Nursing administration; nursing education. *Clinical nurse specialist programs in:* community health, family health, gerontology, psychiatric/mental health. *Nurse practitioner programs in:* community health, family health, gerontology, psychiatric/mental health.
**Study Options** Full-time and part-time.
**Program Entrance Requirements** Computer literacy, minimum overall college GPA of 3.0, transcript of college record, written essay, 2 letters of recommendation, resume, statistics course, GRE General Test. *Application deadline:* 6/15 (fall), 11/15 (spring). Applications may be processed on a rolling basis for some programs. *Application fee:* $60.
**Advanced Placement** Credit given for nursing courses completed elsewhere dependent upon specific evaluations.
**Degree Requirements** 48 total credit hours, thesis or project, comprehensive exam.

#### POST-MASTER'S PROGRAM

**Areas of Study** *Nurse practitioner programs in:* community health, family health, gerontology, psychiatric/mental health.

#### DOCTORAL DEGREE PROGRAM

**Degree** DNP
**Available Programs** Doctorate, Post-Baccalaureate Doctorate.
**Areas of Study** Community health, family health, gerontology, psychiatric/mental health.
**Online Degree Options** Yes (Post-MS to DNP is online).
**Program Entrance Requirements** Minimum overall college GPA of 3.0. Application requirements differ between programs; please contact school for complete requirements. *Application deadline:* 6/1 (fall). Applications may be processed on a rolling basis for some programs. *Application fee:* $60.
**Degree Requirements** 77 credits for Post-BS to DNP, 38 credits for Post-MS to DNP, dissertation, oral exam, residency, written exam.

**Degree** PhD
**Available Programs** Doctorate; Post-Baccalaureate Doctorate.
**Areas of Study** Nursing research.
**Online Degree Options** Yes.
**Program Entrance Requirements** Clinical experience, minimum overall college GPA of 3.0, interview by faculty committee, interview, 3 letters of recommendation, MSN or equivalent, scholarly papers, statistics course, vita, writing sample. *Application deadline:* 6/15 (fall), 11/15 (spring). Applications may be processed on a rolling basis for some programs. *Application fee:* $60.
**Degree Requirements** 55 total credit hours, dissertation, written exam.

### CONTINUING EDUCATION PROGRAM

**Contact** *Telephone:* 607-777-4954. *Fax:* 607-777-4440.

# The College at Brockport, State University of New York

## Department of Nursing
## Brockport, New York

*http://www.brockport.edu/*
Founded in 1867

**DEGREE • BSN**

**Nursing Program Faculty** 24 (50% with doctorates).
**Baccalaureate Enrollment** 200 **Women** 93% **Men** 7% **Minority** 15% **International** 2% **Part-time** 9%
**Distance Learning Courses** Available.
**Nursing Student Activities** Nursing Honor Society, Sigma Theta Tau, Student Nurses' Association.
**Nursing Student Resources** Academic advising; academic or career counseling; assistance for students with disabilities; bookstore; campus computer network; career placement assistance; computer lab; computer-assisted instruction; daycare for children of students; e-mail services; interactive nursing skills videos; Internet; learning resource lab; library services; nursing audiovisuals; remedial services; resume preparation assistance; skills, simulation, or other laboratory; tutoring.
**Library Facilities** 18,952 volumes in health, 1,065 volumes in nursing; 257 periodical subscriptions health-care related.

### BACCALAUREATE PROGRAMS

**Degree** BSN
**Available Programs** ADN to Baccalaureate; Generic Baccalaureate.
**Site Options** Rochester, NY.
**Study Options** Full-time and part-time.
**Program Entrance Requirements** Minimum overall college GPA of 2.75, transcript of college record, CPR certification, health exam, health insurance, high school transcript, immunizations, minimum GPA in nursing prerequisites of 2.0, prerequisite course work. Transfer students are accepted. *Application deadline:* 1/20 (fall).
**Advanced Placement** Credit given for nursing courses completed elsewhere dependent upon specific evaluations.
**Contact** *Telephone:* 585-395-2355. *Fax:* 585-395-5312.

# College of Mount Saint Vincent

## Department of Nursing
## Riverdale, New York

*http://www.mountsaintvincent.edu/408.htm*
Founded in 1911

**DEGREES • BS • MSN**

**Nursing Program Faculty** 30 (90% with doctorates).
**Baccalaureate Enrollment** 520 **Women** 80% **Men** 20% **Minority** 80% **International** 10% **Part-time** 10%
**Graduate Enrollment** 100 **Women** 90% **Men** 10% **Minority** 80% **International** 10% **Part-time** 100%
**Nursing Student Activities** Sigma Theta Tau, Student Nurses' Association.
**Nursing Student Resources** Academic advising; academic or career counseling; bookstore; campus computer network; computer lab; com-

puter-assisted instruction; e-mail services; employment services for current students; housing assistance; interactive nursing skills videos; Internet; learning resource lab; library services; nursing audiovisuals; paid internships; remedial services; resume preparation assistance; skills, simulation, or other laboratory; tutoring.
**Library Facilities** 102,479 volumes (5,304 in nursing).

## BACCALAUREATE PROGRAMS

**Degree** BS
**Available Programs** Baccalaureate for Second Degree; Generic Baccalaureate; International Nurse to Baccalaureate; LPN to Baccalaureate; LPN to RN Baccalaureate.
**Site Options** Manhattan, NY.
**Study Options** Full-time and part-time.
**Program Entrance Requirements** Minimum overall college GPA of 2.7, transcript of college record, CPR certification, written essay, health exam, health insurance, high school biology, high school chemistry, high school foreign language, 3 years high school math, 3 years high school science, high school transcript, immunizations, 1 letter of recommendation, minimum high school GPA of 2.7, minimum GPA in nursing prerequisites of 3.0, prerequisite course work. Transfer students are accepted. *Application deadline:* 8/1 (fall), 1/5 (spring). Applications may be processed on a rolling basis for some programs. *Application fee:* $35.
**Contact** *Telephone:* 718-405-3365. *Fax:* 718-405-3286.

## GRADUATE PROGRAMS

**Contact** *Telephone:* 718-405-3351. *Fax:* 718-405-3286.

### MASTER'S DEGREE PROGRAM

**Degree** MSN
**Available Programs** Master's.

# The College of New Rochelle

## School of Nursing
## New Rochelle, New York

Founded in 1904

### DEGREES • BSN • MS

**Nursing Program Faculty** 15 (75% with doctorates).
**Baccalaureate Enrollment** 521 **Women** 90% **Men** 10% **Minority** 67% **International** 1% **Part-time** 50%
**Graduate Enrollment** 121 **Women** 90% **Men** 10% **Minority** 18% **International** 1% **Part-time** 100%
**Nursing Student Activities** Nursing Honor Society, Sigma Theta Tau, Student Nurses' Association, nursing club.
**Nursing Student Resources** Academic advising; academic or career counseling; assistance for students with disabilities; bookstore; campus computer network; career placement assistance; computer lab; computer-assisted instruction; e-mail services; housing assistance; interactive nursing skills videos; Internet; learning resource lab; library services; nursing audiovisuals; other; remedial services; resume preparation assistance; skills, simulation, or other laboratory; tutoring.
**Library Facilities** 220,000 volumes (8,700 in health, 8,700 in nursing); 1,450 periodical subscriptions (165 health-care related).

## BACCALAUREATE PROGRAMS

**Degree** BSN
**Available Programs** Accelerated Baccalaureate for Second Degree; Accelerated RN Baccalaureate; Baccalaureate for Second Degree; Generic Baccalaureate; RN Baccalaureate.
**Site Options** Bronx, NY.
**Study Options** Full-time and part-time.
**Program Entrance Requirements** Transcript of college record, CPR certification, written essay, health exam, health insurance, high school biology, high school chemistry, high school transcript, immunizations. Transfer students are accepted. *Application deadline:* 3/1 (fall), 10/1 (spring). *Application fee:* $35.
**Advanced Placement** Credit by examination available. Credit given for nursing courses completed elsewhere dependent upon specific evaluations.
**Contact** *Telephone:* 914-654-5803. *Fax:* 914-654-5994.

## GRADUATE PROGRAMS

**Contact** *Telephone:* 914-654-5803. *Fax:* 914-654-5994.

### MASTER'S DEGREE PROGRAM

**Degree** MS
**Available Programs** Master's; RN to Master's.
**Concentrations Available** Health-care administration; nursing administration; nursing education. *Nurse practitioner programs in:* family health.
**Site Options** New Rochelle, NY.
**Study Options** Full-time and part-time.
**Program Entrance Requirements** Clinical experience, minimum overall college GPA of 3.0, transcript of college record, written essay, immunizations, interview, 2 letters of recommendation, physical assessment course, professional liability insurance/malpractice insurance, resume, statistics course. *Application fee:* $35.
**Advanced Placement** Credit given for nursing courses completed elsewhere dependent upon specific evaluations.
**Degree Requirements** 40 total credit hours, thesis or project.

### POST-MASTER'S PROGRAM

**Areas of Study** Health-care administration; nursing administration; nursing education. *Clinical nurse specialist programs in:* palliative care. *Nurse practitioner programs in:* family health.

# College of Staten Island of the City University of New York

## Department of Nursing
## Staten Island, New York

***http://www.csi.cuny.edu/nursing***
Founded in 1955

### DEGREES • BS • MS

**Nursing Program Faculty** 61 (23% with doctorates).
**Baccalaureate Enrollment** 182 **Women** 87% **Men** 13% **Minority** 40% **Part-time** 74%
**Graduate Enrollment** 52 **Women** 99% **Men** 1% **Minority** 43% **International** 7% **Part-time** 93%
**Nursing Student Activities** Nursing Honor Society, Sigma Theta Tau.
**Nursing Student Resources** Academic advising; academic or career counseling; assistance for students with disabilities; bookstore; campus computer network; career placement assistance; computer lab; computer-assisted instruction; daycare for children of students; e-mail services; externships; Internet; learning resource lab; library services; nursing audiovisuals; remedial services; resume preparation assistance; skills, simulation, or other laboratory; tutoring.
**Library Facilities** 3,700 volumes in health, 1,500 volumes in nursing; 58,025 periodical subscriptions (4,900 health-care related).

## BACCALAUREATE PROGRAMS

**Degree** BS
**Available Programs** RN Baccalaureate.
**Site Options** Brooklyn, NY.
**Study Options** Full-time and part-time.
**Program Entrance Requirements** Minimum overall college GPA of 2.5, transcript of college record, CPR certification, health exam, health insurance, high school transcript, immunizations, minimum GPA in nursing prerequisites, professional liability insurance/malpractice insurance, prerequisite course work, RN licensure. Transfer students are accepted. *Application fee:* $65.
**Advanced Placement** Credit given for nursing courses completed elsewhere dependent upon specific evaluations.
**Contact** *Telephone:* 718-982-3810. *Fax:* 718-982-3813.

## GRADUATE PROGRAMS

**Contact** *Telephone:* 718-982-3845. *Fax:* 718-982-3813.

### MASTER'S DEGREE PROGRAM

**Degree** MS
**Available Programs** Master's.
**Concentrations Available** *Clinical nurse specialist programs in:* adult health, gerontology. *Nurse practitioner programs in:* adult health, gerontology.
**Site Options** Brooklyn, NY.
**Study Options** Full-time and part-time.
**Program Entrance Requirements** Clinical experience, minimum overall college GPA of 3.0, transcript of college record, written essay, immunizations, interview, 2 letters of recommendation, nursing research

course, physical assessment course, professional liability insurance/malpractice insurance, prerequisite course work, statistics course. *Application deadline:* Applications may be processed on a rolling basis for some programs. *Application fee:* $65.
**Advanced Placement** Credit given for nursing courses completed elsewhere dependent upon specific evaluations.
**Degree Requirements** 48 total credit hours, thesis or project.

### POST-MASTER'S PROGRAM
**Areas of Study** *Nurse practitioner programs in:* adult health, gerontology.

# Columbia University
## School of Nursing
## New York, New York

*http://www.nursing.columbia.edu/*
Founded in 1754
**DEGREES • BS • MS • MSN/MBA • MSN/MPH • PHD**
**Nursing Program Faculty** 77 (92% with doctorates).
**Baccalaureate Enrollment** 171 **Women** 90% **Men** 10% **Minority** 28% **International** 1%
**Graduate Enrollment** 401 **Women** 92% **Men** 8% **Minority** 33% **International** 2% **Part-time** 62%
**Nursing Student Activities** Sigma Theta Tau, Student Nurses' Association, nursing club.
**Nursing Student Resources** Academic advising; academic or career counseling; assistance for students with disabilities; bookstore; campus computer network; computer lab; computer-assisted instruction; daycare for children of students; e-mail services; employment services for current students; housing assistance; interactive nursing skills videos; Internet; learning resource lab; library services; resume preparation assistance; skills, simulation, or other laboratory.
**Library Facilities** 9.5 million volumes (469,000 in health, 8,220 in nursing); 117,264 periodical subscriptions.

### BACCALAUREATE PROGRAMS
**Degree** BS
**Available Programs** Accelerated Baccalaureate; Accelerated Baccalaureate for Second Degree; Accelerated RN Baccalaureate; Baccalaureate for Second Degree.
**Study Options** Full-time.
**Program Entrance Requirements** Transcript of college record, written essay, 3 letters of recommendation, prerequisite course work. *Application deadline:* 11/15 (summer). *Application fee:* $65.
**Advanced Placement** Credit by examination available. Credit given for nursing courses completed elsewhere dependent upon specific evaluations.
**Expenses (2013–14)** *Tuition:* full-time $75,480. *International tuition:* $75,480 full-time. *Room and board:* room only: $8000 per academic year. *Required fees:* full-time $1300.
**Financial Aid** 90% of baccalaureate students in nursing programs received some form of financial aid in 2012–13. *Gift aid (need-based):* Federal Pell, FSEOG, state, private, college/university gift aid from institutional funds. *Loans:* Perkins, alternative loans. *Work-study:* Federal Work-Study, part-time campus jobs. *Financial aid application deadline:* 3/1.
**Contact** Office of Admissions, School of Nursing, Columbia University, 617 West 168th Street, Suite 134, New York, NY 10032. *Telephone:* 212-305-5756. *Fax:* 212-305-3680. *E-mail:* nursing@columbia.edu.

### GRADUATE PROGRAMS
**Expenses (2013–14)** *Tuition:* part-time $1325 per credit hour. *Room and board:* room only: $8000 per academic year.
**Financial Aid** 98% of graduate students in nursing programs received some form of financial aid in 2012–13. Research assistantships, teaching assistantships, Federal Work-Study, institutionally sponsored loans, and scholarships available. Aid available to part-time students. *Financial aid application deadline:* 2/1.
**Contact** Office of Admissions, School of Nursing, Columbia University, 630 West 168th Street, Box 6, New York, NY 10032. *Telephone:* 212-305-5756. *Fax:* 212-305-3680. *E-mail:* nursing@columbia.edu.

### MASTER'S DEGREE PROGRAM
**Degrees** MS; MSN/MBA; MSN/MPH
**Available Programs** Accelerated Master's for Non-Nursing College Graduates; Accelerated Master's for Nurses with Non-Nursing Degrees; Master's; Master's for Non-Nursing College Graduates; Master's for Nurses with Non-Nursing Degrees.
**Concentrations Available** Nurse anesthesia; nurse-midwifery. *Nurse practitioner programs in:* acute care, adult health, family health, pediatric, psychiatric/mental health.
**Study Options** Full-time and part-time.
**Program Entrance Requirements** Clinical experience, minimum overall college GPA of 3.0, transcript of college record, written essay, interview, 3 letters of recommendation, physical assessment course, prerequisite course work, resume, statistics course, GRE General Test. *Application deadline:* 4/15 (fall), 1/15 (summer). *Application fee:* $65.
**Advanced Placement** Credit by examination available. Credit given for nursing courses completed elsewhere dependent upon specific evaluations.
**Degree Requirements** 45 total credit hours, thesis or project, comprehensive exam.

### POST-MASTER'S PROGRAM
**Areas of Study** Nurse anesthesia. *Nurse practitioner programs in:* acute care, adult health, family health, pediatric, psychiatric/mental health.

### DOCTORAL DEGREE PROGRAM
**Degree** PhD
**Available Programs** Doctorate; Doctorate for Nurses with Non-Nursing Degrees; Post-Baccalaureate Doctorate.
**Areas of Study** Addiction/substance abuse, advanced practice nursing, clinical practice, clinical research, community health, family health, health policy, health promotion/disease prevention, information systems, maternity-newborn, nursing education, nursing policy, nursing research, nursing science, urban health,women's health.
**Program Entrance Requirements** Minimum overall college GPA of 3.0, interview by faculty committee, interview, 3 letters of recommendation, statistics course, vita, writing sample, GRE General Test. *Application deadline:* 1/2 (fall). *Application fee:* $75.
**Degree Requirements** 60 total credit hours, dissertation, written exam.

### POSTDOCTORAL PROGRAM
**Areas of Study** Nursing informatics, nursing research.
**Postdoctoral Program Contact** Office of Scholarship and Research, School of Nursing, Columbia University, 630 West 168th Street, Box 6, New York, NY 10032. *Telephone:* 212-305-5495. *E-mail:* sonosr@columbia.edu.

### CONTINUING EDUCATION PROGRAM
**Contact** William Enlow, Director, School of Nursing, Columbia University, 630 West 168th Street, Box 6, New York, NY 10032. *Telephone:* 212-305-1175. *E-mail:* wme2001@columbia.edu.

# Concordia College–New York
## Nursing Program
## Bronxville, New York

*http://www.concordia-ny.edu/*
Founded in 1881
**DEGREE • BS**
**Nursing Program Faculty** 6 (50% with doctorates).
**Baccalaureate Enrollment** 40 **Women** 80% **Men** 20% **Minority** 48% **International** 2%
**Nursing Student Activities** Student Nurses' Association.
**Nursing Student Resources** Academic advising; academic or career counseling; assistance for students with disabilities; bookstore; campus computer network; career placement assistance; computer lab; computer-assisted instruction; e-mail services; housing assistance; interactive nursing skills videos; Internet; learning resource lab; library services; nursing audiovisuals; resume preparation assistance; skills, simulation, or other laboratory; tutoring.
**Library Facilities** 71,500 volumes; 467 periodical subscriptions.

### BACCALAUREATE PROGRAMS
**Degree** BS
**Available Programs** Accelerated Baccalaureate for Second Degree; Generic Baccalaureate.
**Study Options** Full-time.

**Program Entrance Requirements** Minimum overall college GPA of 3.2, transcript of college record, written essay, health exam, health insurance, high school biology, high school chemistry, 3 years high school science, high school transcript, immunizations, interview, 2 letters of recommendation, minimum high school GPA, minimum GPA in nursing prerequisites of 3.0, professional liability insurance/malpractice insurance, prerequisite course work. Transfer students are accepted. *Application deadline:* 4/1 (winter). *Application fee:* $50.
**Advanced Placement** Credit given for nursing courses completed elsewhere dependent upon specific evaluations.
**Contact** *Telephone:* 914-337-9300.

# Daemen College
## Department of Nursing
## Amherst, New York

*http://www.daemen.edu/*
Founded in 1947

**DEGREES • BS • DNP • MS**
**Nursing Program Faculty** 34 (53% with doctorates).
**Baccalaureate Enrollment** 351 **Women** 96% **Men** 4% **Minority** 3% **International** 2% **Part-time** 60%
**Graduate Enrollment** 175 **Women** 96% **Men** 4% **Minority** 8% **International** 6% **Part-time** 79%
**Distance Learning Courses** Available.
**Nursing Student Activities** Sigma Theta Tau, nursing club.
**Nursing Student Resources** Academic advising; academic or career counseling; assistance for students with disabilities; bookstore; campus computer network; career placement assistance; computer lab; computer-assisted instruction; e-mail services; Internet; learning resource lab; library services; nursing audiovisuals; placement services for program completers; remedial services; resume preparation assistance; skills, simulation, or other laboratory; tutoring.
**Library Facilities** 181,410 volumes (10,000 in health, 4,000 in nursing); 53,175 periodical subscriptions (250 health-care related).

### BACCALAUREATE PROGRAMS

**Degree** BS
**Available Programs** ADN to Baccalaureate; Accelerated RN Baccalaureate; International Nurse to Baccalaureate; RN Baccalaureate.
**Site Options** Jamestown, NY; Olean, NY.
**Study Options** Full-time.
**Program Entrance Requirements** Minimum overall college GPA of 2.0, transcript of college record, 2 years high school math, 2 years high school science, high school transcript, immunizations, minimum high school GPA of 3.0. Transfer students are accepted. *Application deadline:* Applications may be processed on a rolling basis for some programs. *Application fee:* $25.
**Advanced Placement** Credit given for nursing courses completed elsewhere dependent upon specific evaluations.
**Expenses (2013–14)** *Tuition:* full-time $11,790; part-time $392 per credit hour. *Room and board:* $11,300 per academic year. *Required fees:* full-time $340; part-time $16 per credit.
**Financial Aid** 100% of baccalaureate students in nursing programs received some form of financial aid in 2012–13.
**Contact** Dr. Mary Lou Rusin, Professor and Chair, Department of Nursing, Daemen College, 4380 Main Street, Amherst, NY 14226. *Telephone:* 716-839-8387. *Fax:* 716-839-8403. *E-mail:* mrusin@daemen.edu.

### GRADUATE PROGRAMS

**Expenses (2013–14)** *Tuition:* part-time $895 per credit hour. *International tuition:* $895 full-time.
**Financial Aid** 75% of graduate students in nursing programs received some form of financial aid in 2012–13. Institutionally sponsored loans and scholarships available. *Financial aid application deadline:* 2/15.
**Contact** Dr. Mary Lou Rusin, Professor and Chair, Department of Nursing, Daemen College, 4380 Main Street, Amherst, NY 14226. *Telephone:* 716-839-8387. *Fax:* 716-839-8403. *E-mail:* mrusin@daemen.edu.

#### MASTER'S DEGREE PROGRAM

**Degree** MS
**Available Programs** Accelerated AD/RN to Master's; Accelerated RN to Master's; Master's; RN to Master's.
**Concentrations Available** Health-care administration; nursing education. *Nurse practitioner programs in:* adult health, gerontology.
**Study Options** Full-time and part-time.
**Program Entrance Requirements** Clinical experience, minimum overall college GPA of 3.25, transcript of college record, written essay, immunizations, interview, 3 letters of recommendation, statistics course. *Application deadline:* Applications may be processed on a rolling basis for some programs. *Application fee:* $25.
**Advanced Placement** Credit given for nursing courses completed elsewhere dependent upon specific evaluations.
**Degree Requirements** 30 total credit hours, thesis or project.

#### POST-MASTER'S PROGRAM

**Areas of Study** Health-care administration; nursing education. *Nurse practitioner programs in:* adult health, gerontology.

#### DOCTORAL DEGREE PROGRAM

**Degree** DNP
**Available Programs** Doctorate.
**Areas of Study** Advanced practice nursing.
**Program Entrance Requirements** Minimum overall college GPA of 3.25, interview, 3 letters of recommendation, statistics course, vita, writing sample. *Application deadline:* Applications may be processed on a rolling basis for some programs. *Application fee:* $25.
**Degree Requirements** 36 total credit hours, dissertation.

# Dominican College
## Department of Nursing
## Orangeburg, New York

Founded in 1952

**DEGREES • BSN • M SC N**
**Nursing Program Faculty** 14 (21% with doctorates).
**Baccalaureate Enrollment** 182 **Women** 87% **Men** 13% **Minority** 44% **International** 40% **Part-time** 43%
**Graduate Enrollment** 37 **Women** 100% **Minority** 66% **International** 60% **Part-time** 100%
**Nursing Student Activities** Nursing Honor Society, Sigma Theta Tau, Student Nurses' Association.
**Nursing Student Resources** Academic advising; academic or career counseling; assistance for students with disabilities; bookstore; campus computer network; career placement assistance; computer lab; computer-assisted instruction; e-mail services; externships; Internet; learning resource lab; library services; nursing audiovisuals; paid internships; remedial services; resume preparation assistance; skills, simulation, or other laboratory; tutoring.
**Library Facilities** 120,000 volumes (5,650 in health); 450 periodical subscriptions (235 health-care related).

### BACCALAUREATE PROGRAMS

**Degree** BSN
**Available Programs** Accelerated Baccalaureate for Second Degree; Accelerated LPN to Baccalaureate; Accelerated RN Baccalaureate; Generic Baccalaureate; LPN to Baccalaureate; RN Baccalaureate.
**Study Options** Full-time and part-time.
**Program Entrance Requirements** Minimum overall college GPA of 2.7, transcript of college record, CPR certification, health exam, health insurance, high school transcript, immunizations, minimum GPA in nursing prerequisites of 2.0, professional liability insurance/malpractice insurance, prerequisite course work. Transfer students are accepted.
**Advanced Placement** Credit by examination available. Credit given for nursing courses completed elsewhere dependent upon specific evaluations.
**Contact** *Telephone:* 845-848-6051. *Fax:* 845-398-4891.

### GRADUATE PROGRAMS

**Contact** *Telephone:* 845-848-6026. *Fax:* 845-398-4891.

#### MASTER'S DEGREE PROGRAM

**Degree** M Sc N
**Available Programs** Master's.
**Concentrations Available** *Nurse practitioner programs in:* family health.
**Study Options** Full-time and part-time.
**Program Entrance Requirements** Clinical experience, minimum overall college GPA of 3.0, transcript of college record, written essay,

immunizations, 3 letters of recommendation, nursing research course, physical assessment course, professional liability insurance/malpractice insurance, prerequisite course work, statistics course.
**Degree Requirements** 42 total credit hours, thesis or project.

# D'Youville College

## School of Nursing
## Buffalo, New York

*http://www.dyc.edu/academics/nursing/*
Founded in 1908

**DEGREES • BSN • MS**
**Nursing Program Faculty** 41 (20% with doctorates).
**Baccalaureate Enrollment** 492 **Women** 90% **Men** 10% **Minority** 20% **International** 10% **Part-time** 30%
**Graduate Enrollment** 115 **Women** 96% **Men** 4% **Minority** 10% **International** 35% **Part-time** 40%
**Distance Learning Courses** Available.
**Nursing Student Activities** Sigma Theta Tau, Student Nurses' Association.
**Nursing Student Resources** Academic advising; academic or career counseling; assistance for students with disabilities; bookstore; campus computer network; career placement assistance; computer lab; computer-assisted instruction; e-mail services; externships; interactive nursing skills videos; Internet; learning resource lab; library services; nursing audiovisuals; paid internships; placement services for program completers; remedial services; resume preparation assistance; skills, simulation, or other laboratory; tutoring.
**Library Facilities** 116,237 volumes (100,000 in health, 17,000 in nursing); 725 periodical subscriptions (171 health-care related).

### BACCALAUREATE PROGRAMS

**Degree** BSN
**Available Programs** Generic Baccalaureate; RN Baccalaureate.
**Site Options** Buffalo, NY.
**Study Options** Full-time and part-time.
**Program Entrance Requirements** Minimum overall college GPA of 2.5, transcript of college record, health exam, health insurance, high school biology, high school chemistry, 1 year of high school math, 1 year of high school science, high school transcript, immunizations, minimum high school GPA of 2.0, minimum high school rank 50%, minimum GPA in nursing prerequisites of 2.0, professional liability insurance/malpractice insurance, prerequisite course work. Transfer students are accepted.
**Advanced Placement** Credit given for nursing courses completed elsewhere dependent upon specific evaluations.
**Contact** *Telephone:* 716-881-7600. *Fax:* 716-515-0679.

### GRADUATE PROGRAMS

**Contact** *Telephone:* 716-881-7744. *Fax:* 716-515-0679.

#### MASTER'S DEGREE PROGRAM

**Degree** MS
**Available Programs** Master's; RN to Master's.
**Concentrations Available** Nursing education. *Clinical nurse specialist programs in:* community health, palliative care. *Nurse practitioner programs in:* family health.
**Study Options** Full-time and part-time.
**Program Entrance Requirements** Clinical experience, computer literacy, minimum overall college GPA of 3.0, transcript of college record, CPR certification, written essay, immunizations, interview, 2 letters of recommendation, nursing research course, physical assessment course, professional liability insurance/malpractice insurance, prerequisite course work, resume, statistics course.
**Advanced Placement** Credit given for nursing courses completed elsewhere dependent upon specific evaluations.
**Degree Requirements** 41 total credit hours, thesis or project.

#### POST-MASTER'S PROGRAM

**Areas of Study** *Nurse practitioner programs in:* family health.

***See display below and full description on page 472.***

# Elmira College
## Program in Nursing Education
## Elmira, New York

***http://www.elmira.edu/***
Founded in 1855

**DEGREE • BS**
**Nursing Program Faculty** 22 (1% with doctorates).
**Baccalaureate Enrollment** 240 **Women** 90% **Men** 10% **Minority** 5% **International** 3% **Part-time** 20%
**Nursing Student Activities** Sigma Theta Tau, Student Nurses' Association, nursing club.
**Nursing Student Resources** Academic advising; academic or career counseling; assistance for students with disabilities; bookstore; campus computer network; career placement assistance; computer lab; computer-assisted instruction; e-mail services; housing assistance; interactive nursing skills videos; Internet; learning resource lab; library services; nursing audiovisuals; placement services for program completers; resume preparation assistance; skills, simulation, or other laboratory; tutoring; unpaid internships.
**Library Facilities** 203,343 volumes (7,461 in health, 5,200 in nursing); 337 periodical subscriptions (72 health-care related).

### BACCALAUREATE PROGRAMS
**Degree** BS
**Available Programs** ADN to Baccalaureate; Generic Baccalaureate; RN Baccalaureate.
**Study Options** Full-time and part-time.
**Program Entrance Requirements** Minimum overall college GPA of 2.0, transcript of college record, CPR certification, written essay, health exam, health insurance, high school biology, high school chemistry, 3 years high school math, 3 years high school science, high school transcript, immunizations, 2 letters of recommendation, minimum high school GPA of 2.5. Transfer students are accepted. *Application deadline:* Applications may be processed on a rolling basis for some programs. *Application fee:* $100.
**Advanced Placement** Credit by examination available. Credit given for nursing courses completed elsewhere dependent upon specific evaluations.
**Expenses (2013–14)** *Tuition:* full-time $36,600; part-time $325 per contact hour. *International tuition:* $36,600 full-time. *Room and board:* room only: $6300 per academic year. *Required fees:* full-time $500.
**Financial Aid** 83% of baccalaureate students in nursing programs received some form of financial aid in 2012–13. *Gift aid (need-based):* Federal Pell, FSEOG, state, private, college/university gift aid from institutional funds. *Loans:* Federal Direct (Subsidized and Unsubsidized Stafford PLUS), Perkins, college/university. *Work-study:* Federal Work-Study, part-time campus jobs. *Financial aid application deadline (priority):* 2/1.
**Contact** Mrs. Julianna Baumann, Dean, Program in Nursing Education, Elmira College, One Park Place, Elmira, NY 14901. *Telephone:* 607-735-1724. *Fax:* 607-735-1718. *E-mail:* admissions@elmira.edu.

### CONTINUING EDUCATION PROGRAM
**Contact** Dr. Kathleen J. Lucke, Dean of Health Sciences and Professor of Nurse Education, Program in Nursing Education, Elmira College, One Park Place, Elmira, NY 14901. *Telephone:* 607-735-1890. *Fax:* 607-735-1159. *E-mail:* klucke@elmira.edu.

# Excelsior College
## School of Nursing
## Albany, New York

Founded in 1970

**DEGREES • BS • MS**
**Distance Learning Courses** Available.
**Nursing Student Activities** Sigma Theta Tau.
**Nursing Student Resources** Academic advising; academic or career counseling; assistance for students with disabilities; bookstore; computer-assisted instruction; e-mail services; Internet; learning resource lab; library services; nursing audiovisuals; other; resume preparation assistance; skills, simulation, or other laboratory; tutoring.

### BACCALAUREATE PROGRAMS
**Degree** BS
**Available Programs** RN Baccalaureate.
**Study Options** Part-time.
**Program Entrance Requirements** Transcript of college record, high school transcript, RN licensure. Transfer students are accepted. *Application deadline:* Applications may be processed on a rolling basis for some programs.
**Advanced Placement** Credit by examination available. Credit given for nursing courses completed elsewhere dependent upon specific evaluations.
**Contact** *Telephone:* 518-464-8500. *Fax:* 518-464-8777.

### GRADUATE PROGRAMS
**Contact** *Telephone:* 518-464-8500. *Fax:* 518-464-8777.

**MASTER'S DEGREE PROGRAM**
**Degree** MS
**Available Programs** Master's; RN to Master's.
**Concentrations Available** Nursing administration; nursing education; nursing informatics.
**Study Options** Full-time and part-time.
**Online Degree Options** Yes (online only).
**Program Entrance Requirements** Computer literacy, minimum overall college GPA of 3, transcript of college record, written essay, resume. *Application deadline:* Applications may be processed on a rolling basis for some programs.
**Advanced Placement** Credit given for nursing courses completed elsewhere dependent upon specific evaluations.
**Degree Requirements** 39 total credit hours, thesis or project.

**POST-MASTER'S PROGRAM**
**Areas of Study** Nursing education.

# Farmingdale State College
## Nursing Department
## Farmingdale, New York

***http://www.farmingdale.edu***
Founded in 1912

**DEGREE • BS**
**Library Facilities** 180,000 volumes; 706 periodical subscriptions.

### BACCALAUREATE PROGRAMS
**Degree** BS
**Available Programs** Generic Baccalaureate; RN Baccalaureate.
**Contact** *Telephone:* 631-420-2229. *Fax:* 631-420-2269.

# Hartwick College
## Department of Nursing
## Oneonta, New York

***http://www.hartwick.edu/***
Founded in 1797

**DEGREE • BS**
**Nursing Program Faculty** 11 (18% with doctorates).
**Baccalaureate Enrollment** 145 **Women** 93% **Men** 7% **Minority** 9% **International** 1% **Part-time** 12%
**Nursing Student Activities** Sigma Theta Tau, Student Nurses' Association.
**Nursing Student Resources** Academic advising; academic or career counseling; assistance for students with disabilities; bookstore; campus computer network; career placement assistance; computer lab; computer-assisted instruction; e-mail services; employment services for current students; externships; housing assistance; interactive nursing skills videos; Internet; learning resource lab; library services; nursing audiovisuals; placement services for program completers; remedial services; resume preparation assistance; skills, simulation, or other laboratory; tutoring; unpaid internships.
**Library Facilities** 300,832 volumes (5,697 in health, 1,199 in nursing); 13,122 periodical subscriptions (30 health-care related).

## BACCALAUREATE PROGRAMS

**Degree** BS
**Available Programs** Accelerated Baccalaureate; Accelerated Baccalaureate for Second Degree; Generic Baccalaureate; RN Baccalaureate.
**Site Options** Cooperstown, NY; Albany, NY.
**Study Options** Full-time and part-time.
**Program Entrance Requirements** Minimum overall college GPA of 2.5, transcript of college record, CPR certification, written essay, health exam, high school biology, high school chemistry, high school foreign language, 3 years high school math, 2 years high school science, high school transcript, immunizations, 2 letters of recommendation, minimum GPA in nursing prerequisites of 2.5, professional liability insurance/malpractice insurance. Transfer students are accepted. *Application deadline:* Applications may be processed on a rolling basis for some programs. *Application fee:* $35.
**Advanced Placement** Credit given for nursing courses completed elsewhere dependent upon specific evaluations.
**Contact** *Telephone:* 607-431-4780. *Fax:* 607-431-4850.

# Hunter College of the City University of New York

### Hunter-Bellevue School of Nursing
### New York, New York

***http://www.hunter.cuny.edu/schoolhp/nursing***
Founded in 1870

**DEGREES • BSN • DNP • MS • MSN/MPA • MSN/MPH**
**Nursing Program Faculty** 124 (31% with doctorates).
**Baccalaureate Enrollment** 418 **Women** 84% **Men** 16% **Minority** 65% **International** 8% **Part-time** 29%
**Graduate Enrollment** 557 **Women** 85% **Men** 15% **Minority** 52% **International** 4% **Part-time** 91%
**Nursing Student Activities** Sigma Theta Tau, Student Nurses' Association.
**Nursing Student Resources** Academic advising; academic or career counseling; assistance for students with disabilities; bookstore; campus computer network; computer lab; computer-assisted instruction; e-mail services; interactive nursing skills videos; Internet; learning resource lab; library services; nursing audiovisuals; skills, simulation, or other laboratory.
**Library Facilities** 865,240 volumes (39,245 in health, 4,295 in nursing); 95,000 periodical subscriptions (375 health-care related).

## BACCALAUREATE PROGRAMS

**Degree** BSN
**Available Programs** Accelerated Baccalaureate; Generic Baccalaureate; RN Baccalaureate.
**Study Options** Full-time.
**Program Entrance Requirements** Minimum overall college GPA of 3.25, transcript of college record, CPR certification, health exam, immunizations, minimum GPA in nursing prerequisites of 3.0, professional liability insurance/malpractice insurance, prerequisite course work. Transfer students are accepted. *Application deadline:* 2/1 (fall). *Application fee:* $75.
**Advanced Placement** Credit given for nursing courses completed elsewhere dependent upon specific evaluations.
**Expenses (2013–14)** *Tuition, state resident:* full-time $2685; part-time $360 per credit. *Tuition, nonresident:* full-time $9180; part-time $760 per credit. *International tuition:* $9180 full-time. *Required fees:* full-time $400; part-time $119 per term.
**Financial Aid** 70% of baccalaureate students in nursing programs received some form of financial aid in 2012–13.
**Contact** Ms. Maria Mendoza, Pre-Nursing Adviser, Hunter-Bellevue School of Nursing, Hunter College of the City University of New York, 425 East 25th Street, New York, NY 10010. *Telephone:* 212-481-4473. *Fax:* 212-481-8237. *E-mail:* prenursingadvising@hunter.cuny.edu.

## GRADUATE PROGRAMS

**Expenses (2013–14)** *Tuition, state resident:* full-time $4585; part-time $385 per credit. *Tuition, nonresident:* full-time $10,650; part-time $710 per credit. *International tuition:* $10,650 full-time. *Required fees:* full-time $356; part-time $78 per term.
**Financial Aid** 50% of graduate students in nursing programs received some form of financial aid in 2012–13. Federal Work-Study, scholarships, traineeships, and tuition waivers (partial) available. Aid available to part-time students. *Financial aid application deadline:* 5/1.
**Contact** Dr. David Keepnews, Director of Graduate Program, Hunter-Bellevue School of Nursing, Hunter College of the City University of New York, 425 East 25th Street, New York, NY 10010. *Telephone:* 212-481-4465. *Fax:* 212-481-4427. *E-mail:* knokes@hunter.cuny.edu.

### MASTER'S DEGREE PROGRAM

**Degrees** MS; MSN/MPA; MSN/MPH
**Available Programs** Master's.
**Concentrations Available** Clinical nurse leader; nursing administration. *Clinical nurse specialist programs in:* adult health, community health, public health. *Nurse practitioner programs in:* community health, family health, gerontology, psychiatric/mental health.
**Study Options** Full-time and part-time.
**Program Entrance Requirements** Clinical experience, minimum overall college GPA of 3.0, transcript of college record, written essay, immunizations, 2 letters of recommendation, resume, statistics course. *Application deadline:* 4/1 (fall), 11/1 (spring). Applications may be processed on a rolling basis for some programs. *Application fee:* $125.
**Advanced Placement** Credit given for nursing courses completed elsewhere dependent upon specific evaluations.
**Degree Requirements** 42 total credit hours, thesis or project.

### POST-MASTER'S PROGRAM

**Areas of Study** Nursing education. *Nurse practitioner programs in:* psychiatric/mental health.

### DOCTORAL DEGREE PROGRAM

**Degree** DNP
**Available Programs** Doctorate; Post-Baccalaureate Doctorate.
**Areas of Study** Community health, family health, gerontology, neurobehavior.
**Program Entrance Requirements** Clinical experience, minimum overall college GPA of 3.5, interview, 2 letters of recommendation, statistics course, vita. *Application deadline:* 4/1 (fall), 11/1 (spring). Applications may be processed on a rolling basis for some programs. *Application fee:* $125.
**Degree Requirements** 90 total credit hours.

## CONTINUING EDUCATION PROGRAM

**Contact** Continuing Education, Hunter-Bellevue School of Nursing, Hunter College of the City University of New York, 695 Park Avenue, East Building, 10th Floor, New York, NY 10021. *Telephone:* 212-650-3850. *Fax:* 212-772-3402. *E-mail:* ce@hunter.cuny.edu.

# Keuka College

### Division of Nursing
### Keuka Park, New York

***http://asap.keuka.edu/programs/bs-nursing/***
Founded in 1890

**DEGREE • BS**
**Nursing Program Faculty** 5 (20% with doctorates).
**Baccalaureate Enrollment** 238 **Women** 94% **Men** 6% **Minority** 4%
**Distance Learning Courses** Available.
**Nursing Student Activities** Sigma Theta Tau.
**Nursing Student Resources** Academic advising; academic or career counseling; assistance for students with disabilities; bookstore; campus computer network; computer lab; computer-assisted instruction; e-mail services; employment services for current students; interactive nursing skills videos; Internet; learning resource lab; library services; nursing audiovisuals; resume preparation assistance; tutoring.
**Library Facilities** 112,541 volumes (986 in health, 532 in nursing); 384 periodical subscriptions (48 health-care related).

## BACCALAUREATE PROGRAMS

**Degree** BS
**Available Programs** Accelerated RN Baccalaureate.
**Site Options** Geneva, NY; Rochester, NY; Canandaigua, NY.
**Study Options** Full-time and part-time.
**Program Entrance Requirements** Minimum overall college GPA of 2.5, transcript of college record, CPR certification, health exam, immunizations, minimum GPA in nursing prerequisites of 2.5, prerequisite course work, RN licensure. Transfer students are accepted.

**Advanced Placement** Credit by examination available. Credit given for nursing courses completed elsewhere dependent upon specific evaluations.
**Contact** *Telephone:* 315-279-5393. *Fax:* 315-279-5407.

# Lehman College of the City University of New York

## Department of Nursing
## Bronx, New York

***http://www.lehman.edu/academics/nursing/***
Founded in 1931

**DEGREES • BS • DNS • MS**
**Nursing Program Faculty** 43 (35% with doctorates).
**Baccalaureate Enrollment** 300 **Women** 80% **Men** 20% **Minority** 85% **International** 40% **Part-time** 50%
**Graduate Enrollment** 200 **Women** 90% **Men** 10% **Minority** 75% **International** 25% **Part-time** 75%
**Distance Learning Courses** Available.
**Nursing Student Activities** Nursing Honor Society, Sigma Theta Tau, Student Nurses' Association, nursing club.
**Nursing Student Resources** Academic advising; academic or career counseling; assistance for students with disabilities; bookstore; campus computer network; career placement assistance; computer lab; computer-assisted instruction; daycare for children of students; e-mail services; employment services for current students; externships; interactive nursing skills videos; Internet; learning resource lab; library services; nursing audiovisuals; paid internships; placement services for program completers; resume preparation assistance; skills, simulation, or other laboratory; tutoring; unpaid internships.
**Library Facilities** 660,616 volumes (1,000 in health, 500 in nursing); 9,370 periodical subscriptions (200 health-care related).

### BACCALAUREATE PROGRAMS

**Degree** BS
**Available Programs** ADN to Baccalaureate; Accelerated Baccalaureate for Second Degree; Accelerated RN Baccalaureate; Baccalaureate for Second Degree; Generic Baccalaureate; International Nurse to Baccalaureate; RN Baccalaureate.
**Site Options** New York, NY; Queens, NY.
**Study Options** Full-time.
**Online Degree Options** Yes.
**Program Entrance Requirements** Minimum overall college GPA of 2.0, transcript of college record, health exam, high school transcript, immunizations, minimum GPA in nursing prerequisites of 2.75, professional liability insurance/malpractice insurance, prerequisite course work. Transfer students are accepted. *Application deadline:* 3/15 (fall).
**Advanced Placement** Credit given for nursing courses completed elsewhere dependent upon specific evaluations.
**Contact** *Telephone:* 718-960-8214. *Fax:* 718-960-8488.

### GRADUATE PROGRAMS

**Contact** *Telephone:* 718-960-8213. *Fax:* 718-960-8488.

#### MASTER'S DEGREE PROGRAM

**Degree** MS
**Available Programs** Master's; Master's for Nurses with Non-Nursing Degrees.
**Concentrations Available** Nursing administration; nursing education. *Clinical nurse specialist programs in:* adult health, gerontology, parent-child. *Nurse practitioner programs in:* family health, pediatric.
**Site Options** New York, NY.
**Study Options** Full-time and part-time.
**Program Entrance Requirements** Clinical experience, minimum overall college GPA of 3.0, transcript of college record, written essay, immunizations, interview, 2 letters of recommendation, professional liability insurance/malpractice insurance, prerequisite course work. *Application deadline:* 4/1 (fall), 11/1 (spring). Applications may be processed on a rolling basis for some programs. *Application fee:* $125.
**Degree Requirements** 43 total credit hours.

#### POST-MASTER'S PROGRAM

**Areas of Study** *Nurse practitioner programs in:* family health, pediatric.

#### DOCTORAL DEGREE PROGRAM

**Degree** DNS
**Available Programs** Doctorate.
**Areas of Study** Urban health.
**Site Options** New York, NY.
**Program Entrance Requirements** Clinical experience, minimum overall college GPA of 3.5, interview by faculty committee, interview, letters of recommendation, MSN or equivalent, statistics course, vita, writing sample. *Application deadline:* 4/1 (fall).
**Degree Requirements** 51 total credit hours, dissertation, oral exam, written exam, residency.

### CONTINUING EDUCATION PROGRAM

**Contact** *Telephone:* 718-960-8799.

# Le Moyne College

## Nursing Programs
## Syracuse, New York

***http://www.lemoyne.edu/nursing***
Founded in 1946

**DEGREES • BS • MS**
**Nursing Program Faculty** 13 (46% with doctorates).
**Baccalaureate Enrollment** 224 **Women** 90% **Men** 10% **Minority** 5% **Part-time** 20%
**Graduate Enrollment** 24 **Women** 96% **Men** 4% **Minority** 12% **Part-time** 100%
**Distance Learning Courses** Available.
**Nursing Student Activities** Nursing Honor Society, Student Nurses' Association.
**Nursing Student Resources** Academic advising; academic or career counseling; assistance for students with disabilities; bookstore; campus computer network; career placement assistance; computer lab; computer-assisted instruction; e-mail services; employment services for current students; housing assistance; interactive nursing skills videos; Internet; learning resource lab; library services; nursing audiovisuals; placement services for program completers; remedial services; resume preparation assistance; skills, simulation, or other laboratory; tutoring.
**Library Facilities** 283,814 volumes (7,003 in health, 665 in nursing); 131,112 periodical subscriptions (6,508 health-care related).

### BACCALAUREATE PROGRAMS

**Degree** BS
**Available Programs** ADN to Baccalaureate; Accelerated Baccalaureate for Second Degree; RN Baccalaureate.
**Site Options** Syracuse, NY.
**Study Options** Full-time and part-time.
**Program Entrance Requirements** Minimum overall college GPA of 2.6, transcript of college record, CPR certification, written essay, health exam, health insurance, high school biology, high school chemistry, high school foreign language, 3 years high school math, 3 years high school science, high school transcript, immunizations, 2 letters of recommendation, minimum high school GPA of 3.0, minimum high school rank 85%, minimum GPA in nursing prerequisites of 2.5, RN licensure. Transfer students are accepted. *Application deadline:* 2/1 (fall), 8/1 (spring), 5/1 (summer). Applications may be processed on a rolling basis for some programs. *Application fee:* $35.
**Advanced Placement** Credit by examination available. Credit given for nursing courses completed elsewhere dependent upon specific evaluations.
**Expenses (2013–14)** *Tuition:* full-time $29,470; part-time $618 per credit hour. *Room and board:* $11,220; room only: $7430 per academic year. *Required fees:* full-time $350; part-time $75 per term.
**Financial Aid** 90% of baccalaureate students in nursing programs received some form of financial aid in 2012–13.
**Contact** Dr. Susan B. Bastable, Chair and Professor, Nursing Programs, Le Moyne College, 1419 Salt Springs Road, Syracuse, NY 13214. *Telephone:* 315-445-5436. *Fax:* 315-445-6024. *E-mail:* bastabsb@lemoyne.edu.

### GRADUATE PROGRAMS

**Expenses (2013–14)** *Tuition:* part-time $644 per credit hour. *Required fees:* part-time $75 per term.
**Financial Aid** 100% of graduate students in nursing programs received some form of financial aid in 2012–13.

**Contact** Mrs. Kristen P. Trapasso, Director of Graduate Admissions, Nursing Programs, Le Moyne College, 1419 Salt Springs Road, Syracuse, NY 13214. *Telephone:* 315-445-4265. *Fax:* 315-445-6027. *E-mail:* trapaskp@lemoyne.edu.

### MASTER'S DEGREE PROGRAM

**Degree** MS
**Available Programs** Master's; Master's for Nurses with Non-Nursing Degrees.
**Concentrations Available** Nursing administration; nursing education; nursing informatics. *Clinical nurse specialist programs in:* gerontology, palliative care.
**Study Options** Full-time and part-time.
**Program Entrance Requirements** Computer literacy, minimum overall college GPA of 3.0, transcript of college record, written essay, immunizations, interview, 2 letters of recommendation, nursing research course, physical assessment course, resume, statistics course. *Application deadline:* 8/1 (fall), 12/15 (spring), 5/1 (summer). Applications may be processed on a rolling basis for some programs. *Application fee:* $50.
**Advanced Placement** Credit given for nursing courses completed elsewhere dependent upon specific evaluations.
**Degree Requirements** 39 total credit hours, thesis or project.

### POST-MASTER'S PROGRAM

**Areas of Study** Nursing administration; nursing education; nursing informatics. *Clinical nurse specialist programs in:* gerontology, palliative care.

# Long Island University–LIU Brooklyn

## School of Nursing
## Brooklyn, New York

***http://www.liunet.edu/***
Founded in 1926

### DEGREES • BS • MS

**Nursing Program Faculty** 85 (30% with doctorates).
**Baccalaureate Enrollment** 868 **Women** 85% **Men** 15% **Minority** 85% **International** 2% **Part-time** 35%
**Graduate Enrollment** 240 **Women** 90% **Men** 10% **Minority** 85% **Part-time** 83%
**Distance Learning Courses** Available.
**Nursing Student Activities** Nursing Honor Society, Student Nurses' Association, nursing club.
**Nursing Student Resources** Academic advising; academic or career counseling; assistance for students with disabilities; bookstore; campus computer network; career placement assistance; computer lab; computer-assisted instruction; daycare for children of students; e-mail services; employment services for current students; externships; interactive nursing skills videos; Internet; learning resource lab; library services; nursing audiovisuals; paid internships; remedial services; resume preparation assistance; skills, simulation, or other laboratory; tutoring; unpaid internships.
**Library Facilities** 431,179 volumes; 129,613 periodical subscriptions.

### BACCALAUREATE PROGRAMS

**Degree** BS
**Available Programs** ADN to Baccalaureate; Accelerated Baccalaureate for Second Degree; Generic Baccalaureate.
**Site Options** Brooklyn, NY.
**Study Options** Full-time and part-time.
**Program Entrance Requirements** Minimum overall college GPA of 2.75, transcript of college record, CPR certification, health exam, health insurance, high school biology, high school chemistry, 2 years high school math, 2 years high school science, high school transcript, immunizations, interview, minimum high school GPA of 3.0, minimum GPA in nursing prerequisites of 2.75, professional liability insurance/malpractice insurance, prerequisite course work. Transfer students are accepted. *Application deadline:* Applications may be processed on a rolling basis for some programs. *Application fee:* $50.
**Advanced Placement** Credit given for nursing courses completed elsewhere dependent upon specific evaluations.
**Expenses (2013–14)** *Tuition:* full-time $33,000; part-time $974 per credit. *Room and board:* $6158; room only: $4008 per academic year. *Required fees:* full-time $33,000.
**Financial Aid** 96% of baccalaureate students in nursing programs received some form of financial aid in 2012–13. *Gift aid (need-based):* Federal Pell, FSEOG, state, private, college/university gift aid from institutional funds, Scholarships for Disadvantaged Students (Nursing and Pharmacy). *Loans:* Federal Direct (Subsidized and Unsubsidized Stafford PLUS), Perkins, alternative loans, Health Professions Student Loans (HPSL). *Work-study:* Federal Work-Study, part-time campus jobs. *Financial aid application deadline:* Continuous.
**Contact** Ms. Letitia Galdamez, Director of Advisement S.O.N. , School of Nursing, Long Island University–LIU Brooklyn, 1 University Plaza, Brooklyn, NY 11201. *Telephone:* 718-488-1059. *Fax:* 718-780-4019. *E-mail:* galdamez@liu.edu.

### GRADUATE PROGRAMS

**Financial Aid** 75% of graduate students in nursing programs received some form of financial aid in 2012–13. Scholarships and unspecified assistantships available. Aid available to part-time students.
**Contact** Dr. Amy Ma, Director, School of Nursing, Long Island University–LIU Brooklyn, 1 University Plaza, Brooklyn, NY 11201. *Telephone:* 718-488-1059. *Fax:* 718-780-4019. *E-mail:* amy.ma@liu.edu.

### MASTER'S DEGREE PROGRAM

**Degree** MS
**Available Programs** Master's; RN to Master's.
**Concentrations Available** Health-care administration; nursing administration; nursing education. *Nurse practitioner programs in:* adult health, family health.
**Site Options** Brooklyn, NY.
**Study Options** Full-time and part-time.
**Program Entrance Requirements** Clinical experience, computer literacy, minimum overall college GPA of 3.0, transcript of college record, CPR certification, immunizations, interview, 3 letters of recommendation, nursing research course, physical assessment course, professional liability insurance/malpractice insurance, prerequisite course work, resume, statistics course. *Application deadline:* Applications may be processed on a rolling basis for some programs. *Application fee:* $50.
**Advanced Placement** Credit given for nursing courses completed elsewhere dependent upon specific evaluations.
**Degree Requirements** 45 total credit hours.

### POST-MASTER'S PROGRAM

**Areas of Study** Nursing education. *Nurse practitioner programs in:* adult health, family health.

# Long Island University–LIU Post

## Department of Nursing
## Brookville, New York

***http://www.liu.edu/post/nursing***
Founded in 1954

### DEGREES • BS • MS

**Nursing Program Faculty** 13 (54% with doctorates).
**Baccalaureate Enrollment** 98 **Women** 94% **Men** 6% **Minority** 43% **Part-time** 100%
**Graduate Enrollment** 133 **Women** 94% **Men** 6% **Minority** 47% **Part-time** 100%
**Nursing Student Activities** Student Nurses' Association.
**Nursing Student Resources** Academic advising; academic or career counseling; assistance for students with disabilities; bookstore; campus computer network; career placement assistance; computer lab; computer-assisted instruction; e-mail services; employment services for current students; housing assistance; interactive nursing skills videos; Internet; learning resource lab; library services; nursing audiovisuals; placement services for program completers; remedial services; resume preparation assistance; skills, simulation, or other laboratory; tutoring.
**Library Facilities** 506,198 volumes (31,381 in health, 1,414 in nursing); 5,518 periodical subscriptions health-care related.

### BACCALAUREATE PROGRAMS

**Degree** BS
**Available Programs** RN Baccalaureate.
**Site Options** Manhasset, NY; Brentwood, NY.
**Study Options** Part-time.
**Program Entrance Requirements** Minimum overall college GPA of 3.0, transcript of college record, health exam, health insurance, immuni-

zations, minimum GPA in nursing prerequisites of 3.0, professional liability insurance/malpractice insurance, prerequisite course work, RN licensure. Transfer students are accepted. *Application deadline:* Applications may be processed on a rolling basis for some programs. *Application fee:* $50.
**Advanced Placement** Credit by examination available. Credit given for nursing courses completed elsewhere dependent upon specific evaluations.
**Expenses (2013–14)** *Tuition:* part-time $1010 per credit. *Room and board:* $12,534; room only: $7834 per academic year. *Required fees:* part-time $425 per term.
**Financial Aid** 15% of baccalaureate students in nursing programs received some form of financial aid in 2012–13. *Gift aid (need-based):* Federal Pell, FSEOG, state, private, college/university gift aid from institutional funds. *Loans:* Federal Direct (Subsidized and Unsubsidized Stafford PLUS), Perkins. *Work-study:* Federal Work-Study, part-time campus jobs. *Financial aid application deadline:* 3/15.
**Contact** Dr. Mary Infantino, Chairperson and Associate Professor, Department of Nursing, Long Island University–LIU Post, Life Science, Room 270, 720 Northern Boulevard, Brookville, NY 11548-1300. *Telephone:* 516-299-2320. *Fax:* 516-299-2352. *E-mail:* mary.infantino@liu.edu.

## GRADUATE PROGRAMS

**Expenses (2013–14)** *Tuition:* part-time $1110 per credit. *Room and board:* $12,534; room only: $7834 per academic year. *Required fees:* part-time $425 per term.
**Financial Aid** 80% of graduate students in nursing programs received some form of financial aid in 2012–13. Federal Work-Study and unspecified assistantships available. Aid available to part-time students. *Financial aid application deadline:* 5/15.
**Contact** Dr. Mary Infantino, Chairperson and Associate Professor, Department of Nursing, Long Island University–LIU Post, Life Science, Room 270, 720 Northern Boulevard, Brookville, NY 11548-1300. *Telephone:* 516-299-2320. *Fax:* 516-299-2352. *E-mail:* mary.infantino@liu.edu.

### MASTER'S DEGREE PROGRAM

**Degree** MS
**Available Programs** Master's.
**Concentrations Available** Nursing education. *Clinical nurse specialist programs in:* adult health. *Nurse practitioner programs in:* family health.
**Site Options** Manhasset, NY.
**Study Options** Part-time.
**Program Entrance Requirements** Clinical experience, computer literacy, minimum overall college GPA of 3.0, transcript of college record, written essay, immunizations, interview, 2 letters of recommendation, physical assessment course, professional liability insurance/malpractice insurance, prerequisite course work. *Application deadline:* Applications may be processed on a rolling basis for some programs. *Application fee:* $50.
**Advanced Placement** Credit given for nursing courses completed elsewhere dependent upon specific evaluations.
**Degree Requirements** 46 total credit hours, thesis or project.

### POST-MASTER'S PROGRAM

**Areas of Study** Nursing education. *Nurse practitioner programs in:* family health.

# Maria College

### RN Baccalaureate Completion Program
### Albany, New York

Founded in 1958

**DEGREE • BSN**

**Library Facilities** 59,245 volumes; 160 periodical subscriptions.

## BACCALAUREATE PROGRAMS

**Degree** BSN
**Available Programs** RN Baccalaureate.
**Contact** Linda Millenbach, Chairperson, RN Baccalaureate Completion Program, Maria College, 700 New Scotland Avenue, Albany, NY 12208. *Telephone:* 518-438-3111 Ext. 2548. *E-mail:* lmillenbach@mariacollege.edu.

# Medgar Evers College of the City University of New York

### Department of Nursing
### Brooklyn, New York

*http://www.mec.cuny.edu/*
Founded in 1969

**DEGREE • BSN**

**Nursing Program Faculty** 7 (85% with doctorates).
**Baccalaureate Enrollment** 60 **Women** 98% **Men** 2% **Minority** 99% **Part-time** 90%
**Nursing Student Activities** Student Nurses' Association, nursing club.
**Nursing Student Resources** Academic advising; academic or career counseling; assistance for students with disabilities; bookstore; campus computer network; computer lab; computer-assisted instruction; daycare for children of students; e-mail services; interactive nursing skills videos; Internet; learning resource lab; library services; nursing audiovisuals; remedial services; resume preparation assistance; skills, simulation, or other laboratory; tutoring; unpaid internships.
**Library Facilities** 120,000 volumes; 24,410 periodical subscriptions.

## BACCALAUREATE PROGRAMS

**Degree** BSN
**Available Programs** ADN to Baccalaureate; Accelerated RN Baccalaureate.
**Study Options** Full-time and part-time.
**Program Entrance Requirements** Minimum overall college GPA of 2.5, transcript of college record, CPR certification, health exam, health insurance, immunizations, professional liability insurance/malpractice insurance, prerequisite course work, RN licensure. Transfer students are accepted.
**Advanced Placement** Credit given for nursing courses completed elsewhere dependent upon specific evaluations.
**Contact** *Telephone:* 718-270-6230. *Fax:* 718-270-6235.

# Mercy College

### Programs in Nursing
### Dobbs Ferry, New York

Founded in 1951

**DEGREES • BS • MS**

**Nursing Program Faculty** 5 (2% with doctorates).
**Baccalaureate Enrollment** 333 **Women** 96% **Men** 4% **Minority** 75% **International** 1% **Part-time** 88%
**Graduate Enrollment** 100 **Women** 99% **Men** 1% **Minority** 50% **International** 10% **Part-time** 75%
**Distance Learning Courses** Available.
**Nursing Student Activities** Sigma Theta Tau, Student Nurses' Association.
**Nursing Student Resources** Academic advising; academic or career counseling; assistance for students with disabilities; bookstore; campus computer network; career placement assistance; computer lab; computer-assisted instruction; e-mail services; employment services for current students; Internet; learning resource lab; library services; nursing audiovisuals; remedial services; resume preparation assistance; skills, simulation, or other laboratory; tutoring.
**Library Facilities** 249,571 volumes (10,000 in health, 550 in nursing); 736 periodical subscriptions (180 health-care related).

## BACCALAUREATE PROGRAMS

**Degree** BS
**Available Programs** Accelerated RN Baccalaureate; RN Baccalaureate.
**Site Options** Dobbs Ferry, NY.
**Study Options** Full-time and part-time.
**Online Degree Options** Yes.
**Program Entrance Requirements** Minimum overall college GPA, transcript of college record, written essay, immunizations, interview, minimum GPA in nursing prerequisites, prerequisite course work, RN licensure. Transfer students are accepted. *Application deadline:* Applications may be processed on a rolling basis for some programs.
**Advanced Placement** Credit given for nursing courses completed elsewhere dependent upon specific evaluations.
**Contact** *Telephone:* 914-674-7865. *Fax:* 914-674-7623.

## GRADUATE PROGRAMS

**Contact** *Telephone:* 914-674-7867. *Fax:* 914-674-7623.

### MASTER'S DEGREE PROGRAM

**Degree** MS
**Available Programs** Accelerated Master's for Non-Nursing College Graduates; Accelerated Master's for Nurses with Non-Nursing Degrees; Accelerated RN to Master's; Master's; Master's for Non-Nursing College Graduates; Master's for Nurses with Non-Nursing Degrees.
**Concentrations Available** Health-care administration; nursing administration; nursing education.
**Site Options** Dobbs Ferry, NY.
**Study Options** Full-time and part-time.
**Online Degree Options** Yes.
**Program Entrance Requirements** Clinical experience, minimum overall college GPA of 3.0, transcript of college record, written essay, immunizations, interview, 2 letters of recommendation, professional liability insurance/malpractice insurance, resume. *Application deadline:* Applications may be processed on a rolling basis for some programs.
**Advanced Placement** Credit given for nursing courses completed elsewhere dependent upon specific evaluations.
**Degree Requirements** 36 total credit hours, thesis or project.

### POST-MASTER'S PROGRAM

**Areas of Study** Nursing administration; nursing education.

# Molloy College

## Division of Nursing
## Rockville Centre, New York

***http://www.molloy.edu***
Founded in 1955

**DEGREES • BS • MS • MS/MBA • PHD**
**Nursing Program Faculty** 213 (20% with doctorates).
**Baccalaureate Enrollment** 1,395 **Women** 88% **Men** 12% **Minority** 40% **Part-time** 31%
**Graduate Enrollment** 555 **Women** 92% **Men** 8% **Minority** 52% **Part-time** 97%
**Nursing Student Activities** Sigma Theta Tau, Student Nurses' Association.
**Nursing Student Resources** Academic advising; academic or career counseling; assistance for students with disabilities; bookstore; campus computer network; career placement assistance; computer lab; computer-assisted instruction; e-mail services; externships; interactive nursing skills videos; Internet; learning resource lab; library services; nursing audiovisuals; remedial services; resume preparation assistance; skills, simulation, or other laboratory; tutoring.
**Library Facilities** 190,629 volumes (2,172 in health, 719 in nursing); 108,090 periodical subscriptions (18 health-care related).

## BACCALAUREATE PROGRAMS

**Degree** BS
**Available Programs** ADN to Baccalaureate; Accelerated Baccalaureate for Second Degree; Accelerated RN Baccalaureate; Baccalaureate for Second Degree; Generic Baccalaureate; LPN to Baccalaureate; LPN to RN Baccalaureate; RN Baccalaureate.
**Site Options** New Hyde Park, NY; Farmingdale, NY.
**Study Options** Full-time and part-time.
**Program Entrance Requirements** Minimum overall college GPA of 3.0, transcript of college record, written essay, health exam, high school biology, high school chemistry, high school foreign language, 3 years high school math, high school transcript, immunizations, minimum high school GPA of 3.0. Transfer students are accepted. *Application deadline:* Applications may be processed on a rolling basis for some programs. *Application fee:* $30.
**Advanced Placement** Credit given for nursing courses completed elsewhere dependent upon specific evaluations.
**Expenses (2013–14)** *Tuition:* full-time $24,700; part-time $815 per credit. *Room and board:* $13,000; room only: $9500 per academic year. *Required fees:* full-time $1000; part-time $365 per term.
**Financial Aid** 81% of baccalaureate students in nursing programs received some form of financial aid in 2012–13.
**Contact** Marguerite Lane, Dean of Admissions, Division of Nursing, Molloy College, 1000 Hempstead Avenue, PO Box 5002, Rockville Centre, NY 11571-5002. *Telephone:* 516-323-4014. *E-mail:* mlane@molloy.edu.

## GRADUATE PROGRAMS

**Expenses (2013–14)** *Tuition:* part-time $940 per credit. *Required fees:* part-time $400 per term.
**Financial Aid** 38% of graduate students in nursing programs received some form of financial aid in 2012–13. Research assistantships with partial tuition reimbursements available, teaching assistantships with partial tuition reimbursements available, institutionally sponsored loans, scholarships, and unspecified assistantships available. Aid available to part-time students. *Financial aid application deadline:* 4/1.
**Contact** Ms. Joanna Forgione, Associate Director of Admissions, Division of Nursing, Molloy College, 1000 Hempstead Avenue, PO Box 5002, Rockville Centre, NY 11571-5002. *Telephone:* 516-323-4013. *E-mail:* jforgione@molloy.edu.

### MASTER'S DEGREE PROGRAM

**Degrees** MS; MS/MBA
**Available Programs** Master's.
**Concentrations Available** Nursing administration; nursing education; nursing informatics. *Clinical nurse specialist programs in:* adult health. *Nurse practitioner programs in:* adult health, family health, pediatric, psychiatric/mental health.
**Site Options** New Hyde Park, NY; Farmingdale, NY.
**Study Options** Full-time and part-time.
**Program Entrance Requirements** Clinical experience, minimum overall college GPA of 3.0, transcript of college record, CPR certification, written essay, immunizations, interview, 3 letters of recommendation, nursing research course, professional liability insurance/malpractice insurance, prerequisite course work, statistics course. *Application deadline:* Applications may be processed on a rolling basis for some programs. *Application fee:* $60.
**Advanced Placement** Credit given for nursing courses completed elsewhere dependent upon specific evaluations.
**Degree Requirements** 48 total credit hours, thesis or project.

### POST-MASTER'S PROGRAM

**Areas of Study** Nursing administration; nursing education; nursing informatics. *Clinical nurse specialist programs in:* adult health. *Nurse practitioner programs in:* adult health, family health, pediatric, psychiatric/mental health.

### DOCTORAL DEGREE PROGRAM

**Degree** PhD
**Available Programs** Doctorate.
**Areas of Study** Health policy, nursing education, nursing research.
**Program Entrance Requirements** Clinical experience, minimum overall college GPA of 3.5, interview by faculty committee, interview, 3 letters of recommendation, MSN or equivalent, scholarly papers, statistics course, vita, writing sample. *Application deadline:* 2/1 (fall). *Application fee:* $75.
**Degree Requirements** 45 total credit hours, dissertation.

## CONTINUING EDUCATION PROGRAM

**Contact** Kathleen Lapkowski, Associate Director, Nursing Continuing Education, Division of Nursing, Molloy College, 1000 Hempstead Avenue, PO Box 5002, Rockville Centre, NY 11571-5002. *Telephone:* 516-323-3555. *E-mail:* klapkowski@molloy.edu.

***See display on next page and full description on page 482.***

# Mount Saint Mary College

## Division of Nursing
## Newburgh, New York

Founded in 1960

**DEGREES • BSN • MS**
**Nursing Program Faculty** 36 (50% with doctorates).
**Nursing Student Activities** Sigma Theta Tau, Student Nurses' Association, nursing club.
**Nursing Student Resources** Academic advising; academic or career counseling; assistance for students with disabilities; bookstore; campus computer network; career placement assistance; computer lab; computer-assisted instruction; e-mail services; employment services for current students; externships; housing assistance; interactive nursing skills videos; Internet; learning resource lab; library services; nursing audiovisuals; paid internships; remedial services; resume preparation assistance; skills, simulation, or other laboratory; tutoring.

**Library Facilities** 80,568 volumes (2,443 in health, 1,723 in nursing); 69,503 periodical subscriptions (114 health-care related).

## BACCALAUREATE PROGRAMS

**Degree** BSN
**Available Programs** Accelerated Baccalaureate; Accelerated RN Baccalaureate; Generic Baccalaureate; RN Baccalaureate.
**Study Options** Full-time and part-time.
**Program Entrance Requirements** Minimum overall college GPA of 2.75, transcript of college record, CPR certification, health exam, high school biology, high school chemistry, 3 years high school math, high school transcript, immunizations, interview. Transfer students are accepted.
**Advanced Placement** Credit by examination available. Credit given for nursing courses completed elsewhere dependent upon specific evaluations.
**Contact** *Telephone:* 845-569-3248.

## GRADUATE PROGRAMS

**Contact** *Telephone:* 845-569-3248.

### MASTER'S DEGREE PROGRAM

**Degree** MS
**Available Programs** Master's.
**Concentrations Available** *Clinical nurse specialist programs in:* adult health. *Nurse practitioner programs in:* adult health.
**Study Options** Full-time and part-time.
**Program Entrance Requirements** Clinical experience, computer literacy, minimum overall college GPA of 3.0, transcript of college record, written essay, immunizations, interview, 3 letters of recommendation, nursing research course, physical assessment course, professional liability insurance/malpractice insurance, resume, statistics course.
**Degree Requirements** 42 total credit hours, thesis or project.

### POST-MASTER'S PROGRAM

**Areas of Study** Nursing administration; nursing education.

# Nazareth College of Rochester

## Department of Nursing
## Rochester, New York

*http://www.naz.edu/*
Founded in 1924

## DEGREE • BS

**Nursing Program Faculty** 20 (50% with doctorates).
**Baccalaureate Enrollment** 20
**Distance Learning Courses** Available.
**Nursing Student Activities** Nursing Honor Society, Sigma Theta Tau, Student Nurses' Association, nursing club.
**Nursing Student Resources** Academic advising; academic or career counseling; assistance for students with disabilities; bookstore; campus computer network; career placement assistance; computer lab; computer-assisted instruction; daycare for children of students; e-mail services; employment services for current students; externships; housing assistance; interactive nursing skills videos; Internet; learning resource lab; library services; nursing audiovisuals; resume preparation assistance; skills, simulation, or other laboratory; tutoring.
**Library Facilities** 283,248 volumes (267,000 in health, 66,000 in nursing); 16,102 periodical subscriptions (44,000 health-care related).

## BACCALAUREATE PROGRAMS

**Degree** BS
**Available Programs** Generic Baccalaureate; LPN to Baccalaureate; RN Baccalaureate.
**Site Options** Rochester, NY.
**Study Options** Full-time and part-time.
**Program Entrance Requirements** Minimum overall college GPA of 2.75, transcript of college record, CPR certification, written essay, health exam, high school chemistry, high school transcript, immunizations, minimum high school GPA of 2.75, minimum GPA in nursing prerequisites of 2.5, prerequisite course work. Transfer students are accepted.
**Advanced Placement** Credit by examination available. Credit given for nursing courses completed elsewhere dependent upon specific evaluations.

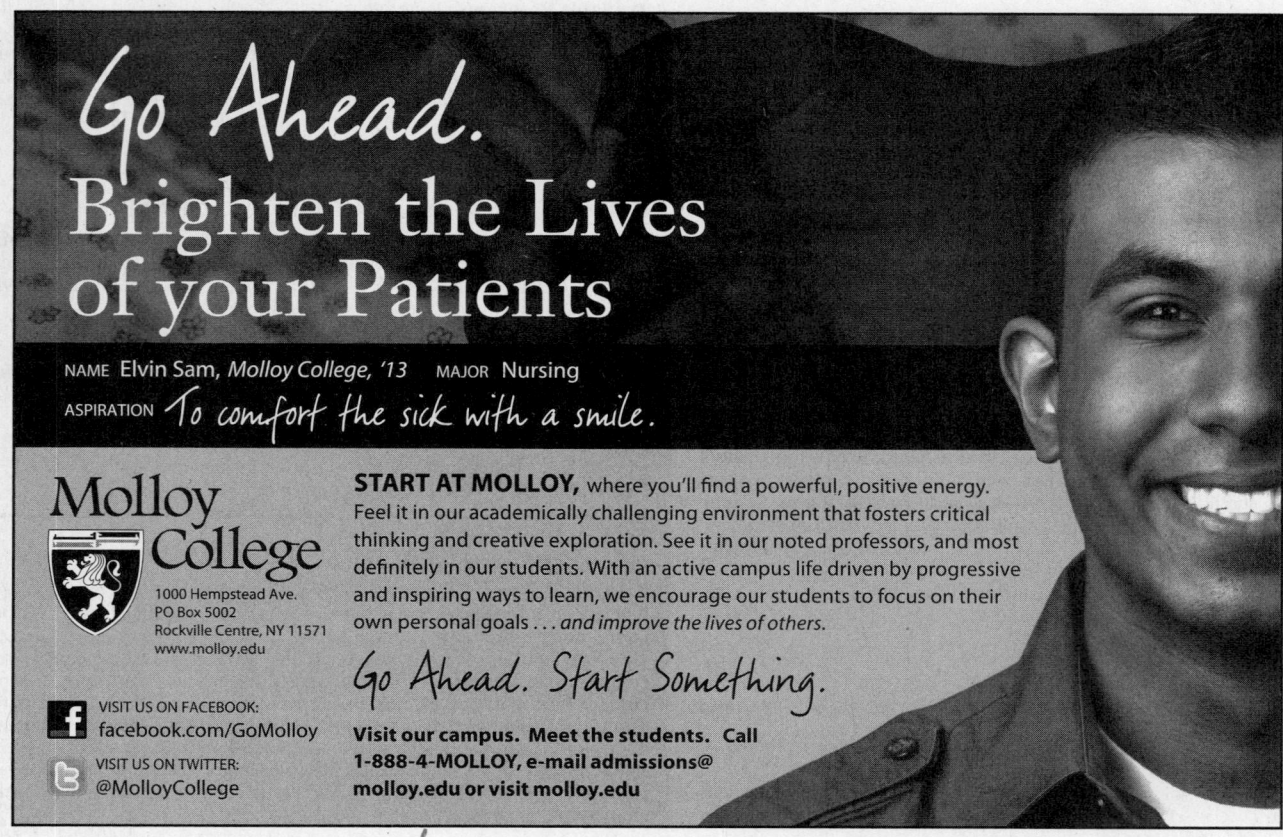

**Contact** Admissions Office, Department of Nursing, Nazareth College of Rochester, 4245 East Avenue, Rochester, NY 14618-3790. *Telephone:* 585-389-2865. *E-mail:* admissions@naz.edu.

# New York City College of Technology of the City University of New York

## Department of Nursing
## Brooklyn, New York

*http://www.citytech.cuny.edu/*
Founded in 1946

**DEGREE • BS**
**Nursing Program Faculty** 22
**Library Facilities** 355,770 volumes; 107,900 periodical subscriptions.

### BACCALAUREATE PROGRAMS

**Degree** BS
**Available Programs** RN Baccalaureate.
**Program Entrance Requirements** Minimum overall college GPA of 2.5, immunizations, professional liability insurance/malpractice insurance, RN licensure. Transfer students are accepted.
**Contact** *Telephone:* 718-260-5660. *Fax:* 718-260-5662.

# New York Institute of Technology

## Department of Nursing
## Old Westbury, New York

Founded in 1955

**DEGREE • BSN**
**Library Facilities** 135,630 volumes; 2,308 periodical subscriptions.

### BACCALAUREATE PROGRAMS

**Degree** BSN
**Available Programs** Generic Baccalaureate.
**Contact** *Telephone:* 516-686-7516.

# New York University

## College of Nursing
## New York, New York

*http://www.nyu.edu/nursing/index.html*
Founded in 1831

**DEGREES • BS • DNP • MS • MS/MPH • MSN/MPA • PHD**
**Nursing Program Faculty** 230 (27% with doctorates).
**Baccalaureate Enrollment** 885 **Women** 86% **Men** 14% **Minority** 49.61% **International** 2.18% **Part-time** 4.86%
**Graduate Enrollment** 696 **Women** 88% **Men** 12% **Minority** 45% **International** 2.87% **Part-time** 94%
**Nursing Student Activities** Nursing Honor Society, Sigma Theta Tau, Student Nurses' Association, nursing club.
**Nursing Student Resources** Academic advising; academic or career counseling; assistance for students with disabilities; bookstore; campus computer network; career placement assistance; computer lab; computer-assisted instruction; e-mail services; employment services for current students; externships; housing assistance; Internet; learning resource lab; library services; nursing audiovisuals; resume preparation assistance; skills, simulation, or other laboratory; tutoring.
**Library Facilities** 149,738 volumes in health, 61,169 volumes in nursing; 39,775 periodical subscriptions health-care related.

### BACCALAUREATE PROGRAMS

**Degree** BS
**Available Programs** Accelerated Baccalaureate for Second Degree; Generic Baccalaureate; RN Baccalaureate.
**Study Options** Full-time and part-time.
**Program Entrance Requirements** Minimum overall college GPA of 3.0, transcript of college record, written essay, high school foreign language, 3 years high school math, 3 years high school science, high school transcript, immunizations, 1 letter of recommendation, minimum GPA in nursing prerequisites of 2.0. Transfer students are accepted. *Application deadline:* 1/1 (fall). *Application fee:* $70.
**Advanced Placement** Credit given for nursing courses completed elsewhere dependent upon specific evaluations.
**Expenses (2013–14)** *Tuition:* full-time $42,472; part-time $1251 per credit. *International tuition:* $42,472 full-time. *Room and board:* $16,622; room only: $14,511 per academic year. *Required fees:* full-time $2373.
**Financial Aid** 83% of baccalaureate students in nursing programs received some form of financial aid in 2012–13.
**Contact** Ms. Titilayo Kuti, Assistant Director for Undergraduate Admissions, College of Nursing, New York University, 726 Broadway, 10th Floor, New York, NY 10003-6677. *Telephone:* 212-998-5336. *Fax:* 212-995-4302. *E-mail:* tok207@nyu.edu.

### GRADUATE PROGRAMS

**Expenses (2013–14)** *Tuition:* part-time $1450 per credit. *Room and board:* $15,181; room only: $10,461 per academic year.
**Financial Aid** 68% of graduate students in nursing programs received some form of financial aid in 2012–13. 2 research assistantships with full and partial tuition reimbursements available (averaging $23,000 per year) were awarded; fellowships with full and partial tuition reimbursements available, career-related internships or fieldwork, institutionally sponsored loans, scholarships, and tuition waivers (partial) also available. Aid available to part-time students. *Financial aid application deadline:* 2/1.
**Contact** Ms. Elizabeth Ensweiler, Assistant Director of Graduate Student Affairs and Admissions, College of Nursing, New York University, 726 Broadway, 10th Floor, New York, NY 10003-6677. *Telephone:* 212-992-7653. *Fax:* 212-995-4302. *E-mail:* ee39@nyu.edu.

#### MASTER'S DEGREE PROGRAM

**Degrees** MS; MS/MPH; MSN/MPA
**Available Programs** Master's; RN to Master's.
**Concentrations Available** Nurse-midwifery; nursing administration; nursing education; nursing informatics. *Nurse practitioner programs in:* acute care, family health, pediatric, primary care, psychiatric/mental health.
**Study Options** Full-time and part-time.
**Program Entrance Requirements** Clinical experience, minimum overall college GPA of 3.0, transcript of college record, CPR certification, written essay, immunizations, 2 letters of recommendation, nursing research course, resume, statistics course. *Application deadline:* 7/1 (fall), 12/1 (spring), 3/1 (summer). Applications may be processed on a rolling basis for some programs. *Application fee:* $80.
**Advanced Placement** Credit given for nursing courses completed elsewhere dependent upon specific evaluations.
**Degree Requirements** 45 total credit hours, thesis or project.

#### POST-MASTER'S PROGRAM

**Areas of Study** Nurse-midwifery; nursing administration; nursing education; nursing informatics. *Nurse practitioner programs in:* acute care, family health, gerontology, pediatric, primary care, psychiatric/mental health.

#### DOCTORAL DEGREE PROGRAM

**Degree** DNP
**Available Programs** Doctorate.
**Areas of Study** Addiction/substance abuse, advanced practice nursing, aging, critical care, family health, gerontology, health promotion/disease prevention, maternity-newborn.
**Program Entrance Requirements** Minimum overall college GPA of 3.5, clinical experience, graduate level research course (taken no more than 5 years ago), 2 letters of recommendation, Miller Analogies Test (MAT), MSN or equivalent, RN license, vita. *Application deadline:* 3/1 (spring). Applications may be processed on a rolling basis for some programs. *Application fee:* $75.
**Degree Requirements** 40 total credit hours, Capstone EBP Clinical Project, oral exam.

**Degree** PhD
**Available Programs** Doctorate; Doctorate for Nurses with Non-Nursing Degrees; Post-Baccalaureate Doctorate.
**Areas of Study** Advanced practice nursing, nursing research.
**Program Entrance Requirements** Clinical experience, minimum overall college GPA of 3.5, interview, 3 letters of recommendation, MSN or equivalent, vita, writing sample, GRE General Test. *Application deadline:* 1/15 (fall). Applications may be processed on a rolling basis for some programs. *Application fee:* $75.

**Degree Requirements** 45 total credit hours, dissertation.

## CONTINUING EDUCATION PROGRAM

**Contact** Dr. Mattia Gilmartin, Continuing Education Director, College of Nursing, New York University, 726 Broadway, 10th Floor, New York, NY 10003-6677. *Telephone:* 212-992-7128. *Fax:* 212-995-3143. *E-mail:* mjg14@nyu.edu.

# Niagara University

## Department of Nursing
## Niagara Falls, Niagara University, New York

***http://www.niagara.edu/nursing***
Founded in 1856

### DEGREE • BS

**Nursing Program Faculty** 15 (47% with doctorates).
**Baccalaureate Enrollment** 187 **Women** 93% **Men** 7% **Minority** 10% **International** 2% **Part-time** 46%
**Distance Learning Courses** Available.
**Nursing Student Activities** Sigma Theta Tau, Student Nurses' Association.
**Nursing Student Resources** Academic advising; academic or career counseling; assistance for students with disabilities; bookstore; campus computer network; career placement assistance; computer lab; computer-assisted instruction; e-mail services; interactive nursing skills videos; Internet; library services; nursing audiovisuals; resume preparation assistance; skills, simulation, or other laboratory; tutoring; unpaid internships.
**Library Facilities** 198,622 volumes; 22,000 periodical subscriptions.

## BACCALAUREATE PROGRAMS

**Degree** BS
**Available Programs** Accelerated Baccalaureate for Second Degree; Generic Baccalaureate; RN Baccalaureate.
**Study Options** Full-time.
**Program Entrance Requirements** Transcript of college record, written essay, health exam, health insurance, high school biology, high school chemistry, 3 years high school science, high school transcript, immunizations, minimum high school GPA of 2.5. Transfer students are accepted. *Application deadline:* 12/20 (fall). *Application fee:* $35.
**Expenses (2013–14)** *Tuition:* part-time $900 per credit hour. *Required fees:* part-time $42 per term.
**Financial Aid** 50% of baccalaureate students in nursing programs received some form of financial aid in 2012–13. *Gift aid (need-based):* Federal Pell, FSEOG, state, private, college/university gift aid from institutional funds. *Loans:* Federal Nursing Student Loans, Federal Direct (Subsidized and Unsubsidized Stafford PLUS), Perkins, college/university. *Work-study:* Federal Work-Study, part-time campus jobs. *Financial aid application deadline (priority):* 2/15.
**Contact** Prof. Frances Crosby, Chairperson, Department of Nursing, Niagara University, PO Box 2203, Niagara University, NY 14109. *Telephone:* 716-286-8155. *Fax:* 716-286-8763. *E-mail:* fcrosby@niagara.edu.

# Pace University

## Lienhard School of Nursing
## New York, New York

***http://www.pace.edu/lienhard***
Founded in 1906

### DEGREES • BS • DNP • MS

**Nursing Program Faculty** 173 (24% with doctorates).
**Baccalaureate Enrollment** 501 **Women** 88% **Men** 12% **Minority** 41% **International** .1% **Part-time** 23%
**Graduate Enrollment** 430 **Women** 91% **Men** 9% **Minority** 47% **International** 1% **Part-time** 99%
**Distance Learning Courses** Available.
**Nursing Student Activities** Nursing Honor Society, Sigma Theta Tau, Student Nurses' Association.
**Nursing Student Resources** Academic advising; academic or career counseling; assistance for students with disabilities; bookstore; campus computer network; career placement assistance; computer lab; computer-assisted instruction; e-mail services; employment services for current students; housing assistance; interactive nursing skills videos; Internet; learning resource lab; library services; nursing audiovisuals; placement services for program completers; resume preparation assistance; skills, simulation, or other laboratory.
**Library Facilities** 809,911 volumes (15,182 in health, 2,844 in nursing); 147,624 periodical subscriptions (7,325 health-care related).

## BACCALAUREATE PROGRAMS

**Degree** BS
**Available Programs** Accelerated Baccalaureate for Second Degree; Generic Baccalaureate; RN Baccalaureate.
**Site Options** Pleasantville, NY; New York, NY.
**Study Options** Full-time and part-time.
**Program Entrance Requirements** Transcript of college record, CPR certification, written essay, health exam, health insurance, high school biology, high school chemistry, high school foreign language, 4 years high school math, 2 years high school science, high school transcript, immunizations, 2 letters of recommendation, minimum GPA in nursing prerequisites of 2.75. Transfer students are accepted. *Application deadline:* 2/15 (fall). *Application fee:* $50.
**Advanced Placement** Credit by examination available. Credit given for nursing courses completed elsewhere dependent upon specific evaluations.
**Expenses (2013–14)** *Tuition:* full-time $36,732; part-time $1054 per credit. *International tuition:* $36,732 full-time. *Room and board:* $13,120 per academic year. *Required fees:* full-time $1337.
**Financial Aid** 90% of baccalaureate students in nursing programs received some form of financial aid in 2012–13. *Gift aid (need-based):* Federal Pell, FSEOG, state, private, college/university gift aid from institutional funds, Federal Nursing, endowed and restricted scholarships and grants. *Loans:* Federal Nursing Student Loans, Federal Direct (Subsidized and Unsubsidized Stafford PLUS), Perkins. *Work-study:* Federal Work-Study. *Financial aid application deadline (priority):* 2/15.
**Contact** Dr. Martha Greenberg, Associate Professor and Chairperson, Undergraduate Department, Lienhard School of Nursing, Pace University, 861 Bedford Road, Pleasantville, NY 10570. *Telephone:* 914-773-3325. *Fax:* 914-773-3345. *E-mail:* mgreenberg@pace.edu.

## GRADUATE PROGRAMS

**Expenses (2013–14)** *Tuition:* part-time $1030 per credit.
**Financial Aid** 58% of graduate students in nursing programs received some form of financial aid in 2012–13. Research assistantships, career-related internships or fieldwork, Federal Work-Study, and tuition waivers (partial) available. Aid available to part-time students.
**Contact** Dr. Joanne K. Singleton, Chair of the Department of Graduate Studies/Director, Doctor of Nursing Program, Lienhard School of Nursing, Pace University, 163 William Street, New York, NY 10038. *Telephone:* 212-618-6010. *E-mail:* jsingleton@pace.edu.

### MASTER'S DEGREE PROGRAM

**Degree** MS
**Available Programs** Master's; Master's for Nurses with Non-Nursing Degrees.
**Concentrations Available** Nursing education. *Nurse practitioner programs in:* family health.
**Site Options** Pleasantville, NY; New York, NY.
**Study Options** Full-time and part-time.
**Online Degree Options** Yes.
**Program Entrance Requirements** Computer literacy, minimum overall college GPA of 3.0, transcript of college record, CPR certification, immunizations, 2 letters of recommendation, nursing research course, professional liability insurance/malpractice insurance, prerequisite course work, resume, statistics course, GRE General Test or MAT. *Application deadline:* 6/1 (fall), 10/15 (spring). *Application fee:* $70.
**Advanced Placement** Credit by examination available. Credit given for nursing courses completed elsewhere dependent upon specific evaluations.
**Degree Requirements** 42 total credit hours, comprehensive exam.

### POST-MASTER'S PROGRAM

**Areas of Study** Nursing education. *Nurse practitioner programs in:* family health.

### DOCTORAL DEGREE PROGRAM

**Degree** DNP
**Available Programs** Doctorate.
**Areas of Study** Family health.
**Site Options** New York, NY.
**Program Entrance Requirements** Clinical experience, minimum overall college GPA of 3.3, 2 letters of recommendation, MSN or equiv-

alent, vita, writing sample. *Application deadline:* 6/1 (fall). *Application fee:* $70.
**Degree Requirements** 37 total credit hours, residency.

***See display below and full description on page 484.***

# Roberts Wesleyan College
## Division of Nursing
## Rochester, New York

***http://www.roberts.edu/Nursing/***
Founded in 1866

**DEGREES • BSCN • M SC N**
**Nursing Program Faculty** 18 (33% with doctorates).
**Baccalaureate Enrollment** 346 **Women** 90% **Men** 10% **Minority** 16% **International** 3% **Part-time** 4%
**Graduate Enrollment** 67 **Women** 94% **Men** 6% **Minority** 13% **International** 12%
**Distance Learning Courses** Available.
**Nursing Student Activities** Sigma Theta Tau, nursing club.
**Nursing Student Resources** Academic advising; academic or career counseling; assistance for students with disabilities; bookstore; campus computer network; career placement assistance; computer lab; computer-assisted instruction; e-mail services; employment services for current students; externships; housing assistance; interactive nursing skills videos; Internet; learning resource lab; library services; nursing audiovisuals; placement services for program completers; remedial services; resume preparation assistance; skills, simulation, or other laboratory; tutoring; unpaid internships.
**Library Facilities** 139,427 volumes (7,669 in health, 6,800 in nursing); 2,148 periodical subscriptions (203 health-care related).

## BACCALAUREATE PROGRAMS

**Degree** BScN
**Available Programs** Generic Baccalaureate; RN Baccalaureate.
**Site Options** Dansville, NY; Buffalo, NY; Rochester, NY; Weedsport, NY; Rochester, NY.
**Study Options** Full-time and part-time.
**Online Degree Options** Yes.
**Program Entrance Requirements** Minimum overall college GPA of 2.5, transcript of college record, CPR certification, written essay, health exam, health insurance, high school biology, high school chemistry, high school transcript, immunizations, 2 letters of recommendation, minimum GPA in nursing prerequisites of 2.5, prerequisite course work. Transfer students are accepted. *Application deadline:* 2/1 (fall). Applications may be processed on a rolling basis for some programs. *Application fee:* $35.
**Expenses (2013–14)** *Tuition:* full-time $26,352; part-time $824 per credit. *International tuition:* $26,352 full-time. *Room and board:* $9630; room only: $6166 per academic year. *Required fees:* full-time $1012; part-time $506 per term.
**Financial Aid** 98% of baccalaureate students in nursing programs received some form of financial aid in 2012–13.
**Contact** Mr. JP Anderson, Associate Vice President for Undergraduate and Seminary Admissions, Division of Nursing, Roberts Wesleyan College, 2301 Westside Drive, Rochester, NY 14624. *Telephone:* 585-594-6400. *Fax:* 585-549-6371. *E-mail:* admissions@roberts.edu.

## GRADUATE PROGRAMS

**Expenses (2013–14)** *Tuition:* full-time $13,626; part-time $757 per credit hour. *International tuition:* $13,626 full-time. *Required fees:* full-time $300.
**Financial Aid** 99% of graduate students in nursing programs received some form of financial aid in 2012–13.
**Contact** Mrs. Brenda Mutton, Graduate Admissions Coordinator, Division of Nursing, Roberts Wesleyan College, 2301 Westside Drive, Rochester, NY 14624-1997. *Telephone:* 585-594-6686. *Fax:* 585-594-6593. *E-mail:* mutton_brenda@roberts.edu.

### MASTER'S DEGREE PROGRAM

**Degree** M Sc N
**Available Programs** Master's.
**Concentrations Available** Nursing administration; nursing education.
**Study Options** Full-time.
**Online Degree Options** Yes.
**Program Entrance Requirements** Clinical experience, computer literacy, minimum overall college GPA of 3.0, transcript of college record, written essay, immunizations, interview, 2 letters of recommendation, nursing research course, physical assessment course, prerequisite course work, resume, statistics course. *Application deadline:* Applications may be processed on a rolling basis for some programs. *Application fee:* $35.

**Degree Requirements** 39 total credit hours, thesis or project.

**POST-MASTER'S PROGRAM**
**Areas of Study** Nursing administration; nursing education.

# The Sage Colleges
## Department of Nursing
## Troy, New York

***http://www.sage.edu/rsc/academics/programs/nursing/***
**DEGREES • BS • DNS • MS • MS/MBA**
**Nursing Program Faculty** 22 (50% with doctorates).
**Baccalaureate Enrollment** 291 **Women** 97% **Men** 3% **Minority** 21% **Part-time** 20%
**Graduate Enrollment** 205 **Women** 93% **Men** 7% **Minority** 16% **International** 1% **Part-time** 84%
**Distance Learning Courses** Available.
**Nursing Student Activities** Nursing Honor Society, Sigma Theta Tau, nursing club.
**Nursing Student Resources** Academic advising; academic or career counseling; assistance for students with disabilities; bookstore; campus computer network; career placement assistance; computer lab; computer-assisted instruction; e-mail services; employment services for current students; externships; interactive nursing skills videos; Internet; learning resource lab; library services; remedial services; resume preparation assistance; skills, simulation, or other laboratory; tutoring.
**Library Facilities** 164,946 volumes; 65,391 periodical subscriptions.

### BACCALAUREATE PROGRAMS

**Degree** BS
**Available Programs** ADN to Baccalaureate; Accelerated Baccalaureate; Accelerated Baccalaureate for Second Degree; Baccalaureate for Second Degree; Generic Baccalaureate; International Nurse to Baccalaureate; LPN to Baccalaureate; RN Baccalaureate.
**Study Options** Full-time and part-time.
**Program Entrance Requirements** Minimum overall college GPA of 3.0, transcript of college record, written essay, health exam, health insurance, high school biology, high school chemistry, 3 years high school math, 3 years high school science, high school transcript, immunizations, interview, 2 letters of recommendation, minimum high school GPA of 3.0, professional liability insurance/malpractice insurance. Transfer students are accepted. *Application deadline:* Applications may be processed on a rolling basis for some programs. *Application fee:* $30.
**Advanced Placement** Credit by examination available. Credit given for nursing courses completed elsewhere dependent upon specific evaluations.
**Expenses (2013–14)** *Tuition:* full-time $27,000; part-time $900 per credit hour. *Room and board:* $11,370; room only: $5970 per academic year. *Required fees:* full-time $1000.
**Financial Aid** 80% of baccalaureate students in nursing programs received some form of financial aid in 2012–13.
**Contact** Toni Sposito, Undergraduate Program Secretary, Department of Nursing, The Sage Colleges, 65 1st Street, Ackerman Hall, Troy, NY 12180-4115. *Telephone:* 518-244-2231. *Fax:* 518-244-2009. *E-mail:* sposia@sage.edu.

### GRADUATE PROGRAMS

**Expenses (2013–14)** *Tuition:* full-time $11,880; part-time $660 per credit hour. *Room and board:* $11,370; room only: $5970 per academic year.
**Financial Aid** Fellowships, research assistantships, Federal Work-Study, scholarships, and unspecified assistantships available.
**Contact** Dr. Madeline Cafiero, MS Program, Department of Nursing, The Sage Colleges, Troy, NY 12180-4115. *Telephone:* 518-244-4574. *Fax:* 518-244-2009. *E-mail:* nursing@sage.edu.

**MASTER'S DEGREE PROGRAM**
**Degrees** MS; MS/MBA
**Available Programs** Accelerated Master's; Accelerated RN to Master's; Master's.
**Concentrations Available** Health-care administration; nursing administration; nursing education. *Clinical nurse specialist programs in:* acute care, adult health, community health, critical care, family health, gerontology, psychiatric/mental health. *Nurse practitioner programs in:* acute care, adult health, community health, family health, gerontology, psychiatric/mental health.
**Study Options** Full-time and part-time.
**Program Entrance Requirements** Minimum overall college GPA of 3.0, transcript of college record, CPR certification, written essay, 2 letters of recommendation, physical assessment course, professional liability insurance/malpractice insurance, resume.
**Advanced Placement** Credit given for nursing courses completed elsewhere dependent upon specific evaluations.
**Degree Requirements** 42 total credit hours, thesis or project.

**POST-MASTER'S PROGRAM**
**Areas of Study** Health-care administration; nursing administration; nursing education. *Clinical nurse specialist programs in:* acute care, adult health, community health, critical care, family health, gerontology, psychiatric/mental health. *Nurse practitioner programs in:* acute care, adult health, community health, family health, gerontology, psychiatric/mental health.

**DOCTORAL DEGREE PROGRAM**
**Degree** DNS
**Available Programs** Doctorate.
**Areas of Study** Faculty preparation, health-care systems, nursing administration, nursing education, nursing policy, nursing research, nursing science.
**Program Entrance Requirements** Minimum overall college GPA of 3.5, interview by faculty committee, 3 letters of recommendation, MSN or equivalent, statistics course, vita, writing sample.
**Degree Requirements** 42 total credit hours, dissertation.

### CONTINUING EDUCATION PROGRAM

**Contact** Graduate & Adult Admission. *E-mail:* spceadm@sage.edu.

# St. Francis College
## Department of Nursing
## Brooklyn Heights, New York

Founded in 1884
**DEGREE • BS**
**Nursing Program Faculty** 9
**Baccalaureate Enrollment** 78 **Women** 90% **Men** 10% **Minority** 50% **International** 2% **Part-time** 60%
**Nursing Student Resources** Academic advising; academic or career counseling; assistance for students with disabilities; bookstore; campus computer network; career placement assistance; computer lab; computer-assisted instruction; e-mail services; employment services for current students; externships; housing assistance; interactive nursing skills videos; Internet; learning resource lab; library services; nursing audiovisuals; remedial services; resume preparation assistance; skills, simulation, or other laboratory; tutoring; unpaid internships.
**Library Facilities** 116,716 volumes; 31,391 periodical subscriptions.

### BACCALAUREATE PROGRAMS

**Degree** BS
**Available Programs** ADN to Baccalaureate; Generic Baccalaureate; International Nurse to Baccalaureate; RN Baccalaureate.
**Study Options** Full-time.
**Program Entrance Requirements** Minimum overall college GPA of 3.0, transcript of college record, CPR certification, written essay, health exam, health insurance, high school transcript, immunizations, interview, 3 letters of recommendation, minimum high school GPA of 3.0, minimum GPA in nursing prerequisites of 3.0, professional liability insurance/malpractice insurance, prerequisite course work. Transfer students are accepted.
**Contact** Dr. Eleanor Kehoe, Associate Professor, Department of Nursing, St. Francis College, 180 Remsen Street, Brooklyn Heights, NY 11201. *Telephone:* 718-489-5497. *Fax:* 718-489-5408. *E-mail:* ekehoe@sfc.edu.

***See display on next page and full description on page 490.***

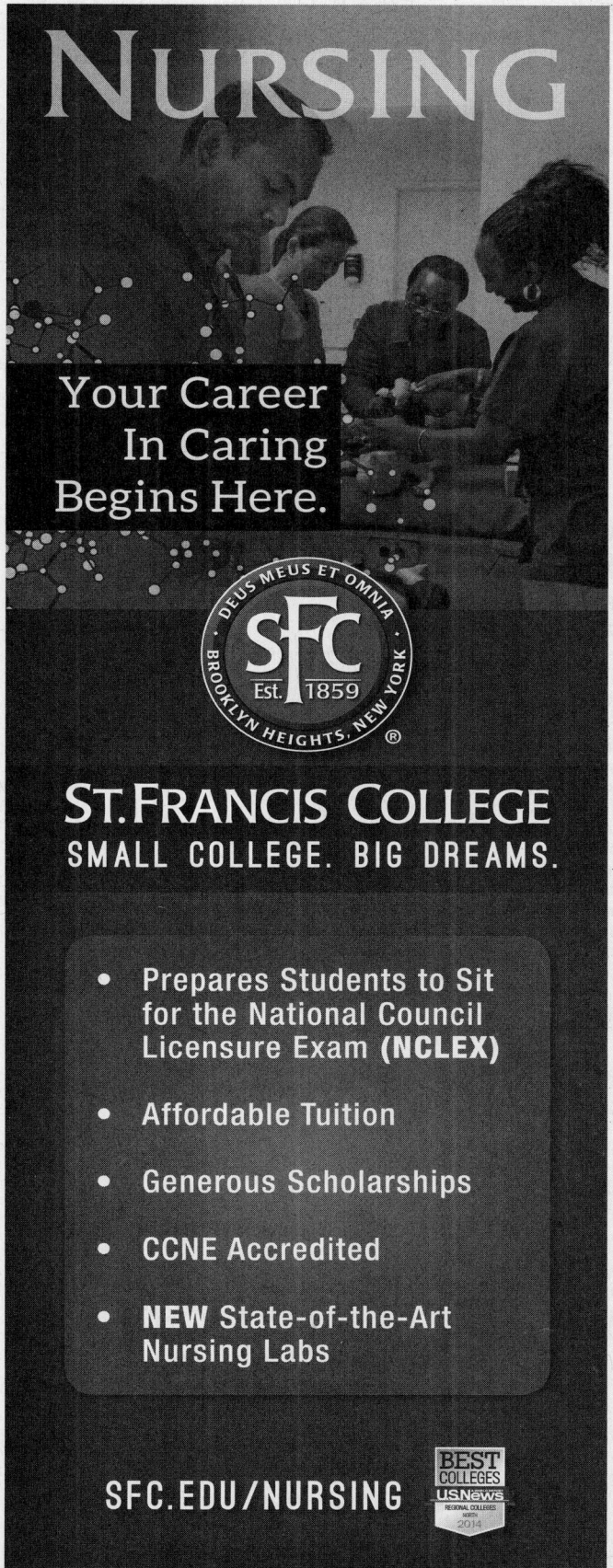


## St. John Fisher College
### Wegmans School of Nursing
### Rochester, New York

*http://www.sjfc.edu/academics/nursing/about/index.dot*
Founded in 1948

**DEGREES • BS • DNP • MS**

**Nursing Program Faculty** 85 (30% with doctorates).
**Baccalaureate Enrollment** 540 **Women** 91% **Men** 9% **Minority** 3% **Part-time** 3%
**Graduate Enrollment** 112 **Women** 90% **Men** 10% **Minority** 3% **Part-time** 99%
**Distance Learning Courses** Available.
**Nursing Student Activities** Sigma Theta Tau, Student Nurses' Association.
**Nursing Student Resources** Academic advising; academic or career counseling; assistance for students with disabilities; bookstore; campus computer network; career placement assistance; computer lab; computer-assisted instruction; daycare for children of students; e-mail services; employment services for current students; interactive nursing skills videos; Internet; learning resource lab; library services; nursing audiovisuals; resume preparation assistance; skills, simulation, or other laboratory; tutoring.
**Library Facilities** 229,031 volumes (30,000 in health, 5,000 in nursing); 48,558 periodical subscriptions (200 health-care related).

### BACCALAUREATE PROGRAMS

**Degree** BS
**Available Programs** ADN to Baccalaureate; Accelerated RN Baccalaureate; Baccalaureate for Second Degree; Generic Baccalaureate; RN Baccalaureate.
**Study Options** Full-time and part-time.
**Program Entrance Requirements** Minimum overall college GPA of 2.75, transcript of college record, CPR certification, written essay, health exam, health insurance, high school transcript, immunizations, 2 letters of recommendation, minimum high school GPA of 2.0, minimum GPA in nursing prerequisites of 2.75, prerequisite course work. Transfer students are accepted. *Application deadline:* 3/1 (fall), 10/1 (spring). Applications may be processed on a rolling basis for some programs. *Application fee:* $30.
**Advanced Placement** Credit given for nursing courses completed elsewhere dependent upon specific evaluations.
**Expenses (2013–14)** *Tuition:* full-time $27,870; part-time $760 per credit hour. *Room and board:* $10,855; room only: $7090 per academic year. *Required fees:* full-time $1220; part-time $720 per term.
**Financial Aid** 95% of baccalaureate students in nursing programs received some form of financial aid in 2012–13. *Gift aid (need-based):* Federal Pell, FSEOG, state, private, college/university gift aid from institutional funds, Federal Nursing. *Loans:* Federal Direct (Subsidized and Unsubsidized Stafford PLUS), Perkins. *Work-study:* Federal Work-Study. *Financial aid application deadline (priority):* 2/15.
**Contact** Dr. Marilyn Dollinger, Chairperson, Wegmans School of Nursing, St. John Fisher College, 3690 East Avenue, Rochester, NY 14618. *Telephone:* 585-385-8476. *Fax:* 585-385-8466. *E-mail:* mdollinger@sjfc.edu.

### GRADUATE PROGRAMS

**Expenses (2013–14)** *Tuition:* part-time $795 per credit hour. *Required fees:* part-time $10 per term.
**Financial Aid** 20% of graduate students in nursing programs received some form of financial aid in 2012–13. Scholarships available.
**Contact** Dr. Cynthia Ricci McCloskey, Graduate Program Director, Wegmans School of Nursing, St. John Fisher College, 3690 East Avenue, Rochester, NY 14618. *Telephone:* 585-385-8471. *Fax:* 585-385-8466. *E-mail:* cmccloskey@sjfc.eud.

#### MASTER'S DEGREE PROGRAM

**Degree** MS
**Available Programs** Master's; RN to Master's.
**Concentrations Available** Nursing education. *Clinical nurse specialist programs in:* adult health, gerontology, pediatric,women's health. *Nurse practitioner programs in:* family health.
**Study Options** Full-time and part-time.
**Program Entrance Requirements** Computer literacy, minimum overall college GPA of 3.0, transcript of college record, CPR certification, written essay, immunizations, 2 letters of recommendation, nursing research course, physical assessment course, resume, statistics course.

*Application deadline:* Applications may be processed on a rolling basis for some programs. *Application fee:* $30.
**Advanced Placement** Credit given for nursing courses completed elsewhere dependent upon specific evaluations.
**Degree Requirements** 46 total credit hours, thesis or project, comprehensive exam.

### POST-MASTER'S PROGRAM

**Areas of Study** Nursing education. *Nurse practitioner programs in:* family health.

### DOCTORAL DEGREE PROGRAM

**Degree** DNP
**Available Programs** Doctorate; Post-Baccalaureate Doctorate.
**Areas of Study** Advanced practice nursing.
**Program Entrance Requirements** Clinical experience, minimum overall college GPA of 3.0, interview by faculty committee, letters of recommendation, scholarly papers, vita, writing sample. *Application deadline:* Applications may be processed on a rolling basis for some programs. *Application fee:* $30.
**Degree Requirements** 48 total credit hours, residency.

# St. Joseph's College, New York

## Department of Nursing
## Brooklyn, New York

***http://www.sjcny.edu/***
Founded in 1916

**DEGREES • BSN • MS**
**Nursing Program Faculty** 17 (47% with doctorates).
**Baccalaureate Enrollment** 263 **Women** 93% **Men** 7% **Minority** 46% **Part-time** 96%
**Graduate Enrollment** 58 **Women** 95% **Men** 5% **Minority** 81% **Part-time** 100%
**Nursing Student Activities** Nursing Honor Society, nursing club.
**Nursing Student Resources** Academic advising; academic or career counseling; assistance for students with disabilities; bookstore; campus computer network; career placement assistance; computer lab; computer-assisted instruction; e-mail services; Internet; learning resource lab; library services; nursing audiovisuals; remedial services; resume preparation assistance; skills, simulation, or other laboratory; tutoring.
**Library Facilities** 156,232 volumes (14,950 in health, 1,545 in nursing); 28,299 periodical subscriptions (3,336 health-care related).

### BACCALAUREATE PROGRAMS

**Degree** BSN
**Available Programs** RN Baccalaureate.
**Site Options** Patchogue, NY.
**Study Options** Full-time and part-time.
**Program Entrance Requirements** Minimum overall college GPA of 2.5, transcript of college record, CPR certification, written essay, health exam, health insurance, immunizations, 2 letters of recommendation, minimum GPA in nursing prerequisites of 2.5, professional liability insurance/malpractice insurance, prerequisite course work, RN licensure. Transfer students are accepted. *Application deadline:* 8/31 (fall), 1/15 (spring). Applications may be processed on a rolling basis for some programs. *Application fee:* $25.
**Advanced Placement** Credit by examination available. Credit given for nursing courses completed elsewhere dependent upon specific evaluations.
**Expenses (2013–14)** *Tuition:* full-time $21,250; part-time $690 per credit. *International tuition:* $21,250 full-time. *Required fees:* full-time $702; part-time $13 per credit; part-time $186 per term.
**Financial Aid** 60% of baccalaureate students in nursing programs received some form of financial aid in 2012–13.
**Contact** Dr. Florence L. Jerdan, Director, Department of Nursing, St. Joseph's College, New York, 245 Clinton Avenue, Brooklyn, NY 11205-3688. *Telephone:* 718-940-5892. *Fax:* 718-638-8839. *E-mail:* fjerdan@sjcny.edu.

### GRADUATE PROGRAMS

**Expenses (2013–14)** *Tuition:* part-time $750 per credit. *Required fees:* part-time $13 per credit; part-time $107 per term.
**Financial Aid** 64% of graduate students in nursing programs received some form of financial aid in 2012–13.
**Contact** Dr. Florence L. Jerdan, Director, Department of Nursing, St. Joseph's College, New York, 245 Clinton Avenue, Brooklyn, NY 11205-3688. *Telephone:* 718-940-5892. *Fax:* 718-638-8839. *E-mail:* fjerdan@sjcny.edu.

### MASTER'S DEGREE PROGRAM

**Degree** MS
**Available Programs** Master's.
**Concentrations Available** Nursing education. *Clinical nurse specialist programs in:* adult health.
**Site Options** Patchogue, NY.
**Study Options** Part-time.
**Program Entrance Requirements** Clinical experience, minimum overall college GPA of 3.0, transcript of college record, CPR certification, written essay, immunizations, interview, 2 letters of recommendation, nursing research course, physical assessment course, professional liability insurance/malpractice insurance, prerequisite course work, resume, statistics course. *Application deadline:* 5/15 (fall). Applications may be processed on a rolling basis for some programs. *Application fee:* $25.
**Advanced Placement** Credit given for nursing courses completed elsewhere dependent upon specific evaluations.
**Degree Requirements** 38 total credit hours, comprehensive exam.

# State University of New York at Plattsburgh

## Department of Nursing
## Plattsburgh, New York

***http://www.plattsburgh.edu/nursing***
Founded in 1889

**DEGREE • BS**
**Nursing Program Faculty** 22 (23% with doctorates).
**Baccalaureate Enrollment** 350 **Women** 90% **Men** 10% **Minority** 25% **International** 4% **Part-time** 25%
**Distance Learning Courses** Available.
**Nursing Student Activities** Sigma Theta Tau, Student Nurses' Association.
**Nursing Student Resources** Academic advising; academic or career counseling; assistance for students with disabilities; bookstore; campus computer network; career placement assistance; computer lab; computer-assisted instruction; e-mail services; employment services for current students; interactive nursing skills videos; Internet; learning resource lab; library services; nursing audiovisuals; remedial services; resume preparation assistance; skills, simulation, or other laboratory; tutoring.
**Library Facilities** 541,609 volumes (19,450 in health, 200 in nursing); 5,222 periodical subscriptions (174 health-care related).

### BACCALAUREATE PROGRAMS

**Degree** BS
**Available Programs** ADN to Baccalaureate; Generic Baccalaureate; RN Baccalaureate.
**Study Options** Full-time.
**Online Degree Options** Yes.
**Program Entrance Requirements** Minimum overall college GPA of 2.5, transcript of college record, high school biology, high school chemistry, 3 years high school math, 3 years high school science, high school transcript, minimum GPA in nursing prerequisites of 2.5. Transfer students are accepted. *Application deadline:* 12/1 (fall), 11/1 (spring). Applications may be processed on a rolling basis for some programs. *Application fee:* $50.
**Expenses (2013–14)** *Tuition, state resident:* full-time $5870; part-time $245 per credit. *Tuition, nonresident:* full-time $15,320; part-time $638 per credit. *International tuition:* $15,320 full-time. *Room and board:* $10,924; room only: $6874 per academic year. *Required fees:* full-time $1289.
**Financial Aid** 82% of baccalaureate students in nursing programs received some form of financial aid in 2012–13. *Gift aid (need-based):* Federal Pell, FSEOG, state, private, college/university gift aid from institutional funds. *Loans:* Federal Nursing Student Loans, Federal Direct (Subsidized and Unsubsidized Stafford PLUS), Perkins, alternative loans. *Work-study:* Federal Work-Study, part-time campus jobs. *Financial aid application deadline (priority):* 2/15.
**Contact** Dr. JoAnn Gleeson-Kreig, Chairperson, Department of Nursing, State University of New York at Plattsburgh, 101 Broad Street,

Plattsburgh, NY 12901. *Telephone:* 518-564-3124. *Fax:* 518-564-3100. *E-mail:* joann.gleeson-kreig@plattsburgh.edu.

# State University of New York College of Technology at Alfred

## Nursing Program
## Alfred, New York

Founded in 1908

**DEGREE • BSN**

**Library Facilities** 61,639 volumes; 68,689 periodical subscriptions.

### BACCALAUREATE PROGRAMS

**Degree** BSN
**Available Programs** Generic Baccalaureate.
**Online Degree Options** Yes.
**Contact** Dr. Kathleen Sellers, Professor and Director of BS-N Program, Nursing Program, State University of New York College of Technology at Alfred, 10 Upper College Drive, Alfred, NY 14802. *Telephone:* 607-587-3680. *Fax:* 315-792-7555. *E-mail:* sellerkf@alfredstate.edu.

# State University of New York College of Technology at Delhi

## Bachelor of Science in Nursing Program
## Delhi, New York

Founded in 1913

**DEGREE • BSN**

**Library Facilities** 48,000 volumes; 248 periodical subscriptions.

### BACCALAUREATE PROGRAMS

**Degree** BSN
**Available Programs** RN Baccalaureate.
**Study Options** Full-time and part-time.
**Online Degree Options** Yes (online only).
**Program Entrance Requirements** RN licensure.
**Contact** *Telephone:* 607-746-4519.

# State University of New York Downstate Medical Center

## College of Nursing
## Brooklyn, New York

***http://www.downstate.edu/nursing/***

Founded in 1858

**DEGREES • BS • MS • MS/MPH**

**Nursing Program Faculty** 19 (79% with doctorates).
**Baccalaureate Enrollment** 133 **Women** 93% **Men** 7% **Minority** 80% **International** 2% **Part-time** 77%
**Graduate Enrollment** 387 **Women** 90% **Men** 10% **Minority** 48% **Part-time** 40%
**Distance Learning Courses** Available.
**Nursing Student Activities** Student Nurses' Association, nursing club.
**Nursing Student Resources** Academic advising; academic or career counseling; assistance for students with disabilities; bookstore; campus computer network; computer lab; computer-assisted instruction; e-mail services; housing assistance; interactive nursing skills videos; Internet; learning resource lab; library services; nursing audiovisuals; paid internships; skills, simulation, or other laboratory; unpaid internships.
**Library Facilities** 357,209 volumes in health, 2,679 volumes in nursing; 619 periodical subscriptions health-care related.

### BACCALAUREATE PROGRAMS

**Degree** BS
**Available Programs** Accelerated Baccalaureate for Second Degree; RN Baccalaureate.
**Study Options** Full-time.
**Program Entrance Requirements** Minimum overall college GPA of 3.0, transcript of college record, written essay, health exam, 2 letters of recommendation, professional liability insurance/malpractice insurance, prerequisite course work. Transfer students are accepted. *Application deadline:* 1/15 (fall), 1/15 (summer). Applications may be processed on a rolling basis for some programs. *Application fee:* $40.
**Advanced Placement** Credit by examination available.
**Expenses (2013–14)** *Tuition, state resident:* full-time $5870; part-time $245 per credit. *Tuition, nonresident:* full-time $15,320; part-time $638 per credit. *International tuition:* $15,320 full-time. *Room and board:* $5329; room only: $870 per academic year. *Required fees:* full-time $330; part-time $12 per credit; part-time $17 per term.
**Financial Aid** 33% of baccalaureate students in nursing programs received some form of financial aid in 2012–13.
**Contact** Dr. Nellie Bailey, Associate Dean, College of Nursing, State University of New York Downstate Medical Center, 450 Clarkson Avenue, Box 22, Brooklyn, NY 11203. *Telephone:* 718-270-7617. *Fax:* 718-270-7641. *E-mail:* nellie.bailey@downstate.edu.

### GRADUATE PROGRAMS

**Expenses (2013–14)** *Tuition, state resident:* full-time $9870; part-time $411 per credit. *Tuition, nonresident:* full-time $18,350; part-time $765 per credit. *International tuition:* $18,350 full-time. *Room and board:* $5329; room only: $870 per academic year. *Required fees:* full-time $305; part-time $12 per credit; part-time $17 per term.
**Financial Aid** 1% of graduate students in nursing programs received some form of financial aid in 2012–13. Traineeships and health workforce retraining available.
**Contact** Dr. Laila N. Sedhom, Associate Dean, College of Nursing, State University of New York Downstate Medical Center, 450 Clarkson Avenue, Box 22, Brooklyn, NY 11203-2098. *Telephone:* 718-270-7605. *Fax:* 718-270-7636. *E-mail:* laila.sedhom@downstate.edu.

#### MASTER'S DEGREE PROGRAM

**Degrees** MS; MS/MPH
**Available Programs** Master's.
**Concentrations Available** Nurse anesthesia; nurse-midwifery. *Clinical nurse specialist programs in:* adult health, maternity-newborn. *Nurse practitioner programs in:* family health,women's health.
**Site Options** Brooklyn, NY.
**Study Options** Full-time and part-time.
**Program Entrance Requirements** Clinical experience, minimum overall college GPA of 3.0, transcript of college record, CPR certification, written essay, interview, 2 letters of recommendation, nursing research course, physical assessment course, professional liability insurance/malpractice insurance, prerequisite course work, resume, statistics course, GRE. *Application deadline:* 1/15 (fall). Applications may be processed on a rolling basis for some programs. *Application fee:* $80.
**Advanced Placement** Credit by examination available. Credit given for nursing courses completed elsewhere dependent upon specific evaluations.
**Degree Requirements** 44 total credit hours, thesis or project.

#### POST-MASTER'S PROGRAM

**Areas of Study** *Nurse practitioner programs in:* family health,women's health.

### CONTINUING EDUCATION PROGRAM

**Contact** Ms. Veronica Arikian, PhD, Director of Continuing Education, College of Nursing, State University of New York Downstate Medical Center, 450 Clarkson Avenue, Box 22, Brooklyn, NY 11203. *Telephone:* 718-270-7488. *Fax:* 718-270-7628. *E-mail:* veronica.arikian@downstate.edu.

# State University of New York Empire State College

## Bachelor of Science in Nursing Program
## Saratoga Springs, New York

***http://www.esc.edu/nursing***

Founded in 1971

**DEGREE • BS**

**Nursing Program Faculty** 6 (33% with doctorates).
**Baccalaureate Enrollment** 485 **Women** 92.4% **Men** 7.6% **Minority** 17.4% **Part-time** 85.9%

**Distance Learning Courses** Available.
**Nursing Student Resources** Academic advising; academic or career counseling; assistance for students with disabilities; bookstore; computer-assisted instruction; e-mail services; interactive nursing skills videos; Internet; library services; nursing audiovisuals; resume preparation assistance; tutoring.
**Library Facilities** 70,000 volumes; 57,000 periodical subscriptions.

## BACCALAUREATE PROGRAMS

**Degree** BS
**Available Programs** RN Baccalaureate.
**Online Degree Options** Yes (online only).
**Program Entrance Requirements** Minimum overall college GPA of 2.0, transcript of college record, written essay, RN licensure. Transfer students are accepted. *Application deadline:* 6/1 (fall), 10/1 (spring). *Application fee:* $50.
**Advanced Placement** Credit by examination available. Credit given for nursing courses completed elsewhere dependent upon specific evaluations.
**Contact** *Telephone:* 518-587-2100 Ext. 2812. *Fax:* 518-587-5126.

# State University of New York Institute of Technology
## School of Nursing and Health Systems
## Utica, New York

***http://www.sunyit.edu/***
Founded in 1966

### DEGREES • BS • MS

**Nursing Program Faculty** 30 (30% with doctorates).
**Baccalaureate Enrollment** 200 **Women** 96% **Men** 4% **Minority** 5% **Part-time** 80%
**Graduate Enrollment** 200 **Women** 90% **Men** 10% **Minority** 10% **Part-time** 70%
**Distance Learning Courses** Available.
**Nursing Student Activities** Nursing Honor Society, Sigma Theta Tau, Student Nurses' Association, nursing club.
**Nursing Student Resources** Academic advising; academic or career counseling; assistance for students with disabilities; bookstore; campus computer network; career placement assistance; computer lab; computer-assisted instruction; e-mail services; employment services for current students; externships; housing assistance; interactive nursing skills videos; Internet; learning resource lab; library services; nursing audiovisuals; other; placement services for program completers; remedial services; resume preparation assistance; skills, simulation, or other laboratory; tutoring; unpaid internships.
**Library Facilities** 148,670 volumes (14,000 in health, 8,500 in nursing); 322 periodical subscriptions (335 health-care related).

## BACCALAUREATE PROGRAMS

**Degree** BS
**Available Programs** ADN to Baccalaureate; Accelerated Baccalaureate; Accelerated RN Baccalaureate; RN Baccalaureate.
**Study Options** Full-time and part-time.
**Online Degree Options** Yes.
**Program Entrance Requirements** Minimum overall college GPA of 3.0, transcript of college record, health exam, health insurance, high school biology, high school chemistry, 3 years high school math, 3 years high school science, high school transcript, immunizations, minimum high school GPA, minimum high school rank 85%, prerequisite course work. Transfer students are accepted. *Application deadline:* 3/15 (fall). *Application fee:* $50.
**Advanced Placement** Credit by examination available. Credit given for nursing courses completed elsewhere dependent upon specific evaluations.
**Expenses (2013–14)** *Tuition, state resident:* full-time $5870; part-time $245 per credit hour. *Tuition, nonresident:* full-time $15,320; part-time $638 per credit hour. *International tuition:* $15,320 full-time. *Room and board:* $11,774; room only: $7664 per academic year. *Required fees:* full-time $1200; part-time $50 per credit.
**Financial Aid** 33% of baccalaureate students in nursing programs received some form of financial aid in 2012–13. *Gift aid (need-based):* Federal Pell, FSEOG, state, private, college/university gift aid from institutional funds. *Loans:* Federal Nursing Student Loans, Federal Direct (Subsidized and Unsubsidized Stafford PLUS), Perkins. *Work-study:* Federal Work-Study, part-time campus jobs. *Financial aid application deadline (priority):* 3/1.
**Contact** Ms. Jennifer Phelan-Ninh, Director of Admissions, School of Nursing and Health Systems, State University of New York Institute of Technology, 100 Seymour Road, Utica, NY 13502. *Telephone:* 315-792-7500. *E-mail:* admissions@sunyit.edu.

## GRADUATE PROGRAMS

**Expenses (2013–14)** *Tuition, state resident:* full-time $9870; part-time $411 per credit hour. *Tuition, nonresident:* full-time $18,350; part-time $765 per credit hour. *International tuition:* $18,350 full-time. *Room and board:* $11,774; room only: $7664 per academic year. *Required fees:* full-time $1160; part-time $50 per credit.
**Financial Aid** 60% of graduate students in nursing programs received some form of financial aid in 2012–13. Federal Work-Study, scholarships, traineeships, and unspecified assistantships available.
**Contact** Ms. Maryrose Raab, Coordinator of Graduate Center, School of Nursing and Health Systems, State University of New York Institute of Technology, 100 Seymour Road, Utica, NY 13502. *Telephone:* 315-792-7297. *Fax:* 315-792-7221. *E-mail:* mb_raab@sunyit.edu.

### MASTER'S DEGREE PROGRAM

**Degree** MS
**Available Programs** Accelerated AD/RN to Master's; Accelerated RN to Master's; Master's; RN to Master's.
**Concentrations Available** Nursing administration; nursing education. *Nurse practitioner programs in:* adult health, family health, gerontology.
**Study Options** Full-time and part-time.
**Online Degree Options** Yes.
**Program Entrance Requirements** Clinical experience, computer literacy, minimum overall college GPA of 3.0, transcript of college record, written essay, immunizations, interview, 2 letters of recommendation, nursing research course, physical assessment course, prerequisite course work, resume, statistics course, GRE General Test (if undergraduate GPA less than 3.3). *Application deadline:* 6/15 (fall), 11/1 (spring). *Application fee:* $50.
**Advanced Placement** Credit given for nursing courses completed elsewhere dependent upon specific evaluations.
**Degree Requirements** 45 total credit hours, comprehensive exam.

### POST-MASTER'S PROGRAM

**Areas of Study** Nursing administration; nursing education. *Nurse practitioner programs in:* adult health, family health, gerontology.

## CONTINUING EDUCATION PROGRAM

**Contact** Dr. Deborah Tyksinski, Associate Provost, Sponsored Research and Continuing Education RF Operations Manager, School of Nursing and Health Systems, State University of New York Institute of Technology, 100 Seymour Road, Utica, NY 13502. *Telephone:* 315-792-7151. *Fax:* 315-792-7278. *E-mail:* debtyk@sunyit.edu.

# State University of New York Upstate Medical University
## College of Nursing
## Syracuse, New York

***http://www.upstate.edu/con***
Founded in 1950

### DEGREES • BS • MS

**Nursing Program Faculty** 21 (40% with doctorates).
**Baccalaureate Enrollment** 136 **Women** 90% **Men** 10% **Minority** 15% **International** 5% **Part-time** 88%
**Graduate Enrollment** 277 **Women** 90% **Men** 10% **Minority** 13% **International** 5% **Part-time** 85%
**Distance Learning Courses** Available.
**Nursing Student Activities** Sigma Theta Tau, Student Nurses' Association.
**Nursing Student Resources** Academic advising; academic or career counseling; assistance for students with disabilities; bookstore; campus computer network; career placement assistance; computer lab; computer-assisted instruction; daycare for children of students; e-mail services; Internet; learning resource lab; library services; skills, simulation, or other laboratory; tutoring.
**Library Facilities** 220,160 volumes (220,382 in health, 1,241 in nursing); 3,200 periodical subscriptions (4,928 health-care related).

## BACCALAUREATE PROGRAMS

**Degree** BS
**Available Programs** ADN to Baccalaureate.
**Site Options** Ithaca, NY.
**Study Options** Full-time and part-time.
**Program Entrance Requirements** Transcript of college record, CPR certification, written essay, health exam, immunizations, 2 letters of recommendation, prerequisite course work, RN licensure. *Application deadline:* 3/15 (fall), 9/15 (spring). *Application fee:* $50.
**Advanced Placement** Credit by examination available. Credit given for nursing courses completed elsewhere dependent upon specific evaluations.
**Contact** *Telephone:* 315-464-4276. *Fax:* 315-464-5168.

## GRADUATE PROGRAMS

**Contact** *Telephone:* 315-464-4276. *Fax:* 315-464-5168.

### MASTER'S DEGREE PROGRAM

**Degree** MS
**Available Programs** Accelerated RN to Master's; Master's; Master's for Nurses with Non-Nursing Degrees; RN to Master's.
**Concentrations Available** *Clinical nurse specialist programs in:* medical-surgical. *Nurse practitioner programs in:* adult health, family health, pediatric, psychiatric/mental health.
**Site Options** Watertown, NY.
**Study Options** Full-time and part-time.
**Program Entrance Requirements** Clinical experience, minimum overall college GPA of 3.0, transcript of college record, CPR certification, written essay, immunizations, 3 letters of recommendation, nursing research course, physical assessment course, statistics course. *Application deadline:* 3/15 (fall), 9/15 (spring). *Application fee:* $50.
**Advanced Placement** Credit by examination available. Credit given for nursing courses completed elsewhere dependent upon specific evaluations.
**Degree Requirements** 47 total credit hours, thesis or project.

### POST-MASTER'S PROGRAM

**Areas of Study** *Clinical nurse specialist programs in:* medical-surgical. *Nurse practitioner programs in:* adult health, family health, pediatric, psychiatric/mental health.

## CONTINUING EDUCATION PROGRAM

**Contact** *Telephone:* 315-464-4276. *Fax:* 315-464-5168.

# Stony Brook University, State University of New York

**School of Nursing**
**Stony Brook, New York**

Founded in 1957

**DEGREES • BS • DNP • MS**

**Nursing Program Faculty** 64 (68% with doctorates).
**Baccalaureate Enrollment** 493 **Women** 83% **Men** 17% **Minority** 46% **International** 12% **Part-time** 71%
**Graduate Enrollment** 557 **Women** 91% **Men** 9% **Minority** 41% **International** 7% **Part-time** 95%
**Distance Learning Courses** Available.
**Nursing Student Activities** Nursing Honor Society, Sigma Theta Tau, Student Nurses' Association, nursing club.
**Nursing Student Resources** Academic advising; academic or career counseling; assistance for students with disabilities; bookstore; campus computer network; career placement assistance; computer lab; computer-assisted instruction; daycare for children of students; e-mail services; employment services for current students; housing assistance; interactive nursing skills videos; Internet; learning resource lab; library services; nursing audiovisuals; placement services for program completers; resume preparation assistance; skills, simulation, or other laboratory.
**Library Facilities** 2.3 million volumes (11,022 in health, 5,075 in nursing); 55,500 periodical subscriptions (280,000 health-care related).

## BACCALAUREATE PROGRAMS

**Degree** BS
**Available Programs** Accelerated Baccalaureate; Generic Baccalaureate; RN Baccalaureate.
**Study Options** Full-time and part-time.
**Program Entrance Requirements** Minimum overall college GPA of 2.5, transcript of college record, CPR certification, written essay, health insurance, immunizations, 3 letters of recommendation, minimum GPA in nursing prerequisites of 2.5, professional liability insurance/malpractice insurance. *Application deadline:* 1/5 (fall), 11/2 (summer). *Application fee:* $40.
**Advanced Placement** Credit by examination available. Credit given for nursing courses completed elsewhere dependent upon specific evaluations.
**Contact** *Telephone:* 631-444-3241. *Fax:* 631-444-3136.

## GRADUATE PROGRAMS

**Contact** *Telephone:* 631-444-2644. *Fax:* 631-444-3136.

### MASTER'S DEGREE PROGRAM

**Degree** MS
**Available Programs** Master's; RN to Master's.
**Concentrations Available** Nurse-midwifery. *Clinical nurse specialist programs in:* adult health, community health, critical care, parent-child, pediatric, perinatal, psychiatric/mental health,women's health. *Nurse practitioner programs in:* adult health, neonatal health, pediatric, psychiatric/mental health,women's health.
**Study Options** Full-time and part-time.
**Program Entrance Requirements** Clinical experience, computer literacy, minimum overall college GPA of 3.0, transcript of college record, CPR certification, written essay, immunizations, interview, 3 letters of recommendation, physical assessment course, professional liability insurance/malpractice insurance, prerequisite course work, resume, statistics course. *Application deadline:* 4/1 (fall), 1/20 (summer). *Application fee:* $40.
**Advanced Placement** Credit given for nursing courses completed elsewhere dependent upon specific evaluations.
**Degree Requirements** 45 total credit hours.

### POST-MASTER'S PROGRAM

**Areas of Study** Nurse-midwifery. *Clinical nurse specialist programs in:* adult health, community health, critical care, parent-child, pediatric, perinatal, psychiatric/mental health,women's health. *Nurse practitioner programs in:* adult health, neonatal health, pediatric, psychiatric/mental health,women's health.

### DOCTORAL DEGREE PROGRAM

**Degree** DNP
**Available Programs** Doctorate.
**Areas of Study** Advanced practice nursing, biology of health and illness, clinical practice, ethics, health policy, health promotion/disease prevention, health-care systems, individualized study, nursing policy, nursing research.
**Program Entrance Requirements** Clinical experience, minimum overall college GPA of 3.0, interview by faculty committee, interview, 3 letters of recommendation, MSN or equivalent, vita, writing sample. *Application deadline:* 12/1 (summer). *Application fee:* $60.
**Degree Requirements** 42 total credit hours.

## CONTINUING EDUCATION PROGRAM

**Contact** *Telephone:* 631-444-3259. *Fax:* 631-444-3136.

# Trocaire College

**Nursing Program**
**Buffalo, New York**

Founded in 1958

**DEGREE • BS**

## BACCALAUREATE PROGRAMS

**Degree** BS
**Available Programs** Generic Baccalaureate.
**Online Degree Options** Yes (online only).
**Contact** Dr. Susan Lombardo, Associate Dean/Director of BSN Program, Nursing Program, Trocaire College, 360 Choate Avenue, Buffalo, NY 14220-2094. *Telephone:* 716-827-2407. *E-mail:* LombardoS@Trocaire.edu.

# University at Buffalo, the State University of New York
## School of Nursing
## Buffalo, New York

*http://www.nursing.buffalo.edu/*
Founded in 1846

**DEGREES • BS • DNP • MS • PHD**

**Nursing Program Faculty** 54 (69% with doctorates).
**Baccalaureate Enrollment** 231 **Women** 85% **Men** 15% **Minority** 34% **International** 4% **Part-time** 11%
**Graduate Enrollment** 177 **Women** 81% **Men** 19% **Minority** 33% **International** 6% **Part-time** 57%
**Distance Learning Courses** Available.
**Nursing Student Activities** Nursing Honor Society, Sigma Theta Tau, nursing club.
**Nursing Student Resources** Academic advising; academic or career counseling; assistance for students with disabilities; bookstore; campus computer network; career placement assistance; computer lab; computer-assisted instruction; daycare for children of students; e-mail services; employment services for current students; externships; housing assistance; interactive nursing skills videos; Internet; learning resource lab; library services; nursing audiovisuals; placement services for program completers; remedial services; resume preparation assistance; skills, simulation, or other laboratory; unpaid internships.
**Library Facilities** 4.1 million volumes (250,000 in health, 25,000 in nursing); 101,758 periodical subscriptions (2,500 health-care related).

### BACCALAUREATE PROGRAMS

**Degree** BS
**Available Programs** Accelerated Baccalaureate for Second Degree; Generic Baccalaureate; RN Baccalaureate.
**Study Options** Full-time.
**Online Degree Options** Yes.
**Program Entrance Requirements** Minimum overall college GPA of 3.0, transcript of college record, CPR certification, written essay, health exam, health insurance, immunizations, minimum GPA in nursing prerequisites of 3.0, prerequisite course work. Transfer students are accepted. *Application deadline:* 2/15 (fall).
**Advanced Placement** Credit given for nursing courses completed elsewhere dependent upon specific evaluations.
**Expenses (2013–14)** *Tuition, state resident:* full-time $5870; part-time $245 per credit hour. *Tuition, nonresident:* full-time $17,810; part-time $742 per credit hour. *International tuition:* $17,810 full-time. *Room and board:* $11,857; room only: $6867 per academic year. *Required fees:* full-time $1747; part-time $106 per credit; part-time $468 per term.
**Financial Aid** 80% of baccalaureate students in nursing programs received some form of financial aid in 2012–13. *Gift aid (need-based):* Federal Pell, FSEOG, state, private, college/university gift aid from institutional funds, Federal Nursing. *Loans:* Federal Nursing Student Loans, Federal Direct (Subsidized and Unsubsidized Stafford PLUS), Perkins, college/university. *Work-study:* Federal Work-Study, part-time campus jobs. *Financial aid application deadline (priority):* 3/1.
**Contact** Dr. David J. Lang, Director of Student Affairs, School of Nursing, University at Buffalo, the State University of New York, 103 Wende Hall, 3435 Main Street, Buffalo, NY 14214. *Telephone:* 716-829-2537. *Fax:* 716-829-2067. *E-mail:* nursing@buffalo.edu.

### GRADUATE PROGRAMS

**Expenses (2013–14)** *Tuition, state resident:* full-time $9870; part-time $411 per credit hour. *Tuition, nonresident:* full-time $18,350; part-time $765 per credit hour. *International tuition:* $18,350 full-time. *Room and board:* $11,144; room only: $8694 per academic year. *Required fees:* full-time $1253; part-time $140 per credit; part-time $308 per term.
**Financial Aid** 80% of graduate students in nursing programs received some form of financial aid in 2012–13. 3 fellowships with full and partial tuition reimbursements available (averaging $17,000 per year), 3 research assistantships with full and partial tuition reimbursements available (averaging $10,600 per year), 7 teaching assistantships with full and partial tuition reimbursements available (averaging $10,600 per year) were awarded; scholarships, traineeships, and unspecified assistantships also available. *Financial aid application deadline:* 3/15.
**Contact** Dr. David J. Lang, Director of Student Affairs, School of Nursing, University at Buffalo, the State University of New York, 103 Wende Hall, 3435 Main Street, Buffalo, NY 14214. *Telephone:* 716-829-2537. *Fax:* 716-829-2067. *E-mail:* nursing@buffalo.edu.

#### MASTER'S DEGREE PROGRAM

**Degree** MS
**Available Programs** Master's.
**Concentrations Available** Nursing administration. *Nurse practitioner programs in:* adult health, family health, psychiatric/mental health.
**Study Options** Full-time and part-time.
**Program Entrance Requirements** Computer literacy, minimum overall college GPA of 3.0, transcript of college record, CPR certification, written essay, immunizations, interview, 3 letters of recommendation, resume, statistics course. *Application deadline:* Applications may be processed on a rolling basis for some programs. *Application fee:* $75.
**Advanced Placement** Credit given for nursing courses completed elsewhere dependent upon specific evaluations.
**Degree Requirements** 44 total credit hours, thesis or project.

#### DOCTORAL DEGREE PROGRAM

**Degree** DNP
**Available Programs** Doctorate; Post-Baccalaureate Doctorate.
**Areas of Study** Addiction/substance abuse, advanced practice nursing, aging, biology of health and illness, clinical nurse leader, clinical practice, community health, critical care, ethics, faculty preparation, family health, gerontology, health policy, health promotion/disease prevention, health-care systems, human health and illness, individualized study, information systems, maternity-newborn, nurse case management, nursing administration, nursing education, nursing policy, nursing research, nursing science, oncology, palliative care, urban health,women's health.
**Online Degree Options** Yes.
**Program Entrance Requirements** Clinical experience, minimum overall college GPA of 3.25, interview by faculty committee, interview, 3 letters of recommendation, statistics course, vita, writing sample, GRE or MAT. *Application deadline:* Applications may be processed on a rolling basis for some programs. *Application fee:* $75.
**Degree Requirements** 93 total credit hours.

**Degree** PhD
**Available Programs** Doctorate, Post-Baccalaureate Doctorate.
**Areas of Study** Addiction/substance abuse, advanced practice nursing, aging, biology of health and illness, clinical nurse leader, clinical practice, community health, critical care, ethics, faculty preparation, gerontology, health policy, health promotion/disease prevention, health-care systems, human health and illness, individualized study, information systems, maternity-newborn, nurse case management, nursing administration, nursing education, nursing policy, nursing research, nursing science, oncology, palliative care, urban health,women's health.
**Online Degree Options** Yes.
**Program Entrance Requirements** Minimum overall college GPA of 3.5, clinical experience, interview, interview by faculty member, 3 letters of recommendation, vita, writing sample. *Application deadline:* Applications processed on a rolling basis. *Application fee:* $75.
**Degree Requirements** 57 total credit hours, dissertation, written exam.

# University of Rochester
## School of Nursing
## Rochester, New York

*http://www.son.rochester.edu/*
Founded in 1850

**DEGREES • BS • DNP • MS • MSN/PHD • PHD**

**Contact** Ms. Elaine M. Andolina, Director of Admissions, School of Nursing, University of Rochester, Box SON, 601 Elmwood Avenue, Rochester, NY 14642. *Telephone:* 585-275-2375. *Fax:* 585-756-8299. *E-mail:* son_admissions@urmc.rochester.edu.

# Utica College
## Department of Nursing
## Utica, New York

*http://www.utica.edu/*
Founded in 1946

**DEGREE • BS**

**Nursing Program Faculty** 83 (6% with doctorates).

**Baccalaureate Enrollment** 668 **Women** 89% **Men** 11% **Minority** 29% **Part-time** 60%
**Distance Learning Courses** Available.
**Nursing Student Activities** Sigma Theta Tau, Student Nurses' Association.
**Nursing Student Resources** Academic advising; academic or career counseling; assistance for students with disabilities; bookstore; campus computer network; career placement assistance; computer lab; computer-assisted instruction; e-mail services; employment services for current students; externships; housing assistance; interactive nursing skills videos; Internet; learning resource lab; library services; nursing audiovisuals; paid internships; placement services for program completers; remedial services; resume preparation assistance; skills, simulation, or other laboratory; tutoring; unpaid internships.
**Library Facilities** 145,412 volumes (2,652 in health, 1,122 in nursing); 657 periodical subscriptions (118 health-care related).

### BACCALAUREATE PROGRAMS

**Degree** BS
**Available Programs** Accelerated Baccalaureate for Second Degree; Generic Baccalaureate; RN Baccalaureate.
**Site Options** Syracuse, NY.
**Study Options** Full-time and part-time.
**Online Degree Options** Yes.
**Program Entrance Requirements** Minimum overall college GPA of 2.8, transcript of college record, written essay, health exam, health insurance, high school biology, high school chemistry, 3 years high school math, 3 years high school science, high school transcript, immunizations, 3 letters of recommendation, minimum high school GPA of 3.0, minimum high school rank 25%, minimum GPA in nursing prerequisites of 2.8. Transfer students are accepted. *Application deadline:* 3/15 (fall), 11/15 (spring). Applications may be processed on a rolling basis for some programs. *Application fee:* $40.
**Advanced Placement** Credit by examination available. Credit given for nursing courses completed elsewhere dependent upon specific evaluations.
**Expenses (2013–14)** *Tuition:* full-time $32,280; part-time $1076 per credit hour. *Room and board:* $12,418 per academic year. *Required fees:* full-time $850; part-time $50 per term.
**Financial Aid** 97% of baccalaureate students in nursing programs received some form of financial aid in 2012–13. *Gift aid (need-based):* Federal Pell, FSEOG, state, private, college/university gift aid from institutional funds. *Loans:* Federal Direct (Subsidized and Unsubsidized Stafford PLUS), Perkins. *Work-study:* Federal Work-Study, part-time campus jobs. *Financial aid application deadline (priority):* 2/15.
**Contact** Mr. Patrick A. Quinn, Vice President for Enrollment Management, Department of Nursing, Utica College, 1600 Burrstone Road, Utica, NY 13502-4892. *Telephone:* 315-792-3006. *Fax:* 315-792-3003. *E-mail:* pquinn@utica.edu.

# Wagner College

## Department of Nursing
## Staten Island, New York

***http://www.wagner.edu/departments/nursing/***
Founded in 1883

### DEGREES • BS • MSN

**Nursing Program Faculty** 17 (90% with doctorates).
**Baccalaureate Enrollment** 60 **Women** 82% **Men** 18% **Minority** 20% **International** 10% **Part-time** 5%
**Graduate Enrollment** 63 **Women** 90% **Men** 10% **Minority** 10% **Part-time** 95%
**Nursing Student Activities** Nursing Honor Society, Sigma Theta Tau, Student Nurses' Association.
**Nursing Student Resources** Academic advising; academic or career counseling; assistance for students with disabilities; bookstore; campus computer network; career placement assistance; computer lab; computer-assisted instruction; e-mail services; externships; housing assistance; interactive nursing skills videos; Internet; learning resource lab; library services; nursing audiovisuals; remedial services; skills, simulation, or other laboratory; tutoring; unpaid internships.
**Library Facilities** 158,160 volumes (4,505 in health, 859 in nursing); 56,399 periodical subscriptions (87 health-care related).

### BACCALAUREATE PROGRAMS

**Degree** BS
**Available Programs** Baccalaureate for Second Degree; Generic Baccalaureate.
**Study Options** Full-time.
**Program Entrance Requirements** Minimum overall college GPA of 3.0, written essay, health exam, health insurance, high school chemistry, high school transcript, immunizations, letters of recommendation, minimum high school GPA of 2.7, minimum GPA in nursing prerequisites of 3.0, prerequisite course work. Transfer students are accepted.
**Advanced Placement** Credit by examination available. Credit given for nursing courses completed elsewhere dependent upon specific evaluations.
**Contact** *Telephone:* 718-390-3452. *Fax:* 718-420-4009.

### GRADUATE PROGRAMS

**Contact** *Telephone:* 718-390-3444. *Fax:* 718-420-4009.

#### MASTER'S DEGREE PROGRAM

**Degree** MSN
**Concentrations Available** Nursing education. *Nurse practitioner programs in:* family health.
**Study Options** Full-time and part-time.
**Program Entrance Requirements** Clinical experience, minimum overall college GPA of 2.7, transcript of college record, CPR certification, immunizations, interview, 2 letters of recommendation, nursing research course, professional liability insurance/malpractice insurance, resume.
**Degree Requirements** 44 total credit hours.

#### POST-MASTER'S PROGRAM

**Areas of Study** *Nurse practitioner programs in:* family health.

# York College of the City University of New York

## Program in Nursing
## Jamaica, New York

***http://www.york.cuny.edu/academics/departments/health-professions/nursing***
Founded in 1967

### DEGREE • BS

**Nursing Program Faculty** 9 (20% with doctorates).
**Baccalaureate Enrollment** 80 **Women** 85% **Men** 15% **Minority** 80% **Part-time** 50%
**Nursing Student Activities** Nursing club.
**Nursing Student Resources** Academic advising; academic or career counseling; assistance for students with disabilities; bookstore; campus computer network; career placement assistance; computer lab; computer-assisted instruction; daycare for children of students; e-mail services; employment services for current students; Internet; library services; resume preparation assistance; skills, simulation, or other laboratory; tutoring.
**Library Facilities** 575,480 volumes (8,714 in health, 567 in nursing); 71,713 periodical subscriptions.

### BACCALAUREATE PROGRAMS

**Degree** BS
**Available Programs** ADN to Baccalaureate; RN Baccalaureate.
**Program Entrance Requirements** Minimum overall college GPA of 3.0, transcript of college record, CPR certification, health exam, immunizations, minimum GPA in nursing prerequisites of 3.0, professional liability insurance/malpractice insurance, prerequisite course work, RN licensure. Transfer students are accepted.
**Advanced Placement** Credit by examination available. Credit given for nursing courses completed elsewhere dependent upon specific evaluations.
**Contact** *Telephone:* 718-262-2165.

# NORTH CAROLINA

## Appalachian State University
### Department of Nursing
### Boone, North Carolina

*http://www.nursing.appstate.edu/*
Founded in 1899

**DEGREE • BSN**
**Nursing Program Faculty** 15 (50% with doctorates).
**Baccalaureate Enrollment** 146 **Women** 90% **Men** 10% **Minority** 5%
**Distance Learning Courses** Available.
**Nursing Student Activities** Nursing Honor Society, Sigma Theta Tau, Student Nurses' Association, nursing club.
**Nursing Student Resources** Academic advising; academic or career counseling; assistance for students with disabilities; bookstore; campus computer network; career placement assistance; computer lab; computer-assisted instruction; e-mail services; interactive nursing skills videos; Internet; learning resource lab; library services; nursing audiovisuals; remedial services; skills, simulation, or other laboratory; tutoring.
**Library Facilities** 937,956 volumes (3.2 million in health, 541,000 in nursing); 23,861 periodical subscriptions (6,764 health-care related).

#### BACCALAUREATE PROGRAMS
**Degree** BSN
**Available Programs** Generic Baccalaureate; RN Baccalaureate.
**Study Options** Full-time.
**Online Degree Options** Yes.
**Program Entrance Requirements** Minimum overall college GPA of 3.0, transcript of college record, CPR certification, health exam, immunizations, minimum GPA in nursing prerequisites of 2.5, professional liability insurance/malpractice insurance, prerequisite course work. Transfer students are accepted. *Application deadline:* 1/15 (fall). *Application fee:* $50.
**Financial Aid** 50% of baccalaureate students in nursing programs received some form of financial aid in 2011–12. *Gift aid (need-based):* Federal Pell, FSEOG, state, private, college/university gift aid from institutional funds. *Loans:* Federal Direct (Subsidized and Unsubsidized Stafford PLUS), Perkins. *Work-study:* Federal Work-Study. *Financial aid application deadline:* Continuous.
**Contact** Ms. Teri Goodman, Administrative Assistant, Department of Nursing, Appalachian State University, Edwin Duncan Hall, Suite 318, 730 River Street, Boone, NC 28608. *Telephone:* 828-262-8039. *Fax:* 828-262-8066. *E-mail:* goodmantk@appstate.edu.

## Barton College
### School of Nursing
### Wilson, North Carolina

*http://www.barton.edu*
Founded in 1902

**DEGREE • BSN**
**Nursing Program Faculty** 10 (30% with doctorates).
**Baccalaureate Enrollment** 98 **Women** 94.8% **Men** 5.2% **Minority** 17.9% **International** 2.5% **Part-time** 3.8%
**Nursing Student Activities** Sigma Theta Tau, Student Nurses' Association, nursing club.
**Nursing Student Resources** Academic advising; academic or career counseling; assistance for students with disabilities; bookstore; campus computer network; career placement assistance; computer lab; computer-assisted instruction; e-mail services; employment services for current students; externships; interactive nursing skills videos; Internet; learning resource lab; library services; nursing audiovisuals; paid internships; placement services for program completers; remedial services; resume preparation assistance; skills, simulation, or other laboratory; tutoring; unpaid internships.
**Library Facilities** 3,500 volumes in health, 2,250 volumes in nursing; 100 periodical subscriptions health-care related.

#### BACCALAUREATE PROGRAMS
**Degree** BSN
**Available Programs** ADN to Baccalaureate; Generic Baccalaureate; RN Baccalaureate.
**Study Options** Full-time and part-time.
**Program Entrance Requirements** Minimum overall college GPA of 2.5, transcript of college record, CPR certification, health exam, health insurance, high school biology, high school chemistry, high school transcript, immunizations, minimum GPA in nursing prerequisites of 2.7, professional liability insurance/malpractice insurance, prerequisite course work. Transfer students are accepted. *Application deadline:* 11/1 (fall).
**Advanced Placement** Credit given for nursing courses completed elsewhere dependent upon specific evaluations.
**Contact** *Telephone:* 252-399-6400. *Fax:* 252-399-6416.

## Cabarrus College of Health Sciences
### Louise Harkey School of Nursing
### Concord, North Carolina

*http://www.cabarruscollege.edu/*
Founded in 1942

**DEGREE • BSN**
**Nursing Program Faculty** 3 (25% with doctorates).
**Baccalaureate Enrollment** 35 **Women** 90% **Men** 10% **Minority** 10% **Part-time** 50%
**Distance Learning Courses** Available.
**Nursing Student Activities** Sigma Theta Tau, Student Nurses' Association, nursing club.
**Nursing Student Resources** Academic advising; academic or career counseling; assistance for students with disabilities; bookstore; campus computer network; career placement assistance; computer lab; computer-assisted instruction; e-mail services; interactive nursing skills videos; Internet; library services; resume preparation assistance; skills, simulation, or other laboratory.
**Library Facilities** 500 volumes in health, 300 volumes in nursing; 300 periodical subscriptions health-care related.

#### BACCALAUREATE PROGRAMS
**Degree** BSN
**Available Programs** RN Baccalaureate.
**Study Options** Full-time and part-time.
**Program Entrance Requirements** Minimum overall college GPA of 2.5, transcript of college record, CPR certification, written essay, health exam, health insurance, 4 years high school math, immunizations, 2 letters of recommendation, RN licensure. Transfer students are accepted. *Application deadline:* 5/1 (fall), 10/1 (spring). Applications may be processed on a rolling basis for some programs. *Application fee:* $35.
**Advanced Placement** Credit by examination available.
**Contact** *Telephone:* 704-403-1756. *Fax:* 704-403-2077.

## Duke University
### School of Nursing
### Durham, North Carolina

*http://www.nursing.duke.edu/*
Founded in 1838

**DEGREES • BSN • MSN • MSN/MBA • PHD**
**Nursing Program Faculty** 81 (94% with doctorates).
**Baccalaureate Enrollment** 214 **Women** 88% **Men** 12% **Minority** 21% **International** 1% **Part-time** 2%
**Graduate Enrollment** 600 **Women** 91% **Men** 9% **Minority** 24% **International** 2% **Part-time** 7%
**Distance Learning Courses** Available.
**Nursing Student Activities** Sigma Theta Tau, Student Nurses' Association.
**Nursing Student Resources** Academic advising; academic or career counseling; assistance for students with disabilities; bookstore; campus computer network; career placement assistance; computer lab; computer-assisted instruction; e-mail services; Internet; library services; nursing audiovisuals; resume preparation assistance; skills, simulation, or other laboratory.
**Library Facilities** 6 million volumes (183,513 in health, 12,366 in nursing); 62,639 periodical subscriptions (4,391 health-care related).

## BACCALAUREATE PROGRAMS

**Degree** BSN
**Available Programs** Accelerated Baccalaureate for Second Degree.
**Site Options** Durham, NC.
**Study Options** Full-time.
**Program Entrance Requirements** Minimum overall college GPA of 3.0, transcript of college record, CPR certification, written essay, health exam, health insurance, immunizations, interview, 3 letters of recommendation, prerequisite course work. *Application deadline:* 12/1 (fall), 6/1 (spring). *Application fee:* $50.
**Expenses (2013–14)** *Tuition:* full-time $39,824; part-time $1111 per credit. *International tuition:* $39,824 full-time. *Required fees:* full-time $1375.
**Financial Aid** 97% of baccalaureate students in nursing programs received some form of financial aid in 2012–13. *Gift aid (need-based):* Federal Pell, FSEOG, state, private, college/university gift aid from institutional funds. *Loans:* Federal Direct (Subsidized and Unsubsidized Stafford PLUS), Perkins, college/university, alternative loans. *Work-study:* Federal Work-Study, part-time campus jobs. *Financial aid application deadline:* 3/1.
**Contact** Mr. Nora Harrington, Admissions Officer, School of Nursing, Duke University, 307 Trent Drive, Box 102400, Durham, NC 27710. *Telephone:* 919-684-4248. *Fax:* 919-668-4693. *E-mail:* SONAdmissions@dm.duke.edu.

## GRADUATE PROGRAMS

**Expenses (2013–14)** *Tuition:* full-time $25,650; part-time $1425 per credit. *Required fees:* full-time $832.
**Financial Aid** 64% of graduate students in nursing programs received some form of financial aid in 2012–13. Career-related internships or fieldwork, institutionally sponsored loans, scholarships, traineeships, and tuition waivers (partial) available. Aid available to part-time students. *Financial aid application deadline:* 4/1.
**Contact** Ms. Nicole Fleming, Admissions Officer, School of Nursing, Duke University, 307 Trent Drive, Box 102400, Durham, NC 27710. *Telephone:* 919-684-4248. *Fax:* 919-668-4693. *E-mail:* SONAdmissions@dm.duke.edu.

### MASTER'S DEGREE PROGRAM

**Degrees** MSN; MSN/MBA
**Available Programs** Master's; RN to Master's.
**Concentrations Available** Health-care administration; nurse anesthesia; nurse case management; nursing administration; nursing education; nursing informatics. *Nurse practitioner programs in:* acute care, adult health, family health, gerontology, neonatal health, oncology, pediatric, primary care.
**Site Options** Durham, NC.
**Study Options** Full-time and part-time.
**Online Degree Options** Yes.
**Program Entrance Requirements** Clinical experience, computer literacy, minimum overall college GPA of 3.0, transcript of college record, CPR certification, written essay, immunizations, interview, 3 letters of recommendation, prerequisite course work, resume, statistics course, GRE General Test. *Application deadline:* 12/1 (fall), 6/1 (spring). *Application fee:* $50.
**Advanced Placement** Credit given for nursing courses completed elsewhere dependent upon specific evaluations.
**Degree Requirements** 39 total credit hours.

### POST-MASTER'S PROGRAM

**Areas of Study** Health-care administration; nurse anesthesia; nurse case management; nursing administration; nursing education; nursing informatics. *Nurse practitioner programs in:* acute care, adult health, family health, gerontology, neonatal health, oncology, pediatric, primary care.

### DOCTORAL DEGREE PROGRAM

**Degree** PhD
**Available Programs** Doctorate; Post-Baccalaureate Doctorate.
**Areas of Study** Health-care systems, illness and transition.
**Site Options** Durham, NC.
**Program Entrance Requirements** Minimum overall college GPA of 3.5, interview by faculty committee, interview, 3 letters of recommendation, MSN or equivalent, statistics course, vita. *Application deadline:* 12/15 (fall). *Application fee:* $75.
**Degree Requirements** 54 total credit hours, dissertation, oral exam.

# East Carolina University
## College of Nursing
## Greenville, North Carolina

*http://www.nursing.ecu.edu/*
Founded in 1907

**DEGREES • BSN • MSN • PHD**
**Nursing Program Faculty** 104 (40% with doctorates).
**Baccalaureate Enrollment** 628 **Women** 90.6% **Men** 9.4% **Minority** 13.4% **International** .4% **Part-time** 16.2%
**Graduate Enrollment** 559 **Women** 90.8% **Men** 9.2% **Minority** 14.6% **Part-time** 73.2%
**Distance Learning Courses** Available.
**Nursing Student Activities** Nursing Honor Society, Sigma Theta Tau, Student Nurses' Association.
**Nursing Student Resources** Academic advising; academic or career counseling; assistance for students with disabilities; bookstore; campus computer network; career placement assistance; computer lab; computer-assisted instruction; e-mail services; employment services for current students; externships; housing assistance; interactive nursing skills videos; Internet; learning resource lab; library services; nursing audiovisuals; remedial services; resume preparation assistance; skills, simulation, or other laboratory; tutoring; unpaid internships.
**Library Facilities** 2.4 million volumes (135,271 in health, 4,000 in nursing); 73,498 periodical subscriptions (16,000 health-care related).

## BACCALAUREATE PROGRAMS

**Degree** BSN
**Available Programs** ADN to Baccalaureate; Generic Baccalaureate.
**Study Options** Full-time.
**Online Degree Options** Yes.
**Program Entrance Requirements** Minimum overall college GPA of 2.5, transcript of college record, CPR certification, health exam, health insurance, immunizations, professional liability insurance/malpractice insurance, prerequisite course work. Transfer students are accepted. *Application deadline:* 2/1 (fall), 9/1 (spring).
**Advanced Placement** Credit given for nursing courses completed elsewhere dependent upon specific evaluations.
**Contact** *Telephone:* 252-744-6477. *Fax:* 252-744-6391.

## GRADUATE PROGRAMS

**Contact** *Telephone:* 252-744-6477. *Fax:* 252-744-6391.

### MASTER'S DEGREE PROGRAM

**Degree** MSN
**Available Programs** Accelerated Master's for Non-Nursing College Graduates; Accelerated Master's for Nurses with Non-Nursing Degrees; Master's; RN to Master's.
**Concentrations Available** Nurse anesthesia; nurse-midwifery; nursing administration; nursing education. *Clinical nurse specialist programs in:* adult health. *Nurse practitioner programs in:* adult health, family health, neonatal health.
**Study Options** Full-time and part-time.
**Online Degree Options** Yes.
**Program Entrance Requirements** Clinical experience, computer literacy, minimum overall college GPA of 3.0, transcript of college record, CPR certification, written essay, immunizations, interview, 3 letters of recommendation, nursing research course, professional liability insurance/malpractice insurance, prerequisite course work, statistics course, GRE General Test or MAT. *Application deadline:* Applications may be processed on a rolling basis for some programs.
**Advanced Placement** Credit given for nursing courses completed elsewhere dependent upon specific evaluations.
**Degree Requirements** Comprehensive exam.

### POST-MASTER'S PROGRAM

**Areas of Study** Nurse anesthesia; nurse-midwifery; nursing administration; nursing education. *Clinical nurse specialist programs in:* adult health. *Nurse practitioner programs in:* adult health, family health, neonatal health.

### DOCTORAL DEGREE PROGRAM

**Degree** PhD
**Available Programs** Doctorate; Post-Baccalaureate Doctorate.
**Areas of Study** Nursing science.
**Program Entrance Requirements** Minimum overall college GPA of 3.2, interview by faculty committee, interview, 3 letters of recommen-

dation, MSN or equivalent, scholarly papers, statistics course, vita, writing sample. *Application deadline:* 3/1 (fall).
**Degree Requirements** 54 total credit hours, dissertation, oral exam, written exam.

# Fayetteville State University

## Program in Nursing
## Fayetteville, North Carolina

***http://www.uncfsu.edu/nursing/***
Founded in 1867

**DEGREE • BSN**
**Library Facilities** 365,783 volumes; 3,488 periodical subscriptions.

### BACCALAUREATE PROGRAMS

**Degree** BSN
**Available Programs** Generic Baccalaureate; RN Baccalaureate.
**Program Entrance Requirements** Minimum overall college GPA of 2.0, transcript of college record, CPR certification, health exam, health insurance, high school biology, 2.0 years high school math, high school transcript, immunizations, minimum high school GPA of 2.0, minimum GPA in nursing prerequisites of 2.0, professional liability insurance/malpractice insurance, prerequisite course work, RN licensure. Transfer students are accepted.
**Contact** Ms. Jacinta Williams, Lecturer/Student Coordinator, Program in Nursing, Fayetteville State University, 1200 Murchison Road, Fayetteville, NC 28301-4298. *Telephone:* 910-672-1925. *E-mail:* jwill126@uncfsu.edu.

# Gardner-Webb University

## School of Nursing
## Boiling Springs, North Carolina

***http://www.gardner-webb.edu/***
Founded in 1905

**DEGREES • BSN • DNP • MSN • MSN/MBA**
**Nursing Program Faculty** 35 (30% with doctorates).
**Baccalaureate Enrollment** 360 **Women** 93% **Men** 7% **Minority** 10% **Part-time** 51%
**Graduate Enrollment** 154 **Women** 96% **Men** 4% **Minority** 94% **International** 1% **Part-time** 38%
**Distance Learning Courses** Available.
**Nursing Student Activities** Sigma Theta Tau, Student Nurses' Association.
**Nursing Student Resources** Academic advising; assistance for students with disabilities; bookstore; campus computer network; computer lab; computer-assisted instruction; e-mail services; housing assistance; interactive nursing skills videos; Internet; learning resource lab; library services; nursing audiovisuals; other; paid internships; remedial services; resume preparation assistance; skills, simulation, or other laboratory; tutoring.
**Library Facilities** 297,291 volumes (6,002 in health, 2,146 in nursing); 230,143 periodical subscriptions (7,808 health-care related).

### BACCALAUREATE PROGRAMS

**Degree** BSN
**Available Programs** ADN to Baccalaureate; Generic Baccalaureate.
**Study Options** Full-time and part-time.
**Online Degree Options** Yes.
**Program Entrance Requirements** Minimum overall college GPA of 3.00, transcript of college record, CPR certification, high school biology, high school chemistry, high school transcript, immunizations, minimum high school GPA of 3.00, minimum GPA in nursing prerequisites of 3.00, professional liability insurance/malpractice insurance, prerequisite course work. Transfer students are accepted. *Application deadline:* 2/15 (fall). *Application fee:* $40.
**Expenses (2013–14)** *Tuition:* full-time $25,440; part-time $406 per credit hour. *Room and board:* $13,000; room only: $8000 per academic year. *Required fees:* full-time $9500.
**Financial Aid** 99% of baccalaureate students in nursing programs received some form of financial aid in 2012–13. *Gift aid (need-based):* Federal Pell, FSEOG, state, private, college/university gift aid from institutional funds. *Loans:* Federal Direct (Subsidized and Unsubsidized Stafford PLUS), Perkins, state, alternative loans. *Work-study:* Federal Work-Study, part-time campus jobs. *Financial aid application deadline (priority):* 3/15.
**Contact** Dr. Reimund Serafica, Chair, School of Nursing, Gardner-Webb University, PO Box 7309, Boiling Springs, NC 28017. *Telephone:* 704-406-2298. *Fax:* 704-406-3919. *E-mail:* rserafica@gardner-webb.edu.

### GRADUATE PROGRAMS

**Expenses (2013–14)** *Tuition:* full-time $4800; part-time $400 per credit hour. *Required fees:* full-time $505.
**Financial Aid** 58% of graduate students in nursing programs received some form of financial aid in 2012–13.
**Contact** Dr. Cindy Miller, Director of MSN Program, School of Nursing, Gardner-Webb University, PO Box 7309, Boiling Springs, NC 28017. *Telephone:* 704-406-4364. *Fax:* 704-406-3919. *E-mail:* mlmiller@gardner-webb.edu.

#### MASTER'S DEGREE PROGRAM

**Degrees** MSN; MSN/MBA
**Available Programs** Master's; Master's for Non-Nursing College Graduates; RN to Master's.
**Concentrations Available** Nursing administration; nursing education. *Nurse practitioner programs in:* family health.
**Study Options** Full-time and part-time.
**Online Degree Options** Yes (online only).
**Program Entrance Requirements** Minimum overall college GPA of 3.0, transcript of college record, immunizations, 3 letters of recommendation, statistics course. *Application deadline:* Applications may be processed on a rolling basis for some programs. *Application fee:* $40.
**Advanced Placement** Credit given for nursing courses completed elsewhere dependent upon specific evaluations.
**Degree Requirements** 36 total credit hours, thesis or project.

#### DOCTORAL DEGREE PROGRAM

**Degree** DNP
**Available Programs** Doctorate.
**Areas of Study** Ethics, faculty preparation, gerontology, health policy, health promotion/disease prevention, health-care systems, human health and illness, information systems, nurse case management, nursing administration, nursing education, nursing policy, nursing research, nursing science.
**Program Entrance Requirements** Clinical experience, minimum overall college GPA of 3.2, interview by faculty committee, 3 letters of recommendation, MSN or equivalent, vita, writing sample. *Application deadline:* 1/15 (summer).
**Degree Requirements** 36 total credit hours, dissertation.

# Lees-McRae College

## Nursing Program
## Banner Elk, North Carolina

***http://www.lmc.edu/academics/programs_of_study/nursing-allied-health/nursing/index.htm***
Founded in 1900

**DEGREE • BSN**
**Nursing Program Faculty** 6
**Baccalaureate Enrollment** 51 **Women** 88% **Men** 12% **Minority** 2% **International** 2%
**Distance Learning Courses** Available.
**Nursing Student Resources** Academic advising; academic or career counseling; bookstore; computer lab; computer-assisted instruction; e-mail services; Internet; learning resource lab; library services; nursing audiovisuals; skills, simulation, or other laboratory.
**Library Facilities** 216,747 volumes; 22,091 periodical subscriptions.

### BACCALAUREATE PROGRAMS

**Degree** BSN
**Available Programs** ADN to Baccalaureate.
**Site Options** Spruce Pine, NC.
**Study Options** Full-time.
**Online Degree Options** Yes.
**Program Entrance Requirements** Transcript of college record, CPR certification, immunizations, 2 letters of recommendation, professional liability insurance/malpractice insurance, RN licensure. Transfer students are accepted. *Application deadline:* 8/1 (fall). Applications may be processed on a rolling basis for some programs.

**Financial Aid** 100% of baccalaureate students in nursing programs received some form of financial aid in 2012–13.

**Contact** Dr. Laura J. Fero, Director of Nursing, Nursing Program, Lees-McRae College, PO Box 128, Banner Elk, NC 28604. *Telephone:* 828-898-2428. *Fax:* 828-898-2598. *E-mail:* ferol@lmc.edu.

# Lenoir-Rhyne University

## Program in Nursing
## Hickory, North Carolina

*http://nur.lr.edu/*
Founded in 1891

### DEGREES • BS • MSN

**Nursing Program Faculty** 30 (4% with doctorates).
**Baccalaureate Enrollment** 300 **Women** 90% **Men** 10% **Minority** 11% **International** 2% **Part-time** 4%
**Distance Learning Courses** Available.
**Nursing Student Activities** Sigma Theta Tau, Student Nurses' Association.
**Nursing Student Resources** Academic advising; academic or career counseling; assistance for students with disabilities; bookstore; campus computer network; career placement assistance; computer lab; computer-assisted instruction; e-mail services; employment services for current students; externships; housing assistance; interactive nursing skills videos; Internet; learning resource lab; library services; nursing audiovisuals; placement services for program completers; remedial services; resume preparation assistance; skills, simulation, or other laboratory; tutoring; unpaid internships.
**Library Facilities** 5,000 volumes in health, 4,200 volumes in nursing; 220 periodical subscriptions health-care related.

### BACCALAUREATE PROGRAMS

**Degree** BS
**Available Programs** ADN to Baccalaureate; Generic Baccalaureate.
**Study Options** Full-time and part-time.
**Program Entrance Requirements** Minimum overall college GPA of 3.0, transcript of college record, CPR certification, written essay, health exam, high school chemistry, high school foreign language, 3 years high school math, high school transcript, immunizations, minimum high school GPA of 3.0, minimum GPA in nursing prerequisites of 2.7, prerequisite course work. Transfer students are accepted. *Application deadline:* 3/1 (fall), 4/1 (summer). Applications may be processed on a rolling basis for some programs. *Application fee:* $35.
**Advanced Placement** Credit by examination available. Credit given for nursing courses completed elsewhere dependent upon specific evaluations.
**Contact** *Telephone:* 828-328-7282. *Fax:* 828-328-7284.

### GRADUATE PROGRAMS

**Contact** *Telephone:* 828-328-7282.

#### MASTER'S DEGREE PROGRAM

**Degree** MSN
**Available Programs** Master's; RN to Master's.
**Concentrations Available** Health-care administration; nursing education.
**Site Options** Asheville, NC.
**Study Options** Full-time and part-time.
**Program Entrance Requirements** Computer literacy, minimum overall college GPA of 3.0, transcript of college record, CPR certification, written essay, immunizations, interview, letters of recommendation, nursing research course, resume, statistics course. *Application deadline:* Applications may be processed on a rolling basis for some programs. *Application fee:* $35.
**Advanced Placement** Credit given for nursing courses completed elsewhere dependent upon specific evaluations.
**Degree Requirements** 36 total credit hours, thesis or project.

# North Carolina Agricultural and Technical State University

## School of Nursing
## Greensboro, North Carolina

*http://www.ncat.edu/academics/schools-colleges1/son/index.html*
Founded in 1891

### DEGREE • BSN

**Nursing Program Faculty** 29 (15% with doctorates).
**Baccalaureate Enrollment** 110 **Women** 91% **Men** 9% **Minority** 95%
**Nursing Student Activities** Sigma Theta Tau, Student Nurses' Association, nursing club.
**Nursing Student Resources** Academic advising; academic or career counseling; assistance for students with disabilities; bookstore; campus computer network; career placement assistance; computer lab; computer-assisted instruction; e-mail services; housing assistance; interactive nursing skills videos; Internet; learning resource lab; library services; nursing audiovisuals; remedial services; resume preparation assistance; skills, simulation, or other laboratory; tutoring.
**Library Facilities** 702,159 volumes; 3,205 periodical subscriptions.

### BACCALAUREATE PROGRAMS

**Degree** BSN
**Available Programs** Accelerated Baccalaureate for Second Degree; Generic Baccalaureate; RN Baccalaureate.
**Site Options** Greensboro, NC.
**Study Options** Full-time.
**Program Entrance Requirements** Minimum overall college GPA of 2.8, transcript of college record, CPR certification, written essay, health exam, health insurance, high school biology, high school foreign language, 3 years high school math, 3 years high school science, high school transcript, immunizations, minimum high school GPA of 3.0, minimum GPA in nursing prerequisites of 2.8, professional liability insurance/malpractice insurance, prerequisite course work. Transfer students are accepted. *Application deadline:* 2/15 (spring). *Application fee:* $45.
**Expenses (2012–13)** *Tuition, area resident:* full-time $3238. *Tuition, state resident:* full-time $8537. *Room and board:* $3077 per academic year. *Required fees:* full-time $1703.
**Financial Aid** ***Gift aid (need-based):*** Federal Pell, FSEOG, state, private, college/university gift aid from institutional funds. *Loans:* Federal Direct (Subsidized and Unsubsidized Stafford PLUS), Perkins. *Work-study:* Federal Work-Study. *Financial aid application deadline (priority):* 3/1.
**Contact** Mrs. Carliss Jacobs, Student Services Director, School of Nursing, North Carolina Agricultural and Technical State University, Noble Hall, 1601 East Market Street, Greensboro, NC 27411. *Telephone:* 336-334-7750. *Fax:* 336-334-7637. *E-mail:* carlissl@ncat.edu.

# North Carolina Central University

## Department of Nursing
## Durham, North Carolina

*http://www.nccu.edu/*
Founded in 1910

### DEGREE • BSN

**Nursing Program Faculty** 30 (4% with doctorates).
**Nursing Student Activities** Sigma Theta Tau.
**Nursing Student Resources** Academic advising; academic or career counseling; assistance for students with disabilities; bookstore; campus computer network; career placement assistance; computer lab; computer-assisted instruction; e-mail services; employment services for current students; externships; housing assistance; interactive nursing skills videos; Internet; learning resource lab; library services; nursing audiovisuals; paid internships; placement services for program completers; resume preparation assistance; skills, simulation, or other laboratory; tutoring.
**Library Facilities** 695,876 volumes; 1,952 periodical subscriptions.

### BACCALAUREATE PROGRAMS

**Degree** BSN
**Available Programs** Generic Baccalaureate.
**Study Options** Full-time.

**Program Entrance Requirements** Minimum overall college GPA of 2.0, transcript of college record, health exam, immunizations, minimum GPA in nursing prerequisites of 2.5, professional liability insurance/malpractice insurance, prerequisite course work. Transfer students are accepted.
**Advanced Placement** Credit given for nursing courses completed elsewhere dependent upon specific evaluations.
**Contact** *Telephone:* 919-530-5336. *Fax:* 919-530-5343.

# Queens University of Charlotte
## Presbyterian School of Nursing
## Charlotte, North Carolina

***http://www.queens.edu/nursing/***
Founded in 1857

**DEGREES • BSN • MSN • MSN/MBA**
**Nursing Program Faculty** 60 (20% with doctorates).
**Baccalaureate Enrollment** 260 **Women** 95% **Men** 5% **Minority** 25% **International** 5% **Part-time** 10%
**Graduate Enrollment** 55 **Women** 95% **Men** 5% **Minority** 25% **International** 5% **Part-time** 50%
**Distance Learning Courses** Available.
**Nursing Student Activities** Nursing Honor Society, Sigma Theta Tau, Student Nurses' Association.
**Nursing Student Resources** Academic advising; academic or career counseling; assistance for students with disabilities; bookstore; campus computer network; career placement assistance; computer lab; computer-assisted instruction; e-mail services; employment services for current students; externships; housing assistance; interactive nursing skills videos; Internet; learning resource lab; library services; nursing audiovisuals; placement services for program completers; remedial services; resume preparation assistance; skills, simulation, or other laboratory; tutoring; unpaid internships.
**Library Facilities** 126,242 volumes (1,703 in health, 713 in nursing); 592 periodical subscriptions (516 health-care related).

### BACCALAUREATE PROGRAMS
**Degree** BSN
**Available Programs** ADN to Baccalaureate; Accelerated Baccalaureate; Accelerated Baccalaureate for Second Degree; Baccalaureate for Second Degree; Generic Baccalaureate; RN Baccalaureate.
**Site Options** Charlotte, NC.
**Study Options** Full-time.
**Online Degree Options** Yes.
**Program Entrance Requirements** Minimum overall college GPA of 3.0, transcript of college record, CPR certification, written essay, health exam, health insurance, high school biology, high school chemistry, 2 years high school math, 1 year of high school science, high school transcript, immunizations, minimum high school GPA of 3.0, minimum GPA in nursing prerequisites of 3.0, prerequisite course work. Transfer students are accepted. *Application deadline:* 3/15 (fall), 9/21 (spring). *Application fee:* $40.
**Advanced Placement** Credit given for nursing courses completed elsewhere dependent upon specific evaluations.
**Expenses (2013–14)** *Tuition:* full-time $28,800.
**Financial Aid** 85% of baccalaureate students in nursing programs received some form of financial aid in 2012–13.
**Contact** Holly Boyd, Senior Director of Admissions, Presbyterian School of Nursing, Queens University of Charlotte, 1900 Selwyn Avenue, Charlotte, NC 28274. *Telephone:* 704-337-2314. *Fax:* 704-337-2415. *E-mail:* psonadmissions@queens.edu.

### GRADUATE PROGRAMS
**Expenses (2013–14)** *Tuition:* part-time $485 per credit hour.
**Financial Aid** 25% of graduate students in nursing programs received some form of financial aid in 2012–13.
**Contact** Holly Boyd, Senior Director of Admissions, Presbyterian School of Nursing, Queens University of Charlotte, 1900 Selwyn Avenue, Charlotte, NC 28274. *Telephone:* 704-337-2314. *Fax:* 704-337-2415. *E-mail:* psonadmissions@queens.edu.

#### MASTER'S DEGREE PROGRAM
**Degrees** MSN; MSN/MBA
**Available Programs** Master's; RN to Master's.
**Concentrations Available** Clinical nurse leader; nursing administration; nursing education.
**Site Options** Charlotte, NC.
**Study Options** Full-time and part-time.
**Online Degree Options** Yes (online only).
**Program Entrance Requirements** Minimum overall college GPA of 3.0, transcript of college record, written essay, professional liability insurance/malpractice insurance, resume. *Application deadline:* Applications may be processed on a rolling basis for some programs. *Application fee:* $40.
**Advanced Placement** Credit given for nursing courses completed elsewhere dependent upon specific evaluations.
**Degree Requirements** 36 total credit hours, thesis or project.

### CONTINUING EDUCATION PROGRAM
**Contact** Julia Walton, Director, Continuing Education. *Telephone:* 704-688-2838. *E-mail:* waltonj@queens.edu.

# The University of North Carolina at Chapel Hill
## School of Nursing
## Chapel Hill, North Carolina

***http://nursing.unc.edu/***
Founded in 1789

**DEGREES • BSN • DNP • MSN • PHD**
**Nursing Program Faculty** 141 (70% with doctorates).
**Baccalaureate Enrollment** 379 **Women** 82.9% **Men** 17.1% **Minority** 28.2% **International** 5% **Part-time** 7.1%
**Graduate Enrollment** 343 **Women** 90% **Men** 10% **Minority** 28.2% **International** 3.3% **Part-time** 46%
**Distance Learning Courses** Available.
**Nursing Student Activities** Sigma Theta Tau, Student Nurses' Association, nursing club.
**Nursing Student Resources** Academic advising; academic or career counseling; assistance for students with disabilities; bookstore; campus computer network; career placement assistance; computer lab; computer-assisted instruction; daycare for children of students; e-mail services; employment services for current students; housing assistance; interactive nursing skills videos; Internet; learning resource lab; library services; nursing audiovisuals; other; remedial services; resume preparation assistance; skills, simulation, or other laboratory; tutoring.
**Library Facilities** 7.4 million volumes (347,000 in health, 9,200 in nursing); 104,885 periodical subscriptions (200,000 health-care related).

### BACCALAUREATE PROGRAMS
**Degree** BSN
**Available Programs** Accelerated Baccalaureate; Accelerated Baccalaureate for Second Degree; Baccalaureate for Second Degree; Generic Baccalaureate.
**Study Options** Full-time.
**Program Entrance Requirements** Minimum overall college GPA of 2.8, transcript of college record, CPR certification, written essay, health exam, health insurance, high school transcript, immunizations, minimum GPA in nursing prerequisites, professional liability insurance/malpractice insurance, prerequisite course work. Transfer students are accepted. *Application deadline:* 8/10 (spring), 12/22 (summer). *Application fee:* $80.
**Advanced Placement** Credit given for nursing courses completed elsewhere dependent upon specific evaluations.
**Contact** Ms. Carlee Meritt, Assistant Director for Undergraduate Admissions, School of Nursing, The University of North Carolina at Chapel Hill, CB #7460, Chapel Hill, NC 27599-7460. *Telephone:* 919-966-4260. *Fax:* 919-966-3540. *E-mail:* carlee_meritt@unc.edu.

### GRADUATE PROGRAMS
**Expenses (2013–14)** *Tuition, state resident:* full-time $12,493. *Tuition, nonresident:* full-time $29,970. *International tuition:* $29,970 full-time. *Room and board:* $13,500 per academic year. *Required fees:* full-time $1922.
**Financial Aid** 8 fellowships, 6 research assistantships (averaging $8,000 per year), 10 teaching assistantships (averaging $8,000 per year) were awarded; scholarships, traineeships, and unspecified assistantships also available.
**Contact** Ms. Jennifer Moore, Assistant Director, Graduate Admissions, School of Nursing, The University of North Carolina at Chapel Hill, CB

#7460, Chapel Hill, NC 27599-7460. *Telephone:* 919-966-4260. *Fax:* 919-966-3540. *E-mail:* jennifer.j.moore@unc.edu.

**MASTER'S DEGREE PROGRAM**
**Degree** MSN
**Available Programs** Master's; RN to Master's.
**Concentrations Available** Clinical nurse leader; nursing education.
**Study Options** Full-time and part-time.
**Program Entrance Requirements** Clinical experience, minimum overall college GPA of 3.0, transcript of college record, CPR certification, written essay, immunizations, 3 letters of recommendation, professional liability insurance/malpractice insurance, resume, statistics course, GRE General Test. *Application deadline:* 1/14 (fall). *Application fee:* $85.
**Advanced Placement** Credit given for nursing courses completed elsewhere dependent upon specific evaluations.
**Degree Requirements** 42 total credit hours, thesis or project, comprehensive exam.

**POST-MASTER'S PROGRAM**
**Areas of Study** Clinical nurse leader; nursing informatics. *Nurse practitioner programs in:* psychiatric/mental health.

**DOCTORAL DEGREE PROGRAM**
**Degree** DNP
**Available Programs** Doctorate.
**Areas of Study** Adult health ,advanced practice nursing, family health, gerontology, health-care systems, nursing administration, nursing informatics, oncology, outcomes, pediatric, primary care, psychiatric/mental health.
**Program Entrance Requirements** Minimum overall college GPA of 3.0, interview, 3 letters of recommendation, statistics course, vita, writing sample. *Application deadline:* 1/14 (fall). Applications may be processed on a rolling basis for some programs. *Application fee:* $85.
**Degree Requirements** 54 total credit hours, dissertation, oral exam, residency, written exam.

**Degree** PhD
**Available Programs** Doctorate; Post-Baccalaureate Doctorate.
**Areas of Study** Addiction/substance abuse, advanced practice nursing, aging, bio-behavioral research, biology of health and illness, clinical nurse leader, clinical practice, clinical research, community health, critical care, ethics, faculty preparation, family health, forensic nursing, gerontology, health policy, health promotion/disease prevention, health-care systems, human health and illness, illness and transition, individualized study, information systems, maternity-newborn, neuro-behavior, nurse case management, nursing administration, nursing education, nursing policy, nursing research, nursing science, oncology, palliative care, urban health,women's health.
**Program Entrance Requirements** Minimum overall college GPA of 3.0, interview, 3 letters of recommendation, statistics course, vita, writing sample, GRE General Test. *Application deadline:* 1/14 (fall). Applications may be processed on a rolling basis for some programs. *Application fee:* $85.
**Degree Requirements** 54 total credit hours, dissertation, oral exam, written exam, residency.

**POSTDOCTORAL PROGRAM**
**Areas of Study** Addiction/substance abuse, adolescent health, aging, cancer care, chronic illness, community health, family health, gerontology, health promotion/disease prevention, individualized study, infection prevention/skin care, information systems, neuro-behavior, nursing informatics, nursing interventions, nursing research, nursing science, outcomes, self-care, vulnerable population,women's health.
**Postdoctoral Program Contact** Dr. Suzanne Thoyre, Director, PhD and Post-Doctoral Programs, School of Nursing, The University of North Carolina at Chapel Hill, Carrington Hall, CB #7460, Chapel Hill, NC 27599-7460. *Telephone:* 919-966-8418. *Fax:* 919-843-9969. *E-mail:* thoyre@email.unc.edu.

## CONTINUING EDUCATION PROGRAM

**Contact** Dr. Sonda Oppewal, Director, Center for Lifelong Learning, School of Nursing, The University of North Carolina at Chapel Hill, L400 Carrington Hall, CB #7460, Chapel Hill, NC 27599-7460. *Telephone:* 919-966-3638. *Fax:* 919-966-7298. *E-mail:* oppewal@email.unc.edu.

# The University of North Carolina at Charlotte

### School of Nursing
### Charlotte, North Carolina

*http://www.nursing.uncc.edu/*
Founded in 1946

**DEGREES • BSN • MSN**
**Nursing Program Faculty** 51 (50% with doctorates).
**Baccalaureate Enrollment** 330 **Women** 92% **Men** 8% **Minority** 8% **Part-time** 5%
**Graduate Enrollment** 200 **Women** 80% **Men** 20% **Minority** 10% **Part-time** 65%
**Distance Learning Courses** Available.
**Nursing Student Activities** Sigma Theta Tau, Student Nurses' Association.
**Nursing Student Resources** Academic advising; academic or career counseling; assistance for students with disabilities; bookstore; campus computer network; career placement assistance; computer lab; computer-assisted instruction; e-mail services; externships; interactive nursing skills videos; Internet; learning resource lab; library services; nursing audiovisuals; resume preparation assistance; skills, simulation, or other laboratory; tutoring.
**Library Facilities** 1.1 million volumes (39,000 in health, 2,400 in nursing); 57,471 periodical subscriptions (160 health-care related).

## BACCALAUREATE PROGRAMS

**Degree** BSN
**Available Programs** ADN to Baccalaureate; Generic Baccalaureate; RN Baccalaureate.
**Study Options** Full-time.
**Program Entrance Requirements** Minimum overall college GPA of 2.5, transcript of college record, CPR certification, written essay, health exam, health insurance, high school biology, high school chemistry, high school foreign language, 3 years high school math, 3 years high school science, high school transcript, immunizations, 3 letters of recommendation, minimum GPA in nursing prerequisites of 2.5, prerequisite course work. Transfer students are accepted. *Application deadline:* 1/31 (fall), 8/31 (winter).
**Contact** *Telephone:* 704-687-4676. *Fax:* 704-687-3180.

## GRADUATE PROGRAMS

**Contact** *Telephone:* 704-687-7992. *Fax:* 704-687-6017.

**MASTER'S DEGREE PROGRAM**
**Degree** MSN
**Available Programs** Master's; RN to Master's.
**Concentrations Available** Nurse anesthesia; nursing administration; nursing education. *Clinical nurse specialist programs in:* community health. *Nurse practitioner programs in:* adult health, family health.
**Study Options** Full-time and part-time.
**Online Degree Options** Yes.
**Program Entrance Requirements** Clinical experience, computer literacy, minimum overall college GPA of 3.0, transcript of college record, CPR certification, written essay, immunizations, interview, 3 letters of recommendation, nursing research course, professional liability insurance/malpractice insurance, resume, statistics course.

**POST-MASTER'S PROGRAM**
**Areas of Study** Nurse anesthesia; nursing administration; nursing education. *Nurse practitioner programs in:* family health.

# The University of North Carolina at Greensboro

### School of Nursing
### Greensboro, North Carolina

*http://www.uncg.edu/nur/*
Founded in 1891

**DEGREES • BSN • MSN • MSN/MBA • PHD**
**Nursing Program Faculty** 58 (53% with doctorates).

**Baccalaureate Enrollment** 740 **Women** 89% **Men** 11% **Minority** 29% **International** 1% **Part-time** 26%
**Graduate Enrollment** 338 **Women** 82% **Men** 18% **Minority** 21% **International** 2% **Part-time** 57%
**Distance Learning Courses** Available.
**Nursing Student Activities** Nursing Honor Society, Sigma Theta Tau, Student Nurses' Association.
**Nursing Student Resources** Academic advising; academic or career counseling; assistance for students with disabilities; bookstore; campus computer network; career placement assistance; computer lab; computer-assisted instruction; e-mail services; externships; Internet; learning resource lab; library services; nursing audiovisuals; paid internships; placement services for program completers; remedial services; resume preparation assistance; skills, simulation, or other laboratory; tutoring; unpaid internships.
**Library Facilities** 1.1 million volumes (933 in health, 92 in nursing); 52,691 periodical subscriptions (80 health-care related).

## BACCALAUREATE PROGRAMS

**Degree** BSN
**Available Programs** ADN to Baccalaureate; Baccalaureate for Second Degree; Generic Baccalaureate; LPN to Baccalaureate; RN Baccalaureate.
**Site Options** Hickory, NC; Greensboro, NC.
**Study Options** Full-time.
**Program Entrance Requirements** Minimum overall college GPA of 2.7, transcript of college record, CPR certification, health exam, immunizations, minimum GPA in nursing prerequisites of 3.0, professional liability insurance/malpractice insurance, prerequisite course work. Transfer students are accepted. *Application deadline:* 2/1 (fall). *Application fee:* $55.
**Expenses (2013–14)** *Tuition, state resident:* full-time $3932; part-time $492 per credit hour. *Tuition, nonresident:* full-time $6880; part-time $2217 per credit hour. *International tuition:* $6880 full-time. *Room and board:* $6179; room only: $4586 per academic year. *Required fees:* full-time $2458; part-time $91 per credit; part-time $102 per term.
**Financial Aid** 71% of baccalaureate students in nursing programs received some form of financial aid in 2012–13. *Gift aid (need-based):* Federal Pell, FSEOG, state, private, college/university gift aid from institutional funds. *Loans:* Federal Direct (Subsidized and Unsubsidized Stafford PLUS), Perkins, state, college/university. *Work-study:* Federal Work-Study. *Financial aid application deadline (priority):* 3/1.
**Contact** Dr. Anita S. Tesh, Associate Dean, School of Nursing, The University of North Carolina at Greensboro, PO Box 26170, Greensboro, NC 27402-6170. *Telephone:* 336-334-5280. *Fax:* 336-334-3628. *E-mail:* astesh@uncg.edu.

## GRADUATE PROGRAMS

**Expenses (2013–14)** *Tuition, state resident:* full-time $4542; part-time $567 per credit hour. *Tuition, nonresident:* full-time $17,990; part-time $2185 per credit hour. *International tuition:* $17,990 full-time. *Room and board:* $6179; room only: $4556 per academic year. *Required fees:* full-time $2454; part-time $97 per credit.
**Financial Aid** 75% of graduate students in nursing programs received some form of financial aid in 2012–13. Research assistantships with full tuition reimbursements available, career-related internships or fieldwork, Federal Work-Study, scholarships, and traineeships available. Aid available to part-time students.
**Contact** Eileen Kohlenberg, Associate Dean and Director of Graduate Studies, School of Nursing, The University of North Carolina at Greensboro, PO Box 26170, Greensboro, NC 27402-6170. *Telephone:* 336-334-5561. *Fax:* 336-334-3628. *E-mail:* eileen_kohlenberg@uncg.edu.

### MASTER'S DEGREE PROGRAM

**Degrees** MSN; MSN/MBA
**Available Programs** Master's.
**Concentrations Available** Nurse anesthesia; nursing administration; nursing education. *Nurse practitioner programs in:* adult health, gerontology.
**Site Options** Hickory, NC; Raleigh, NC.
**Study Options** Full-time and part-time.
**Online Degree Options** Yes.
**Program Entrance Requirements** Clinical experience, minimum overall college GPA of 3.0, transcript of college record, CPR certification, immunizations, 3 letters of recommendation, physical assessment course, professional liability insurance/malpractice insurance, prerequisite course work, statistics course, GRE General Test or MAT. *Application deadline:* Applications may be processed on a rolling basis for some programs. *Application fee:* $60.
**Advanced Placement** Credit given for nursing courses completed elsewhere dependent upon specific evaluations.
**Degree Requirements** 36 total credit hours, thesis or project, comprehensive exam.

### POST-MASTER'S PROGRAM

**Areas of Study** Nurse anesthesia. *Nurse practitioner programs in:* adult health, gerontology.

### DOCTORAL DEGREE PROGRAM

**Degree** PhD
**Available Programs** Doctorate.
**Areas of Study** Aging, faculty preparation, gerontology, health policy, health promotion/disease prevention, nursing administration, nursing education, nursing research, nursing science,women's health.
**Program Entrance Requirements** Minimum overall college GPA of 3.0, interview by faculty committee, interview, 3 letters of recommendation, MSN or equivalent, writing sample. *Application deadline:* Applications may be processed on a rolling basis for some programs. *Application fee:* $60.
**Degree Requirements** 57 total credit hours, dissertation, oral exam, written exam, residency.

# The University of North Carolina at Pembroke

### Nursing Program
### Pembroke, North Carolina

***http://www.uncp.edu/nursing/***
Founded in 1887

**DEGREE • BSN**
**Nursing Program Faculty** 20 (5% with doctorates).
**Baccalaureate Enrollment** 139
**Distance Learning Courses** Available.
**Nursing Student Activities** Student Nurses' Association.
**Nursing Student Resources** Academic advising; academic or career counseling; assistance for students with disabilities; bookstore; campus computer network; computer lab; computer-assisted instruction; e-mail services; housing assistance; interactive nursing skills videos; Internet; learning resource lab; library services; nursing audiovisuals; remedial services; resume preparation assistance; skills, simulation, or other laboratory; tutoring.
**Library Facilities** 517,987 volumes; 65,210 periodical subscriptions.

## BACCALAUREATE PROGRAMS

**Degree** BSN
**Available Programs** Generic Baccalaureate; RN Baccalaureate.
**Site Options** Southern Pines, NC; Fayetteville, NC; Hamlet, NC.
**Study Options** Full-time.
**Program Entrance Requirements** Minimum overall college GPA, health exam, minimum GPA in nursing prerequisites, prerequisite course work, RN licensure. Transfer students are accepted. *Application deadline:* 1/15 (spring).
**Advanced Placement** Credit given for nursing courses completed elsewhere dependent upon specific evaluations.
**Contact** *Telephone:* 910-521-6522. *Fax:* 910-521-6178.

# The University of North Carolina Wilmington

### School of Nursing
### Wilmington, North Carolina

***http://www.uncw.edu/son***
Founded in 1947

**DEGREES • BS • MSN**
**Nursing Program Faculty** 45 (53% with doctorates).
**Baccalaureate Enrollment** 317 **Women** 93% **Men** 7% **Minority** 14% **Part-time** 22%
**Graduate Enrollment** 90 **Women** 90% **Men** 10% **Minority** 17% **Part-time** 49%

**Distance Learning Courses** Available.

**Nursing Student Activities** Sigma Theta Tau, Student Nurses' Association.

**Nursing Student Resources** Academic advising; academic or career counseling; assistance for students with disabilities; bookstore; campus computer network; career placement assistance; computer lab; computer-assisted instruction; e-mail services; employment services for current students; externships; housing assistance; interactive nursing skills videos; Internet; learning resource lab; library services; nursing audiovisuals; remedial services; resume preparation assistance; skills, simulation, or other laboratory; tutoring; unpaid internships.

**Library Facilities** 1 million volumes (16,535 in health, 989 in nursing); 34,029 periodical subscriptions (3,823 health-care related).

## BACCALAUREATE PROGRAMS

**Degree** BS

**Available Programs** Generic Baccalaureate; RN Baccalaureate.

**Site Options** Jacksonville, NC.

**Study Options** Full-time.

**Online Degree Options** Yes.

**Program Entrance Requirements** Minimum overall college GPA of 2.7, transcript of college record, CPR certification, written essay, health exam, health insurance, immunizations, minimum GPA in nursing prerequisites of 2.7, professional liability insurance/malpractice insurance, prerequisite course work. Transfer students are accepted. *Application deadline:* 12/15 (fall), 7/1 (spring).

**Advanced Placement** Credit given for nursing courses completed elsewhere dependent upon specific evaluations.

**Expenses (2013–14)** *Tuition, state resident:* full-time $4026; part-time $136 per credit. *Tuition, nonresident:* full-time $16,163; part-time $546 per credit. *Room and board:* $8624 per academic year. *Required fees:* full-time $2317; part-time $27 per credit.

**Financial Aid** ***Gift aid (need-based):*** Federal Pell, FSEOG, state, private, college/university gift aid from institutional funds. *Loans:* Federal Direct (Subsidized and Unsubsidized Stafford PLUS), Perkins, state. *Work-study:* Federal Work-Study. *Financial aid application deadline (priority):* 3/1.

**Contact** Mr. Mark Werbeach, Student Service Coordinator, School of Nursing, The University of North Carolina Wilmington, 601 South College Road, Wilmington, NC 28403-5995. *Telephone:* 910-962-7211. *Fax:* 910-962-7656. *E-mail:* werbeachm@uncw.edu.

## GRADUATE PROGRAMS

**Expenses (2013–14)** *Tuition, state resident:* full-time $4163. *Tuition, nonresident:* full-time $16,098. *Room and board:* $9490 per academic year. *Required fees:* full-time $2317.

**Financial Aid** 2 teaching assistantships (averaging $9,500 per year) were awarded.

**Contact** Dr. Julie S. Taylor, Graduate Coordinator, School of Nursing, The University of North Carolina Wilmington, 601 South College Road, Wilmington, NC 28403-5995. *Telephone:* 910-962-7927. *Fax:* 910-962-4921. *E-mail:* taylorjs@uncw.edu.

### MASTER'S DEGREE PROGRAM

**Degree** MSN

**Available Programs** Master's.

**Concentrations Available** *Nurse practitioner programs in:* family health.

**Study Options** Full-time and part-time.

**Program Entrance Requirements** Clinical experience, computer literacy, minimum overall college GPA of 3.0, transcript of college record, CPR certification, written essay, immunizations, 3 letters of recommendation, physical assessment course, professional liability insurance/malpractice insurance, prerequisite course work, resume, statistics course, GRE General Test. *Application deadline:* 3/1 (fall). *Application fee:* $60.

**Advanced Placement** Credit given for nursing courses completed elsewhere dependent upon specific evaluations.

**Degree Requirements** 47 total credit hours, thesis or project, comprehensive exam.

### POST-MASTER'S PROGRAM

**Areas of Study** *Nurse practitioner programs in:* family health.

# Western Carolina University

## School of Nursing
## Cullowhee, North Carolina

***http://www.wcu.edu/***

Founded in 1889

## DEGREES • BSN • MS

**Nursing Program Faculty** 31 (50% with doctorates).

**Baccalaureate Enrollment** 200 **Women** 94% **Men** 6% **Minority** 2%

**Graduate Enrollment** 122 **Women** 90% **Men** 10% **Minority** 2%

**Distance Learning Courses** Available.

**Nursing Student Activities** Sigma Theta Tau, Student Nurses' Association.

**Nursing Student Resources** Academic advising; academic or career counseling; assistance for students with disabilities; bookstore; campus computer network; career placement assistance; computer lab; computer-assisted instruction; daycare for children of students; e-mail services; externships; housing assistance; interactive nursing skills videos; Internet; learning resource lab; library services; nursing audiovisuals; resume preparation assistance; skills, simulation, or other laboratory; tutoring.

**Library Facilities** 626,918 volumes (10,000 in health, 900 in nursing); 12,465 periodical subscriptions (70 health-care related).

## BACCALAUREATE PROGRAMS

**Degree** BSN

**Available Programs** Accelerated Baccalaureate; Generic Baccalaureate; RN Baccalaureate.

**Site Options** Enka, NC.

**Study Options** Full-time.

**Online Degree Options** Yes.

**Program Entrance Requirements** Minimum overall college GPA of 3.0, transcript of college record, CPR certification, health exam, high school transcript, immunizations, minimum GPA in nursing prerequisites of 2.0, professional liability insurance/malpractice insurance, prerequisite course work. Transfer students are accepted. *Application deadline:* 2/1 (fall), 7/1 (spring). *Application fee:* $45.

**Contact** *Telephone:* 828-227-7467. *Fax:* 828-227-7052.

## GRADUATE PROGRAMS

**Contact** *Telephone:* 828-670-8810 Ext. 247.

### MASTER'S DEGREE PROGRAM

**Degree** MS

**Available Programs** Master's.

**Concentrations Available** Nurse anesthesia; nursing administration; nursing education. *Nurse practitioner programs in:* family health.

**Site Options** Enka, NC.

**Study Options** Full-time and part-time.

**Online Degree Options** Yes.

**Program Entrance Requirements** Clinical experience, minimum overall college GPA of 3.0, transcript of college record, CPR certification, written essay, immunizations, interview, 3 letters of recommendation, nursing research course, physical assessment course, professional liability insurance/malpractice insurance, resume, statistics course. *Application deadline:* 4/15 (fall), 10/15 (winter). *Application fee:* $45.

**Advanced Placement** Credit given for nursing courses completed elsewhere dependent upon specific evaluations.

**Degree Requirements** Thesis or project, comprehensive exam.

### POST-MASTER'S PROGRAM

**Areas of Study** Nursing administration; nursing education. *Nurse practitioner programs in:* family health.

### POSTDOCTORAL PROGRAM

**Postdoctoral Program Contact***Telephone:* 828-227-7467. *Fax:* 828-227-7071.

## Winston-Salem State University

### Department of Nursing
### Winston-Salem, North Carolina

***http://www.wssu.edu/***
Founded in 1892

**DEGREES • BSN • MSN**
**Nursing Program Faculty** 34 (13% with doctorates).
**Baccalaureate Enrollment** 252 **Women** 77% **Men** 23% **Minority** 61%
**Graduate Enrollment** 15
**Nursing Student Activities** Nursing Honor Society, Sigma Theta Tau, Student Nurses' Association.
**Nursing Student Resources** Academic advising; academic or career counseling; assistance for students with disabilities; bookstore; campus computer network; computer lab; interactive nursing skills videos; learning resource lab; nursing audiovisuals; skills, simulation, or other laboratory.
**Library Facilities** 4,381 volumes in health, 2,691 volumes in nursing; 2,205 periodical subscriptions health-care related.

#### BACCALAUREATE PROGRAMS

**Degree** BSN
**Available Programs** ADN to Baccalaureate; Accelerated RN Baccalaureate; Baccalaureate for Second Degree; Generic Baccalaureate; LPN to Baccalaureate; RN Baccalaureate.
**Site Options** Wilkesboro, NC; Salisbury, NC; Boone, NC.
**Study Options** Full-time.
**Program Entrance Requirements** Minimum overall college GPA of 2.6, transcript of college record, CPR certification, health exam, immunizations, professional liability insurance/malpractice insurance, prerequisite course work. Transfer students are accepted.
**Advanced Placement** Credit by examination available. Credit given for nursing courses completed elsewhere dependent upon specific evaluations.
**Contact** *Telephone:* 336-750-2560. *Fax:* 336-750-2599.

#### GRADUATE PROGRAMS

**Contact** *Telephone:* 336-750-2275. *Fax:* 336-750-2007.

**MASTER'S DEGREE PROGRAM**
**Degree** MSN
**Available Programs** Master's.
**Concentrations Available** Nursing education. *Nurse practitioner programs in:* family health, psychiatric/mental health.
**Study Options** Full-time and part-time.
**Program Entrance Requirements** Clinical experience, transcript of college record, CPR certification, immunizations, interview, 3 letters of recommendation, nursing research course, physical assessment course, professional liability insurance/malpractice insurance, resume, statistics course.
**Advanced Placement** Credit given for nursing courses completed elsewhere dependent upon specific evaluations.
**Degree Requirements** 50 total credit hours, thesis or project.

#### CONTINUING EDUCATION PROGRAM

**Contact** *Telephone:* 336-750-2665. *Fax:* 336-750-2599.

# NORTH DAKOTA

## Dickinson State University

### Department of Nursing
### Dickinson, North Dakota

***http://www.dickinsonstate.edu/***
Founded in 1918

**DEGREE • BSN**
**Nursing Program Faculty** 6 (33% with doctorates).
**Baccalaureate Enrollment** 34 **Women** 94% **Men** 6% **Minority** 3%
**International** 12% **Part-time** 9%
**Nursing Student Activities** Student Nurses' Association.
**Nursing Student Resources** Academic advising; academic or career counseling; assistance for students with disabilities; bookstore; campus computer network; career placement assistance; computer lab; computer-assisted instruction; e-mail services; employment services for current students; externships; housing assistance; interactive nursing skills videos; Internet; learning resource lab; library services; nursing audiovisuals; other; placement services for program completers; remedial services; resume preparation assistance; skills, simulation, or other laboratory; tutoring; unpaid internships.
**Library Facilities** 105,713 volumes (2,319 in health, 912 in nursing); 823 periodical subscriptions (4,540 health-care related).

#### BACCALAUREATE PROGRAMS

**Degree** BSN
**Available Programs** ADN to Baccalaureate; LPN to Baccalaureate; LPN to RN Baccalaureate; RN Baccalaureate.
**Study Options** Full-time and part-time.
**Program Entrance Requirements** Minimum overall college GPA of 2.5, transcript of college record, CPR certification, health exam, health insurance, immunizations, minimum GPA in nursing prerequisites of 2.5, prerequisite course work. Transfer students are accepted. *Application deadline:* 2/1 (fall).
**Advanced Placement** Credit given for nursing courses completed elsewhere dependent upon specific evaluations.
**Expenses (2013–14)** *Tuition, state resident:* full-time $4704; part-time $196 per credit hour. *Tuition, nonresident:* full-time $7022; part-time $294 per credit hour. *International tuition:* $7022 full-time. *Room and board:* $5582; room only: $2146 per academic year. *Required fees:* full-time $600; part-time $48 per credit.
**Financial Aid** 100% of baccalaureate students in nursing programs received some form of financial aid in 2012–13.
**Contact** Dr. Mary Anne Marsh, Chair, Department of Nursing, Dickinson State University, 291 Campus Drive, Dickinson, ND 58601-4896. *Telephone:* 701-483-2133. *Fax:* 701-483-2524. *E-mail:* maryanne.marsh@dickinsonstate.edu.

## Minot State University

### Department of Nursing
### Minot, North Dakota

***http://www.minotstateu.edu/nursing/***
Founded in 1913

**DEGREE • BSN**
**Nursing Program Faculty** 22 (27% with doctorates).
**Baccalaureate Enrollment** 179 **Women** 92% **Men** 8% **Minority** 23%
**International** 5% **Part-time** 20%
**Distance Learning Courses** Available.
**Nursing Student Activities** Sigma Theta Tau, Student Nurses' Association.
**Nursing Student Resources** Academic advising; academic or career counseling; assistance for students with disabilities; bookstore; campus computer network; career placement assistance; computer lab; computer-assisted instruction; e-mail services; housing assistance; interactive nursing skills videos; Internet; learning resource lab; library services; nursing audiovisuals; paid internships; remedial services; resume preparation assistance; skills, simulation, or other laboratory; tutoring; unpaid internships.
**Library Facilities** 8,500 volumes in health, 1,750 volumes in nursing; 37 periodical subscriptions health-care related.

#### BACCALAUREATE PROGRAMS

**Degree** BSN
**Available Programs** Generic Baccalaureate; RN Baccalaureate.
**Study Options** Full-time.
**Online Degree Options** Yes.
**Program Entrance Requirements** Minimum overall college GPA of 2.75, transcript of college record, CPR certification, written essay, immunizations, 2 letters of recommendation, minimum GPA in nursing prerequisites of 2.8, prerequisite course work. Transfer students are accepted. *Application deadline:* 9/15 (fall), 2/1 (spring). *Application fee:* $25.
**Advanced Placement** Credit given for nursing courses completed elsewhere dependent upon specific evaluations.
**Expenses (2012–13)** *Tuition, state resident:* full-time $6000; part-time $190 per credit. *Tuition, nonresident:* full-time $6000; part-time $190 per credit. *International tuition:* $6000 full-time. *Required fees:* full-time $900.

**Financial Aid** 70% of baccalaureate students in nursing programs received some form of financial aid in 2011–12.
**Contact** Ms. Nicola J. Roed, Chair, Department of Nursing, Department of Nursing, Minot State University, 500 University Avenue West, Minot, ND 58707-0002. *Telephone:* 701-858-3526. *Fax:* 701-858-4309. *E-mail:* nicola.roed@minotstateu.edu.

# North Dakota State University

## Department of Nursing
## Fargo, North Dakota

***http://www.ndsu.edu/ndsu/nursing/***
Founded in 1890

### DEGREES • BSN • DNP • MS

**Nursing Program Faculty** 15 (49% with doctorates).
**Baccalaureate Enrollment** 195 **Women** 90% **Men** 10% **Minority** 5% **International** 3% **Part-time** 10%
**Graduate Enrollment** 24 **Women** 95% **Men** 5% **Minority** 1% **Part-time** 45%
**Nursing Student Activities** Sigma Theta Tau, Student Nurses' Association.
**Nursing Student Resources** Academic advising; academic or career counseling; assistance for students with disabilities; bookstore; campus computer network; career placement assistance; computer lab; computer-assisted instruction; daycare for children of students; e-mail services; employment services for current students; interactive nursing skills videos; Internet; learning resource lab; library services; nursing audiovisuals; paid internships; placement services for program completers; remedial services; resume preparation assistance; skills, simulation, or other laboratory; tutoring.
**Library Facilities** 8,631 volumes in health, 1,841 volumes in nursing; 121 periodical subscriptions health-care related.

### BACCALAUREATE PROGRAMS

**Degree** BSN
**Available Programs** ADN to Baccalaureate; Generic Baccalaureate; LPN to Baccalaureate.
**Study Options** Full-time.
**Program Entrance Requirements** Minimum overall college GPA of 3.0, transcript of college record, CPR certification, health exam, health insurance, immunizations, 2 letters of recommendation, minimum GPA in nursing prerequisites of 3.0, prerequisite course work. Transfer students are accepted.
**Advanced Placement** Credit by examination available. Credit given for nursing courses completed elsewhere dependent upon specific evaluations.
**Contact** *Telephone:* 701-231-7395. *Fax:* 701-231-7606.

### GRADUATE PROGRAMS

**Contact** *Telephone:* 701-231-8355. *Fax:* 701-231-7606.

#### MASTER'S DEGREE PROGRAM

**Degree** MS
**Available Programs** Master's.
**Concentrations Available** Nursing education. *Clinical nurse specialist programs in:* adult health. *Nurse practitioner programs in:* family health.
**Study Options** Full-time and part-time.
**Program Entrance Requirements** Computer literacy, minimum overall college GPA of 3.0, transcript of college record, CPR certification, immunizations, interview, 3 letters of recommendation, nursing research course, physical assessment course, professional liability insurance/malpractice insurance, resume, statistics course.
**Advanced Placement** Credit given for nursing courses completed elsewhere dependent upon specific evaluations.
**Degree Requirements** 58 total credit hours, thesis or project, comprehensive exam.

#### DOCTORAL DEGREE PROGRAM

**Degree** DNP
**Available Programs** Post-Baccalaureate Doctorate.
**Areas of Study** Advanced practice nursing, family health.
**Online Degree Options** Yes.
**Program Entrance Requirements** Clinical experience, minimum overall college GPA of 3.0, interview by faculty committee, 2 letters of recommendation, statistics course, vita, writing sample.
**Degree Requirements** 86 total credit hours, dissertation, oral exam.

# Sanford College of Nursing

## Sanford College of Nursing
## Bismarck, North Dakota

***http://www.bismarck.sanfordhealth.org/collegeofnursing/***
Founded in 1988

### DEGREE • BSN

**Nursing Program Faculty** 15 (7% with doctorates).
**Baccalaureate Enrollment** 109 **Women** 89% **Men** 11% **Minority** 15%
**Nursing Student Activities** Sigma Theta Tau, Student Nurses' Association.
**Nursing Student Resources** Academic advising; bookstore; computer lab; computer-assisted instruction; e-mail services; Internet; library services; nursing audiovisuals; paid internships; placement services for program completers; resume preparation assistance; skills, simulation, or other laboratory; tutoring.
**Library Facilities** 5,049 volumes (1,485 in health, 1,335 in nursing); 630 periodical subscriptions (655 health-care related).

### BACCALAUREATE PROGRAMS

**Degree** BSN
**Available Programs** RN Baccalaureate.
**Study Options** Full-time and part-time.
**Program Entrance Requirements** Minimum overall college GPA of 2.5, transcript of college record, written essay, health exam, high school transcript, immunizations, interview, minimum GPA in nursing prerequisites of 2.5, prerequisite course work. Transfer students are accepted. *Application deadline:* 11/1 (fall), 2/1 (spring). *Application fee:* $40.
**Advanced Placement** Credit by examination available. Credit given for nursing courses completed elsewhere dependent upon specific evaluations.
**Expenses (2012–13)** *Tuition:* full-time $10,312; part-time $430 per credit. *Required fees:* full-time $855.
**Financial Aid** 98% of baccalaureate students in nursing programs received some form of financial aid in 2011–12.
**Contact** Ms. Mary Smith, Director of Student Services, Sanford College of Nursing, 512 North 7th Street, Bismarck, ND 58501. *Telephone:* 701-323-6271. *Fax:* 701-323-6289. *E-mail:* msmith@mocn.edu.

# University of Jamestown

## Department of Nursing
## Jamestown, North Dakota

Founded in 1883

### DEGREE • BSN

**Nursing Program Faculty** 11 (9% with doctorates).
**Baccalaureate Enrollment** 80
**Nursing Student Activities** Sigma Theta Tau, Student Nurses' Association.
**Nursing Student Resources** Academic advising; academic or career counseling; bookstore; campus computer network; computer lab; computer-assisted instruction; e-mail services; externships; interactive nursing skills videos; Internet; learning resource lab; library services; nursing audiovisuals; resume preparation assistance; skills, simulation, or other laboratory; tutoring.
**Library Facilities** 104,952 volumes (990 in health, 983 in nursing); 22,010 periodical subscriptions (163 health-care related).

### BACCALAUREATE PROGRAMS

**Degree** BSN
**Study Options** Full-time and part-time.
**Program Entrance Requirements** Minimum overall college GPA of 3.0, transcript of college record, written essay, high school transcript, immunizations, prerequisite course work. Transfer students are accepted.
**Advanced Placement** Credit given for nursing courses completed elsewhere dependent upon specific evaluations.
**Contact** *Telephone:* 701-252-3467 Ext. 2562. *Fax:* 701-253-4318.

# University of Mary
## Division of Nursing
## Bismarck, North Dakota

***http://www.umary.edu/templates/template_degrees.php?degree=Nursing***
Founded in 1959

**DEGREES • BSN • MSN**
**Nursing Program Faculty** 45 (31% with doctorates).
**Baccalaureate Enrollment** 123 **Women** 88% **Men** 12% **Minority** 7%
**Graduate Enrollment** 198 **Women** 98% **Men** 2% **Minority** 14% **Part-time** 23%
**Distance Learning Courses** Available.
**Nursing Student Activities** Sigma Theta Tau, Student Nurses' Association.
**Nursing Student Resources** Academic advising; academic or career counseling; assistance for students with disabilities; bookstore; campus computer network; career placement assistance; computer lab; computer-assisted instruction; e-mail services; employment services for current students; externships; housing assistance; interactive nursing skills videos; Internet; library services; nursing audiovisuals; placement services for program completers; resume preparation assistance; skills, simulation, or other laboratory; unpaid internships.
**Library Facilities** 64,524 volumes (4,350 in health, 800 in nursing); 210 periodical subscriptions (70 health-care related).

### BACCALAUREATE PROGRAMS
**Degree** BSN
**Available Programs** Generic Baccalaureate; LPN to Baccalaureate; RN Baccalaureate.
**Study Options** Full-time and part-time.
**Online Degree Options** Yes.
**Program Entrance Requirements** Minimum overall college GPA of 2.75, transcript of college record, CPR certification, written essay, health exam, high school transcript, immunizations, interview, 2 letters of recommendation, minimum GPA in nursing prerequisites of 2.0, professional liability insurance/malpractice insurance, prerequisite course work. Transfer students are accepted.
**Advanced Placement** Credit by examination available. Credit given for nursing courses completed elsewhere dependent upon specific evaluations.
**Contact** *Telephone:* 701-255-7500. *Fax:* 701-255-7687.

### GRADUATE PROGRAMS
**Contact** *Telephone:* 701-355-8266. *Fax:* 701-255-7687.

#### MASTER'S DEGREE PROGRAM
**Degree** MSN
**Available Programs** Master's; RN to Master's.
**Concentrations Available** Nursing administration; nursing education. *Nurse practitioner programs in:* family health.
**Site Options** Billings, MT; Gillette, WY; Kansas City, MO.
**Study Options** Full-time and part-time.
**Online Degree Options** Yes.
**Program Entrance Requirements** Clinical experience, minimum overall college GPA of 2.75, transcript of college record, CPR certification, written essay, immunizations, interview, 2 letters of recommendation, physical assessment course, prerequisite course work, resume. *Application deadline:* Applications may be processed on a rolling basis for some programs.
**Advanced Placement** Credit given for nursing courses completed elsewhere dependent upon specific evaluations.
**Degree Requirements** 45 total credit hours, thesis or project, comprehensive exam.

# University of North Dakota
## College of Nursing
## Grand Forks, North Dakota

***http://www.nursing.und.edu/***
Founded in 1883

**DEGREES • BSN • MS • PHD**
**Nursing Program Faculty** 75 (30% with doctorates).
**Baccalaureate Enrollment** 304 **Women** 84% **Men** 16% **Minority** 8% **International** 1% **Part-time** 9%
**Graduate Enrollment** 264 **Women** 88.1% **Men** 11.9% **Minority** 12.8% **International** 1% **Part-time** 52.3%
**Distance Learning Courses** Available.
**Nursing Student Activities** Nursing Honor Society, Sigma Theta Tau, Student Nurses' Association.
**Nursing Student Resources** Academic advising; academic or career counseling; assistance for students with disabilities; bookstore; career placement assistance; computer lab; computer-assisted instruction; daycare for children of students; e-mail services; employment services for current students; externships; housing assistance; interactive nursing skills videos; Internet; learning resource lab; library services; nursing audiovisuals; paid internships; placement services for program completers; remedial services; resume preparation assistance; skills, simulation, or other laboratory; tutoring.
**Library Facilities** 1.2 million volumes (81,000 in health, 10,200 in nursing); 44,704 periodical subscriptions (30,000 health-care related).

### BACCALAUREATE PROGRAMS
**Degree** BSN
**Available Programs** ADN to Baccalaureate; Accelerated Baccalaureate for Second Degree; Baccalaureate for Second Degree; Generic Baccalaureate; LPN to Baccalaureate.
**Study Options** Full-time and part-time.
**Program Entrance Requirements** Minimum overall college GPA of 2.5, transcript of college record, CPR certification, written essay, health insurance, immunizations, minimum GPA in nursing prerequisites of 2.5, prerequisite course work. Transfer students are accepted. *Application deadline:* 2/1 (fall), 7/1 (spring).
**Advanced Placement** Credit by examination available. Credit given for nursing courses completed elsewhere dependent upon specific evaluations.
**Expenses (2012–13)** *Tuition, state resident:* full-time $7254; part-time $302 per credit. *Tuition, nonresident:* full-time $10,223; part-time $426 per credit. *International tuition:* $17,170 full-time. *Room and board:* $6084; room only: $5942 per academic year. *Required fees:* full-time $1000; part-time $45 per credit; part-time $500 per term.
**Financial Aid** 82% of baccalaureate students in nursing programs received some form of financial aid in 2011–12.
**Contact** Ms. Lucy Heintz, Director of the Office of Student Services, College of Nursing, University of North Dakota, UND Nursing Building, 430 Oxford Street, Stop 9025, Grand Forks, ND 58202-9025. *Telephone:* 701-777-4534. *Fax:* 701-777-4096. *E-mail:* lucy.heintz@email.und.edu.

### GRADUATE PROGRAMS
**Expenses (2012–13)** *Tuition, state resident:* full-time $7704; part-time $361 per credit. *Tuition, nonresident:* full-time $7704; part-time $361 per credit. *International tuition:* $7704 full-time. *Room and board:* $6084; room only: $3627 per academic year. *Required fees:* full-time $1000; part-time $42 per credit.
**Financial Aid** 84% of graduate students in nursing programs received some form of financial aid in 2011–12. 3 research assistantships with full and partial tuition reimbursements available (averaging $10,498 per year), 6 teaching assistantships with full and partial tuition reimbursements available (averaging $10,669 per year) were awarded; fellowships with full and partial tuition reimbursements available, Federal Work-Study, institutionally sponsored loans, scholarships, traineeships, and tuition waivers (full and partial) also available. Aid available to part-time students. *Financial aid application deadline:* 3/15.
**Contact** Dr. Laurel Shepherd, Chair, Graduate Nursing Department, College of Nursing, University of North Dakota, 430 Oxford Street, Stop 9025, Room 361, Grand Forks, ND 58202-9025. *Telephone:* 701-777-4543. *Fax:* 701-777-4096. *E-mail:* laurel.shepherd@und.edu.

#### MASTER'S DEGREE PROGRAM
**Degree** MS
**Available Programs** Master's.
**Concentrations Available** Nurse anesthesia; nursing education. *Clinical nurse specialist programs in:* gerontology, psychiatric/mental health, public health. *Nurse practitioner programs in:* family health, gerontology, primary care, psychiatric/mental health.
**Study Options** Full-time and part-time.
**Online Degree Options** Yes.
**Program Entrance Requirements** Clinical experience, minimum overall college GPA of 3.0, transcript of college record, CPR certification, written essay, immunizations, interview, 3 letters of recommendation, prerequisite course work, resume, statistics course. *Application deadline:* 1/15 (fall). *Application fee:* $35.

**Advanced Placement** Credit given for nursing courses completed elsewhere dependent upon specific evaluations.
**Degree Requirements** 57 total credit hours, thesis or project.

### POST-MASTER'S PROGRAM

**Areas of Study** Nurse anesthesia; nursing education. *Clinical nurse specialist programs in:* gerontology, psychiatric/mental health. *Nurse practitioner programs in:* family health, gerontology, primary care, psychiatric/mental health.

### DOCTORAL DEGREE PROGRAM

**Degree** PhD
**Available Programs** Doctorate.
**Areas of Study** Bio-behavioral research, nursing research.
**Online Degree Options** Yes (online only).
**Program Entrance Requirements** Minimum overall college GPA of 3.5, interview by faculty committee, 3 letters of recommendation, MSN or equivalent, statistics course, vita, GRE or MAT. *Application deadline:* 2/1 (fall). *Application fee:* $35.
**Degree Requirements** 90 total credit hours, dissertation, oral exam, written exam.

# OHIO

## Ashland University

### Dwight Schar College of Nursing and Health Sciences
### Ashland, Ohio

***http://www.ashland.edu/nursing***
Founded in 1878

**DEGREE • BSN**
**Nursing Program Faculty** 24 (33% with doctorates).
**Baccalaureate Enrollment** 368 **Women** 84% **Men** 16% **Minority** 6% **Part-time** 3%
**Distance Learning Courses** Available.
**Nursing Student Activities** Nursing Honor Society, Sigma Theta Tau, Student Nurses' Association, nursing club.
**Nursing Student Resources** Academic advising; academic or career counseling; assistance for students with disabilities; bookstore; campus computer network; career placement assistance; computer lab; computer-assisted instruction; e-mail services; employment services for current students; interactive nursing skills videos; Internet; learning resource lab; library services; nursing audiovisuals; remedial services; resume preparation assistance; skills, simulation, or other laboratory; tutoring; unpaid internships.
**Library Facilities** 205,200 volumes; 1,625 periodical subscriptions.

### BACCALAUREATE PROGRAMS

**Degree** BSN
**Available Programs** ADN to Baccalaureate; Accelerated Baccalaureate; Accelerated Baccalaureate for Second Degree; Baccalaureate for Second Degree; Generic Baccalaureate; RN Baccalaureate.
**Study Options** Full-time and part-time.
**Online Degree Options** Yes.
**Program Entrance Requirements** Minimum overall college GPA of 3.0, transcript of college record, CPR certification, health exam, health insurance, high school transcript, immunizations, minimum high school GPA. Transfer students are accepted. *Application deadline:* Applications may be processed on a rolling basis for some programs.
**Advanced Placement** Credit given for nursing courses completed elsewhere dependent upon specific evaluations.
**Financial Aid** 95% of baccalaureate students in nursing programs received some form of financial aid in 2012–13. *Gift aid (need-based):* Federal Pell, FSEOG, state, private, college/university gift aid from institutional funds. *Loans:* Federal Direct (Subsidized and Unsubsidized Stafford PLUS), Perkins, college/university. *Work-study:* Federal Work-Study. *Financial aid application deadline:* Continuous.
**Contact** Mr. Kyle Vaughn, Admission Representative, Dwight Schar College of Nursing and Health Sciences, Ashland University, 401 College Avenue, Ashland, OH 44805. *Telephone:* 419-289-5086. *E-mail:* cvaughn2@ashland.edu.

## Capital University

### School of Nursing
### Columbus, Ohio

***http://www.capital.edu/***
Founded in 1830

**DEGREES • BSN • MN/MBA • MSN • MSN/JD • MSN/MDIV**
**Nursing Program Faculty** 45 (30% with doctorates).
**Baccalaureate Enrollment** 464 **Women** 82% **Men** 18% **Minority** 9% **International** 1% **Part-time** 19%
**Graduate Enrollment** 45 **Women** 87% **Men** 13% **Minority** 31% **International** 2% **Part-time** 98%
**Nursing Student Activities** Sigma Theta Tau, Student Nurses' Association.
**Nursing Student Resources** Academic advising; academic or career counseling; assistance for students with disabilities; bookstore; campus computer network; computer lab; computer-assisted instruction; e-mail services; interactive nursing skills videos; Internet; learning resource lab; library services; nursing audiovisuals; remedial services; resume preparation assistance; skills, simulation, or other laboratory; tutoring; unpaid internships.
**Library Facilities** 220,594 volumes (6,209 in health); 163,236 periodical subscriptions (82 health-care related).

### BACCALAUREATE PROGRAMS

**Degree** BSN
**Available Programs** ADN to Baccalaureate; Accelerated Baccalaureate for Second Degree; Generic Baccalaureate; RN Baccalaureate.
**Study Options** Full-time and part-time.
**Program Entrance Requirements** Minimum overall college GPA of 3.0, transcript of college record, health exam, health insurance, high school biology, high school chemistry, high school foreign language, 3 years high school math, 3 years high school science, high school transcript, immunizations, minimum high school GPA of 3.0. Transfer students are accepted. *Application deadline:* 5/1 (fall). Applications may be processed on a rolling basis for some programs. *Application fee:* $25.
**Advanced Placement** Credit by examination available. Credit given for nursing courses completed elsewhere dependent upon specific evaluations.
**Expenses (2013–14)** *Tuition:* full-time $31,990; part-time $1066 per credit hour. *International tuition:* $31,990 full-time. *Room and board:* $9060 per academic year.
**Financial Aid** 100% of baccalaureate students in nursing programs received some form of financial aid in 2012–13. *Gift aid (need-based):* Federal Pell, FSEOG, state, private, college/university gift aid from institutional funds, Federal Nursing. *Loans:* Federal Nursing Student Loans, Federal Direct (Subsidized and Unsubsidized Stafford PLUS), Perkins, college/university. *Work-study:* Federal Work-Study, part-time campus jobs. *Financial aid application deadline (priority):* 3/1.
**Contact** Dr. Judi Macke, Program Coordinator, School of Nursing, Capital University, 1 College and Main, Columbus, OH 43209-2394. *Telephone:* 614-236-6339. *Fax:* 614-236-6157. *E-mail:* jmacke@capital.edu.

### GRADUATE PROGRAMS

**Financial Aid** 30% of graduate students in nursing programs received some form of financial aid in 2012–13. Career-related internships or fieldwork and traineeships available.
**Contact** Dr. Sharon Stout-Shaffer, Program Coordinator, School of Nursing, Capital University, 1 College and Main, Columbus, OH 43209-2394. *Telephone:* 614-236-6363. *Fax:* 614-236-6703. *E-mail:* sstoutsh@capital.edu.

### MASTER'S DEGREE PROGRAM

**Degrees** MN/MBA; MSN; MSN/JD; MSN/MDIV
**Available Programs** Master's; RN to Master's.
**Concentrations Available** Legal nurse consultant; nursing administration; nursing education. *Clinical nurse specialist programs in:* adult health, gerontology.
**Study Options** Full-time and part-time.
**Program Entrance Requirements** Computer literacy, minimum overall college GPA of 3.0, transcript of college record, CPR certification, written essay, immunizations, 3 letters of recommendation, nursing research course, physical assessment course, professional liability insurance/malpractice insurance, resume, statistics course. *Application deadline:* 8/1 (fall), 12/1 (winter), 12/1 (spring), 5/1 (summer). Applica-

tions may be processed on a rolling basis for some programs. *Application fee:* $25.
**Advanced Placement** Credit given for nursing courses completed elsewhere dependent upon specific evaluations.
**Degree Requirements** 36 total credit hours, comprehensive exam.

**POST-MASTER'S PROGRAM**
**Areas of Study** Legal nurse consultant; nursing education. *Clinical nurse specialist programs in:* adult health, gerontology.

# Case Western Reserve University
## Frances Payne Bolton School of Nursing
## Cleveland, Ohio

*http://fpb.case.edu/*
Founded in 1826

### DEGREES • BSN • MSN • MSN/MA • MSN/MBA • MSN/PHD • PHD

**Nursing Program Faculty** 95 (76% with doctorates).
**Baccalaureate Enrollment** 323 **Women** 91% **Men** 9% **Minority** 34% **International** 2.7% **Part-time** .9%
**Graduate Enrollment** 503 **Women** 86% **Men** 14% **Minority** 14% **International** 6.3% **Part-time** 42%
**Distance Learning Courses** Available.
**Nursing Student Activities** Nursing Honor Society, Sigma Theta Tau, Student Nurses' Association, nursing club.
**Nursing Student Resources** Academic advising; academic or career counseling; assistance for students with disabilities; bookstore; campus computer network; career placement assistance; computer lab; computer-assisted instruction; e-mail services; employment services for current students; housing assistance; interactive nursing skills videos; Internet; learning resource lab; library services; nursing audiovisuals; other; paid internships; placement services for program completers; remedial services; resume preparation assistance; skills, simulation, or other laboratory; tutoring.
**Library Facilities** 2.9 million volumes (475,000 in health); 111,270 periodical subscriptions (2,500 health-care related).

### BACCALAUREATE PROGRAMS

**Degree** BSN
**Available Programs** Generic Baccalaureate.
**Study Options** Full-time.
**Program Entrance Requirements** CPR certification, written essay, health insurance, high school biology, high school chemistry, 2 years high school science, high school transcript, immunizations, 2 letters of recommendation, minimum high school GPA of 3.0. Transfer students are accepted. *Application deadline:* 1/15 (fall). *Application fee:* $35.
**Advanced Placement** Credit given for nursing courses completed elsewhere dependent upon specific evaluations.
**Expenses (2013–14)** *Tuition:* full-time $41,420. *Room and board:* $12,898 per academic year. *Required fees:* full-time $1368.
**Financial Aid** 100% of baccalaureate students in nursing programs received some form of financial aid in 2012–13. *Gift aid (need-based):* Federal Pell, FSEOG, state, private, college/university gift aid from institutional funds. *Loans:* Federal Nursing Student Loans, Federal Direct (Subsidized and Unsubsidized Stafford PLUS), Perkins, college/university, alternative loans. *Work-study:* Federal Work-Study. *Financial aid application deadline (priority):* 2/15.
**Contact** Office of Student Services, Frances Payne Bolton School of Nursing, Case Western Reserve University, 10900 Euclid Avenue, Cleveland, OH 44106-4904. *Telephone:* 216-368-2529. *Fax:* 216-368-0124. *E-mail:* admissions@fpb.case.edu.

### GRADUATE PROGRAMS

**Expenses (2013–14)** *Tuition:* full-time $41,964; part-time $1749 per credit hour. *Room and board:* $12,310 per academic year. *Required fees:* full-time $820.
**Financial Aid** 90% of graduate students in nursing programs received some form of financial aid in 2012–13. 4 research assistantships (averaging $13,932 per year), 31 teaching assistantships (averaging $15,120 per year) were awarded; fellowships, Federal Work-Study, institutionally sponsored loans, scholarships, and tuition waivers (partial) also available. Aid available to part-time students. *Financial aid application deadline:* 5/15.
**Contact** Office of Student Services, Frances Payne Bolton School of Nursing, Case Western Reserve University, 10900 Euclid Avenue, Cleveland, OH 44106-4904. *Telephone:* 216-368-2529. *Fax:* 216-368-0124. *E-mail:* admissions@fbp.case.edu.

**MASTER'S DEGREE PROGRAM**
**Degrees** MSN; MSN/MA; MSN/MBA; MSN/PhD
**Available Programs** Accelerated AD/RN to Master's; Master's; Master's for Non-Nursing College Graduates; RN to Master's.
**Concentrations Available** Nurse anesthesia; nurse-midwifery; nursing education. *Clinical nurse specialist programs in:* oncology, palliative care, psychiatric/mental health. *Nurse practitioner programs in:* acute care, adult health, family health, gerontology, neonatal health, oncology, pediatric, psychiatric/mental health,women's health.
**Study Options** Full-time and part-time.
**Program Entrance Requirements** Minimum overall college GPA of 3.0, transcript of college record, written essay, immunizations, 3 letters of recommendation, professional liability insurance/malpractice insurance, resume, statistics course, MAT or GRE General Test. *Application deadline:* 6/1 (fall), 10/1 (spring), 3/1 (summer). Applications may be processed on a rolling basis for some programs. *Application fee:* $75.
**Advanced Placement** Credit given for nursing courses completed elsewhere dependent upon specific evaluations.
**Degree Requirements** 40 total credit hours.

**POST-MASTER'S PROGRAM**
**Areas of Study** Nurse anesthesia; nurse-midwifery; nursing education. *Clinical nurse specialist programs in:* oncology, palliative care, psychiatric/mental health. *Nurse practitioner programs in:* acute care, adult health, family health, gerontology, neonatal health, oncology, pediatric, psychiatric/mental health,women's health.

**DOCTORAL DEGREE PROGRAM**
**Degree** PhD
**Available Programs** Doctorate; Doctorate for Nurses with Non-Nursing Degrees; Post-Baccalaureate Doctorate.
**Areas of Study** Aging, bio-behavioral research, biology of health and illness, community health, critical care, ethics, family health, gerontology, health policy, health promotion/disease prevention, health-care systems, human health and illness, illness and transition, information systems, maternity-newborn, neuro-behavior, nursing administration, nursing policy, nursing research, nursing science, oncology, palliative care, urban health,women's health.
**Program Entrance Requirements** Minimum overall college GPA of 3.0, interview by faculty committee, 3 letters of recommendation, statistics course, vita, writing sample, GRE General Test, MAT (for DNP). *Application deadline:* 3/1 (fall), 10/1 (spring). Applications may be processed on a rolling basis for some programs. *Application fee:* $75.
**Degree Requirements** 57 total credit hours, dissertation, oral exam, residency.

**POSTDOCTORAL PROGRAM**
**Areas of Study** Adolescent health, aging, cancer care, chronic illness, community health, family health, gerontology, health promotion/disease prevention, infection prevention/skin care, information systems, neurobehavior, nursing informatics, nursing interventions, nursing research, nursing science, outcomes, self-care, vulnerable population,women's health.
**Postdoctoral Program Contact** Dr. Shirley M. Moore, Professor and Associate Dean for Research, Frances Payne Bolton School of Nursing, Case Western Reserve University, 10900 Euclid Avenue, Cleveland, OH 44106-4904. *Telephone:* 216-368-5978. *Fax:* 216-368-3542. *E-mail:* shirley.moore@case.edu.

### CONTINUING EDUCATION PROGRAM

**Contact** Ms. Mary Variath, Instructor in Nursing, Frances Payne Bolton School of Nursing, Case Western Reserve University, 10900 Euclid Avenue, Cleveland, OH 44106-4904. *Telephone:* 216-368-2202. *Fax:* 216-368-5303. *E-mail:* mary.variath@case.edu.

# Cedarville University
## School of Nursing
## Cedarville, Ohio

*http://www.cedarville.edu/academics/nursing*
Founded in 1887

### DEGREES • BSN • MSN

**Nursing Program Faculty** 22 (36% with doctorates).

**Baccalaureate Enrollment** 408 **Women** 88.5% **Men** 11.5% **Minority** 4% **International** .5% **Part-time** .01%
**Graduate Enrollment** 45 **Women** 90% **Men** 10% **Minority** 18% **International** 16% **Part-time** 47%
**Distance Learning Courses** Available.
**Nursing Student Activities** Nursing Honor Society, Student Nurses' Association.
**Nursing Student Resources** Academic advising; academic or career counseling; assistance for students with disabilities; bookstore; campus computer network; career placement assistance; computer lab; computer-assisted instruction; e-mail services; employment services for current students; housing assistance; interactive nursing skills videos; Internet; library services; nursing audiovisuals; paid internships; resume preparation assistance; skills, simulation, or other laboratory; tutoring.
**Library Facilities** 239,169 volumes (6,386 in health, 1,160 in nursing); 9,094 periodical subscriptions (70 health-care related).

## BACCALAUREATE PROGRAMS

**Degree** BSN
**Available Programs** ADN to Baccalaureate; RN Baccalaureate.
**Study Options** Full-time and part-time.
**Program Entrance Requirements** Minimum overall college GPA of 2.8, transcript of college record, CPR certification, written essay, health exam, health insurance, high school biology, high school chemistry, high school foreign language, 4 years high school math, 4 years high school science, high school transcript, immunizations, 1 letter of recommendation, minimum high school GPA of 3.0, minimum high school rank 50%, minimum GPA in nursing prerequisites of 2.8, professional liability insurance/malpractice insurance, prerequisite course work. Transfer students are accepted. *Application deadline:* Applications may be processed on a rolling basis for some programs. *Application fee:* $30.
**Advanced Placement** Credit given for nursing courses completed elsewhere dependent upon specific evaluations.
**Expenses (2013–14)** *Tuition:* full-time $26,220; part-time $992 per credit. *International tuition:* $26,220 full-time. *Room and board:* $5750; room only: $3300 per academic year. *Required fees:* full-time $200.
**Financial Aid** 95% of baccalaureate students in nursing programs received some form of financial aid in 2012–13.
**Contact** Ms. Amy Holderby, Director of Admissions, School of Nursing, Cedarville University, 251 North Main Street, Cedarville, OH 45314-0601. *Telephone:* 800-233-2784. *Fax:* 937-766-7700. *E-mail:* admissions@cedarville.edu.

## GRADUATE PROGRAMS

**Expenses (2013–14)** *Tuition:* full-time $8576; part-time $536 per hour. *International tuition:* $8576 full-time.
**Financial Aid** 67% of graduate students in nursing programs received some form of financial aid in 2012–13.
**Contact** Ashley Wasserman, MSN Representative, School of Nursing, Cedarville University, 251 North Main Street, Cedarville, OH 45314. *Telephone:* 937-766-3151. *E-mail:* awasserman@cedarville.edu.

### MASTER'S DEGREE PROGRAM

**Degree** MSN
**Available Programs** Master's.
**Concentrations Available** *Clinical nurse specialist programs in:* community health, family health. *Nurse practitioner programs in:* family health.
**Study Options** Full-time and part-time.
**Online Degree Options** Yes.
**Program Entrance Requirements** Clinical experience, computer literacy, minimum overall college GPA of 3.0, transcript of college record, written essay, interview, 3 letters of recommendation, prerequisite course work, resume. *Application deadline:* Applications may be processed on a rolling basis for some programs. *Application fee:* $30.
**Degree Requirements** 42 total credit hours, thesis or project.

# Chamberlain College of Nursing

**Chamberlain College of Nursing**
**Columbus, Ohio**

**DEGREES • BSN • MSN**
**Distance Learning Courses** Available.

## BACCALAUREATE PROGRAMS

**Degree** BSN
**Available Programs** Accelerated Baccalaureate; Accelerated Baccalaureate for Second Degree; RN Baccalaureate.
**Contact** *Telephone:* 888-556-8226.

## GRADUATE PROGRAMS

**Contact** *Telephone:* 888-556-8226.

### MASTER'S DEGREE PROGRAM

**Degree** MSN
**Available Programs** Master's.

# Cleveland State University

**School of Nursing**
**Cleveland, Ohio**

***http://www.csuohio.edu/nursing***
Founded in 1964

**DEGREES • BSN • MSN • MSN/MBA • PHD**
**Nursing Program Faculty** 54 (13% with doctorates).
**Baccalaureate Enrollment** 307 **Women** 83% **Men** 17% **Minority** 21% **International** 6%
**Graduate Enrollment** 72 **Women** 94% **Men** 6% **Minority** 29% **Part-time** 100%
**Distance Learning Courses** Available.
**Nursing Student Activities** Sigma Theta Tau, Student Nurses' Association.
**Nursing Student Resources** Academic advising; academic or career counseling; assistance for students with disabilities; bookstore; campus computer network; computer lab; computer-assisted instruction; daycare for children of students; e-mail services; employment services for current students; interactive nursing skills videos; Internet; learning resource lab; library services; nursing audiovisuals; remedial services; resume preparation assistance; skills, simulation, or other laboratory; tutoring.
**Library Facilities** 539,684 volumes (6,000 in health, 300 in nursing); 11,153 periodical subscriptions (70 health-care related).

## BACCALAUREATE PROGRAMS

**Degree** BSN
**Available Programs** Accelerated Baccalaureate for Second Degree; Generic Baccalaureate; RN Baccalaureate.
**Study Options** Full-time.
**Online Degree Options** Yes.
**Program Entrance Requirements** Minimum overall college GPA of 2.5, transcript of college record, CPR certification, written essay, health exam, health insurance, immunizations, interview, 2 letters of recommendation, minimum GPA in nursing prerequisites of 2.75, prerequisite course work. Transfer students are accepted. *Application deadline:* 3/1 (fall). *Application fee:* $25.
**Advanced Placement** Credit given for nursing courses completed elsewhere dependent upon specific evaluations.
**Expenses (2013–14)** *Tuition, state resident:* full-time $9449. *Tuition, nonresident:* full-time $12,628. *International tuition:* $12,628 full-time. *Room and board:* $11,858; room only: $8108 per academic year.
**Financial Aid** 80% of baccalaureate students in nursing programs received some form of financial aid in 2012–13. *Gift aid (need-based):* Federal Pell, FSEOG, state, private, college/university gift aid from institutional funds. *Loans:* Federal Direct (Subsidized and Unsubsidized Stafford PLUS), Perkins, state, alternative loans. *Work-study:* Federal Work-Study, part-time campus jobs. *Financial aid application deadline (priority):* 2/15.
**Contact** Mrs. Mary Leanza Manzuk, Recruiter/Advisor, School of Nursing, Cleveland State University, 2121 Euclid Avenue, JH 238, Cleveland, OH 44115-2214. *Telephone:* 216-687-3810. *Fax:* 216-687-3556. *E-mail:* sonadvising@csuohio.edu.

## GRADUATE PROGRAMS

**Expenses (2013–14)** *Tuition, state resident:* part-time $521 per credit hour. *Tuition, nonresident:* part-time $531 per credit hour.
**Financial Aid** 50% of graduate students in nursing programs received some form of financial aid in 2012–13.
**Contact** Ms. Mary Leanza Manzuk, Recruiter/Advisor, School of Nursing, Cleveland State University, 2121 Euclid Avenue, JH 238, Cleveland, OH 44115-2214. *Telephone:* 216-687-3598. *Fax:* 216-687-3556. *E-mail:* sonadvising@csuohio.edu.

**MASTER'S DEGREE PROGRAM**
**Degrees** MSN; MSN/MBA
**Available Programs** Master's.
**Concentrations Available** Clinical nurse leader; nursing education. *Clinical nurse specialist programs in:* community health, forensic nursing.
**Study Options** Part-time.
**Online Degree Options** Yes (online only).
**Program Entrance Requirements** Computer literacy, minimum overall college GPA of 3.0, transcript of college record, CPR certification, written essay, immunizations, 2 letters of recommendation, professional liability insurance/malpractice insurance, resume, statistics course. *Application deadline:* 3/1 (fall). *Application fee:* $55.
**Advanced Placement** Credit given for nursing courses completed elsewhere dependent upon specific evaluations.
**Degree Requirements** 31 total credit hours.

**POST-MASTER'S PROGRAM**
**Areas of Study** Nursing education.

**DOCTORAL DEGREE PROGRAM**
**Degree** PhD
**Available Programs** Doctorate.
**Areas of Study** Nursing education.
**Program Entrance Requirements** Clinical experience, minimum overall college GPA of 3.25, interview by faculty committee, 2 letters of recommendation, MSN or equivalent, statistics course, vita, writing sample. *Application deadline:* 2/1 (fall). *Application fee:* $30.
**Degree Requirements** 67 total credit hours, dissertation, written exam, residency.

### CONTINUING EDUCATION PROGRAM

**Contact** Noelle Muscatello, Program Assistant, Continuing Education Programs for Health Care Professionals, School of Nursing, Cleveland State University, 2121 Euclid Avenue, Julka Hall, Room 238, Cleveland, OH 44115. *Telephone:* 216-687-3867. *Fax:* 216-687-3556. *E-mail:* j.n.muscatello@csuohio.edu.

## College of Mount St. Joseph
### Department of Nursing
### Cincinnati, Ohio

***http://www.msj.edu/***
Founded in 1920

**DEGREES • BSN • MN**
**Nursing Program Faculty** 32 (4% with doctorates).
**Baccalaureate Enrollment** 287 **Women** 97% **Men** 3% **Minority** 5% **Part-time** 60%
**Graduate Enrollment** 21 **Women** 90% **Men** 10% **Minority** 5%
**Nursing Student Activities** Nursing Honor Society, Sigma Theta Tau, Student Nurses' Association.
**Nursing Student Resources** Academic advising; academic or career counseling; assistance for students with disabilities; bookstore; campus computer network; career placement assistance; computer lab; computer-assisted instruction; daycare for children of students; e-mail services; employment services for current students; externships; housing assistance; interactive nursing skills videos; Internet; learning resource lab; library services; nursing audiovisuals; placement services for program completers; remedial services; resume preparation assistance; skills, simulation, or other laboratory; tutoring.
**Library Facilities** 95,428 volumes (1,800 in health, 1,200 in nursing); 9,306 periodical subscriptions (300 health-care related).

### BACCALAUREATE PROGRAMS

**Degree** BSN
**Available Programs** Accelerated RN Baccalaureate; Generic Baccalaureate.
**Site Options** Cincinnati, OH; Covington, KY.
**Study Options** Full-time and part-time.
**Program Entrance Requirements** Minimum overall college GPA of 2.75, transcript of college record, CPR certification, health exam, health insurance, high school chemistry, 2 years high school math, 2 years high school science, high school transcript, immunizations, interview, minimum high school GPA of 2.75, minimum high school rank 60%, minimum GPA in nursing prerequisites of 2.75, professional liability insurance/malpractice insurance, prerequisite course work. Transfer students are accepted. *Application deadline:* Applications may be processed on a rolling basis for some programs. *Application fee:* $25.
**Advanced Placement** Credit by examination available. Credit given for nursing courses completed elsewhere dependent upon specific evaluations.
**Contact** *Telephone:* 513-244-4511. *Fax:* 513-451-2547.

### GRADUATE PROGRAMS

**Contact** *Telephone:* 513-244-4503. *Fax:* 513-451-2547.

**MASTER'S DEGREE PROGRAM**
**Degree** MN
**Available Programs** Accelerated Master's for Non-Nursing College Graduates.
**Study Options** Full-time.
**Program Entrance Requirements** Minimum overall college GPA of 3.0, transcript of college record, CPR certification, written essay, immunizations, interview, professional liability insurance/malpractice insurance, prerequisite course work, statistics course. *Application deadline:* Applications may be processed on a rolling basis for some programs. *Application fee:* $50.
**Advanced Placement** Credit by examination available. Credit given for nursing courses completed elsewhere dependent upon specific evaluations.
**Degree Requirements** 64 total credit hours, thesis or project.

## Defiance College
### Bachelor's Degree in Nursing
### Defiance, Ohio

Founded in 1850

**DEGREE • BSN**
**Nursing Program Faculty** 3
**Baccalaureate Enrollment** 41 **Women** 63.6% **Men** 36.4% **Minority** 21% **Part-time** 51.5%
**Distance Learning Courses** Available.
**Nursing Student Resources** Academic advising; academic or career counseling; assistance for students with disabilities; bookstore; campus computer network; career placement assistance; computer lab; e-mail services; employment services for current students; housing assistance; Internet; library services; remedial services; resume preparation assistance; tutoring.
**Library Facilities** 175,083 volumes (151,961 in health, 32,588 in nursing); 38,108 periodical subscriptions (1,962 health-care related).

### BACCALAUREATE PROGRAMS

**Degree** BSN
**Available Programs** ADN to Baccalaureate; Accelerated RN Baccalaureate; RN Baccalaureate.
**Site Options** Lima, OH.
**Study Options** Full-time and part-time.
**Program Entrance Requirements** Minimum overall college GPA of 2.5, transcript of college record, CPR certification, health insurance, high school biology, high school chemistry, 3 years high school math, 3 years high school science, high school transcript, immunizations, interview, minimum high school GPA of 2.25, minimum GPA in nursing prerequisites of 2.75, professional liability insurance/malpractice insurance, prerequisite course work, RN licensure. Transfer students are accepted. *Application deadline:* Applications may be processed on a rolling basis for some programs.
**Advanced Placement** Credit given for nursing courses completed elsewhere dependent upon specific evaluations.
**Expenses (2013–14)** *Tuition:* full-time $28,050; part-time $450 per contact hour. *Room and board:* $9260 per academic year. *Required fees:* full-time $590; part-time $95 per term.
**Financial Aid** 87% of baccalaureate students in nursing programs received some form of financial aid in 2012–13. *Gift aid (need-based):* Federal Pell, FSEOG, state, private, college/university gift aid from institutional funds. *Loans:* Federal Direct (Subsidized and Unsubsidized Stafford PLUS), Perkins, alternative loans. *Work-study:* Federal Work-Study, part-time campus jobs. *Financial aid application deadline (priority):* 4/1.
**Contact** Gloria Arps, RN, Assistant Professor of Practice of Nursing/Director of Nursing, Bachelor's Degree in Nursing, Defiance College, 701 North Clinton Street, Tenzer 101, Defiance, OH 43512.

*Telephone:* 419-783-2448. *Fax:* 419-783-2448. *E-mail:* garps@defiance.edu.

# Franciscan University of Steubenville

## Department of Nursing
## Steubenville, Ohio

Founded in 1946

**DEGREES • BSN • MSN**

**Nursing Program Faculty** 15 (20% with doctorates).
**Baccalaureate Enrollment** 177 **Women** 91% **Men** 9% **Minority** 5% **International** 1% **Part-time** 5%
**Graduate Enrollment** 23 **Women** 78% **Men** 22% **Minority** 4% **Part-time** 83%
**Nursing Student Activities** Student Nurses' Association.
**Nursing Student Resources** Academic advising; academic or career counseling; assistance for students with disabilities; bookstore; campus computer network; computer lab; e-mail services; Internet; learning resource lab; library services; resume preparation assistance; tutoring.
**Library Facilities** 29,761 volumes in health, 8,946 volumes in nursing; 178 periodical subscriptions health-care related.

### BACCALAUREATE PROGRAMS

**Degree** BSN
**Available Programs** Generic Baccalaureate; RN Baccalaureate; RPN to Baccalaureate.
**Study Options** Full-time and part-time.
**Program Entrance Requirements** Minimum overall college GPA of 2.5, transcript of college record, health exam, health insurance, high school biology, high school chemistry, 2 years high school science, high school transcript, immunizations, 2 letters of recommendation, minimum high school GPA of 2.4, minimum GPA in nursing prerequisites of 2.5, professional liability insurance/malpractice insurance, prerequisite course work. Transfer students are accepted.
**Advanced Placement** Credit by examination available. Credit given for nursing courses completed elsewhere dependent upon specific evaluations.
**Contact** *Telephone:* 740-283-6324. *Fax:* 740-283-6449.

### GRADUATE PROGRAMS

**Contact** *Telephone:* 740-284-7245. *Fax:* 740-283-6449.

**MASTER'S DEGREE PROGRAM**
**Degree** MSN
**Available Programs** Master's; RN to Master's.
**Concentrations Available** Nursing education. *Nurse practitioner programs in:* family health.
**Study Options** Full-time and part-time.
**Program Entrance Requirements** Clinical experience, minimum overall college GPA of 3.0, transcript of college record, interview, 2 letters of recommendation, nursing research course, physical assessment course, professional liability insurance/malpractice insurance, prerequisite course work, statistics course.
**Advanced Placement** Credit given for nursing courses completed elsewhere dependent upon specific evaluations.
**Degree Requirements** 48 total credit hours, thesis or project.

# Franklin University

## Nursing Program
## Columbus, Ohio

Founded in 1902

**DEGREE • BSN**

**Library Facilities** 102,000 volumes.

### BACCALAUREATE PROGRAMS

**Degree** BSN
**Available Programs** Accelerated Baccalaureate; Generic Baccalaureate.
**Contact** Gail Baumlein, Program Chair, Nursing Program, Franklin University, 201 South Grant Avenue, Columbus, OH 43215. *Telephone:* 614-947-6209. *Fax:* 614-255-9678. *E-mail:* gail.baumlein@franklin.edu.

# Hiram College

## Nursing Department
## Hiram, Ohio

***http://www.hiram.edu/nursing***
Founded in 1850

**DEGREE • BSN**

**Nursing Program Faculty** 18 (20% with doctorates).
**Baccalaureate Enrollment** 83 **Women** 88% **Men** 12% **Minority** 18% **International** 2% **Part-time** 1%
**Nursing Student Activities** Sigma Theta Tau, Student Nurses' Association.
**Nursing Student Resources** Academic advising; academic or career counseling; assistance for students with disabilities; bookstore; campus computer network; career placement assistance; computer lab; computer-assisted instruction; e-mail services; employment services for current students; externships; interactive nursing skills videos; Internet; learning resource lab; library services; nursing audiovisuals; remedial services; resume preparation assistance; skills, simulation, or other laboratory; tutoring.
**Library Facilities** 506,792 volumes (3,846 in health, 869 in nursing); 8,890 periodical subscriptions (555 health-care related).

### BACCALAUREATE PROGRAMS

**Degree** BSN
**Available Programs** Generic Baccalaureate.
**Study Options** Full-time.
**Program Entrance Requirements** Transcript of college record, written essay, health exam, high school biology, high school chemistry, high school foreign language, high school transcript, immunizations, minimum high school GPA of 2.75. Transfer students are accepted. *Application deadline:* Applications may be processed on a rolling basis for some programs.
**Advanced Placement** Credit given for nursing courses completed elsewhere dependent upon specific evaluations.
**Contact** *Telephone:* 330-569-6104. *Fax:* 330-569-6136.

# Hondros College

## Nursing Programs
## Westerville, Ohio

Founded in 1981

**DEGREE • BSN**

### BACCALAUREATE PROGRAMS

**Degree** BSN
**Available Programs** Generic Baccalaureate.
**Study Options** Full-time and part-time.
**Online Degree Options** Yes (online only).
**Program Entrance Requirements** Transfer students are accepted.
**Contact** Admissions Office, Nursing Programs, Hondros College, 4140 Executive Parkway, Westerville, OH 43081. *Telephone:* 614-508-7277. *E-mail:* customercare@hondros.edu.

# Kent State University

## College of Nursing
## Kent, Ohio

***http://www.kent.edu/nursing***
Founded in 1910

**DEGREES • BSN • DNP • MSN • MSN/MBA • MSN/MPA • PHD**

**Nursing Program Faculty** 140 (20% with doctorates).
**Baccalaureate Enrollment** 1,260 **Women** 85% **Men** 15% **Minority** 11% **International** 1% **Part-time** 19%
**Graduate Enrollment** 504 **Women** 87% **Men** 13% **Minority** 30% **International** 3% **Part-time** 91%
**Distance Learning Courses** Available.
**Nursing Student Activities** Nursing Honor Society, Sigma Theta Tau, Student Nurses' Association.
**Nursing Student Resources** Academic advising; academic or career counseling; assistance for students with disabilities; bookstore; campus

computer network; career placement assistance; computer lab; computer-assisted instruction; e-mail services; employment services for current students; externships; housing assistance; interactive nursing skills videos; Internet; learning resource lab; library services; nursing audiovisuals; other; paid internships; placement services for program completers; remedial services; resume preparation assistance; skills, simulation, or other laboratory; tutoring.
**Library Facilities** 2.3 million volumes; 12,000 periodical subscriptions (300 health-care related).

## BACCALAUREATE PROGRAMS

**Degree** BSN
**Available Programs** ADN to Baccalaureate; Accelerated Baccalaureate; Accelerated Baccalaureate for Second Degree; Baccalaureate for Second Degree; Generic Baccalaureate; RN Baccalaureate.
**Site Options** Salem, OH; Burton, OH, OH; Canton, OH; Warren, OH.
**Study Options** Full-time and part-time.
**Program Entrance Requirements** Minimum overall college GPA of 2.75, transcript of college record, CPR certification, written essay, health exam, high school biology, high school transcript, immunizations, 2 letters of recommendation, minimum high school GPA of 2.75, minimum GPA in nursing prerequisites of 2.75, prerequisite course work. Transfer students are accepted. *Application deadline:* 5/2 (fall), 11/30 (spring).
**Advanced Placement** Credit given for nursing courses completed elsewhere dependent upon specific evaluations.
**Expenses (2013–14)** *Tuition, area resident:* full-time $9816; part-time $447 per credit hour. *Tuition, state resident:* full-time $5554; part-time $253 per credit hour. *Tuition, nonresident:* full-time $17,776; part-time $809 per credit hour. *International tuition:* $17,776 full-time. *Room and board:* $9536 per academic year. *Required fees:* full-time $794; part-time $72 per credit.
**Financial Aid** 95% of baccalaureate students in nursing programs received some form of financial aid in 2012–13. *Gift aid (need-based):* Federal Pell, FSEOG, state, private, college/university gift aid from institutional funds. *Loans:* Federal Nursing Student Loans, Federal Direct (Subsidized and Unsubsidized Stafford PLUS), Perkins, state, college/university, alternative loans. *Work-study:* Federal Work-Study. *Financial aid application deadline (priority):* 3/1.
**Contact** Mr. Curtis Good, Director of Student Services, College of Nursing, Kent State University, Henderson Hall, Kent, OH 44242-0001. *Telephone:* 330-672-9972. *Fax:* 330-672-7911. *E-mail:* cjgood@kent.edu.

## GRADUATE PROGRAMS

**Expenses (2013–14)** *Tuition, state resident:* part-time $475 per credit hour. *Tuition, nonresident:* part-time $817 per credit hour. *Room and board:* $10,000 per academic year.
**Financial Aid** 85% of graduate students in nursing programs received some form of financial aid in 2012–13. 10 research assistantships with full tuition reimbursements available, 10 teaching assistantships with full tuition reimbursements available were awarded; Federal Work-Study, institutionally sponsored loans, traineeships, tuition waivers (full), and unspecified assistantships also available. *Financial aid application deadline:* 2/1.
**Contact** Dr. Gail Bromley, Associate Dean, Academics, College of Nursing, Kent State University, 214 Henderson Hall, PO Box 5190, Kent, OH 44242-0001. *Telephone:* 330-672-8761. *Fax:* 330-672-6387. *E-mail:* gbromley@kent.edu.

### MASTER'S DEGREE PROGRAM

**Degrees** MSN; MSN/MBA; MSN/MPA
**Available Programs** Accelerated RN to Master's; Master's.
**Concentrations Available** Health-care administration; nursing education. *Clinical nurse specialist programs in:* adult health, pediatric. *Nurse practitioner programs in:* acute care, adult health, family health, pediatric, primary care, psychiatric/mental health,women's health.
**Study Options** Full-time and part-time.
**Online Degree Options** Yes.
**Program Entrance Requirements** Clinical experience, computer literacy, minimum overall college GPA of 3.0, transcript of college record, CPR certification, written essay, immunizations, interview, 3 letters of recommendation, professional liability insurance/malpractice insurance, resume, statistics course, GRE (if undergraduate GPA less than 3.0). *Application deadline:* 4/1 (fall), 11/1 (spring). Applications may be processed on a rolling basis for some programs. *Application fee:* $30.
**Advanced Placement** Credit given for nursing courses completed elsewhere dependent upon specific evaluations.
**Degree Requirements** 40 total credit hours.

### POST-MASTER'S PROGRAM

**Areas of Study** Health-care administration; nursing education. *Clinical nurse specialist programs in:* adult health, pediatric. *Nurse practitioner programs in:* acute care, adult health, family health, pediatric, primary care, psychiatric/mental health,women's health.

### DOCTORAL DEGREE PROGRAM

**Degree** DNP
**Available Programs** Doctorate.
**Areas of Study** Aging, clinical practice, ethics, family health, gerontology, health policy, health promotion/disease prevention, human health and illness, maternity-newborn, nurse case management, nursing administration, nursing education, nursing research, nursing science, palliative care,women's health.
**Online Degree Options** Yes.
**Program Entrance Requirements** Minimum overall college GPA of 3.0, clinical experience, interview, interview by faculty committee, 2 letters of recommendation, MSN or equivalent, scholarly papers, statistics course, vita, writing sample. *Application deadline:* 7/15 (fall). Applications may be processed on a rolling basis for some programs. *Application fee:* $30.
**Degree Requirements** 72 total credit hours, dissertation, oral exam, written exam.

**Degree** PhD
**Available Programs** Doctorate.
**Areas of Study** Aging, clinical practice, ethics, family health, gerontology, health policy, health promotion/disease prevention, human health and illness, maternity-newborn, nurse case management, nursing administration, nursing education, nursing research, nursing science, palliative care,women's health.
**Online Degree Options** Yes.
**Program Entrance Requirements** Clinical experience, minimum overall college GPA of 3.0, interview by faculty committee, interview, 2 letters of recommendation, MSN or equivalent, scholarly papers, statistics course, vita, writing sample, GRE. *Application deadline:* 7/15 (fall). Applications may be processed on a rolling basis for some programs. *Application fee:* $30.
**Degree Requirements** 72 total credit hours, dissertation, oral exam, written exam.

## CONTINUING EDUCATION PROGRAM

**Contact** Shirley Hemminger, Coordinator of Continuing Nursing Education, College of Nursing, Kent State University, PO Box 5190, Kent, OH 44242-0001. *Telephone:* 330-672-8812. *Fax:* 330-672-2433. *E-mail:* shemming@kent.edu.

# Kettering College
## Division of Nursing
## Kettering, Ohio

***http://www.kc.edu/nursing***
Founded in 1967

**DEGREE • BSN**
**Nursing Program Faculty** 17 (15% with doctorates).
**Baccalaureate Enrollment** 60 **Women** 95% **Part-time** 100%
**Distance Learning Courses** Available.
**Nursing Student Activities** Student Nurses' Association.
**Nursing Student Resources** Academic advising; academic or career counseling; assistance for students with disabilities; bookstore; campus computer network; computer lab; computer-assisted instruction; e-mail services; externships; interactive nursing skills videos; Internet; learning resource lab; library services; nursing audiovisuals; remedial services; resume preparation assistance; skills, simulation, or other laboratory; tutoring.
**Library Facilities** 29,390 volumes (4,060 in health, 1,073 in nursing); 266 periodical subscriptions (173 health-care related).

## BACCALAUREATE PROGRAMS

**Degree** BSN
**Available Programs** Generic Baccalaureate; RN Baccalaureate.
**Study Options** Full-time.
**Online Degree Options** Yes (online only).
**Program Entrance Requirements** Minimum overall college GPA of 2.5, transcript of college record, CPR certification, health insurance, immunizations, minimum GPA in nursing prerequisites of 2.5, prereq-

uisite course work. Transfer students are accepted. *Application deadline:* 5/25 (spring).
**Advanced Placement** Credit given for nursing courses completed elsewhere dependent upon specific evaluations.
**Expenses (2013–14)** *Tuition:* full-time $11,110; part-time $418 per credit. *Room and board:* $3675 per academic year. *Required fees:* full-time $1200; part-time $400 per term.
**Financial Aid** 42% of baccalaureate students in nursing programs received some form of financial aid in 2012–13. *Gift aid (need-based):* Federal Pell, state, private, college/university gift aid from institutional funds. *Loans:* Federal Nursing Student Loans, Federal Direct (Subsidized and Unsubsidized Stafford PLUS), Perkins, college/university. *Work-study:* Federal Work-Study, part-time campus jobs. *Financial aid application deadline (priority):* 3/31.
**Contact** Dr. Cherie R. Rebar, Director, Division of Nursing/Chair, Prelicensure Nursing Programs, Division of Nursing, Kettering College, 3737 Southern Boulevard, Kettering, OH 45429. *Telephone:* 937-395-8642. *Fax:* 937-395-8810. *E-mail:* cherie.rebar@kc.edu.

# Lourdes University

## School of Nursing
## Sylvania, Ohio

***http://www.lourdes.edu/***
Founded in 1958

**DEGREES • BSN • MSN**
**Nursing Program Faculty** 25 (32% with doctorates).
**Baccalaureate Enrollment** 236 **Women** 83% **Men** 17% **Minority** 23% **Part-time** 39%
**Graduate Enrollment** 144 **Women** 88% **Men** 12% **Minority** 13% **Part-time** 15%
**Nursing Student Activities** Nursing Honor Society, Sigma Theta Tau, Student Nurses' Association.
**Nursing Student Resources** Academic advising; academic or career counseling; assistance for students with disabilities; bookstore; campus computer network; career placement assistance; computer lab; computer-assisted instruction; e-mail services; employment services for current students; housing assistance; interactive nursing skills videos; Internet; learning resource lab; library services; nursing audiovisuals; placement services for program completers; remedial services; resume preparation assistance; skills, simulation, or other laboratory; tutoring.
**Library Facilities** 187,314 volumes (1,200 in health, 700 in nursing); 68,916 periodical subscriptions (101 health-care related).

### BACCALAUREATE PROGRAMS

**Degree** BSN
**Available Programs** ADN to Baccalaureate; Generic Baccalaureate; LPN to Baccalaureate; LPN to RN Baccalaureate; RN Baccalaureate.
**Study Options** Full-time and part-time.
**Program Entrance Requirements** Minimum overall college GPA of 2.5, transcript of college record, CPR certification, health exam, high school transcript, immunizations, minimum GPA in nursing prerequisites of 2.5, prerequisite course work, RN licensure. Transfer students are accepted. *Application deadline:* 1/2 (fall), 8/1 (winter).
**Advanced Placement** Credit by examination available. Credit given for nursing courses completed elsewhere dependent upon specific evaluations.
**Expenses (2013–14)** *Tuition:* full-time $17,455; part-time $582 per credit. *Room and board:* $7800; room only: $4600 per academic year. *Required fees:* full-time $1200; part-time $50 per credit.
**Financial Aid** 98% of baccalaureate students in nursing programs received some form of financial aid in 2012–13.
**Contact** Ms. Pat Yancy, Nursing Advisor/Recruiter, School of Nursing, Lourdes University, 6832 Convent Boulevard, Sylvania, OH 43560. *Telephone:* 419-824-8919. *Fax:* 419-824-3985. *E-mail:* pyancy@lourdes.edu.

### GRADUATE PROGRAMS

**Expenses (2013–14)** *Tuition:* full-time $9375; part-time $625 per credit. *Room and board:* $7800; room only: $4600 per academic year.
**Financial Aid** 50% of graduate students in nursing programs received some form of financial aid in 2012–13.
**Contact** Dr. Deborah Vargo, MSN Director, School of Nursing, Lourdes University, 6832 Convent Boulevard, Sylvania, OH 43560. *Telephone:* 419-824-3792. *Fax:* 419-824-3985. *E-mail:* dvargo@lourdes.edu.

**MASTER'S DEGREE PROGRAM**
**Degree** MSN
**Available Programs** Master's; RN to Master's.
**Concentrations Available** Nurse anesthesia; nursing administration; nursing education.
**Study Options** Full-time and part-time.
**Program Entrance Requirements** Transcript of college record, written essay, interview, letters of recommendation, nursing research course. *Application deadline:* 8/1 (fall), 1/2 (winter). Applications may be processed on a rolling basis for some programs.
**Degree Requirements** 33 total credit hours, thesis or project.

# Malone University

## School of Nursing
## Canton, Ohio

***http://www.malone.edu/***
Founded in 1892

**DEGREES • BSN • MSN**
**Nursing Program Faculty** 35 (21% with doctorates).
**Baccalaureate Enrollment** 241 **Women** 82% **Men** 18% **Minority** 6% **Part-time** 7.4%
**Graduate Enrollment** 64 **Women** 95% **Men** 5% **Minority** 7% **Part-time** 100%
**Nursing Student Activities** Sigma Theta Tau, Student Nurses' Association.
**Nursing Student Resources** Academic advising; academic or career counseling; assistance for students with disabilities; bookstore; campus computer network; career placement assistance; computer lab; computer-assisted instruction; e-mail services; employment services for current students; interactive nursing skills videos; Internet; learning resource lab; library services; nursing audiovisuals; remedial services; resume preparation assistance; skills, simulation, or other laboratory; tutoring; unpaid internships.
**Library Facilities** 250,747 volumes; 50,713 periodical subscriptions.

### BACCALAUREATE PROGRAMS

**Degree** BSN
**Available Programs** ADN to Baccalaureate; Generic Baccalaureate; RN Baccalaureate.
**Study Options** Full-time and part-time.
**Program Entrance Requirements** Minimum overall college GPA of 2.5, transcript of college record, CPR certification, health exam, health insurance, high school biology, high school chemistry, 2 years high school math, 3 years high school science, high school transcript, immunizations, 2 letters of recommendation, minimum high school GPA of 2.5, minimum GPA in nursing prerequisites of 2.0, professional liability insurance/malpractice insurance, prerequisite course work. Transfer students are accepted. *Application deadline:* Applications may be processed on a rolling basis for some programs. *Application fee:* $20.
**Advanced Placement** Credit given for nursing courses completed elsewhere dependent upon specific evaluations.
**Expenses (2013–14)** *Tuition:* full-time $24,934; part-time $445 per credit hour. *Room and board:* $8438; room only: $4412 per academic year. *Required fees:* full-time $385.
**Contact** Vice President for Enrollment Management, School of Nursing, Malone University, 2600 Cleveland Avenue NW, Canton, OH 44709. *Telephone:* 330-471-8145. *Fax:* 330-471-8149. *E-mail:* admissions@malone.edu.

### GRADUATE PROGRAMS

**Expenses (2013–14)** *Tuition:* full-time $21,865; part-time $645 per hour. *Required fees:* full-time $4050.
**Contact** Ms. Jean Yanok, Administrative Assistant, School of Nursing, Malone University, 2600 Cleveland Avenue NW, Canton, OH 44709. *Telephone:* 330-471-8366. *Fax:* 330-471-8607. *E-mail:* jyanok@malone.edu.

**MASTER'S DEGREE PROGRAM**
**Degree** MSN
**Available Programs** Master's.
**Concentrations Available** *Nurse practitioner programs in:* family health.
**Study Options** Full-time and part-time.
**Program Entrance Requirements** Clinical experience, computer literacy, minimum overall college GPA of 3.0, transcript of college record,

CPR certification, written essay, immunizations, interview, 2 letters of recommendation, nursing research course, physical assessment course, professional liability insurance/malpractice insurance, resume, statistics course. *Application deadline:* Applications may be processed on a rolling basis for some programs. *Application fee:* $150.
**Advanced Placement** Credit given for nursing courses completed elsewhere dependent upon specific evaluations.
**Degree Requirements** 56 total credit hours, thesis or project.

# Mercy College of Ohio
## Division of Nursing
## Toledo, Ohio

***http://www.mercycollege.edu/***
Founded in 1993

**DEGREE • BSN**
**Nursing Program Faculty** 89 (6% with doctorates).
**Baccalaureate Enrollment** 312 **Women** 86% **Men** 14% **Minority** 15% **Part-time** 34%
**Distance Learning Courses** Available.
**Nursing Student Activities** Sigma Theta Tau, Student Nurses' Association.
**Nursing Student Resources** Academic advising; academic or career counseling; assistance for students with disabilities; campus computer network; career placement assistance; computer lab; computer-assisted instruction; e-mail services; employment services for current students; housing assistance; interactive nursing skills videos; Internet; learning resource lab; library services; nursing audiovisuals; remedial services; resume preparation assistance; skills, simulation, or other laboratory; tutoring.
**Library Facilities** 6,000 volumes (3,580 in health, 800 in nursing); 128 periodical subscriptions (325 health-care related).

### BACCALAUREATE PROGRAMS
**Degree** BSN
**Available Programs** Generic Baccalaureate; RN Baccalaureate.
**Study Options** Full-time and part-time.
**Online Degree Options** Yes.
**Program Entrance Requirements** Minimum overall college GPA of 2.7, transcript of college record, CPR certification, health exam, health insurance, high school biology, high school chemistry, 2 years high school math, high school transcript, immunizations, minimum high school GPA of 2.7. Transfer students are accepted. *Application deadline:* 8/1 (fall). *Application fee:* $25.
**Advanced Placement** Credit by examination available.
**Expenses (2013–14)** *Tuition:* full-time $10,770; part-time $396 per credit hour. *Required fees:* full-time $660; part-time $22 per credit.
**Financial Aid** 85% of baccalaureate students in nursing programs received some form of financial aid in 2012–13. *Gift aid (need-based):* Federal Pell, FSEOG, state, private, college/university gift aid from institutional funds, Federal Nursing. *Loans:* Federal Direct (Subsidized and Unsubsidized Stafford PLUS), state, college/university. *Work-study:* Federal Work-Study. *Financial aid application deadline:* Continuous.
**Contact** Ms. Aimee Bishop-Stuart, Director of Admissions, Division of Nursing, Mercy College of Ohio, 2221 Madison Avenue, Toledo, OH 43604. *Telephone:* 888-806-3729. *Fax:* 419-251-1462. *E-mail:* aimee.bishop-stuart@mercycollege.edu.

# Miami University
## Department of Nursing
## Hamilton, Ohio

***http://www.regionals.miamioh.edu/nsg/***
Founded in 1809

**DEGREE • BSN**
**Nursing Program Faculty** 13 (23% with doctorates).
**Baccalaureate Enrollment** 106 **Women** 98% **Men** 2% **Minority** 7% **Part-time** 56%
**Distance Learning Courses** Available.
**Nursing Student Activities** Sigma Theta Tau, Student Nurses' Association.
**Nursing Student Resources** Academic advising; academic or career counseling; assistance for students with disabilities; bookstore; campus computer network; computer lab; daycare for children of students; e-mail services; interactive nursing skills videos; Internet; learning resource lab; library services; nursing audiovisuals; resume preparation assistance; tutoring.
**Library Facilities** 4.2 million volumes (29,000 in nursing); 109,477 periodical subscriptions (852 health-care related).

### BACCALAUREATE PROGRAMS
**Degree** BSN
**Available Programs** ADN to Baccalaureate; Generic Baccalaureate; RN Baccalaureate.
**Site Options** Hamilton, OH; Middletown, OH.
**Study Options** Full-time and part-time.
**Program Entrance Requirements** Minimum overall college GPA of 2.5, transcript of college record, health exam, health insurance, high school chemistry, 2 years high school math, 1 year of high school science, high school transcript, immunizations, minimum high school GPA of 3.0, minimum GPA in nursing prerequisites of 2.5, professional liability insurance/malpractice insurance. Transfer students are accepted.
**Advanced Placement** Credit given for nursing courses completed elsewhere dependent upon specific evaluations.
**Contact** *Telephone:* 513-785-7751. *Fax:* 513-785-7767.

# Miami University Hamilton
## Bachelor of Science in Nursing Program
## Hamilton, Ohio

Founded in 1968

**DEGREE • BSN**
**Nursing Program Faculty** 27 (15% with doctorates).
**Baccalaureate Enrollment** 116
**Distance Learning Courses** Available.
**Nursing Student Activities** Sigma Theta Tau, Student Nurses' Association.
**Nursing Student Resources** Academic advising; academic or career counseling; assistance for students with disabilities; bookstore; campus computer network; career placement assistance; computer lab; computer-assisted instruction; daycare for children of students; e-mail services; employment services for current students; interactive nursing skills videos; Internet; learning resource lab; library services; nursing audiovisuals; placement services for program completers; remedial services; resume preparation assistance; skills, simulation, or other laboratory; tutoring.
**Library Facilities** 68,000 volumes; 400 periodical subscriptions.

### BACCALAUREATE PROGRAMS
**Degree** BSN
**Available Programs** Generic Baccalaureate; RN Baccalaureate.
**Site Options** West Chester, OH; Middletown, OH.
**Contact** *Telephone:* 513-785-7772. *Fax:* 513-785-7767.

# Mount Carmel College of Nursing
## Nursing Programs
## Columbus, Ohio

***http://www.mccn.edu/***
Founded in 1903

**DEGREES • BSN • MS**
**Nursing Program Faculty** 117 (18% with doctorates).
**Baccalaureate Enrollment** 947 **Women** 90% **Men** 10% **Minority** 11% **Part-time** 31%
**Graduate Enrollment** 174 **Women** 94% **Men** 6% **Minority** 21% **Part-time** 44%
**Distance Learning Courses** Available.
**Nursing Student Activities** Sigma Theta Tau, Student Nurses' Association.
**Nursing Student Resources** Academic advising; academic or career counseling; assistance for students with disabilities; bookstore; campus computer network; computer lab; computer-assisted instruction; e-mail services; housing assistance; interactive nursing skills videos; Internet; learning resource lab; library services; nursing audiovisuals; resume preparation assistance; skills, simulation, or other laboratory; tutoring.
**Library Facilities** 95,090 volumes (4,755 in health, 2,282 in nursing); 8,830 periodical subscriptions (5,677 health-care related).

## BACCALAUREATE PROGRAMS

**Degree** BSN
**Available Programs** Accelerated Baccalaureate for Second Degree; Generic Baccalaureate; RN Baccalaureate.
**Site Options** Lancaster, OH.
**Study Options** Full-time.
**Online Degree Options** Yes.
**Program Entrance Requirements** Minimum overall college GPA of 2.8, transcript of college record, written essay, health exam, high school biology, high school chemistry, high school foreign language, 3 years high school math, 3 years high school science, high school transcript, immunizations, minimum high school GPA of 3.0. Transfer students are accepted. *Application deadline:* 4/1 (fall), 11/1 (spring). Applications may be processed on a rolling basis for some programs. *Application fee:* $30.
**Advanced Placement** Credit given for nursing courses completed elsewhere dependent upon specific evaluations.
**Expenses (2013–14)** *Tuition:* full-time $16,897; part-time $528 per credit hour. *Room and board:* room only: $5000 per academic year. *Required fees:* full-time $851.
**Financial Aid** 88% of baccalaureate students in nursing programs received some form of financial aid in 2012–13. *Gift aid (need-based):* Federal Pell, FSEOG, state, private, college/university gift aid from institutional funds. *Loans:* Federal Nursing Student Loans, Federal Direct (Subsidized and Unsubsidized Stafford PLUS), college/university. *Work-study:* part-time campus jobs. *Financial aid application deadline:* Continuous.
**Contact** Kim M. Campbell, Director, Admissions and Recruitment, Nursing Programs, Mount Carmel College of Nursing, 127 South Davis Avenue, Columbus, OH 43222-1504. *Telephone:* 614-234-5144. *Fax:* 614-234-2875. *E-mail:* kcampbell@mccn.edu.

## GRADUATE PROGRAMS

**Expenses (2013–14)** *Tuition:* full-time $8560; part-time $428 per credit hour. *Room and board:* room only: $5000 per academic year. *Required fees:* full-time $98.
**Financial Aid** 86% of graduate students in nursing programs received some form of financial aid in 2012–13.
**Contact** Kathy Walters, MS Program Coordinator, Nursing Programs, Mount Carmel College of Nursing, 127 South Davis Avenue, Columbus, OH 43222-1504. *Telephone:* 614-234-5408. *Fax:* 614-234-5403. *E-mail:* kwalters@mccn.edu.

### MASTER'S DEGREE PROGRAM

**Degree** MS
**Available Programs** Master's.
**Concentrations Available** Nursing administration; nursing education. *Clinical nurse specialist programs in:* adult health. *Nurse practitioner programs in:* family health, gerontology.
**Study Options** Full-time and part-time.
**Program Entrance Requirements** Minimum overall college GPA of 3.0, transcript of college record, CPR certification, written essay, 3 letters of recommendation, professional liability insurance/malpractice insurance, resume. *Application deadline:* 7/1 (fall), 11/1 (spring), 4/1 (summer). Applications may be processed on a rolling basis for some programs. *Application fee:* $30.
**Degree Requirements** 34 total credit hours, thesis or project.

### POST-MASTER'S PROGRAM

**Areas of Study** Nursing administration; nursing education. *Nurse practitioner programs in:* family health, gerontology.

# Mount Vernon Nazarene University

### School of Nursing and Health Sciences
### Mount Vernon, Ohio

*http://www.mvnu.edu/*
Founded in 1964

**DEGREE • BS**
**Nursing Program Faculty** 12 (8% with doctorates).
**Baccalaureate Enrollment** 109
**Nursing Student Activities** Sigma Theta Tau, nursing club.
**Nursing Student Resources** Academic advising; academic or career counseling; assistance for students with disabilities; bookstore; campus computer network; computer lab; computer-assisted instruction; e-mail services; employment services for current students; interactive nursing skills videos; Internet; learning resource lab; library services; nursing audiovisuals; remedial services; resume preparation assistance; skills, simulation, or other laboratory; tutoring.
**Library Facilities** 105,420 volumes; 17,271 periodical subscriptions.

## BACCALAUREATE PROGRAMS

**Degree** BS
**Available Programs** ADN to Baccalaureate; Generic Baccalaureate.
**Study Options** Full-time and part-time.
**Program Entrance Requirements** Transcript of college record, CPR certification, health exam, health insurance, immunizations, minimum GPA in nursing prerequisites of 2.0, professional liability insurance/malpractice insurance, prerequisite course work. Transfer students are accepted. *Application deadline:* Applications may be processed on a rolling basis for some programs.
**Contact** Nursing Program, School of Nursing and Health Sciences, Mount Vernon Nazarene University, 800 Martinsburg Road, Mount Vernon, OH 43050. *Telephone:* 740-392-6868.

# Muskingum University

### Department of Nursing
### New Concord, Ohio

Founded in 1837

**DEGREE • BSN**
**Library Facilities** 233,000 volumes; 900 periodical subscriptions.

## BACCALAUREATE PROGRAMS

**Degree** BSN
**Available Programs** Generic Baccalaureate.
**Contact** *Telephone:* 740-826-6151.

# Notre Dame College

### Nursing Department
### South Euclid, Ohio

Founded in 1922

**DEGREE • BSN**

## BACCALAUREATE PROGRAMS

**Degree** BSN
**Available Programs** Generic Baccalaureate; RN Baccalaureate.
**Contact** *Telephone:* 216-373-5183.

# Ohio Northern University

### Nursing Program
### Ada, Ohio

Founded in 1871

**DEGREE • BSN**

## BACCALAUREATE PROGRAMS

**Degree** BSN
**Available Programs** Accelerated RN Baccalaureate; RN Baccalaureate.
**Study Options** Full-time.
**Program Entrance Requirements** High school biology, high school chemistry, 2 years high school math, high school transcript, minimum high school GPA of 3.3. Transfer students are accepted.
**Contact** Admissions Undergraduate, Admissions Office, Nursing Program, Ohio Northern University, 525 North Main Street, Ada, OH 45810. *Telephone:* 888-408-4668. *Fax:* 419-772-2821. *E-mail:* admissions-ug@onu.edu.

# The Ohio State University
## College of Nursing
## Columbus, Ohio

*http://www.nursing.osu.edu/*
Founded in 1870

### DEGREES • BSN • DNP • MS • MS/MPH • PHD

**Nursing Program Faculty** 110 (20% with doctorates).
**Baccalaureate Enrollment** 710 **Women** 85% **Men** 15% **Minority** 11% **International** 1% **Part-time** 33%
**Graduate Enrollment** 580 **Women** 85% **Men** 15% **Minority** 13% **International** 2% **Part-time** 33%
**Distance Learning Courses** Available.
**Nursing Student Activities** Nursing Honor Society, Sigma Theta Tau, Student Nurses' Association, nursing club.
**Nursing Student Resources** Academic advising; academic or career counseling; assistance for students with disabilities; bookstore; campus computer network; career placement assistance; computer lab; computer-assisted instruction; daycare for children of students; e-mail services; employment services for current students; externships; housing assistance; interactive nursing skills videos; Internet; learning resource lab; library services; nursing audiovisuals; other; paid internships; placement services for program completers; remedial services; resume preparation assistance; skills, simulation, or other laboratory; tutoring; unpaid internships.
**Library Facilities** 6.2 million volumes (112,764 in health, 12,534 in nursing); 26,297 periodical subscriptions (6,297 health-care related).

### BACCALAUREATE PROGRAMS

**Degree** BSN
**Available Programs** Generic Baccalaureate; RN Baccalaureate.
**Study Options** Full-time.
**Online Degree Options** Yes.
**Program Entrance Requirements** Minimum overall college GPA of 3.2, transcript of college record, written essay, high school biology, high school chemistry, high school foreign language, 3 years high school math, 2 years high school science, high school transcript, minimum GPA in nursing prerequisites of 3.2, prerequisite course work. *Application deadline:* 1/15 (fall), 9/1 (summer). *Application fee:* $60.
**Advanced Placement** Credit by examination available. Credit given for nursing courses completed elsewhere dependent upon specific evaluations.
**Expenses (2013–14)** *Tuition, state resident:* full-time $9170; part-time $4585 per semester. *Tuition, nonresident:* full-time $25,430; part-time $12,715 per semester. *International tuition:* $25,430 full-time. *Room and board:* $10,800; room only: $6000 per academic year. *Required fees:* full-time $2400; part-time $200 per credit; part-time $1200 per term.
**Financial Aid** 80% of baccalaureate students in nursing programs received some form of financial aid in 2012–13. *Gift aid (need-based):* Federal Pell, FSEOG, state, private, college/university gift aid from institutional funds. *Loans:* Federal Nursing Student Loans, Federal Direct (Subsidized and Unsubsidized Stafford PLUS), Perkins, college/university. *Work-study:* Federal Work-Study, part-time campus jobs. *Financial aid application deadline (priority):* 2/15.
**Contact** Ms. Jennifer Marinello, Associate Director, College of Nursing, The Ohio State University, Graduate and Professional Admissions, 105 Student Academic Services Building, Columbus, OH 43210. *Telephone:* 614-292-9444. *Fax:* 614-292-3895. *E-mail:* marinello.1@osu.edu.

### GRADUATE PROGRAMS

**Expenses (2013–14)** *Tuition, state resident:* full-time $11,560; part-time $5780 per semester. *Tuition, nonresident:* full-time $29,225; part-time $14,613 per semester. *International tuition:* $29,225 full-time. *Room and board:* $10,800; room only: $6000 per academic year. *Required fees:* full-time $3240; part-time $405 per credit; part-time $1620 per term.
**Financial Aid** 90% of graduate students in nursing programs received some form of financial aid in 2012–13. Fellowships, research assistantships, teaching assistantships, Federal Work-Study, institutionally sponsored loans, and unspecified assistantships available. Aid available to part-time students.
**Contact** Ms. Jackie Min, Graduate Outreach Coordinator, College of Nursing, The Ohio State University, 1585 Neil Avenue, 212 Newton Hall, Columbus, OH 43210-1289. *Telephone:* 614-688-8145. *Fax:* 614-292-9399. *E-mail:* min.37@osu.edu.

#### MASTER'S DEGREE PROGRAM

**Degrees** MS; MS/MPH
**Available Programs** Master's; Master's for Non-Nursing College Graduates; Master's for Nurses with Non-Nursing Degrees; RN to Master's.
**Concentrations Available** Clinical nurse leader; health-care administration; nurse-midwifery; nursing administration. *Clinical nurse specialist programs in:* adult health, community health, public health. *Nurse practitioner programs in:* acute care, adult health, community health, family health, gerontology, neonatal health, pediatric, primary care, psychiatric/mental health,women's health.
**Study Options** Full-time and part-time.
**Online Degree Options** Yes.
**Program Entrance Requirements** Minimum overall college GPA of 3.5, transcript of college record, written essay, 3 letters of recommendation, prerequisite course work, resume. *Application deadline:* 1/15 (fall), 10/12 (summer). *Application fee:* $60.
**Advanced Placement** Credit given for nursing courses completed elsewhere dependent upon specific evaluations.
**Degree Requirements** 30 total credit hours, thesis or project, comprehensive exam.

#### POST-MASTER'S PROGRAM

**Areas of Study** Clinical nurse leader; health-care administration; nurse-midwifery; nursing administration. *Clinical nurse specialist programs in:* adult health, community health, public health. *Nurse practitioner programs in:* acute care, adult health, community health, family health, gerontology, neonatal health, pediatric, primary care, psychiatric/mental health,women's health.

#### DOCTORAL DEGREE PROGRAM

**Degree** DNP
**Available Programs** Doctorate, Post-Baccalaureate Doctorate.
**Areas of Study** Addiction/substance abuse, advanced practice nursing, aging, bio-behavioral research, biology of health and illness, clinical nurse leader, clinical practice, clinical research, community health, critical care, ethics, faculty preparation, family health, forensic nursing, gerontology, health policy, health promotion/disease prevention, health-care systems, human health and illness, illness and transition, individualized study, information systems, maternity-newborn, neuro-behavior, nurse case management, nursing administration, nursing education, nursing policy, nursing research, nursing science, oncology, palliative care, urban health,women's health.
**Online Degree Options** Yes (online only).
**Program Entrance Requirements** Minimum overall college GPA of 3.5, clinical experience, interview by faculty committee, 3 letters of recommendation, MSN or equivalent, vita, writing sample. *Application deadline:* 3/1 (fall). *Application fee:* $60.
**Degree Requirements** 54 total credit hours, oral exam, residency, written exam.

**Degree** PhD
**Available Programs** Doctorate; Post-Baccalaureate Doctorate.
**Areas of Study** Addiction/substance abuse, advanced practice nursing, aging, bio-behavioral research, biology of health and illness, clinical practice, clinical research, community health, critical care, ethics, faculty preparation, family health, forensic nursing, gerontology, health policy, health promotion/disease prevention, health-care systems, human health and illness, illness and transition, individualized study, information systems, maternity-newborn, neuro-behavior, nurse case management, nursing administration, nursing education, nursing policy, nursing research, nursing science, oncology, palliative care, urban health,women's health.
**Program Entrance Requirements** Clinical experience, minimum overall college GPA of 3.5, 3 letters of recommendation, MSN or equivalent, vita, writing sample. *Application deadline:* 3/1 (fall). *Application fee:* $60.
**Degree Requirements** 54 total credit hours, dissertation, oral exam, written exam, residency.

### CONTINUING EDUCATION PROGRAM

**Contact** Ms. Jackie Loversidge, Director of Continuing Education, College of Nursing, The Ohio State University, 1585 Neil Avenue, Columbus, OH 43210-1289. *Telephone:* 614-292-6379. *Fax:* 614-292-7976. *E-mail:* loversidge.1@osu.edu.

# Ohio University
## School of Nursing
## Athens, Ohio

*http://www.ohio.edu/chsp/nrse/*
Founded in 1804

**DEGREES • BSN • MSN**
**Nursing Program Faculty** 9 (89% with doctorates).
**Nursing Student Activities** Nursing Honor Society, Sigma Theta Tau.
**Nursing Student Resources** Academic or career counseling; career placement assistance; computer lab; e-mail services; Internet; library services.
**Library Facilities** 3.3 million volumes; 62,042 periodical subscriptions.

### BACCALAUREATE PROGRAMS
**Degree** BSN
**Available Programs** Generic Baccalaureate; RN Baccalaureate.
**Online Degree Options** Yes.
**Program Entrance Requirements** Transfer students are accepted.
**Contact** *Telephone:* 740-593-4494. *Fax:* 740-593-0286.

### GRADUATE PROGRAMS
**Contact** *Telephone:* 740-593-4494. *Fax:* 740-593-0144.

**MASTER'S DEGREE PROGRAM**
**Degree** MSN
**Available Programs** Master's.
**Concentrations Available** Nursing administration; nursing education. *Nurse practitioner programs in:* family health.
**Study Options** Full-time and part-time.
**Program Entrance Requirements** Minimum overall college GPA of 3.0, transcript of college record, written essay, 3 letters of recommendation, resume, statistics course.
**Advanced Placement** Credit given for nursing courses completed elsewhere dependent upon specific evaluations.
**Degree Requirements** 55 total credit hours.

# Otterbein University
## Department of Nursing
## Westerville, Ohio

*http://www.otterbein.edu/*
Founded in 1847

**DEGREES • BSN • MSN**
**Nursing Student Activities** Nursing Honor Society, Sigma Theta Tau.
**Library Facilities** 182,629 volumes; 1,012 periodical subscriptions.

### BACCALAUREATE PROGRAMS
**Degree** BSN
**Available Programs** Accelerated RN Baccalaureate; Generic Baccalaureate; LPN to Baccalaureate; RN Baccalaureate.
**Program Entrance Requirements** Transfer students are accepted.
**Advanced Placement** Credit by examination available. Credit given for nursing courses completed elsewhere dependent upon specific evaluations.
**Contact** *Telephone:* 614-823-1614. *Fax:* 614-823-3131.

### GRADUATE PROGRAMS
**Contact** *Telephone:* 614-823-1614.

**MASTER'S DEGREE PROGRAM**
**Degree** MSN
**Available Programs** Master's.
**Concentrations Available** Nursing administration; nursing education. *Clinical nurse specialist programs in:* adult health. *Nurse practitioner programs in:* adult health, family health.
**Study Options** Part-time.

**POST-MASTER'S PROGRAM**
**Areas of Study** Nursing education. *Nurse practitioner programs in:* adult health, family health.

### CONTINUING EDUCATION PROGRAM
**Contact** *Telephone:* 614-823-1614.

# Shawnee State University
## Department of Nursing
## Portsmouth, Ohio

*http://www.shawnee.edu/*
Founded in 1986

**DEGREE • BSN**
**Nursing Program Faculty** 9
**Nursing Student Activities** Student Nurses' Association.
**Nursing Student Resources** Academic advising; academic or career counseling; assistance for students with disabilities; bookstore; campus computer network; career placement assistance; computer lab; computer-assisted instruction; daycare for children of students; e-mail services; employment services for current students; housing assistance; interactive nursing skills videos; Internet; learning resource lab; library services; nursing audiovisuals; other; placement services for program completers; remedial services; resume preparation assistance; skills, simulation, or other laboratory; tutoring.
**Library Facilities** 135,302 volumes (8,273 in health, 870 in nursing); 58,868 periodical subscriptions (1,798 health-care related).

### BACCALAUREATE PROGRAMS
**Degree** BSN
**Available Programs** ADN to Baccalaureate; RN Baccalaureate.
**Study Options** Full-time and part-time.
**Program Entrance Requirements** Minimum overall college GPA of 2.5, transcript of college record, CPR certification, health exam, health insurance, high school transcript, immunizations, professional liability insurance/malpractice insurance, prerequisite course work, RN licensure. Transfer students are accepted.
**Advanced Placement** Credit given for nursing courses completed elsewhere dependent upon specific evaluations.
**Contact** *Telephone:* 740-351-3378. *Fax:* 740-351-3354.

### CONTINUING EDUCATION PROGRAM
**Contact** *Telephone:* 740-351-3281.

# The University of Akron
## School of Nursing
## Akron, Ohio

*http://www.uakron.edu/nursing/*
Founded in 1870

**DEGREES • BSN • MSN • PHD**
**Nursing Program Faculty** 98 (25% with doctorates).
**Baccalaureate Enrollment** 551 **Women** 78% **Men** 22% **Minority** 10% **Part-time** 1%
**Graduate Enrollment** 329 **Women** 87% **Men** 13% **Minority** 9% **Part-time** 74%
**Distance Learning Courses** Available.
**Nursing Student Activities** Sigma Theta Tau, Student Nurses' Association, nursing club.
**Nursing Student Resources** Academic advising; academic or career counseling; assistance for students with disabilities; bookstore; campus computer network; career placement assistance; computer lab; computer-assisted instruction; daycare for children of students; e-mail services; employment services for current students; interactive nursing skills videos; Internet; learning resource lab; library services; nursing audiovisuals; remedial services; resume preparation assistance; skills, simulation, or other laboratory; tutoring.
**Library Facilities** 1.3 million volumes (36,800 in health, 10,258 in nursing); 481,872 periodical subscriptions (7,804 health-care related).

### BACCALAUREATE PROGRAMS
**Degree** BSN
**Available Programs** ADN to Baccalaureate; Accelerated Baccalaureate for Second Degree; Accelerated RN Baccalaureate; Generic Baccalaureate; LPN to Baccalaureate; LPN to RN Baccalaureate.
**Site Options** Lorain, OH; Orville, OH; Medina, OH; Lakewood (UA Lakewood), OH; Kirtland (Lakeland Community College), OH.

**Study Options** Full-time and part-time.
**Online Degree Options** Yes.
**Program Entrance Requirements** Transcript of college record, CPR certification, health exam, immunizations, minimum GPA in nursing prerequisites of 2.75, prerequisite course work. Transfer students are accepted. *Application deadline:* Applications may be processed on a rolling basis for some programs. *Application fee:* $40.
**Advanced Placement** Credit given for nursing courses completed elsewhere dependent upon specific evaluations.
**Expenses (2012–13)** *Tuition, state resident:* full-time $9552; part-time $345 per credit hour. *Tuition, nonresident:* full-time $17,753; part-time $687 per credit hour. *International tuition:* $17,753 full-time. *Room and board:* $11,878; room only: $6306 per academic year. *Required fees:* full-time $634; part-time $53 per credit; part-time $317 per term.
**Financial Aid** 80% of baccalaureate students in nursing programs received some form of financial aid in 2011–12. *Gift aid (need-based):* Federal Pell, FSEOG, state, college/university gift aid from institutional funds. *Loans:* Federal Nursing Student Loans, Federal Direct (Subsidized and Unsubsidized Stafford PLUS), Perkins, college/university. *Work-study:* Federal Work-Study, part-time campus jobs. *Financial aid application deadline (priority):* 2/1.
**Contact** School of Nursing, School of Nursing, The University of Akron, Mary Gladwin Hall, 209 Carroll Street, Akron, OH 44325-3701. *Telephone:* 330-972-7551. *Fax:* 330-972-5737.

## GRADUATE PROGRAMS

**Expenses (2012–13)** *Tuition, state resident:* full-time $7285; part-time $405 per credit hour. *Tuition, nonresident:* full-time $12,473; part-time $693 per credit hour. *Room and board:* $11,878; room only: $6306 per academic year. *Required fees:* full-time $613; part-time $34 per credit; part-time $306 per term.
**Financial Aid** 80% of graduate students in nursing programs received some form of financial aid in 2011–12. 4 research assistantships with full tuition reimbursements available, 14 teaching assistantships with full tuition reimbursements available were awarded; career-related internships or fieldwork and Federal Work-Study also available.
**Contact** Dr. Marlene S. Huff, Coordinator, Educational Progression and Graduate Programs, School of Nursing, The University of Akron, Akron, OH 44325-3701. *Telephone:* 330-972-5930. *Fax:* 330-972-5737. *E-mail:* mhuff@uakron.edu.

### MASTER'S DEGREE PROGRAM

**Degree** MSN
**Available Programs** Master's; RN to Master's.
**Concentrations Available** Nurse anesthesia; nursing administration. *Clinical nurse specialist programs in:* adult health, gerontology, pediatric, psychiatric/mental health. *Nurse practitioner programs in:* acute care, adult health, gerontology, pediatric, primary .care, psychiatric/mental health.
**Site Options** Lorain, OH; Orville, OH.
**Study Options** Full-time and part-time.
**Program Entrance Requirements** Clinical experience, computer literacy, minimum overall college GPA of 3.0, transcript of college record, CPR certification, written essay, immunizations, interview, 3 letters of recommendation, physical assessment course, professional liability insurance/malpractice insurance, prerequisite course work, resume, statistics course. *Application deadline:* Applications may be processed on a rolling basis for some programs. *Application fee:* $40.
**Advanced Placement** Credit given for nursing courses completed elsewhere dependent upon specific evaluations.
**Degree Requirements** 53 total credit hours.

### POST-MASTER'S PROGRAM

**Areas of Study** Nurse anesthesia. *Clinical nurse specialist programs in:* adult health, gerontology, pediatric, psychiatric/mental health. *Nurse practitioner programs in:* acute care, adult health, family health, gerontology, pediatric, primary care, psychiatric/mental health.

### DOCTORAL DEGREE PROGRAM

**Degree** PhD
**Available Programs** Doctorate.
**Areas of Study** Advanced practice nursing, aging, clinical practice, community health, critical care, ethics, family health, gerontology, health policy, health promotion/disease prevention, health-care systems, human health and illness, illness and transition, individualized study, maternity-newborn, nursing administration, nursing policy, nursing research, nursing science,women's health.
**Program Entrance Requirements** Minimum overall college GPA of 3.0, interview by faculty committee, interview, 3 letters of recommendation, MSN or equivalent, vita, writing sample, GRE. *Application deadline:* Applications may be processed on a rolling basis for some programs. *Application fee:* $40.
**Degree Requirements** 72 total credit hours, dissertation, oral exam, written exam, residency.

## CONTINUING EDUCATION PROGRAM

**Contact** Dr. Marlene S. Huff, Coordinator, Educational Progression and Graduate Programs, School of Nursing, The University of Akron, Akron, OH 44325-3701. *Telephone:* 330-972-5930. *Fax:* 330-972-5737. *E-mail:* mhuff@uakron.edu.

# University of Cincinnati
## College of Nursing
## Cincinnati, Ohio

***http://www.nursing.uc.edu/***
Founded in 1819

**DEGREES • BSN • MSN • MSN/MBA • MSN/PHD • PHD**
**Nursing Program Faculty** 143 (31% with doctorates).
**Baccalaureate Enrollment** 631 **Women** 90% **Men** 10% **Minority** 14% **Part-time** 13%
**Graduate Enrollment** 360 **Women** 86% **Men** 14% **Minority** 14% **International** 2%
**Distance Learning Courses** Available.
**Nursing Student Activities** Sigma Theta Tau, Student Nurses' Association.
**Nursing Student Resources** Academic advising; academic or career counseling; assistance for students with disabilities; bookstore; campus computer network; computer lab; computer-assisted instruction; e-mail services; employment services for current students; externships; housing assistance; interactive nursing skills videos; Internet; learning resource lab; library services; nursing audiovisuals; paid internships; remedial services; resume preparation assistance; skills, simulation, or other laboratory; tutoring; unpaid internships.
**Library Facilities** 4.3 million volumes (221,630 in health, 21,306 in nursing); 123,795 periodical subscriptions (2,384 health-care related).

## BACCALAUREATE PROGRAMS

**Degree** BSN
**Available Programs** ADN to Baccalaureate; Accelerated Baccalaureate for Second Degree; Generic Baccalaureate; RN Baccalaureate.
**Site Options** Cincinnati, OH.
**Study Options** Full-time.
**Program Entrance Requirements** Minimum overall college GPA of 2.5, transcript of college record, CPR certification, health insurance, high school biology, high school chemistry, 3 years high school math, high school transcript, immunizations, prerequisite course work. Transfer students are accepted. *Application deadline:* 6/30 (fall).
**Advanced Placement** Credit by examination available. Credit given for nursing courses completed elsewhere dependent upon specific evaluations.
**Contact** *Telephone:* 513-558-5070. *Fax:* 513-558-7523.

## GRADUATE PROGRAMS

**Contact** *Telephone:* 513-558-5072. *Fax:* 513-558-7523.

### MASTER'S DEGREE PROGRAM

**Degrees** MSN; MSN/MBA; MSN/PhD
**Available Programs** Accelerated Master's for Non-Nursing College Graduates; Master's.
**Concentrations Available** Nurse anesthesia; nurse-midwifery; nursing administration. *Clinical nurse specialist programs in:* adult health, critical care, gerontology, medical-surgical, occupational health, public health. *Nurse practitioner programs in:* adult health, family health, neonatal health, occupational health, pediatric,women's health.
**Site Options** Cincinnati, OH.
**Study Options** Full-time and part-time.
**Online Degree Options** Yes.
**Program Entrance Requirements** Clinical experience, computer literacy, transcript of college record, CPR certification, written essay, immunizations, interview, 3 letters of recommendation, physical assessment course, professional liability insurance/malpractice insurance, resume, statistics course, GRE General Test. *Application deadline:* 10/1 (fall), 9/1 (winter), 1/1 (spring), 3/1 (summer). Applications may be processed on a rolling basis for some programs. *Application fee:* $40.

**Advanced Placement** Credit given for nursing courses completed elsewhere dependent upon specific evaluations.
**Degree Requirements** 65 total credit hours, thesis or project.

**POST-MASTER'S PROGRAM**
**Areas of Study** Nursing education. *Nurse practitioner programs in:* adult health, family health, neonatal health, occupational health, pediatric, psychiatric/mental health,women's health.

**DOCTORAL DEGREE PROGRAM**
**Degree** PhD
**Available Programs** Doctorate; Post-Baccalaureate Doctorate.
**Areas of Study** Addiction/substance abuse, community health, critical care, ethics, faculty preparation, family health, health promotion/disease prevention, health-care systems, human health and illness, illness and transition, individualized study, maternity-newborn, nursing administration, nursing research, nursing science, oncology,women's health.
**Site Options** Cincinnati, OH.
**Program Entrance Requirements** Minimum overall college GPA of 3.0, interview by faculty committee, interview, 3 letters of recommendation, statistics course, vita, writing sample, GRE General Test. *Application deadline:* 8/15 (fall). Applications may be processed on a rolling basis for some programs. *Application fee:* $40.
**Degree Requirements** 135 total credit hours, dissertation, oral exam, written exam, residency.

### CONTINUING EDUCATION PROGRAM
**Contact** *Telephone:* 513-558-5311. *Fax:* 513-558-5054.

## University of Phoenix–Cleveland Campus
### College of Nursing
### Independence, Ohio

Founded in 2000
**DEGREES • BSN • MSN**
**Nursing Program Faculty** 10 (20% with doctorates).
**Baccalaureate Enrollment** 17 **Women** 82.4% **Men** 17.6% **Minority** 11.8%
**Graduate Enrollment** 4 **Women** 100%
**Nursing Student Activities** Sigma Theta Tau.
**Nursing Student Resources** Academic advising; academic or career counseling; assistance for students with disabilities; bookstore; campus computer network; computer lab; computer-assisted instruction; e-mail services; interactive nursing skills videos; Internet; learning resource lab; library services; nursing audiovisuals; remedial services; skills, simulation, or other laboratory; tutoring.
**Library Facilities** 16,781 periodical subscriptions (1,300 health-care related).

### BACCALAUREATE PROGRAMS
**Degree** BSN
**Available Programs** Accelerated Baccalaureate.
**Site Options** Beachwood, OH.
**Study Options** Full-time.
**Program Entrance Requirements** Transcript of college record, CPR certification, immunizations, 1 letter of recommendation, RN licensure. Transfer students are accepted. *Application deadline:* Applications may be processed on a rolling basis for some programs.
**Advanced Placement** Credit by examination available. Credit given for nursing courses completed elsewhere dependent upon specific evaluations.
**Contact** *Telephone:* 216-447-8807.

### GRADUATE PROGRAMS
**Contact** *Telephone:* 216-447-8807.

**MASTER'S DEGREE PROGRAM**
**Degree** MSN
**Available Programs** Master's.
**Concentrations Available** Nursing administration.
**Site Options** Beachwood, OH.
**Study Options** Full-time.
**Program Entrance Requirements** Clinical experience, computer literacy, minimum overall college GPA of 2.5, transcript of college record. *Application deadline:* Applications may be processed on a rolling basis for some programs. *Application fee:* $45.
**Advanced Placement** Credit given for nursing courses completed elsewhere dependent upon specific evaluations.
**Degree Requirements** 39 total credit hours, thesis or project.

## University of Rio Grande
### Holzer School of Nursing
### Rio Grande, Ohio

Founded in 1876
**DEGREE • BSN**
**Nursing Program Faculty** 9
**Library Facilities** 96,731 volumes; 850 periodical subscriptions.

### BACCALAUREATE PROGRAMS
**Degree** BSN
**Available Programs** RN Baccalaureate.
**Study Options** Full-time and part-time.
**Contact** *Telephone:* 800-282-7201 Ext. 7308. *Fax:* 740-245-7177.

## The University of Toledo
### College of Nursing
### Toledo, Ohio

***http://www.utoledo.edu/nursing***
Founded in 1872
**DEGREES • BSN • DNP • MSN**
**Nursing Program Faculty** 51 (51% with doctorates).
**Baccalaureate Enrollment** 474 **Women** 90% **Men** 10% **Minority** 10% **International** 1% **Part-time** 17%
**Graduate Enrollment** 306 **Women** 80% **Men** 20% **Minority** 13% **International** 1% **Part-time** 65%
**Distance Learning Courses** Available.
**Nursing Student Activities** Sigma Theta Tau, Student Nurses' Association.
**Nursing Student Resources** Academic advising; academic or career counseling; assistance for students with disabilities; bookstore; campus computer network; computer lab; computer-assisted instruction; daycare for children of students; e-mail services; employment services for current students; interactive nursing skills videos; Internet; learning resource lab; library services; nursing audiovisuals; remedial services; resume preparation assistance; skills, simulation, or other laboratory; tutoring.
**Library Facilities** 1.9 million volumes (33,000 in health, 4,000 in nursing); 95,498 periodical subscriptions (10,000 health-care related).

### BACCALAUREATE PROGRAMS
**Degree** BSN
**Available Programs** ADN to Baccalaureate; Generic Baccalaureate; RN Baccalaureate.
**Site Options** Toledo, OH.
**Study Options** Full-time.
**Online Degree Options** Yes.
**Program Entrance Requirements** Minimum overall college GPA of 3.0, transcript of college record, CPR certification, health exam, health insurance, high school biology, high school chemistry, high school foreign language, 3 years high school math, 3 years high school science, high school transcript, immunizations, minimum high school GPA of 2.75, minimum GPA in nursing prerequisites of 2.0, professional liability insurance/malpractice insurance, prerequisite course work. Transfer students are accepted. *Application deadline:* 5/1 (fall), 9/1 (spring), 1/15 (summer). *Application fee:* $45.
**Advanced Placement** Credit given for nursing courses completed elsewhere dependent upon specific evaluations.
**Expenses (2013–14)** *Tuition, state resident:* full-time $7864; part-time $328 per credit hour. *Tuition, nonresident:* full-time $16,984; part-time $708 per credit hour. *International tuition:* $16,984 full-time. *Room and board:* $10,912; room only: $7312 per academic year. *Required fees:* full-time $1190; part-time $50 per credit.
**Financial Aid** 95% of baccalaureate students in nursing programs received some form of financial aid in 2012–13. *Gift aid (need-based):* Federal Pell, FSEOG, state, private, college/university gift aid from institutional funds, Academic Competitiveness Grants, National SMART

Grants, TEACH Grants. *Loans:* Federal Direct (Subsidized and Unsubsidized Stafford PLUS), Perkins, alternative loans. *Work-study:* Federal Work-Study. *Financial aid application deadline (priority):* 4/1.
**Contact** Ms. Kathleen Mitchell, Assistant Dean for Student Services, College of Nursing, The University of Toledo, Mail Stop #1026, 3000 Arlington Avenue, Toledo, OH 43614-2598. *Telephone:* 419-383-5839. *Fax:* 419-383-5894. *E-mail:* kathleen.mitchell@utoledo.edu.

## GRADUATE PROGRAMS

**Expenses (2013–14)** *Tuition, state resident:* full-time $13,036; part-time $543 per credit hour. *Tuition, nonresident:* full-time $23,270; part-time $969 per credit hour. *International tuition:* $23,270 full-time. *Room and board:* $12,842; room only: $7312 per academic year. *Required fees:* full-time $1798; part-time $50 per credit.
**Financial Aid** 91% of graduate students in nursing programs received some form of financial aid in 2012–13. Research assistantships with full and partial tuition reimbursements available, Federal Work-Study, institutionally sponsored loans, scholarships, traineeships, and tuition waivers (full and partial) available.
**Contact** Mr. David Lymanstall, Director, Graduate Advising, College of Nursing, The University of Toledo, Mail Stop #1026, 3000 Arlington Avenue, Toledo, OH 43614-2598. *Telephone:* 419-383-5841. *Fax:* 419-383-5894. *E-mail:* david.lymanstall@utoledo.edu.

### MASTER'S DEGREE PROGRAM

**Degree** MSN
**Available Programs** Master's; Master's for Non-Nursing College Graduates; Master's for Nurses with Non-Nursing Degrees.
**Concentrations Available** Clinical nurse leader; nursing education. *Nurse practitioner programs in:* family health, pediatric.
**Site Options** Toledo, OH.
**Study Options** Full-time and part-time.
**Program Entrance Requirements** Computer literacy, minimum overall college GPA of 3.0, transcript of college record, CPR certification, written essay, immunizations, 3 letters of recommendation, resume, GRE. *Application deadline:* 12/15 (fall), 9/1 (spring). *Application fee:* $110.
**Advanced Placement** Credit given for nursing courses completed elsewhere dependent upon specific evaluations.
**Degree Requirements** 55 total credit hours, thesis or project, comprehensive exam.

### POST-MASTER'S PROGRAM

**Areas of Study** Nursing education. *Nurse practitioner programs in:* family health, pediatric.

### DOCTORAL DEGREE PROGRAM

**Degree** DNP
**Available Programs** Doctorate; Post-Baccalaureate Doctorate.
**Areas of Study** Advanced practice nursing, nursing administration.
**Site Options** Toledo, OH.
**Online Degree Options** Yes.
**Program Entrance Requirements** Clinical experience, minimum overall college GPA of 3.0, interview by faculty committee, interview, 3 letters of recommendation, MSN or equivalent, statistics course, vita, writing sample. *Application deadline:* 12/15 (fall). *Application fee:* $110.
**Degree Requirements** 89 total credit hours.

## CONTINUING EDUCATION PROGRAM

**Contact** Dr. Deborah Mattin, Director, Continuing Nursing Education, College of Nursing, The University of Toledo, Mail Stop #1026, 3000 Arlington Avenue, Toledo, OH 43614-2598. *Telephone:* 419-383-5812. *Fax:* 419-383-5894. *E-mail:* deborah.mattin@utoledo.edu.

# Urbana University

## College of Nursing and Allied Health
## Urbana, Ohio

***http://www.urbana.edu/academics/college-of-nursing-and-allied-health/***
Founded in 1850

**DEGREES • BSN • MSN**

**Nursing Program Faculty** 4 (100% with doctorates).
**Baccalaureate Enrollment** 30 **Women** 98% **Men** 2% **Minority** 2% **Part-time** 100%
**Graduate Enrollment** 60 **Women** 100% **Minority** 8% **Part-time** 100%
**Distance Learning Courses** Available.
**Nursing Student Activities** Nursing Honor Society.
**Nursing Student Resources** Academic advising; academic or career counseling; assistance for students with disabilities; bookstore; campus computer network; career placement assistance; computer lab; e-mail services; Internet; learning resource lab; library services; nursing audiovisuals; placement services for program completers; remedial services; resume preparation assistance; tutoring.
**Library Facilities** 61,600 volumes (320 in health, 250 in nursing); 800 periodical subscriptions (1,000 health-care related).

## BACCALAUREATE PROGRAMS

**Degree** BSN
**Available Programs** ADN to Baccalaureate.
**Site Options** Springfield, OH; Dayton, OH.
**Study Options** Full-time and part-time.
**Online Degree Options** Yes.
**Program Entrance Requirements** Minimum overall college GPA of 2.0, transcript of college record, CPR certification, health exam, health insurance, immunizations, 3 letters of recommendation, minimum GPA in nursing prerequisites of 3.0, professional liability insurance/malpractice insurance, RN licensure. Transfer students are accepted. *Application deadline:* Applications may be processed on a rolling basis for some programs.
**Expenses (2013–14)** *Tuition:* part-time $445 per credit hour. *Required fees:* part-time $300 per term.
**Financial Aid** 10% of baccalaureate students in nursing programs received some form of financial aid in 2012–13.
**Contact** Dr. Sue Z. Green, BSN Program Chair, College of Nursing and Allied Health, Urbana University, Losch Hall, Suite #6, 579 College Way, Urbana, OH 43078. *Telephone:* 937-652-6734. *E-mail:* sgreen@urbana.edu.

## GRADUATE PROGRAMS

**Expenses (2013–14)** *Tuition:* part-time $510 per credit hour. *Required fees:* part-time $300 per term.
**Financial Aid** 10% of graduate students in nursing programs received some form of financial aid in 2012–13.
**Contact** Dr. Barbara Miville, MSN Program Chair, College of Nursing and Allied Health, Urbana University, Losch Hall, Suite #6, 579 College Way, Urbana, OH 43078. *Telephone:* 937-652-6735. *Fax:* 937-484-1251. *E-mail:* bmiville@urbana.edu.

### MASTER'S DEGREE PROGRAM

**Degree** MSN
**Available Programs** Master's; Master's for Nurses with Non-Nursing Degrees; RN to Master's.
**Concentrations Available** Nursing administration; nursing education.
**Site Options** Springfield, OH; Dayton, OH.
**Study Options** Full-time and part-time.
**Program Entrance Requirements** Computer literacy, minimum overall college GPA of 3.0, transcript of college record, CPR certification, written essay, immunizations, interview, 3 letters of recommendation, professional liability insurance/malpractice insurance, resume. *Application deadline:* 8/1 (fall), 12/1 (spring), 5/1 (summer). Applications may be processed on a rolling basis for some programs.
**Advanced Placement** Credit given for nursing courses completed elsewhere dependent upon specific evaluations.
**Degree Requirements** 47 total credit hours, thesis or project.

## CONTINUING EDUCATION PROGRAM

**Contact** Ms. Renee Crabill, Administrative Assistant, College of Nursing and Allied Health, Urbana University, 579 College Way, Urbana, OH 43078. *Telephone:* 937-484-1374. *E-mail:* rcrabill@urbana.edu.

# Ursuline College

## The Breen School of Nursing
## Pepper Pike, Ohio

Founded in 1871

**DEGREES • BSN • DNP • MSN • MSN/MBA**

**Nursing Program Faculty** 25 (35% with doctorates).
**Baccalaureate Enrollment** 350 **Women** 92% **Men** 8% **Minority** 28% **International** 1%
**Graduate Enrollment** 280 **Women** 90% **Men** 10% **Minority** 28% **International** 2% **Part-time** 75%
**Distance Learning Courses** Available.

**Nursing Student Activities** Nursing Honor Society, Sigma Theta Tau, Student Nurses' Association.
**Nursing Student Resources** Academic advising; academic or career counseling; assistance for students with disabilities; bookstore; campus computer network; career placement assistance; computer lab; computer-assisted instruction; e-mail services; employment services for current students; externships; interactive nursing skills videos; Internet; learning resource lab; library services; nursing audiovisuals; placement services for program completers; remedial services; resume preparation assistance; skills, simulation, or other laboratory; tutoring; unpaid internships.
**Library Facilities** 208,262 volumes; 47,869 periodical subscriptions.

## BACCALAUREATE PROGRAMS

**Degree** BSN
**Available Programs** ADN to Baccalaureate; Accelerated Baccalaureate; Accelerated Baccalaureate for Second Degree; Accelerated RN Baccalaureate; Baccalaureate for Second Degree; Generic Baccalaureate; RN Baccalaureate.
**Study Options** Full-time.
**Program Entrance Requirements** Minimum overall college GPA of 2.5, transcript of college record, written essay, health exam, health insurance, high school biology, high school chemistry, 2 years high school math, 2 years high school science, high school transcript, immunizations, 1 letter of recommendation, minimum high school GPA of 2.75, minimum GPA in nursing prerequisites of 2.75. Transfer students are accepted. *Application deadline:* Applications may be processed on a rolling basis for some programs. *Application fee:* $100.
**Advanced Placement** Credit given for nursing courses completed elsewhere dependent upon specific evaluations.
**Expenses (2013–14)** *Tuition:* full-time $28,000; part-time $880 per credit hour.
**Financial Aid** ***Gift aid (need-based):*** Federal Pell, FSEOG, state, private, college/university gift aid from institutional funds, United Negro College Fund. *Loans:* Federal Direct (Subsidized and Unsubsidized Stafford PLUS), Perkins, state, college/university. *Work-study:* Federal Work-Study. *Financial aid application deadline:* Continuous.
**Contact** Elizabeth Beach, Coordinator, BSN Enrollment, The Breen School of Nursing, Ursuline College, 2550 Lander Road, Pepper Pike, OH 44124-4398. *Telephone:* 440-449-4200. *Fax:* 440-449-4267.

## GRADUATE PROGRAMS

**Contact** Dr. Janet R. Baker, Director, Graduate Program, The Breen School of Nursing, Ursuline College, 2550 Lander Road, Pepper Pike, OH 44124-4398. *Telephone:* 440-449-4200 Ext. 8172. *Fax:* 440-684-6053. *E-mail:* jbaker@ursuline.edu.

### MASTER'S DEGREE PROGRAM

**Degrees** MSN; MSN/MBA
**Available Programs** Accelerated Master's; Master's.
**Concentrations Available** Nurse case management; nursing education; nursing informatics. *Clinical nurse specialist programs in:* adult health, palliative care. *Nurse practitioner programs in:* adult health, family health.
**Study Options** Full-time and part-time.
**Program Entrance Requirements** Clinical experience, minimum overall college GPA of 3.0, transcript of college record, CPR certification, written essay, immunizations, 3 letters of recommendation, resume. *Application deadline:* 6/15 (fall), 12/15 (spring). Applications may be processed on a rolling basis for some programs.
**Advanced Placement** Credit given for nursing courses completed elsewhere dependent upon specific evaluations.
**Degree Requirements** 43 total credit hours, thesis or project.

### POST-MASTER'S PROGRAM

**Areas of Study** Nurse case management; nursing education; nursing informatics. *Clinical nurse specialist programs in:* adult health, palliative care. *Nurse practitioner programs in:* adult health, family health.

### DOCTORAL DEGREE PROGRAM

**Degree** DNP
**Available Programs** Doctorate.
**Program Entrance Requirements** Clinical experience, minimum overall college GPA of 3.0, 2 letters of recommendation, MSN or equivalent, vita, writing sample. *Application deadline:* 5/15 (fall). Applications may be processed on a rolling basis for some programs. *Application fee:* $25.
**Degree Requirements** 38 total credit hours, dissertation.

# Walsh University

## Department of Nursing
## North Canton, Ohio

***http://www.walsh.edu/***
Founded in 1958

**DEGREES • BSN • DNP • MSN**
**Nursing Program Faculty** 18 (40% with doctorates).
**Baccalaureate Enrollment** 271 **Women** 77% **Men** 23% **Minority** 5% **International** 1% **Part-time** 10%
**Graduate Enrollment** 32 **Women** 100% **Part-time** 80%
**Distance Learning Courses** Available.
**Nursing Student Activities** Sigma Theta Tau, Student Nurses' Association.
**Nursing Student Resources** Academic advising; academic or career counseling; assistance for students with disabilities; bookstore; campus computer network; career placement assistance; computer lab; computer-assisted instruction; e-mail services; employment services for current students; housing assistance; interactive nursing skills videos; Internet; learning resource lab; library services; nursing audiovisuals; placement services for program completers; remedial services; resume preparation assistance; skills, simulation, or other laboratory; tutoring.
**Library Facilities** 277,307 volumes (4,000 in health, 2,000 in nursing); 61,193 periodical subscriptions (114 health-care related).

## BACCALAUREATE PROGRAMS

**Degree** BSN
**Available Programs** Accelerated Baccalaureate; Accelerated Baccalaureate for Second Degree; Generic Baccalaureate; RN Baccalaureate.
**Site Options** Akron, OH; Canton, OH.
**Study Options** Full-time and part-time.
**Program Entrance Requirements** Transcript of college record, CPR certification, health exam, health insurance, high school chemistry, high school foreign language, 3 years high school math, 3 years high school science, high school transcript, immunizations, minimum high school GPA of 2.3, minimum GPA in nursing prerequisites of 2.75, professional liability insurance/malpractice insurance, prerequisite course work. Transfer students are accepted. *Application deadline:* 8/15 (fall), 12/31 (spring), 4/15 (summer). Applications may be processed on a rolling basis for some programs. *Application fee:* $25.
**Advanced Placement** Credit by examination available. Credit given for nursing courses completed elsewhere dependent upon specific evaluations.
**Expenses (2012–13)** *Tuition:* full-time $23,550; part-time $785 per credit. *International tuition:* $23,550 full-time. *Room and board:* $10,200; room only: $6000 per academic year. *Required fees:* full-time $1140; part-time $38 per credit.
**Financial Aid** 94% of baccalaureate students in nursing programs received some form of financial aid in 2011–12.
**Contact** Dr. Linda G. Linc, Professor and Chair, Department of Nursing, Walsh University, 2020 East Maple Street, North Canton, OH 44720-3336. *Telephone:* 330-490-7251. *Fax:* 330-490-7206. *E-mail:* llinc@walsh.edu.

## GRADUATE PROGRAMS

**Expenses (2012–13)** *Tuition:* full-time $5265; part-time $585 per credit. *International tuition:* $5265 full-time. *Room and board:* $10,200; room only: $6000 per academic year.
**Financial Aid** 40% of graduate students in nursing programs received some form of financial aid in 2011–12.
**Contact** Dr. Karen Gehrling, Director, Graduate Programs, Department of Nursing, Walsh University, 2020 East Maple Street, North Canton, OH 44720. *Telephone:* 330-490-7251. *Fax:* 330-490-7206. *E-mail:* kgehrling@walsh.edu.

### MASTER'S DEGREE PROGRAM

**Degree** MSN
**Available Programs** Accelerated AD/RN to Master's; Master's.
**Concentrations Available** Clinical nurse leader; nursing education.
**Study Options** Full-time and part-time.
**Online Degree Options** Yes (online only).
**Program Entrance Requirements** Minimum overall college GPA of 3.0, transcript of college record, written essay, interview, statistics course. *Application deadline:* Applications may be processed on a rolling basis for some programs. *Application fee:* $25.
**Advanced Placement** Credit given for nursing courses completed elsewhere dependent upon specific evaluations.

**Degree Requirements** 36 total credit hours, thesis or project.

**DOCTORAL DEGREE PROGRAM**
**Degree** DNP
**Available Programs** Post-Baccalaureate Doctorate.
**Areas of Study** Ethics, health policy, health promotion/disease prevention, health-care systems, information systems, nurse case management, nursing administration, nursing policy, nursing research, nursing science.
**Online Degree Options** Yes (online only).
**Program Entrance Requirements** Minimum overall college GPA of 3.0, interview by faculty committee, interview, 2 letters of recommendation, MSN or equivalent, statistics course, writing sample. *Application deadline:* Applications may be processed on a rolling basis for some programs. *Application fee:* $25.
**Degree Requirements** 38 total credit hours, residency.

# Wright State University
## College of Nursing and Health
## Dayton, Ohio

*http://nursing.wright.edu/*
Founded in 1964

**DEGREES • BSN • DNP • MS • MS/MBA**
**Nursing Program Faculty** 68 (33% with doctorates).
**Baccalaureate Enrollment** 787 **Women** 84% **Men** 16% **Minority** 16% **International** 1% **Part-time** 35%
**Graduate Enrollment** 257 **Women** 94% **Men** 6% **Minority** 14% **Part-time** 86%
**Distance Learning Courses** Available.
**Nursing Student Activities** Nursing Honor Society, Sigma Theta Tau, Student Nurses' Association, nursing club.
**Nursing Student Resources** Academic advising; academic or career counseling; assistance for students with disabilities; bookstore; campus computer network; career placement assistance; computer lab; computer-assisted instruction; daycare for children of students; e-mail services; employment services for current students; externships; housing assistance; interactive nursing skills videos; Internet; learning resource lab; library services; nursing audiovisuals; remedial services; resume preparation assistance; skills, simulation, or other laboratory; tutoring.
**Library Facilities** 910,287 volumes (111,826 in health, 7,646 in nursing); 36,138 periodical subscriptions (1,279 health-care related).

### BACCALAUREATE PROGRAMS

**Degree** BSN
**Available Programs** Accelerated Baccalaureate for Second Degree; Baccalaureate for Second Degree; Generic Baccalaureate; RN Baccalaureate.
**Site Options** Dayton, OH; Chillicothe, OH; Celina, OH.
**Study Options** Full-time and part-time.
**Program Entrance Requirements** Minimum overall college GPA of 2.5, transcript of college record, written essay, high school transcript, minimum GPA in nursing prerequisites of 2.5, prerequisite course work. Transfer students are accepted. *Application deadline:* 6/30 (fall), 12/30 (spring).
**Advanced Placement** Credit by examination available. Credit given for nursing courses completed elsewhere dependent upon specific evaluations.
**Contact** *Telephone:* 937-775-3132. *Fax:* 937-775-4571.

### GRADUATE PROGRAMS

**Contact** *Telephone:* 937-775-3577. *Fax:* 937-775-4571.

**MASTER'S DEGREE PROGRAM**
**Degrees** MS; MS/MBA
**Available Programs** Master's; Master's for Nurses with Non-Nursing Degrees.
**Concentrations Available** Clinical nurse leader; health-care administration; nursing administration. *Clinical nurse specialist programs in:* adult health, community health, pediatric, public health, school health. *Nurse practitioner programs in:* acute care, family health, pediatric.
**Study Options** Full-time and part-time.
**Online Degree Options** Yes.
**Program Entrance Requirements** Clinical experience, computer literacy, minimum overall college GPA of 3.0, transcript of college record, written essay, interview, physical assessment course, statistics course, GRE General Test. *Application deadline:* Applications may be processed on a rolling basis for some programs. *Application fee:* $30.
**Advanced Placement** Credit given for nursing courses completed elsewhere dependent upon specific evaluations.
**Degree Requirements** 48 total credit hours, thesis or project.

**POST-MASTER'S PROGRAM**
**Areas of Study** *Clinical nurse specialist programs in:* school health. *Nurse practitioner programs in:* acute care, family health, pediatric.

**DOCTORAL DEGREE PROGRAM**
**Degree** DNP
**Available Programs** Doctorate.
**Areas of Study** Advanced practice nursing, biology of health and illness, clinical practice, community health, family health, health policy, health promotion/disease prevention, health-care systems, information systems, nursing administration, nursing policy, nursing science.
**Online Degree Options** Yes (online only).
**Program Entrance Requirements** Clinical experience, minimum overall college GPA of 3.3, interview by faculty committee, 3 letters of recommendation, MSN or equivalent, statistics course, vita, writing sample.
**Degree Requirements** 54 total credit hours, dissertation.

### CONTINUING EDUCATION PROGRAM

**Contact** *Telephone:* 937-775-3577. *Fax:* 937-775-4571.

# Xavier University
## School of Nursing
## Cincinnati, Ohio

Founded in 1831

**DEGREES • BSN • MSN • MSN/ED D • MSN/MBA**
**Nursing Program Faculty** 72 (11% with doctorates).
**Baccalaureate Enrollment** 317 **Women** 90% **Men** 10% **Minority** 10% **Part-time** 18%
**Graduate Enrollment** 235 **Women** 96% **Men** 4% **Minority** 10% **Part-time** 72%
**Nursing Student Activities** Sigma Theta Tau, nursing club.
**Nursing Student Resources** Academic advising; academic or career counseling; assistance for students with disabilities; bookstore; campus computer network; career placement assistance; computer lab; computer-assisted instruction; e-mail services; employment services for current students; externships; housing assistance; interactive nursing skills videos; Internet; learning resource lab; library services; nursing audiovisuals; remedial services; resume preparation assistance; skills, simulation, or other laboratory; tutoring.
**Library Facilities** 479,256 volumes (8,900 in health, 1,160 in nursing); 58,509 periodical subscriptions (200 health-care related).

### BACCALAUREATE PROGRAMS

**Degree** BSN
**Available Programs** Generic Baccalaureate.
**Study Options** Full-time and part-time.
**Program Entrance Requirements** Minimum overall college GPA of 2.7, transcript of college record, written essay, high school chemistry, high school foreign language, 3 years high school math, 2 years high school science, high school transcript, minimum high school GPA of 3.0. Transfer students are accepted. *Application deadline:* Applications may be processed on a rolling basis for some programs. *Application fee:* $35.
**Advanced Placement** Credit given for nursing courses completed elsewhere dependent upon specific evaluations.
**Financial Aid** 90% of baccalaureate students in nursing programs received some form of financial aid in 2012–13. *Gift aid (need-based):* Federal Pell, FSEOG, state, private, college/university gift aid from institutional funds. *Loans:* Federal Direct (Subsidized and Unsubsidized Stafford PLUS), Perkins. *Work-study:* Federal Work-Study, part-time campus jobs. *Financial aid application deadline (priority):* 2/15.
**Contact** Ms. Marilyn Volk Gomez, Director of Nursing Student Services, School of Nursing, Xavier University, 3800 Victory Parkway, Cincinnati, OH 45207-7351. *Telephone:* 513-745-4392. *Fax:* 513-745-1087. *E-mail:* gomez@xavier.edu.

### GRADUATE PROGRAMS

**Financial Aid** 30% of graduate students in nursing programs received some form of financial aid in 2012–13.

**Contact** Ms. Marilyn Volk Gomez, Director of Nursing Student Services, School of Nursing, Xavier University, 3800 Victory Parkway, Cincinnati, OH 45207-7351. *Telephone:* 513-745-4392. *Fax:* 513-745-1087. *E-mail:* gomez@xavier.edu.

**MASTER'S DEGREE PROGRAM**

**Degrees** MSN; MSN/Ed D; MSN/MBA

**Available Programs** Accelerated Master's for Non-Nursing College Graduates; Master's; Master's for Nurses with Non-Nursing Degrees; RN to Master's.

**Concentrations Available** Clinical nurse leader; nursing administration; nursing education; nursing informatics. *Clinical nurse specialist programs in:* forensic nursing, school health.

**Study Options** Full-time and part-time.

**Program Entrance Requirements** Minimum overall college GPA of 2.8, transcript of college record, written essay, 3 letters of recommendation, statistics course, GRE. *Application deadline:* Applications may be processed on a rolling basis for some programs.

**Degree Requirements** 36 total credit hours, thesis or project.

## Youngstown State University

### Department of Nursing
### Youngstown, Ohio

Founded in 1908

**DEGREES • BSN • MSN**

**Nursing Program Faculty** 22 (18% with doctorates).

**Baccalaureate Enrollment** 22

**Graduate Enrollment** 24 **Women** 75% **Men** 25% **Minority** 13%

**Nursing Student Activities** Sigma Theta Tau, Student Nurses' Association.

**Nursing Student Resources** Academic advising; academic or career counseling; assistance for students with disabilities; bookstore; campus computer network; career placement assistance; computer lab; computer-assisted instruction; e-mail services; housing assistance; interactive nursing skills videos; Internet; learning resource lab; library services; nursing audiovisuals; placement services for program completers; resume preparation assistance; skills, simulation, or other laboratory; tutoring.

**Library Facilities** 931,931 volumes; 44,724 periodical subscriptions.

#### BACCALAUREATE PROGRAMS

**Degree** BSN

**Site Options** Boardman, OH.

**Study Options** Full-time.

**Program Entrance Requirements** Minimum overall college GPA of 2.0, transcript of college record, CPR certification, health exam, health insurance, high school biology, high school chemistry, high school foreign language, 3 years high school math, 3 years high school science, high school transcript, immunizations, minimum high school GPA, minimum high school rank, minimum GPA in nursing prerequisites of 2.5, prerequisite course work. Transfer students are accepted.

**Advanced Placement** Credit by examination available. Credit given for nursing courses completed elsewhere dependent upon specific evaluations.

**Contact** *Telephone:* 330-941-2328. *Fax:* 330-941-2309.

#### GRADUATE PROGRAMS

**Contact** *Telephone:* 330-941-1796. *Fax:* 330-941-2309.

**MASTER'S DEGREE PROGRAM**

**Degree** MSN

**Concentrations Available** Nurse anesthesia; nursing education.

**Study Options** Full-time and part-time.

**Program Entrance Requirements** Clinical experience, computer literacy, transcript of college record, CPR certification, written essay, immunizations, nursing research course, physical assessment course, prerequisite course work, resume, GRE General Test.

**Advanced Placement** Credit given for nursing courses completed elsewhere dependent upon specific evaluations.

**Degree Requirements** Thesis or project.

# OKLAHOMA

## Bacone College

### Department of Nursing
### Muskogee, Oklahoma

Founded in 1880

**DEGREE • BSN**

**Nursing Program Faculty** 8

**Baccalaureate Enrollment** 16 **Women** 100% **Minority** 65%

**Nursing Student Activities** Student Nurses' Association, nursing club.

**Nursing Student Resources** Academic advising; bookstore; campus computer network; computer lab; computer-assisted instruction; interactive nursing skills videos; Internet; learning resource lab; library services; nursing audiovisuals; remedial services; skills, simulation, or other laboratory.

**Library Facilities** 34,564 volumes; 121 periodical subscriptions.

#### BACCALAUREATE PROGRAMS

**Degree** BSN

**Available Programs** Accelerated RN Baccalaureate.

**Program Entrance Requirements** Transcript of college record, CPR certification, health exam, health insurance, immunizations, 2 letters of recommendation, minimum GPA in nursing prerequisites of 2.5, prerequisite course work, RN licensure.

**Contact** *Telephone:* 888-682-5514.

## East Central University

### Department of Nursing
### Ada, Oklahoma

*http://www.ecok.edu*

Founded in 1909

**DEGREE • BS**

**Nursing Program Faculty** 17 (31% with doctorates).

**Baccalaureate Enrollment** 495 **Women** 86% **Men** 14% **Minority** 44% **International** 1% **Part-time** 14%

**Distance Learning Courses** Available.

**Nursing Student Activities** Student Nurses' Association.

**Nursing Student Resources** Academic advising; academic or career counseling; assistance for students with disabilities; bookstore; campus computer network; career placement assistance; computer lab; computer-assisted instruction; daycare for children of students; e-mail services; employment services for current students; externships; housing assistance; interactive nursing skills videos; Internet; learning resource lab; library services; nursing audiovisuals; other; placement services for program completers; resume preparation assistance; skills, simulation, or other laboratory; tutoring.

**Library Facilities** 264,524 volumes (2,236 in health, 893 in nursing); 40,969 periodical subscriptions (266 health-care related).

#### BACCALAUREATE PROGRAMS

**Degree** BS

**Available Programs** ADN to Baccalaureate; Generic Baccalaureate.

**Site Options** Ardmore, OK; McAlester, OK; Durant, OK.

**Study Options** Full-time and part-time.

**Program Entrance Requirements** Minimum overall college GPA of 2.5, transcript of college record, CPR certification, health exam, immunizations, minimum GPA in nursing prerequisites of 2.5, professional liability insurance/malpractice insurance, prerequisite course work. Transfer students are accepted. *Application deadline:* 9/17 (spring).

**Advanced Placement** Credit given for nursing courses completed elsewhere dependent upon specific evaluations.

**Contact** *Telephone:* 580-310-5434. *Fax:* 580-310-5785.

## Langston University
### School of Nursing and Health Professions
### Langston, Oklahoma

*http://www.langston.edu/academics/colleges/nursing-health-professions/nursing-health-professions*
Founded in 1897

**DEGREE • BSN**
**Nursing Program Faculty** 16 (13% with doctorates).
**Nursing Student Activities** Student Nurses' Association, nursing club.
**Nursing Student Resources** Academic advising; academic or career counseling; assistance for students with disabilities; bookstore; campus computer network; career placement assistance; computer lab; computer-assisted instruction; daycare for children of students; e-mail services; housing assistance; interactive nursing skills videos; Internet; learning resource lab; library services; nursing audiovisuals; remedial services; resume preparation assistance; skills, simulation, or other laboratory; tutoring.
**Library Facilities** 97,565 volumes (35,397 in health, 2,664 in nursing); 1,235 periodical subscriptions (978 health-care related).

**BACCALAUREATE PROGRAMS**
**Degree** BSN
**Available Programs** Generic Baccalaureate; LPN to Baccalaureate; RN Baccalaureate.
**Site Options** Tulsa, OK.
**Study Options** Full-time and part-time.
**Program Entrance Requirements** Minimum overall college GPA of 2.5, transcript of college record, written essay, health exam, immunizations, minimum GPA in nursing prerequisites of 2.5, professional liability insurance/malpractice insurance, prerequisite course work. Transfer students are accepted.
**Advanced Placement** Credit by examination available. Credit given for nursing courses completed elsewhere dependent upon specific evaluations.
**Contact** *Telephone:* 405-466-3411. *Fax:* 405-466-2195.

## Northeastern State University
### Department of Nursing
### Tahlequah, Oklahoma

*http://academics.nsuok.edu/healthprofessions/HealthProHome.aspx*
Founded in 1846

**DEGREES • BSN • MSN**
**Nursing Program Faculty** 6 (33% with doctorates).
**Baccalaureate Enrollment** 120 **Women** 92% **Men** 8% **Minority** 29% **Part-time** 94%
**Graduate Enrollment** 15 **Women** 93% **Men** 7% **Minority** 27% **Part-time** 100%
**Distance Learning Courses** Available.
**Nursing Student Activities** Sigma Theta Tau, Student Nurses' Association.
**Nursing Student Resources** Academic advising; academic or career counseling; assistance for students with disabilities; bookstore; campus computer network; career placement assistance; computer lab; computer-assisted instruction; e-mail services; employment services for current students; housing assistance; Internet; library services; nursing audiovisuals; placement services for program completers; resume preparation assistance; tutoring.
**Library Facilities** 429,808 volumes (21,000 in health, 15,500 in nursing); 5,758 periodical subscriptions (1,000 health-care related).

**BACCALAUREATE PROGRAMS**
**Degree** BSN
**Available Programs** Accelerated RN Baccalaureate; RN Baccalaureate.
**Site Options** Broken Arrow, OK; Miami, OK; Muskogee, OK.
**Online Degree Options** Yes (online only).
**Program Entrance Requirements** Minimum overall college GPA of 2.0, transcript of college record, CPR certification, health exam, immunizations, 3 letters of recommendation, minimum GPA in nursing prerequisites of 2.0, professional liability insurance/malpractice insurance, prerequisite course work, RN licensure. Transfer students are accepted.
**Contact** *Telephone:* 918-781-5410. *Fax:* 918-781-5411.

**GRADUATE PROGRAMS**
**Contact** *Telephone:* 918-781-5410. *Fax:* 918-781-5411.

**MASTER'S DEGREE PROGRAM**
**Degree** MSN
**Available Programs** Master's.
**Concentrations Available** Nursing education.
**Site Options** Broken Arrow, OK; Miami, OK; Muskogee, OK.
**Study Options** Full-time and part-time.
**Online Degree Options** Yes (online only).
**Program Entrance Requirements** Minimum overall college GPA of 3.0, transcript of college record, CPR certification, immunizations, 3 letters of recommendation, nursing research course, professional liability insurance/malpractice insurance, statistics course. *Application deadline:* 8/1 (fall), 1/2 (spring).
**Advanced Placement** Credit given for nursing courses completed elsewhere dependent upon specific evaluations.
**Degree Requirements** 32 total credit hours, thesis or project.

## Northwestern Oklahoma State University
### Division of Nursing
### Alva, Oklahoma

*http://www.nwosu.edu/nursing*
Founded in 1897

**DEGREE • BSN**
**Nursing Program Faculty** 15 (.02% with doctorates).
**Baccalaureate Enrollment** 60 **Women** 98% **Men** 2% **Minority** 2% **International** 2% **Part-time** 1%
**Distance Learning Courses** Available.
**Nursing Student Activities** Nursing Honor Society, Student Nurses' Association.
**Nursing Student Resources** Academic advising; academic or career counseling; assistance for students with disabilities; bookstore; campus computer network; career placement assistance; computer lab; computer-assisted instruction; e-mail services; housing assistance; interactive nursing skills videos; Internet; learning resource lab; library services; nursing audiovisuals; remedial services; skills, simulation, or other laboratory; tutoring.
**Library Facilities** 169,232 volumes; 17,100 periodical subscriptions (59 health-care related).

**BACCALAUREATE PROGRAMS**
**Degree** BSN
**Available Programs** ADN to Baccalaureate; Accelerated Baccalaureate; Accelerated LPN to Baccalaureate; Accelerated RN Baccalaureate; Baccalaureate for Second Degree; Generic Baccalaureate; LPN to Baccalaureate; LPN to RN Baccalaureate; RN Baccalaureate.
**Site Options** Enid, OK; Woodward, OK; Alva, OK.
**Study Options** Full-time and part-time.
**Program Entrance Requirements** Minimum overall college GPA of 2.5, transcript of college record, CPR certification, health exam, high school transcript, immunizations, 3 letters of recommendation, minimum high school GPA of 2.5, minimum GPA in nursing prerequisites of 2.5, professional liability insurance/malpractice insurance, prerequisite course work. Transfer students are accepted. *Application deadline:* 2/2 (spring).
**Advanced Placement** Credit by examination available. Credit given for nursing courses completed elsewhere dependent upon specific evaluations.
**Contact** *Telephone:* 580-327-8489. *Fax:* 580-327-8434.

## Oklahoma Baptist University
### School of Nursing
### Shawnee, Oklahoma

*http://www.okbu.edu/*
Founded in 1910

**DEGREES • BSN • MSN**
**Nursing Program Faculty** 18 (16% with doctorates).
**Baccalaureate Enrollment** 235 **Women** 95% **Men** 5% **Minority** 8% **International** 1% **Part-time** 4%

**Graduate Enrollment** 26 **Women** 94% **Men** 6% **Minority** 8% **International** 6%
**Nursing Student Activities** Sigma Theta Tau, Student Nurses' Association.
**Nursing Student Resources** Academic advising; academic or career counseling; assistance for students with disabilities; bookstore; campus computer network; career placement assistance; computer lab; computer-assisted instruction; e-mail services; externships; interactive nursing skills videos; Internet; learning resource lab; library services; nursing audiovisuals; remedial services; resume preparation assistance; skills, simulation, or other laboratory; tutoring; unpaid internships.
**Library Facilities** 230,000 volumes (10,000 in health, 5,500 in nursing); 1,800 periodical subscriptions (65 health-care related).

## BACCALAUREATE PROGRAMS

**Degree** BSN
**Available Programs** ADN to Baccalaureate; Accelerated LPN to Baccalaureate; Baccalaureate for Second Degree; Generic Baccalaureate; LPN to Baccalaureate; LPN to RN Baccalaureate; RN Baccalaureate.
**Study Options** Full-time and part-time.
**Program Entrance Requirements** Minimum overall college GPA of 2.25, transcript of college record, CPR certification, health exam, health insurance, high school chemistry, high school transcript, immunizations, minimum GPA in nursing prerequisites of 2.8, prerequisite course work. Transfer students are accepted. *Application deadline:* 4/1 (fall), 4/1 (winter), 4/1 (spring), 6/30 (summer). *Application fee:* $50.
**Advanced Placement** Credit by examination available.
**Expenses (2013–14)** *Tuition:* full-time $19,830; part-time $644 per credit hour. *Required fees:* full-time $2012; part-time $85 per term.
**Financial Aid** 93% of baccalaureate students in nursing programs received some form of financial aid in 2012–13.
**Contact** Dr. Lana Bolhouse, Dean, School of Nursing, Oklahoma Baptist University, 500 West University, Shawnee, OK 74804. *Telephone:* 405-878-2081. *Fax:* 405-878-2083. *E-mail:* lana.bolhouse@okbu.edu.

## GRADUATE PROGRAMS

**Expenses (2013–14)** *Tuition:* part-time $450 per credit hour.
**Financial Aid** 100% of graduate students in nursing programs received some form of financial aid in 2012–13.
**Contact** Mrs. Lana Melton, Administrative Assistant, School of Nursing, Oklahoma Baptist University, 111 Harrison, Oklahoma City, OK 73104. *Telephone:* 405-319-8470. *E-mail:* Lana.Melton@okbu.edu.

### MASTER'S DEGREE PROGRAM

**Degree** MSN
**Available Programs** Master's.
**Concentrations Available** Nursing education.
**Site Options** Oklahoma City, OK.
**Study Options** Full-time.
**Program Entrance Requirements** Clinical experience, minimum overall college GPA of 3.0, transcript of college record, written essay, resume, statistics course. *Application deadline:* 7/30 (fall), 12/20 (winter), 7/30 (spring), 7/30 (summer). Applications may be processed on a rolling basis for some programs.
**Degree Requirements** 39 total credit hours, thesis or project.

# Oklahoma Christian University

## Nursing Program
## Oklahoma City, Oklahoma

Founded in 1950

**DEGREE • BSN**
**Library Facilities** 194,874 volumes; 36,384 periodical subscriptions.

## BACCALAUREATE PROGRAMS

**Degree** BSN
**Available Programs** Generic Baccalaureate.
**Program Entrance Requirements** Minimum overall college GPA of 2.75, 3 letters of recommendation.
**Contact** *Telephone:* 405-425-1921.

# Oklahoma City University

## Kramer School of Nursing
## Oklahoma City, Oklahoma

*http://www.okcu.edu/nursing*
Founded in 1904

**DEGREES • BSN • DNP • MSN • MSN/MBA • PHD**
**Nursing Program Faculty** 49 (31% with doctorates).
**Baccalaureate Enrollment** 321 **Women** 83% **Men** 17% **Minority** 40% **International** 20% **Part-time** 10%
**Graduate Enrollment** 46 **Women** 70% **Men** 30% **Minority** 52% **International** 37% **Part-time** 65%
**Distance Learning Courses** Available.
**Nursing Student Activities** Sigma Theta Tau, Student Nurses' Association.
**Nursing Student Resources** Academic advising; academic or career counseling; assistance for students with disabilities; bookstore; campus computer network; career placement assistance; computer lab; computer-assisted instruction; e-mail services; employment services for current students; housing assistance; interactive nursing skills videos; Internet; learning resource lab; library services; nursing audiovisuals; placement services for program completers; remedial services; resume preparation assistance; skills, simulation, or other laboratory; tutoring.
**Library Facilities** 522,263 volumes (2,714 in health, 590 in nursing); 51 periodical subscriptions (234 health-care related).

## BACCALAUREATE PROGRAMS

**Degree** BSN
**Available Programs** ADN to Baccalaureate; Accelerated Baccalaureate; Accelerated Baccalaureate for Second Degree; Baccalaureate for Second Degree; Generic Baccalaureate; International Nurse to Baccalaureate; RN Baccalaureate.
**Site Options** Lawton, OK; Ardmore , OK.
**Study Options** Full-time and part-time.
**Program Entrance Requirements** Minimum overall college GPA of 3.0, transcript of college record, CPR certification, health insurance, high school transcript, immunizations, minimum GPA in nursing prerequisites of 3.0, prerequisite course work. Transfer students are accepted. *Application deadline:* 8/1 (fall), 12/1 (spring), 4/1 (summer). Applications may be processed on a rolling basis for some programs. *Application fee:* $50.
**Advanced Placement** Credit by examination available. Credit given for nursing courses completed elsewhere dependent upon specific evaluations.
**Expenses (2013–14)** *Tuition:* full-time $24,740; part-time $840 per credit hour. *International tuition:* $24,740 full-time. *Room and board:* $9210 per academic year. *Required fees:* full-time $6720; part-time $210 per credit.
**Financial Aid** 85% of baccalaureate students in nursing programs received some form of financial aid in 2012–13. *Gift aid (need-based):* Federal Pell, FSEOG, state, private, college/university gift aid from institutional funds, United Negro College Fund, Federal Nursing, Native American Grants. *Loans:* Federal Nursing Student Loans, Federal Direct (Subsidized and Unsubsidized Stafford PLUS), Perkins. *Work-study:* Federal Work-Study, part-time campus jobs. *Financial aid application deadline (priority):* 3/1.
**Contact** Ms. Debbie Taber, Intake Specialist, Kramer School of Nursing, Oklahoma City University, 2501 North Blackwelder Avenue, Oklahoma City, OK 73106-1493. *Telephone:* 405-208-5924. *Fax:* 405-208-5914. *E-mail:* djtaber@okcu.edu.

## GRADUATE PROGRAMS

**Expenses (2013–14)** *Tuition:* full-time $11,232; part-time $936 per credit hour. *International tuition:* $11,232 full-time. *Room and board:* $9210 per academic year. *Required fees:* full-time $2520; part-time $210 per credit.
**Financial Aid** 92% of graduate students in nursing programs received some form of financial aid in 2012–13.
**Contact** Mrs. Shelley Cassada, Graduate Specialist, Kramer School of Nursing, Oklahoma City University, 2501 North Blackwelder Avenue, Oklahoma City, OK 73106-1493. *Telephone:* 405-208-5960. *Fax:* 405-208-5914. *E-mail:* neallisoncatalfu@okcu.edu.

### MASTER'S DEGREE PROGRAM

**Degrees** MSN; MSN/MBA
**Available Programs** Accelerated AD/RN to Master's; Accelerated Master's; Accelerated Master's for Nurses with Non-Nursing Degrees;

Accelerated RN to Master's; Master's; Master's for Nurses with Non-Nursing Degrees; RN to Master's.
**Concentrations Available** Nursing administration; nursing education.
**Study Options** Full-time and part-time.
**Program Entrance Requirements** Minimum overall college GPA of 3.0, transcript of college record, written essay, nursing research course, physical assessment course, statistics course. *Application deadline:* 8/1 (fall), 12/1 (spring), 4/1 (summer). Applications may be processed on a rolling basis for some programs. *Application fee:* $50.
**Advanced Placement** Credit given for nursing courses completed elsewhere dependent upon specific evaluations.
**Degree Requirements** 33 total credit hours, thesis or project.

### DOCTORAL DEGREE PROGRAM

**Degree** DNP
**Available Programs** Doctorate, Doctorate for Nurses with Non-Nursing Degrees, Post-Baccalaureate Doctorate.
**Areas of Study** Clinical practice, nursing administration, nursing education.
**Program Entrance Requirements** Minimum overall college GPA of 3.5, clinical experience, interview by faculty committee, MSN or equivalent, statistics course, vita, writing sample. *Application deadline:* 4/1 (fall). *Application fee:* $50.
**Degree Requirements** 90 total credit hours, dissertation, oral exam, residency, written exam.

**Degree** PhD
**Available Programs** Doctorate; Doctorate for Nurses with Non-Nursing Degrees; Post-Baccalaureate Doctorate.
**Areas of Study** Nursing administration, nursing education.
**Program Entrance Requirements** Clinical experience, minimum overall college GPA of 3.5, interview by faculty committee, MSN or equivalent, statistics course, vita, writing sample. *Application deadline:* 4/1 (fall). *Application fee:* $50.
**Degree Requirements** 90 total credit hours, dissertation, oral exam, written exam, residency.

### CONTINUING EDUCATION PROGRAM

**Contact** Mr. Christopher Black, Director of Communications and Outreach, Kramer School of Nursing, Oklahoma City University, 2501 North Blackwelder Avenue, Oklahoma City, OK 73106-1493. *Telephone:* 405-208-5832. *Fax:* 405-208-5914. *E-mail:* cblack@okcu.edu.

## Oklahoma Panhandle State University

### Bachelor of Science in Nursing Program
### Goodwell, Oklahoma

*http://www.opsu.edu/*
Founded in 1909

**DEGREE • BSN**
**Nursing Program Faculty** 4
**Baccalaureate Enrollment** 57 **Women** 90% **Men** 10% **Minority** 19% **Part-time** 73%
**Distance Learning Courses** Available.
**Nursing Student Activities** Student Nurses' Association.
**Nursing Student Resources** Academic advising; academic or career counseling; assistance for students with disabilities; bookstore; campus computer network; computer-assisted instruction; e-mail services; Internet; library services.
**Library Facilities** 1,019 volumes in health, 380 volumes in nursing; 2,032 periodical subscriptions health-care related.

### BACCALAUREATE PROGRAMS

**Degree** BSN
**Available Programs** ADN to Baccalaureate.
**Study Options** Full-time and part-time.
**Online Degree Options** Yes (online only).
**Program Entrance Requirements** Minimum overall college GPA of 2.0, transcript of college record, CPR certification, immunizations, minimum GPA in nursing prerequisites of 2.0, RN licensure. Transfer students are accepted. *Application deadline:* 8/1 (fall), 1/10 (spring), 5/20 (summer).
**Advanced Placement** Credit given for nursing courses completed elsewhere dependent upon specific evaluations.
**Contact** *Telephone:* 580-349-1520. *Fax:* 580-349-1529.

## Oklahoma Wesleyan University

### School of Nursing
### Bartlesville, Oklahoma

*http://www.okwu.edu/*
Founded in 1909

**DEGREE • BSN**
**Nursing Program Faculty** 31 (35% with doctorates).
**Baccalaureate Enrollment** 140 **Women** 96% **Men** 4% **Minority** 23%
**Nursing Student Resources** Academic advising; academic or career counseling; assistance for students with disabilities; bookstore; campus computer network; computer lab; computer-assisted instruction; interactive nursing skills videos; Internet; learning resource lab; library services; nursing audiovisuals; skills, simulation, or other laboratory.
**Library Facilities** 108,717 volumes (946 in health, 483 in nursing); 82 periodical subscriptions (40 health-care related).

### BACCALAUREATE PROGRAMS

**Degree** BSN
**Available Programs** ADN to Baccalaureate; Accelerated RN Baccalaureate; Baccalaureate for Second Degree; Generic Baccalaureate; International Nurse to Baccalaureate; LPN to Baccalaureate; RN Baccalaureate.
**Study Options** Full-time.
**Program Entrance Requirements** Minimum overall college GPA of 2.3, transcript of college record, CPR certification, health exam, health insurance, immunizations, 2 letters of recommendation, minimum GPA in nursing prerequisites of 2.75, professional liability insurance/malpractice insurance, prerequisite course work, RN licensure. Transfer students are accepted.
**Advanced Placement** Credit by examination available. Credit given for nursing courses completed elsewhere dependent upon specific evaluations.
**Contact** *Telephone:* 918-335-6254. *Fax:* 918-335-6204.

## Oral Roberts University

### Anna Vaughn School of Nursing
### Tulsa, Oklahoma

*http://www.oru.edu/*
Founded in 1963

**DEGREE • BSN**
**Nursing Program Faculty** 29 (10% with doctorates).
**Baccalaureate Enrollment** 209 **Women** 88% **Men** 12% **Minority** 26% **International** 6%
**Nursing Student Activities** Student Nurses' Association.
**Nursing Student Resources** Academic advising; academic or career counseling; assistance for students with disabilities; bookstore; campus computer network; computer lab; computer-assisted instruction; e-mail services; employment services for current students; housing assistance; interactive nursing skills videos; Internet; learning resource lab; library services; nursing audiovisuals; remedial services; resume preparation assistance; skills, simulation, or other laboratory; tutoring.
**Library Facilities** 8,099 volumes in health, 2,763 volumes in nursing; 56 periodical subscriptions health-care related.

### BACCALAUREATE PROGRAMS

**Degree** BSN
**Available Programs** ADN to Baccalaureate; Generic Baccalaureate; RN Baccalaureate.
**Study Options** Full-time and part-time.
**Program Entrance Requirements** Minimum overall college GPA of 3.3, transcript of college record, CPR certification, health exam, health insurance, high school biology, high school chemistry, 2 years high school math, 2 years high school science, high school transcript, immunizations, minimum high school GPA of 2.5, minimum GPA in nursing prerequisites of 2.5. Transfer students are accepted. *Application deadline:* 7/31 (fall), 11/20 (spring). *Application fee:* $35.
**Advanced Placement** Credit given for nursing courses completed elsewhere dependent upon specific evaluations.
**Expenses (2013–14)** *Tuition:* full-time $21,696; part-time $906 per credit hour. *International tuition:* $21,696 full-time. *Room and board:*

$9296; room only: $4534 per academic year. *Required fees:* full-time $1162; part-time $1162 per term.
**Financial Aid** 98% of baccalaureate students in nursing programs received some form of financial aid in 2012–13.
**Contact** Dr. Kenda Jezek, Dean, Anna Vaughn School of Nursing, Oral Roberts University, 7777 South Lewis Avenue, Tulsa, OK 74171. *Telephone:* 918-495-6198. *Fax:* 918-495-6020. *E-mail:* kjezek@oru.edu.

# Rogers State University
## Nursing Program
## Claremore, Oklahoma

Founded in 1909

**DEGREE • BSN**
**Baccalaureate Enrollment** 18 **Women** 94% **Men** 6% **Minority** 38% **International** 11%
**Distance Learning Courses** Available.
**Nursing Student Activities** Student Nurses' Association.
**Nursing Student Resources** Academic advising; academic or career counseling; assistance for students with disabilities; bookstore; campus computer network; career placement assistance; computer lab; computer-assisted instruction; daycare for children of students; e-mail services; housing assistance; interactive nursing skills videos; Internet; learning resource lab; library services; nursing audiovisuals; placement services for program completers; remedial services; resume preparation assistance; skills, simulation, or other laboratory.
**Library Facilities** 216,655 volumes; 46,559 periodical subscriptions.

### BACCALAUREATE PROGRAMS

**Degree** BSN
**Available Programs** ADN to Baccalaureate.
**Site Options** Bartlesville, OK.
**Program Entrance Requirements** Minimum overall college GPA, CPR certification, health exam, health insurance, immunizations, minimum GPA in nursing prerequisites, RN licensure. Transfer students are accepted.
**Contact** *Telephone:* 918-343-7885. *Fax:* 918-343-7628.

# Southern Nazarene University
## School of Nursing
## Bethany, Oklahoma

***http://www.snu.edu/***
Founded in 1899

**DEGREES • BS • MS**
**Nursing Program Faculty** 35 (40% with doctorates).
**Baccalaureate Enrollment** 101 **Women** 90% **Men** 10% **Minority** 35% **International** 2% **Part-time** 10%
**Graduate Enrollment** 34 **Women** 90% **Men** 10% **Minority** 10%
**Distance Learning Courses** Available.
**Nursing Student Activities** Sigma Theta Tau, Student Nurses' Association.
**Nursing Student Resources** Academic advising; academic or career counseling; assistance for students with disabilities; bookstore; campus computer network; career placement assistance; computer lab; computer-assisted instruction; e-mail services; employment services for current students; externships; housing assistance; interactive nursing skills videos; Internet; learning resource lab; library services; nursing audiovisuals; paid internships; remedial services; skills, simulation, or other laboratory; tutoring.
**Library Facilities** 101,117 volumes; 41,048 periodical subscriptions.

### BACCALAUREATE PROGRAMS

**Degree** BS
**Available Programs** ADN to Baccalaureate; Baccalaureate for Second Degree; Generic Baccalaureate; LPN to Baccalaureate.
**Study Options** Full-time.
**Program Entrance Requirements** Minimum overall college GPA of 2.75, transcript of college record, CPR certification, health exam, health insurance, immunizations, minimum GPA in nursing prerequisites of 2.75, professional liability insurance/malpractice insurance, prerequisite course work. Transfer students are accepted. *Application deadline:* 12/5 (fall). Applications may be processed on a rolling basis for some programs.
**Advanced Placement** Credit by examination available. Credit given for nursing courses completed elsewhere dependent upon specific evaluations.
**Contact** *Telephone:* 405-717-6217. *Fax:* 405-717-6264.

### GRADUATE PROGRAMS

**Contact** *Telephone:* 405-717-6217. *Fax:* 405-717-6264.

**MASTER'S DEGREE PROGRAM**
**Degree** MS
**Available Programs** Accelerated Master's; Accelerated Master's for Nurses with Non-Nursing Degrees.
**Concentrations Available** Nursing administration; nursing education.
**Site Options** Tulsa, OK.
**Study Options** Full-time.
**Program Entrance Requirements** Clinical experience, computer literacy, minimum overall college GPA of 3.0, transcript of college record, immunizations, interview, 3 letters of recommendation, nursing research course, physical assessment course, resume, statistics course. *Application deadline:* Applications may be processed on a rolling basis for some programs.
**Advanced Placement** Credit given for nursing courses completed elsewhere dependent upon specific evaluations.
**Degree Requirements** 39 total credit hours, thesis or project.

# Southwestern Oklahoma State University
## School of Nursing
## Weatherford, Oklahoma

***http://www.swosu.edu/academics/nursing/index.asp***
Founded in 1901

**DEGREE • BSN**
**Nursing Program Faculty** 9 (15% with doctorates).
**Baccalaureate Enrollment** 80 **Women** 90% **Men** 10% **Minority** 12% **International** 1%
**Distance Learning Courses** Available.
**Nursing Student Activities** Sigma Theta Tau, Student Nurses' Association, nursing club.
**Nursing Student Resources** Academic advising; academic or career counseling; assistance for students with disabilities; bookstore; campus computer network; computer lab; computer-assisted instruction; e-mail services; externships; housing assistance; interactive nursing skills videos; Internet; learning resource lab; library services; nursing audiovisuals; remedial services; skills, simulation, or other laboratory; tutoring.
**Library Facilities** 284 periodical subscriptions health-care related.

### BACCALAUREATE PROGRAMS

**Degree** BSN
**Available Programs** ADN to Baccalaureate; Generic Baccalaureate; RN Baccalaureate.
**Site Options** Oklahoma City, OK; Weatherford, OK; Elk City, OK.
**Study Options** Full-time.
**Online Degree Options** Yes.
**Program Entrance Requirements** Minimum overall college GPA of 2.25, transcript of college record, CPR certification, immunizations, 2 letters of recommendation, minimum GPA in nursing prerequisites of 2.25, professional liability insurance/malpractice insurance, prerequisite course work. Transfer students are accepted. *Application deadline:* 2/1 (fall).
**Advanced Placement** Credit given for nursing courses completed elsewhere dependent upon specific evaluations.
**Contact** *Telephone:* 580-774-3261. *Fax:* 580-774-7075.

# University of Central Oklahoma

## Department of Nursing
## Edmond, Oklahoma

***http://www.uco.edu/cms/nursing***
Founded in 1890

**DEGREES • BSN • MS**

**Nursing Program Faculty** 54 (2% with doctorates).

**Baccalaureate Enrollment** 265 **Women** 90% **Men** 10% **Minority** 19% **International** 5% **Part-time** 1%

**Graduate Enrollment** 22

**Nursing Student Activities** Nursing Honor Society, Sigma Theta Tau, Student Nurses' Association.

**Nursing Student Resources** Academic advising; academic or career counseling; assistance for students with disabilities; bookstore; campus computer network; career placement assistance; computer lab; computer-assisted instruction; e-mail services; externships; interactive nursing skills videos; Internet; learning resource lab; library services; nursing audiovisuals; remedial services; skills, simulation, or other laboratory; tutoring.

**Library Facilities** 526,153 volumes (3,000 in health, 1,661 in nursing); 125,692 periodical subscriptions.

## BACCALAUREATE PROGRAMS

**Degree** BSN

**Available Programs** Generic Baccalaureate; LPN to Baccalaureate; RN Baccalaureate.

**Site Options** Oklahoma City, OK; Midwest City, OK.

**Study Options** Full-time and part-time.

**Program Entrance Requirements** Minimum overall college GPA of 2.5, transcript of college record, CPR certification, immunizations, professional liability insurance/malpractice insurance, prerequisite course work. Transfer students are accepted. *Application deadline:* 9/13 (fall), 1/31 (spring). *Application fee:* $25.

**Advanced Placement** Credit given for nursing courses completed elsewhere dependent upon specific evaluations.

**Expenses (2013–14)** *Tuition, area resident:* full-time $7061; part-time $252 per credit hour. *International tuition:* $14,384 full-time. *Room and board:* $6940; room only: $3362 per academic year. *Required fees:* full-time $1988.

**Financial Aid** 35% of baccalaureate students in nursing programs received some form of financial aid in 2012–13.

**Contact** Vicki Addison, Administrative Assistant, Department of Nursing, University of Central Oklahoma, 100 North University Drive, Edmond, OK 73034-5209. *Telephone:* 405-974-5000. *E-mail:* vaddison@uco.edu.

## GRADUATE PROGRAMS

**Expenses (2013–14)** *Tuition, area resident:* full-time $7245; part-time $302 per credit hour. *International tuition:* $14,711 full-time. *Room and board:* $6940; room only: $3362 per academic year. *Required fees:* full-time $1987.

**Contact** Dr. Nancy Dentlinger, Masters Coordinator, Department of Nursing, University of Central Oklahoma, 100 North University Drive, Edmond, OK 73034. *Telephone:* 405-974-5379. *Fax:* 405-974-3848. *E-mail:* ndentlinger@uco.edu.

### MASTER'S DEGREE PROGRAM

**Degree** MS

**Available Programs** Master's.

**Concentrations Available** Nursing education.

**Study Options** Full-time and part-time.

**Program Entrance Requirements** Minimum overall college GPA of 3.0, transcript of college record, CPR certification, immunizations, 3 letters of recommendation, professional liability insurance/malpractice insurance, prerequisite course work, statistics course. *Application deadline:* 4/1 (fall), 11/1 (spring). *Application fee:* $50.

**Advanced Placement** Credit given for nursing courses completed elsewhere dependent upon specific evaluations.

**Degree Requirements** 34 total credit hours, thesis or project, comprehensive exam.

# University of Oklahoma Health Sciences Center

## College of Nursing
## Oklahoma City, Oklahoma

***http://www.nursing.ouhsc.edu/***
Founded in 1890

**DEGREES • BSN • MS • PHD**

**Nursing Program Faculty** 185 (16% with doctorates).

**Baccalaureate Enrollment** 892 **Women** 85% **Men** 15% **Minority** 37% **International** 1% **Part-time** 4%

**Graduate Enrollment** 256 **Women** 93% **Men** 7% **Minority** 26% **International** 1% **Part-time** 71%

**Distance Learning Courses** Available.

**Nursing Student Activities** Sigma Theta Tau, Student Nurses' Association.

**Nursing Student Resources** Academic advising; academic or career counseling; assistance for students with disabilities; bookstore; campus computer network; computer lab; computer-assisted instruction; e-mail services; employment services for current students; housing assistance; Internet; learning resource lab; library services; nursing audiovisuals; skills, simulation, or other laboratory; tutoring.

**Library Facilities** 335,340 volumes; 4,941 periodical subscriptions.

## BACCALAUREATE PROGRAMS

**Degree** BSN

**Available Programs** ADN to Baccalaureate; Accelerated Baccalaureate for Second Degree; Generic Baccalaureate; LPN to RN Baccalaureate.

**Site Options** Lawton, OK; Tulsa, OK.

**Study Options** Full-time.

**Program Entrance Requirements** Minimum overall college GPA of 2.5, transcript of college record, high school transcript, minimum GPA in nursing prerequisites of 2.5, prerequisite course work. Transfer students are accepted. *Application deadline:* 1/15 (fall). *Application fee:* $65.

**Advanced Placement** Credit by examination available. Credit given for nursing courses completed elsewhere dependent upon specific evaluations.

**Contact** *Telephone:* 405-271-2128. *Fax:* 405-271-7341.

## GRADUATE PROGRAMS

**Contact** *Telephone:* 405-271-2128. *Fax:* 405-271-7341.

### MASTER'S DEGREE PROGRAM

**Degree** MS

**Available Programs** Master's; Master's for Non-Nursing College Graduates.

**Concentrations Available** Clinical nurse leader; health-care administration; nursing education. *Clinical nurse specialist programs in:* acute care. *Nurse practitioner programs in:* adult health, family health, neonatal health, pediatric.

**Site Options** Lawton, OK; Tulsa, OK.

**Study Options** Full-time and part-time.

**Online Degree Options** Yes.

**Program Entrance Requirements** Computer literacy, minimum overall college GPA of 3.0, transcript of college record, 3 letters of recommendation, nursing research course, professional liability insurance/malpractice insurance, prerequisite course work, statistics course. *Application deadline:* 3/1 (fall), 8/1 (spring), 1/15 (summer). *Application fee:* $65.

**Advanced Placement** Credit given for nursing courses completed elsewhere dependent upon specific evaluations.

**Degree Requirements** 38 total credit hours, thesis or project, comprehensive exam.

### POST-MASTER'S PROGRAM

**Areas of Study** Clinical nurse leader; health-care administration; nursing education. *Nurse practitioner programs in:* adult health, family health, neonatal health, pediatric.

### DOCTORAL DEGREE PROGRAM

**Degree** PhD

**Available Programs** Doctorate.

**Areas of Study** Nursing education.

**Program Entrance Requirements** Minimum overall college GPA of 3.5, interview by faculty committee, 3 letters of recommendation,

scholarly papers, statistics course, vita, writing sample. *Application deadline:* 4/14 (fall). *Application fee:* $65.
**Degree Requirements** 90 total credit hours, dissertation, oral exam, written exam.

### CONTINUING EDUCATION PROGRAM

**Contact** *Telephone:* 405-271-2428. *Fax:* 405-271-7341.

## University of Phoenix–Oklahoma City Campus

### College of Health and Human Services
### Oklahoma City, Oklahoma

Founded in 1976
**Nursing Program Faculty** 1
**Nursing Student Activities** Sigma Theta Tau.
**Nursing Student Resources** Academic advising; academic or career counseling; assistance for students with disabilities; bookstore; campus computer network; computer lab; computer-assisted instruction; e-mail services; interactive nursing skills videos; Internet; learning resource lab; library services; nursing audiovisuals; skills, simulation, or other laboratory; tutoring.
**Library Facilities** 16,781 periodical subscriptions (1,300 health-care related).

## University of Phoenix–Tulsa Campus

### College of Health and Human Services
### Tulsa, Oklahoma

Founded in 1998
**Nursing Student Activities** Sigma Theta Tau.
**Nursing Student Resources** Academic advising; academic or career counseling; assistance for students with disabilities; bookstore; campus computer network; computer lab; computer-assisted instruction; e-mail services; interactive nursing skills videos; Internet; learning resource lab; library services; nursing audiovisuals; remedial services; skills, simulation, or other laboratory; tutoring.
**Library Facilities** 16,781 periodical subscriptions (1,300 health-care related).

## University of Tulsa

### School of Nursing
### Tulsa, Oklahoma

***http://www.utulsa.edu/nursing***
Founded in 1894

**DEGREE • BSN**
**Nursing Program Faculty** 13 (33% with doctorates).
**Baccalaureate Enrollment** 80 **Women** 88% **Men** 12% **Minority** 20% **International** 1% **Part-time** 2%
**Nursing Student Activities** Sigma Theta Tau, Student Nurses' Association.
**Nursing Student Resources** Academic advising; academic or career counseling; assistance for students with disabilities; bookstore; campus computer network; career placement assistance; computer lab; computer-assisted instruction; daycare for children of students; e-mail services; employment services for current students; externships; housing assistance; interactive nursing skills videos; Internet; learning resource lab; library services; nursing audiovisuals; placement services for program completers; remedial services; resume preparation assistance; skills, simulation, or other laboratory; tutoring.
**Library Facilities** 1.4 million volumes (4,300 in nursing); 53,504 periodical subscriptions (118 health-care related).

### BACCALAUREATE PROGRAMS

**Degree** BSN
**Available Programs** Generic Baccalaureate; LPN to RN Baccalaureate; RN Baccalaureate.
**Study Options** Full-time.
**Program Entrance Requirements** Minimum overall college GPA of 2.5, transcript of college record, CPR certification, written essay, health exam, immunizations, minimum GPA in nursing prerequisites. Transfer students are accepted. *Application deadline:* 2/1 (fall). Applications may be processed on a rolling basis for some programs.
**Advanced Placement** Credit by examination available. Credit given for nursing courses completed elsewhere dependent upon specific evaluations.
**Expenses (2012–13)** *Tuition:* full-time $32,410; part-time $1035 per credit hour. *International tuition:* $32,410 full-time. *Room and board:* $9934; room only: $5524 per academic year. *Required fees:* full-time $400.
**Financial Aid** 90% of baccalaureate students in nursing programs received some form of financial aid in 2011–12. *Gift aid (need-based):* Federal Pell, FSEOG, state, private, college/university gift aid from institutional funds. *Loans:* Federal Direct (Subsidized and Unsubsidized Stafford PLUS), Perkins. *Work-study:* Federal Work-Study, part-time campus jobs. *Financial aid application deadline (priority):* 3/1.
**Contact** Dr. Susan Kathleen Gaston, Director, School of Nursing, University of Tulsa, 800 South Tucker Drive, Tulsa, OK 74104-9700. *Telephone:* 918-631-3116. *Fax:* 918-631-2068. *E-mail:* susan-gaston@utulsa.edu.

# OREGON

## George Fox University

### Nursing Department
### Newberg, Oregon

***http://www.georgefox.edu/academics/undergrad/departments/nursing/index.html***
Founded in 1891

**DEGREE • BSN**
**Nursing Program Faculty** 15 (20% with doctorates).
**Baccalaureate Enrollment** 110 **Women** 91% **Men** 9% **Minority** 8%
**Nursing Student Activities** Nursing club.
**Nursing Student Resources** Academic advising; academic or career counseling; assistance for students with disabilities; bookstore; campus computer network; career placement assistance; computer lab; computer-assisted instruction; e-mail services; employment services for current students; housing assistance; interactive nursing skills videos; Internet; learning resource lab; library services; nursing audiovisuals; remedial services; resume preparation assistance; skills, simulation, or other laboratory; tutoring.
**Library Facilities** 251,000 volumes (490 in health, 100 in nursing); 57,509 periodical subscriptions (5,600 health-care related).

### BACCALAUREATE PROGRAMS

**Degree** BSN
**Available Programs** Generic Baccalaureate.
**Study Options** Full-time.
**Program Entrance Requirements** Minimum overall college GPA of 2.8, transcript of college record, CPR certification, written essay, immunizations, 2 letters of recommendation, minimum GPA in nursing prerequisites of 2.8, prerequisite course work. Transfer students are accepted. *Application deadline:* 10/2 (fall). *Application fee:* $50.
**Contact** *Telephone:* 503-554-2950. *Fax:* 503-554-3900.

## Linfield College

### School of Nursing
### McMinnville, Oregon

***http://www.linfield.edu/portland***
Founded in 1849

**DEGREE • BSN**
**Nursing Program Faculty** 64 (22% with doctorates).
**Baccalaureate Enrollment** 314 **Women** 85.4% **Men** 14.6% **Minority** 17.8% **International** .3% **Part-time** 3.5%
**Nursing Student Activities** Sigma Theta Tau, Student Nurses' Association, nursing club.

**Nursing Student Resources** Academic advising; academic or career counseling; bookstore; campus computer network; computer lab; e-mail services; Internet; learning resource lab; library services; nursing audio-visuals; resume preparation assistance; skills, simulation, or other laboratory.
**Library Facilities** 184,441 volumes (7,201 in health, 1,482 in nursing); 985 periodical subscriptions (249 health-care related).

### BACCALAUREATE PROGRAMS

**Degree** BSN
**Available Programs** ADN to Baccalaureate; Accelerated Baccalaureate for Second Degree; Baccalaureate for Second Degree; Generic Baccalaureate.
**Site Options** Portland, OR.
**Study Options** Full-time.
**Program Entrance Requirements** Minimum overall college GPA of 2.9, transcript of college record, CPR certification, written essay, health exam, health insurance, immunizations, 1 letter of recommendation, minimum GPA in nursing prerequisites of 2.75, professional liability insurance/malpractice insurance, prerequisite course work. Transfer students are accepted.
**Advanced Placement** Credit given for nursing courses completed elsewhere dependent upon specific evaluations.
**Contact** *Telephone:* 503-413-8481. *Fax:* 503-413-6283.

### CONTINUING EDUCATION PROGRAM

**Contact** *Telephone:* 503-413-7163. *Fax:* 503-413-6846.

## Oregon Health & Science University
### School of Nursing
### Portland, Oregon

*http://www.ohsu.edu/xd/education/schools/school-of-nursing/*
Founded in 1974

**DEGREES • BS • MN/MPH • MS • PHD**
**Nursing Program Faculty** 138 (40% with doctorates).
**Baccalaureate Enrollment** 573 **Women** 83% **Men** 17% **Minority** 7% **International** 1% **Part-time** 68%
**Graduate Enrollment** 219 **Women** 74% **Men** 26% **Minority** 4% **International** 2% **Part-time** 56%
**Distance Learning Courses** Available.
**Nursing Student Activities** Nursing Honor Society, Sigma Theta Tau, Student Nurses' Association, nursing club.
**Nursing Student Resources** Academic advising; assistance for students with disabilities; bookstore; campus computer network; computer lab; e-mail services; externships; interactive nursing skills videos; Internet; learning resource lab; library services; nursing audiovisuals; resume preparation assistance; skills, simulation, or other laboratory.
**Library Facilities** 315,470 volumes (227,344 in health, 7,666 in nursing); 2,121 periodical subscriptions (2,357 health-care related).

### BACCALAUREATE PROGRAMS

**Degree** BS
**Available Programs** Accelerated Baccalaureate; Generic Baccalaureate; RN Baccalaureate.
**Site Options** Klamath Falls, OR; Ashland, OR; La Grande, OR.
**Study Options** Full-time.
**Program Entrance Requirements** Transcript of college record, written essay, minimum GPA in nursing prerequisites of 3.0, prerequisite course work. Transfer students are accepted. *Application deadline:* 2/15 (fall). *Application fee:* $120.
**Advanced Placement** Credit given for nursing courses completed elsewhere dependent upon specific evaluations.
**Contact** *Telephone:* 503-494-7725. *Fax:* 503-494-6433.

### GRADUATE PROGRAMS

**Contact** *Telephone:* 503-494-7725. *Fax:* 503-494-4350.

#### MASTER'S DEGREE PROGRAM

**Degrees** MN/MPH; MS
**Available Programs** Accelerated Master's for Non-Nursing College Graduates; Master's.
**Concentrations Available** Nurse anesthesia; nurse-midwifery; nursing education. *Nurse practitioner programs in:* family health, psychiatric/mental health.
**Site Options** Klamath Falls, OR; Ashland, OR; La Grande, OR.
**Study Options** Full-time and part-time.
**Program Entrance Requirements** Clinical experience, computer literacy, minimum overall college GPA of 3.0, transcript of college record, CPR certification, written essay, immunizations, interview, 3 letters of recommendation, resume, statistics course, GRE General Test. *Application deadline:* 12/1 (fall). Applications may be processed on a rolling basis for some programs. *Application fee:* $120.
**Advanced Placement** Credit given for nursing courses completed elsewhere dependent upon specific evaluations.
**Degree Requirements** 45 total credit hours, comprehensive exam.

#### POST-MASTER'S PROGRAM

**Areas of Study** Nurse-midwifery; nursing education. *Nurse practitioner programs in:* family health, gerontology, psychiatric/mental health.

#### DOCTORAL DEGREE PROGRAM

**Degree** PhD
**Available Programs** Doctorate; Post-Baccalaureate Doctorate.
**Areas of Study** Advanced practice nursing, aging, clinical practice, ethics, faculty preparation, family health, gerontology, health policy, health promotion/disease prevention, health-care systems, human health and illness, illness and transition, nursing policy, nursing research, nursing science,women's health.
**Program Entrance Requirements** Clinical experience, minimum overall college GPA of 3.0, interview by faculty committee, 3 letters of recommendation, MSN or equivalent, scholarly papers, statistics course, vita, writing sample, GRE General Test. *Application deadline:* 12/1 (fall). Applications may be processed on a rolling basis for some programs. *Application fee:* $120.
**Degree Requirements** 90 total credit hours, dissertation, oral exam, written exam, residency.

#### POSTDOCTORAL PROGRAM

**Areas of Study** Adolescent health, aging, chronic illness, family health, gerontology, health promotion/disease prevention, nursing interventions, nursing research, nursing science, outcomes, self-care, vulnerable population,women's health.
**Postdoctoral Program Contact***Telephone:* 503-494-7725. *Fax:* 503-494-4350.

### CONTINUING EDUCATION PROGRAM

**Contact** *Telephone:* 503-494-6772. *Fax:* 503-494-4350.

## University of Portland
### School of Nursing
### Portland, Oregon

*http://www.nursing.up.edu/*
Founded in 1901

**DEGREES • BSN • DNP • MS**
**Nursing Program Faculty** 48 (36% with doctorates).
**Baccalaureate Enrollment** 613 **Women** 88% **Men** 12% **Minority** 32% **International** 1%
**Graduate Enrollment** 58 **Women** 84% **Men** 16% **Minority** 14% **International** 3%
**Distance Learning Courses** Available.
**Nursing Student Activities** Sigma Theta Tau, Student Nurses' Association, nursing club.
**Nursing Student Resources** Academic advising; academic or career counseling; assistance for students with disabilities; bookstore; campus computer network; career placement assistance; computer lab; computer-assisted instruction; daycare for children of students; e-mail services; employment services for current students; housing assistance; interactive nursing skills videos; Internet; learning resource lab; library services; nursing audiovisuals; remedial services; resume preparation assistance; skills, simulation, or other laboratory; tutoring.
**Library Facilities** 219,693 volumes (4,488 in health, 1,135 in nursing); 6,830 periodical subscriptions (1,698 health-care related).

### BACCALAUREATE PROGRAMS

**Degree** BSN
**Available Programs** Generic Baccalaureate.

**Study Options** Full-time.
**Program Entrance Requirements** Minimum overall college GPA of 2.7, transcript of college record, CPR certification, written essay, health exam, health insurance, high school chemistry, high school transcript, immunizations, 1 letter of recommendation, minimum high school GPA of 2.7, minimum GPA in nursing prerequisites of 2.7, prerequisite course work. Transfer students are accepted. *Application deadline:* 1/15 (fall), 2/1 (spring). *Application fee:* $50.
**Advanced Placement** Credit by examination available. Credit given for nursing courses completed elsewhere dependent upon specific evaluations.
**Expenses (2013–14)** *Tuition:* full-time $43,378. *Room and board:* $11,004 per academic year. *Required fees:* full-time $2315.
**Financial Aid** 95% of baccalaureate students in nursing programs received some form of financial aid in 2012–13.
**Contact** Mr. Jason McDonald, Dean of Admissions, School of Nursing, University of Portland, 5000 North Willamette Boulevard, Portland, OR 97203-5798. *Telephone:* 503-943-7147. *E-mail:* mcdonaja@up.edu.

## GRADUATE PROGRAMS

**Expenses (2013–14)** *Tuition:* part-time $1025 per credit. *Room and board:* $12,512 per academic year. *Required fees:* part-time $50 per credit.
**Financial Aid** 84% of graduate students in nursing programs received some form of financial aid in 2012–13. Fellowships, research assistantships, Federal Work-Study and scholarships available. Aid available to part-time students. *Financial aid application deadline:* 3/1.
**Contact** Ms. Sally Peters, Graduate Program Counselor, School of Nursing, University of Portland, 5000 North Willamette Boulevard, MSC-153, Portland, OR 97203-5798. *Telephone:* 503-943-7423. *Fax:* 503-943-7729. *E-mail:* Peterss@up.edu.

### MASTER'S DEGREE PROGRAM

**Degree** MS
**Available Programs** Master's.
**Concentrations Available** Clinical nurse leader; nursing education.
**Study Options** Part-time.
**Program Entrance Requirements** Computer literacy, minimum overall college GPA of 3.0, transcript of college record, written essay, interview, 2 letters of recommendation, resume, statistics course, GRE General Test or MAT. *Application deadline:* 1/15 (summer). Applications may be processed on a rolling basis for some programs. *Application fee:* $50.
**Advanced Placement** Credit given for nursing courses completed elsewhere dependent upon specific evaluations.
**Degree Requirements** 42 total credit hours, thesis or project.

### DOCTORAL DEGREE PROGRAM

**Degree** DNP
**Available Programs** Doctorate; Post-Baccalaureate Doctorate.
**Areas of Study** Advanced practice nursing.
**Program Entrance Requirements** Minimum overall college GPA of 3.0, interview by faculty committee, 3 letters of recommendation, statistics course, vita, writing sample, GRE General Test or MAT. *Application deadline:* 1/15 (summer). Applications may be processed on a rolling basis for some programs. *Application fee:* $50.
**Degree Requirements** 83 total credit hours, oral exam, residency.

# PENNSYLVANIA

## Alvernia University

### Nursing
### Reading, Pennsylvania

*http://www.alvernia.edu/*
Founded in 1958

**DEGREES • BSN • MSN**
**Nursing Program Faculty** 13 (6% with doctorates).
**Baccalaureate Enrollment** 227 **Women** 96% **Men** 4% **Minority** 10% **International** 3% **Part-time** 10%
**Nursing Student Activities** Nursing Honor Society, Sigma Theta Tau, Student Nurses' Association.
**Nursing Student Resources** Academic advising; academic or career counseling; assistance for students with disabilities; bookstore; campus computer network; computer lab; computer-assisted instruction; e-mail services; employment services for current students; externships; interactive nursing skills videos; Internet; learning resource lab; library services; nursing audiovisuals; remedial services; resume preparation assistance; skills, simulation, or other laboratory; tutoring.
**Library Facilities** 89,361 volumes (3,015 in health, 995 in nursing); 41,005 periodical subscriptions (89 health-care related).

## BACCALAUREATE PROGRAMS

**Degree** BSN
**Available Programs** Generic Baccalaureate; LPN to Baccalaureate; LPN to RN Baccalaureate; RN Baccalaureate.
**Site Options** Reading, PA.
**Study Options** Full-time.
**Program Entrance Requirements** Minimum overall college GPA of 2.7, transcript of college record, CPR certification, written essay, health exam, health insurance, high school biology, high school chemistry, 2 years high school math, 2 years high school science, high school transcript, immunizations, 2 letters of recommendation, minimum high school GPA of 2.7, minimum GPA in nursing prerequisites of 2.7. Transfer students are accepted.
**Advanced Placement** Credit by examination available. Credit given for nursing courses completed elsewhere dependent upon specific evaluations.
**Financial Aid** 75% of baccalaureate students in nursing programs received some form of financial aid in 2012–13.
**Contact** Dr. Mary Ellen Symanski, Nursing Department Chair, Nursing, Alvernia University, 400 Saint Bernardine Street, Reading, PA 19607. *Telephone:* 610-796-8217. *Fax:* 610-796-8464. *E-mail:* maryellen.symanski@alvernia.edu.

## GRADUATE PROGRAMS

**Contact** Dr. Kathleen Wisser, RN to BSN and MSN Coordinator, Nursing, Alvernia University, 400 Saint Bernardine Street, Reading, PA 19607. *Telephone:* 610-790-2853. *Fax:* 610-796-8464. *E-mail:* kathleen.wisser@alvernia.edu.

### MASTER'S DEGREE PROGRAM

**Degree** MSN
**Available Programs** Master's; RN to Master's.
**Concentrations Available** *Clinical nurse specialist programs in:* acute care, adult health, cardiovascular, critical care, family health, forensic nursing, gerontology, home health care, medical-surgical, oncology.
**Site Options** Reading, PA; Schuylkill Haven, PA.
**Study Options** Part-time.
**Program Entrance Requirements** Clinical experience, computer literacy, minimum overall college GPA of 3.0, transcript of college record, CPR certification, immunizations, interview, physical assessment course, professional liability insurance/malpractice insurance, resume, statistics course.
**Advanced Placement** Credit given for nursing courses completed elsewhere dependent upon specific evaluations.
**Degree Requirements** 36 total credit hours.

## CONTINUING EDUCATION PROGRAM

**Contact** Ms. Mary Arbogast, Nursing Outreach Coordinator, Nursing, Alvernia University, 400 Saint Bernardine Street, Reading, PA 19607. *Telephone:* 610-796-8429. *Fax:* 610-796-8367. *E-mail:* mary.arbogast@alvernia.edu.

## Bloomsburg University of Pennsylvania

### Department of Nursing
### Bloomsburg, Pennsylvania

*http://www.bloomu.edu/*
Founded in 1839

**DEGREES • BSN • MSN • MSN/MBA**
**Nursing Program Faculty** 42 (40% with doctorates).
**Baccalaureate Enrollment** 357 **Women** 87.7% **Men** 12.3% **Minority** 6.4% **Part-time** 11.2%
**Graduate Enrollment** 89 **Women** 78.7% **Men** 21.3% **Minority** 9% **Part-time** 69.7%
**Distance Learning Courses** Available.

**Nursing Student Activities** Sigma Theta Tau, Student Nurses' Association, nursing club.
**Nursing Student Resources** Academic advising; academic or career counseling; assistance for students with disabilities; bookstore; campus computer network; career placement assistance; computer lab; computer-assisted instruction; daycare for children of students; e-mail services; employment services for current students; externships; housing assistance; interactive nursing skills videos; Internet; learning resource lab; library services; nursing audiovisuals; paid internships; placement services for program completers; remedial services; resume preparation assistance; skills, simulation, or other laboratory; tutoring; unpaid internships.
**Library Facilities** 552,492 volumes (3,329 in health, 2,427 in nursing); 7,994 periodical subscriptions health-care related.

## BACCALAUREATE PROGRAMS

**Degree** BSN
**Available Programs** ADN to Baccalaureate; Baccalaureate for Second Degree; Generic Baccalaureate; LPN to RN Baccalaureate.
**Site Options** Danville, PA.
**Study Options** Full-time.
**Program Entrance Requirements** Minimum overall college GPA of 2.5, transcript of college record, CPR certification, written essay, health exam, health insurance, high school biology, high school chemistry, 2 years high school math, 3 years high school science, high school transcript, immunizations, interview, 3 letters of recommendation, minimum high school GPA of 3.0, minimum high school rank 80%, minimum GPA in nursing prerequisites of 2.5, professional liability insurance/malpractice insurance, prerequisite course work, RN licensure. Transfer students are accepted. *Application deadline:* 11/15 (fall). *Application fee:* $35.
**Advanced Placement** Credit by examination available. Credit given for nursing courses completed elsewhere dependent upon specific evaluations.
**Expenses (2013–14)** *Tuition, area resident:* full-time $6622; part-time $276 per credit. *Tuition, state resident:* full-time $6622; part-time $376. *Tuition, nonresident:* full-time $16,556; part-time $690 per credit. *Room and board:* $7848; room only: $4886 per academic year. *Required fees:* full-time $1960; part-time $72 per credit; part-time $55 per term.
**Financial Aid** 61% of baccalaureate students in nursing programs received some form of financial aid in 2012–13. *Gift aid (need-based):* Federal Pell, FSEOG, state, private, college/university gift aid from institutional funds. *Loans:* Federal Direct (Subsidized and Unsubsidized Stafford PLUS), Perkins, state, alternative loans. *Work-study:* Federal Work-Study, part-time campus jobs. *Financial aid application deadline (priority):* 3/15.
**Contact** Dr. Michelle Ficca, Department Chairperson, Department of Nursing, Bloomsburg University of Pennsylvania, 400 East 2nd Street, Room 3109, MCHS, Bloomsburg, PA 17815. *Telephone:* 570-389-4615. *Fax:* 570-389-5008. *E-mail:* mficca@bloomu.edu.

## GRADUATE PROGRAMS

**Expenses (2013–14)** *Tuition, state resident:* part-time $442 per credit hour. *Tuition, nonresident:* part-time $663 per credit hour. *Required fees:* part-time $96 per credit; part-time $55 per term.
**Financial Aid** 35% of graduate students in nursing programs received some form of financial aid in 2012–13. Unspecified assistantships available.
**Contact** Dr. Michelle Ficca, Coordinator of Graduate Program, Department of Nursing, Bloomsburg University of Pennsylvania, 400 East Second Street, Room 3136, MCHS, Bloomsburg, PA 17815. *Telephone:* 570-389-4615. *Fax:* 570-389-5008. *E-mail:* mficca@bloomu.edu.

### MASTER'S DEGREE PROGRAM

**Degrees** MSN; MSN/MBA
**Available Programs** Master's; Master's for Nurses with Non-Nursing Degrees; RN to Master's.
**Concentrations Available** Nurse anesthesia; nursing administration. *Clinical nurse specialist programs in:* community health, school health. *Nurse practitioner programs in:* adult health, family health, gerontology.
**Study Options** Full-time and part-time.
**Program Entrance Requirements** Clinical experience, minimum overall college GPA of 3.0, transcript of college record, CPR certification, written essay, immunizations, interview, 3 letters of recommendation, nursing research course, physical assessment course, professional liability insurance/malpractice insurance, resume, statistics course. *Application deadline:* 7/1 (fall). *Application fee:* $35.
**Advanced Placement** Credit by examination available. Credit given for nursing courses completed elsewhere dependent upon specific evaluations.
**Degree Requirements** 39 total credit hours, comprehensive exam.

# California University of Pennsylvania

## Department of Nursing
## California, Pennsylvania

***http://www.calu.edu/academics/colleges/eberly/nursing/index.htm***
Founded in 1852

### DEGREE • BSN

**Nursing Program Faculty** 5 (60% with doctorates).
**Baccalaureate Enrollment** 145 **Women** 83% **Men** 17% **Minority** 3% **Part-time** 92%
**Nursing Student Activities** Sigma Theta Tau.
**Nursing Student Resources** Academic advising; academic or career counseling; assistance for students with disabilities; bookstore; campus computer network; career placement assistance; computer lab; computer-assisted instruction; daycare for children of students; e-mail services; employment services for current students; Internet; library services; nursing audiovisuals; placement services for program completers; remedial services; resume preparation assistance; tutoring.
**Library Facilities** 3,840 volumes in health, 2,010 volumes in nursing; 80 periodical subscriptions health-care related.

## BACCALAUREATE PROGRAMS

**Degree** BSN
**Available Programs** RN Baccalaureate.
**Site Options** West Mifflin, PA.
**Study Options** Full-time and part-time.
**Program Entrance Requirements** Minimum overall college GPA of 2.0, transcript of college record, CPR certification, health exam, health insurance, immunizations, 2 letters of recommendation, professional liability insurance/malpractice insurance, prerequisite course work, RN licensure. Transfer students are accepted.
**Advanced Placement** Credit by examination available. Credit given for nursing courses completed elsewhere dependent upon specific evaluations.
**Contact** *Telephone:* 724-938-5739. *Fax:* 724-938-1612.

# Carlow University

## School of Nursing
## Pittsburgh, Pennsylvania

***http://www3.carlow.edu/academics/schools/sch-nurs/index.html***
Founded in 1929

### DEGREES • BSN • MSN

**Nursing Program Faculty** 31 (23% with doctorates).
**Baccalaureate Enrollment** 333 **Women** 99% **Men** 1% **Minority** 13% **Part-time** 21%
**Graduate Enrollment** 54 **Women** 94% **Men** 6% **Minority** 11% **Part-time** 94%
**Nursing Student Activities** Nursing Honor Society, Sigma Theta Tau, Student Nurses' Association.
**Nursing Student Resources** Academic advising; academic or career counseling; assistance for students with disabilities; bookstore; campus computer network; career placement assistance; computer lab; computer-assisted instruction; daycare for children of students; e-mail services; employment services for current students; externships; housing assistance; Internet; learning resource lab; library services; nursing audiovisuals; other; paid internships; placement services for program completers; remedial services; resume preparation assistance; skills, simulation, or other laboratory; tutoring; unpaid internships.
**Library Facilities** 132,930 volumes (14,100 in health, 5,450 in nursing); 60 periodical subscriptions health-care related.

## BACCALAUREATE PROGRAMS

**Degree** BSN

**Available Programs** Accelerated RN Baccalaureate; Baccalaureate for Second Degree; Generic Baccalaureate.
**Site Options** Cranberry Township, PA; Greensburg, PA.
**Study Options** Full-time and part-time.
**Program Entrance Requirements** Minimum overall college GPA of 3.0, transcript of college record, CPR certification, health exam, health insurance, high school biology, high school chemistry, 2 years high school math, 2 years high school science, high school transcript, immunizations, interview, minimum high school GPA of 3.0, minimum GPA in nursing prerequisites of 2.0, professional liability insurance/malpractice insurance, prerequisite course work. Transfer students are accepted.
**Advanced Placement** Credit by examination available. Credit given for nursing courses completed elsewhere dependent upon specific evaluations.
**Contact** *Telephone:* 412-578-6059. *Fax:* 412-578-6668.

## GRADUATE PROGRAMS

**Contact** *Telephone:* 412-578-8764. *Fax:* 412-578-6321.

### MASTER'S DEGREE PROGRAM

**Degree** MSN
**Available Programs** Accelerated Master's; Master's; RN to Master's.
**Concentrations Available** Nurse case management; nursing administration; nursing education. *Clinical nurse specialist programs in:* home health care. *Nurse practitioner programs in:* family health.
**Site Options** Cranberry Township, PA; Greensburg, PA.
**Study Options** Full-time and part-time.
**Program Entrance Requirements** Clinical experience, computer literacy, minimum overall college GPA of 3.0, transcript of college record, CPR certification, written essay, immunizations, interview, 3 letters of recommendation, professional liability insurance/malpractice insurance, prerequisite course work, resume, statistics course.
**Advanced Placement** Credit by examination available. Credit given for nursing courses completed elsewhere dependent upon specific evaluations.
**Degree Requirements** 56 total credit hours, thesis or project, comprehensive exam.

### POST-MASTER'S PROGRAM

**Areas of Study** *Clinical nurse specialist programs in:* home health care. *Nurse practitioner programs in:* family health.

## CONTINUING EDUCATION PROGRAM

**Contact** *Telephone:* 412-578-8764. *Fax:* 412-578-6321.

# Cedar Crest College

## Department of Nursing
## Allentown, Pennsylvania

***http://www.cedarcrest.edu/***
Founded in 1867

**DEGREES • BS • MSN**
**Nursing Program Faculty** 21 (24% with doctorates).
**Baccalaureate Enrollment** 287 **Women** 96% **Men** 4% **Minority** 23% **International** 8% **Part-time** 68%
**Graduate Enrollment** 23 **Women** 96% **Men** 4% **Minority** 4% **Part-time** 100%
**Nursing Student Activities** Nursing Honor Society, Sigma Theta Tau, Student Nurses' Association.
**Nursing Student Resources** Academic advising; academic or career counseling; assistance for students with disabilities; bookstore; campus computer network; career placement assistance; computer lab; computer-assisted instruction; e-mail services; interactive nursing skills videos; Internet; learning resource lab; library services; nursing audiovisuals; remedial services; skills, simulation, or other laboratory; tutoring.
**Library Facilities** 149,853 volumes; 28,278 periodical subscriptions.

## BACCALAUREATE PROGRAMS

**Degree** BS
**Available Programs** Baccalaureate for Second Degree; Generic Baccalaureate; LPN to Baccalaureate; RN Baccalaureate.
**Study Options** Full-time and part-time.
**Program Entrance Requirements** Minimum overall college GPA of 2.5, CPR certification, written essay, health exam, health insurance, high school biology, high school chemistry, 3 years high school math, 2 years high school science, high school transcript, immunizations, minimum GPA in nursing prerequisites of 2.7, prerequisite course work. Transfer students are accepted. *Application deadline:* Applications may be processed on a rolling basis for some programs.
**Advanced Placement** Credit given for nursing courses completed elsewhere dependent upon specific evaluations.
**Contact** *Telephone:* 610-740-3780. *Fax:* 610-606-4647.

## GRADUATE PROGRAMS

**Contact** *Telephone:* 610-606-4666 Ext. 3480.

### MASTER'S DEGREE PROGRAM

**Degree** MSN
**Available Programs** Master's.
**Study Options** Part-time.
**Program Entrance Requirements** Clinical experience, minimum overall college GPA of 3.0, transcript of college record, CPR certification, immunizations, interview, 3 letters of recommendation, nursing research course, physical assessment course, resume, statistics course. *Application deadline:* Applications may be processed on a rolling basis for some programs. *Application fee:* $30.
**Advanced Placement** Credit given for nursing courses completed elsewhere dependent upon specific evaluations.
**Degree Requirements** 38 total credit hours, thesis or project.

# Chatham University

## Nursing Programs
## Pittsburgh, Pennsylvania

***http://www.chatham.edu/***
Founded in 1869

**DEGREES • BSN • DNP • MSN**
**Nursing Program Faculty** 27 (80% with doctorates).
**Baccalaureate Enrollment** 99 **Women** 83% **Men** 17% **Minority** 5% **Part-time** 80%
**Graduate Enrollment** 116 **Women** 86% **Men** 14% **Minority** 28% **Part-time** 63%
**Distance Learning Courses** Available.
**Nursing Student Activities** Nursing Honor Society, Sigma Theta Tau.
**Nursing Student Resources** Academic advising; academic or career counseling; assistance for students with disabilities; bookstore; campus computer network; career placement assistance; computer lab; e-mail services; employment services for current students; housing assistance; Internet; library services; other; placement services for program completers; remedial services; resume preparation assistance; tutoring.
**Library Facilities** 91,318 volumes (1,747 in health, 1,732 in nursing); 31,656 periodical subscriptions (967 health-care related).

## BACCALAUREATE PROGRAMS

**Degree** BSN
**Available Programs** RN Baccalaureate; RPN to Baccalaureate.
**Study Options** Full-time and part-time.
**Program Entrance Requirements** Written essay, health insurance, high school transcript, immunizations, 2 letters of recommendation. Transfer students are accepted. *Application deadline:* 4/15 (fall), 11/1 (spring). Applications may be processed on a rolling basis for some programs.
**Advanced Placement** Credit by examination available. Credit given for nursing courses completed elsewhere dependent upon specific evaluations.
**Expenses (2013–14)** *Tuition:* part-time $759 per credit.
**Financial Aid** *Gift aid (need-based):* Federal Pell, FSEOG, state, private, college/university gift aid from institutional funds. *Loans:* Federal Direct (Subsidized and Unsubsidized Stafford PLUS), Perkins. *Work-study:* Federal Work-Study, part-time campus jobs. *Financial aid application deadline:* Continuous.
**Contact** Ms. Leah Albert, Admission Counselor, Nursing Programs, Chatham University, Berry Hall, Woodland Road, Pittsburgh, PA 15232. *Telephone:* 412-365-1296. *Fax:* 412-365-1609. *E-mail:* lalbert@chatham.edu.

## GRADUATE PROGRAMS

**Expenses (2013–14)** *Tuition:* part-time $827 per credit. *Required fees:* part-time $22 per credit.
**Financial Aid** 75% of graduate students in nursing programs received some form of financial aid in 2012–13.
**Contact** Mr. David A. Vey, Assistant Director of Online Admission, Nursing Programs, Chatham University, Admission Office, Woodland

Road, Pittsburgh, PA 15232. *Telephone:* 412-365-1498. *Fax:* 412-365-1609. *E-mail:* dvey@chatham.edu.

**MASTER'S DEGREE PROGRAM**
**Degree** MSN
**Available Programs** Master's.
**Concentrations Available** Nursing administration; nursing education; nursing informatics.
**Study Options** Full-time and part-time.
**Online Degree Options** Yes (online only).
**Program Entrance Requirements** Minimum overall college GPA of 3.0, transcript of college record, written essay, resume. *Application deadline:* 8/15 (fall). Applications may be processed on a rolling basis for some programs.
**Advanced Placement** Credit given for nursing courses completed elsewhere dependent upon specific evaluations.
**Degree Requirements** 36 total credit hours, thesis or project.

**DOCTORAL DEGREE PROGRAM**
**Degree** DNP
**Available Programs** Doctorate.
**Online Degree Options** Yes (online only).
**Program Entrance Requirements** Clinical experience, minimum overall college GPA of 3.0, 2 letters of recommendation, MSN or equivalent, vita, writing sample. *Application deadline:* 4/15 (fall), 9/15 (spring).
**Degree Requirements** 27 total credit hours, residency.

# Clarion University of Pennsylvania
## School of Nursing
## Oil City, Pennsylvania

*http://www.clarion.edu/*
Founded in 1867

**DEGREES • BSN • MSN**
**Nursing Program Faculty** 25 (25% with doctorates).
**Baccalaureate Enrollment** 163 **Women** 85.9% **Men** 14.1% **Minority** 4.3% **Part-time** 91.4%
**Graduate Enrollment** 69 **Women** 85.5% **Men** 14.5% **Minority** 2.9% **Part-time** 100%
**Distance Learning Courses** Available.
**Nursing Student Activities** Nursing Honor Society, Sigma Theta Tau, Student Nurses' Association, nursing club.
**Nursing Student Resources** Academic advising; academic or career counseling; assistance for students with disabilities; bookstore; campus computer network; career placement assistance; computer lab; computer-assisted instruction; daycare for children of students; e-mail services; employment services for current students; externships; housing assistance; interactive nursing skills videos; Internet; learning resource lab; library services; nursing audiovisuals; placement services for program completers; remedial services; resume preparation assistance; skills, simulation, or other laboratory; tutoring.
**Library Facilities** 474,723 volumes (12,000 in health, 7,000 in nursing); 33,515 periodical subscriptions (300 health-care related).

**BACCALAUREATE PROGRAMS**
**Degree** BSN
**Available Programs** ADN to Baccalaureate; RN Baccalaureate.
**Study Options** Full-time and part-time.
**Online Degree Options** Yes (online only).
**Program Entrance Requirements** Minimum overall college GPA of 2.5, transcript of college record, CPR certification, health exam, health insurance, high school transcript, immunizations, minimum GPA in nursing prerequisites of 2.0, professional liability insurance/malpractice insurance, RN licensure. Transfer students are accepted. *Application deadline:* 8/1 (fall), 12/1 (winter). Applications may be processed on a rolling basis for some programs. *Application fee:* $30.
**Expenses (2013–14)** *Tuition, state resident:* part-time $276 per credit. *Tuition, nonresident:* part-time $282 per credit. *Required fees:* part-time $70 per credit.
**Financial Aid** 80% of baccalaureate students in nursing programs received some form of financial aid in 2012–13.
**Contact** Ms. Angela West, PhD, Chairperson, Nursing Department, School of Nursing, Clarion University of Pennsylvania, 1801 West First Street, Oil City, PA 16301. *Telephone:* 814-393-1258. *Fax:* 814-676-0251. *E-mail:* awest@clarion.edu.

**GRADUATE PROGRAMS**
**Expenses (2013–14)** *Tuition, state resident:* part-time $442 per credit. *Tuition, nonresident:* part-time $451 per credit. *Required fees:* part-time $132 per credit.
**Financial Aid** 90% of graduate students in nursing programs received some form of financial aid in 2012–13. 2 research assistantships with full tuition reimbursements available (averaging $4,660 per year) were awarded. *Financial aid application deadline:* 3/1.
**Contact** Dr. Deborah Ciesielka, Coordinator, MSN Family Nurse Practitioner Program, School of Nursing, Clarion University of Pennsylvania, 4900 Friendship Avenue, Pittsburgh, PA 15224. *Telephone:* 412-578-7277. *E-mail:* dciesielka@clarion.edu.

**MASTER'S DEGREE PROGRAM**
**Degree** MSN
**Available Programs** Master's; RN to Master's.
**Concentrations Available** *Nurse practitioner programs in:* family health.
**Site Options** Pittsburgh, PA; Edinboro, PA.
**Study Options** Full-time and part-time.
**Program Entrance Requirements** Clinical experience, computer literacy, minimum overall college GPA of 3.0, transcript of college record, CPR certification, written essay, immunizations, interview, 3 letters of recommendation, professional liability insurance/malpractice insurance, statistics course. *Application deadline:* 4/1 (fall), 11/1 (winter), 11/1 (spring), 4/1 (summer). *Application fee:* $50.
**Advanced Placement** Credit given for nursing courses completed elsewhere dependent upon specific evaluations.
**Degree Requirements** 45 total credit hours, thesis or project, comprehensive exam.

**POST-MASTER'S PROGRAM**
**Areas of Study** *Nurse practitioner programs in:* family health.

# DeSales University
## Department of Nursing and Health
## Center Valley, Pennsylvania

*http://www.desales.edu/*
Founded in 1964

**DEGREES • BSN • MSN • MSN/MBA**
**Nursing Program Faculty** 74 (23% with doctorates).
**Baccalaureate Enrollment** 193 **Women** 88% **Men** 12% **Minority** 4% **International** 2% **Part-time** 23%
**Graduate Enrollment** 85 **Women** 93% **Men** 7% **Minority** 2% **Part-time** 95%
**Nursing Student Activities** Nursing Honor Society, Sigma Theta Tau, Student Nurses' Association.
**Nursing Student Resources** Academic advising; academic or career counseling; bookstore; campus computer network; career placement assistance; computer lab; computer-assisted instruction; e-mail services; employment services for current students; externships; interactive nursing skills videos; Internet; learning resource lab; library services; nursing audiovisuals; paid internships; placement services for program completers; remedial services; resume preparation assistance; skills, simulation, or other laboratory; tutoring; unpaid internships.
**Library Facilities** 163,208 volumes (1,215 in health, 100 in nursing); 251 periodical subscriptions (100 health-care related).

**BACCALAUREATE PROGRAMS**
**Degree** BSN
**Available Programs** ADN to Baccalaureate; Accelerated Baccalaureate; Accelerated RN Baccalaureate; Baccalaureate for Second Degree; Generic Baccalaureate; RN Baccalaureate.
**Study Options** Full-time and part-time.
**Program Entrance Requirements** Minimum overall college GPA of 2.5, transcript of college record, written essay, high school biology, high school chemistry, high school foreign language, 2 years high school math, 3 years high school science, high school transcript, 2 letters of recommendation, minimum high school GPA of 2.5, minimum high school rank 33%, minimum GPA in nursing prerequisites of 2.0. Transfer students are accepted. *Application deadline:* Applications may be processed on a rolling basis for some programs. *Application fee:* $30.

**Advanced Placement** Credit by examination available. Credit given for nursing courses completed elsewhere dependent upon specific evaluations.
**Contact** *Telephone:* 610-282-1100 Ext. 1285. *Fax:* 610-282-2091.

## GRADUATE PROGRAMS

**Contact** *Telephone:* 610-282-1100 Ext. 1664. *Fax:* 610-282-2091.

### MASTER'S DEGREE PROGRAM

**Degrees** MSN; MSN/MBA
**Available Programs** Accelerated AD/RN to Master's; Master's; RN to Master's.
**Concentrations Available** Nursing administration; nursing education. *Clinical nurse specialist programs in:* adult health. *Nurse practitioner programs in:* family health.
**Study Options** Full-time and part-time.
**Program Entrance Requirements** Minimum overall college GPA of 3.0, transcript of college record, written essay, interview, 3 letters of recommendation, prerequisite course work, statistics course. *Application deadline:* Applications may be processed on a rolling basis for some programs. *Application fee:* $35.
**Advanced Placement** Credit given for nursing courses completed elsewhere dependent upon specific evaluations.
**Degree Requirements** 47 total credit hours.

### POST-MASTER'S PROGRAM

**Areas of Study** Nursing education. *Clinical nurse specialist programs in:* adult health. *Nurse practitioner programs in:* family health.

## CONTINUING EDUCATION PROGRAM

**Contact** *Telephone:* 610-282-1100 Ext. 1271. *Fax:* 610-282-2091.

# Drexel University

## College of Nursing and Health Professions
## Philadelphia, Pennsylvania

***http://www.drexel.edu/cnhp***
Founded in 1891

### DEGREES • BSN • DR NP • MSN

**Nursing Program Faculty** 73 (52% with doctorates).
**Baccalaureate Enrollment** 1,696 **Women** 87% **Men** 13% **Minority** 21% **International** 1% **Part-time** 46%
**Graduate Enrollment** 1,010 **Women** 89% **Men** 11% **Minority** 19% **International** 2% **Part-time** 96%
**Distance Learning Courses** Available.
**Nursing Student Activities** Nursing Honor Society, Sigma Theta Tau, Student Nurses' Association, nursing club.
**Nursing Student Resources** Academic advising; academic or career counseling; assistance for students with disabilities; bookstore; campus computer network; career placement assistance; computer lab; computer-assisted instruction; e-mail services; housing assistance; interactive nursing skills videos; Internet; learning resource lab; library services; nursing audiovisuals; paid internships; placement services for program completers; remedial services; resume preparation assistance; skills, simulation, or other laboratory; tutoring.
**Library Facilities** 625,531 volumes (51,000 in health, 5,015 in nursing); 32,850 periodical subscriptions (63,000 health-care related).

## BACCALAUREATE PROGRAMS

**Degree** BSN
**Available Programs** Accelerated Baccalaureate; Accelerated Baccalaureate for Second Degree; Generic Baccalaureate; RN Baccalaureate.
**Site Options** Philadelphia, PA.
**Study Options** Full-time.
**Program Entrance Requirements** CPR certification, written essay, health insurance, high school biology, high school chemistry, 3 years high school math, 2 years high school science, high school transcript, immunizations, 2 letters of recommendation. Transfer students are accepted. *Application deadline:* 1/15 (fall). *Application fee:* $75.
**Expenses (2012–13)** *Tuition:* full-time $33,800; part-time $930 per credit. *International tuition:* $33,800 full-time. *Room and board:* $11,200; room only: $5625 per academic year. *Required fees:* full-time $3170; part-time $145 per term.
**Financial Aid** 66% of baccalaureate students in nursing programs received some form of financial aid in 2011–12.
**Contact** Ms. Vanessa Thomas, Director of Undergraduate Admissions, College of Nursing and Health Professions, Drexel University, 3141 Chestnut Street, Enrollment Management, Philadelphia, PA 19104. *Telephone:* 215-895-6732. *Fax:* 215-895-5939. *E-mail:* VMT26@drexel.edu.

## GRADUATE PROGRAMS

**Expenses (2012–13)** *Tuition:* part-time $800 per credit.
**Financial Aid** 44% of graduate students in nursing programs received some form of financial aid in 2011–12. Fellowships, research assistantships, teaching assistantships, career-related internships or fieldwork, Federal Work-Study, institutionally sponsored loans, and tuition waivers (partial) available. Aid available to part-time students. *Financial aid application deadline:* 5/1.
**Contact** Mr. Redian Furxhui, Academic Advisor, MSN Programs, College of Nursing and Health Professions, Drexel University, 1505 Race Street, Mail Stop 501, Philadelphia, PA 19102-1192. *Telephone:* 215-762-3999. *Fax:* 215-762-1259. *E-mail:* rf53@drexel.edu.

### MASTER'S DEGREE PROGRAM

**Degree** MSN
**Available Programs** Master's; RN to Master's.
**Concentrations Available** Clinical nurse leader; nurse anesthesia; nursing administration; nursing education. *Clinical nurse specialist programs in:*women's health. *Nurse practitioner programs in:* acute care, adult health, family health, pediatric, psychiatric/mental health,women's health.
**Site Options** Philadelphia, PA.
**Study Options** Full-time and part-time.
**Online Degree Options** Yes.
**Program Entrance Requirements** Clinical experience, computer literacy, minimum overall college GPA of 3.0, transcript of college record, CPR certification, written essay, immunizations, 2 letters of recommendation, resume. *Application deadline:* 1/1 (fall). Applications may be processed on a rolling basis for some programs. *Application fee:* $75.
**Advanced Placement** Credit given for nursing courses completed elsewhere dependent upon specific evaluations.
**Degree Requirements** 55 total credit hours, thesis or project, comprehensive exam.

### POST-MASTER'S PROGRAM

**Areas of Study** Nursing administration; nursing education. *Nurse practitioner programs in:* family health, pediatric.

### DOCTORAL DEGREE PROGRAM

**Degree** Dr NP
**Available Programs** Doctorate.
**Areas of Study** Clinical practice, faculty preparation, nursing administration, nursing education, nursing research, nursing science.
**Site Options** Philadelphia, PA.
**Online Degree Options** Yes (online only).
**Program Entrance Requirements** Clinical experience, minimum overall college GPA of 3.25, interview by faculty committee, interview, 2 letters of recommendation, vita, writing sample, GRE General Test. *Application deadline:* 6/1 (fall).
**Degree Requirements** 48 total credit hours, dissertation, oral exam, written exam, residency.

## CONTINUING EDUCATION PROGRAM

**Contact** Mr. Wayne Miller, Director of Continuing Nursing Education, College of Nursing and Health Professions, Drexel University, 245 North 15th Street, Mail Stop #501, Philadelphia, PA 19102. *Telephone:* 215-762-8521. *Fax:* 215-762-7778. *E-mail:* wdm22@drexel.edu.

# Duquesne University

## School of Nursing
## Pittsburgh, Pennsylvania

***http://www.duq.edu/nursing***
Founded in 1878

### DEGREES • BSN • MSN • PHD

**Nursing Program Faculty** 86 (78% with doctorates).
**Baccalaureate Enrollment** 565 **Women** 90% **Men** 10% **Minority** 10% **International** 1% **Part-time** 1%
**Graduate Enrollment** 252 **Women** 94% **Men** 6% **Minority** 20% **International** 1% **Part-time** 37%

**Distance Learning Courses** Available.
**Nursing Student Activities** Nursing Honor Society, Sigma Theta Tau, Student Nurses' Association, nursing club.
**Nursing Student Resources** Academic advising; academic or career counseling; assistance for students with disabilities; bookstore; campus computer network; career placement assistance; computer lab; computer-assisted instruction; daycare for children of students; e-mail services; employment services for current students; externships; housing assistance; interactive nursing skills videos; Internet; learning resource lab; library services; nursing audiovisuals; paid internships; placement services for program completers; remedial services; resume preparation assistance; skills, simulation, or other laboratory; tutoring; unpaid internships.
**Library Facilities** 739,768 volumes (27,613 in health, 1,951 in nursing); 101,861 periodical subscriptions (1,779 health-care related).

## BACCALAUREATE PROGRAMS

**Degree** BSN
**Available Programs** Accelerated Baccalaureate for Second Degree; Generic Baccalaureate.
**Study Options** Full-time and part-time.
**Program Entrance Requirements** Minimum overall college GPA of 3.0, transcript of college record, written essay, high school biology, high school chemistry, high school foreign language, 2 years high school math, 3 years high school science, high school transcript, 2 letters of recommendation, minimum high school GPA of 3.0, minimum high school rank 40%. Transfer students are accepted. *Application deadline:* 5/1 (fall), 11/1 (spring). Applications may be processed on a rolling basis for some programs. *Application fee:* $50.
**Advanced Placement** Credit by examination available.
**Expenses (2013–14)** *Tuition:* full-time $28,913; part-time $943 per credit. *International tuition:* $28,913 full-time. *Room and board:* $10,632 per academic year. *Required fees:* full-time $2472; part-time $96 per credit.
**Financial Aid** 89% of baccalaureate students in nursing programs received some form of financial aid in 2012–13.
**Contact** Ms. Susan Hardner, Nursing Recruiter, School of Nursing, Duquesne University, 600 Forbes Avenue, Pittsburgh, PA 15282-1760. *Telephone:* 412-396-4945. *Fax:* 412-396-6346. *E-mail:* hardnersue@duq.edu.

## GRADUATE PROGRAMS

**Expenses (2013–14)** *Tuition:* part-time $1036 per credit. *Required fees:* part-time $96 per credit.
**Financial Aid** 48% of graduate students in nursing programs received some form of financial aid in 2012–13. 18 research assistantships with partial tuition reimbursements available (averaging $1,170 per year), 3 teaching assistantships with partial tuition reimbursements available (averaging $1,170 per year) were awarded; institutionally sponsored loans, scholarships, traineeships, tuition waivers (partial), and unspecified assistantships also available. Aid available to part-time students. *Financial aid application deadline:* 7/1.
**Contact** Ms. Susan Hardner, Nursing Recruiter, School of Nursing, Duquesne University, 600 Forbes Avenue, Pittsburgh, PA 15282-1760. *Telephone:* 412-396-4945. *Fax:* 412-396-6346. *E-mail:* hardnersue@duq.edu.

### MASTER'S DEGREE PROGRAM

**Degree** MSN
**Available Programs** Master's.
**Concentrations Available** Nursing education. *Clinical nurse specialist programs in:* forensic nursing. *Nurse practitioner programs in:* family health.
**Study Options** Full-time and part-time.
**Online Degree Options** Yes (online only).
**Program Entrance Requirements** Clinical experience, computer literacy, minimum overall college GPA of 3.0, transcript of college record, written essay, interview, 2 letters of recommendation, nursing research course, physical assessment course, prerequisite course work, resume, statistics course. *Application deadline:* 3/1 (summer).
**Advanced Placement** Credit given for nursing courses completed elsewhere dependent upon specific evaluations.
**Degree Requirements** 47 total credit hours, thesis or project.

### POST-MASTER'S PROGRAM

**Areas of Study** *Clinical nurse specialist programs in:* forensic nursing. *Nurse practitioner programs in:* family health.

### DOCTORAL DEGREE PROGRAM

**Degree** PhD
**Available Programs** Doctorate.
**Areas of Study** Nursing research.
**Online Degree Options** Yes (online only).
**Program Entrance Requirements** Minimum overall college GPA of 3.5, interview by faculty committee, 3 letters of recommendation, MSN or equivalent, scholarly papers, statistics course, vita, writing sample. *Application deadline:* 1/15 (summer).
**Degree Requirements** 58 total credit hours, dissertation, oral exam, written exam, residency.

## CONTINUING EDUCATION PROGRAM

**Contact** Miss Kellie Collier, Administrative Assistant, School of Nursing, Duquesne University, 600 Forbes Avenue, Pittsburgh, PA 15282-1760. *Telephone:* 412-396-5203. *Fax:* 412-396-6346. *E-mail:* collier1@duq.edu.

***See display on next page and full description on page 470.***

# Eastern University
## Program in Nursing
## St. Davids, Pennsylvania

***http://www.eastern.edu/academics/programs/nursing-department-undergraduate***
Founded in 1952

**DEGREE • BSN**
**Nursing Program Faculty** 7 (43% with doctorates).
**Baccalaureate Enrollment** 100 **Women** 92% **Men** 8% **Minority** 25% **International** 32%
**Distance Learning Courses** Available.
**Nursing Student Activities** Sigma Theta Tau, Student Nurses' Association.
**Nursing Student Resources** Academic advising; academic or career counseling; assistance for students with disabilities; bookstore; campus computer network; career placement assistance; computer lab; computer-assisted instruction; e-mail services; employment services for current students; Internet; learning resource lab; library services; nursing audiovisuals; placement services for program completers; remedial services; resume preparation assistance; skills, simulation, or other laboratory; tutoring; unpaid internships.
**Library Facilities** 473,190 volumes (5,858 in health, 3,000 in nursing); 79,525 periodical subscriptions (821 health-care related).

## BACCALAUREATE PROGRAMS

**Degree** BSN
**Available Programs** Accelerated RN Baccalaureate; Baccalaureate for Second Degree; Generic Baccalaureate; International Nurse to Baccalaureate.
**Site Options** Wynnewood, PA; West Chester, PA; Harrisburg, PA.
**Study Options** Full-time.
**Program Entrance Requirements** Minimum overall college GPA of 3.0, transcript of college record, CPR certification, written essay, health exam, health insurance, high school chemistry, high school transcript, immunizations, interview, 2 letters of recommendation, minimum GPA in nursing prerequisites of 3.0, professional liability insurance/malpractice insurance, prerequisite course work, RN licensure. Transfer students are accepted. *Application deadline:* Applications may be processed on a rolling basis for some programs. *Application fee:* $40.
**Contact** *Telephone:* 800-732-7669. *Fax:* 610-341-1468.

# East Stroudsburg University of Pennsylvania
## Department of Nursing
## East Stroudsburg, Pennsylvania

***http://www4.esu.edu/***
Founded in 1893

**DEGREE • BS**
**Nursing Program Faculty** 14 (77% with doctorates).
**Baccalaureate Enrollment** 166 **Women** 75% **Men** 25%

**Nursing Student Activities** Nursing Honor Society, Sigma Theta Tau, Student Nurses' Association, nursing club.

**Nursing Student Resources** Academic advising; academic or career counseling; assistance for students with disabilities; bookstore; campus computer network; career placement assistance; computer lab; computer-assisted instruction; daycare for children of students; e-mail services; employment services for current students; externships; housing assistance; interactive nursing skills videos; Internet; learning resource lab; library services; nursing audiovisuals; other; placement services for program completers; remedial services; resume preparation assistance; skills, simulation, or other laboratory; tutoring; unpaid internships.

**Library Facilities** 569,096 volumes (16,810 in health, 2,035 in nursing); 3,900 periodical subscriptions (495 health-care related).

## BACCALAUREATE PROGRAMS

**Degree** BS

**Available Programs** Generic Baccalaureate; RN Baccalaureate.

**Study Options** Full-time.

**Program Entrance Requirements** Minimum overall college GPA of 2.75, transcript of college record, health exam, 2 years high school math, 2 years high school science, high school transcript, immunizations, minimum high school GPA of 3.0, minimum high school rank 75%, minimum GPA in nursing prerequisites of 2.75. Transfer students are accepted. *Application deadline:* 5/1 (fall), 1/1 (winter), 1/1 (spring). Applications may be processed on a rolling basis for some programs. *Application fee:* $100.

**Advanced Placement** Credit by examination available. Credit given for nursing courses completed elsewhere dependent upon specific evaluations.

**Contact** *Telephone:* 570-422-3569. *Fax:* 570-422-3848.

# Edinboro University of Pennsylvania

## Department of Nursing
## Edinboro, Pennsylvania

*http://www.edinboro.edu/*
Founded in 1857

**DEGREE • BSN**

**Nursing Program Faculty** 23 (56% with doctorates).
**Baccalaureate Enrollment** 315 **Women** 87.4% **Men** 12.6% **Minority** 9.4% **International** 4.2% **Part-time** .4%
**Nursing Student Activities** Sigma Theta Tau, Student Nurses' Association, nursing club.
**Nursing Student Resources** Academic advising; academic or career counseling; assistance for students with disabilities; bookstore; campus computer network; career placement assistance; computer lab; computer-assisted instruction; e-mail services; employment services for current students; housing assistance; interactive nursing skills videos; Internet; learning resource lab; library services; nursing audiovisuals; remedial services; resume preparation assistance; skills, simulation, or other laboratory; tutoring.
**Library Facilities** 485,338 volumes (500,000 in health, 100 in nursing); 1,024 periodical subscriptions (105 health-care related).

## BACCALAUREATE PROGRAMS

**Degree** BSN
**Available Programs** ADN to Baccalaureate; Accelerated Baccalaureate; Accelerated Baccalaureate for Second Degree; Baccalaureate for Second Degree; Generic Baccalaureate; International Nurse to Baccalaureate.
**Site Options** Erie, PA.
**Study Options** Full-time and part-time.
**Program Entrance Requirements** Minimum overall college GPA of 2.75, CPR certification, health exam, high school biology, high school chemistry, 2 years high school math, 2 years high school science, high school transcript, immunizations, minimum high school rank 40%, minimum GPA in nursing prerequisites of 2.75, professional liability insurance/malpractice insurance. *Application deadline:* Applications may be processed on a rolling basis for some programs. *Application fee:* $30.
**Advanced Placement** Credit by examination available.

**Expenses (2013–14)** *Tuition, state resident:* full-time $4425; part-time $276 per credit. *Tuition, nonresident:* full-time $6351; part-time $414 per credit. *International tuition:* $6351 full-time. *Room and board:* $11,496; room only: $8070 per academic year. *Required fees:* full-time $137.
**Financial Aid** 75% of baccalaureate students in nursing programs received some form of financial aid in 2012–13.
**Contact** Dr. Thomas R. White, Chairperson, Department of Nursing, Department of Nursing, Edinboro University of Pennsylvania, Human Services Building, #125, 215 Scotland Road, Edinboro, PA 16444. *Telephone:* 814-732-2900. *Fax:* 814-732-2536. *E-mail:* twhite@edinboro.edu.

# Gannon University
## Villa Maria School of Nursing
## Erie, Pennsylvania

*http://www.gannon.edu/Academic-Offerings/Health-Professions-and-Sciences/Villa-Maria-School-of-Nursing/*
Founded in 1925

**DEGREES • BSN • DNP • MSN**
**Nursing Program Faculty** 16 (20% with doctorates).
**Baccalaureate Enrollment** 350 **Women** 88% **Men** 12% **Minority** 4% **International** 3% **Part-time** 5%
**Graduate Enrollment** 97 **Women** 68% **Men** 32% **Minority** 6% **Part-time** 38%
**Distance Learning Courses** Available.
**Nursing Student Activities** Nursing Honor Society, Sigma Theta Tau.
**Nursing Student Resources** Academic advising; academic or career counseling; assistance for students with disabilities; bookstore; campus computer network; career placement assistance; computer lab; computer-assisted instruction; e-mail services; employment services for current students; externships; housing assistance; interactive nursing skills videos; Internet; learning resource lab; library services; nursing audiovisuals; other; paid internships; placement services for program completers; remedial services; resume preparation assistance; skills, simulation, or other laboratory; tutoring; unpaid internships.
**Library Facilities** 266,136 volumes (140,000 in health, 20,000 in nursing); 58,039 periodical subscriptions (3,000 health-care related).

### BACCALAUREATE PROGRAMS
**Degree** BSN
**Available Programs** ADN to Baccalaureate; Baccalaureate for Second Degree; Generic Baccalaureate; International Nurse to Baccalaureate; RN Baccalaureate.
**Study Options** Full-time and part-time.
**Online Degree Options** Yes.
**Program Entrance Requirements** Minimum overall college GPA of 2.7, transcript of college record, CPR certification, written essay, health exam, health insurance, high school biology, high school chemistry, 4 years high school math, 2 years high school science, high school transcript, immunizations, 1 letter of recommendation, minimum high school GPA of 2.5, minimum high school rank 40%, minimum GPA in nursing prerequisites of 2.7. Transfer students are accepted. *Application deadline:* Applications may be processed on a rolling basis for some programs. *Application fee:* $25.
**Expenses (2012–13)** *Tuition:* full-time $27,550; part-time $675 per credit. *Room and board:* $9600; room only: $7000 per academic year. *Required fees:* full-time $700; part-time $18 per credit.
**Financial Aid** 40% of baccalaureate students in nursing programs received some form of financial aid in 2011–12. *Gift aid (need-based):* Federal Pell, FSEOG, state, private, college/university gift aid from institutional funds. *Loans:* Federal Nursing Student Loans, Federal Direct (Subsidized and Unsubsidized Stafford PLUS), Perkins. *Work-study:* Federal Work-Study, part-time campus jobs. *Financial aid application deadline (priority):* 3/15.
**Contact** Ms. Patricia Ann Marshall, Director, Undergraduate Programs in Nursing, Villa Maria School of Nursing, Gannon University, 109 University Square, Morosky Academic Center, Erie, PA 16541-0001. *Telephone:* 814-871-5470. *Fax:* 814-871-5662. *E-mail:* marshall001@gannon.edu.

### GRADUATE PROGRAMS
**Expenses (2012–13)** *Tuition:* part-time $850 per credit. *Required fees:* part-time $18 per credit.
**Financial Aid** Scholarships available.
**Contact** Dr. Kathleen Patterson, School and Graduate Program Director, Villa Maria School of Nursing, Gannon University, 109 University Square, Erie, PA 16541-0001. *Telephone:* 814-871-5547. *Fax:* 814-871-5662. *E-mail:* patterso018@gannon.edu.

#### MASTER'S DEGREE PROGRAM
**Degree** MSN
**Available Programs** Accelerated AD/RN to Master's; Accelerated RN to Master's; Master's; RN to Master's.
**Concentrations Available** Nurse anesthesia; nursing administration. *Nurse practitioner programs in:* family health.
**Study Options** Full-time and part-time.
**Program Entrance Requirements** Clinical experience, computer literacy, minimum overall college GPA of 3.0, transcript of college record, CPR certification, written essay, immunizations, interview, 3 letters of recommendation, nursing research course, professional liability insurance/malpractice insurance, prerequisite course work, statistics course, GRE General Test. *Application deadline:* Applications may be processed on a rolling basis for some programs. *Application fee:* $50.
**Advanced Placement** Credit given for nursing courses completed elsewhere dependent upon specific evaluations.
**Degree Requirements** 46 total credit hours, thesis or project.

#### POST-MASTER'S PROGRAM
**Areas of Study** Nurse anesthesia; nursing administration. *Nurse practitioner programs in:* family health.

#### DOCTORAL DEGREE PROGRAM
**Degree** DNP
**Available Programs** Doctorate.
**Areas of Study** Clinical practice, family health.
**Program Entrance Requirements** Clinical experience, minimum overall college GPA of 3.0, interview by faculty committee, 3 letters of recommendation, MSN or equivalent, statistics course, vita, writing sample. *Application deadline:* Applications may be processed on a rolling basis for some programs. *Application fee:* $50.
**Degree Requirements** 42 total credit hours, dissertation, residency.

# Gwynedd Mercy University
## School of Nursing
## Gwynedd Valley, Pennsylvania

Founded in 1948

**DEGREES • BSN • MSN**
**Nursing Program Faculty** 21 (43% with doctorates).
**Baccalaureate Enrollment** 85 **Women** 95% **Men** 5% **Minority** 5% **Part-time** 28%
**Graduate Enrollment** 40 **Women** 85% **Men** 15% **Minority** 10% **International** 5% **Part-time** 80%
**Nursing Student Activities** Sigma Theta Tau, Student Nurses' Association.
**Nursing Student Resources** Academic advising; bookstore; campus computer network; computer lab; computer-assisted instruction; daycare for children of students; e-mail services; interactive nursing skills videos; learning resource lab; library services; nursing audiovisuals; resume preparation assistance; skills, simulation, or other laboratory; tutoring.
**Library Facilities** 105,070 volumes; 667 periodical subscriptions.

### BACCALAUREATE PROGRAMS
**Degree** BSN
**Available Programs** ADN to Baccalaureate; Accelerated RN Baccalaureate; RN Baccalaureate.
**Site Options** Fort Washington, PA.
**Study Options** Full-time and part-time.
**Program Entrance Requirements** Minimum overall college GPA of 2.8, transcript of college record, CPR certification, health exam, health insurance, high school biology, high school chemistry, 2 years high school math, high school transcript, immunizations, letters of recommendation, minimum high school rank 33%, minimum GPA in nursing prerequisites, professional liability insurance/malpractice insurance, RN licensure. Transfer students are accepted.
**Advanced Placement** Credit by examination available. Credit given for nursing courses completed elsewhere dependent upon specific evaluations.
**Contact** *Telephone:* 215-646-7300 Ext. 425. *Fax:* 215-641-5556 Ext. 528.

## GRADUATE PROGRAMS

**Contact** *Telephone:* 215-646-7300 Ext. 407. *Fax:* 215-542-5789.

### MASTER'S DEGREE PROGRAM

**Degree** MSN
**Available Programs** Master's; RN to Master's.
**Concentrations Available** *Clinical nurse specialist programs in:* gerontology, oncology, pediatric. *Nurse practitioner programs in:* adult health, pediatric.
**Study Options** Full-time and part-time.
**Program Entrance Requirements** Clinical experience, minimum overall college GPA of 3.0, transcript of college record, written essay, immunizations, interview, 2 letters of recommendation, physical assessment course, professional liability insurance/malpractice insurance, statistics course, GRE General Test or MAT.
**Advanced Placement** Credit by examination available. Credit given for nursing courses completed elsewhere dependent upon specific evaluations.
**Degree Requirements** 43 total credit hours.

### POST-MASTER'S PROGRAM

**Areas of Study** *Nurse practitioner programs in:* adult health, pediatric.

# Holy Family University

## School of Nursing and Allied Health Professions
## Philadelphia, Pennsylvania

***http://www.holyfamily.edu/sn/index.shtml***
Founded in 1954

**DEGREES • BSN • MSN**
**Nursing Program Faculty** 17 (67% with doctorates).
**Baccalaureate Enrollment** 700 **Women** 90% **Men** 10% **Minority** 40% **International** 5% **Part-time** 14%
**Graduate Enrollment** 80 **Women** 97% **Men** 3% **Minority** 27% **Part-time** 100%
**Distance Learning Courses** Available.
**Nursing Student Activities** Nursing Honor Society, Sigma Theta Tau, Student Nurses' Association, nursing club.
**Nursing Student Resources** Academic advising; academic or career counseling; assistance for students with disabilities; bookstore; campus computer network; career placement assistance; computer lab; computer-assisted instruction; daycare for children of students; e-mail services; employment services for current students; externships; housing assistance; interactive nursing skills videos; Internet; learning resource lab; library services; nursing audiovisuals; other; remedial services; resume preparation assistance; skills, simulation, or other laboratory; tutoring; unpaid internships.
**Library Facilities** 145,442 volumes (8,159 in health, 2,177 in nursing); 21,932 periodical subscriptions (279 health-care related).

## BACCALAUREATE PROGRAMS

**Degree** BSN
**Available Programs** ADN to Baccalaureate; Accelerated Baccalaureate for Second Degree; Accelerated RN Baccalaureate; Generic Baccalaureate; International Nurse to Baccalaureate.
**Site Options** Bensalem, PA; Newtown, PA; Philadelphia, PA.
**Study Options** Full-time.
**Program Entrance Requirements** Minimum overall college GPA of 3.0, transcript of college record, CPR certification, health exam, health insurance, high school biology, high school chemistry, high school foreign language, 3 years high school math, 3 years high school science, high school transcript, immunizations, 2 letters of recommendation, minimum high school GPA of 3.0, minimum high school rank 60%, minimum GPA in nursing prerequisites of 2.75, prerequisite course work. Transfer students are accepted. *Application deadline:* 8/1 (fall), 1/5 (spring), 4/30 (summer). Applications may be processed on a rolling basis for some programs. *Application fee:* $25.
**Expenses (2013–14)** *Tuition:* full-time $26,200; part-time $560 per credit hour. *International tuition:* $26,200 full-time. *Room and board:* $6800; room only: $3400 per academic year. *Required fees:* full-time $900; part-time $100 per term.
**Financial Aid** 85% of baccalaureate students in nursing programs received some form of financial aid in 2012–13.
**Contact** Lauren A. Campbell, Director of Undergraduate Admissions, School of Nursing and Allied Health Professions, Holy Family University, 9801 Frankford Avenue, Philadelphia, PA 19114-2094. *Telephone:* 215-637-3050. *Fax:* 215-281-1022. *E-mail:* admissions@holyfamily.edu.

## GRADUATE PROGRAMS

**Expenses (2013–14)** *Tuition:* part-time $670 per credit hour. *International tuition:* $670 full-time. *Required fees:* part-time $125 per term.
**Financial Aid** 85% of graduate students in nursing programs received some form of financial aid in 2012–13.
**Contact** Gidget Montelibano, Graduate Admissions, School of Nursing and Allied Health Professions, Holy Family University, 9701 Frankford Avenue, Philadelphia, PA 19114-2094. *Telephone:* 267-341-3358. *E-mail:* gmontelibano@holyfamily.edu.

### MASTER'S DEGREE PROGRAM

**Degree** MSN
**Available Programs** Master's; Master's for Nurses with Non-Nursing Degrees.
**Concentrations Available** Nursing administration; nursing education.
**Study Options** Part-time.
**Program Entrance Requirements** Minimum overall college GPA of 3.0, transcript of college record, CPR certification, written essay, immunizations, 2 letters of recommendation, nursing research course, professional liability insurance/malpractice insurance, prerequisite course work, resume, statistics course. *Application deadline:* 8/1 (fall), 12/20 (spring), 5/10 (summer). Applications may be processed on a rolling basis for some programs. *Application fee:* $25.
**Advanced Placement** Credit given for nursing courses completed elsewhere dependent upon specific evaluations.
**Degree Requirements** 30 total credit hours, thesis or project, comprehensive exam.

### POST-MASTER'S PROGRAM

**Areas of Study** Health-care administration; nursing administration; nursing education. *Clinical nurse specialist programs in:* public health. *Nurse practitioner programs in:* community health.

## CONTINUING EDUCATION PROGRAM

**Contact** Dr. Mary Wombwell, Professor, School of Nursing and Allied Health Professions, Holy Family University, 9801 Frankford Avenue, Philadelphia, PA 19114. *Telephone:* 267-341-3300. *Fax:* 215-637-6598. *E-mail:* mwombwell@holyfamily.edu.

# Immaculata University

## Division of Nursing
## Immaculata, Pennsylvania

***http://www.immaculata.edu/nursing/***
Founded in 1920

**DEGREES • BSN • MSN**
**Nursing Program Faculty** 80 (50% with doctorates).
**Baccalaureate Enrollment** 1,125 **Women** 92% **Men** 8% **Minority** 13% **International** 2% **Part-time** 90%
**Graduate Enrollment** 105 **Women** 97% **Men** 3% **Minority** 15% **Part-time** 100%
**Nursing Student Activities** Sigma Theta Tau, nursing club.
**Nursing Student Resources** Academic advising; academic or career counseling; assistance for students with disabilities; bookstore; campus computer network; career placement assistance; computer lab; computer-assisted instruction; e-mail services; employment services for current students; externships; interactive nursing skills videos; Internet; learning resource lab; library services; nursing audiovisuals; placement services for program completers; resume preparation assistance; skills, simulation, or other laboratory; tutoring.
**Library Facilities** 1,500 volumes in health, 1,500 volumes in nursing; 115 periodical subscriptions health-care related.

## BACCALAUREATE PROGRAMS

**Degree** BSN
**Available Programs** Accelerated RN Baccalaureate; Generic Baccalaureate; RN Baccalaureate.
**Site Options** Philadelphia, PA; Abington, PA; Christiana, DE.
**Study Options** Full-time.
**Program Entrance Requirements** Transcript of college record, CPR certification, written essay, health exam, high school chemistry, high school foreign language, 2 years high school math, 3 years high school science, high school transcript, immunizations, interview, 2 letters of rec-

ommendation, minimum high school GPA of 3.0, prerequisite course work. Transfer students are accepted. *Application deadline:* 1/31 (fall). *Application fee:* $35.
**Advanced Placement** Credit by examination available.
**Expenses (2013–14)** *Tuition:* full-time $29,000; part-time $470 per credit. *International tuition:* $29,000 full-time. *Room and board:* $10,000; room only: $5330 per academic year. *Required fees:* full-time $600; part-time $100 per term.
**Financial Aid** 75% of baccalaureate students in nursing programs received some form of financial aid in 2012–13.
**Contact** Ms. Gwen Dreibelbis, Admissions Counselor, Division of Nursing, Immaculata University, 1145 King Road, Immaculata, PA 19345. *Telephone:* 610-647-4400 Ext. 3013. *Fax:* 610-640-0836. *E-mail:* gdreibelbis@immaculata.edu.

## GRADUATE PROGRAMS

**Expenses (2013–14)** *Tuition:* part-time $620 per credit.
**Financial Aid** 25% of graduate students in nursing programs received some form of financial aid in 2012–13.
**Contact** Dr. Jane Tang, Coordinator, MSN Program, Division of Nursing, Immaculata University, 1145 King Road, Immaculata, PA 19345-0691. *Telephone:* 610-647-4400 Ext. 3309. *Fax:* 610-640-0286. *E-mail:* jtang@immaculata.edu.

### MASTER'S DEGREE PROGRAM

**Degree** MSN
**Available Programs** Master's; Master's for Non-Nursing College Graduates.
**Concentrations Available** Nursing administration; nursing education.
**Site Options** Abington, PA; Christiana, DE.
**Study Options** Part-time.
**Program Entrance Requirements** Minimum overall college GPA of 3.0, transcript of college record, written essay, interview, 3 letters of recommendation, physical assessment course, statistics course. *Application deadline:* Applications may be processed on a rolling basis for some programs. *Application fee:* $50.
**Advanced Placement** Credit given for nursing courses completed elsewhere dependent upon specific evaluations.
**Degree Requirements** 39 total credit hours, thesis or project.

# Indiana University of Pennsylvania

## Department of Nursing and Allied Health
## Indiana, Pennsylvania

***http://www.iup.edu/rn-alliedhealth/default.aspx***
Founded in 1875

### DEGREES • BSN • MS • PHD

**Nursing Program Faculty** 39 (54% with doctorates).
**Baccalaureate Enrollment** 112 **Women** 87.57% **Men** 12.43% **Minority** 4.02% **International** 4.39%
**Graduate Enrollment** 44 **Women** 93.18% **Men** 6.82% **Minority** 2.27% **Part-time** 100%
**Distance Learning Courses** Available.
**Nursing Student Activities** Nursing Honor Society, Sigma Theta Tau, Student Nurses' Association, nursing club.
**Nursing Student Resources** Academic advising; academic or career counseling; assistance for students with disabilities; bookstore; campus computer network; career placement assistance; computer lab; computer-assisted instruction; e-mail services; employment services for current students; housing assistance; interactive nursing skills videos; Internet; learning resource lab; library services; nursing audiovisuals; remedial services; resume preparation assistance; skills, simulation, or other laboratory; tutoring.
**Library Facilities** 888,056 volumes (5,758 in health, 3,395 in nursing); 32,718 periodical subscriptions (225 health-care related).

## BACCALAUREATE PROGRAMS

**Degree** BSN
**Available Programs** Baccalaureate for Second Degree; Generic Baccalaureate; LPN to Baccalaureate.
**Study Options** Full-time and part-time.
**Program Entrance Requirements** Minimum overall college GPA of 3.0, transcript of college record, high school chemistry, 3 years high school math, high school transcript, minimum high school GPA of 3.0, prerequisite course work. Transfer students are accepted. *Application deadline:* Applications may be processed on a rolling basis for some programs. *Application fee:* $50.
**Expenses (2012–13)** *Tuition, state resident:* full-time $6428; part-time $268 per credit. *Tuition, nonresident:* full-time $16,070; part-time $670 per credit. *International tuition:* $16,070 full-time. *Room and board:* $10,466; room only: $7740 per academic year. *Required fees:* full-time $2244; part-time $52 per credit; part-time $203 per term.
**Financial Aid** 85% of baccalaureate students in nursing programs received some form of financial aid in 2011–12.
**Contact** Mr. Chris Kitas, Associate Director of Institutional Research, Planning and Assessment, Department of Nursing and Allied Health, Indiana University of Pennsylvania, Institutional Research Planning and Assessment, 404 Sutton Hall, Indiana, PA 15705. *Telephone:* 724-357-5562. *Fax:* 724-357-3833. *E-mail:* Chris.Kitas@iup.edu.

## GRADUATE PROGRAMS

**Expenses (2012–13)** *Tuition, state resident:* full-time $8136; part-time $452 per credit. *Tuition, nonresident:* full-time $12,204; part-time $678 per credit. *International tuition:* $12,204 full-time. *Room and board:* $10,466; room only: $7740 per academic year. *Required fees:* full-time $2232.
**Financial Aid** 68% of graduate students in nursing programs received some form of financial aid in 2011–12. 2 fellowships (averaging $1,750 per year), 4 research assistantships with full and partial tuition reimbursements available (averaging $3,060 per year), 2 teaching assistantships (averaging $22,398 per year) were awarded; career-related internships or fieldwork, Federal Work-Study, scholarships, and unspecified assistantships also available. Aid available to part-time students. *Financial aid application deadline:* 4/15.
**Contact** Dr. Elizabeth A. Palmer, Department Chair, Department of Nursing and Allied Health, Indiana University of Pennsylvania, 1010 Oakland Avenue, Indiana, PA 15705-1087. *Telephone:* 724-357-2557. *Fax:* 724-357-3267. *E-mail:* lpalmer@iup.edu.

### MASTER'S DEGREE PROGRAM

**Degree** MS
**Available Programs** Master's; Master's for Nurses with Non-Nursing Degrees.
**Concentrations Available** Nursing administration; nursing education.
**Site Options** Monroeville, PA.
**Study Options** Part-time.
**Program Entrance Requirements** Clinical experience, minimum overall college GPA of 3.0, transcript of college record, written essay, 2 letters of recommendation, nursing research course, resume, statistics course. *Application deadline:* Applications may be processed on a rolling basis for some programs. *Application fee:* $50.
**Advanced Placement** Credit given for nursing courses completed elsewhere dependent upon specific evaluations.
**Degree Requirements** 36 total credit hours.

### DOCTORAL DEGREE PROGRAM

**Degree** PhD
**Available Programs** Doctorate.
**Areas of Study** Nursing education.
**Program Entrance Requirements** Minimum overall college GPA of 3.5, interview by faculty committee, 2 letters of recommendation, MSN or equivalent, statistics course, vita, writing sample, GRE. *Application deadline:* Applications may be processed on a rolling basis for some programs. *Application fee:* $50.
**Degree Requirements** 60 total credit hours, dissertation, oral exam, written exam, residency.

# La Roche College

## Department of Nursing and Nursing Management
## Pittsburgh, Pennsylvania

***http://www.laroche.edu/***
Founded in 1963

### DEGREES • BSN • MSN

**Nursing Program Faculty** 11 (90% with doctorates).
**Baccalaureate Enrollment** 84 **Women** 90% **Men** 10% **Minority** 2% **Part-time** 80%
**Graduate Enrollment** 25 **Women** 90% **Men** 10% **Part-time** 90%
**Distance Learning Courses** Available.

**Nursing Student Activities** Sigma Theta Tau.

**Nursing Student Resources** Academic advising; academic or career counseling; assistance for students with disabilities; bookstore; campus computer network; computer lab; e-mail services; externships; Internet; library services; resume preparation assistance; tutoring.

**Library Facilities** 153,338 volumes; 548 periodical subscriptions (850 health-care related).

## BACCALAUREATE PROGRAMS

**Degree** BSN

**Available Programs** Accelerated RN Baccalaureate; LPN to RN Baccalaureate; RN Baccalaureate.

**Study Options** Full-time and part-time.

**Online Degree Options** Yes (online only).

**Program Entrance Requirements** Minimum overall college GPA of 3.0, transcript of college record, CPR certification, written essay, health exam, health insurance, high school chemistry, high school transcript, immunizations, interview, 2 letters of recommendation, minimum high school GPA of 3.0, professional liability insurance/malpractice insurance, RN licensure. Transfer students are accepted. *Application deadline:* Applications may be processed on a rolling basis for some programs. *Application fee:* $50.

**Advanced Placement** Credit by examination available. Credit given for nursing courses completed elsewhere dependent upon specific evaluations.

**Expenses (2013–14)** *Tuition:* full-time $11,664; part-time $595 per credit hour. *Room and board:* $3200 per academic year. *Required fees:* full-time $45; part-time $25 per credit.

**Financial Aid** 90% of baccalaureate students in nursing programs received some form of financial aid in 2012–13. *Gift aid (need-based):* Federal Pell, FSEOG, state, private, college/university gift aid from institutional funds. *Loans:* Federal Direct (Subsidized and Unsubsidized Stafford PLUS), Perkins, state. *Work-study:* Federal Work-Study. *Financial aid application deadline (priority):* 5/1.

**Contact** Ms. Hope A. Schiffgens, Director, Graduate Studies and Adult Education, Department of Nursing and Nursing Management, La Roche College, 9000 Babcock Boulevard, Pittsburgh, PA 15237. *Telephone:* 412-536-1266. *Fax:* 412-536-1283. *E-mail:* hope.schiffgens@laroche.edu.

## GRADUATE PROGRAMS

**Expenses (2013–14)** *Tuition:* full-time $5625; part-time $525 per credit hour. *Room and board:* $3370 per academic year.

**Financial Aid** 85% of graduate students in nursing programs received some form of financial aid in 2012–13.

**Contact** Ms. Hope A. Schiffgens, Director, Graduate Studies and Adult Education, Department of Nursing and Nursing Management, La Roche College, 9000 Babcock Boulevard, Pittsburgh, PA 15237. *Telephone:* 412-536-1262. *Fax:* 412-536-1283. *E-mail:* hope.schiffgens@laroche.edu.

### MASTER'S DEGREE PROGRAM

**Degree** MSN

**Available Programs** Master's; RN to Master's.

**Concentrations Available** Nurse anesthesia; nursing administration; nursing education.

**Study Options** Full-time and part-time.

**Online Degree Options** Yes (online only).

**Program Entrance Requirements** Clinical experience, minimum overall college GPA of 3.0, transcript of college record, immunizations, interview, 2 letters of recommendation, professional liability insurance/malpractice insurance, resume. *Application deadline:* Applications may be processed on a rolling basis for some programs. *Application fee:* $50.

**Advanced Placement** Credit given for nursing courses completed elsewhere dependent upon specific evaluations.

**Degree Requirements** 36 total credit hours, thesis or project.

## CONTINUING EDUCATION PROGRAM

**Contact** Ms. Hope A. Schiffgens, Director, Graduate Studies and Adult Education, Department of Nursing and Nursing Management, La Roche College, 9000 Babcock Boulevard, Pittsburgh, PA 15237. *Telephone:* 412-536-1260. *Fax:* 412-536-1283. *E-mail:* hope.schiffgens@laroche.edu.

# La Salle University

### School of Nursing and Health Sciences
### Philadelphia, Pennsylvania

*http://www.lasalle.edu/schools/snhs/*

Founded in 1863

**DEGREES • BSN • MSN • MSN/MBA**

**Nursing Program Faculty** 45 (32% with doctorates).

**Nursing Student Activities** Sigma Theta Tau, Student Nurses' Association, nursing club.

**Nursing Student Resources** Academic advising; academic or career counseling; assistance for students with disabilities; bookstore; campus computer network; career placement assistance; computer lab; computer-assisted instruction; e-mail services; employment services for current students; externships; housing assistance; interactive nursing skills videos; Internet; learning resource lab; library services; nursing audiovisuals; placement services for program completers; remedial services; resume preparation assistance; skills, simulation, or other laboratory; tutoring.

**Library Facilities** 420,000 volumes (8,350 in nursing); 60,705 periodical subscriptions (310 health-care related).

## BACCALAUREATE PROGRAMS

**Degree** BSN

**Available Programs** Baccalaureate for Second Degree; Generic Baccalaureate; LPN to Baccalaureate; RN Baccalaureate.

**Site Options** Newtown, PA.

**Study Options** Full-time and part-time.

**Program Entrance Requirements** Minimum overall college GPA of 2.75, transcript of college record, CPR certification, written essay, health exam, health insurance, high school biology, high school chemistry, 3 years high school math, 3 years high school science, high school transcript, immunizations, interview, 2 letters of recommendation, minimum high school GPA of 3.0, minimum high school rank 25%, minimum GPA in nursing prerequisites of 2.75, professional liability insurance/malpractice insurance, prerequisite course work. Transfer students are accepted.

**Advanced Placement** Credit by examination available. Credit given for nursing courses completed elsewhere dependent upon specific evaluations.

**Contact** *Telephone:* 215-951-1430. *Fax:* 215-951-1896.

## GRADUATE PROGRAMS

**Contact** *Telephone:* 215-951-1413. *Fax:* 215-951-1896.

### MASTER'S DEGREE PROGRAM

**Degrees** MSN; MSN/MBA

**Available Programs** Master's; RN to Master's.

**Concentrations Available** Nurse anesthesia; nursing administration. *Clinical nurse specialist programs in:* adult health, public health. *Nurse practitioner programs in:* adult health, family health.

**Site Options** Newtown, PA.

**Study Options** Full-time and part-time.

**Program Entrance Requirements** Clinical experience, minimum overall college GPA of 3.0, transcript of college record, CPR certification, written essay, immunizations, interview, 2 letters of recommendation, nursing research course, physical assessment course, professional liability insurance/malpractice insurance, resume, statistics course.

**Advanced Placement** Credit given for nursing courses completed elsewhere dependent upon specific evaluations.

**Degree Requirements** 41 total credit hours.

### POST-MASTER'S PROGRAM

**Areas of Study** Nurse anesthesia; nursing administration; nursing education. *Clinical nurse specialist programs in:* adult health, public health. *Nurse practitioner programs in:* adult health, family health.

## CONTINUING EDUCATION PROGRAM

**Contact** *Telephone:* 215-951-1432. *Fax:* 215-951-1896.

## Lock Haven University of Pennsylvania

### Nursing Program
### Lock Haven, Pennsylvania

Founded in 1870

**DEGREE • BSN**

#### BACCALAUREATE PROGRAMS

**Degree** BSN
**Available Programs** Accelerated Baccalaureate; RN Baccalaureate.
**Study Options** Full-time and part-time.
**Program Entrance Requirements** RN licensure.
**Contact** Kim Owens, Department Chair, Nursing Program, Lock Haven University of Pennsylvania, 201 University Drive, Lock Haven, PA 16830. *Telephone:* 814-768-3430. *E-mail:* kowens@lhup.edu.

## Mansfield University of Pennsylvania

### Department of Health Sciences–Nursing
### Mansfield, Pennsylvania

***http://www.mansfield.edu/***
Founded in 1857

**DEGREES • BSN • MSN**

**Nursing Program Faculty** 12 (50% with doctorates).
**Baccalaureate Enrollment** 186 **Women** 95% **Men** 5% **Minority** 4% **International** 1% **Part-time** 5%
**Graduate Enrollment** 52 **Women** 98% **Men** 2% **Minority** 1% **Part-time** 100%
**Distance Learning Courses** Available.
**Nursing Student Activities** Nursing Honor Society, Student Nurses' Association, nursing club.
**Nursing Student Resources** Academic advising; academic or career counseling; assistance for students with disabilities; bookstore; campus computer network; career placement assistance; computer lab; daycare for children of students; e-mail services; employment services for current students; housing assistance; Internet; learning resource lab; library services; nursing audiovisuals; remedial services; resume preparation assistance; skills, simulation, or other laboratory; tutoring.
**Library Facilities** 1,300 volumes in health, 500 volumes in nursing; 550 periodical subscriptions health-care related.

#### BACCALAUREATE PROGRAMS

**Degree** BSN
**Available Programs** Generic Baccalaureate; RN Baccalaureate.
**Site Options** Sayre, PA.
**Study Options** Full-time and part-time.
**Program Entrance Requirements** Minimum overall college GPA of 2.7, transcript of college record, CPR certification, health exam, health insurance, high school biology, high school chemistry, 2 years high school math, 2 years high school science, high school transcript, immunizations, minimum high school GPA of 2.7, minimum high school rank 60%, professional liability insurance/malpractice insurance. Transfer students are accepted. *Application deadline:* Applications may be processed on a rolling basis for some programs. *Application fee:* $25.
**Advanced Placement** Credit by examination available. Credit given for nursing courses completed elsewhere dependent upon specific evaluations.
**Expenses (2012–13)** *Tuition, area resident:* full-time $6428; part-time $268 per credit. *Tuition, state resident:* full-time $10,608; part-time $429 per credit. *Tuition, nonresident:* full-time $16,070; part-time $429 per credit. *Room and board:* $9974 per academic year. *Required fees:* full-time $2498.
**Financial Aid** 90% of baccalaureate students in nursing programs received some form of financial aid in 2011–12. *Gift aid (need-based):* Federal Pell, FSEOG, state, private, college/university gift aid from institutional funds. *Loans:* Federal Direct (Subsidized and Unsubsidized Stafford PLUS), Perkins. *Work-study:* Federal Work-Study, part-time campus jobs. *Financial aid application deadline:* 6/30(priority: 2/15).
**Contact** Admissions Office, Department of Health Sciences–Nursing, Mansfield University of Pennsylvania, Alumni Hall, Mansfield, PA 16933. *Telephone:* 570-662-4243. *Fax:* 570-662-4121. *E-mail:* admissions@mansfield.edu.

#### GRADUATE PROGRAMS

**Expenses (2012–13)** *Tuition, area resident:* part-time $429 per credit. *Tuition, state resident:* part-time $644 per credit. *Tuition, nonresident:* part-time $644 per credit. *Required fees:* part-time $84 per credit.
**Financial Aid** 50% of graduate students in nursing programs received some form of financial aid in 2011–12.
**Contact** Dr. Janeen Bartlett Sheehe, Department Chair and Nursing Program Director, Department of Health Sciences–Nursing, Mansfield University of Pennsylvania, 212C Elliott Hall, Mansfield, PA 16933. *Telephone:* 570-662-4522. *Fax:* 570-662-4137. *E-mail:* jsheehe@mansfield.edu.

**MASTER'S DEGREE PROGRAM**

**Degree** MSN
**Available Programs** Master's.
**Concentrations Available** Nursing administration; nursing education.
**Study Options** Part-time.
**Online Degree Options** Yes (online only).
**Program Entrance Requirements** Minimum overall college GPA of 3.0, transcript of college record, 1 letter of recommendation, nursing research course, prerequisite course work. *Application deadline:* Applications may be processed on a rolling basis for some programs. *Application fee:* $25.
**Advanced Placement** Credit given for nursing courses completed elsewhere dependent upon specific evaluations.
**Degree Requirements** 33 total credit hours, thesis or project.

## Marywood University

### Department of Nursing
### Scranton, Pennsylvania

***http://www.marywood.edu/nursing/index.html***
Founded in 1915

**DEGREES • BSN • MSN • MSN/MPH**

**Nursing Program Faculty** 16 (50% with doctorates).
**Baccalaureate Enrollment** 117 **Women** 90% **Men** 10% **Minority** 5% **International** 3% **Part-time** 5%
**Graduate Enrollment** 17 **Women** 100% **Part-time** 90%
**Distance Learning Courses** Available.
**Nursing Student Activities** Sigma Theta Tau, Student Nurses' Association.
**Nursing Student Resources** Academic advising; academic or career counseling; assistance for students with disabilities; bookstore; campus computer network; computer lab; daycare for children of students; e-mail services; employment services for current students; interactive nursing skills videos; Internet; learning resource lab; library services; nursing audiovisuals; skills, simulation, or other laboratory; tutoring.
**Library Facilities** 7,400 volumes in health, 3,006 volumes in nursing; 750 periodical subscriptions health-care related.

#### BACCALAUREATE PROGRAMS

**Degree** BSN
**Available Programs** ADN to Baccalaureate; Generic Baccalaureate; International Nurse to Baccalaureate; LPN to Baccalaureate; RN Baccalaureate.
**Study Options** Full-time and part-time.
**Program Entrance Requirements** Transcript of college record, high school biology, high school chemistry, 1 year of high school math, high school transcript, 1 letter of recommendation. Transfer students are accepted.
**Advanced Placement** Credit given for nursing courses completed elsewhere dependent upon specific evaluations.
**Contact** *Telephone:* 570-348-6211 Ext. 2374. *Fax:* 570-961-4761.

#### GRADUATE PROGRAMS

**Contact** *Telephone:* 570-348-6211 Ext. 2475. *Fax:* 570-961-4761.

**MASTER'S DEGREE PROGRAM**

**Degrees** MSN; MSN/MPH
**Available Programs** Master's.
**Concentrations Available** Nursing administration.
**Study Options** Full-time and part-time.

**Program Entrance Requirements** Clinical experience, minimum overall college GPA of 3.0, transcript of college record, written essay, 2 letters of recommendation, nursing research course, physical assessment course, statistics course.
**Degree Requirements** 39 total credit hours, thesis or project.

### CONTINUING EDUCATION PROGRAM

**Contact** *Telephone:* 570-340-6060. *Fax:* 570-961-4776.

## Messiah College

### Department of Nursing
### Mechanicsburg, Pennsylvania

*http://www.messiah.edu/*
Founded in 1909

**DEGREES • BSN • MSN**
**Nursing Program Faculty** 33 (18% with doctorates).
**Baccalaureate Enrollment** 207 **Women** 94% **Men** 6% **Minority** 7% **International** 1% **Part-time** 2%
**Graduate Enrollment** 20 **Women** 95% **Men** 5% **Part-time** 20%
**Nursing Student Activities** Nursing Honor Society, Sigma Theta Tau, Student Nurses' Association, nursing club.
**Nursing Student Resources** Academic advising; academic or career counseling; assistance for students with disabilities; bookstore; campus computer network; career placement assistance; computer lab; computer-assisted instruction; e-mail services; employment services for current students; interactive nursing skills videos; Internet; learning resource lab; library services; nursing audiovisuals; remedial services; resume preparation assistance; skills, simulation, or other laboratory; tutoring.
**Library Facilities** 253,484 volumes (6,649 in health, 644 in nursing); 98,644 periodical subscriptions (7,799 health-care related).

### BACCALAUREATE PROGRAMS

**Degree** BSN
**Available Programs** Generic Baccalaureate.
**Study Options** Full-time and part-time.
**Program Entrance Requirements** Minimum overall college GPA of 3.0, transcript of college record, CPR certification, health exam, health insurance, high school foreign language, 2 years high school math, 2 years high school science, high school transcript, immunizations, minimum high school rank, minimum GPA in nursing prerequisites of 2.7, prerequisite course work. Transfer students are accepted. *Application deadline:* Applications may be processed on a rolling basis for some programs. *Application fee:* $30.
**Advanced Placement** Credit given for nursing courses completed elsewhere dependent upon specific evaluations.
**Expenses (2013–14)** *Tuition:* full-time $29,650; part-time $1240 per credit hour. *Room and board:* $9070; room only: $4800 per academic year. *Required fees:* full-time $940.
**Financial Aid** 100% of baccalaureate students in nursing programs received some form of financial aid in 2012–13.
**Contact** Dana Britton, Director of Admissions, Department of Nursing, Messiah College, Suite 3005, One College Avenue, Mechanicsburg, PA 17055. *Telephone:* 800-233-4220. *Fax:* 717-796-5374. *E-mail:* admiss@messiah.edu.

### GRADUATE PROGRAMS

**Expenses (2013–14)** *Tuition:* part-time $575 per credit.
**Contact** Jackie Gehman, Graduate Enrollment Coordinator, Department of Nursing, Messiah College, Graduate Admissions Office, One College Avenue, Suite 3060, Mechanicsburg, PA 17055. *Telephone:* 717-796-5061. *Fax:* 717-691-2307. *E-mail:* GradPrograms@messiah.edu.

#### MASTER'S DEGREE PROGRAM

**Degree** MSN
**Available Programs** RN to Master's.
**Concentrations Available** Nursing education.
**Study Options** Full-time and part-time.
**Online Degree Options** Yes (online only).
**Program Entrance Requirements** Clinical experience, minimum overall college GPA of 3.0, transcript of college record, written essay, 3 letters of recommendation, nursing research course, physical assessment course, prerequisite course work, resume, statistics course. *Application deadline:* 6/15 (fall), 11/1 (winter), 11/1 (spring), 3/15 (summer). Applications may be processed on a rolling basis for some programs. *Application fee:* $30.
**Degree Requirements** 39 total credit hours, comprehensive exam.

## Millersville University of Pennsylvania

### Department of Nursing
### Millersville, Pennsylvania

*http://www.millersville.edu/nursing/*
Founded in 1855

**DEGREES • BSN • MSN**
**Nursing Program Faculty** 10 (60% with doctorates).
**Baccalaureate Enrollment** 101 **Women** 95% **Men** 5% **Minority** 18% **Part-time** 90%
**Graduate Enrollment** 110 **Women** 86% **Men** 14% **Minority** 3% **Part-time** 100%
**Nursing Student Activities** Sigma Theta Tau.
**Nursing Student Resources** Academic advising; academic or career counseling; assistance for students with disabilities; bookstore; computer lab; e-mail services; interactive nursing skills videos; Internet; library services; nursing audiovisuals; resume preparation assistance.
**Library Facilities** 363,250 volumes; 77,665 periodical subscriptions (82 health-care related).

### BACCALAUREATE PROGRAMS

**Degree** BSN
**Available Programs** RN Baccalaureate.
**Site Options** Harrisburg, PA.
**Study Options** Full-time and part-time.
**Program Entrance Requirements** Minimum overall college GPA of 2.0, transcript of college record, RN licensure. Transfer students are accepted. *Application deadline:* Applications may be processed on a rolling basis for some programs. *Application fee:* $40.
**Expenses (2012–13)** *Tuition, state resident:* part-time $358 per credit. *Tuition, nonresident:* part-time $768 per credit.
**Financial Aid** 50% of baccalaureate students in nursing programs received some form of financial aid in 2011–12.
**Contact** Dr. Barbara Zimmerman, Chairperson, Department of Nursing, Millersville University of Pennsylvania, Caputo Hall, PO Box 1002, Millersville, PA 17551-0302. *Telephone:* 717-872-3376. *Fax:* 717-871-4877. *E-mail:* barbara.zimmerman@millersville.edu.

### GRADUATE PROGRAMS

**Expenses (2012–13)** *Tuition, state resident:* part-time $548 per credit. *Tuition, nonresident:* part-time $773 per credit.
**Financial Aid** 50% of graduate students in nursing programs received some form of financial aid in 2011–12. 3 research assistantships with partial tuition reimbursements available (averaging $5,000 per year) were awarded; institutionally sponsored loans and unspecified assistantships also available. Aid available to part-time students. *Financial aid application deadline:* 3/15.
**Contact** Dr. Deborah Castellucci, Graduate Program Coordinator, Department of Nursing, Millersville University of Pennsylvania, Caputo Hall, PO Box 1002, Millersville, PA 17551-0302. *Telephone:* 717-871-5341. *Fax:* 717-871-4887. *E-mail:* deborah.castellucci@millersville.edu.

#### MASTER'S DEGREE PROGRAM

**Degree** MSN
**Available Programs** Master's.
**Concentrations Available** Nursing education. *Nurse practitioner programs in:* family health.
**Study Options** Part-time.
**Program Entrance Requirements** Clinical experience, minimum overall college GPA of 3.0, transcript of college record, interview, 3 letters of recommendation, nursing research course, physical assessment course, resume, statistics course. *Application deadline:* 1/15 (spring). *Application fee:* $40.
**Degree Requirements** Thesis or project.

#### POST-MASTER'S PROGRAM

**Areas of Study** Nursing education. *Nurse practitioner programs in:* family health.

# Misericordia University

## Department of Nursing
## Dallas, Pennsylvania

***http://www.misericordia.edu/nursing***
Founded in 1924

**DEGREES • BSN • MSN**
**Nursing Program Faculty** 34 (5% with doctorates).
**Baccalaureate Enrollment** 243 **Women** 89% **Men** 11% **Minority** 3% **Part-time** 35%
**Graduate Enrollment** 45 **Women** 95% **Men** 5% **Part-time** 100%
**Distance Learning Courses** Available.
**Nursing Student Activities** Nursing Honor Society, Sigma Theta Tau, Student Nurses' Association, nursing club.
**Nursing Student Resources** Academic advising; academic or career counseling; assistance for students with disabilities; bookstore; campus computer network; career placement assistance; computer lab; computer-assisted instruction; e-mail services; employment services for current students; externships; housing assistance; interactive nursing skills videos; Internet; learning resource lab; library services; nursing audiovisuals; placement services for program completers; remedial services; resume preparation assistance; skills, simulation, or other laboratory; tutoring.
**Library Facilities** 550,890 volumes (6 in health, 5 in nursing); 24,992 periodical subscriptions (15 health-care related).

### BACCALAUREATE PROGRAMS

**Degree** BSN
**Available Programs** Accelerated RN Baccalaureate; Baccalaureate for Second Degree; Generic Baccalaureate; RN Baccalaureate.
**Study Options** Full-time and part-time.
**Program Entrance Requirements** Minimum overall college GPA of 3.0, transcript of college record, CPR certification, health exam, health insurance, high school biology, high school chemistry, 1 year of high school math, high school transcript, immunizations, letters of recommendation, minimum high school GPA of 2.5, minimum high school rank 33%, minimum GPA in nursing prerequisites of 3.0, professional liability insurance/malpractice insurance. Transfer students are accepted. *Application deadline:* 8/1 (fall), 8/1 (winter), 12/1 (spring), 4/1 (summer). Applications may be processed on a rolling basis for some programs. *Application fee:* $200.
**Advanced Placement** Credit by examination available. Credit given for nursing courses completed elsewhere dependent upon specific evaluations.
**Expenses (2013–14)** *Tuition:* full-time $12,943; part-time $495 per credit. *Room and board:* $3785 per academic year. *Required fees:* full-time $970; part-time $450 per term.
**Financial Aid** 75% of baccalaureate students in nursing programs received some form of financial aid in 2012–13. *Gift aid (need-based):* Federal Pell, FSEOG, state, private, college/university gift aid from institutional funds, Federal Nursing. *Loans:* Federal Nursing Student Loans, Perkins, state. *Work-study:* Federal Work-Study. *Financial aid application deadline (priority):* 3/1.
**Contact** Mr. Glenn Bozinski, Admissions, Department of Nursing, Misericordia University, 301 Lake Street, Dallas, PA 18612. *Telephone:* 570-674-6434. *E-mail:* gbozinsk@misericordia.edu.

### GRADUATE PROGRAMS

**Expenses (2013–14)** *Tuition:* part-time $575 per credit.
**Financial Aid** 90% of graduate students in nursing programs received some form of financial aid in 2012–13. Teaching assistantships, career-related internships or fieldwork, scholarships, traineeships, tuition waivers (partial), and unspecified assistantships available. Aid available to part-time students. *Financial aid application deadline:* 6/30.
**Contact** Ms. Maureen Sheridan, Adult Education Counselor, Graduate Programs, Department of Nursing, Misericordia University, 301 Lake Street, Dallas, PA 18612. *Telephone:* 570-674-6451. *Fax:* 570-674-8902. *E-mail:* msherida@misericordia.edu.

#### MASTER'S DEGREE PROGRAM

**Degree** MSN
**Available Programs** Master's; RN to Master's.
**Concentrations Available** Nursing education. *Clinical nurse specialist programs in:* family health. *Nurse practitioner programs in:* family health.
**Study Options** Part-time.
**Program Entrance Requirements** Clinical experience, computer literacy, minimum overall college GPA of 3.0, transcript of college record, written essay, 3 letters of recommendation, nursing research course, physical assessment course, professional liability insurance/malpractice insurance, statistics course. *Application deadline:* 7/18 (fall), 7/18 (winter), 12/1 (spring), 4/1 (summer). Applications may be processed on a rolling basis for some programs. *Application fee:* $200.
**Advanced Placement** Credit given for nursing courses completed elsewhere dependent upon specific evaluations.
**Degree Requirements** 46 total credit hours, thesis or project.

#### POST-MASTER'S PROGRAM

**Areas of Study** Nursing education. *Clinical nurse specialist programs in:* family health. *Nurse practitioner programs in:* family health.

# Moravian College

## Department of Nursing
## Bethlehem, Pennsylvania

***http://www.moravian.edu/***
Founded in 1742

**DEGREES • BS • MS**
**Nursing Program Faculty** 28 (46% with doctorates).
**Baccalaureate Enrollment** 244 **Women** 90% **Men** 10% **Minority** 15% **International** 1% **Part-time** 35%
**Graduate Enrollment** 39 **Women** 100% **Minority** 3% **Part-time** 100%
**Nursing Student Activities** Sigma Theta Tau, Student Nurses' Association.
**Nursing Student Resources** Academic advising; academic or career counseling; assistance for students with disabilities; bookstore; campus computer network; career placement assistance; computer lab; computer-assisted instruction; e-mail services; employment services for current students; externships; housing assistance; interactive nursing skills videos; Internet; learning resource lab; library services; nursing audiovisuals; placement services for program completers; remedial services; resume preparation assistance; skills, simulation, or other laboratory; tutoring.
**Library Facilities** 337,468 volumes (4,600 in health, 1,900 in nursing); 49,280 periodical subscriptions (275 health-care related).

### BACCALAUREATE PROGRAMS

**Degree** BS
**Available Programs** Accelerated Baccalaureate; Generic Baccalaureate; RN Baccalaureate.
**Study Options** Full-time.
**Program Entrance Requirements** CPR certification, written essay, health exam, health insurance, high school biology, high school foreign language, 3 years high school math, 3 years high school science, high school transcript, immunizations, 1 letter of recommendation, minimum GPA in nursing prerequisites of 3.0, prerequisite course work. Transfer students are accepted. *Application deadline:* 3/1 (fall). *Application fee:* $40.
**Advanced Placement** Credit by examination available. Credit given for nursing courses completed elsewhere dependent upon specific evaluations.
**Expenses (2013–14)** *Tuition:* full-time $34,938. *International tuition:* $34,938 full-time. *Room and board:* $10,854; room only: $6160 per academic year. *Required fees:* full-time $720.
**Financial Aid** 90% of baccalaureate students in nursing programs received some form of financial aid in 2012–13. *Gift aid (need-based):* Federal Pell, FSEOG, state, private, college/university gift aid from institutional funds. *Loans:* Federal Direct (Subsidized and Unsubsidized Stafford PLUS), Perkins. *Work-study:* Federal Work-Study, part-time campus jobs. *Financial aid application deadline (priority):* 2/14.
**Contact** Ms. Carole Reese, Interim Vice President of Enrollment, Department of Nursing, Moravian College, 1200 Main Street, Bethlehem, PA 18018. *Telephone:* 800-441-3191. *E-mail:* creese@moravian.edu.

### GRADUATE PROGRAMS

**Expenses (2013–14)** *Tuition:* part-time $2247 per course. *Required fees:* part-time $33 per credit; part-time $45 per term.
**Contact** Dr. Lori Hoffman, RN, MS Program Coordinator, Department of Nursing, Moravian College, 1200 Main Street, Bethlehem, PA 18018. *Telephone:* 610-625-7769. *Fax:* 610-625-7861. *E-mail:* lorihoffman@moravian.edu.

#### MASTER'S DEGREE PROGRAM

**Degree** MS

**Available Programs** Master's; Master's for Nurses with Non-Nursing Degrees.
**Concentrations Available** Clinical nurse leader; nursing administration; nursing education.
**Study Options** Part-time.
**Program Entrance Requirements** Computer literacy, minimum overall college GPA of 3.0, transcript of college record, written essay, 2 letters of recommendation, prerequisite course work, resume, statistics course. *Application deadline:* Applications may be processed on a rolling basis for some programs. *Application fee:* $40.
**Advanced Placement** Credit given for nursing courses completed elsewhere dependent upon specific evaluations.
**Degree Requirements** 36 total credit hours, thesis or project.

### CONTINUING EDUCATION PROGRAM

**Contact** Dr. Dawn Goodolf, RN, Comenius Center BS Program in Nursing Coordinator, Department of Nursing, Moravian College, 1200 Main Street, Bethlehem, PA 18018. *Telephone:* 610-625-7764. *Fax:* 610-625-7861. *E-mail:* medmg01@moravian.edu.

## Mount Aloysius College

**Division of Nursing**
**Cresson, Pennsylvania**

*http://www.mtaloy.edu/*
Founded in 1939

### DEGREE • BSN

**Nursing Program Faculty** 8 (25% with doctorates).
**Baccalaureate Enrollment** 72 **Women** 88% **Men** 12% **Minority** 1% **Part-time** 89%
**Distance Learning Courses** Available.
**Nursing Student Activities** Student Nurses' Association.
**Nursing Student Resources** Academic advising; academic or career counseling; assistance for students with disabilities; bookstore; campus computer network; computer lab; computer-assisted instruction; daycare for children of students; e-mail services; interactive nursing skills videos; Internet; learning resource lab; library services; nursing audiovisuals; remedial services; resume preparation assistance; skills, simulation, or other laboratory; tutoring.
**Library Facilities** 90,750 volumes (6,000 in health, 900 in nursing); 164 periodical subscriptions (42 health-care related).

### BACCALAUREATE PROGRAMS

**Degree** BSN
**Available Programs** ADN to Baccalaureate; Accelerated RN Baccalaureate.
**Site Options** Johnstown, PA; Altoona, PA.
**Study Options** Full-time.
**Online Degree Options** Yes.
**Program Entrance Requirements** Transcript of college record, health exam, high school transcript, immunizations, RN licensure. Transfer students are accepted. *Application deadline:* Applications may be processed on a rolling basis for some programs. *Application fee:* $30.
**Advanced Placement** Credit by examination available. Credit given for nursing courses completed elsewhere dependent upon specific evaluations.
**Contact** *Telephone:* 814-886-6401. *Fax:* 814-886-6374.

### CONTINUING EDUCATION PROGRAM

**Contact** *Telephone:* 814-886-6403. *Fax:* 814-886-2978.

## Neumann University

**Program in Nursing and Health Sciences**
**Aston, Pennsylvania**

*http://www.neumann.edu/*
Founded in 1965

### DEGREES • BS • MS

**Nursing Program Faculty** 37 (14% with doctorates).
**Baccalaureate Enrollment** 585 **Women** 87.9% **Men** 12.1% **Minority** 23.8% **International** .3% **Part-time** 40.2%
**Graduate Enrollment** 34 **Women** 100% **Minority** 23.5% **Part-time** 100%
**Nursing Student Activities** Nursing Honor Society, Sigma Theta Tau, Student Nurses' Association.
**Nursing Student Resources** Academic advising; academic or career counseling; assistance for students with disabilities; bookstore; campus computer network; career placement assistance; computer lab; computer-assisted instruction; e-mail services; employment services for current students; externships; housing assistance; interactive nursing skills videos; Internet; learning resource lab; library services; nursing audiovisuals; paid internships; remedial services; resume preparation assistance; skills, simulation, or other laboratory; tutoring; unpaid internships.
**Library Facilities** 64,000 volumes (600 in health, 540 in nursing); 94,000 periodical subscriptions (6,500 health-care related).

### BACCALAUREATE PROGRAMS

**Degree** BS
**Available Programs** ADN to Baccalaureate; Accelerated RN Baccalaureate; Baccalaureate for Second Degree; Generic Baccalaureate; International Nurse to Baccalaureate; LPN to Baccalaureate; LPN to RN Baccalaureate.
**Study Options** Full-time and part-time.
**Program Entrance Requirements** Minimum overall college GPA of 2.5, transcript of college record, health exam, health insurance, high school biology, high school chemistry, high school foreign language, 2 years high school math, 4 years high school science, high school transcript, immunizations, minimum high school GPA of 2.5, minimum GPA in nursing prerequisites of 2.5, prerequisite course work. Transfer students are accepted. *Application deadline:* Applications may be processed on a rolling basis for some programs.
**Advanced Placement** Credit by examination available. Credit given for nursing courses completed elsewhere dependent upon specific evaluations.
**Financial Aid** 95% of baccalaureate students in nursing programs received some form of financial aid in 2012–13.
**Contact** Ms. Casey Downie, Admissions Counselor, Program in Nursing and Health Sciences, Neumann University, One Neumann Drive, Aston, PA 19014-1298. *Telephone:* 800-963-8626 Ext. 5614. *Fax:* 610-558-5652. *E-mail:* downiec@neumann.edu.

### GRADUATE PROGRAMS

**Financial Aid** 50% of graduate students in nursing programs received some form of financial aid in 2012–13. Available to part-time students. *Application deadline:* 3/15.
**Contact** Ms. Kittie Pain, Associate Director, Admissions, Program in Nursing and Health Sciences, Neumann University, One Neumann Drive, Aston, PA 19014-1298. *Telephone:* 800-963-8626 Ext. 5613. *Fax:* 610-558-5652. *E-mail:* nursediv@neumann.edu.

#### MASTER'S DEGREE PROGRAM

**Degree** MS
**Available Programs** Master's.
**Concentrations Available** Nursing education. *Nurse practitioner programs in:* adult health.
**Study Options** Full-time and part-time.
**Program Entrance Requirements** Computer literacy, minimum overall college GPA of 3.0, transcript of college record, CPR certification, immunizations, interview, 2 letters of recommendation, nursing research course, physical assessment course, professional liability insurance/malpractice insurance, prerequisite course work, statistics course, GRE or MAT. *Application deadline:* Applications may be processed on a rolling basis for some programs.
**Advanced Placement** Credit given for nursing courses completed elsewhere dependent upon specific evaluations.
**Degree Requirements** 43 total credit hours, thesis or project.

#### POST-MASTER'S PROGRAM

**Areas of Study** Nursing education. *Nurse practitioner programs in:* adult health.

## Penn State University Park

**School of Nursing**
**State College, University Park, Pennsylvania**

*http://www.nursing.psu.edu/*
Founded in 1855

### DEGREES • BS • MS • MSN/PHD • PHD

**Nursing Program Faculty** 110 (20% with doctorates).

**Baccalaureate Enrollment** 824 **Women** 95% **Men** 5% **Minority** 7% **Part-time** 43%
**Graduate Enrollment** 61 **Women** 92% **Men** 8% **Minority** 10% **Part-time** 59%
**Distance Learning Courses** Available.
**Nursing Student Activities** Sigma Theta Tau, Student Nurses' Association.
**Nursing Student Resources** Academic advising; academic or career counseling; assistance for students with disabilities; bookstore; campus computer network; career placement assistance; computer lab; computer-assisted instruction; daycare for children of students; e-mail services; employment services for current students; externships; housing assistance; interactive nursing skills videos; Internet; learning resource lab; library services; nursing audiovisuals; paid internships; remedial services; resume preparation assistance; skills, simulation, or other laboratory; tutoring.
**Library Facilities** 5.4 million volumes (244,000 in health); 131,358 periodical subscriptions (3,500 health-care related).

### BACCALAUREATE PROGRAMS

**Degree** BS
**Available Programs** ADN to Baccalaureate; Generic Baccalaureate; RN Baccalaureate.
**Site Options** Uniontown, PA; New Kensington, PA; Harrisburg, PA; Hershey, PA; University Park, PA; Altoona, PA; Mont Alto, PA; Sharon, PA: Scranton, PA.
**Study Options** Full-time.
**Online Degree Options** Yes.
**Program Entrance Requirements** Transcript of college record, 3 years high school math, 3 years high school science, high school transcript. Transfer students are accepted. *Application deadline:* 11/30 (fall). *Application fee:* $50.
**Advanced Placement** Credit given for nursing courses completed elsewhere dependent upon specific evaluations.
**Contact** *Telephone:* 814-863-8185. *Fax:* 814-863-2925.

### GRADUATE PROGRAMS

**Contact** *Telephone:* 814-863-2211. *Fax:* 814-865-2925.

#### MASTER'S DEGREE PROGRAM

**Degrees** MS; MSN/PhD
**Available Programs** Master's.
**Concentrations Available** Nursing administration. *Clinical nurse specialist programs in:* adult health, community health, gerontology. *Nurse practitioner programs in:* adult health, family health.
**Site Options** Hershey, PA; University Park, PA.
**Study Options** Full-time and part-time.
**Online Degree Options** Yes.
**Program Entrance Requirements** Computer literacy, minimum overall college GPA of 3.0, transcript of college record, CPR certification, written essay, immunizations, 2 letters of recommendation, professional liability insurance/malpractice insurance. *Application deadline:* Applications may be processed on a rolling basis for some programs. *Application fee:* $65.
**Advanced Placement** Credit given for nursing courses completed elsewhere dependent upon specific evaluations.
**Degree Requirements** 43 total credit hours, thesis or project.

#### POST-MASTER'S PROGRAM

**Areas of Study** *Nurse practitioner programs in:* family health.

#### DOCTORAL DEGREE PROGRAM

**Degree** PhD
**Available Programs** Doctorate.
**Areas of Study** Bio-behavioral research, faculty preparation, gerontology, human health and illness, illness and transition, individualized study, nursing research, nursing science.
**Site Options** Hershey, PA; University Park, PA.
**Program Entrance Requirements** Minimum overall college GPA of 3.5, interview, 3 letters of recommendation, MSN or equivalent, writing sample. *Application deadline:* Applications may be processed on a rolling basis for some programs. *Application fee:* $65.
**Degree Requirements** 58 total credit hours, dissertation, oral exam, written exam, residency.

#### POSTDOCTORAL PROGRAM

**Areas of Study** Gerontology.
**Postdoctoral Program Contact***Telephone:* 814-865-9337. *Fax:* 814-865-2925.

### CONTINUING EDUCATION PROGRAM

**Contact** *Telephone:* 814-865-8469. *Fax:* 814-865-3779.

## Pennsylvania College of Health Sciences

### Bachelor of Science in Nursing Program
### Lancaster, Pennsylvania

Founded in 1903
**DEGREE • BSN**
**Library Facilities** 60,590 volumes; 17,719 periodical subscriptions.

### BACCALAUREATE PROGRAMS

**Degree** BSN
**Available Programs** RN Baccalaureate.
**Program Entrance Requirements** Minimum overall college GPA of 2.0, RN licensure.
**Expenses (2012–13)** *Tuition:* part-time $425 per credit hour.
**Contact** Program Chair, Bachelor of Science in Nursing Program, Pennsylvania College of Health Sciences, 410 North Lime Street, Lancaster, PA 17602. *Telephone:* 800-622-5443. *E-mail:* jlhershe@lancastergeneralcollege.edu.

## Pennsylvania College of Technology

### School of Health Sciences
### Williamsport, Pennsylvania

Founded in 1965
**DEGREE • BSN**
**Nursing Program Faculty** 37 (5% with doctorates).
**Baccalaureate Enrollment** 12 **Women** 100% **International** 1% **Part-time** 92%
**Nursing Student Activities** Student Nurses' Association.
**Nursing Student Resources** Academic advising; academic or career counseling; assistance for students with disabilities; bookstore; campus computer network; career placement assistance; computer lab; computer-assisted instruction; daycare for children of students; e-mail services; employment services for current students; externships; housing assistance; interactive nursing skills videos; Internet; learning resource lab; library services; nursing audiovisuals; placement services for program completers; remedial services; resume preparation assistance; skills, simulation, or other laboratory; tutoring.
**Library Facilities** 140,885 volumes; 62,601 periodical subscriptions.

### BACCALAUREATE PROGRAMS

**Degree** BSN
**Available Programs** RN Baccalaureate.
**Program Entrance Requirements** Transfer students are accepted.
**Contact** *Telephone:* 800-367-9222 Ext. 4525.

## Robert Morris University

### School of Nursing and Health Sciences
### Moon Township, Pennsylvania

***http://www.rmu.edu/web/cms/schools/snhs/nursing/Pages/default.aspx***
Founded in 1921
**DEGREES • BSN • DNP • MSN**
**Nursing Program Faculty** 30 (50% with doctorates).
**Baccalaureate Enrollment** 462 **Women** 87% **Men** 13% **Minority** 8% **Part-time** 24%
**Graduate Enrollment** 161 **Women** 86% **Men** 14% **Minority** 17% **Part-time** 100%
**Distance Learning Courses** Available.
**Nursing Student Activities** Nursing Honor Society, Sigma Theta Tau, Student Nurses' Association.
**Nursing Student Resources** Academic advising; academic or career counseling; assistance for students with disabilities; bookstore; campus

computer network; career placement assistance; computer lab; computer-assisted instruction; e-mail services; employment services for current students; externships; housing assistance; interactive nursing skills videos; Internet; learning resource lab; library services; nursing audiovisuals; paid internships; placement services for program completers; remedial services; resume preparation assistance; skills, simulation, or other laboratory; tutoring; unpaid internships.

**Library Facilities** 112,707 volumes; 195 periodical subscriptions.

## BACCALAUREATE PROGRAMS

**Degree** BSN

**Available Programs** Baccalaureate for Second Degree; Generic Baccalaureate; RN Baccalaureate.

**Study Options** Full-time and part-time.

**Online Degree Options** Yes.

**Program Entrance Requirements** Minimum overall college GPA of 3.0, transcript of college record, written essay, health exam, health insurance, high school biology, high school chemistry, 2 years high school math, 2 years high school science, high school transcript, immunizations, 2 letters of recommendation, minimum high school GPA of 3.0, minimum GPA in nursing prerequisites of 2.0, prerequisite course work. Transfer students are accepted. *Application deadline:* 5/1 (fall), 11/1 (spring). Applications may be processed on a rolling basis for some programs. *Application fee:* $30.

**Advanced Placement** Credit given for nursing courses completed elsewhere dependent upon specific evaluations.

**Expenses (2013–14)** *Tuition:* full-time $26,910; part-time $850 per credit. *International tuition:* $26,910 full-time. *Room and board:* $11,585; room only: $5505 per academic year. *Required fees:* full-time $654; part-time $30 per credit.

**Financial Aid** 72% of baccalaureate students in nursing programs received some form of financial aid in 2012–13.

**Contact** Enrollment Services, School of Nursing and Health Sciences, Robert Morris University, 6001 University Boulevard, Moon Township, PA 15108-1189. *Telephone:* 412-397-5200. *Fax:* 412-397-2425. *E-mail:* admissionsoffice@rmu.edu.

## GRADUATE PROGRAMS

**Expenses (2013–14)** *Tuition:* part-time $470 per credit.

**Financial Aid** 80% of graduate students in nursing programs received some form of financial aid in 2012–13. Federal Work-Study, institutionally sponsored loans, and unspecified assistantships available. *Financial aid application deadline:* 5/1.

**Contact** Enrollment Services, School of Nursing and Health Sciences, Robert Morris University, 6001 University Boulevard, Moon Township, PA 15108-1189. *Telephone:* 412-397-5200. *Fax:* 412-397-2425. *E-mail:* GraduateAdmissions@rmu.edu.

### MASTER'S DEGREE PROGRAM

**Degree** MSN

**Available Programs** Master's.

**Concentrations Available** Nursing education.

**Study Options** Part-time.

**Program Entrance Requirements** Clinical experience, minimum overall college GPA of 3.25, transcript of college record, CPR certification, written essay, interview, 2 letters of recommendation, statistics course. *Application deadline:* Applications may be processed on a rolling basis for some programs. *Application fee:* $35.

**Degree Requirements** 36 total credit hours, thesis or project.

### DOCTORAL DEGREE PROGRAM

**Degree** DNP

**Available Programs** Doctorate; Post-Baccalaureate Doctorate.

**Areas of Study** Advanced practice nursing.

**Program Entrance Requirements** Clinical experience, minimum overall college GPA of 3.25, interview by faculty committee, 2 letters of recommendation, vita, writing sample. *Application deadline:* Applications may be processed on a rolling basis for some programs. *Application fee:* $35.

# Saint Francis University

## Department of Nursing
## Loretto, Pennsylvania

***http://www.francis.edu/nursing/***

Founded in 1847

### DEGREE • BSN

**Nursing Program Faculty** 7 (1% with doctorates).

**Baccalaureate Enrollment** 85 **Women** 90% **Men** 10% **Minority** 2%

**Nursing Student Activities** Student Nurses' Association, nursing club.

**Nursing Student Resources** Academic advising; academic or career counseling; assistance for students with disabilities; bookstore; campus computer network; career placement assistance; computer lab; computer-assisted instruction; e-mail services; employment services for current students; externships; interactive nursing skills videos; Internet; learning resource lab; library services; nursing audiovisuals; resume preparation assistance; skills, simulation, or other laboratory; tutoring.

**Library Facilities** 99,500 volumes (150,000 in health, 120,000 in nursing); 39,800 periodical subscriptions (25 health-care related).

## BACCALAUREATE PROGRAMS

**Degree** BSN

**Available Programs** Generic Baccalaureate.

**Study Options** Full-time and part-time.

**Program Entrance Requirements** Transcript of college record, high school biology, high school chemistry, 2 years high school math, 2 years high school science, high school transcript, minimum high school GPA of 3.0, minimum high school rank 50%, minimum GPA in nursing prerequisites of 2.7, prerequisite course work. Transfer students are accepted. *Application deadline:* Applications may be processed on a rolling basis for some programs. *Application fee:* $30.

**Advanced Placement** Credit by examination available. Credit given for nursing courses completed elsewhere dependent upon specific evaluations.

**Contact** *Telephone:* 814-472-3027. *Fax:* 814-472-3849.

# Slippery Rock University of Pennsylvania

## Department of Nursing
## Slippery Rock, Pennsylvania

***http://www.sru.edu/academics/colleges/ches/nursing/Pages/Welcome.aspx***

Founded in 1889

### DEGREE • BSN

**Nursing Program Faculty** 7 (100% with doctorates).

**Baccalaureate Enrollment** 230 **Women** 95% **Men** 5% **Minority** 1% **Part-time** 97%

**Distance Learning Courses** Available.

**Nursing Student Activities** Sigma Theta Tau.

**Nursing Student Resources** Academic advising; academic or career counseling; assistance for students with disabilities; bookstore; campus computer network; career placement assistance; computer lab; computer-assisted instruction; daycare for children of students; e-mail services; employment services for current students; housing assistance; Internet; library services; nursing audiovisuals; placement services for program completers; resume preparation assistance; tutoring.

**Library Facilities** 747,585 volumes (7,214 in health, 925 in nursing); 74,495 periodical subscriptions (1,299 health-care related).

## BACCALAUREATE PROGRAMS

**Degree** BSN

**Available Programs** ADN to Baccalaureate; RN Baccalaureate.

**Study Options** Full-time and part-time.

**Online Degree Options** Yes (online only).

**Program Entrance Requirements** Minimum overall college GPA of 2.5, transcript of college record, minimum GPA in nursing prerequisites of 2.5, professional liability insurance/malpractice insurance, RN licensure. Transfer students are accepted. *Application deadline:* Applications may be processed on a rolling basis for some programs. *Application fee:* $30.

**Advanced Placement** Credit by examination available. Credit given for nursing courses completed elsewhere dependent upon specific evaluations.
**Contact** *Telephone:* 724-738-4921. *Fax:* 724-738-2509.

# Temple University
## Department of Nursing
## Philadelphia, Pennsylvania

*http://www.temple.edu/nursing*
Founded in 1884

### DEGREES • BSN • DNP • MSN

**Nursing Program Faculty** 37 (50% with doctorates).
**Baccalaureate Enrollment** 400 **Women** 85% **Men** 15% **Minority** 49% **Part-time** 62%
**Graduate Enrollment** 120 **Women** 95% **Men** 5% **Minority** 16% **Part-time** 100%
**Distance Learning Courses** Available.
**Nursing Student Activities** Nursing Honor Society, Sigma Theta Tau, Student Nurses' Association, nursing club.
**Nursing Student Resources** Academic advising; academic or career counseling; assistance for students with disabilities; bookstore; campus computer network; career placement assistance; computer lab; computer-assisted instruction; e-mail services; externships; housing assistance; interactive nursing skills videos; Internet; learning resource lab; library services; nursing audiovisuals; remedial services; resume preparation assistance; skills, simulation, or other laboratory; tutoring.
**Library Facilities** 60,374 volumes in health, 1,350 volumes in nursing; 67,942 periodical subscriptions (1,350 health-care related).

### BACCALAUREATE PROGRAMS

**Degree** BSN
**Available Programs** Generic Baccalaureate; RN Baccalaureate.
**Study Options** Full-time.
**Program Entrance Requirements** Minimum overall college GPA of 3.0, transcript of college record, CPR certification, written essay, health exam, health insurance, high school biology, high school chemistry, high school foreign language, 3 years high school math, 3 years high school science, high school transcript, immunizations, interview, minimum high school GPA of 3.0, minimum GPA in nursing prerequisites of 3.0, prerequisite course work. Transfer students are accepted. *Application deadline:* 2/15 (fall). *Application fee:* $50.
**Advanced Placement** Credit given for nursing courses completed elsewhere dependent upon specific evaluations.
**Contact** *Telephone:* 215-707-4618. *Fax:* 215-707-1599.

### GRADUATE PROGRAMS

**Contact** *Telephone:* 215-707-3789. *Fax:* 215-707-1599.

#### MASTER'S DEGREE PROGRAM

**Degree** MSN
**Available Programs** Master's.
**Concentrations Available** Nursing education. *Clinical nurse specialist programs in:* psychiatric/mental health. *Nurse practitioner programs in:* adult health, family health, pediatric.
**Study Options** Full-time and part-time.
**Program Entrance Requirements** Clinical experience, minimum overall college GPA of 3.0, transcript of college record, CPR certification, written essay, immunizations, interview, 2 letters of recommendation, nursing research course, physical assessment course, professional liability insurance/malpractice insurance, statistics course, GRE General Test.
**Advanced Placement** Credit given for nursing courses completed elsewhere dependent upon specific evaluations.
**Degree Requirements** 36 total credit hours.

#### POST-MASTER'S PROGRAM

**Areas of Study** Nursing education. *Clinical nurse specialist programs in:* psychiatric/mental health. *Nurse practitioner programs in:* adult health, family health, pediatric.

#### DOCTORAL DEGREE PROGRAM

**Degree** DNP
**Available Programs** Doctorate.

# Thomas Jefferson University
## Department of Nursing
## Philadelphia, Pennsylvania

*http://www.tju.edu/*
Founded in 1824

### DEGREES • BSN • DNP • MSN

**Nursing Program Faculty** 38 (42% with doctorates).
**Nursing Student Activities** Nursing Honor Society, Sigma Theta Tau, Student Nurses' Association.
**Nursing Student Resources** Academic advising; academic or career counseling; assistance for students with disabilities; bookstore; campus computer network; career placement assistance; computer lab; computer-assisted instruction; e-mail services; interactive nursing skills videos; Internet; learning resource lab; library services; nursing audiovisuals; paid internships; placement services for program completers; remedial services; resume preparation assistance; skills, simulation, or other laboratory; tutoring.
**Library Facilities** 146,000 volumes in health, 4,700 volumes in nursing; 2,100 periodical subscriptions health-care related.

### BACCALAUREATE PROGRAMS

**Degree** BSN
**Available Programs** ADN to Baccalaureate; Accelerated Baccalaureate; Accelerated Baccalaureate for Second Degree; Accelerated RN Baccalaureate; Baccalaureate for Second Degree; Generic Baccalaureate; RN Baccalaureate.
**Site Options** Atlantic City, NJ; Philadelphia, PA.
**Study Options** Full-time and part-time.
**Program Entrance Requirements** Minimum overall college GPA of 2.9, transcript of college record, CPR certification, written essay, health exam, health insurance, high school transcript, immunizations, 2 letters of recommendation, prerequisite course work. Transfer students are accepted.
**Advanced Placement** Credit by examination available. Credit given for nursing courses completed elsewhere dependent upon specific evaluations.
**Contact** *Telephone:* 215-503-8104. *Fax:* 215-503-0376.

### GRADUATE PROGRAMS

**Contact** *Telephone:* 215-503-8057. *Fax:* 215-932-1468.

#### MASTER'S DEGREE PROGRAM

**Degree** MSN
**Available Programs** Accelerated Master's; Accelerated RN to Master's; Master's; Master's for Non-Nursing College Graduates; Master's for Nurses with Non-Nursing Degrees; RN to Master's.
**Concentrations Available** Nurse anesthesia; nursing education; nursing informatics. *Clinical nurse specialist programs in:* acute care, adult health, community health, critical care, home health care, medical-surgical, oncology, pediatric, public health. *Nurse practitioner programs in:* acute care, adult health, family health, neonatal health, oncology, pediatric.
**Site Options** Philadelphia, PA.
**Study Options** Full-time and part-time.
**Program Entrance Requirements** Clinical experience, computer literacy, minimum overall college GPA of 3.0, transcript of college record, CPR certification, written essay, interview, 3 letters of recommendation, nursing research course, physical assessment course, professional liability insurance/malpractice insurance, resume, statistics course.
**Advanced Placement** Credit given for nursing courses completed elsewhere dependent upon specific evaluations.
**Degree Requirements** 36 total credit hours.

#### POST-MASTER'S PROGRAM

**Areas of Study** Nursing education; nursing informatics. *Nurse practitioner programs in:* acute care, adult health, family health, neonatal health, oncology, pediatric.

#### DOCTORAL DEGREE PROGRAM

**Degree** DNP
**Available Programs** Doctorate.
**Areas of Study** Advanced practice nursing, clinical practice, individualized study.
**Program Entrance Requirements** Clinical experience, minimum overall college GPA of 3.2, interview by faculty committee, interview, 3

letters of recommendation, MSN or equivalent, scholarly papers, statistics course, vita, writing sample.
**Degree Requirements** 36 total credit hours, written exam, residency.

### CONTINUING EDUCATION PROGRAM

**Contact** *Telephone:* 215-503-8057. *Fax:* 215-503-0376.

# University of Pennsylvania

## School of Nursing
## Philadelphia, Pennsylvania

***http://www.nursing.upenn.edu/***
Founded in 1740

### DEGREES • BSN • MSN • MSN/MBA • MSN/MPH • MSN/PHD • PHD

**Nursing Program Faculty** 339 (21% with doctorates).
**Baccalaureate Enrollment** 556 **Women** 88% **Men** 12% **Minority** 39.3% **International** 1.4% **Part-time** .7%
**Graduate Enrollment** 528 **Women** 88% **Men** 12% **Minority** 21.4% **International** 3.2% **Part-time** 58.3%
**Nursing Student Activities** Nursing Honor Society, Sigma Theta Tau, Student Nurses' Association.
**Nursing Student Resources** Academic advising; academic or career counseling; assistance for students with disabilities; bookstore; campus computer network; career placement assistance; computer lab; computer-assisted instruction; daycare for children of students; e-mail services; employment services for current students; externships; housing assistance; interactive nursing skills videos; Internet; learning resource lab; library services; nursing audiovisuals; other; paid internships; placement services for program completers; remedial services; resume preparation assistance; skills, simulation, or other laboratory; tutoring; unpaid internships.
**Library Facilities** 6.1 million volumes; 109,467 periodical subscriptions.

### BACCALAUREATE PROGRAMS

**Degree** BSN
**Available Programs** ADN to Baccalaureate; Accelerated Baccalaureate; Accelerated Baccalaureate for Second Degree; Accelerated RN Baccalaureate; Baccalaureate for Second Degree; Generic Baccalaureate; RN Baccalaureate.
**Study Options** Full-time and part-time.
**Program Entrance Requirements** Minimum overall college GPA of 3.0, transcript of college record, written essay, health exam, health insurance, high school biology, high school chemistry, high school foreign language, 4 years high school math, 4 years high school science, high school transcript, immunizations, interview, 2 letters of recommendation, minimum high school GPA of 3.0, minimum high school rank 10%. Transfer students are accepted. *Application deadline:* 1/1 (fall). *Application fee:* $75.
**Advanced Placement** Credit given for nursing courses completed elsewhere dependent upon specific evaluations.
**Financial Aid** 96% of baccalaureate students in nursing programs received some form of financial aid in 2012–13.
**Contact** Office of Enrollment Management, School of Nursing, University of Pennsylvania, 418 Curie Boulevard, Philadelphia, PA 19104-4217. *Telephone:* 215-898-4271. *Fax:* 215-573-8439. *E-mail:* admissions@nursing.upenn.edu.

### GRADUATE PROGRAMS

**Financial Aid** 94% of graduate students in nursing programs received some form of financial aid in 2012–13. Fellowships, research assistantships, teaching assistantships, institutionally sponsored loans, scholarships, traineeships, and unspecified assistantships available. *Financial aid application deadline:* 12/15.
**Contact** Carol Ladden, Director, Graduate Enrollment, School of Nursing, University of Pennsylvania, 418 Curie Boulevard, Philadelphia, PA 19104-4217. *Telephone:* 215-898-4271. *Fax:* 215-573-8439. *E-mail:* admissions@nursing.upenn.edu.

#### MASTER'S DEGREE PROGRAM

**Degrees** MSN; MSN/MBA; MSN/MPH; MSN/PhD
**Available Programs** Accelerated Master's for Non-Nursing College Graduates; Accelerated Master's for Nurses with Non-Nursing Degrees; Master's.
**Concentrations Available** Health-care administration; nurse anesthesia; nurse-midwifery; nursing administration. *Clinical nurse specialist programs in:* acute care, adult health, pediatric. *Nurse practitioner programs in:* acute care, adult health, family health, gerontology, neonatal health, pediatric, primary care, psychiatric/mental health,women's health.
**Study Options** Full-time and part-time.
**Program Entrance Requirements** Clinical experience, computer literacy, minimum overall college GPA of 3.0, transcript of college record, CPR certification, written essay, immunizations, interview, 3 letters of recommendation, prerequisite course work, resume, statistics course, GRE General Test. *Application deadline:* 7/1 (fall), 11/1 (winter), 11/1 (spring), 3/15 (summer). Applications may be processed on a rolling basis for some programs. *Application fee:* $80.
**Advanced Placement** Credit given for nursing courses completed elsewhere dependent upon specific evaluations.
**Degree Requirements** 36 total credit hours.

#### POST-MASTER'S PROGRAM

**Areas of Study** Health-care administration; nurse anesthesia; nurse-midwifery; nursing administration; nursing education. *Clinical nurse specialist programs in:* acute care, adult health, maternity-newborn, medical-surgical, pediatric. *Nurse practitioner programs in:* acute care, adult health, family health, gerontology, neonatal health, oncology, pediatric, primary care, psychiatric/mental health,women's health.

#### DOCTORAL DEGREE PROGRAM

**Degree** PhD
**Available Programs** Doctorate; Doctorate for Nurses with Non-Nursing Degrees; Post-Baccalaureate Doctorate.
**Areas of Study** Addiction/substance abuse, aging, bio-behavioral research, biology of health and illness, clinical practice, community health, critical care, ethics, faculty preparation, family health, gerontology, health policy, health promotion/disease prevention, health-care systems, human health and illness, illness and transition, individualized study, information systems, maternity-newborn, neuro-behavior, nursing administration, nursing policy, nursing research, nursing science, oncology, palliative care, urban health,women's health.
**Program Entrance Requirements** Minimum overall college GPA of 3.5, interview by faculty committee, interview, 3 letters of recommendation, MSN or equivalent, statistics course, vita, writing sample, GRE General Test. *Application deadline:* 11/1 (fall). *Application fee:* $80.
**Degree Requirements** 42 total credit hours, dissertation, oral exam, written exam, residency.

#### POSTDOCTORAL PROGRAM

**Areas of Study** Adolescent health, aging, cancer care, chronic illness, community health, family health, gerontology, health promotion/disease prevention, individualized study, nursing informatics, nursing interventions, nursing research, nursing science, outcomes, self-care, vulnerable population,women's health.
**Postdoctoral Program Contact** Dr. Yvonne Paterson, Associate Dean for Nursing Research, School of Nursing, University of Pennsylvania, 418 Curie Boulevard, Claire M. Fagin Hall, 4th Floor, Philadelphia, PA 19104-4271. *Telephone:* 215-898-3151. *E-mail:* research@nursing.upenn.edu.

### CONTINUING EDUCATION PROGRAM

**Contact** Janet L. Tomcavage, Program Management, School of Nursing, University of Pennsylvania, 418 Curie Boulevard, Philadelphia, PA 19104-4271. *Telephone:* 215-898-5422. *E-mail:* tomcavag@nursing.upenn.edu.

# University of Pittsburgh

## School of Nursing
## Pittsburgh, Pennsylvania

***http://www.nursing.pitt.edu/***
Founded in 1787

### DEGREES • BSN • MSN • PHD

**Nursing Program Faculty** 117 (80% with doctorates).
**Baccalaureate Enrollment** 607 **Women** 89% **Men** 11% **Minority** 13% **International** .6% **Part-time** 1%
**Graduate Enrollment** 418 **Women** 86% **Men** 14% **Minority** 11% **International** 3% **Part-time** 48%
**Distance Learning Courses** Available.

**Nursing Student Activities** Nursing Honor Society, Sigma Theta Tau, Student Nurses' Association.
**Nursing Student Resources** Academic advising; academic or career counseling; assistance for students with disabilities; bookstore; campus computer network; career placement assistance; computer lab; computer-assisted instruction; daycare for children of students; e-mail services; employment services for current students; externships; housing assistance; interactive nursing skills videos; Internet; learning resource lab; library services; nursing audiovisuals; other; paid internships; placement services for program completers; remedial services; resume preparation assistance; skills, simulation, or other laboratory; tutoring.
**Library Facilities** 6.1 million volumes (310,683 in health, 8,651 in nursing); 87,417 periodical subscriptions (4,738 health-care related).

## BACCALAUREATE PROGRAMS

**Degree** BSN
**Available Programs** Accelerated Baccalaureate for Second Degree; Generic Baccalaureate; RN Baccalaureate.
**Site Options** Johnstown, PA.
**Study Options** Full-time.
**Program Entrance Requirements** Minimum overall college GPA of 3.0, transcript of college record, written essay, health exam, health insurance, high school biology, high school chemistry, 4 years high school math, 3 years high school science, high school transcript, immunizations, 1 letter of recommendation, minimum high school GPA of 3.3, minimum GPA in nursing prerequisites of 3.0. Transfer students are accepted. *Application deadline:* Applications may be processed on a rolling basis for some programs. *Application fee:* $45.
**Advanced Placement** Credit by examination available.
**Expenses (2013–14)** *Tuition, state resident:* full-time $20,444; part-time $851 per credit. *Tuition, nonresident:* full-time $33,358; part-time $1389 per credit. *International tuition:* $33,358 full-time. *Room and board:* $8150; room only: $5950 per academic year. *Required fees:* full-time $884; part-time $226 per term.
**Financial Aid** 58% of baccalaureate students in nursing programs received some form of financial aid in 2012–13.
**Contact** Mrs. Suzanne Brody, Associate Director of Student Services Recruitment, School of Nursing, University of Pittsburgh, 239 Victoria Building, 3500 Victoria Street, Pittsburgh, PA 15261. *Telephone:* 412-624-1291. *Fax:* 412-624-2409. *E-mail:* brodys@pitt.edu.

## GRADUATE PROGRAMS

**Expenses (2013–14)** *Tuition, state resident:* full-time $23,408; part-time $955 per credit. *Tuition, nonresident:* full-time $26,996; part-time $1103 per credit. *International tuition:* $26,996 full-time. *Required fees:* full-time $764; part-time $212 per term.
**Financial Aid** 58% of graduate students in nursing programs received some form of financial aid in 2012–13. 19 fellowships with full and partial tuition reimbursements available (averaging $16,063 per year), 13 research assistantships with full and partial tuition reimbursements available (averaging $9,927 per year), 19 teaching assistantships with full and partial tuition reimbursements available (averaging $14,358 per year) were awarded; scholarships, traineeships, and unspecified assistantships also available. Aid available to part-time students. *Financial aid application deadline:* 7/1.
**Contact** Mrs. Suzanne Brody, Associate Director of Student Services Recruitment, School of Nursing, University of Pittsburgh, 239 Victoria Building, 3500 Victoria Street, Pittsburgh, PA 15261. *Telephone:* 412-624-1291. *Fax:* 412-624-2409. *E-mail:* brodys@pitt.edu.

### MASTER'S DEGREE PROGRAM

**Degree** MSN
**Available Programs** Master's; RN to Master's.
**Concentrations Available** Clinical nurse leader; nurse anesthesia; nursing administration; nursing informatics. *Nurse practitioner programs in:* neonatal health.
**Site Options** Bradford, PA; Johnstown, PA; Greensburg, PA.
**Study Options** Full-time and part-time.
**Online Degree Options** Yes.
**Program Entrance Requirements** Clinical experience, minimum overall college GPA of 3.0, transcript of college record, CPR certification, written essay, immunizations, interview, 3 letters of recommendation, professional liability insurance/malpractice insurance, resume, statistics course, GRE or MAT. *Application deadline:* Applications may be processed on a rolling basis for some programs. *Application fee:* $50.
**Advanced Placement** Credit by examination available. Credit given for nursing courses completed elsewhere dependent upon specific evaluations.
**Degree Requirements** 52 total credit hours, comprehensive exam.

### POST-MASTER'S PROGRAM

**Areas of Study** Nurse case management; nursing education; nursing informatics. *Nurse practitioner programs in:* acute care, gerontology, neonatal health.

### DOCTORAL DEGREE PROGRAM

**Degree** PhD
**Available Programs** Doctorate; Post-Baccalaureate Doctorate.
**Areas of Study** Nursing research, nursing science.
**Program Entrance Requirements** Minimum overall college GPA of 3.5, interview by faculty committee, interview, 3 letters of recommendation, MSN or equivalent, statistics course, vita, writing sample, GRE. *Application deadline:* Applications may be processed on a rolling basis for some programs. *Application fee:* $50.
**Degree Requirements** 64 total credit hours, dissertation.

### POSTDOCTORAL PROGRAM

**Areas of Study** Nursing research, nursing science.
**Postdoctoral Program Contact** Dr. Judith A. Erlen, PhD Program Coordinator/Associate Director of Center for Research in Chronic Disorders, School of Nursing, University of Pittsburgh, 3500 Victoria Street, Pittsburgh, PA 15261. *Telephone:* 412-624-1905. *Fax:* 412-624-8521. *E-mail:* jae001@pitt.edu.

## CONTINUING EDUCATION PROGRAM

**Contact** Mrs. Mary Rodgers Schubert, Interim Director of Continuing Education Program, School of Nursing, University of Pittsburgh, 226 Victoria Building, 3500 Victoria Street, Pittsburgh, PA 15261. *Telephone:* 412-624-3156. *E-mail:* mschuber@pitt.edu.

# University of Pittsburgh at Bradford

## Department of Nursing
## Bradford, Pennsylvania

***http://www.upb.pitt.edu/***
Founded in 1963

**DEGREE • BSN**
**Nursing Program Faculty** 10 (30% with doctorates).
**Baccalaureate Enrollment** 6 **Women** 83% **Men** 17% **Minority** 17% **Part-time** 17%
**Distance Learning Courses** Available.
**Nursing Student Activities** Nursing club.
**Nursing Student Resources** Academic advising; academic or career counseling; assistance for students with disabilities; bookstore; campus computer network; career placement assistance; computer lab; computer-assisted instruction; e-mail services; employment services for current students; externships; housing assistance; Internet; learning resource lab; library services; nursing audiovisuals; remedial services; resume preparation assistance; skills, simulation, or other laboratory; tutoring; unpaid internships.
**Library Facilities** 99,223 volumes (629 in health, 296 in nursing); 231 periodical subscriptions (13 health-care related).

## BACCALAUREATE PROGRAMS

**Degree** BSN
**Available Programs** Generic Baccalaureate; RN Baccalaureate.
**Study Options** Full-time and part-time.
**Program Entrance Requirements** Transcript of college record, CPR certification, health exam, health insurance, high school transcript, immunizations, minimum high school GPA of 2.5, minimum GPA in nursing prerequisites of 2.5, professional liability insurance/malpractice insurance, prerequisite course work, RN licensure. Transfer students are accepted. *Application deadline:* Applications may be processed on a rolling basis for some programs. *Application fee:* $45.
**Advanced Placement** Credit by examination available. Credit given for nursing courses completed elsewhere dependent upon specific evaluations.
**Expenses (2013–14)** *Tuition, state resident:* full-time $15,640; part-time $651 per credit. *Tuition, nonresident:* full-time $29,092; part-time $1212 per credit. *International tuition:* $29,092 full-time. *Room and board:* $8238; room only: $5092 per academic year. *Required fees:* full-time $852; part-time $312 per credit.
**Financial Aid** 83% of baccalaureate students in nursing programs received some form of financial aid in 2012–13.

**Contact** Mr. Alexander Nazemetz, Nursing Admissions, Department of Nursing, University of Pittsburgh at Bradford, 300 Campus Drive, Bradford, PA 16701. *Telephone:* 800-872-1787. *Fax:* 814-362-5150. *E-mail:* nazemetz@pitt.edu.

# The University of Scranton
## Department of Nursing
## Scranton, Pennsylvania

***http://www.scranton.edu/academics/pcps/nursing/index.shtml***
Founded in 1888

**DEGREES • BSN • MSN**
**Nursing Program Faculty** 50 (85% with doctorates).
**Baccalaureate Enrollment** 265 **Women** 92% **Men** 8% **Minority** 7% **Part-time** 8%
**Graduate Enrollment** 95 **Women** 70% **Men** 30% **Minority** 6% **Part-time** 50%
**Nursing Student Activities** Nursing Honor Society, Sigma Theta Tau, Student Nurses' Association, nursing club.
**Nursing Student Resources** Academic advising; academic or career counseling; bookstore; campus computer network; career placement assistance; computer lab; computer-assisted instruction; e-mail services; employment services for current students; interactive nursing skills videos; Internet; learning resource lab; library services; nursing audiovisuals; placement services for program completers; remedial services; resume preparation assistance; skills, simulation, or other laboratory; tutoring.
**Library Facilities** 486,650 volumes (28,400 in health, 8,484 in nursing); 45,972 periodical subscriptions (106 health-care related).

### BACCALAUREATE PROGRAMS

**Degree** BSN
**Available Programs** Baccalaureate for Second Degree; Generic Baccalaureate; LPN to RN Baccalaureate; RN Baccalaureate.
**Study Options** Full-time and part-time.
**Program Entrance Requirements** Minimum overall college GPA of 2.5, transcript of college record, written essay, health exam, health insurance, high school biology, high school chemistry, high school foreign language, 3 years high school math, 3 years high school science, high school transcript, immunizations, minimum high school rank 30%, minimum GPA in nursing prerequisites. Transfer students are accepted. *Application deadline:* 3/1 (fall). Applications may be processed on a rolling basis for some programs. *Application fee:* $75.
**Advanced Placement** Credit by examination available. Credit given for nursing courses completed elsewhere dependent upon specific evaluations.
**Expenses (2013–14)** *Tuition:* full-time $38,404; part-time $988 per credit. *Room and board:* $6000; room only: $4000 per academic year. *Required fees:* full-time $350; part-time $50 per credit.
**Financial Aid** 80% of baccalaureate students in nursing programs received some form of financial aid in 2012–13.
**Contact** Dr. Patricia Harrington, Chairperson, Department of Nursing, The University of Scranton, 800 Linden Street, McGurrin Hall, Scranton, PA 18510-4595. *Telephone:* 570-941-7673. *Fax:* 570-941-7903. *E-mail:* harringtonp1@scranton.edu.

### GRADUATE PROGRAMS

**Expenses (2013–14)** *Tuition:* part-time $988 per credit.
**Financial Aid** 90% of graduate students in nursing programs received some form of financial aid in 2012–13. 6 teaching assistantships with full and partial tuition reimbursements available (averaging $6,600 per year) were awarded; career-related internships or fieldwork, Federal Work-Study, and unspecified assistantships also available. Aid available to part-time students. *Financial aid application deadline:* 3/1.
**Contact** Dr. Mary Jane Hanson, Director, Graduate Nursing Program, Department of Nursing, The University of Scranton, 800 Linden Street, McGurrin Hall, Scranton, PA 18510-4595. *Telephone:* 570-941-4060. *Fax:* 570-941-7903. *E-mail:* hansonm2@scranton.edu.

### MASTER'S DEGREE PROGRAM

**Degree** MSN
**Available Programs** Accelerated AD/RN to Master's; Accelerated RN to Master's; Master's; RN to Master's.
**Concentrations Available** Nurse anesthesia; nursing education. *Clinical nurse specialist programs in:* adult health. *Nurse practitioner programs in:* family health.
**Site Options** Wilkes-Barre, PA.
**Study Options** Full-time and part-time.
**Program Entrance Requirements** Clinical experience, minimum overall college GPA of 3.0, transcript of college record, CPR certification, written essay, immunizations, interview, 3 letters of recommendation, nursing research course, physical assessment course, professional liability insurance/malpractice insurance, prerequisite course work, statistics course. *Application deadline:* 8/1 (fall), 1/1 (spring). Applications may be processed on a rolling basis for some programs. *Application fee:* $50.
**Advanced Placement** Credit given for nursing courses completed elsewhere dependent upon specific evaluations.
**Degree Requirements** 46 total credit hours, comprehensive exam.

### POST-MASTER'S PROGRAM

**Areas of Study** Nurse anesthesia; nursing education. *Clinical nurse specialist programs in:* adult health. *Nurse practitioner programs in:* family health.

# Villanova University
## College of Nursing
## Villanova, Pennsylvania

***http://www.nursing.villanova.edu/***
Founded in 1842

**DEGREES • BSN • MSN • PHD**
**Nursing Program Faculty** 90 (57% with doctorates).
**Baccalaureate Enrollment** 528 **Women** 94% **Men** 6% **Minority** 19% **International** .4% **Part-time** 1%
**Graduate Enrollment** 213 **Women** 91% **Men** 9% **Minority** 2.3% **International** 1.4% **Part-time** 88%
**Distance Learning Courses** Available.
**Nursing Student Activities** Nursing Honor Society, Sigma Theta Tau, Student Nurses' Association, nursing club.
**Nursing Student Resources** Academic advising; academic or career counseling; assistance for students with disabilities; bookstore; campus computer network; career placement assistance; computer lab; computer-assisted instruction; e-mail services; employment services for current students; housing assistance; interactive nursing skills videos; Internet; learning resource lab; library services; nursing audiovisuals; remedial services; resume preparation assistance; skills, simulation, or other laboratory; tutoring.
**Library Facilities** 755,000 volumes (15,235 in health, 1,806 in nursing); 12,000 periodical subscriptions (1,586 health-care related).

### BACCALAUREATE PROGRAMS

**Degree** BSN
**Available Programs** ADN to Baccalaureate; Accelerated Baccalaureate for Second Degree; Baccalaureate for Second Degree; Generic Baccalaureate; International Nurse to Baccalaureate; RN Baccalaureate.
**Study Options** Full-time and part-time.
**Online Degree Options** Yes.
**Program Entrance Requirements** Minimum overall college GPA of 3.00, transcript of college record, CPR certification, written essay, health exam, health insurance, high school biology, high school chemistry, high school foreign language, 3 years high school math, 3 years high school science, high school transcript, immunizations, 2 letters of recommendation, minimum high school GPA of 3.0, minimum GPA in nursing prerequisites. Transfer students are accepted. *Application deadline:* 11/1 (fall), 1/15 (winter). *Application fee:* $80.
**Advanced Placement** Credit given for nursing courses completed elsewhere dependent upon specific evaluations.
**Expenses (2013–14)** *Tuition:* full-time $43,380; part-time $1830 per credit hour. *International tuition:* $43,380 full-time. *Room and board:* $12,290; room only: $6750 per academic year. *Required fees:* full-time $320; part-time $30 per credit; part-time $90 per term.
**Financial Aid** 72% of baccalaureate students in nursing programs received some form of financial aid in 2012–13. *Gift aid (need-based):* Federal Pell, FSEOG, state, private, college/university gift aid from institutional funds, endowed and restricted scholarships and grants. *Loans:* Federal Nursing Student Loans, Federal Direct (Subsidized and Unsubsidized Stafford PLUS), Perkins, alternative loans. *Work-study:* Federal Work-Study, part-time campus jobs. *Financial aid application deadline:* 2/7(priority: 2/7).
**Contact** Dr. Angelina A. Arcamone, Assistant Dean and Director, Undergraduate Program, College of Nursing, Villanova University,

Driscoll Hall, 800 Lancaster Avenue, Villanova, PA 19085-1690. *Telephone:* 610-519-4926. *Fax:* 610-519-7650. *E-mail:* angelina.arcamone@villanova.edu.

## GRADUATE PROGRAMS

**Expenses (2013–14)** *Tuition:* full-time $7065; part-time $785 per credit hour. *International tuition:* $7065 full-time. *Required fees:* full-time $90; part-time $30 per credit; part-time $90 per term.

**Financial Aid** 47% of graduate students in nursing programs received some form of financial aid in 2012–13. 5 teaching assistantships with full tuition reimbursements available (averaging $14,475 per year) were awarded; institutionally sponsored loans, scholarships, traineeships, tuition waivers (full), and unspecified assistantships also available. *Financial aid application deadline:* 7/1.

**Contact** Dr. Marguerite K. Schlag, Assistant Dean and Director, Graduate Program, College of Nursing, Villanova University, Driscoll Hall, 800 Lancaster Avenue, Villanova, PA 19085-1690. *Telephone:* 610-519-4934. *Fax:* 610-519-7997. *E-mail:* marguerite.schlag@villanova.edu.

### MASTER'S DEGREE PROGRAM

**Degree** MSN

**Available Programs** Master's.

**Concentrations Available** Health-care administration; nurse anesthesia; nursing education. *Nurse practitioner programs in:* adult health, family health, pediatric.

**Site Options** Philadelphia, PA.

**Study Options** Full-time and part-time.

**Program Entrance Requirements** Clinical experience, computer literacy, minimum overall college GPA of 3.0, transcript of college record, CPR certification, written essay, immunizations, 3 letters of recommendation, nursing research course, physical assessment course, professional liability insurance/malpractice insurance, resume, statistics course, GRE or MAT. *Application deadline:* 7/1 (fall), 11/1 (spring), 4/1 (summer). Applications may be processed on a rolling basis for some programs. *Application fee:* $50.

**Advanced Placement** Credit given for nursing courses completed elsewhere dependent upon specific evaluations.

**Degree Requirements** 45 total credit hours, thesis or project.

### POST-MASTER'S PROGRAM

**Areas of Study** Health-care administration; nurse anesthesia; nursing education. *Nurse practitioner programs in:* adult health, family health, pediatric.

### DOCTORAL DEGREE PROGRAM

**Degree** PhD

**Available Programs** Doctorate.

**Areas of Study** Faculty preparation, nursing education, nursing research.

**Program Entrance Requirements** Clinical experience, minimum overall college GPA of 3.5, interview, 3 letters of recommendation, MSN or equivalent, scholarly papers, vita, writing sample, GRE. *Application deadline:* 12/1 (fall), 12/1 (summer). *Application fee:* $70.

**Degree Requirements** 51 total credit hours, dissertation, oral exam, written exam.

## CONTINUING EDUCATION PROGRAM

**Contact** Dr. Lynore DeSilets, Assistant Dean and Director, Continuing Education, College of Nursing, Villanova University, Driscoll Hall, 800 Lancaster Avenue, Villanova, PA 19085-1690. *Telephone:* 610-519-4931. *Fax:* 610-519-6780. *E-mail:* lyn.desilets@villanova.edu.

# Waynesburg University

**Department of Nursing**
**Waynesburg, Pennsylvania**

***http://www.waynesburg.edu/***
Founded in 1849

## DEGREES • BSN • DNP • MSN • MSN/MBA

**Nursing Program Faculty** 48 (39% with doctorates).

**Baccalaureate Enrollment** 337 **Women** 91% **Men** 9% **Minority** 1%

**Graduate Enrollment** 240 **Women** 95% **Men** 5% **Minority** 1% **Part-time** 95%

**Nursing Student Activities** Sigma Theta Tau, Student Nurses' Association.

**Nursing Student Resources** Academic advising; academic or career counseling; assistance for students with disabilities; bookstore; campus computer network; career placement assistance; computer lab; computer-assisted instruction; e-mail services; employment services for current students; externships; Internet; learning resource lab; library services; nursing audiovisuals; paid internships; placement services for program completers; remedial services; resume preparation assistance; skills, simulation, or other laboratory; tutoring.

**Library Facilities** 100,000 volumes (4,500 in nursing); 1,206 periodical subscriptions (46 health-care related).

## BACCALAUREATE PROGRAMS

**Degree** BSN

**Available Programs** Accelerated Baccalaureate; Accelerated Baccalaureate for Second Degree; Generic Baccalaureate; LPN to Baccalaureate.

**Site Options** Monroeville, PA; Canonsburg, PA; Wexford, PA.

**Study Options** Full-time.

**Program Entrance Requirements** Minimum overall college GPA of 3.0, transcript of college record, CPR certification, health exam, health insurance, high school biology, high school chemistry, 2 years high school math, 2 years high school science, high school transcript, immunizations, minimum high school GPA of 3.0, minimum GPA in nursing prerequisites of 3.0, professional liability insurance/malpractice insurance, prerequisite course work. Transfer students are accepted. *Application deadline:* Applications may be processed on a rolling basis for some programs. *Application fee:* $75.

**Advanced Placement** Credit by examination available.

**Expenses (2013–14)** *Tuition:* full-time $20,180; part-time $840 per credit hour. *International tuition:* $20,180 full-time. *Room and board:* $8350; room only: $4330 per academic year. *Required fees:* full-time $1160.

**Financial Aid** 90% of baccalaureate students in nursing programs received some form of financial aid in 2012–13.

**Contact** Dr. Nancy R. Mosser, Director/Chairperson, Department of Nursing, Waynesburg University, 51 West College Street, Waynesburg, PA 15370-1222. *Telephone:* 724-852-3356. *Fax:* 724-852-3220. *E-mail:* nmosser@waynesburg.edu.

## GRADUATE PROGRAMS

**Financial Aid** 50% of graduate students in nursing programs received some form of financial aid in 2012–13.

**Contact** Dr. Kimberly Stephens, Co-Chair of Graduate and Professional Studies Program, Department of Nursing, Waynesburg University, Monroeville Center, Penn Center, Building 3, Pittsburgh, PA 15235. *Telephone:* 412-824-3700. *E-mail:* kpstephe@waynesburg.edu.

### MASTER'S DEGREE PROGRAM

**Degrees** MSN; MSN/MBA

**Available Programs** Accelerated Master's; Accelerated Master's for Nurses with Non-Nursing Degrees; Accelerated RN to Master's.

**Concentrations Available** Nursing administration; nursing education; nursing informatics.

**Site Options** Monroeville, PA; Canonsburg, PA; Wexford, PA.

**Study Options** Part-time.

**Program Entrance Requirements** Clinical experience, computer literacy, minimum overall college GPA of 3.0, transcript of college record, written essay, 2 letters of recommendation, resume, statistics course. *Application deadline:* Applications may be processed on a rolling basis for some programs. *Application fee:* $75.

**Degree Requirements** 36 total credit hours, thesis or project.

### DOCTORAL DEGREE PROGRAM

**Degree** DNP

**Available Programs** Doctorate; Post-Baccalaureate Doctorate.

**Areas of Study** Advanced practice nursing, health-care systems, nursing administration.

**Site Options** Monroeville, PA.

**Program Entrance Requirements** Minimum overall college GPA of 3.0, interview by faculty committee, interview, letters of recommendation, MSN or equivalent, statistics course, vita, writing sample. *Application deadline:* Applications may be processed on a rolling basis for some programs.

**Degree Requirements** 80 total credit hours, oral exam, written exam, residency.

# West Chester University of Pennsylvania

## Department of Nursing
## West Chester, Pennsylvania

*http://www.wcupa.edu/_academics/Healthsciences/nursing/*
Founded in 1871

**DEGREES • BSN • MSN**

**Nursing Program Faculty** 40 (28% with doctorates).
**Baccalaureate Enrollment** 384 **Women** 88% **Men** 12% **Minority** 11% **International** .5% **Part-time** 28%
**Graduate Enrollment** 42 **Women** 93% **Men** 7% **Minority** 19% **International** 1% **Part-time** 81%
**Distance Learning Courses** Available.
**Nursing Student Activities** Nursing Honor Society, Sigma Theta Tau, Student Nurses' Association.
**Nursing Student Resources** Academic advising; academic or career counseling; assistance for students with disabilities; bookstore; campus computer network; career placement assistance; computer lab; computer-assisted instruction; e-mail services; employment services for current students; externships; housing assistance; interactive nursing skills videos; Internet; learning resource lab; library services; nursing audiovisuals; remedial services; resume preparation assistance; skills, simulation, or other laboratory; tutoring.
**Library Facilities** 1.4 million volumes (88 in nursing); 7,090 periodical subscriptions (173 health-care related).

### BACCALAUREATE PROGRAMS

**Degree** BSN
**Available Programs** Accelerated Baccalaureate for Second Degree; Generic Baccalaureate; RN Baccalaureate.
**Study Options** Full-time and part-time.
**Program Entrance Requirements** Written essay, health exam, health insurance, high school biology, high school chemistry, 3 years high school math, 3 years high school science, high school transcript, minimum high school GPA, minimum high school rank. *Application deadline:* Applications may be processed on a rolling basis for some programs. *Application fee:* $45.
**Advanced Placement** Credit given for nursing courses completed elsewhere dependent upon specific evaluations.
**Expenses (2012–13)** *Tuition, state resident:* full-time $6428; part-time $268 per credit. *Tuition, nonresident:* full-time $16,070; part-time $670 per credit. *International tuition:* $16,070 full-time. *Room and board:* $7784; room only: $4848 per academic year. *Required fees:* full-time $2192; part-time $91 per credit.
**Financial Aid** 85% of baccalaureate students in nursing programs received some form of financial aid in 2011–12. *Gift aid (need-based):* Federal Pell, FSEOG, state, private, college/university gift aid from institutional funds. *Loans:* Federal Nursing Student Loans, Federal Direct (Subsidized and Unsubsidized Stafford PLUS), Perkins. *Work-study:* Federal Work-Study, part-time campus jobs. *Financial aid application deadline (priority):* 3/1.
**Contact** Dr. Cheryl Monturo, Interim Chairperson, Department of Nursing, West Chester University of Pennsylvania, 855 South New Street, West Chester, PA 19383. *Telephone:* 610-436-2693. *Fax:* 610-436-3083. *E-mail:* cmonturo@wcupa.edu.

### GRADUATE PROGRAMS

**Expenses (2012–13)** *Tuition, state resident:* full-time $8494; part-time $429 per credit. *Tuition, nonresident:* full-time $12,750; part-time $644 per credit. *International tuition:* $12,750 full-time. *Required fees:* part-time $105 per credit; part-time $865 per term.
**Financial Aid** 60% of graduate students in nursing programs received some form of financial aid in 2011–12. Unspecified assistantships available. Aid available to part-time students. *Financial aid application deadline:* 2/15.
**Contact** Dr. Ann C. Stowe, Graduate Program Coordinator, Department of Nursing, West Chester University of Pennsylvania, 855 South New Street, Sturzebecker Health Sciences Center, West Chester, PA 19383. *Telephone:* 610-436-2331. *Fax:* 610-436-3083. *E-mail:* astowe@wcupa.edu.

#### MASTER'S DEGREE PROGRAM

**Degree** MSN
**Available Programs** Master's.
**Concentrations Available** Nursing administration; nursing education. *Clinical nurse specialist programs in:* public health.
**Study Options** Full-time and part-time.
**Program Entrance Requirements** Clinical experience, minimum overall college GPA of 2.8, transcript of college record, written essay, interview, 2 letters of recommendation, physical assessment course, resume, statistics course. *Application deadline:* Applications may be processed on a rolling basis for some programs. *Application fee:* $45.
**Advanced Placement** Credit given for nursing courses completed elsewhere dependent upon specific evaluations.
**Degree Requirements** 39 total credit hours, comprehensive exam.

# Widener University

## School of Nursing
## Chester, Pennsylvania

*http://www.widener.edu/*
Founded in 1821

**DEGREES • BSN • MSN • MSN/PHD • PHD**

**Nursing Program Faculty** 93 (31% with doctorates).
**Baccalaureate Enrollment** 578 **Women** 90% **Men** 10% **Minority** 23% **International** 1% **Part-time** 1%
**Graduate Enrollment** 267 **Women** 94% **Men** 6% **Minority** 15% **Part-time** 88%
**Distance Learning Courses** Available.
**Nursing Student Activities** Nursing Honor Society, Sigma Theta Tau, Student Nurses' Association.
**Nursing Student Resources** Academic advising; academic or career counseling; assistance for students with disabilities; bookstore; campus computer network; career placement assistance; computer lab; computer-assisted instruction; e-mail services; employment services for current students; housing assistance; interactive nursing skills videos; Internet; learning resource lab; library services; nursing audiovisuals; placement services for program completers; remedial services; resume preparation assistance; skills, simulation, or other laboratory; tutoring.
**Library Facilities** 208,847 volumes (14,890 in health, 2,639 in nursing); 2,695 periodical subscriptions (451 health-care related).

### BACCALAUREATE PROGRAMS

**Degree** BSN
**Available Programs** ADN to Baccalaureate; Generic Baccalaureate; RN Baccalaureate.
**Study Options** Full-time.
**Program Entrance Requirements** Transcript of college record, health exam, health insurance, high school biology, high school chemistry, high school foreign language, 3 years high school math, 3 years high school science, high school transcript, immunizations, minimum high school GPA of 2.85, minimum GPA in nursing prerequisites of 3.0. Transfer students are accepted. *Application deadline:* Applications may be processed on a rolling basis for some programs.
**Advanced Placement** Credit by examination available. Credit given for nursing courses completed elsewhere dependent upon specific evaluations.
**Expenses (2012–13)** *Tuition:* full-time $35,764; part-time $1190 per credit. *International tuition:* $35,764 full-time. *Room and board:* $11,300; room only: $6300 per academic year. *Required fees:* full-time $795; part-time $349 per term.
**Financial Aid** 98% of baccalaureate students in nursing programs received some form of financial aid in 2011–12. *Gift aid (need-based):* Federal Pell, FSEOG, state, private, college/university gift aid from institutional funds, Federal Nursing. *Loans:* Federal Direct (Subsidized and Unsubsidized Stafford PLUS), Perkins. *Work-study:* Federal Work-Study, part-time campus jobs. *Financial aid application deadline (priority):* 2/15.
**Contact** Dr. Rose Schwartz, RN, Director, Prelicensure BSN, School of Nursing, Widener University, One University Place, Chester, PA 19013-5892. *Telephone:* 610-499-4211. *Fax:* 610-499-4216. *E-mail:* raschwartz@widener.edu.

### GRADUATE PROGRAMS

**Expenses (2012–13)** *Tuition:* part-time $840 per credit. *Required fees:* part-time $111 per credit.
**Financial Aid** 49% of graduate students in nursing programs received some form of financial aid in 2011–12. Career-related internships or fieldwork, Federal Work-Study, and traineeships available. Aid available to part-time students. *Financial aid application deadline:* 4/1.

**Contact** Mrs. Betty Boyles, Administrative Assistant for Graduate Programs, School of Nursing, Widener University, One University Place, Chester, PA 19013-5892. *Telephone:* 610-499-4208. *Fax:* 610-499-4216. *E-mail:* eaboyles@widener.edu.

### MASTER'S DEGREE PROGRAM

**Degrees** MSN; MSN/PhD
**Available Programs** Master's; Master's for Nurses with Non-Nursing Degrees.
**Concentrations Available** Nursing education. *Clinical nurse specialist programs in:* acute care, adult health, critical care, gerontology. *Nurse practitioner programs in:* family health.
**Site Options** Harrisburg, PA.
**Study Options** Full-time and part-time.
**Program Entrance Requirements** Clinical experience, computer literacy, minimum overall college GPA of 3.0, transcript of college record, immunizations, interview, 2 letters of recommendation, nursing research course, resume, statistics course, GRE General Test. *Application deadline:* 7/15 (fall), 11/15 (spring), 3/16 (summer). Applications may be processed on a rolling basis for some programs.
**Advanced Placement** Credit given for nursing courses completed elsewhere dependent upon specific evaluations.
**Degree Requirements** 42 total credit hours.

### POST-MASTER'S PROGRAM

**Areas of Study** Nursing education. *Clinical nurse specialist programs in:* acute care, adult health, critical care, gerontology. *Nurse practitioner programs in:* family health.

### DOCTORAL DEGREE PROGRAM

**Degree** PhD
**Available Programs** Doctorate.
**Areas of Study** Faculty preparation, nursing education, nursing research, nursing science.
**Program Entrance Requirements** Minimum overall college GPA of 3.5, interview, 2 letters of recommendation, MSN or equivalent, statistics course, vita, writing sample, GRE General Test. *Application deadline:* 7/15 (fall), 11/15 (spring), 3/17 (summer). Applications may be processed on a rolling basis for some programs.
**Degree Requirements** 63 total credit hours, dissertation, written exam.

### CONTINUING EDUCATION PROGRAM

**Contact** Ms. Marcia Bowers, Director for Community Relations and Continuing Education, School of Nursing, Widener University, One University Place, Chester, PA 19013. *Telephone:* 610-499-1327. *Fax:* 610-499-4216. *E-mail:* mdbowers@widener.edu.

# Wilkes University

## Department of Nursing
## Wilkes-Barre, Pennsylvania

*http://www.wilkes.edu/*
Founded in 1933

### DEGREES • BS • MS

**Nursing Program Faculty** 25 (20% with doctorates).
**Baccalaureate Enrollment** 300 **Women** 90% **Men** 10% **Minority** 5% **Part-time** 15%
**Graduate Enrollment** 65 **Women** 85% **Men** 15% **Minority** 5% **Part-time** 75%
**Distance Learning Courses** Available.
**Nursing Student Activities** Sigma Theta Tau, Student Nurses' Association, nursing club.
**Nursing Student Resources** Academic advising; academic or career counseling; assistance for students with disabilities; bookstore; campus computer network; career placement assistance; computer lab; computer-assisted instruction; daycare for children of students; e-mail services; employment services for current students; externships; housing assistance; interactive nursing skills videos; Internet; learning resource lab; library services; nursing audiovisuals; paid internships; placement services for program completers; remedial services; resume preparation assistance; skills, simulation, or other laboratory; tutoring; unpaid internships.
**Library Facilities** 13,450 volumes in health, 13,000 volumes in nursing; 70 periodical subscriptions health-care related.

### BACCALAUREATE PROGRAMS

**Degree** BS
**Available Programs** ADN to Baccalaureate; Accelerated Baccalaureate for Second Degree; Accelerated LPN to Baccalaureate; Accelerated RN Baccalaureate; Generic Baccalaureate; LPN to RN Baccalaureate; RN Baccalaureate.
**Study Options** Full-time and part-time.
**Program Entrance Requirements** Minimum overall college GPA of 2.0, transcript of college record, CPR certification, health exam, health insurance, high school biology, high school chemistry, 2 years high school math, 3 years high school science, high school transcript, immunizations, minimum high school GPA, professional liability insurance/malpractice insurance. Transfer students are accepted.
**Advanced Placement** Credit by examination available. Credit given for nursing courses completed elsewhere dependent upon specific evaluations.
**Contact** *Telephone:* 570-408-4074. *Fax:* 570-408-7807.

### GRADUATE PROGRAMS

**Contact** *Telephone:* 570-408-4078. *Fax:* 570-408-7807.

### MASTER'S DEGREE PROGRAM

**Degree** MS
**Available Programs** Accelerated AD/RN to Master's; Accelerated RN to Master's; Master's; Master's for Non-Nursing College Graduates; RN to Master's.
**Concentrations Available** Nursing administration; nursing education. *Clinical nurse specialist programs in:* gerontology, psychiatric/mental health.
**Study Options** Full-time and part-time.
**Program Entrance Requirements** Clinical experience, minimum overall college GPA of 3.0, transcript of college record, CPR certification, immunizations, interview, 3 letters of recommendation, nursing research course, physical assessment course, professional liability insurance/malpractice insurance, statistics course.
**Advanced Placement** Credit given for nursing courses completed elsewhere dependent upon specific evaluations.
**Degree Requirements** 37 total credit hours, thesis or project.

### POST-MASTER'S PROGRAM

**Areas of Study** Nursing administration; nursing education. *Clinical nurse specialist programs in:* gerontology, psychiatric/mental health.

### CONTINUING EDUCATION PROGRAM

**Contact** *Telephone:* 570-408-4462.

# York College of Pennsylvania

## Department of Nursing
## York, Pennsylvania

*http://www.ycp.edu/academics/academic-departments/nursing/*
Founded in 1787

### DEGREES • BS • DNP • MS

**Nursing Program Faculty** 74 (26% with doctorates).
**Baccalaureate Enrollment** 614 **Women** 94% **Men** 6% **Minority** 4% **Part-time** 6%
**Graduate Enrollment** 94 **Women** 92% **Men** 8% **Minority** 6% **International** 1% **Part-time** 47%
**Distance Learning Courses** Available.
**Nursing Student Activities** Sigma Theta Tau, Student Nurses' Association, nursing club.
**Nursing Student Resources** Academic advising; academic or career counseling; assistance for students with disabilities; bookstore; campus computer network; career placement assistance; computer lab; computer-assisted instruction; e-mail services; employment services for current students; externships; housing assistance; interactive nursing skills videos; Internet; learning resource lab; library services; nursing audiovisuals; paid internships; placement services for program completers; remedial services; resume preparation assistance; skills, simulation, or other laboratory; tutoring.
**Library Facilities** 429,072 volumes (6,681 in health, 1,226 in nursing); 40,557 periodical subscriptions (83 health-care related).

## BACCALAUREATE PROGRAMS

**Degree** BS
**Available Programs** ADN to Baccalaureate; Generic Baccalaureate; LPN to Baccalaureate; RN Baccalaureate.
**Study Options** Full-time and part-time.
**Program Entrance Requirements** Minimum overall college GPA of 2.8, transcript of college record, CPR certification, health exam, health insurance, high school biology, high school chemistry, 1 year of high school math, 3 years high school science, high school transcript, immunizations, 2 letters of recommendation, minimum high school GPA of 3.4, minimum high school rank 40%, minimum GPA in nursing prerequisites of 2.8, professional liability insurance/malpractice insurance, prerequisite course work. *Application deadline:* Applications may be processed on a rolling basis for some programs.
**Advanced Placement** Credit by examination available. Credit given for nursing courses completed elsewhere dependent upon specific evaluations.
**Expenses (2012–13)** *Tuition:* full-time $14,900. *Room and board:* $9300; room only: $5220 per academic year. *Required fees:* full-time $1620.
**Financial Aid** 90% of baccalaureate students in nursing programs received some form of financial aid in 2011–12. *Gift aid (need-based):* Federal Pell, FSEOG, state, private, college/university gift aid from institutional funds. *Loans:* Federal Nursing Student Loans, Federal Direct (Subsidized and Unsubsidized Stafford PLUS), Perkins, college/university. *Work-study:* Federal Work-Study, part-time campus jobs. *Financial aid application deadline:* Continuous.
**Contact** Karen S. March, Chairperson and Professor, Department of Nursing, York College of Pennsylvania, 441 Country Club Road, York, PA 17405-7199. *Telephone:* 717-815-1243. *Fax:* 717-849-1651. *E-mail:* kmarch@ycp.edu.

## GRADUATE PROGRAMS

**Expenses (2012–13)** *Tuition:* part-time $670 per credit. *Required fees:* part-time $340 per term.
**Financial Aid** 8% of graduate students in nursing programs received some form of financial aid in 2011–12.
**Contact** Dr. Linda Coniff Pugh, Director, Department of Nursing, York College of Pennsylvania, York, PA 17405-7199. *Telephone:* 717-815-6592. *Fax:* 717-849-1659. *E-mail:* lpugh@ycp.edu.

### MASTER'S DEGREE PROGRAM

**Degree** MS
**Available Programs** Master's; RN to Master's.
**Concentrations Available** Nurse anesthesia; nursing education. *Clinical nurse specialist programs in:* adult health. *Nurse practitioner programs in:* adult health.
**Study Options** Part-time.
**Program Entrance Requirements** Clinical experience, computer literacy, minimum overall college GPA of 3.0, transcript of college record, CPR certification, written essay, immunizations, interview, 2 letters of recommendation, nursing research course, physical assessment course, professional liability insurance/malpractice insurance, resume, statistics course. *Application deadline:* 6/30 (fall). Applications may be processed on a rolling basis for some programs. *Application fee:* $50.
**Advanced Placement** Credit given for nursing courses completed elsewhere dependent upon specific evaluations.
**Degree Requirements** 41 total credit hours, thesis or project.

### POST-MASTER'S PROGRAM

**Areas of Study** *Nurse practitioner programs in:* adult health.

### DOCTORAL DEGREE PROGRAM

**Degree** DNP
**Available Programs** Doctorate.
**Areas of Study** Advanced practice nursing, clinical practice, health policy, health-care systems, individualized study, information systems, nursing policy, nursing science.
**Program Entrance Requirements** Clinical experience, minimum overall college GPA of 3.5, interview by faculty committee, 2 letters of recommendation, MSN or equivalent, statistics course, vita, writing sample. *Application deadline:* 3/1 (fall). Applications may be processed on a rolling basis for some programs. *Application fee:* $50.
**Degree Requirements** 37 total credit hours, residency.

# PUERTO RICO

## Inter American University of Puerto Rico, Aguadilla Campus

### Nursing Program
### Aguadilla, Puerto Rico

Founded in 1957

**DEGREE • BSN**
**Nursing Program Faculty** 20 (20% with doctorates).
**Baccalaureate Enrollment** 397 **Women** 69% **Men** 31%
**Nursing Student Activities** Student Nurses' Association.
**Nursing Student Resources** Academic advising; assistance for students with disabilities; campus computer network; computer lab; computer-assisted instruction; e-mail services; interactive nursing skills videos; Internet; learning resource lab; library services; nursing audiovisuals; skills, simulation, or other laboratory; tutoring.
**Library Facilities** 61,452 volumes; 215 periodical subscriptions (36 health-care related).

### BACCALAUREATE PROGRAMS

**Degree** BSN
**Available Programs** RN Baccalaureate.
**Site Options** Aguadilla, PR.
**Study Options** Full-time.
**Program Entrance Requirements** Minimum overall college GPA of 2.50, transcript of college record, CPR certification, high school transcript, immunizations, minimum high school GPA of 2.50. Transfer students are accepted.
**Advanced Placement** Credit given for nursing courses completed elsewhere dependent upon specific evaluations.
**Financial Aid** ***Loans:*** Perkins. *Work-study:* Federal Work-Study.
**Contact** Admissions, Nursing Program, Inter American University of Puerto Rico, Aguadilla Campus, PO Box 20000, Aguadilla, PR 00605. *Telephone:* 787-891-0925. *E-mail:* dperez@aguadilla.inter.edu.

## Inter American University of Puerto Rico, Arecibo Campus

### Nursing Program
### Arecibo, Puerto Rico

Founded in 1957

**DEGREE • BS**
**Library Facilities** 73,642 volumes; 640 periodical subscriptions.

### BACCALAUREATE PROGRAMS

**Degree** BS
**Available Programs** Generic Baccalaureate.
**Contact** *Telephone:* 787-878-5475.

## Inter American University of Puerto Rico, Metropolitan Campus

### Carmen Torres de Tiburcio School of Nursing
### San Juan, Puerto Rico

***http://www.metro.inter.edu/index.asp***
Founded in 1960

**DEGREE • BSN**
**Nursing Program Faculty** 26 (27% with doctorates).
**Baccalaureate Enrollment** 312 **Women** 57% **Men** 43%
**Nursing Student Activities** Student Nurses' Association.
**Nursing Student Resources** Academic advising; academic or career counseling; assistance for students with disabilities; bookstore; campus computer network; career placement assistance; computer lab; computer-assisted instruction; daycare for children of students; e-mail services; employment services for current students; externships; interactive

nursing skills videos; Internet; learning resource lab; library services; nursing audiovisuals; paid internships; placement services for program completers; remedial services; skills, simulation, or other laboratory; tutoring.
**Library Facilities** 171,173 volumes (36,000 in health, 21,759 in nursing); 41,660 periodical subscriptions (2,090 health-care related).

### BACCALAUREATE PROGRAMS

**Degree** BSN
**Available Programs** ADN to Baccalaureate; Accelerated Baccalaureate; Generic Baccalaureate.
**Study Options** Full-time and part-time.
**Program Entrance Requirements** Minimum overall college GPA of 2.0, transcript of college record, CPR certification, health exam, health insurance, high school transcript, immunizations, 2 letters of recommendation, minimum high school rank 4%, minimum GPA in nursing prerequisites of 2. Transfer students are accepted.
**Advanced Placement** Credit by examination available. Credit given for nursing courses completed elsewhere dependent upon specific evaluations.
**Contact** *Telephone:* 787-763-3066. *Fax:* 787-250-1242 Ext. 2159.

## Pontifical Catholic University of Puerto Rico

**Department of Nursing**
**Ponce, Puerto Rico**

*http://www.pucpr.edu/*
Founded in 1948

**DEGREE • BSN**

**Library Facilities** 1,499 volumes in nursing.

### BACCALAUREATE PROGRAMS

**Degree** BSN
**Available Programs** Generic Baccalaureate.
**Program Entrance Requirements** Minimum overall college GPA of 2.0, CPR certification, health exam, health insurance, immunizations, interview, letters of recommendation, minimum high school GPA of 2.5, prerequisite course work.
**Contact** *Telephone:* 787-841-2000 Ext. 1604.

## Universidad Adventista de las Antillas

**Department of Nursing**
**Mayagüez, Puerto Rico**

Founded in 1957

**DEGREE • BSN**

**Nursing Program Faculty** 11 (18% with doctorates).
**Baccalaureate Enrollment** 257 **Women** 69% **Men** 31% **Minority** 100%
**International** 13% **Part-time** 1%
**Nursing Student Activities** Nursing club.
**Nursing Student Resources** Academic advising; academic or career counseling; assistance for students with disabilities; campus computer network; computer lab; computer-assisted instruction; e-mail services; employment services for current students; housing assistance; interactive nursing skills videos; Internet; learning resource lab; library services; nursing audiovisuals; remedial services; resume preparation assistance; skills, simulation, or other laboratory; tutoring; unpaid internships.
**Library Facilities** 67,345 volumes (2,488 in health, 1,556 in nursing); 105 periodical subscriptions (29 health-care related).

### BACCALAUREATE PROGRAMS

**Degree** BSN
**Available Programs** Generic Baccalaureate; RN Baccalaureate.
**Study Options** Full-time.
**Program Entrance Requirements** Minimum overall college GPA of 2.3, transcript of college record, health exam, health insurance, high school transcript, immunizations, interview, 2 letters of recommendation, minimum high school GPA of 2.5. Transfer students are accepted.
**Advanced Placement** Credit given for nursing courses completed elsewhere dependent upon specific evaluations.
**Contact** *Telephone:* 787-834-9595 Ext. 2209. *Fax:* 787-834-9597.

### CONTINUING EDUCATION PROGRAM

**Contact** *Telephone:* 787-834-9595 Ext. 2284. *Fax:* 787-834-9597.

## Universidad del Turabo

**Nursing Program**
**Gurabo, Puerto Rico**

Founded in 1972

**DEGREE • BS**

### BACCALAUREATE PROGRAMS

**Degree** BS
**Available Programs** Generic Baccalaureate.
**Contact** *Telephone:* 787-743-7979.

## Universidad Metropolitana

**Department of Nursing**
**San Juan, Puerto Rico**

*http://www.suagm.edu/umet/oa_pe_cs_programas.asp?cn_id=686*
Founded in 1980

**DEGREE • BSN**

**Library Facilities** 5,438 volumes in health; 110 periodical subscriptions health-care related.

### BACCALAUREATE PROGRAMS

**Degree** BSN
**Contact** *Telephone:* 787-766-1717 Ext. 6422. *Fax:* 787-769-7663.

## University of Puerto Rico in Arecibo

**Department of Nursing**
**Arecibo, Puerto Rico**

*http://www.upra.edu/*
Founded in 1967

**DEGREE • BSN**

**Nursing Program Faculty** 21
**Library Facilities** 65,000 volumes; 3,660 periodical subscriptions.

### BACCALAUREATE PROGRAMS

**Degree** BSN
**Available Programs** Generic Baccalaureate.
**Contact** *Telephone:* 787-878-2830. *Fax:* 787-880-4972.

## University of Puerto Rico in Humacao

**Department of Nursing**
**Humacao, Puerto Rico**

*http://www1.uprh.edu/enfe/*
Founded in 1962

**DEGREE • BS**

**Nursing Program Faculty** 16 (12% with doctorates).
**Nursing Student Activities** Student Nurses' Association.
**Nursing Student Resources** Skills, simulation, or other laboratory.
**Library Facilities** 75,518 volumes; 57,383 periodical subscriptions.

### BACCALAUREATE PROGRAMS

**Degree** BS

**Available Programs** Generic Baccalaureate.
**Study Options** Full-time and part-time.
**Program Entrance Requirements** Minimum overall college GPA, transcript of college record, health exam, health insurance, high school transcript, immunizations, minimum high school GPA of 2.0, minimum GPA in nursing prerequisites of 2.5. Transfer students are accepted.
**Advanced Placement** Credit by examination available. Credit given for nursing courses completed elsewhere dependent upon specific evaluations.
**Contact** *Telephone:* 787-850-9346. *Fax:* 787-850-9411.

## University of Puerto Rico, Mayagüez Campus

### Department of Nursing
### Mayagüez, Puerto Rico

***http://www.uprm.edu/enfe/***
Founded in 1911

**DEGREE • BSN**
**Nursing Program Faculty** 21 (10% with doctorates).
**Nursing Student Activities** Nursing Honor Society, Sigma Theta Tau, Student Nurses' Association.
**Nursing Student Resources** Academic advising; academic or career counseling; assistance for students with disabilities; bookstore; campus computer network; career placement assistance; computer lab; computer-assisted instruction; e-mail services; employment services for current students; interactive nursing skills videos; Internet; learning resource lab; library services; nursing audiovisuals; paid internships; placement services for program completers; remedial services; resume preparation assistance; skills, simulation, or other laboratory; tutoring.
**Library Facilities** 68 periodical subscriptions health-care related.

#### BACCALAUREATE PROGRAMS

**Degree** BSN
**Available Programs** Generic Baccalaureate.
**Study Options** Full-time.
**Program Entrance Requirements** High school transcript, immunizations. Transfer students are accepted.
**Advanced Placement** Credit by examination available.
**Contact** *Telephone:* 787-263-3482. *Fax:* 787-832-3875.

#### CONTINUING EDUCATION PROGRAM

**Contact** *Telephone:* 787-265-3842. *Fax:* 787-832-3875.

## University of Puerto Rico, Medical Sciences Campus

### School of Nursing
### San Juan, Puerto Rico

***http://www.md.rcm.upr.edu/***
Founded in 1950

**DEGREES • BSN • MSN**
**Nursing Program Faculty** 37 (25% with doctorates).
**Baccalaureate Enrollment** 241 **Women** 85% **Men** 15% **Part-time** 12%
**Graduate Enrollment** 158 **Women** 79% **Men** 21% **Part-time** 6%
**Nursing Student Activities** Sigma Theta Tau, Student Nurses' Association.
**Nursing Student Resources** Academic advising; academic or career counseling; assistance for students with disabilities; computer lab; computer-assisted instruction; e-mail services; employment services for current students; interactive nursing skills videos; Internet; library services; nursing audiovisuals; skills, simulation, or other laboratory; tutoring.
**Library Facilities** 7,830 volumes in health, 1,143 volumes in nursing; 1,215 periodical subscriptions health-care related.

#### BACCALAUREATE PROGRAMS

**Degree** BSN
**Available Programs** ADN to Baccalaureate; Generic Baccalaureate.
**Study Options** Full-time and part-time.
**Program Entrance Requirements** Minimum overall college GPA of 2.0, transcript of college record, health exam, immunizations, interview, minimum high school GPA of 2.0, prerequisite course work. Transfer students are accepted.
**Contact** *Telephone:* 787-758-2525 Ext. 1984. *Fax:* 787-281-0721.

#### GRADUATE PROGRAMS

**Contact** *Telephone:* 787-758-2525 Ext. 3105. *Fax:* 787-281-0721.

**MASTER'S DEGREE PROGRAM**
**Degree** MSN
**Available Programs** Master's.
**Concentrations Available** Nurse anesthesia; nursing administration; nursing education. *Clinical nurse specialist programs in:* adult health, community health, critical care, gerontology, maternity-newborn, pediatric, psychiatric/mental health.
**Site Options** Mayaguez, PR.
**Study Options** Full-time and part-time.
**Program Entrance Requirements** Clinical experience, minimum overall college GPA of 2.5, transcript of college record, immunizations, interview, resume, statistics course, GRE or EXADEP.
**Degree Requirements** 48 total credit hours, thesis or project.

#### CONTINUING EDUCATION PROGRAM

**Contact** *Telephone:* 787-758-2525 Ext. 2102. *Fax:* 787-281-0721.

## University of the Sacred Heart

### Program in Nursing
### San Juan, Puerto Rico

Founded in 1935

**DEGREES • BSN • MSN**
**Nursing Student Resources** Skills, simulation, or other laboratory.

#### BACCALAUREATE PROGRAMS

**Degree** BSN
**Available Programs** Generic Baccalaureate.
**Contact** *Telephone:* 787-728-1515. *Fax:* 787-727-1250.

#### GRADUATE PROGRAMS

**Contact** *Telephone:* 787-728-1515 Ext. 2427. *Fax:* 787-727-1250.

**MASTER'S DEGREE PROGRAM**
**Degree** MSN
**Available Programs** Master's.
**Concentrations Available** *Nurse practitioner programs in:* occupational health.
**Degree Requirements** 37 total credit hours.

# RHODE ISLAND

## Rhode Island College

### Department of Nursing
### Providence, Rhode Island

***http://www.ric.edu/nursing***
Founded in 1854

**DEGREES • BSN • MSN**
**Nursing Program Faculty** 49 (39% with doctorates).
**Baccalaureate Enrollment** 415 **Women** 89% **Men** 11% **Minority** 36% **Part-time** 38%
**Graduate Enrollment** 43 **Women** 98% **Men** 2% **Minority** 19% **Part-time** 98%
**Distance Learning Courses** Available.
**Nursing Student Activities** Sigma Theta Tau, Student Nurses' Association, nursing club.
**Nursing Student Resources** Academic advising; academic or career counseling; assistance for students with disabilities; bookstore; campus computer network; career placement assistance; computer lab; computer-assisted instruction; daycare for children of students; e-mail services;

employment services for current students; housing assistance; interactive nursing skills videos; Internet; learning resource lab; library services; nursing audiovisuals; paid internships; placement services for program completers; remedial services; resume preparation assistance; skills, simulation, or other laboratory; tutoring.
**Library Facilities** 714,853 volumes (574 in nursing); 1.3 million periodical subscriptions (63 health-care related).

## BACCALAUREATE PROGRAMS

**Degree** BSN
**Available Programs** Baccalaureate for Second Degree; Generic Baccalaureate; RN Baccalaureate.
**Site Options** Providence, RI.
**Study Options** Full-time and part-time.
**Program Entrance Requirements** Minimum overall college GPA of 2.7, CPR certification, health exam, health insurance, high school biology, high school chemistry, high school foreign language, 4 years high school math, 2 years high school science, high school transcript, immunizations, letters of recommendation, minimum GPA in nursing prerequisites of 3.0, prerequisite course work. Transfer students are accepted. *Application deadline:* 10/15 (fall), 4/15 (spring).
**Advanced Placement** Credit given for nursing courses completed elsewhere dependent upon specific evaluations.
**Contact** *Telephone:* 401-456-8014. *Fax:* 401-456-8206.

## GRADUATE PROGRAMS

**Contact** *Telephone:* 401-456-9720. *Fax:* 401-456-8206.

### MASTER'S DEGREE PROGRAM

**Degree** MSN
**Available Programs** Master's.
**Concentrations Available** *Clinical nurse specialist programs in:* acute care, adult health, community health. *Nurse practitioner programs in:* acute care, adult health.
**Site Options** Providence, RI.
**Study Options** Full-time and part-time.
**Program Entrance Requirements** Minimum overall college GPA of 3.0, transcript of college record, written essay, letters of recommendation, resume, statistics course. *Application deadline:* 2/15 (fall). *Application fee:* $50.
**Advanced Placement** Credit given for nursing courses completed elsewhere dependent upon specific evaluations.
**Degree Requirements** 45 total credit hours, thesis or project.

# Salve Regina University

## Department of Nursing
## Newport, Rhode Island

***http://www.salve.edu/academics/departments/nur/***
Founded in 1934

### DEGREE • BS

**Nursing Program Faculty** 23 (18% with doctorates).
**Baccalaureate Enrollment** 314 **Women** 91% **Men** 9% **Minority** 10% **International** 1% **Part-time** 15%
**Nursing Student Activities** Sigma Theta Tau, Student Nurses' Association, nursing club.
**Nursing Student Resources** Academic advising; academic or career counseling; assistance for students with disabilities; bookstore; campus computer network; career placement assistance; computer lab; computer-assisted instruction; e-mail services; housing assistance; interactive nursing skills videos; Internet; learning resource lab; library services; nursing audiovisuals; paid internships; resume preparation assistance; skills, simulation, or other laboratory; tutoring; unpaid internships.
**Library Facilities** 6,882 volumes in health, 1,081 volumes in nursing; 76 periodical subscriptions health-care related.

## BACCALAUREATE PROGRAMS

**Degree** BS
**Available Programs** Generic Baccalaureate; RN Baccalaureate.
**Site Options** Warwick, RI.
**Study Options** Full-time and part-time.
**Program Entrance Requirements** Minimum overall college GPA of 2.7, transcript of college record, written essay, high school biology, high school chemistry, high school foreign language, 3 years high school math, 3 years high school science, high school transcript, 2 letters of recommendation, minimum GPA in nursing prerequisites of 2.0, prerequisite course work. Transfer students are accepted. *Application deadline:* 2/1 (fall). Applications may be processed on a rolling basis for some programs. *Application fee:* $50.
**Advanced Placement** Credit by examination available. Credit given for nursing courses completed elsewhere dependent upon specific evaluations.
**Expenses (2012–13)** *Tuition:* full-time $33,450; part-time $1115 per credit. *International tuition:* $33,450 full-time. *Room and board:* $11,950; room only: $7000 per academic year. *Required fees:* full-time $500; part-time $40 per term.
**Financial Aid** 85% of baccalaureate students in nursing programs received some form of financial aid in 2011–12. *Gift aid (need-based):* Federal Pell, FSEOG, state, private, college/university gift aid from institutional funds. *Loans:* Federal Nursing Student Loans, Federal Direct (Subsidized and Unsubsidized Stafford PLUS), Perkins, college/university, alternative loans. *Work-study:* Federal Work-Study, part-time campus jobs. *Financial aid application deadline (priority):* 3/1.
**Contact** Mrs. Colleen Emerson, Dean of Undergraduate Admissions, Department of Nursing, Salve Regina University, 100 Ochre Point Avenue, Newport, RI 02840-4192. *Telephone:* 888-467-2583. *Fax:* 401-848-2823. *E-mail:* sruadmis@salve.edu.

## CONTINUING EDUCATION PROGRAM

**Contact** Ms. Kelly Alverson, Director of Continuing Education and Graduate Enrollment, Department of Nursing, Salve Regina University, Graduate Studies and Continuing Education Office, Newport, RI 02840-4192. *Telephone:* 800-637-0002. *Fax:* 401-341-2973. *E-mail:* kelly.alverson@salve.edu.

# University of Rhode Island

## College of Nursing
## Kingston, Rhode Island

***http://www.uri.edu/nursing***
Founded in 1892

### DEGREES • BS • MS • PHD

**Nursing Program Faculty** 47 (50% with doctorates).
**Baccalaureate Enrollment** 851 **Women** 87% **Men** 13% **Minority** 24% **International** 1% **Part-time** 10%
**Graduate Enrollment** 110 **Women** 95% **Men** 5% **Minority** 5% **International** 6% **Part-time** 75%
**Nursing Student Activities** Sigma Theta Tau, Student Nurses' Association.
**Nursing Student Resources** Academic advising; academic or career counseling; assistance for students with disabilities; bookstore; campus computer network; career placement assistance; computer lab; computer-assisted instruction; e-mail services; externships; housing assistance; interactive nursing skills videos; Internet; learning resource lab; library services; nursing audiovisuals; remedial services; resume preparation assistance; skills, simulation, or other laboratory; tutoring.
**Library Facilities** 1.4 million volumes.

## BACCALAUREATE PROGRAMS

**Degree** BS
**Available Programs** ADN to Baccalaureate; Generic Baccalaureate; RN Baccalaureate.
**Site Options** Providence, RI.
**Study Options** Full-time and part-time.
**Program Entrance Requirements** Minimum overall college GPA of 2.5, transcript of college record, CPR certification, written essay, health exam, health insurance, high school foreign language, 3 years high school math, 2 years high school science, high school transcript, immunizations, 2 letters of recommendation, minimum high school rank 30%, minimum GPA in nursing prerequisites of 2.2. Transfer students are accepted.
**Advanced Placement** Credit given for nursing courses completed elsewhere dependent upon specific evaluations.
**Contact** *Telephone:* 401-874-7100.

## GRADUATE PROGRAMS

**Contact** *Telephone:* 401-874-2766. *Fax:* 401-874-2061.

### MASTER'S DEGREE PROGRAM

**Degree** MS
**Available Programs** Master's; RN to Master's.

**Concentrations Available** Clinical nurse leader; nursing administration; nursing education. *Clinical nurse specialist programs in:* gerontology, psychiatric/mental health. *Nurse practitioner programs in:* family health, gerontology.
**Site Options** Providence, RI.
**Study Options** Full-time and part-time.
**Program Entrance Requirements** Clinical experience, minimum overall college GPA of 3.0, transcript of college record, written essay, immunizations, 3 letters of recommendation, nursing research course, professional liability insurance/malpractice insurance, resume, statistics course, GRE or MAT.
**Degree Requirements** 41 total credit hours, thesis or project, comprehensive exam.

**POST-MASTER'S PROGRAM**
**Areas of Study** Nursing administration; nursing education. *Clinical nurse specialist programs in:* gerontology, psychiatric/mental health. *Nurse practitioner programs in:* family health, gerontology.

**DOCTORAL DEGREE PROGRAM**
**Degree** PhD
**Available Programs** Doctorate.
**Areas of Study** Nursing research, nursing science.
**Program Entrance Requirements** Clinical experience, minimum overall college GPA of 3.0, interview by faculty committee, 3 letters of recommendation, MSN or equivalent, scholarly papers, statistics course, vita, writing sample, GRE.
**Degree Requirements** 61 total credit hours, dissertation, oral exam, written exam, residency.

# SOUTH CAROLINA

## Charleston Southern University
### Wingo School of Nursing
### Charleston, South Carolina

***http://www.csuniv.edu/***
Founded in 1964

**DEGREES • BSN • MSN**
**Nursing Program Faculty** 18 (22% with doctorates).
**Baccalaureate Enrollment** 111 **Women** 90% **Men** 10% **Minority** 25%
**Graduate Enrollment** 16 **Women** 99% **Men** 1% **Minority** 10%
**Distance Learning Courses** Available.
**Nursing Student Activities** Sigma Theta Tau, Student Nurses' Association.
**Nursing Student Resources** Academic advising; academic or career counseling; assistance for students with disabilities; bookstore; campus computer network; career placement assistance; computer lab; computer-assisted instruction; e-mail services; externships; interactive nursing skills videos; Internet; learning resource lab; library services; nursing audiovisuals; remedial services; resume preparation assistance; skills, simulation, or other laboratory; tutoring.
**Library Facilities** 192,600 volumes (2,400 in health, 250 in nursing); 1,111 periodical subscriptions (55 health-care related).

#### BACCALAUREATE PROGRAMS
**Degree** BSN
**Available Programs** ADN to Baccalaureate; Generic Baccalaureate; RN Baccalaureate.
**Study Options** Full-time.
**Online Degree Options** Yes.
**Program Entrance Requirements** Minimum overall college GPA of 2.75, transcript of college record, CPR certification, written essay, health exam, health insurance, immunizations, minimum GPA in nursing prerequisites of 3.0, professional liability insurance/malpractice insurance, prerequisite course work. Transfer students are accepted. *Application deadline:* 3/15 (fall).
**Advanced Placement** Credit given for nursing courses completed elsewhere dependent upon specific evaluations.
**Contact** *Telephone:* 843-863-7075. *Fax:* 843-863-7540.

#### GRADUATE PROGRAMS
**Contact** *Telephone:* 843-863-7075. *Fax:* 843-863-7540.

**MASTER'S DEGREE PROGRAM**
**Degree** MSN
**Available Programs** Master's; RN to Master's.
**Concentrations Available** Nursing education.
**Study Options** Full-time.
**Online Degree Options** Yes (online only).
**Program Entrance Requirements** Clinical experience, minimum overall college GPA of 3.0, transcript of college record, written essay, 3 letters of recommendation, resume. *Application deadline:* 6/31 (fall). *Application fee:* $20.
**Advanced Placement** Credit given for nursing courses completed elsewhere dependent upon specific evaluations.
**Degree Requirements** 39 total credit hours, thesis or project.

## Clemson University
### School of Nursing
### Clemson, South Carolina

***http://www.clemson.edu/hehd/departments/nursing/***
Founded in 1889

**DEGREES • BS • MS**
**Nursing Program Faculty** 22 (71% with doctorates).
**Baccalaureate Enrollment** 402 **Women** 99% **Men** 1% **Minority** 11%
**Graduate Enrollment** 82 **Women** 90% **Men** 10% **Minority** 8% **Part-time** 54%
**Distance Learning Courses** Available.
**Nursing Student Activities** Nursing Honor Society, Sigma Theta Tau, Student Nurses' Association.
**Nursing Student Resources** Academic advising; academic or career counseling; assistance for students with disabilities; bookstore; campus computer network; career placement assistance; computer lab; computer-assisted instruction; e-mail services; employment services for current students; externships; housing assistance; interactive nursing skills videos; Internet; learning resource lab; library services; nursing audiovisuals; other; remedial services; resume preparation assistance; skills, simulation, or other laboratory; tutoring; unpaid internships.
**Library Facilities** 1.2 million volumes (29,800 in health, 5,548 in nursing); 5,587 periodical subscriptions (877 health-care related).

#### BACCALAUREATE PROGRAMS
**Degree** BS
**Available Programs** Accelerated Baccalaureate; Generic Baccalaureate; RN Baccalaureate.
**Site Options** Greenville, SC.
**Study Options** Full-time and part-time.
**Program Entrance Requirements** Minimum overall college GPA of 2.5, transcript of college record, CPR certification, health insurance, high school biology, high school chemistry, 3 years high school math, 3 years high school science, high school transcript, immunizations, minimum high school GPA of 2.5, professional liability insurance/malpractice insurance, prerequisite course work. Transfer students are accepted.
**Advanced Placement** Credit by examination available. Credit given for nursing courses completed elsewhere dependent upon specific evaluations.
**Financial Aid** 90% of baccalaureate students in nursing programs received some form of financial aid in 2011–12. *Gift aid (need-based):* Federal Pell, FSEOG, state, private, college/university gift aid from institutional funds. *Loans:* Federal Direct (Subsidized and Unsubsidized Stafford PLUS), Perkins, state, college/university, private loans. *Work-study:* Federal Work-Study, part-time campus jobs. *Financial aid application deadline (priority):* 3/1.
**Contact** Mr. Robert S. Barkley, Director of Admissions, School of Nursing, Clemson University, 106 Sikes Hall, Clemson, SC 29634. *Telephone:* 864-656-5463. *Fax:* 864-656-2464. *E-mail:* rbrtbkl@clemson.edu.

#### GRADUATE PROGRAMS
**Financial Aid** 75% of graduate students in nursing programs received some form of financial aid in 2011–12. 2 fellowships with partial tuition reimbursements available (averaging $11,000 per year), 1 research assistantship with partial tuition reimbursement available (averaging $6,900 per year), 24 teaching assistantships with partial tuition reimbursements available (averaging $5,001 per year) were awarded; career-related internships or fieldwork, institutionally sponsored loans, scholarships, and unspecified assistantships also available.

Contact Mr. Patrick R. Harris, Student Services Program Coordinator, School of Nursing, Clemson University, 225 South Pleasantburg Drive, Greenville, SC 29606. *Telephone:* 864-250-8881. *Fax:* 864-250-6711. *E-mail:* pharri4@clemson.edu.

**MASTER'S DEGREE PROGRAM**
**Degree** MS
**Available Programs** Master's.
**Concentrations Available** Nursing administration; nursing education. *Nurse practitioner programs in:* adult health, family health, gerontology.
**Site Options** Greenville, SC.
**Study Options** Full-time and part-time.
**Program Entrance Requirements** Clinical experience, computer literacy, minimum overall college GPA of 3.0, transcript of college record, CPR certification, written essay, immunizations, 2 letters of recommendation, nursing research course, physical assessment course, professional liability insurance/malpractice insurance, prerequisite course work, resume, statistics course, GRE General Test. *Application deadline:* 4/1 (fall), 10/1 (spring).
**Advanced Placement** Credit given for nursing courses completed elsewhere dependent upon specific evaluations.
**Degree Requirements** 45 total credit hours, thesis or project, comprehensive exam.

**POST-MASTER'S PROGRAM**
**Areas of Study** Nursing administration; nursing education. *Nurse practitioner programs in:* adult health, family health, gerontology.

**DOCTORAL DEGREE PROGRAM**
**Program Entrance Requirements** GRE General Test.

## Coastal Carolina University
### Nursing Completion Program
### Conway, South Carolina

Founded in 1954
**DEGREE • BSN**
**Library Facilities** 265,069 volumes; 52,430 periodical subscriptions.

**BACCALAUREATE PROGRAMS**
**Degree** BSN
**Available Programs** RN Baccalaureate.
**Program Entrance Requirements** Immunizations, professional liability insurance/malpractice insurance, prerequisite course work, RN licensure.
**Contact** Director of the Nursing Completion Program, Nursing Completion Program, Coastal Carolina University, PO Box 261954, Conway, SC 29528-6054. *Telephone:* 843-349-4112. *E-mail:* pbohanna@coastal.edu.

## Francis Marion University
### Department of Nursing
### Florence, South Carolina

***http://www.fmarion.edu/***
Founded in 1970
**DEGREE • BSN**
**Nursing Program Faculty** 13 (38% with doctorates).
**Baccalaureate Enrollment** 213 **Women** 86% **Men** 14% **Minority** 26%
**Distance Learning Courses** Available.
**Nursing Student Activities** Nursing Honor Society, Sigma Theta Tau, Student Nurses' Association.
**Nursing Student Resources** Academic advising; academic or career counseling; assistance for students with disabilities; bookstore; campus computer network; career placement assistance; computer lab; computer-assisted instruction; daycare for children of students; e-mail services; externships; housing assistance; interactive nursing skills videos; Internet; learning resource lab; library services; nursing audiovisuals; paid internships; placement services for program completers; remedial services; resume preparation assistance; skills, simulation, or other laboratory; tutoring; unpaid internships.
**Library Facilities** 415,592 volumes; 860 periodical subscriptions.

**BACCALAUREATE PROGRAMS**
**Degree** BSN
**Available Programs** ADN to Baccalaureate; Generic Baccalaureate.
**Study Options** Full-time.
**Online Degree Options** Yes.
**Program Entrance Requirements** Transcript of college record, CPR certification, written essay, health insurance, immunizations, 3 letters of recommendation, minimum GPA in nursing prerequisites of 3.0, prerequisite course work. Transfer students are accepted. *Application deadline:* 3/1 (fall), 10/1 (spring). *Application fee:* $78.
**Contact** *Telephone:* 843-661-1226. *Fax:* 843-661-1696.

## Lander University
### School of Nursing
### Greenwood, South Carolina

***http://www.lander.edu/nursing/***
Founded in 1872
**DEGREE • BSN**
**Nursing Program Faculty** 21 (10% with doctorates).
**Baccalaureate Enrollment** 273 **Women** 92% **Men** 8% **Minority** 21% **Part-time** 16%
**Distance Learning Courses** Available.
**Nursing Student Activities** Sigma Theta Tau, Student Nurses' Association.
**Nursing Student Resources** Academic advising; academic or career counseling; assistance for students with disabilities; bookstore; campus computer network; career placement assistance; computer lab; computer-assisted instruction; e-mail services; externships; housing assistance; interactive nursing skills videos; Internet; learning resource lab; library services; nursing audiovisuals; resume preparation assistance; skills, simulation, or other laboratory.
**Library Facilities** 186,690 volumes (6,209 in health, 1,145 in nursing); 657 periodical subscriptions (36 health-care related).

**BACCALAUREATE PROGRAMS**
**Degree** BSN
**Available Programs** Accelerated Baccalaureate; Accelerated Baccalaureate for Second Degree; Accelerated RN Baccalaureate; Baccalaureate for Second Degree; Generic Baccalaureate; RN Baccalaureate.
**Site Options** Greenwood, SC.
**Study Options** Full-time and part-time.
**Online Degree Options** Yes.
**Program Entrance Requirements** Minimum overall college GPA of 2.6, transcript of college record, CPR certification, health exam, health insurance, immunizations, professional liability insurance/malpractice insurance, prerequisite course work. Transfer students are accepted. *Application deadline:* Applications may be processed on a rolling basis for some programs. *Application fee:* $35.
**Advanced Placement** Credit given for nursing courses completed elsewhere dependent upon specific evaluations.
**Contact** *Telephone:* 864-388-8307. *Fax:* 864-388-8125.

## Medical University of South Carolina
### College of Nursing
### Charleston, South Carolina

***http://www.musc.edu/nursing***
Founded in 1824
**DEGREES • BSN • MSN • PHD**
**Nursing Program Faculty** 47 (83% with doctorates).
**Baccalaureate Enrollment** 191 **Women** 84% **Men** 16% **Minority** 14% **Part-time** 1%
**Graduate Enrollment** 217 **Women** 93% **Men** 7% **Minority** 20% **Part-time** 28%
**Distance Learning Courses** Available.
**Nursing Student Activities** Sigma Theta Tau, Student Nurses' Association.
**Nursing Student Resources** Academic advising; academic or career counseling; bookstore; campus computer network; computer lab; computer-assisted instruction; e-mail services; interactive nursing skills videos; Internet; learning resource lab; library services; nursing audiovisuals; other; resume preparation assistance; skills, simulation, or other laboratory; tutoring.

**Library Facilities** 151,763 volumes (40,000 in health, 1,677 in nursing); 20,173 periodical subscriptions (19,000 health-care related).

## BACCALAUREATE PROGRAMS

**Degree** BSN
**Available Programs** Accelerated Baccalaureate; Accelerated Baccalaureate for Second Degree.
**Site Options** Charleston, SC.
**Study Options** Full-time.
**Program Entrance Requirements** Minimum overall college GPA of 3.0, transcript of college record, CPR certification, written essay, health exam, health insurance, immunizations, 3 letters of recommendation, minimum GPA in nursing prerequisites of 3.0, prerequisite course work. Transfer students are accepted. *Application deadline:* 1/15 (fall), 9/15 (spring). *Application fee:* $95.
**Advanced Placement** Credit by examination available. Credit given for nursing courses completed elsewhere dependent upon specific evaluations.
**Expenses (2013–14)** *Tuition, state resident:* full-time $21,876; part-time $660 per credit hour. *Tuition, nonresident:* full-time $33,000; part-time $1124 per credit hour. *Required fees:* full-time $1410.
**Financial Aid** 87% of baccalaureate students in nursing programs received some form of financial aid in 2012–13. *Gift aid (need-based):* Federal Pell, FSEOG, state, private, college/university gift aid from institutional funds, Federal Nursing, Scholarships for Disadvantaged Students (SDS). *Loans:* Federal Nursing Student Loans, Federal Direct (Subsidized and Unsubsidized Stafford PLUS), Perkins, state, alternative loans, Health Professions Student Loans (HPSL), Loans for Disadvantaged Students program, Primary Care Loans. *Work-study:* Federal Work-Study.
**Contact** Mrs. Mardi Long, Program Coordinator, College of Nursing, Medical University of South Carolina, 99 Jonathan Lucas Street, MSC 160, Charleston, SC 29425-1600. *Telephone:* 843-792-6683. *Fax:* 843-792-9258. *E-mail:* longm@musc.edu.

## GRADUATE PROGRAMS

**Expenses (2013–14)** *Tuition, state resident:* full-time $23,871; part-time $819 per credit hour. *Tuition, nonresident:* full-time $28,659; part-time $985 per credit hour. *Required fees:* full-time $1355; part-time $510 per credit; part-time $845 per term.
**Financial Aid** 84% of graduate students in nursing programs received some form of financial aid in 2012–13. Federal Work-Study, scholarships, and traineeships available. Aid available to part-time students. *Financial aid application deadline:* 3/10.
**Contact** Dr. Robin L. Bissinger, Associate Dean for Academics, College of Nursing, Medical University of South Carolina, 99 Jonathan Lucas Street, Room 209, MSC 160, Charleston, SC 29425-1600. *Telephone:* 843-792-0531. *Fax:* 843-792-1741. *E-mail:* bissinrl@musc.edu.

### MASTER'S DEGREE PROGRAM

**Degree** MSN
**Available Programs** Master's.
**Concentrations Available** *Nurse practitioner programs in:* adult health, family health, gerontology, pediatric, primary care.
**Site Options** Charleston, SC.
**Study Options** Full-time and part-time.
**Online Degree Options** Yes (online only).
**Program Entrance Requirements** Minimum overall college GPA of 3.0, transcript of college record, CPR certification, written essay, immunizations, 3 letters of recommendation, prerequisite course work, resume, statistics course. *Application deadline:* 3/1 (fall). *Application fee:* $95.
**Advanced Placement** Credit given for nursing courses completed elsewhere dependent upon specific evaluations.
**Degree Requirements** 60 total credit hours.

### DOCTORAL DEGREE PROGRAM

**Degree** PhD
**Available Programs** Doctorate; Post-Baccalaureate Doctorate.
**Areas of Study** Community health, family health, nursing administration, nursing education, nursing policy, nursing research, nursing science.
**Site Options** Charleston, SC.
**Online Degree Options** Yes (online only).
**Program Entrance Requirements** Minimum overall college GPA of 3.5, interview by faculty committee, interview, 3 letters of recommendation, MSN or equivalent, statistics course, vita, writing sample. *Application deadline:* 3/1 (fall). Applications may be processed on a rolling basis for some programs. *Application fee:* $95.
**Degree Requirements** 62 total credit hours, dissertation, oral exam, written exam.

### POSTDOCTORAL PROGRAM

**Areas of Study** Gerontology, nursing interventions, nursing research, vulnerable population.
**Postdoctoral Program Contact** Dr. William Basco, Program Director, College of Nursing, Medical University of South Carolina, Rutledge Towers, MSC 106, Charleston, SC 29425. *Telephone:* 843-876-6512. *Fax:* 843-876-8709. *E-mail:* bascob@musc.edu.

# Newberry College
## Department of Nursing
## Newberry, South Carolina

Founded in 1856

**DEGREE • BSN**
**Nursing Program Faculty** 7 (14% with doctorates).
**Baccalaureate Enrollment** 39 **Women** 90% **Men** 10% **Minority** 8% **International** 3% **Part-time** 3%
**Nursing Student Activities** Student Nurses' Association.
**Nursing Student Resources** Academic advising; academic or career counseling; assistance for students with disabilities; bookstore; campus computer network; career placement assistance; computer-assisted instruction; e-mail services; Internet; learning resource lab; library services; nursing audiovisuals; resume preparation assistance; skills, simulation, or other laboratory; tutoring.
**Library Facilities** 62,171 volumes; 102 periodical subscriptions.

## BACCALAUREATE PROGRAMS

**Degree** BSN
**Available Programs** ADN to Baccalaureate; Generic Baccalaureate.
**Study Options** Full-time.
**Program Entrance Requirements** Minimum overall college GPA of 2.75, prerequisite course work.
**Advanced Placement** Credit given for nursing courses completed elsewhere dependent upon specific evaluations.
**Expenses (2013–14)** *Tuition:* full-time $22,050; part-time $525 per credit hour. *Room and board:* $12,100; room only: $7600 per academic year. *Required fees:* full-time $1750; part-time $125 per credit.
**Financial Aid** ***Gift aid (need-based):*** Federal Pell, FSEOG, state, private, college/university gift aid from institutional funds. *Loans:* Federal Direct (Subsidized and Unsubsidized Stafford PLUS), Perkins. *Work-study:* Federal Work-Study, part-time campus jobs. *Financial aid application deadline (priority):* 3/15.
**Contact** Department Chair, Department of Nursing, Newberry College, 2100 College Street, Newberry, SC 29108. *Telephone:* 800-845-4955. *E-mail:* mcdowell@newberry.edu.

# South Carolina State University
## Department of Nursing
## Orangeburg, South Carolina

Founded in 1896

**DEGREE • BSN**
**Library Facilities** 313,329 volumes; 3,031 periodical subscriptions.

## BACCALAUREATE PROGRAMS

**Degree** BSN
**Available Programs** Generic Baccalaureate; RN Baccalaureate.
**Program Entrance Requirements** Minimum overall college GPA of 2.8, immunizations, minimum high school GPA of 2.8.
**Contact** *Telephone:* 803-536-7063. *Fax:* 803-536-8593.

# University of South Carolina
## College of Nursing
## Columbia, South Carolina

***http://www.sc.edu/nursing***
Founded in 1801

**DEGREES • BSN • DNP • MSN • PHD**
**Nursing Program Faculty** 109 (29% with doctorates).
**Baccalaureate Enrollment** 1,159 **Women** 92.23% **Men** 7.77% **Minority** 21.14% **International** .51% **Part-time** 1.29%

**Graduate Enrollment** 185 **Women** 92% **Men** 8% **Minority** 21% **Part-time** 75%
**Distance Learning Courses** Available.
**Nursing Student Activities** Sigma Theta Tau, Student Nurses' Association, nursing club.
**Nursing Student Resources** Academic advising; academic or career counseling; assistance for students with disabilities; bookstore; campus computer network; career placement assistance; computer lab; computer-assisted instruction; e-mail services; Internet; learning resource lab; library services; nursing audiovisuals; remedial services; skills, simulation, or other laboratory; tutoring.
**Library Facilities** 4.5 million volumes (74,730 in health, 6,799 in nursing); 1,400 periodical subscriptions health-care related.

## BACCALAUREATE PROGRAMS

**Degree** BSN
**Available Programs** Generic Baccalaureate.
**Site Options** Allendale, SC; Lancaster, SC; Walterboro, SC.
**Study Options** Full-time and part-time.
**Program Entrance Requirements** Minimum overall college GPA of 3.0, transcript of college record, high school biology, high school chemistry, high school foreign language, 4 years high school math, 3 years high school science, high school transcript, immunizations, minimum GPA in nursing prerequisites of 3.0. Transfer students are accepted. *Application deadline:* 12/1 (fall), 11/1 (spring), 12/1 (summer). *Application fee:* $50.
**Advanced Placement** Credit by examination available. Credit given for nursing courses completed elsewhere dependent upon specific evaluations.
**Expenses (2013–14)** *Tuition, state resident:* full-time $11,716; part-time $519 per credit hour. *Tuition, nonresident:* full-time $30,528; part-time $1322 per credit hour. *International tuition:* $30,528 full-time. *Room and board:* $8537; room only: $5988 per academic year. *Required fees:* full-time $2880.
**Financial Aid** 94% of baccalaureate students in nursing programs received some form of financial aid in 2012–13. *Gift aid (need-based):* Federal Pell, FSEOG, state, private, college/university gift aid from institutional funds, United Negro College Fund, Federal Nursing, USC Opportunity Grants, Gamecock Guarantee. *Loans:* Federal Nursing Student Loans, Federal Direct (Subsidized and Unsubsidized Stafford PLUS), Perkins. *Work-study:* Federal Work-Study, part-time campus jobs. *Financial aid application deadline (priority):* 4/1.
**Contact** Mrs. Gail Vereen, Student Services Manager, College of Nursing, University of South Carolina, College of Nursing, 1601 Greene Street, Columbia, SC 29208. *Telephone:* 803-777-7412. *Fax:* 803-777-0616. *E-mail:* gsveree@mailbox.sc.edu.

## GRADUATE PROGRAMS

**Expenses (2013–14)** *Tuition, state resident:* full-time $13,140; part-time $560 per credit hour. *Tuition, nonresident:* full-time $26,960; part-time $1140 per credit hour. *International tuition:* $26,960 full-time. *Room and board:* room only: $10,920 per academic year. *Required fees:* full-time $2680.
**Financial Aid** 59% of graduate students in nursing programs received some form of financial aid in 2012–13. 1 fellowship (averaging $1,200 per year), 3 research assistantships with partial tuition reimbursements available (averaging $2,790 per year), 11 teaching assistantships (averaging $5,533 per year) were awarded; scholarships, traineeships, and unspecified assistantships also available. *Financial aid application deadline:* 4/1.
**Contact** Ms. Christine Hodgson, Graduate Student Advisor, College of Nursing, University of South Carolina, College of Nursing, 1601 Greene Street, Columbia, SC 29208. *Telephone:* 803-777-8437. *Fax:* 803-777-2305. *E-mail:* hodgsonc@mailbox.sc.edu.

### MASTER'S DEGREE PROGRAM

**Degree** MSN
**Available Programs** Master's.
**Concentrations Available** *Nurse practitioner programs in:* acute care, family health.
**Study Options** Full-time and part-time.
**Program Entrance Requirements** Minimum overall college GPA of 3.0, transcript of college record, written essay, immunizations, 2 letters of recommendation, resume, GRE General Test, MAT. *Application deadline:* 5/1 (fall). *Application fee:* $50.
**Advanced Placement** Credit given for nursing courses completed elsewhere dependent upon specific evaluations.
**Degree Requirements** 45 total credit hours, comprehensive exam.

### POST-MASTER'S PROGRAM

**Areas of Study** *Nurse practitioner programs in:* acute care, family health.

### DOCTORAL DEGREE PROGRAM

**Degree** DNP
**Available Programs** Doctorate, Post-Baccalaureate Doctorate.
**Areas of Study** Advanced practice nursing.
**Online Degree Options** Yes.
**Program Entrance Requirements** Minimum overall college GPA of 3.0, interview by faculty committee, 3 letters of recommendation, vita, writing sample. *Application deadline:* 5/1 (fall). *Application fee:* $50.
**Degree Requirements** 33 total credit hours, dissertation, residency.

**Degree** PhD
**Available Programs** Doctorate; Post-Baccalaureate Doctorate.
**Areas of Study** Health promotion/disease prevention, health-care systems, individualized study, nursing science.
**Program Entrance Requirements** Minimum overall college GPA of 3.0, interview by faculty committee, 3 letters of recommendation, scholarly papers, statistics course, vita, writing sample, GRE General Test. *Application deadline:* 2/1 (fall). *Application fee:* $50.
**Degree Requirements** 60 total credit hours, dissertation, oral exam, written exam, residency.

### POSTDOCTORAL PROGRAM

**Areas of Study** Individualized study.
**Postdoctoral Program Contact** Dr. Sue Heiney, Interim Associate Dean for Research, College of Nursing, University of South Carolina, 1601 Greene Street, Columbia, SC 29208. *Telephone:* 803-777-8214. *Fax:* 803-777-5561. *E-mail:* heineys@mailbox.sc.edu.

## CONTINUING EDUCATION PROGRAM

**Contact** Dr. Peggy Hewlett, Director, Center for Nursing Leadership, College of Nursing, University of South Carolina, 1601 Greene Street, Columbia, SC 29208. *Telephone:* 803-777-3039. *Fax:* 803-777-6800. *E-mail:* hewlett@mailbox.sc.edu.

# University of South Carolina Aiken

### School of Nursing
### Aiken, South Carolina

***http://www.usca.edu/nursing/***
Founded in 1961

### DEGREE • BSN

**Nursing Program Faculty** 15 (40% with doctorates).
**Baccalaureate Enrollment** 250 **Women** 88% **Men** 12% **Minority** 30% **International** 1% **Part-time** 2%
**Distance Learning Courses** Available.
**Nursing Student Activities** Sigma Theta Tau, Student Nurses' Association.
**Nursing Student Resources** Academic advising; academic or career counseling; assistance for students with disabilities; bookstore; campus computer network; career placement assistance; computer lab; computer-assisted instruction; daycare for children of students; e-mail services; employment services for current students; housing assistance; interactive nursing skills videos; Internet; learning resource lab; library services; nursing audiovisuals; placement services for program completers; resume preparation assistance; skills, simulation, or other laboratory; tutoring.
**Library Facilities** 283,111 volumes (200 in health, 100 in nursing); 4,425 periodical subscriptions (100 health-care related).

## BACCALAUREATE PROGRAMS

**Degree** BSN
**Available Programs** ADN to Baccalaureate; Generic Baccalaureate; RN Baccalaureate.
**Study Options** Full-time.
**Online Degree Options** Yes.
**Program Entrance Requirements** Transcript of college record, CPR certification, written essay, health exam, immunizations, 2 letters of recommendation, minimum GPA in nursing prerequisites of 3.00, prerequisite course work. Transfer students are accepted. *Application deadline:* 3/15 (fall), 10/15 (spring).

**Advanced Placement** Credit by examination available. Credit given for nursing courses completed elsewhere dependent upon specific evaluations.

**Expenses (2013–14)** *Tuition, state resident:* full-time $9018; part-time $384 per credit hour. *Tuition, nonresident:* full-time $18,050; part-time $768 per credit hour. *International tuition:* $18,050 full-time. *Room and board:* $6550; room only: $4550 per academic year. *Required fees:* full-time $1070; part-time $30 per credit; part-time $18 per term.

**Financial Aid** 50% of baccalaureate students in nursing programs received some form of financial aid in 2012–13.

**Contact** Ms. Kathy Simmons, Administrative Assistant, School of Nursing, University of South Carolina Aiken, 471 University Parkway, Aiken, SC 29801. *Telephone:* 803-648-3392. *Fax:* 803-641-3725. *E-mail:* kathers@usca.edu.

## University of South Carolina Beaufort

### Nursing Program
### Bluffton, South Carolina

*http://www.uscb.edu/*

Founded in 1959

**DEGREE • BSN**

**Nursing Program Faculty** 13 (54% with doctorates).

**Baccalaureate Enrollment** 74 **Women** 92% **Men** 8% **Minority** 23% **Part-time** 25%

**Distance Learning Courses** Available.

**Nursing Student Activities** Student Nurses' Association.

**Nursing Student Resources** Academic advising; academic or career counseling; assistance for students with disabilities; bookstore; campus computer network; career placement assistance; computer lab; computer-assisted instruction; e-mail services; employment services for current students; externships; housing assistance; interactive nursing skills videos; Internet; learning resource lab; library services; nursing audiovisuals; paid internships; remedial services; resume preparation assistance; skills, simulation, or other laboratory; tutoring; unpaid internships.

**Library Facilities** 84,865 volumes (2,273 in health, 198 in nursing); 146 periodical subscriptions (120 health-care related).

#### BACCALAUREATE PROGRAMS

**Degree** BSN

**Available Programs** Generic Baccalaureate; RN Baccalaureate.

**Site Options** Beaufort, SC.

**Study Options** Full-time.

**Program Entrance Requirements** Minimum overall college GPA of 3.0, transcript of college record, CPR certification, health exam, health insurance, immunizations, 2 letters of recommendation, minimum GPA in nursing prerequisites of 2.75, prerequisite course work. Transfer students are accepted. *Application deadline:* 8/1 (spring). *Application fee:* $25.

**Advanced Placement** Credit by examination available. Credit given for nursing courses completed elsewhere dependent upon specific evaluations.

**Expenses (2013–14)** *Tuition, state resident:* full-time $8586; part-time $358 per credit hour. *Tuition, nonresident:* full-time $18,438; part-time $768 per credit hour. *Room and board:* $18,152 per academic year. *Required fees:* full-time $550.

**Financial Aid** 90% of baccalaureate students in nursing programs received some form of financial aid in 2012–13.

**Contact** Dr. Rose Kearney-Nunnery, Professor and Chair, Department of Nursing, Nursing Program, University of South Carolina Beaufort, 1 University Boulevard, Bluffton, SC 29909. *Telephone:* 843-208-8124. *E-mail:* nursing@uscb.edu.

## University of South Carolina Upstate

### Mary Black School of Nursing
### Spartanburg, South Carolina

*https://www.uscupstate.edu/academics/nursing/default.aspx?id=2287*

Founded in 1967

**DEGREE • BSN**

**Nursing Program Faculty** 80 (15% with doctorates).

**Baccalaureate Enrollment** 448 **Women** 90% **Men** 10% **Minority** 28% **International** 2% **Part-time** 6%

**Distance Learning Courses** Available.

**Nursing Student Activities** Nursing Honor Society, Sigma Theta Tau, Student Nurses' Association.

**Nursing Student Resources** Academic advising; academic or career counseling; assistance for students with disabilities; bookstore; campus computer network; career placement assistance; computer lab; computer-assisted instruction; daycare for children of students; e-mail services; employment services for current students; externships; housing assistance; interactive nursing skills videos; Internet; learning resource lab; library services; nursing audiovisuals; paid internships; resume preparation assistance; skills, simulation, or other laboratory; tutoring; unpaid internships.

**Library Facilities** 426,268 volumes (214,998 in health, 23,359 in nursing); 89,799 periodical subscriptions.

#### BACCALAUREATE PROGRAMS

**Degree** BSN

**Available Programs** Generic Baccalaureate; RN Baccalaureate.

**Site Options** Greenville, SC.

**Study Options** Full-time and part-time.

**Online Degree Options** Yes.

**Program Entrance Requirements** Transcript of college record, CPR certification, health exam, health insurance, immunizations, minimum GPA in nursing prerequisites of 2.75, professional liability insurance/malpractice insurance, prerequisite course work. Transfer students are accepted. *Application deadline:* 1/15 (fall), 5/1 (spring).

**Advanced Placement** Credit by examination available. Credit given for nursing courses completed elsewhere dependent upon specific evaluations.

**Contact** *Telephone:* 864-503-5444. *Fax:* 864-503-5405.

# SOUTH DAKOTA

## Augustana College

### Department of Nursing
### Sioux Falls, South Dakota

*http://www.augie.edu/*

Founded in 1860

**DEGREE • BA**

**Nursing Program Faculty** 9 (44% with doctorates).

**Baccalaureate Enrollment** 210 **Women** 85% **Men** 15% **Minority** 6% **Part-time** 4%

**Nursing Student Activities** Sigma Theta Tau, Student Nurses' Association.

**Nursing Student Resources** Academic advising; academic or career counseling; assistance for students with disabilities; bookstore; campus computer network; career placement assistance; computer lab; computer-assisted instruction; daycare for children of students; e-mail services; employment services for current students; housing assistance; interactive nursing skills videos; Internet; learning resource lab; library services; nursing audiovisuals; remedial services; resume preparation assistance; skills, simulation, or other laboratory; tutoring; unpaid internships.

**Library Facilities** 233,000 volumes; 20,385 periodical subscriptions.

#### BACCALAUREATE PROGRAMS

**Degree** BA

**Available Programs** Generic Baccalaureate.

**Study Options** Full-time and part-time.
**Program Entrance Requirements** Minimum overall college GPA of 2.7, transcript of college record, CPR certification, written essay, health exam, health insurance, high school transcript, immunizations, 2 letters of recommendation, minimum high school GPA of 3.0, minimum GPA in nursing prerequisites of 2.7, prerequisite course work. Transfer students are accepted. *Application deadline:* 2/15 (fall). Applications may be processed on a rolling basis for some programs.
**Advanced Placement** Credit given for nursing courses completed elsewhere dependent upon specific evaluations.
**Expenses (2013–14)** *Tuition:* full-time $28,200. *International tuition:* $28,200 full-time. *Room and board:* $6920; room only: $3651 per academic year. *Required fees:* full-time $500.
**Financial Aid** 98% of baccalaureate students in nursing programs received some form of financial aid in 2012–13.
**Contact** Debbie Anderson, Office Assistant, Department of Nursing, Augustana College, 2001 South Summit Avenue, Sioux Falls, SD 57197. *Telephone:* 605-274-4721. *Fax:* 605-274-4723. *E-mail:* debbie.anderson@augie.edu.

# Mount Marty College
## Nursing Program
## Yankton, South Dakota

*http://www.mtmc.edu/*
Founded in 1936

### DEGREE • BSN
**Nursing Program Faculty** 13 (15% with doctorates).
**Baccalaureate Enrollment** 89 **Women** 89% **Men** 11% **Minority** 7% **Part-time** 2%
**Nursing Student Activities** Sigma Theta Tau, Student Nurses' Association, nursing club.
**Nursing Student Resources** Academic advising; academic or career counseling; assistance for students with disabilities; bookstore; campus computer network; career placement assistance; computer lab; computer-assisted instruction; daycare for children of students; e-mail services; employment services for current students; externships; housing assistance; interactive nursing skills videos; Internet; learning resource lab; library services; nursing audiovisuals; paid internships; placement services for program completers; remedial services; resume preparation assistance; skills, simulation, or other laboratory; tutoring; unpaid internships.
**Library Facilities** 79,898 volumes (8,750 in health, 5,350 in nursing); 298 periodical subscriptions (85 health-care related).

### BACCALAUREATE PROGRAMS
**Degree** BSN
**Available Programs** ADN to Baccalaureate; Accelerated LPN to Baccalaureate; Generic Baccalaureate; International Nurse to Baccalaureate; LPN to Baccalaureate; LPN to RN Baccalaureate; RN Baccalaureate.
**Site Options** Watertown, SD.
**Study Options** Full-time and part-time.
**Program Entrance Requirements** Minimum overall college GPA of 2.7, transcript of college record, CPR certification, health exam, health insurance, high school transcript, immunizations, minimum GPA in nursing prerequisites of 2.0, prerequisite course work. Transfer students are accepted. *Application deadline:* Applications may be processed on a rolling basis for some programs.
**Advanced Placement** Credit given for nursing courses completed elsewhere dependent upon specific evaluations.
**Contact** *Telephone:* 605-668-1594. *Fax:* 605-668-1607.

# National American University
## School of Nursing
## Rapid City, South Dakota

Founded in 1941

### DEGREE • BSN
**Library Facilities** 31,018 volumes; 268 periodical subscriptions.

### BACCALAUREATE PROGRAMS
**Degree** BSN
**Available Programs** Generic Baccalaureate.
**Contact** *Telephone:* 303-876-7181. *Fax:* 303-876-7105.

# Presentation College
## Department of Nursing
## Aberdeen, South Dakota

*http://www.presentation.edu/*
Founded in 1951

### DEGREE • BSN
**Nursing Program Faculty** 21 (9% with doctorates).
**Baccalaureate Enrollment** 185 **Women** 95% **Men** 5% **Minority** 4% **Part-time** 24%
**Distance Learning Courses** Available.
**Nursing Student Activities** Nursing Honor Society, Sigma Theta Tau, Student Nurses' Association, nursing club.
**Nursing Student Resources** Academic advising; academic or career counseling; assistance for students with disabilities; bookstore; campus computer network; career placement assistance; computer lab; computer-assisted instruction; e-mail services; employment services for current students; externships; interactive nursing skills videos; Internet; learning resource lab; library services; nursing audiovisuals; placement services for program completers; remedial services; resume preparation assistance; skills, simulation, or other laboratory; tutoring; unpaid internships.
**Library Facilities** 87,546 volumes (378 in health, 353 in nursing); 86,106 periodical subscriptions (2,172 health-care related).

### BACCALAUREATE PROGRAMS
**Degree** BSN
**Available Programs** ADN to Baccalaureate; Baccalaureate for Second Degree; Generic Baccalaureate; LPN to RN Baccalaureate; RN Baccalaureate.
**Site Options** Fargo , ND; Fairmont, MN.
**Study Options** Full-time and part-time.
**Online Degree Options** Yes.
**Program Entrance Requirements** Minimum overall college GPA of 2.5, transcript of college record, CPR certification, written essay, health exam, high school biology, high school chemistry, 2 years high school math, high school transcript, immunizations, 2 letters of recommendation, minimum high school GPA of 2.7, minimum GPA in nursing prerequisites of 2.5, prerequisite course work. Transfer students are accepted. *Application deadline:* 3/1 (fall).
**Advanced Placement** Credit by examination available. Credit given for nursing courses completed elsewhere dependent upon specific evaluations.
**Contact** *Telephone:* 605-229-8492. *Fax:* 605-229-8489.

# South Dakota State University
## College of Nursing
## Brookings, South Dakota

*http://www.sdstate.edu/nurs/*
Founded in 1881

### DEGREES • BS • MS • PHD
**Nursing Program Faculty** 127 (22% with doctorates).
**Baccalaureate Enrollment** 553 **Women** 82% **Men** 18% **Minority** 4%
**Graduate Enrollment** 166 **Women** 96% **Men** 4% **Minority** 2% **Part-time** 100%
**Distance Learning Courses** Available.
**Nursing Student Activities** Sigma Theta Tau, Student Nurses' Association, nursing club.
**Nursing Student Resources** Academic advising; academic or career counseling; assistance for students with disabilities; bookstore; campus computer network; career placement assistance; computer lab; computer-assisted instruction; e-mail services; employment services for current students; externships; interactive nursing skills videos; Internet; learning resource lab; library services; nursing audiovisuals; paid internships; placement services for program completers; remedial services; resume preparation assistance; skills, simulation, or other laboratory; tutoring.
**Library Facilities** 790,900 volumes (20,000 in health, 5,700 in nursing); 32,900 periodical subscriptions (4,402 health-care related).

### BACCALAUREATE PROGRAMS
**Degree** BS

**Available Programs** Accelerated Baccalaureate; Generic Baccalaureate; RN Baccalaureate.
**Site Options** Rapid City, SD; Sioux Falls, SD.
**Study Options** Full-time.
**Online Degree Options** Yes.
**Program Entrance Requirements** Minimum overall college GPA of 2.7, transcript of college record, CPR certification, health exam, health insurance, immunizations, interview, minimum GPA in nursing prerequisites of 2.7, professional liability insurance/malpractice insurance, prerequisite course work. Transfer students are accepted. *Application deadline:* 1/25 (fall), 9/25 (spring).
**Advanced Placement** Credit given for nursing courses completed elsewhere dependent upon specific evaluations.
**Contact** *Telephone:* 605-688-6153. *Fax:* 605-688-6523.

## GRADUATE PROGRAMS

**Contact** *Telephone:* 605-688-4114. *Fax:* 605-688-5827.

### MASTER'S DEGREE PROGRAM

**Degree** MS
**Available Programs** Master's; RN to Master's.
**Concentrations Available** Clinical nurse leader; nursing administration; nursing education. *Nurse practitioner programs in:* family health, neonatal health, psychiatric/mental health.
**Site Options** Rapid City, SD; Sioux Falls, SD.
**Study Options** Full-time and part-time.
**Online Degree Options** Yes.
**Program Entrance Requirements** Clinical experience, minimum overall college GPA of 3.0, transcript of college record, CPR certification, written essay, immunizations, 3 letters of recommendation, professional liability insurance/malpractice insurance, statistics course. *Application deadline:* 3/1 (fall). *Application fee:* $200.
**Advanced Placement** Credit given for nursing courses completed elsewhere dependent upon specific evaluations.
**Degree Requirements** 48 total credit hours, thesis or project, comprehensive exam.

### POST-MASTER'S PROGRAM

**Areas of Study** Nursing education. *Nurse practitioner programs in:* family health.

### DOCTORAL DEGREE PROGRAM

**Degree** PhD
**Available Programs** Doctorate.
**Areas of Study** Nursing research.
**Site Options** Sioux Falls, SD.
**Program Entrance Requirements** Minimum overall college GPA of 3.3, interview by faculty committee, 4 letters of recommendation, MSN or equivalent, scholarly papers, vita, writing sample. *Application deadline:* 3/1 (fall).
**Degree Requirements** 60 total credit hours, dissertation, oral exam, written exam.

## CONTINUING EDUCATION PROGRAM

**Contact** *Telephone:* 605-688-5178. *Fax:* 605-688-5745.

# University of Sioux Falls

## School of Nursing
## Sioux Falls, South Dakota

***http://www.usiouxfalls.edu/nursing***
Founded in 1883

**DEGREE • BSN**
**Nursing Program Faculty** 5 (20% with doctorates).
**Baccalaureate Enrollment** 169
**Distance Learning Courses** Available.
**Nursing Student Activities** Nursing Honor Society, Sigma Theta Tau, Student Nurses' Association.
**Nursing Student Resources** Academic advising; academic or career counseling; assistance for students with disabilities; bookstore; campus computer network; career placement assistance; computer lab; computer-assisted instruction; e-mail services; employment services for current students; interactive nursing skills videos; Internet; learning resource lab; library services; nursing audiovisuals; other; placement services for program completers; remedial services; resume preparation assistance; skills, simulation, or other laboratory; tutoring.
**Library Facilities** 85,713 volumes; 378 periodical subscriptions.

## BACCALAUREATE PROGRAMS

**Degree** BSN
**Available Programs** Accelerated Baccalaureate; Generic Baccalaureate; RN Baccalaureate.
**Online Degree Options** Yes.
**Program Entrance Requirements** Minimum overall college GPA of 2.75, written essay, letters of recommendation, minimum high school GPA of 2.75, prerequisite course work, RN licensure.
**Contact** School of Nursing, School of Nursing, University of Sioux Falls, 1101 West 22nd Street, Sioux Falls, SD 57105. *Telephone:* 605-331-6697. *E-mail:* Nursing@usiouxfalls.edu.

# The University of South Dakota

## Department of Nursing
## Vermillion, South Dakota

***http://www.usd.edu/health-sciences/nursing/***
Founded in 1862

**DEGREE • BSN**
**Nursing Program Faculty** 43 (5% with doctorates).
**Baccalaureate Enrollment** 275 **Women** 87% **Men** 13% **Minority** 7% **Part-time** 70%
**Nursing Student Activities** Student Nurses' Association.
**Nursing Student Resources** Academic advising; assistance for students with disabilities; bookstore; campus computer network; computer lab; e-mail services; Internet; library services; skills, simulation, or other laboratory; tutoring.
**Library Facilities** 863,292 volumes; 64,575 periodical subscriptions.

## BACCALAUREATE PROGRAMS

**Degree** BSN
**Available Programs** Generic Baccalaureate; RN Baccalaureate.
**Site Options** Sioux Falls, SD; Vermillion, SD.
**Study Options** Full-time and part-time.
**Program Entrance Requirements** Minimum overall college GPA of 2.7, health exam, health insurance, immunizations, 3 letters of recommendation, minimum GPA in nursing prerequisites of 2.7, professional liability insurance/malpractice insurance, prerequisite course work. Transfer students are accepted. *Application deadline:* 2/1 (fall), 8/1 (spring).
**Advanced Placement** Credit given for nursing courses completed elsewhere dependent upon specific evaluations.
**Expenses (2013–14)** *Tuition, state resident:* part-time $139 per credit hour. *Tuition, nonresident:* part-time $208 per credit hour. *Room and board:* $13,388; room only: $7570 per academic year. *Required fees:* part-time $200 per term.
**Financial Aid** 78% of baccalaureate students in nursing programs received some form of financial aid in 2012–13. *Gift aid (need-based):* Federal Pell, FSEOG, private, college/university gift aid from institutional funds, Federal Nursing. *Loans:* Federal Nursing Student Loans, Federal Direct (Subsidized and Unsubsidized Stafford PLUS), Perkins, college/university. *Work-study:* Federal Work-Study. *Financial aid application deadline (priority):* 3/15.
**Contact** USD Nursing Program Office, Department of Nursing, The University of South Dakota, 414 East Clark Street, Vermillion, SD 57069. *Telephone:* 605-677-5006. *E-mail:* nursing@usd.edu.

# TENNESSEE

# Aquinas College

## School of Nursing
## Nashville, Tennessee

***http://www.aquinas.edu/nursing/***
Founded in 1961

**DEGREES • BSN • MSN**
**Nursing Program Faculty** 6 (33% with doctorates).

**Baccalaureate Enrollment** 14 **Women** 93% **Men** 7% **Minority** 12% **Part-time** 100%

**Graduate Enrollment** 14 **Women** 100% **Part-time** 11%

**Nursing Student Activities** Nursing Honor Society.

**Nursing Student Resources** Academic advising; academic or career counseling; assistance for students with disabilities; bookstore; campus computer network; career placement assistance; computer lab; computer-assisted instruction; e-mail services; employment services for current students; interactive nursing skills videos; Internet; learning resource lab; library services; nursing audiovisuals; remedial services; resume preparation assistance; skills, simulation, or other laboratory; tutoring.

**Library Facilities** 2,290 volumes in health, 1,220 volumes in nursing; 85 periodical subscriptions health-care related.

## BACCALAUREATE PROGRAMS

**Degree** BSN

**Available Programs** Accelerated RN Baccalaureate.

**Study Options** Part-time.

**Program Entrance Requirements** Transcript of college record, CPR certification, health exam, health insurance, high school chemistry, immunizations, interview, minimum high school GPA of 2.5, minimum GPA in nursing prerequisites of 2.5, professional liability insurance/malpractice insurance, prerequisite course work, RN licensure. Transfer students are accepted. *Application deadline:* Applications may be processed on a rolling basis for some programs. *Application fee:* $25.

**Advanced Placement** Credit by examination available. Credit given for nursing courses completed elsewhere dependent upon specific evaluations.

**Expenses (2013–14)** *Tuition:* full-time $19,950; part-time $665 per credit hour. *Required fees:* full-time $600.

**Financial Aid** 100% of baccalaureate students in nursing programs received some form of financial aid in 2012–13.

**Contact** Dr. Ignatius Perkins OP, PhD, RN, FAAN, RN to BSN Program Director, School of Nursing, Aquinas College, 4210 Harding Pike, Nashville, TN 37205. *Telephone:* 615-297-2008. *Fax:* 615-783-0562. *E-mail:* perkinsi@aquinascollege.edu.

## GRADUATE PROGRAMS

**Expenses (2013–14)** *Tuition:* part-time $690 per credit.

**Financial Aid** 70% of graduate students in nursing programs received some form of financial aid in 2012–13.

**Contact** Br. Ignatius Perkins, OP, PhD, RN, FAAN, Dean, School of Nursing/Director, MSN Program, School of Nursing, Aquinas College, 4210 Harding Pike, Nashville, TN 37205. *Telephone:* 615-297-2008. *Fax:* 615-783-0562. *E-mail:* perkinsi@aquinascollege.edu.

### MASTER'S DEGREE PROGRAM

**Degree** MSN

**Available Programs** Master's.

**Concentrations Available** Nursing education.

**Study Options** Part-time.

**Program Entrance Requirements** Computer literacy, minimum overall college GPA of 3.0, transcript of college record, CPR certification, written essay, immunizations, interview, 2 letters of recommendation, professional liability insurance/malpractice insurance, resume. *Application deadline:* Applications may be processed on a rolling basis for some programs. *Application fee:* $25.

**Advanced Placement** Credit by examination available. Credit given for nursing courses completed elsewhere dependent upon specific evaluations.

**Degree Requirements** 40 total credit hours, thesis or project.

### POST-MASTER'S PROGRAM

**Areas of Study** Nursing education.

# Austin Peay State University

**School of Nursing**
**Clarksville, Tennessee**

***http://www.apsu.edu/nursing01***
Founded in 1927

**DEGREES • BSN • MSN**

**Nursing Program Faculty** 39 (26% with doctorates).

**Baccalaureate Enrollment** 260 **Women** 89.23% **Men** 10.77% **Minority** 23.46%

**Graduate Enrollment** 181 **Women** 94% **Men** 6% **Minority** 17.68% **Part-time** 71.82%

**Distance Learning Courses** Available.

**Nursing Student Activities** Nursing Honor Society, Sigma Theta Tau, Student Nurses' Association.

**Nursing Student Resources** Academic advising; academic or career counseling; assistance for students with disabilities; bookstore; campus computer network; computer lab; computer-assisted instruction; daycare for children of students; e-mail services; employment services for current students; interactive nursing skills videos; Internet; library services; nursing audiovisuals; remedial services; resume preparation assistance; skills, simulation, or other laboratory; tutoring.

**Library Facilities** 370,064 volumes (4,700 in health, 800 in nursing); 47,758 periodical subscriptions (80 health-care related).

## BACCALAUREATE PROGRAMS

**Degree** BSN

**Available Programs** ADN to Baccalaureate; Baccalaureate for Second Degree; Generic Baccalaureate; RN Baccalaureate.

**Study Options** Full-time.

**Program Entrance Requirements** Minimum overall college GPA of 3.0, transcript of college record, immunizations, minimum GPA in nursing prerequisites of 3.0, prerequisite course work. Transfer students are accepted. *Application deadline:* 5/1 (fall), 9/1 (spring).

**Expenses (2013–14)** *Tuition, state resident:* full-time $6876; part-time $297 per credit hour. *Tuition, nonresident:* full-time $23,513; part-time $901 per credit hour. *Room and board:* $4587; room only: $3100 per academic year. *Required fees:* full-time $390; part-time $25 per credit.

**Financial Aid** 64% of baccalaureate students in nursing programs received some form of financial aid in 2012–13. *Gift aid (need-based):* Federal Pell, FSEOG, state, private, college/university gift aid from institutional funds. *Loans:* Federal Direct (Subsidized and Unsubsidized Stafford PLUS), Perkins. *Work-study:* Federal Work-Study, part-time campus jobs. *Financial aid application deadline (priority):* 2/3.

**Contact** Ms. Debbie Cochener, Administrative Specialist/Pre-Nursing Advisor, School of Nursing, Austin Peay State University, PO Box 4658, Clarksville, TN 37044. *Telephone:* 931-221-7708. *Fax:* 931-221-7595. *E-mail:* cochenerd@apsu.edu.

## GRADUATE PROGRAMS

**Expenses (2013–14)** *Tuition, state resident:* full-time $8424; part-time $468 per credit hour. *Tuition, nonresident:* full-time $11,808; part-time $656 per credit hour. *Room and board:* $4587; room only: $3100 per academic year. *Required fees:* full-time $200; part-time $25 per credit.

**Financial Aid** 63% of graduate students in nursing programs received some form of financial aid in 2012–13.

**Contact** Dr. Michele Robertson, Coordinator of the MSN RODP, School of Nursing, Austin Peay State University, PO Box 4658, Clarksville, TN 37044. *Telephone:* 931-221-7489. *Fax:* 931-221-7595. *E-mail:* robertsonm@apsu.edu.

### MASTER'S DEGREE PROGRAM

**Degree** MSN

**Available Programs** Master's.

**Concentrations Available** Nursing administration; nursing education; nursing informatics. *Nurse practitioner programs in:* family health.

**Study Options** Full-time and part-time.

**Online Degree Options** Yes (online only).

**Program Entrance Requirements** Minimum overall college GPA of 3.0, transcript of college record, statistics course. *Application deadline:* 7/1 (fall), 11/1 (spring), 4/1 (summer). Applications may be processed on a rolling basis for some programs. *Application fee:* $25.

**Advanced Placement** Credit given for nursing courses completed elsewhere dependent upon specific evaluations.

**Degree Requirements** 46 total credit hours.

### POST-MASTER'S PROGRAM

**Areas of Study** Nursing administration; nursing education; nursing informatics. *Nurse practitioner programs in:* family health.

# Baptist College of Health Sciences
## Nursing Division
## Memphis, Tennessee

*http://www.bchs.edu/*
Founded in 1994

### DEGREE • BSN

**Nursing Program Faculty** 40 (20% with doctorates).
**Baccalaureate Enrollment** 731 **Women** 89% **Men** 11% **Minority** 43% **Part-time** 45%
**Distance Learning Courses** Available.
**Nursing Student Activities** Sigma Theta Tau, Student Nurses' Association.
**Nursing Student Resources** Academic advising; academic or career counseling; assistance for students with disabilities; bookstore; campus computer network; computer lab; computer-assisted instruction; e-mail services; employment services for current students; externships; housing assistance; interactive nursing skills videos; Internet; learning resource lab; library services; nursing audiovisuals; paid internships; placement services for program completers; resume preparation assistance; skills, simulation, or other laboratory; tutoring.
**Library Facilities** 2,573 volumes in health, 1,790 volumes in nursing; 213 periodical subscriptions health-care related.

### BACCALAUREATE PROGRAMS

**Degree** BSN
**Available Programs** Generic Baccalaureate; LPN to Baccalaureate; RN Baccalaureate.
**Study Options** Full-time and part-time.
**Program Entrance Requirements** Minimum overall college GPA of 2.5, CPR certification, health exam, health insurance, 2 years high school math, 2 years high school science, high school transcript, immunizations, 3 letters of recommendation, minimum high school GPA of 2.75. Transfer students are accepted. *Application deadline:* 6/1 (fall), 11/1 (spring). *Application fee:* $25.
**Contact** *Telephone:* 901-572-2441. *Fax:* 901-572-2461.

# Belmont University
## School of Nursing
## Nashville, Tennessee

*http://www.belmont.edu/nursing*
Founded in 1951

### DEGREES • BSN • MSN

**Nursing Program Faculty** 65 (19% with doctorates).
**Baccalaureate Enrollment** 406 **Women** 84% **Men** 16% **Minority** 6% **International** 3% **Part-time** 8%
**Graduate Enrollment** 43 **Women** 98% **Men** 2% **Minority** 12% **International** 2% **Part-time** 63%
**Nursing Student Activities** Nursing Honor Society, Sigma Theta Tau, Student Nurses' Association.
**Nursing Student Resources** Academic advising; academic or career counseling; assistance for students with disabilities; bookstore; campus computer network; career placement assistance; computer lab; computer-assisted instruction; e-mail services; employment services for current students; externships; housing assistance; interactive nursing skills videos; Internet; learning resource lab; library services; nursing audiovisuals; placement services for program completers; remedial services; resume preparation assistance; skills, simulation, or other laboratory; tutoring.
**Library Facilities** 232,140 volumes (6,000 in health, 800 in nursing); 788 periodical subscriptions (7,500 health-care related).

### BACCALAUREATE PROGRAMS

**Degree** BSN
**Available Programs** ADN to Baccalaureate; Accelerated Baccalaureate; Accelerated Baccalaureate for Second Degree; Baccalaureate for Second Degree; Generic Baccalaureate; LPN to RN Baccalaureate; RN Baccalaureate.
**Study Options** Full-time and part-time.
**Program Entrance Requirements** Minimum overall college GPA of 2.5, transcript of college record, CPR certification, written essay, health exam, health insurance, high school biology, high school chemistry, 3 years high school math, 3 years high school science, high school transcript, immunizations, 1 letter of recommendation, minimum high school GPA of 2.5, minimum GPA in nursing prerequisites of 3.0. Transfer students are accepted. *Application deadline:* Applications may be processed on a rolling basis for some programs. *Application fee:* $50.
**Advanced Placement** Credit by examination available. Credit given for nursing courses completed elsewhere dependent upon specific evaluations.
**Contact** *Telephone:* 615-460-6120. *Fax:* 615-460-6125.

### GRADUATE PROGRAMS

**Contact** *Telephone:* 615-460-6027. *Fax:* 615-460-6125.

#### MASTER'S DEGREE PROGRAM

**Degree** MSN
**Available Programs** Master's.
**Concentrations Available** Nursing education. *Nurse practitioner programs in:* family health.
**Study Options** Full-time and part-time.
**Program Entrance Requirements** Clinical experience, minimum overall college GPA of 3.0, transcript of college record, CPR certification, written essay, immunizations, interview, 2 letters of recommendation, resume, GRE. *Application fee:* $50.
**Advanced Placement** Credit given for nursing courses completed elsewhere dependent upon specific evaluations.
**Degree Requirements** 41 total credit hours, comprehensive exam.

#### POST-MASTER'S PROGRAM

**Areas of Study** Nursing education. *Nurse practitioner programs in:* family health.

# Bethel University
## Nursing Program
## McKenzie, Tennessee

*http://www.bethelu.edu/*
Founded in 1842

### DEGREE • BSN

**Nursing Program Faculty** 7
**Baccalaureate Enrollment** 46 **Women** 83% **Men** 17% **Minority** 17% **International** 4%
**Distance Learning Courses** Available.
**Nursing Student Activities** Student Nurses' Association.
**Nursing Student Resources** Academic advising; academic or career counseling; assistance for students with disabilities; bookstore; campus computer network; career placement assistance; computer lab; computer-assisted instruction; e-mail services; housing assistance; interactive nursing skills videos; Internet; learning resource lab; library services; nursing audiovisuals; remedial services; resume preparation assistance; skills, simulation, or other laboratory; tutoring.
**Library Facilities** 45,000 volumes (1,146 in nursing); 111,700 periodical subscriptions (99 health-care related).

### BACCALAUREATE PROGRAMS

**Degree** BSN
**Available Programs** ADN to Baccalaureate; Generic Baccalaureate.
**Study Options** Full-time.
**Program Entrance Requirements** Minimum overall college GPA of 2.75, transcript of college record, CPR certification, health exam, health insurance, immunizations, minimum GPA in nursing prerequisites of 2.0, professional liability insurance/malpractice insurance, prerequisite course work. Transfer students are accepted. *Application deadline:* 3/1 (spring). *Application fee:* $25.
**Advanced Placement** Credit given for nursing courses completed elsewhere dependent upon specific evaluations.
**Expenses (2012–13)** *Tuition:* full-time $12,900; part-time $398 per credit. *Required fees:* full-time $1070; part-time $535 per term.
**Financial Aid** 80% of baccalaureate students in nursing programs received some form of financial aid in 2011–12.
**Contact** Ms. Mary Bess Griffith, Director, Nursing Program, Bethel University, 325 Cherry Avenue, McKenzie, TN 38201. *Telephone:* 731-352-6768. *Fax:* 731-352-2771. *E-mail:* griffithmb@bethelu.edu.

# Carson-Newman University

## Department of Nursing
## Jefferson City, Tennessee

***http://www.cn.edu/***
Founded in 1851

**DEGREES • BSN • MSN**
**Nursing Program Faculty** 21 (42% with doctorates).
**Baccalaureate Enrollment** 101 **Women** 83% **Men** 17% **Minority** 1% **Part-time** 1%
**Graduate Enrollment** 58 **Women** 98% **Men** 2% **Minority** 1% **Part-time** 84%
**Distance Learning Courses** Available.
**Nursing Student Activities** Sigma Theta Tau, Student Nurses' Association.
**Nursing Student Resources** Academic advising; academic or career counseling; assistance for students with disabilities; bookstore; campus computer network; career placement assistance; computer lab; computer-assisted instruction; daycare for children of students; e-mail services; employment services for current students; housing assistance; interactive nursing skills videos; Internet; learning resource lab; library services; nursing audiovisuals; placement services for program completers; remedial services; resume preparation assistance; skills, simulation, or other laboratory; tutoring.
**Library Facilities** 283,517 volumes (6,492 in health, 4,780 in nursing); 3,966 periodical subscriptions (8,447 health-care related).

### BACCALAUREATE PROGRAMS

**Degree** BSN
**Available Programs** Accelerated Baccalaureate; Generic Baccalaureate; LPN to Baccalaureate; RN Baccalaureate.
**Study Options** Full-time.
**Online Degree Options** Yes.
**Program Entrance Requirements** Minimum overall college GPA of 2.75, transcript of college record, health exam, health insurance, high school transcript, immunizations, minimum GPA in nursing prerequisites of 2.75, prerequisite course work. Transfer students are accepted. *Application deadline:* Applications may be processed on a rolling basis for some programs.
**Advanced Placement** Credit by examination available. Credit given for nursing courses completed elsewhere dependent upon specific evaluations.
**Expenses (2013–14)** *Tuition:* full-time $22,640; part-time $944 per credit hour. *International tuition:* $22,640 full-time. *Room and board:* $8450; room only: $4470 per academic year. *Required fees:* full-time $1040; part-time $345 per term.
**Financial Aid** 95% of baccalaureate students in nursing programs received some form of financial aid in 2012–13. *Gift aid (need-based):* Federal Pell, FSEOG, state, private, college/university gift aid from institutional funds. *Loans:* Perkins, state, college/university, alternative loans. *Work-study:* Federal Work-Study, part-time campus jobs. *Financial aid application deadline (priority):* 4/1.
**Contact** Dr. Angela F. Wood, RN, Interim Chair, Department of Nursing, Department of Nursing, Carson-Newman University, 1646 Russell Avenue, C-N Box 71883, Jefferson City, TN 37760. *Telephone:* 865-471-3442. *Fax:* 865-471-4574. *E-mail:* awood@cn.edu.

### GRADUATE PROGRAMS

**Expenses (2013–14)** *Tuition:* part-time $514 per credit hour. *Room and board:* $8256; room only: $4416 per academic year. *Required fees:* part-time $44 per term.
**Financial Aid** 95% of graduate students in nursing programs received some form of financial aid in 2012–13.
**Contact** Dr. Kimberly S. Bolton, Graduate Program Director, Graduate Studies in Nursing, Department of Nursing, Carson-Newman University, 1646 Russell Avenue, C-N Box 71883, Jefferson City, TN 37760. *Telephone:* 865-471-4056. *Fax:* 865-471-4574. *E-mail:* kbolton@cn.edu.

#### MASTER'S DEGREE PROGRAM

**Degree** MSN
**Available Programs** Accelerated AD/RN to Master's; Master's.
**Concentrations Available** Nursing education. *Nurse practitioner programs in:* family health.
**Study Options** Full-time and part-time.
**Program Entrance Requirements** Minimum overall college GPA of 3.0, transcript of college record, written essay, interview, 3 letters of recommendation. *Application deadline:* Applications may be processed on a rolling basis for some programs. *Application fee:* $50.
**Advanced Placement** Credit given for nursing courses completed elsewhere dependent upon specific evaluations.
**Degree Requirements** 45 total credit hours, thesis or project, comprehensive exam.

#### POST-MASTER'S PROGRAM

**Areas of Study** Nursing education. *Nurse practitioner programs in:* family health.

# Christian Brothers University

## RN to BSN Program
## Memphis, Tennessee

***http://www.cbu.edu/nursing***
Founded in 1871

**DEGREE • BSN**
**Nursing Program Faculty** 4 (50% with doctorates).
**Baccalaureate Enrollment** 61
**Nursing Student Activities** Sigma Theta Tau.
**Nursing Student Resources** Academic advising; academic or career counseling; assistance for students with disabilities; bookstore; campus computer network; career placement assistance; computer lab; computer-assisted instruction; e-mail services; housing assistance; interactive nursing skills videos; Internet; learning resource lab; library services; nursing audiovisuals; remedial services; resume preparation assistance; skills, simulation, or other laboratory; tutoring.
**Library Facilities** 101,898 volumes; 371 periodical subscriptions.

### BACCALAUREATE PROGRAMS

**Degree** BSN
**Available Programs** RN Baccalaureate.
**Study Options** Full-time and part-time.
**Program Entrance Requirements** Minimum overall college GPA, transcript of college record, CPR certification, written essay, immunizations, interview, 2 letters of recommendation, RN licensure. Transfer students are accepted. *Application deadline:* 8/1 (fall), 12/5 (spring). Applications may be processed on a rolling basis for some programs. *Application fee:* $25.
**Advanced Placement** Credit given for nursing courses completed elsewhere dependent upon specific evaluations.
**Expenses (2013–14)** *Tuition:* part-time $405 per credit hour.
**Financial Aid** 78% of baccalaureate students in nursing programs received some form of financial aid in 2012–13.
**Contact** Dr. Peggy Veeser, Director and Professor, RN to BSN Program, Christian Brothers University, 650 East Parkway South, Box 89, Memphis, TN 38104. *Telephone:* 901-321-3339. *Fax:* 901-321-3324. *E-mail:* pveeser@cbu.edu.

# Cumberland University

## Rudy School of Nursing and Health Professions
## Lebanon, Tennessee

***http://www.cumberland.edu/Nursing/***
Founded in 1842

**DEGREE • BSN**
**Nursing Program Faculty** 17 (12% with doctorates).
**Baccalaureate Enrollment** 345 **Women** 87% **Men** 13% **Minority** 12% **International** .05% **Part-time** 23%
**Distance Learning Courses** Available.
**Nursing Student Activities** Sigma Theta Tau, Student Nurses' Association.
**Nursing Student Resources** Academic advising; academic or career counseling; assistance for students with disabilities; bookstore; campus computer network; career placement assistance; computer lab; computer-assisted instruction; e-mail services; externships; housing assistance; interactive nursing skills videos; Internet; learning resource lab; library services; nursing audiovisuals; remedial services; resume preparation assistance; skills, simulation, or other laboratory; tutoring.
**Library Facilities** 112,112 volumes (125 in health, 66 in nursing); 232 periodical subscriptions (25 health-care related).

## BACCALAUREATE PROGRAMS

**Degree** BSN
**Available Programs** ADN to Baccalaureate; Accelerated Baccalaureate; Accelerated Baccalaureate for Second Degree; Accelerated RN Baccalaureate; Baccalaureate for Second Degree; Generic Baccalaureate; RN Baccalaureate.
**Site Options** Mt. Juliet, TN.
**Study Options** Full-time and part-time.
**Online Degree Options** Yes.
**Program Entrance Requirements** Minimum overall college GPA of 3.0, transcript of college record, CPR certification, written essay, health exam, health insurance, high school transcript, immunizations, minimum high school GPA of 2.75, minimum GPA in nursing prerequisites of 3.0, professional liability insurance/malpractice insurance, prerequisite course work. Transfer students are accepted. *Application deadline:* 6/6 (fall), 10/3 (spring), 2/7 (summer). Applications may be processed on a rolling basis for some programs. *Application fee:* $25.
**Advanced Placement** Credit by examination available. Credit given for nursing courses completed elsewhere dependent upon specific evaluations.
**Expenses (2013–14)** *Tuition:* full-time $19,200; part-time $800 per credit hour. *Room and board:* $3500; room only: $3000 per academic year. *Required fees:* full-time $1000; part-time $150 per credit; part-time $500 per term.
**Financial Aid** 95% of baccalaureate students in nursing programs received some form of financial aid in 2012–13.
**Contact** Dr. Carole Ann Bach, Professor and Dean, Rudy School of Nursing and Health Professions, Cumberland University, One Cumberland Square, McFarland Campus, Lebanon, TN 37087-3554. *Telephone:* 615-547-1200. *Fax:* 615-449-1368. *E-mail:* cbach@cumberland.edu.

# East Tennessee State University

### College of Nursing
### Johnson City, Tennessee

***http://www.etsu.edu/nursing***
Founded in 1911

**DEGREES • BSN • DNP • MSN • PHD**
**Nursing Program Faculty** 70 (36% with doctorates).
**Baccalaureate Enrollment** 780 **Women** 80% **Men** 20% **Minority** 6% **Part-time** 10%
**Graduate Enrollment** 397 **Women** 90% **Men** 10% **Minority** 2% **International** 1% **Part-time** 50%
**Distance Learning Courses** Available.
**Nursing Student Activities** Nursing Honor Society, Sigma Theta Tau, Student Nurses' Association.
**Nursing Student Resources** Academic advising; academic or career counseling; assistance for students with disabilities; bookstore; campus computer network; career placement assistance; computer lab; computer-assisted instruction; daycare for children of students; e-mail services; employment services for current students; externships; housing assistance; interactive nursing skills videos; Internet; learning resource lab; library services; nursing audiovisuals; remedial services; resume preparation assistance; skills, simulation, or other laboratory; tutoring.
**Library Facilities** 1.1 million volumes; 3,714 periodical subscriptions.

## BACCALAUREATE PROGRAMS

**Degree** BSN
**Available Programs** ADN to Baccalaureate; Accelerated Baccalaureate for Second Degree; Accelerated RN Baccalaureate; Generic Baccalaureate; LPN to Baccalaureate; RN Baccalaureate.
**Site Options** Cleveland, TN; Kingsport, TN; Sevierville, TN; Pellissippi, TN.
**Study Options** Full-time and part-time.
**Online Degree Options** Yes.
**Program Entrance Requirements** Minimum overall college GPA of 2.6, transcript of college record, minimum GPA in nursing prerequisites of 2.6, prerequisite course work. Transfer students are accepted. *Application deadline:* 10/1 (fall), 2/1 (spring). *Application fee:* $45.
**Advanced Placement** Credit given for nursing courses completed elsewhere dependent upon specific evaluations.
**Expenses (2013–14)** *Tuition, area resident:* full-time $3772. *Room and board:* $2910; room only: $1630 per academic year.
**Financial Aid** 93% of baccalaureate students in nursing programs received some form of financial aid in 2012–13.
**Contact** Mr. Scott Vaughn, Director, Student Services, College of Nursing, East Tennessee State University, PO Box 70664, Office of Student Services, Johnson City, TN 37614. *Telephone:* 423-439-4578. *Fax:* 423-439-4522. *E-mail:* nursing@etsu.edu.

## GRADUATE PROGRAMS

**Expenses (2013–14)** *Tuition, area resident:* full-time $4108. *Room and board:* $2910; room only: $1630 per academic year.
**Financial Aid** 90% of graduate students in nursing programs received some form of financial aid in 2012–13. 2 research assistantships with full and partial tuition reimbursements available (averaging $4,000 per year) were awarded; career-related internships or fieldwork, institutionally sponsored loans, scholarships, and unspecified assistantships also available. *Financial aid application deadline:* 7/1.
**Contact** Ms. Amy Bower, Coordinator, College of Nursing, East Tennessee State University, PO Box 70664, Office of Student Services, Johnson City, TN 37614. *Telephone:* 423-439-4578. *Fax:* 423-439-4522. *E-mail:* bowera@etsu.edu.

### MASTER'S DEGREE PROGRAM

**Degree** MSN
**Available Programs** Master's; Master's for Nurses with Non-Nursing Degrees.
**Concentrations Available** Clinical nurse leader; nursing administration; nursing education; nursing informatics. *Nurse practitioner programs in:* family health.
**Study Options** Full-time and part-time.
**Online Degree Options** Yes.
**Program Entrance Requirements** Minimum overall college GPA of 3.0, transcript of college record, written essay, 3 letters of recommendation, resume, statistics course. *Application deadline:* 2/1 (fall), 7/1 (spring), 12/1 (summer). *Application fee:* $35.
**Advanced Placement** Credit given for nursing courses completed elsewhere dependent upon specific evaluations.
**Degree Requirements** 46 total credit hours, comprehensive exam.

### POST-MASTER'S PROGRAM

**Areas of Study** Nursing administration; nursing education; nursing informatics. *Nurse practitioner programs in:* family health.

### DOCTORAL DEGREE PROGRAM

**Degree** DNP
**Available Programs** Doctorate, Doctorate for Nurses with Non-Nursing Degrees, Post-Baccalaureate Doctorate.
**Areas of Study** Advanced practice nursing, nursing administration.
**Program Entrance Requirements** Minimum overall college GPA of 3.0, clinical experience, interview by faculty committee, letters of recommendation, MSN or equivalent, vita, writing sample. *Application deadline:* 2/1 (fall), 10/1 (spring). *Application fee:* $35.
**Degree Requirements** 79-85 total credit hours, residency.

**Degree** PhD
**Available Programs** Doctorate.
**Areas of Study** Individualized study.
**Program Entrance Requirements** Clinical experience, minimum overall college GPA of 3.0, interview by faculty committee, 3 letters of recommendation, MSN or equivalent, statistics course, vita, writing sample, GRE General Test. *Application deadline:* 2/1 (spring). *Application fee:* $35.
**Degree Requirements** 62 total credit hours, dissertation, written exam, residency.

## CONTINUING EDUCATION PROGRAM

**Contact** Dr. Wendy Nehring, Dean, College of Nursing, East Tennessee State University, PO Box 70629, 807 University Parkway, Johnson City, TN 37614-1709. *Telephone:* 423-439-4052. *E-mail:* nehringw@etsu.edu.

# King College

### School of Nursing
### Bristol, Tennessee

***http://www.king.edu/***
Founded in 1867

**DEGREES • BSN • MSN • MSN/MBA**
**Nursing Program Faculty** 31 (26% with doctorates).

**Baccalaureate Enrollment** 366 **Women** 96% **Men** 4% **Minority** 1% **International** 1%
**Graduate Enrollment** 35 **Women** 99% **Men** 1% **Minority** 1%
**Distance Learning Courses** Available.
**Nursing Student Activities** Student Nurses' Association.
**Nursing Student Resources** Academic advising; academic or career counseling; assistance for students with disabilities; bookstore; campus computer network; career placement assistance; computer lab; computer-assisted instruction; e-mail services; employment services for current students; externships; interactive nursing skills videos; Internet; learning resource lab; library services; nursing audiovisuals; paid internships; remedial services; resume preparation assistance; skills, simulation, or other laboratory; tutoring.
**Library Facilities** 94,486 volumes (929 in health, 158 in nursing); 347 periodical subscriptions (87 health-care related).

## BACCALAUREATE PROGRAMS

**Degree** BSN
**Available Programs** Accelerated RN Baccalaureate; Generic Baccalaureate.
**Site Options** Kingsport, TN.
**Study Options** Full-time.
**Program Entrance Requirements** Minimum overall college GPA of 2.0, transcript of college record, CPR certification, written essay, health exam, health insurance, high school biology, high school chemistry, high school foreign language, 2 years high school math, 2 years high school science, high school transcript, immunizations, minimum high school GPA of 2.6, minimum high school rank 25%, minimum GPA in nursing prerequisites of 2.75. Transfer students are accepted. *Application deadline:* 6/1 (fall). *Application fee:* $100.
**Contact** *Telephone:* 423-652-4841. *Fax:* 423-652-4833.

## GRADUATE PROGRAMS

**Contact** *Telephone:* 423-652-4841. *Fax:* 423-652-4833.

### MASTER'S DEGREE PROGRAM

**Degrees** MSN; MSN/MBA
**Available Programs** Accelerated RN to Master's; Master's.
**Concentrations Available** *Clinical nurse specialist programs in:* acute care, adult health, oncology.
**Study Options** Full-time.
**Program Entrance Requirements** Clinical experience, computer literacy, minimum overall college GPA of 3.0, transcript of college record, CPR certification, written essay, immunizations, 2 letters of recommendation, nursing research course, physical assessment course, resume, statistics course. *Application deadline:* 4/15 (fall). *Application fee:* $100.
**Degree Requirements** 39 total credit hours, thesis or project.

# Lincoln Memorial University

**Caylor School of Nursing**
**Harrogate, Tennessee**

*http://www.lmunet.edu/academics/nursing/index2.shtml*
Founded in 1897

**DEGREES • BSN • MSN**

**Nursing Program Faculty** 50 (57% with doctorates).
**Baccalaureate Enrollment** 70 **Women** 80% **Men** 20% **Minority** 3% **International** 3%
**Graduate Enrollment** 65
**Nursing Student Activities** Student Nurses' Association.
**Nursing Student Resources** Academic advising; academic or career counseling; bookstore; campus computer network; career placement assistance; computer lab; e-mail services; externships; interactive nursing skills videos; Internet; learning resource lab; library services; nursing audiovisuals; other; placement services for program completers; skills, simulation, or other laboratory; tutoring.
**Library Facilities** 323,046 volumes (1,230 in health, 630 in nursing); 334 periodical subscriptions (36 health-care related).

## BACCALAUREATE PROGRAMS

**Degree** BSN
**Available Programs** ADN to Baccalaureate; Accelerated Baccalaureate; Generic Baccalaureate; RN Baccalaureate.
**Site Options** Knoxville, TN.
**Study Options** Full-time.
**Program Entrance Requirements** Minimum overall college GPA of 2.75, transcript of college record, CPR certification, immunizations, professional liability insurance/malpractice insurance, prerequisite course work, RN licensure. Transfer students are accepted. *Application deadline:* Applications may be processed on a rolling basis for some programs.
**Contact** *Telephone:* 423-869-3611. *Fax:* 423-869-6444.

## GRADUATE PROGRAMS

**Contact** *Telephone:* 423-869-6283. *Fax:* 423-869-6244.

### MASTER'S DEGREE PROGRAM

**Degree** MSN
**Available Programs** Master's.
**Concentrations Available** Nurse anesthesia. *Nurse practitioner programs in:* family health, psychiatric/mental health.
**Site Options** Knoxville, TN.
**Study Options** Full-time and part-time.
**Program Entrance Requirements** Clinical experience, computer literacy, transcript of college record, CPR certification, written essay, immunizations, interview, 3 letters of recommendation, professional liability insurance/malpractice insurance, prerequisite course work, statistics course. *Application deadline:* Applications may be processed on a rolling basis for some programs.

### POST-MASTER'S PROGRAM

**Areas of Study** *Nurse practitioner programs in:* family health, psychiatric/mental health.

# Lipscomb University

**Department of Nursing**
**Nashville, Tennessee**

Founded in 1891

**DEGREE • BSN**

**Library Facilities** 274,396 volumes; 712 periodical subscriptions.

## BACCALAUREATE PROGRAMS

**Degree** BSN
**Available Programs** Generic Baccalaureate.
**Contact** *Telephone:* 615-996-6650.

# Martin Methodist College

**Division of Nursing**
**Pulaski, Tennessee**

*http://www.martinmethodist.edu/*
Founded in 1870

**DEGREE • BSN**

**Nursing Program Faculty** 7 (43% with doctorates).
**Baccalaureate Enrollment** 71 **Women** 96% **Men** 4% **Minority** 2%
**Distance Learning Courses** Available.
**Nursing Student Activities** Student Nurses' Association.
**Nursing Student Resources** Academic advising; academic or career counseling; bookstore; campus computer network; career placement assistance; computer lab; computer-assisted instruction; e-mail services; employment services for current students; housing assistance; interactive nursing skills videos; Internet; learning resource lab; library services; nursing audiovisuals; placement services for program completers; remedial services; resume preparation assistance; skills, simulation, or other laboratory; tutoring; unpaid internships.
**Library Facilities** 84,000 volumes (875 in nursing); 664 periodical subscriptions (400 health-care related).

## BACCALAUREATE PROGRAMS

**Degree** BSN
**Available Programs** Generic Baccalaureate.
**Study Options** Full-time.
**Program Entrance Requirements** Transcript of college record, CPR certification, health insurance, immunizations, minimum GPA in nursing prerequisites, prerequisite course work. Transfer students are accepted. *Application deadline:* 2/1 (fall), 2/1 (winter). *Application fee:* $30.

**Expenses (2012–13)** *Tuition:* full-time $20,000. *Room and board:* $10,000; room only: $7000 per academic year. *Required fees:* full-time $700; part-time $350 per term.
**Financial Aid** 100% of baccalaureate students in nursing programs received some form of financial aid in 2011–12.
**Contact** Dr. Kenneth R. Burns, Professor and Chair, Division of Nursing, Martin Methodist College, 433 West Madison Street, Pulaski, TN 38478. *Telephone:* 931-424-7395. *Fax:* 931-363-9891. *E-mail:* kburns@martinmethodist.edu.

# Middle Tennessee State University

## School of Nursing
## Murfreesboro, Tennessee

***http://www.mtsu.edu/***
Founded in 1911

**DEGREES • BSN • MSN**
**Nursing Program Faculty** 45 (65% with doctorates).
**Baccalaureate Enrollment** 300 **Women** 85% **Men** 15% **Minority** 15%
**Graduate Enrollment** 100 **Women** 80% **Men** 20% **Minority** 15% **Part-time** 50%
**Distance Learning Courses** Available.
**Nursing Student Activities** Sigma Theta Tau, Student Nurses' Association.
**Nursing Student Resources** Academic advising; academic or career counseling; assistance for students with disabilities; bookstore; campus computer network; career placement assistance; computer lab; computer-assisted instruction; e-mail services; interactive nursing skills videos; Internet; learning resource lab; library services; nursing audiovisuals; remedial services; resume preparation assistance; skills, simulation, or other laboratory; tutoring.
**Library Facilities** 100 volumes in health, 45 volumes in nursing; 100 periodical subscriptions health-care related.

### BACCALAUREATE PROGRAMS

**Degree** BSN
**Available Programs** Generic Baccalaureate; LPN to RN Baccalaureate; RN Baccalaureate.
**Study Options** Full-time.
**Online Degree Options** Yes.
**Program Entrance Requirements** Minimum overall college GPA of 2.8, transcript of college record, CPR certification, health exam, health insurance, immunizations, interview, minimum GPA in nursing prerequisites of 2.75, professional liability insurance/malpractice insurance, prerequisite course work. Transfer students are accepted. *Application deadline:* 2/1 (fall), 10/1 (spring).
**Advanced Placement** Credit by examination available. Credit given for nursing courses completed elsewhere dependent upon specific evaluations.
**Financial Aid** ***Gift aid (need-based):*** Federal Pell, FSEOG, state, private, college/university gift aid from institutional funds. *Loans:* Federal Direct (Subsidized and Unsubsidized Stafford PLUS), Perkins, college/university. *Work-study:* Federal Work-Study. *Financial aid application deadline (priority):* 3/1.
**Contact** Dr. Karen S. Ward, Interim Director, School of Nursing, Middle Tennessee State University, PO Box 81, 1301 East Main Street, Murfreesboro, TN 37132-0001. *Telephone:* 615-898-2437. *Fax:* 615-898-5441. *E-mail:* karen.ward@mtsu.edu.

### GRADUATE PROGRAMS

**Contact** Dr. Karen S. Ward, Interim Director, School of Nursing, Middle Tennessee State University, PO Box 81, 1301 East Main Street, Murfreesboro, TN 37132-0001. *Telephone:* 615-898-2437. *Fax:* 615-898-5441. *E-mail:* karen.ward@mtsu.edu.

#### MASTER'S DEGREE PROGRAM

**Degree** MSN
**Available Programs** Accelerated AD/RN to Master's; Master's.
**Concentrations Available** Nursing administration; nursing education; nursing informatics. *Nurse practitioner programs in:* family health.
**Site Options** multiple cities.
**Study Options** Full-time and part-time.
**Online Degree Options** Yes.
**Program Entrance Requirements** Minimum overall college GPA of 3.0, transcript of college record, 3 letters of recommendation, prerequisite course work, resume. *Application deadline:* Applications may be processed on a rolling basis for some programs.
**Degree Requirements** 43 total credit hours, thesis or project.

#### POST-MASTER'S PROGRAM

**Areas of Study** *Nurse practitioner programs in:* family health.

# Milligan College

## Department of Nursing
## Milligan College, Tennessee

***http://www.milligan.edu/BSN/***
Founded in 1866

**DEGREE • BSN**
**Nursing Program Faculty** 10 (25% with doctorates).
**Baccalaureate Enrollment** 195 **Women** 90% **Men** 10% **Minority** 2%
**Nursing Student Activities** Nursing Honor Society, Student Nurses' Association.
**Nursing Student Resources** Academic advising; academic or career counseling; assistance for students with disabilities; bookstore; campus computer network; career placement assistance; computer lab; computer-assisted instruction; e-mail services; employment services for current students; externships; interactive nursing skills videos; Internet; learning resource lab; library services; nursing audiovisuals; placement services for program completers; remedial services; resume preparation assistance; skills, simulation, or other laboratory; tutoring; unpaid internships.
**Library Facilities** 145,605 volumes (2,430 in health, 184 in nursing); 11,097 periodical subscriptions (340 health-care related).

### BACCALAUREATE PROGRAMS

**Degree** BSN
**Available Programs** ADN to Baccalaureate; Baccalaureate for Second Degree; Generic Baccalaureate; LPN to Baccalaureate; LPN to RN Baccalaureate; RN Baccalaureate.
**Study Options** Full-time and part-time.
**Program Entrance Requirements** Minimum overall college GPA of 2.5, transcript of college record, CPR certification, written essay, health exam, immunizations, letters of recommendation, minimum GPA in nursing prerequisites of 2.5, professional liability insurance/malpractice insurance, prerequisite course work. Transfer students are accepted. *Application deadline:* Applications may be processed on a rolling basis for some programs. *Application fee:* $30.
**Advanced Placement** Credit given for nursing courses completed elsewhere dependent upon specific evaluations.
**Contact** *Telephone:* 423-461-8655. *Fax:* 423-461-8982.

# South College

## Department of Nursing
## Knoxville, Tennessee

Founded in 1882

**DEGREE • BSN**
**Nursing Program Faculty** 14 (25% with doctorates).
**Baccalaureate Enrollment** 75 **Women** 90% **Men** 10% **Minority** 10%
**Nursing Student Activities** Student Nurses' Association.
**Nursing Student Resources** Academic advising; academic or career counseling; assistance for students with disabilities; bookstore; campus computer network; career placement assistance; computer lab; computer-assisted instruction; e-mail services; externships; interactive nursing skills videos; Internet; learning resource lab; library services; nursing audiovisuals; placement services for program completers; resume preparation assistance; skills, simulation, or other laboratory; tutoring.

### BACCALAUREATE PROGRAMS

**Degree** BSN
**Available Programs** Generic Baccalaureate.
**Study Options** Full-time.
**Program Entrance Requirements** CPR certification, written essay, health exam, immunizations, interview, 2 letters of recommendation, minimum GPA in nursing prerequisites of 2.5. Transfer students are accepted. *Application fee:* $25.

**Advanced Placement** Credit by examination available. Credit given for nursing courses completed elsewhere dependent upon specific evaluations.
**Expenses (2013–14)** *Tuition:* full-time $9000. *International tuition:* $9000 full-time. *Required fees:* full-time $150.
**Financial Aid** ***Gift aid (need-based):*** Federal Pell, FSEOG, state, private, college/university gift aid from institutional funds. *Loans:* Perkins. *Work-study:* Federal Work-Study. *Financial aid application deadline:* Continuous.
**Contact** Nursing Contact, Department of Nursing, South College, Knoxville, TN 37909. *Telephone:* 865-251-1800.

# Southern Adventist University
## School of Nursing
## Collegedale, Tennessee

***http://www.southern.edu/nursing***
Founded in 1892

### DEGREES • BS • DNP • MSN • MSN/MBA

**Nursing Program Faculty** 28 (29% with doctorates).
**Baccalaureate Enrollment** 131 **Women** 80% **Men** 20% **Minority** 40% **International** 6% **Part-time** 51%
**Graduate Enrollment** 192 **Women** 82% **Men** 18% **Minority** 20% **International** 4% **Part-time** 51%
**Distance Learning Courses** Available.
**Nursing Student Activities** Sigma Theta Tau, nursing club.
**Nursing Student Resources** Academic advising; academic or career counseling; assistance for students with disabilities; bookstore; campus computer network; career placement assistance; computer lab; computer-assisted instruction; e-mail services; employment services for current students; housing assistance; interactive nursing skills videos; Internet; learning resource lab; library services; nursing audiovisuals; remedial services; resume preparation assistance; skills, simulation, or other laboratory; tutoring.
**Library Facilities** 170,176 volumes (7,029 in health, 1,603 in nursing); 56,047 periodical subscriptions.

### BACCALAUREATE PROGRAMS

**Degree** BS
**Available Programs** ADN to Baccalaureate.
**Site Options** Chattanooga, TN.
**Study Options** Full-time and part-time.
**Online Degree Options** Yes.
**Program Entrance Requirements** Minimum overall college GPA of 2.5, transcript of college record, CPR certification, health exam, high school transcript, immunizations, 2 letters of recommendation, minimum GPA in nursing prerequisites of 2.0, prerequisite course work, RN licensure. Transfer students are accepted. *Application deadline:* 2/1 (fall), 9/1 (winter). Applications may be processed on a rolling basis for some programs.
**Advanced Placement** Credit given for nursing courses completed elsewhere dependent upon specific evaluations.
**Expenses (2013–14)** *Tuition:* full-time $18,990; part-time $800 per credit. *International tuition:* $18,990 full-time. *Room and board:* $5700; room only: $3700 per academic year.
**Financial Aid** 80% of baccalaureate students in nursing programs received some form of financial aid in 2012–13. *Gift aid (need-based):* Federal Pell, FSEOG, state, private, college/university gift aid from institutional funds. *Loans:* Federal Nursing Student Loans, Federal Direct (Subsidized and Unsubsidized Stafford PLUS), Perkins, college/university. *Work-study:* Federal Work-Study, part-time campus jobs. *Financial aid application deadline (priority):* 3/1.
**Contact** Mrs. Linda Marlowe, Admissions and Progression Coordinator, School of Nursing, Southern Adventist University, PO Box 370, Collegedale, TN 37315-0370. *Telephone:* 423-236-2941. *Fax:* 423-236-1940. *E-mail:* lmarlowe@southern.edu.

### GRADUATE PROGRAMS

**Expenses (2013–14)** *Tuition:* full-time $10,000; part-time $570 per hour. *International tuition:* $10,000 full-time. *Required fees:* full-time $300; part-time $100 per credit.
**Financial Aid** 85% of graduate students in nursing programs received some form of financial aid in 2012–13.
**Contact** Mrs. Diane Proffitt, Applications Manager, School of Nursing, Southern Adventist University, PO Box 370, Collegedale, TN 37315-0370. *Telephone:* 423-236-2957. *Fax:* 423-236-1940. *E-mail:* dproffit@southern.edu.

#### MASTER'S DEGREE PROGRAM

**Degrees** MSN; MSN/MBA
**Available Programs** Accelerated RN to Master's; Master's.
**Concentrations Available** Nursing education. *Nurse practitioner programs in:* acute care, adult health, family health.
**Study Options** Full-time and part-time.
**Online Degree Options** Yes (online only).
**Program Entrance Requirements** Clinical experience, minimum overall college GPA of 3.0, transcript of college record, CPR certification, written essay, immunizations, interview, 2 letters of recommendation, prerequisite course work, statistics course. *Application deadline:* 7/1 (fall), 11/1 (winter). Applications may be processed on a rolling basis for some programs. *Application fee:* $25.
**Advanced Placement** Credit given for nursing courses completed elsewhere dependent upon specific evaluations.
**Degree Requirements** 46 total credit hours, thesis or project.

#### POST-MASTER'S PROGRAM

**Areas of Study** *Nurse practitioner programs in:* acute care, adult health, family health.

#### DOCTORAL DEGREE PROGRAM

**Degree** DNP
**Available Programs** Doctorate.
**Areas of Study** Advanced practice nursing, aging, biology of health and illness, health promotion/disease prevention.
**Online Degree Options** Yes (online only).
**Program Entrance Requirements** Clinical experience, minimum overall college GPA of 3.0, interview by faculty committee, interview, 3 letters of recommendation, MSN or equivalent, scholarly papers, statistics course, vita, writing sample. *Application deadline:* 5/1 (fall). Applications may be processed on a rolling basis for some programs. *Application fee:* $25.
**Degree Requirements** 42 total credit hours.

### CONTINUING EDUCATION PROGRAM

**Contact** Mrs. Sylvia Mayer, Director of Admissions and Progressions, School of Nursing, Southern Adventist University, PO Box 370, Collegedale, TN 37315-0370. *Telephone:* 423-236-2941. *Fax:* 423-236-1940. *E-mail:* smayer@southern.edu.

# Tennessee State University
## Division of Nursing
## Nashville, Tennessee

***http://www.tnstate.edu/nursing/***
Founded in 1912

### DEGREES • BSN • MSN

**Nursing Program Faculty** 49 (33% with doctorates).
**Baccalaureate Enrollment** 107 **Women** 81% **Men** 19% **Minority** 66% **Part-time** 21%
**Graduate Enrollment** 285 **Women** 89% **Men** 11% **Minority** 48% **International** 10% **Part-time** 45%
**Distance Learning Courses** Available.
**Nursing Student Activities** Sigma Theta Tau.
**Nursing Student Resources** Academic advising; academic or career counseling; assistance for students with disabilities; bookstore; campus computer network; computer lab; e-mail services; interactive nursing skills videos; Internet; learning resource lab; library services; nursing audiovisuals; skills, simulation, or other laboratory; tutoring.
**Library Facilities** 630,890 volumes (50,000 in health, 25,000 in nursing); 300 periodical subscriptions health-care related.

### BACCALAUREATE PROGRAMS

**Degree** BSN
**Available Programs** Generic Baccalaureate; RN Baccalaureate.
**Site Options** Nashville, TN.
**Study Options** Full-time.
**Program Entrance Requirements** Minimum overall college GPA of 2.8, transcript of college record, CPR certification, health exam, immunizations, minimum high school GPA of 2.8, minimum GPA in nursing prerequisites of 2.8, professional liability insurance/malpractice insurance,

prerequisite course work. Transfer students are accepted. *Application deadline:* 3/1 (fall).
**Expenses (2013–14)** *Tuition, state resident:* full-time $6774; part-time $290 per credit hour. *Tuition, nonresident:* full-time $20,190; part-time $820 per credit hour. *International tuition:* $20,250 full-time. *Room and board:* $9250; room only: $6460 per academic year. *Required fees:* full-time $750; part-time $25 per credit.
**Financial Aid** 80% of baccalaureate students in nursing programs received some form of financial aid in 2012–13. *Gift aid (need-based):* Federal Pell, FSEOG, state, private, college/university gift aid from institutional funds. *Loans:* Federal Direct (Subsidized and Unsubsidized Stafford PLUS), Perkins. *Work-study:* Federal Work-Study. *Financial aid application deadline (priority):* 4/1.
**Contact** Dr. Pamela D. Ark, BSN Program Director, Division of Nursing, Tennessee State University, 3500 John A. Merritt Boulevard, Box 9590, Nashville, TN 37209-1561. *Telephone:* 615-963-7615. *Fax:* 615-963-5593. *E-mail:* park@tnstate.edu.

## GRADUATE PROGRAMS

**Expenses (2013–14)** *Tuition, state resident:* full-time $8730; part-time $433 per credit hour. *Tuition, nonresident:* full-time $20,834; part-time $1015 per credit hour.
**Financial Aid** 80% of graduate students in nursing programs received some form of financial aid in 2012–13. Research assistantships, teaching assistantships available.
**Contact** Dr. Jane C. Norman, MSN Program Director, Division of Nursing, Tennessee State University, 3500 John A. Merritt Boulevard, Box 9590, Nashville, TN 37209-1561. *Telephone:* 615-963-5255. *Fax:* 615-963-7614. *E-mail:* jnorman@tnstate.edu.

### MASTER'S DEGREE PROGRAM

**Degree** MSN
**Available Programs** RN to Master's.
**Concentrations Available** Nursing administration; nursing education; nursing informatics. *Nurse practitioner programs in:* family health.
**Site Options** Nashville, TN.
**Study Options** Full-time and part-time.
**Online Degree Options** Yes.
**Program Entrance Requirements** Computer literacy, minimum overall college GPA of 3.0, transcript of college record, CPR certification, written essay, immunizations, 3 letters of recommendation, nursing research course, physical assessment course, professional liability insurance/malpractice insurance, resume, GRE General Test or MAT. *Application deadline:* 7/15 (fall), 11/15 (spring), 3/15 (summer). Applications may be processed on a rolling basis for some programs. *Application fee:* $25.
**Advanced Placement** Credit given for nursing courses completed elsewhere dependent upon specific evaluations.
**Degree Requirements** 45 total credit hours, thesis or project, comprehensive exam.

### POST-MASTER'S PROGRAM

**Areas of Study** Nursing administration; nursing education; nursing informatics. *Nurse practitioner programs in:* family health.

## CONTINUING EDUCATION PROGRAM

**Contact** Dr. Kathy L. Martin, Associate Dean, Health Sciences/Executive Director, Nursing, Division of Nursing, Tennessee State University, 3500 John A. Merritt Boulevard, Box 9590, Nashville, TN 37209-1561. *Telephone:* 615-963-5251. *Fax:* 615-963-5049. *E-mail:* kmartin3@tnstate.edu.

# Tennessee Technological University

### Whitson-Hester School of Nursing
### Cookeville, Tennessee

***http://www.tntech.edu/nursing***
Founded in 1915

**DEGREES • BSN • M SC N • MSN**
**Nursing Program Faculty** 21 (19% with doctorates).
**Baccalaureate Enrollment** 187 **Women** 91% **Men** 9% **Minority** 3% **Part-time** 1%
**Graduate Enrollment** 47 **Women** 89% **Men** 11% **Minority** 4% **Part-time** 94%
**Distance Learning Courses** Available.
**Nursing Student Activities** Sigma Theta Tau, Student Nurses' Association.
**Nursing Student Resources** Academic advising; academic or career counseling; assistance for students with disabilities; bookstore; campus computer network; career placement assistance; computer lab; computer-assisted instruction; daycare for children of students; e-mail services; employment services for current students; externships; housing assistance; Internet; learning resource lab; library services; nursing audiovisuals; paid internships; placement services for program completers; remedial services; resume preparation assistance; skills, simulation, or other laboratory; tutoring; unpaid internships.
**Library Facilities** 704,377 volumes (312,892 in health, 11,893 in nursing); 1,636 periodical subscriptions (96 health-care related).

## BACCALAUREATE PROGRAMS

**Degree** BSN
**Available Programs** ADN to Baccalaureate; Baccalaureate for Second Degree; Generic Baccalaureate; RN Baccalaureate.
**Study Options** Full-time.
**Program Entrance Requirements** Minimum overall college GPA of 2.5, transcript of college record, CPR certification, written essay, health exam, high school biology, high school foreign language, 4 years high school math, 2 years high school science, high school transcript, immunizations, minimum high school GPA of 3.0, minimum GPA in nursing prerequisites of 2.5, professional liability insurance/malpractice insurance, prerequisite course work. Transfer students are accepted. *Application deadline:* 2/1 (fall), 6/1 (spring).
**Advanced Placement** Credit given for nursing courses completed elsewhere dependent upon specific evaluations.
**Contact** *Telephone:* 931-372-3229. *Fax:* 931-372-6244.

## GRADUATE PROGRAMS

**Contact** *Telephone:* 931-372-3229. *Fax:* 931-372-6244.

### MASTER'S DEGREE PROGRAM

**Degrees** M Sc N; MSN
**Available Programs** Master's; Master's for Nurses with Non-Nursing Degrees.
**Concentrations Available** Nursing administration; nursing education; nursing informatics. *Nurse practitioner programs in:* family health.
**Study Options** Full-time and part-time.
**Online Degree Options** Yes (online only).
**Program Entrance Requirements** Computer literacy, minimum overall college GPA of 3.0, transcript of college record, CPR certification, written essay, immunizations, 3 letters of recommendation, nursing research course, professional liability insurance/malpractice insurance, resume. *Application deadline:* 8/1 (fall), 12/1 (spring), 5/1 (summer). Applications may be processed on a rolling basis for some programs. *Application fee:* $25.
**Advanced Placement** Credit given for nursing courses completed elsewhere dependent upon specific evaluations.
**Degree Requirements** 46 total credit hours, thesis or project.

# Tennessee Wesleyan College

### Fort Sanders Nursing Department
### Knoxville, Tennessee

***http://www.twcnet.edu/admissions/nursing-program/***
Founded in 1857

**DEGREE • BSN**
**Nursing Program Faculty** 18 (6% with doctorates).
**Baccalaureate Enrollment** 128 **Women** 89% **Men** 11% **Minority** 3% **International** 2% **Part-time** 3%
**Distance Learning Courses** Available.
**Nursing Student Activities** Nursing Honor Society, Sigma Theta Tau, Student Nurses' Association.
**Nursing Student Resources** Academic advising; assistance for students with disabilities; bookstore; campus computer network; computer lab; e-mail services; Internet; library services; nursing audiovisuals; other; skills, simulation, or other laboratory.
**Library Facilities** 5,000 volumes in health, 4,000 volumes in nursing; 135 periodical subscriptions health-care related.

## BACCALAUREATE PROGRAMS

**Degree** BSN

**Available Programs** ADN to Baccalaureate; Generic Baccalaureate; RN Baccalaureate.
**Site Options** Knoxville, TN.
**Study Options** Full-time.
**Program Entrance Requirements** Minimum overall college GPA of 2.7, transcript of college record, CPR certification, written essay, health exam, high school transcript, immunizations, interview, minimum GPA in nursing prerequisites of 2.7, prerequisite course work. Transfer students are accepted. *Application deadline:* 1/15 (fall). *Application fee:* $25.
**Advanced Placement** Credit given for nursing courses completed elsewhere dependent upon specific evaluations.
**Contact** *Telephone:* 865-777-5100. *Fax:* 865-777-5114.

# Union University

## School of Nursing
## Jackson, Tennessee

***http://www.uu.edu/academics/son/***
Founded in 1823

### DEGREES • BSN • MSN

**Nursing Program Faculty** 28 (36% with doctorates).
**Baccalaureate Enrollment** 285 **Women** 93% **Men** 7% **Minority** 27% **International** 2% **Part-time** 56%
**Graduate Enrollment** 55 **Women** 80% **Men** 20% **Minority** 25% **Part-time** 4%
**Nursing Student Activities** Nursing Honor Society, Sigma Theta Tau, Student Nurses' Association.
**Nursing Student Resources** Academic advising; academic or career counseling; assistance for students with disabilities; bookstore; campus computer network; career placement assistance; computer lab; computer-assisted instruction; e-mail services; employment services for current students; housing assistance; Internet; learning resource lab; library services; nursing audiovisuals; resume preparation assistance; skills, simulation, or other laboratory; tutoring.
**Library Facilities** 218,154 volumes (6,005 in nursing); 20,585 periodical subscriptions (1,284 health-care related).

### BACCALAUREATE PROGRAMS

**Degree** BSN
**Available Programs** Accelerated Baccalaureate for Second Degree; Generic Baccalaureate; LPN to Baccalaureate; RN Baccalaureate.
**Site Options** Germantown, TN.
**Study Options** Full-time.
**Program Entrance Requirements** Minimum overall college GPA of 2.8, transcript of college record, CPR certification, health exam, immunizations, minimum GPA in nursing prerequisites of 2.8, prerequisite course work. Transfer students are accepted.
**Advanced Placement** Credit by examination available. Credit given for nursing courses completed elsewhere dependent upon specific evaluations.
**Contact** *Telephone:* 731-661-5538. *Fax:* 731-661-5504.

### GRADUATE PROGRAMS

**Contact** *Telephone:* 731-661-5538. *Fax:* 901-661-5504.

#### MASTER'S DEGREE PROGRAM

**Degree** MSN
**Available Programs** Master's.
**Concentrations Available** Nurse anesthesia; nursing administration; nursing education. *Clinical nurse specialist programs in:* adult health, pediatric. *Nurse practitioner programs in:* family health.
**Site Options** Germantown, TN.
**Study Options** Full-time and part-time.
**Program Entrance Requirements** Minimum overall college GPA of 3.0, transcript of college record, CPR certification, written essay, immunizations, interview, 3 letters of recommendation, professional liability insurance/malpractice insurance, GRE.
**Advanced Placement** Credit given for nursing courses completed elsewhere dependent upon specific evaluations.
**Degree Requirements** 46 total credit hours.

#### POST-MASTER'S PROGRAM

**Areas of Study** Nursing administration; nursing education. *Clinical nurse specialist programs in:* adult health, pediatric. *Nurse practitioner programs in:* family health.

### CONTINUING EDUCATION PROGRAM

**Contact** *Telephone:* 731-661-5152. *Fax:* 731-661-5504.

# University of Memphis

## Loewenberg School of Nursing
## Memphis, Tennessee

***http://www.nursing.memphis.edu/***
Founded in 1912

### DEGREES • BSN • MSN

**Nursing Program Faculty** 65 (22% with doctorates).
**Baccalaureate Enrollment** 441 **Women** 91% **Men** 9% **Minority** 23% **Part-time** 15%
**Graduate Enrollment** 124 **Women** 92% **Men** 8% **Minority** 30% **Part-time** 75%
**Distance Learning Courses** Available.
**Nursing Student Activities** Sigma Theta Tau, Student Nurses' Association.
**Nursing Student Resources** Academic advising; academic or career counseling; assistance for students with disabilities; bookstore; campus computer network; career placement assistance; computer lab; computer-assisted instruction; daycare for children of students; e-mail services; externships; housing assistance; interactive nursing skills videos; Internet; learning resource lab; library services; nursing audiovisuals; paid internships; remedial services; resume preparation assistance; skills, simulation, or other laboratory; tutoring.
**Library Facilities** 1.5 million volumes (74,513 in health); 6,771 periodical subscriptions (878 health-care related).

### BACCALAUREATE PROGRAMS

**Degree** BSN
**Available Programs** ADN to Baccalaureate; Accelerated Baccalaureate; Accelerated Baccalaureate for Second Degree; Accelerated RN Baccalaureate; Baccalaureate for Second Degree; Generic Baccalaureate; RN Baccalaureate.
**Site Options** Jackson, TN.
**Study Options** Full-time.
**Program Entrance Requirements** Minimum overall college GPA of 2.7, transcript of college record, CPR certification, health exam, high school biology, high school chemistry, high school foreign language, 3 years high school math, 2 years high school science, high school transcript, immunizations, minimum high school GPA of 3.0, minimum GPA in nursing prerequisites of 2.4, prerequisite course work. Transfer students are accepted.
**Advanced Placement** Credit by examination available. Credit given for nursing courses completed elsewhere dependent upon specific evaluations.
**Contact** *Telephone:* 901-678-2003. *Fax:* 901-678-4906.

### GRADUATE PROGRAMS

**Contact** *Telephone:* 901-678-2003. *Fax:* 901-678-4906.

#### MASTER'S DEGREE PROGRAM

**Degree** MSN
**Available Programs** Accelerated Master's for Nurses with Non-Nursing Degrees; Master's; Master's for Non-Nursing College Graduates; Master's for Nurses with Non-Nursing Degrees.
**Concentrations Available** Nursing administration; nursing education. *Nurse practitioner programs in:* family health.
**Site Options** Jackson, TN.
**Study Options** Full-time and part-time.
**Online Degree Options** Yes.
**Program Entrance Requirements** Minimum overall college GPA of 2.8, CPR certification, immunizations, 3 letters of recommendation, professional liability insurance/malpractice insurance.
**Advanced Placement** Credit given for nursing courses completed elsewhere dependent upon specific evaluations.
**Degree Requirements** 45 total credit hours, comprehensive exam.

#### POST-MASTER'S PROGRAM

**Areas of Study** *Nurse practitioner programs in:* family health.

# The University of Tennessee
## College of Nursing
## Knoxville, Tennessee

***https://nursing.utk.edu/Pages/default.aspx***
Founded in 1794

**DEGREES • BSN • MSN • MSN/PHD • PHD**
**Nursing Program Faculty** 58 (64% with doctorates).
**Baccalaureate Enrollment** 523 **Women** 88% **Men** 12% **Minority** 19.1% **International** .5% **Part-time** 8%
**Graduate Enrollment** 160 **Women** 85% **Men** 15% **Minority** 10% **International** .6% **Part-time** 40.6%
**Distance Learning Courses** Available.
**Nursing Student Activities** Sigma Theta Tau, Student Nurses' Association.
**Nursing Student Resources** Academic advising; academic or career counseling; assistance for students with disabilities; bookstore; campus computer network; computer lab; computer-assisted instruction; e-mail services; employment services for current students; externships; interactive nursing skills videos; Internet; learning resource lab; library services; nursing audiovisuals; remedial services; skills, simulation, or other laboratory; tutoring.
**Library Facilities** 3.1 million volumes (59,214 in health, 3,711 in nursing); 58,765 periodical subscriptions (572 health-care related).

### BACCALAUREATE PROGRAMS

**Degree** BSN
**Available Programs** Accelerated Baccalaureate; Generic Baccalaureate; RN Baccalaureate.
**Study Options** Full-time and part-time.
**Program Entrance Requirements** Transcript of college record, CPR certification, written essay, health exam, health insurance, high school biology, high school chemistry, 3 years high school math, 2 years high school science, high school transcript, immunizations, interview, minimum high school GPA of 3.2, minimum GPA in nursing prerequisites of 3.2, professional liability insurance/malpractice insurance, prerequisite course work. Transfer students are accepted. *Application deadline:* 12/1 (fall), 12/1 (summer). *Application fee:* $30.
**Advanced Placement** Credit given for nursing courses completed elsewhere dependent upon specific evaluations.
**Expenses (2013–14)** *Tuition, state resident:* full-time $9684. *Tuition, nonresident:* full-time $28,174. *International tuition:* $28,174 full-time. *Room and board:* $9170 per academic year. *Required fees:* full-time $600.
**Financial Aid** 90% of baccalaureate students in nursing programs received some form of financial aid in 2012–13. *Gift aid (need-based):* Federal Pell, FSEOG, state, private, college/university gift aid from institutional funds. *Loans:* Federal Direct (Subsidized and Unsubsidized Stafford PLUS), Perkins, state, college/university. *Work-study:* Federal Work-Study. *Financial aid application deadline (priority):* 2/15.
**Contact** Katie McCay, Director, Student Services, College of Nursing, The University of Tennessee, 1200 Volunteer Boulevard, Knoxville, TN 37996-4180. *Telephone:* 865-974-7604. *Fax:* 865-974-3569. *E-mail:* katie.mccay@utk.edu.

### GRADUATE PROGRAMS

**Expenses (2013–14)** *Tuition, area resident:* full-time $10,944; part-time $598 per credit hour. *Tuition, state resident:* full-time $10,944; part-time $531 per credit hour. *Tuition, nonresident:* full-time $29,432; part-time $1542 per credit hour. *Room and board:* $12,008 per academic year. *Required fees:* full-time $427; part-time $36 per credit.
**Financial Aid** 25% of graduate students in nursing programs received some form of financial aid in 2012–13. 3 fellowships, 1 research assistantship were awarded; teaching assistantships, Federal Work-Study, institutionally sponsored loans, and unspecified assistantships also available. *Financial aid application deadline:* 2/1.
**Contact** Dr. Mary Gunther, Chair, Masters Program/Director, Graduate Studies, College of Nursing, The University of Tennessee, 1200 Volunteer Boulevard, Knoxville, TN 37996-4180. *Telephone:* 865-974-4151. *Fax:* 865-974-3569. *E-mail:* mgunther@utk.edu.

### MASTER'S DEGREE PROGRAM

**Degrees** MSN; MSN/PhD
**Available Programs** Master's.
**Concentrations Available** Nurse anesthesia; nursing administration. *Clinical nurse specialist programs in:* pediatric, psychiatric/mental health. *Nurse practitioner programs in:* family health, pediatric, psychiatric/mental health.
**Study Options** Full-time and part-time.
**Program Entrance Requirements** Minimum overall college GPA of 3.0, transcript of college record, CPR certification, written essay, immunizations, 3 letters of recommendation, physical assessment course, professional liability insurance/malpractice insurance, prerequisite course work, statistics course, GRE General Test. *Application deadline:* 2/1 (fall), 10/1 (spring), 10/1 (summer). *Application fee:* $30.
**Advanced Placement** Credit given for nursing courses completed elsewhere dependent upon specific evaluations.
**Degree Requirements** 41 total credit hours, comprehensive exam.

### POST-MASTER'S PROGRAM

**Areas of Study** Nurse anesthesia; nursing administration; nursing education. *Clinical nurse specialist programs in:* pediatric, psychiatric/mental health. *Nurse practitioner programs in:* family health, pediatric, psychiatric/mental health.

### DOCTORAL DEGREE PROGRAM

**Degree** PhD
**Available Programs** Doctorate; Post-Baccalaureate Doctorate.
**Areas of Study** Advanced practice nursing, bio-behavioral research, biology of health and illness, faculty preparation, family health, health policy, health promotion/disease prevention, health-care systems, human health and illness, individualized study, neuro-behavior, nursing administration, nursing education, nursing policy, nursing research, nursing science,women's health.
**Online Degree Options** Yes (online only).
**Program Entrance Requirements** Minimum overall college GPA of 3.0, interview by faculty committee, interview, 3 letters of recommendation, writing sample, GRE General Test. *Application deadline:* 2/1 (fall), 10/1 (summer). *Application fee:* $30.
**Degree Requirements** 67 total credit hours, dissertation, oral exam, written exam, residency.

### CONTINUING EDUCATION PROGRAM

**Contact** Maureen Nalle, Coordinator, Continuing Education, College of Nursing, The University of Tennessee, 1200 Volunteer Boulevard, Knoxville, TN 37996-4180. *Telephone:* 865-974-7598. *Fax:* 865-974-3569. *E-mail:* mnalle@utk.edu.

# The University of Tennessee at Chattanooga
## School of Nursing
## Chattanooga, Tennessee

***http://www.utc.edu/Academic/Nursing***
Founded in 1886

**DEGREES • BSN • DNP • MSN**
**Nursing Program Faculty** 27 (48% with doctorates).
**Baccalaureate Enrollment** 172 **Women** 90% **Men** 10% **Minority** 8%
**Graduate Enrollment** 107 **Women** 70% **Men** 30% **Minority** 15% **Part-time** 32%
**Distance Learning Courses** Available.
**Nursing Student Activities** Sigma Theta Tau, Student Nurses' Association.
**Nursing Student Resources** Academic advising; academic or career counseling; assistance for students with disabilities; bookstore; campus computer network; career placement assistance; computer lab; computer-assisted instruction; daycare for children of students; e-mail services; employment services for current students; interactive nursing skills videos; Internet; learning resource lab; library services; nursing audiovisuals; skills, simulation, or other laboratory; tutoring.
**Library Facilities** 19,370 volumes in health, 3,100 volumes in nursing; 200 periodical subscriptions health-care related.

### BACCALAUREATE PROGRAMS

**Degree** BSN
**Available Programs** ADN to Baccalaureate; Baccalaureate for Second Degree; Generic Baccalaureate.
**Study Options** Full-time.
**Online Degree Options** Yes (online only).
**Program Entrance Requirements** Minimum overall college GPA of 2.75, transcript of college record, CPR certification, health exam, health

insurance, high school foreign language, 3 years high school math, high school transcript, immunizations, 2 letters of recommendation, minimum high school GPA of 2.0, minimum GPA in nursing prerequisites of 2.75, professional liability insurance/malpractice insurance, prerequisite course work. Transfer students are accepted. *Application deadline:* 3/1 (fall).
**Advanced Placement** Credit given for nursing courses completed elsewhere dependent upon specific evaluations.
**Contact** *Telephone:* 423-425-4750. *Fax:* 423-425-4668.

## GRADUATE PROGRAMS

**Contact** *Telephone:* 423-425-4750. *Fax:* 423-425-4668.

### MASTER'S DEGREE PROGRAM

**Degree** MSN
**Available Programs** Master's.
**Concentrations Available** Nurse anesthesia. *Nurse practitioner programs in:* family health.
**Site Options** Tupelo, MS.
**Study Options** Full-time and part-time.
**Program Entrance Requirements** Clinical experience, computer literacy, minimum overall college GPA of 3.0, transcript of college record, CPR certification, written essay, immunizations, interview, 3 letters of recommendation, nursing research course, physical assessment course, professional liability insurance/malpractice insurance, resume, statistics course, GRE General Test, MAT. *Application deadline:* 1/31 (winter), 8/1 (summer). *Application fee:* $30.
**Advanced Placement** Credit given for nursing courses completed elsewhere dependent upon specific evaluations.
**Degree Requirements** 48 total credit hours, comprehensive exam.

### POST-MASTER'S PROGRAM

**Areas of Study** Nurse anesthesia. *Nurse practitioner programs in:* family health.

### DOCTORAL DEGREE PROGRAM

**Degree** DNP
**Available Programs** Doctorate.
**Online Degree Options** Yes (online only).
**Program Entrance Requirements** Clinical experience, minimum overall college GPA of 3.0, interview by faculty committee, 3.0 letters of recommendation, MSN or equivalent, vita. *Application deadline:* 9/1 (winter). *Application fee:* $30.
**Degree Requirements** 36 total credit hours.

# The University of Tennessee at Martin

## Department of Nursing
## Martin, Tennessee

*http://www.utm.edu/*
Founded in 1900

## DEGREE • BSN

**Nursing Program Faculty** 15 (20% with doctorates).
**Baccalaureate Enrollment** 198 **Women** 88% **Men** 12% **Minority** 6% **Part-time** 27%
**Distance Learning Courses** Available.
**Nursing Student Activities** Nursing Honor Society, Sigma Theta Tau, Student Nurses' Association, nursing club.
**Nursing Student Resources** Academic advising; academic or career counseling; assistance for students with disabilities; bookstore; campus computer network; career placement assistance; computer lab; computer-assisted instruction; daycare for children of students; e-mail services; employment services for current students; housing assistance; interactive nursing skills videos; Internet; learning resource lab; library services; nursing audiovisuals; remedial services; resume preparation assistance; skills, simulation, or other laboratory; tutoring.
**Library Facilities** 379,072 volumes (1,772 in health, 1,645 in nursing); 10,803 periodical subscriptions health-care related.

## BACCALAUREATE PROGRAMS

**Degree** BSN
**Available Programs** ADN to Baccalaureate; Generic Baccalaureate; LPN to RN Baccalaureate.
**Site Options** Ripley, TN; Selmer, TN; Parsons, TN.
**Study Options** Full-time.
**Program Entrance Requirements** Minimum overall college GPA of 2.0, transcript of college record, CPR certification, written essay, health exam, health insurance, high school biology, high school chemistry, high school foreign language, 3 years high school math, 2 years high school science, high school transcript, immunizations, interview, minimum high school GPA of 3.0, minimum GPA in nursing prerequisites of 2.0, professional liability insurance/malpractice insurance, prerequisite course work. Transfer students are accepted. *Application deadline:* 2/1 (fall).
**Advanced Placement** Credit by examination available. Credit given for nursing courses completed elsewhere dependent upon specific evaluations.
**Contact** *Telephone:* 731-881-7138. *Fax:* 731-881-7939.

# The University of Tennessee Health Science Center

## College of Nursing
## Memphis, Tennessee

*http://www.uthsc.edu/*
Founded in 1911

## DEGREES • BSN • DNP • MSN

**Nursing Program Faculty** 51 (87% with doctorates).
**Distance Learning Courses** Available.
**Nursing Student Activities** Student Nurses' Association, nursing club.
**Nursing Student Resources** Academic advising; academic or career counseling; assistance for students with disabilities; bookstore; campus computer network; computer lab; computer-assisted instruction; e-mail services; externships; interactive nursing skills videos; Internet; learning resource lab; library services; nursing audiovisuals; other; resume preparation assistance; skills, simulation, or other laboratory; tutoring.
**Library Facilities** 165,200 volumes; 1,784 periodical subscriptions.

## BACCALAUREATE PROGRAMS

**Degree** BSN
**Available Programs** ADN to Baccalaureate; Accelerated Baccalaureate; Accelerated Baccalaureate for Second Degree; RN Baccalaureate.
**Study Options** Full-time and part-time.
**Online Degree Options** Yes.
**Program Entrance Requirements** Written essay, minimum GPA in nursing prerequisites. Transfer students are accepted. *Application fee:* $45.
**Contact** Jamie Overton, Director, Student Affairs, College of Nursing, The University of Tennessee Health Science Center, 920 Madison Avenue, Suite 1021, Memphis, TN 38163. *Telephone:* 901-448-6139. *Fax:* 901-448-4121. *E-mail:* joverton@uthsc.edu.

## GRADUATE PROGRAMS

**Financial Aid** Fellowships, teaching assistantships, Federal Work-Study, institutionally sponsored loans, scholarships, and traineeships available.
**Contact** Jamie Overton, Director, Student Affairs, College of Nursing, The University of Tennessee Health Science Center, 920 Madison Avenue, Suite 1021, Memphis, TN 38163. *Telephone:* 901-448-6139. *Fax:* 901-448-4121. *E-mail:* joverton@uthsc.edu.

### MASTER'S DEGREE PROGRAM

**Degree** MSN
**Available Programs** Master's.
**Concentrations Available** Clinical nurse leader.
**Study Options** Full-time and part-time.
**Program Entrance Requirements** Computer literacy, transcript of college record, CPR certification, written essay, immunizations, interview, 3 letters of recommendation, prerequisite course work, statistics course, GRE General Test. *Application deadline:* 1/15 (fall), 1/15 (summer).

### DOCTORAL DEGREE PROGRAM

**Degree** DNP
**Available Programs** Doctorate; Post-Baccalaureate Doctorate.
**Areas of Study** Advanced practice nursing, clinical practice, critical care, family health, gerontology.
**Online Degree Options** Yes (online only).
**Program Entrance Requirements** Minimum overall college GPA of 3.0, interview by faculty committee, interview, 3 letters of recommendation, writing sample. *Application deadline:* 1/15 (fall). *Application fee:* $65.
**Degree Requirements** Residency.

# Vanderbilt University
## Vanderbilt University School of Nursing
## Nashville, Tennessee

***http://www.nursing.vanderbilt.edu/***
Founded in 1873

**DEGREES • DNP • MSN • MSN/MDIV • MSN/MTS • PHD**
**Nursing Program Faculty** 161 (65% with doctorates).
**Baccalaureate Enrollment** 894
**Graduate Enrollment** 894 **Women** 89% **Men** 11% **Minority** 13% **International** 1% **Part-time** 41%
**Distance Learning Courses** Available.
**Nursing Student Activities** Nursing Honor Society, Sigma Theta Tau.
**Nursing Student Resources** Academic advising; academic or career counseling; assistance for students with disabilities; bookstore; campus computer network; career placement assistance; computer lab; computer-assisted instruction; e-mail services; housing assistance; interactive nursing skills videos; Internet; learning resource lab; library services; nursing audiovisuals; remedial services; resume preparation assistance; skills, simulation, or other laboratory; tutoring.
**Library Facilities** 2.6 million volumes (190,156 in health); 78,041 periodical subscriptions (3,816 health-care related).

### GRADUATE PROGRAMS

**Expenses (2013–14)** *Tuition:* full-time $43,899; part-time $1126 per credit hour. *International tuition:* $43,899 full-time. *Required fees:* full-time $1321; part-time $440 per credit.
**Financial Aid** 85% of graduate students in nursing programs received some form of financial aid in 2012–13. Scholarships available. Aid available to part-time students. *Financial aid application deadline:* 3/15.
**Contact** Patricia Peerman, Assistant Dean of Enrollment Management, Vanderbilt University School of Nursing, Vanderbilt University, 207 Godchaux Hall, Nashville, TN 37240. *Telephone:* 615-322-3800. *Fax:* 615-343-0333. *E-mail:* paddy.peerman@vanderbilt.edu.

#### MASTER'S DEGREE PROGRAM
**Degrees** MSN; MSN/MDIV; MSN/MTS
**Available Programs** Master's; Master's for Non-Nursing College Graduates; RN to Master's.
**Concentrations Available** Health-care administration; nurse-midwifery; nursing administration; nursing informatics. *Nurse practitioner programs in:* acute care, adult health, family health, neonatal health, pediatric, psychiatric/mental health,women's health.
**Study Options** Full-time and part-time.
**Online Degree Options** Yes (online only).
**Program Entrance Requirements** Computer literacy, minimum overall college GPA of 3.0, transcript of college record, CPR certification, written essay, immunizations, 3 letters of recommendation, prerequisite course work, statistics course, GRE General Test (within the past 5 years). *Application deadline:* 12/1 (fall). Applications may be processed on a rolling basis for some programs. *Application fee:* $50.
**Advanced Placement** Credit by examination available. Credit given for nursing courses completed elsewhere dependent upon specific evaluations.
**Degree Requirements** 39 total credit hours.

#### POST-MASTER'S PROGRAM
**Areas of Study** Health-care administration; nurse-midwifery; nursing administration; nursing informatics. *Nurse practitioner programs in:* acute care, adult health, family health, neonatal health, pediatric, psychiatric/mental health,women's health.

#### DOCTORAL DEGREE PROGRAM
**Degree** DNP
**Available Programs** Doctorate.
**Areas of Study** Biology of health and illness, clinical practice, community health, critical care, family health, gerontology, health policy, health promotion/disease prevention, health-care systems, human health and illness, information systems, maternity-newborn, nursing administration, nursing policy, palliative care,women's health.
**Program Entrance Requirements** Minimum overall college GPA of 3.5, interview by faculty committee, 3 letters of recommendation, MSN or equivalent, statistics course, vita, writing sample, GRE General Test. *Application deadline:* 1/15 (fall). Applications may be processed on a rolling basis for some programs. *Application fee:* $50.
**Degree Requirements** 74 total credit hours, oral exam.

**Degree** PhD
**Available Programs** Doctorate.
**Areas of Study** Clinical research, nursing research.
**Program Entrance Requirements** Minimum overall college GPA of 3.5, interview by faculty committee, 3 letters of recommendation, MSN or equivalent, statistics course, vita, writing sample. *Application deadline:* 1/15 (fall).
**Degree Requirements** 72 semester credit hours, dissertation, oral exam.

#### POSTDOCTORAL PROGRAM
**Areas of Study** Individualized study.
**Postdoctoral Program Contact** Dr. Ann Minnick, Director, Vanderbilt University School of Nursing, Vanderbilt University, 415 Godchaux Hall, Nashville, TN 37240. *Telephone:* 615-343-2998. *Fax:* 615-343-5898. *E-mail:* ann.minnick@vanderbilt.edu.

# TEXAS

# Abilene Christian University
## Patty Hanks Shelton School of Nursing
## Abilene, Texas

***See description of programs under Patty Hanks Shelton School of Nursing (Abilene, Texas)***

# Angelo State University
## Department of Nursing and Rehabilitation Sciences
## San Angelo, Texas

***http://www.angelo.edu/dept/nursing***
Founded in 1928

**DEGREES • BSN • MSN**
**Nursing Program Faculty** 31 (35% with doctorates).
**Baccalaureate Enrollment** 257 **Women** 83% **Men** 17% **Minority** 34% **Part-time** 38%
**Graduate Enrollment** 109 **Women** 87% **Men** 13% **Minority** 24% **Part-time** 80%
**Distance Learning Courses** Available.
**Nursing Student Activities** Nursing Honor Society, Sigma Theta Tau, Student Nurses' Association.
**Nursing Student Resources** Academic advising; academic or career counseling; assistance for students with disabilities; bookstore; campus computer network; computer lab; computer-assisted instruction; e-mail services; housing assistance; interactive nursing skills videos; Internet; learning resource lab; library services; nursing audiovisuals; remedial services; skills, simulation, or other laboratory; tutoring.
**Library Facilities** 584,809 volumes (8,865 in health, 5,190 in nursing); 45,713 periodical subscriptions (160 health-care related).

### BACCALAUREATE PROGRAMS

**Degree** BSN
**Available Programs** Generic Baccalaureate; RN Baccalaureate.
**Study Options** Full-time.
**Online Degree Options** Yes.
**Program Entrance Requirements** Minimum overall college GPA of 2.5, transcript of college record, CPR certification, health insurance, immunizations, 2 letters of recommendation, prerequisite course work. Transfer students are accepted. *Application deadline:* 2/15 (fall), 10/1 (spring).
**Expenses (2013–14)** *Tuition, state resident:* full-time $5734; part-time $156 per credit hour. *Tuition, nonresident:* full-time $18,442; part-time $510 per credit hour. *Room and board:* $7352; room only: $4552 per academic year. *Required fees:* full-time $4036; part-time $481 per credit; part-time $1412 per term.

**Financial Aid** 74% of baccalaureate students in nursing programs received some form of financial aid in 2012–13.
**Contact** Ms. Crystal M. Nelms, Academic College Advisor, Department of Nursing and Rehabilitation Sciences, Angelo State University, ASU Station #10911, San Angelo, TX 76909. *Telephone:* 325-942-2630. *Fax:* 325-942-2631. *E-mail:* chhs@angelo.edu.

## GRADUATE PROGRAMS

**Expenses (2013–14)** *Tuition, state resident:* full-time $7354; part-time $201 per credit hour. *Tuition, nonresident:* full-time $20,062; part-time $555 per credit hour. *Room and board:* $7352; room only: $4552 per academic year. *Required fees:* full-time $3920; part-time $455 per credit; part-time $1372 per term.
**Financial Aid** 67% of graduate students in nursing programs received some form of financial aid in 2012–13. 1 research assistantship (averaging $7,490 per year) was awarded; career-related internships or fieldwork, Federal Work-Study, and scholarships also available. Aid available to part-time students. *Financial aid application deadline:* 3/1.
**Contact** Dr. Molly Walker, Graduate Adviser, MSN Program, Department of Nursing and Rehabilitation Sciences, Angelo State University, ASU Station #10902, San Angelo, TX 76909. *Telephone:* 325-942-2224. *Fax:* 325-942-2236. *E-mail:* molly.walker@angelo.edu.

### MASTER'S DEGREE PROGRAM

**Degree** MSN
**Available Programs** Master's; Master's for Non-Nursing College Graduates; RN to Master's.
**Concentrations Available** Nursing education. *Clinical nurse specialist programs in:* adult health, medical-surgical. *Nurse practitioner programs in:* family health.
**Study Options** Full-time and part-time.
**Online Degree Options** Yes (online only).
**Program Entrance Requirements** Computer literacy, minimum overall college GPA of 3.0, transcript of college record, CPR certification, written essay, immunizations, 3 letters of recommendation, physical assessment course, prerequisite course work, statistics course. *Application deadline:* 4/1 (fall), 9/1 (spring), 4/1 (summer). *Application fee:* $40.
**Advanced Placement** Credit given for nursing courses completed elsewhere dependent upon specific evaluations.
**Degree Requirements** 34 total credit hours, comprehensive exam.

# Baylor University

## Louise Herrington School of Nursing
## Dallas, Texas

***http://www.baylor.edu/nursing***
Founded in 1845

**DEGREES • BSN • DNP • MSN**
**Nursing Program Faculty** 74 (28% with doctorates).
**Baccalaureate Enrollment** 360 **Women** 89% **Men** 11% **Minority** 37% **International** 1.5% **Part-time** 5%
**Graduate Enrollment** 66 **Women** 92% **Men** 8% **Minority** 23% **Part-time** 20%
**Distance Learning Courses** Available.
**Nursing Student Activities** Sigma Theta Tau, Student Nurses' Association.
**Nursing Student Resources** Academic advising; academic or career counseling; assistance for students with disabilities; campus computer network; career placement assistance; computer lab; e-mail services; employment services for current students; housing assistance; interactive nursing skills videos; Internet; learning resource lab; library services; nursing audiovisuals; placement services for program completers; resume preparation assistance; skills, simulation, or other laboratory; tutoring.
**Library Facilities** 3 million volumes (4,800 in health, 4,800 in nursing); 82,294 periodical subscriptions (101 health-care related).

## BACCALAUREATE PROGRAMS

**Degree** BSN
**Available Programs** Accelerated Baccalaureate for Second Degree; Generic Baccalaureate.
**Study Options** Full-time.
**Program Entrance Requirements** Transcript of college record, CPR certification, health exam, health insurance, immunizations, interview, minimum GPA in nursing prerequisites of 3.0, prerequisite course work. Transfer students are accepted. *Application deadline:* 1/15 (fall), 5/31 (spring), 12/5 (summer). *Application fee:* $45.
**Advanced Placement** Credit by examination available. Credit given for nursing courses completed elsewhere dependent upon specific evaluations.
**Expenses (2013–14)** *Tuition:* full-time $32,574; part-time $1357 per contact hour. *International tuition:* $32,574 full-time. *Room and board:* $9330; room only: $5000 per academic year. *Required fees:* full-time $3398; part-time $142 per credit.
**Financial Aid** 90% of baccalaureate students in nursing programs received some form of financial aid in 2012–13. *Gift aid (need-based):* Federal Pell, FSEOG, state, college/university gift aid from institutional funds. *Loans:* Federal Nursing Student Loans, Federal Direct (Subsidized and Unsubsidized Stafford PLUS), Perkins, state, private loans. *Work-study:* Federal Work-Study, part-time campus jobs. *Financial aid application deadline (priority):* 3/1.
**Contact** Recruiter, Louise Herrington School of Nursing, Baylor University, 3700 Worth Street, Dallas, TX 75246. *Telephone:* 214-820-3361. *Fax:* 214-820-3835. *E-mail:* BU_Nursing@baylor.edu.

## GRADUATE PROGRAMS

**Expenses (2013–14)** *Tuition:* full-time $24,426; part-time $1357 per contact hour. *International tuition:* $24,426 full-time. *Room and board:* $9330; room only: $5000 per academic year. *Required fees:* full-time $3398; part-time $142 per credit.
**Financial Aid** 100% of graduate students in nursing programs received some form of financial aid in 2012–13. 13 teaching assistantships (averaging $4,932 per year) were awarded; Federal Work-Study, scholarships, and unspecified assistantships also available. Aid available to part-time students. *Financial aid application deadline:* 6/30.
**Contact** Dr. Barbara Camune, Director, Graduate Program, Louise Herrington School of Nursing, Baylor University, 3700 Worth Street, Dallas, TX 75246. *Telephone:* 214-820-3361. *Fax:* 214-820-4770. *E-mail:* barvara_camune@baylor.edu.

### MASTER'S DEGREE PROGRAM

**Degree** MSN
**Available Programs** Master's.
**Concentrations Available** Health-care administration.
**Study Options** Full-time.
**Online Degree Options** Yes (online only).
**Program Entrance Requirements** Clinical experience, minimum overall college GPA of 3.0, transcript of college record, CPR certification, written essay, immunizations, interview, 3 letters of recommendation, prerequisite course work, statistics course, GRE General Test or MAT. *Application deadline:* 2/1 (fall). *Application fee:* $50.
**Advanced Placement** Credit given for nursing courses completed elsewhere dependent upon specific evaluations.
**Degree Requirements** 36 total credit hours, thesis or project.

### DOCTORAL DEGREE PROGRAM

**Degree** DNP
**Available Programs** Doctorate.
**Areas of Study** Advanced practice nursing, family health, maternity-newborn.
**Program Entrance Requirements** Minimum overall college GPA of 3.0, interview by faculty committee, interview, 3 letters of recommendation, MSN or equivalent, statistics course, writing sample, GRE General Test. *Application deadline:* 2/1 (fall). *Application fee:* $50.
**Degree Requirements** 75 total credit hours, residency.

# Concordia University Texas

## School of Nursing
## Austin, Texas

Founded in 1926

**DEGREE • BSN**
**Library Facilities** 80,000 volumes; 21,000 periodical subscriptions.

## BACCALAUREATE PROGRAMS

**Degree** BSN
**Available Programs** Generic Baccalaureate.
**Program Entrance Requirements** *Application deadline:* 5/15 (fall), 10/1 (spring).
**Contact** Kathryn Lauchner, PhD, Director of School of Nursing and Assistant Dean College of Science, School of Nursing, Concordia

University Texas, 11400 Concordia University Drive, Austin, TX 78726. *Telephone:* 512-313-5514. *E-mail:* kathy.lauchner@concordia.edu.

# East Texas Baptist University

## Department of Nursing
## Marshall, Texas

***http://www.etbu.edu/nursing/***
Founded in 1912

**DEGREE • BSN**

**Nursing Program Faculty** 8 (25% with doctorates).
**Baccalaureate Enrollment** 43 **Women** 95% **Men** 5% **Minority** 10%
**Nursing Student Activities** Student Nurses' Association.
**Nursing Student Resources** Academic advising; academic or career counseling; assistance for students with disabilities; bookstore; campus computer network; computer lab; computer-assisted instruction; e-mail services; employment services for current students; housing assistance; interactive nursing skills videos; Internet; learning resource lab; library services; nursing audiovisuals; remedial services; resume preparation assistance; skills, simulation, or other laboratory; tutoring.
**Library Facilities** 5.2 million volumes (568 in health, 291 in nursing); 28,752 periodical subscriptions (2,100 health-care related).

### BACCALAUREATE PROGRAMS

**Degree** BSN
**Available Programs** Generic Baccalaureate.
**Study Options** Full-time.
**Program Entrance Requirements** Transcript of college record, CPR certification, health insurance, immunizations, 2 letters of recommendation, minimum GPA in nursing prerequisites of 2.8, prerequisite course work. Transfer students are accepted. *Application deadline:* 1/15 (fall).
**Advanced Placement** Credit given for nursing courses completed elsewhere dependent upon specific evaluations.
**Financial Aid** 99% of baccalaureate students in nursing programs received some form of financial aid in 2012–13. *Gift aid (need-based):* Federal Pell, FSEOG, state, private, college/university gift aid from institutional funds, Federal Nursing. *Loans:* Federal Direct (Subsidized and Unsubsidized Stafford PLUS), Perkins, state. *Work-study:* Federal Work-Study, part-time campus jobs. *Financial aid application deadline (priority):* 6/1.
**Contact** Alysce Parish, Enrollment and Clinical Excellence Specialist, Department of Nursing, East Texas Baptist University, One Tiger Drive, Marshall, TX 75670-1498. *Telephone:* 903-923-2210. *Fax:* 903-938-9225. *E-mail:* aparish@etbu.edu.

# Hardin-Simmons University

## Patty Hanks Shelton School of Nursing
## Abilene, Texas

***See description of programs under Patty Hanks Shelton School of Nursing (Abilene, Texas).***

# Houston Baptist University

## School of Nursing and Allied Health
## Houston, Texas

Founded in 1960

**DEGREE • BSN**

**Nursing Program Faculty** 19 (15% with doctorates).
**Baccalaureate Enrollment** 190 **Women** 95% **Men** 5% **Minority** 78% **International** 2% **Part-time** 20%
**Nursing Student Activities** Nursing Honor Society, Sigma Theta Tau, Student Nurses' Association.
**Nursing Student Resources** Academic advising; academic or career counseling; assistance for students with disabilities; bookstore; career placement assistance; computer lab; e-mail services; employment services for current students; externships; housing assistance; interactive nursing skills videos; Internet; learning resource lab; library services; nursing audiovisuals; paid internships; placement services for program completers; remedial services; resume preparation assistance; skills, simulation, or other laboratory; tutoring; unpaid internships.
**Library Facilities** 322,277 volumes (4,276 in health, 1,200 in nursing); 74,186 periodical subscriptions (117 health-care related).

### BACCALAUREATE PROGRAMS

**Degree** BSN
**Available Programs** Generic Baccalaureate; RN Baccalaureate.
**Site Options** Houston, TX.
**Study Options** Full-time.
**Program Entrance Requirements** Minimum overall college GPA of 3.0, transcript of college record, CPR certification, health exam, health insurance, immunizations, minimum GPA in nursing prerequisites of 3.0, prerequisite course work. Transfer students are accepted. *Application deadline:* 3/1 (fall), 10/1 (spring).
**Advanced Placement** Credit by examination available.
**Expenses (2013–14)** *Tuition:* full-time $29,000. *Room and board:* $8000 per academic year. *Required fees:* full-time $12,000.
**Financial Aid** 80% of baccalaureate students in nursing programs received some form of financial aid in 2012–13. *Gift aid (need-based):* Federal Pell, FSEOG, state, private, college/university gift aid from institutional funds. *Loans:* Federal Direct (Subsidized and Unsubsidized Stafford PLUS). *Work-study:* Federal Work-Study, part-time campus jobs. *Financial aid application deadline:* 4/15(priority: 3/1).
**Contact** Dr. Renae Schumann, Dean, School of Nursing and Allied Health, School of Nursing and Allied Health, Houston Baptist University, Houston Baptist University, 7502 Fondren, Houston, TX 77074. *Telephone:* 281-649-3680. *Fax:* 281-649-3340. *E-mail:* rschumann@hbu.edu.

# Lamar University

## Department of Nursing
## Beaumont, Texas

***http://www.dept.lamar.edu/nursing/***
Founded in 1923

**DEGREES • BSN • MSN • MSN/MBA**

**Nursing Program Faculty** 43 (28% with doctorates).
**Baccalaureate Enrollment** 537 **Women** 83% **Men** 17% **Minority** 40%
**Graduate Enrollment** 71 **Women** 93% **Men** 7% **Minority** 46% **Part-time** 77%
**Distance Learning Courses** Available.
**Nursing Student Activities** Sigma Theta Tau, Student Nurses' Association.
**Nursing Student Resources** Academic advising; academic or career counseling; assistance for students with disabilities; bookstore; campus computer network; computer lab; computer-assisted instruction; e-mail services; employment services for current students; housing assistance; interactive nursing skills videos; Internet; learning resource lab; library services; nursing audiovisuals; remedial services; resume preparation assistance; skills, simulation, or other laboratory; tutoring.
**Library Facilities** 526,180 volumes (7,166 in health, 3,318 in nursing); 26,618 periodical subscriptions (1,059 health-care related).

### BACCALAUREATE PROGRAMS

**Degree** BSN
**Available Programs** ADN to Baccalaureate; Generic Baccalaureate; RN Baccalaureate.
**Study Options** Full-time.
**Online Degree Options** Yes.
**Program Entrance Requirements** Minimum overall college GPA of 2.0, transcript of college record, CPR certification, health exam, immunizations, minimum GPA in nursing prerequisites of 2.5, professional liability insurance/malpractice insurance, prerequisite course work. Transfer students are accepted. *Application deadline:* 3/1 (fall), 10/1 (spring). *Application fee:* $25.
**Advanced Placement** Credit given for nursing courses completed elsewhere dependent upon specific evaluations.
**Expenses (2013–14)** *Tuition, state resident:* full-time $7498; part-time $208 per credit hour. *Tuition, nonresident:* full-time $15,923; part-time $559 per credit hour. *Room and board:* $7966; room only: $5098 per academic year. *Required fees:* full-time $300; part-time $150 per term.
**Financial Aid** 64% of baccalaureate students in nursing programs received some form of financial aid in 2012–13.
**Contact** Nursing Advisor, Academic Advisor, Department of Nursing, Lamar University, PO Box 10079, Beaumont, TX 77710. *Telephone:* 409-880-8822. *E-mail:* nursing@lamar.edu.

## GRADUATE PROGRAMS

**Expenses (2013–14)** *Tuition, state resident:* full-time $4500; part-time $250 per credit hour. *Tuition, nonresident:* full-time $5256; part-time $292 per credit hour. *Room and board:* $7966; room only: $5098 per academic year.

**Financial Aid** 64% of graduate students in nursing programs received some form of financial aid in 2012–13.

**Contact** Dr. Nancy Bume, Director of Graduate Nursing Studies, Department of Nursing, Lamar University, PO Box 10081, Beaumont, TX 77710. *Telephone:* 409-880-7720. *Fax:* 409-880-8698. *E-mail:* nancy.blume@lamar.edu.

### MASTER'S DEGREE PROGRAM

**Degrees** MSN; MSN/MBA

**Available Programs** Master's.

**Concentrations Available** Nursing administration; nursing education.

**Study Options** Full-time and part-time.

**Online Degree Options** Yes (online only).

**Program Entrance Requirements** Computer literacy, minimum overall college GPA of 3.0, transcript of college record, CPR certification, immunizations, professional liability insurance/malpractice insurance, prerequisite course work, statistics course. *Application deadline:* Applications may be processed on a rolling basis for some programs. *Application fee:* $25.

**Advanced Placement** Credit given for nursing courses completed elsewhere dependent upon specific evaluations.

**Degree Requirements** 37 total credit hours, thesis or project.

### POST-MASTER'S PROGRAM

**Areas of Study** Nursing administration; nursing education.

## CONTINUING EDUCATION PROGRAM

**Contact** Dr. Cindy Stinson, Coordinator of Continuing Education, Department of Nursing, Lamar University, PO Box 10081, Beaumont, TX 77710. *Telephone:* 409-880-8833. *Fax:* 409-880-1865. *E-mail:* cynthia.stinson@lamar.edu.

# Lubbock Christian University

**Department of Nursing**
**Lubbock, Texas**

Founded in 1957

### DEGREE • BSN

**Nursing Program Faculty** 5 (40% with doctorates).

**Library Facilities** 128,890 volumes; 404 periodical subscriptions.

## BACCALAUREATE PROGRAMS

**Degree** BSN

**Available Programs** RN Baccalaureate.

**Study Options** Part-time.

**Program Entrance Requirements** Minimum overall college GPA of 2.5, transcript of college record, CPR certification, health exam, immunizations, interview, 2 letters of recommendation, minimum high school GPA, minimum GPA in nursing prerequisites of 2.5, professional liability insurance/malpractice insurance, prerequisite course work, RN licensure. Transfer students are accepted.

# McMurry University

**Patty Hanks Shelton School of Nursing**
**Abilene, Texas**

*See description of programs under Patty Hanks Shelton School of Nursing (Abilene, Texas).*

# Midwestern State University

**Nursing Program**
**Wichita Falls, Texas**

*http://www.mwsu.edu/academics/hs2/nursing/*

Founded in 1922

### DEGREES • BSN • MSN

**Nursing Program Faculty** 20 (35% with doctorates).

**Baccalaureate Enrollment** 482 **Women** 83% **Men** 17% **Minority** 54% **International** 6% **Part-time** 23%

**Graduate Enrollment** 122 **Women** 82% **Men** 18% **Minority** 30% **International** 3% **Part-time** 34%

**Distance Learning Courses** Available.

**Nursing Student Activities** Nursing Honor Society, Sigma Theta Tau, Student Nurses' Association.

**Nursing Student Resources** Academic advising; academic or career counseling; assistance for students with disabilities; bookstore; campus computer network; career placement assistance; computer lab; computer-assisted instruction; e-mail services; employment services for current students; externships; housing assistance; interactive nursing skills videos; Internet; learning resource lab; library services; nursing audiovisuals; other; placement services for program completers; remedial services; resume preparation assistance; skills, simulation, or other laboratory; tutoring.

**Library Facilities** 462,657 volumes (10,000 in health, 5,000 in nursing); 884 periodical subscriptions (6,000 health-care related).

## BACCALAUREATE PROGRAMS

**Degree** BSN

**Available Programs** ADN to Baccalaureate; Generic Baccalaureate.

**Study Options** Full-time and part-time.

**Program Entrance Requirements** Transcript of college record, CPR certification, health exam, health insurance, immunizations, minimum GPA in nursing prerequisites of 3.0, professional liability insurance/malpractice insurance, prerequisite course work. Transfer students are accepted. *Application deadline:* 3/15 (fall), 9/30 (spring). *Application fee:* $25.

**Advanced Placement** Credit given for nursing courses completed elsewhere dependent upon specific evaluations.

**Contact** *Telephone:* 940-397-3254. *Fax:* 940-397-4911.

## GRADUATE PROGRAMS

**Contact** *Telephone:* 940-397-4600. *Fax:* 940-397-4911.

### MASTER'S DEGREE PROGRAM

**Degree** MSN

**Available Programs** Master's; RN to Master's.

**Concentrations Available** Nursing education. *Nurse practitioner programs in:* family health, psychiatric/mental health.

**Study Options** Full-time and part-time.

**Online Degree Options** Yes.

**Program Entrance Requirements** Clinical experience, minimum overall college GPA of 3.0, transcript of college record, CPR certification, immunizations, interview, professional liability insurance/malpractice insurance, statistics course, GRE General Test or MAT. *Application deadline:* 7/1 (fall), 11/1 (spring), 4/15 (summer). Applications may be processed on a rolling basis for some programs. *Application fee:* $35.

**Advanced Placement** Credit by examination available. Credit given for nursing courses completed elsewhere dependent upon specific evaluations.

**Degree Requirements** 40 total credit hours, thesis or project.

### POST-MASTER'S PROGRAM

**Areas of Study** Nursing education. *Nurse practitioner programs in:* family health, psychiatric/mental health.

## CONTINUING EDUCATION PROGRAM

**Contact** *Telephone:* 940-397-4048. *Fax:* 940-397-4513.

# Patty Hanks Shelton School of Nursing

## Patty Hanks Shelton School of Nursing
## Abilene, Texas

*http://www.phssn.edu/*

**DEGREES • BSN • MSN**

**Nursing Program Faculty** 17 (30% with doctorates).

**Baccalaureate Enrollment** 131 **Women** 89% **Men** 11% **Minority** 25% **International** 2% **Part-time** 9%

**Graduate Enrollment** 18 **Women** 73% **Men** 27% **Minority** 17%

**Distance Learning Courses** Available.

**Nursing Student Activities** Nursing Honor Society, Sigma Theta Tau, Student Nurses' Association.

**Nursing Student Resources** Academic advising; academic or career counseling; assistance for students with disabilities; bookstore; campus computer network; career placement assistance; computer lab; computer-assisted instruction; e-mail services; employment services for current students; externships; interactive nursing skills videos; Internet; learning resource lab; library services; nursing audiovisuals; remedial services; resume preparation assistance; skills, simulation, or other laboratory; tutoring.

**Library Facilities** 9,200 volumes in health, 1,300 volumes in nursing; 140 periodical subscriptions health-care related.

### BACCALAUREATE PROGRAMS

**Degree** BSN

**Available Programs** Generic Baccalaureate; RN Baccalaureate.

**Study Options** Full-time.

**Program Entrance Requirements** Minimum overall college GPA of 3.0, transcript of college record, CPR certification, health exam, health insurance, immunizations, 2 letters of recommendation, minimum GPA in nursing prerequisites of 3.0, professional liability insurance/malpractice insurance, prerequisite course work. Transfer students are accepted. *Application deadline:* 6/13 (fall), 10/13 (spring).

**Advanced Placement** Credit by examination available. Credit given for nursing courses completed elsewhere dependent upon specific evaluations.

**Financial Aid** 80% of baccalaureate students in nursing programs received some form of financial aid in 2011–12.

**Contact** Mrs. Sharon Eichhorst, Director of Student Development, Patty Hanks Shelton School of Nursing, 2149 Hickory Street, Abilene, TX 79601. *Telephone:* 325-671-2353. *Fax:* 325-671-2386. *E-mail:* seichhorst@phssn.edu.

### GRADUATE PROGRAMS

**Expenses (2012–13)** *Tuition:* part-time $725 per credit hour.

**Financial Aid** 50% of graduate students in nursing programs received some form of financial aid in 2011–12.

**Contact** Dr. Indira Tyler, Associate Dean, Patty Hanks Shelton School of Nursing, 2149 Hickory Street, Abilene, TX 79601. *Telephone:* 325-671-2367. *Fax:* 325-671-2386. *E-mail:* Indira.D. Tyler@phssn.edu.

#### MASTER'S DEGREE PROGRAM

**Degree** MSN

**Available Programs** Master's.

**Concentrations Available** Nursing education. *Nurse practitioner programs in:* family health.

**Study Options** Full-time and part-time.

**Program Entrance Requirements** Clinical experience, minimum overall college GPA of 3.5, transcript of college record, CPR certification, written essay, immunizations, interview, 3 letters of recommendation, physical assessment course, professional liability insurance/malpractice insurance, resume, statistics course. *Application deadline:* 8/12 (fall).

**Advanced Placement** Credit given for nursing courses completed elsewhere dependent upon specific evaluations.

**Degree Requirements** 49 total credit hours.

#### POST-MASTER'S PROGRAM

**Areas of Study** *Nurse practitioner programs in:* family health.

### CONTINUING EDUCATION PROGRAM

**Contact** Dr. Nina Ouimette, Dean and Professor, Patty Hanks Shelton School of Nursing, 2149 Hickory Street, Abilene, TX 79601. *Telephone:* 325-671-2399. *Fax:* 325-671-2386. *E-mail:* nouimette@phssn.edu.

# Prairie View A&M University

## College of Nursing
## Houston, Texas

*http://www.pvamu.edu/nursing*

Founded in 1878

**DEGREES • BSN • MSN**

**Nursing Program Faculty** 66 (26% with doctorates).

**Baccalaureate Enrollment** 447 **Women** 85% **Men** 15% **Minority** 38% **International** 2% **Part-time** 19%

**Graduate Enrollment** 103 **Women** 95% **Men** 5% **Minority** 25% **International** 2% **Part-time** 78%

**Distance Learning Courses** Available.

**Nursing Student Activities** Nursing Honor Society, Sigma Theta Tau, Student Nurses' Association, nursing club.

**Nursing Student Resources** Academic advising; academic or career counseling; assistance for students with disabilities; bookstore; campus computer network; career placement assistance; computer lab; computer-assisted instruction; e-mail services; employment services for current students; interactive nursing skills videos; Internet; learning resource lab; library services; nursing audiovisuals; placement services for program completers; resume preparation assistance; skills, simulation, or other laboratory; tutoring.

**Library Facilities** 355,707 volumes in health, 7,899 volumes in nursing; 9,283 periodical subscriptions health-care related.

### BACCALAUREATE PROGRAMS

**Degree** BSN

**Available Programs** Generic Baccalaureate; LPN to Baccalaureate; RN Baccalaureate.

**Site Options** Woodlands, TX; College Station, TX.

**Study Options** Full-time and part-time.

**Program Entrance Requirements** Minimum overall college GPA of 2.5, transcript of college record, CPR certification, health exam, immunizations, minimum GPA in nursing prerequisites of 2.0, professional liability insurance/malpractice insurance, prerequisite course work. Transfer students are accepted. *Application deadline:* 3/1 (fall), 10/1 (spring). *Application fee:* $25.

**Advanced Placement** Credit given for nursing courses completed elsewhere dependent upon specific evaluations.

**Contact** *Telephone:* 713-797-7031. *Fax:* 713-797-7092.

### GRADUATE PROGRAMS

**Contact** *Telephone:* 713-797-7015. *Fax:* 713-797-7011.

#### MASTER'S DEGREE PROGRAM

**Degree** MSN

**Available Programs** Master's.

**Concentrations Available** Nursing administration; nursing education. *Nurse practitioner programs in:* family health.

**Study Options** Full-time and part-time.

**Program Entrance Requirements** Clinical experience, minimum overall college GPA of 2.75, transcript of college record, CPR certification, immunizations, interview, 3 letters of recommendation, physical assessment course, prerequisite course work, resume, statistics course, MAT or GRE. *Application deadline:* 6/1 (fall), 10/1 (spring), 4/1 (summer). *Application fee:* $25.

**Advanced Placement** Credit by examination available. Credit given for nursing courses completed elsewhere dependent upon specific evaluations.

**Degree Requirements** 53 total credit hours, thesis or project.

#### POST-MASTER'S PROGRAM

**Areas of Study** Nursing administration; nursing education. *Nurse practitioner programs in:* family health.

## Sam Houston State University

### Nursing Program
### Huntsville, Texas

Founded in 1879

**DEGREE • BSN**

**Library Facilities** 1.3 million volumes.

#### BACCALAUREATE PROGRAMS

**Degree** BSN
**Available Programs** Generic Baccalaureate.
**Contact** Anne S. Stiles, PhD, Professor and Chair, Nursing Program, Sam Houston State University, Huntsville, TX 77341. *Telephone:* 936-294-2379. *E-mail:* kberry@shsu.edu.

## Southwestern Adventist University

### Department of Nursing
### Keene, Texas

*http://www.swau.edu/*
Founded in 1894

**DEGREE • BS**

**Nursing Program Faculty** 10 (38% with doctorates).
**Baccalaureate Enrollment** 93 **Women** 82% **Men** 18% **Minority** 67% **International** 9% **Part-time** 28%
**Nursing Student Activities** Student Nurses' Association.
**Nursing Student Resources** Academic advising; academic or career counseling; assistance for students with disabilities; bookstore; campus computer network; computer lab; computer-assisted instruction; e-mail services; externships; interactive nursing skills videos; Internet; learning resource lab; library services; nursing audiovisuals; remedial services; resume preparation assistance; skills, simulation, or other laboratory; tutoring.
**Library Facilities** 135,453 volumes (1,791 in health, 847 in nursing); 4,500 periodical subscriptions (5,168 health-care related).

#### BACCALAUREATE PROGRAMS

**Degree** BS
**Available Programs** Generic Baccalaureate; LPN to RN Baccalaureate; RN Baccalaureate.
**Study Options** Full-time and part-time.
**Program Entrance Requirements** Transcript of college record, CPR certification, health exam, health insurance, immunizations, 3 letters of recommendation, minimum GPA in nursing prerequisites of 2.75, prerequisite course work. *Application deadline:* 8/15 (spring).
**Advanced Placement** Credit by examination available.
**Expenses (2013–14)** *Tuition:* full-time $18,240; part-time $760 per credit hour. *International tuition:* $18,240 full-time. *Room and board:* $72,201; room only: $3520 per academic year. *Required fees:* full-time $700; part-time $150 per term.
**Financial Aid** 88% of baccalaureate students in nursing programs received some form of financial aid in 2012–13.
**Contact** Dr. Lenora D. Follett, Chair, Department of Nursing, Department of Nursing, Southwestern Adventist University, 300 West Magnolia, PO Box 567, Keene, TX 76059. *Telephone:* 817-202-6670. *Fax:* 817-202-6713. *E-mail:* lenora.follett@swau.edu.

## Stephen F. Austin State University

### Richard and Lucille Dewitt School of Nursing
### Nacogdoches, Texas

*http://www.fp.sfasu.edu/nursing/*
Founded in 1923

**DEGREE • BSN**

**Nursing Program Faculty** 34 (38% with doctorates).
**Baccalaureate Enrollment** 285
**Distance Learning Courses** Available.
**Nursing Student Activities** Sigma Theta Tau, Student Nurses' Association.
**Nursing Student Resources** Academic advising; academic or career counseling; assistance for students with disabilities; bookstore; campus computer network; career placement assistance; computer lab; computer-assisted instruction; e-mail services; employment services for current students; housing assistance; interactive nursing skills videos; Internet; learning resource lab; library services; nursing audiovisuals; resume preparation assistance; skills, simulation, or other laboratory; tutoring.
**Library Facilities** 745,807 volumes; 827 periodical subscriptions.

#### BACCALAUREATE PROGRAMS

**Degree** BSN
**Available Programs** Generic Baccalaureate; RN Baccalaureate.
**Site Options** Nacogdoches, TX.
**Study Options** Full-time.
**Program Entrance Requirements** Minimum overall college GPA of 2.75, transcript of college record, CPR certification, health insurance, high school transcript, immunizations, minimum GPA in nursing prerequisites of 2.5, professional liability insurance/malpractice insurance, prerequisite course work. Transfer students are accepted. *Application deadline:* 2/1 (fall), 9/12 (spring).
**Advanced Placement** Credit given for nursing courses completed elsewhere dependent upon specific evaluations.
**Contact** Dr. Sara E. Bishop, Interim Director, Richard and Lucille Dewitt School of Nursing, Stephen F. Austin State University, SFA Box 6156, Nacogdoches, TX 75962. *Telephone:* 936-468-7704. *Fax:* 936-468-7752.

## Tarleton State University

### Department of Nursing
### Stephenville, Texas

*http://www.tarleton.edu/~nursing*
Founded in 1899

**DEGREE • BSN**

**Nursing Program Faculty** 19 (14% with doctorates).
**Baccalaureate Enrollment** 230 **Women** 95% **Men** 5% **Minority** 15% **International** 2% **Part-time** 25%
**Nursing Student Activities** Sigma Theta Tau, Student Nurses' Association.
**Nursing Student Resources** Academic advising; academic or career counseling; assistance for students with disabilities; bookstore; computer lab; computer-assisted instruction; daycare for children of students; e-mail services; employment services for current students; externships; learning resource lab; library services; nursing audiovisuals; remedial services; resume preparation assistance; skills, simulation, or other laboratory; tutoring; unpaid internships.
**Library Facilities** 400,000 volumes; 25,800 periodical subscriptions.

#### BACCALAUREATE PROGRAMS

**Degree** BSN
**Available Programs** ADN to Baccalaureate; Generic Baccalaureate; LPN to Baccalaureate.
**Study Options** Full-time and part-time.
**Program Entrance Requirements** Transcript of college record, CPR certification, written essay, health exam, high school transcript, immunizations, 3 letters of recommendation, minimum GPA in nursing prerequisites of 2.75, professional liability insurance/malpractice insurance, prerequisite course work. Transfer students are accepted.
**Advanced Placement** Credit by examination available. Credit given for nursing courses completed elsewhere dependent upon specific evaluations.
**Contact** *Telephone:* 254-968-9139. *Fax:* 254-968-9716.

#### CONTINUING EDUCATION PROGRAM

**Contact** *Telephone:* 325-649-8058. *Fax:* 325-649-8959.

# Texas A&M Health Science Center

## College of Nursing
## College Station, Texas

*http://www.tamhsc.edu*
Founded in 1999

### DEGREE • BSN

**Nursing Program Faculty** 28 (33% with doctorates).
**Baccalaureate Enrollment** 145 **Women** 89% **Men** 11% **Minority** 7% **Part-time** 2%
**Distance Learning Courses** Available.
**Nursing Student Activities** Sigma Theta Tau, Student Nurses' Association, nursing club.
**Nursing Student Resources** Academic advising; assistance for students with disabilities; bookstore; campus computer network; career placement assistance; computer lab; computer-assisted instruction; e-mail services; externships; interactive nursing skills videos; Internet; learning resource lab; library services; nursing audiovisuals; remedial services; resume preparation assistance; skills, simulation, or other laboratory; tutoring.

### BACCALAUREATE PROGRAMS

**Degree** BSN
**Available Programs** ADN to Baccalaureate; Accelerated Baccalaureate for Second Degree; Generic Baccalaureate; RN Baccalaureate.
**Site Options** Round Rock, TX.
**Study Options** Full-time.
**Online Degree Options** Yes.
**Program Entrance Requirements** Minimum overall college GPA of 3.0, transcript of college record, CPR certification, written essay, health exam, health insurance, high school foreign language, immunizations, 1 letter of recommendation, minimum GPA in nursing prerequisites of 2.75, professional liability insurance/malpractice insurance, prerequisite course work. Transfer students are accepted. *Application deadline:* 8/1 (winter), 2/1 (summer). *Application fee:* $50.
**Advanced Placement** Credit by examination available. Credit given for nursing courses completed elsewhere dependent upon specific evaluations.
**Financial Aid** 89% of baccalaureate students in nursing programs received some form of financial aid in 2011–12.
**Contact** Kathryn Willis Cochran, Associate Dean for Student Affairs, College of Nursing, Texas A&M Health Science Center, 8447 State Highway 47, Bryan, TX 77807-3260. *Telephone:* 979-436-0110. *Fax:* 979-436-0098. *E-mail:* cochran@tamhsc.edu.

# Texas A&M International University

## Canseco School of Nursing
## Laredo, Texas

Founded in 1969

### DEGREES • BSN • MSN

**Nursing Program Faculty** 24 (17% with doctorates).
**Baccalaureate Enrollment** 117 **Women** 74.4% **Men** 25.6% **Minority** 95.7% **Part-time** 1%
**Graduate Enrollment** 40 **Women** 82.5% **Men** 17.5% **Minority** 100% **International** 1% **Part-time** 100%
**Distance Learning Courses** Available.
**Nursing Student Activities** Nursing Honor Society, Student Nurses' Association.
**Nursing Student Resources** Academic advising; academic or career counseling; assistance for students with disabilities; bookstore; campus computer network; career placement assistance; computer lab; computer-assisted instruction; daycare for children of students; e-mail services; employment services for current students; externships; housing assistance; interactive nursing skills videos; Internet; learning resource lab; library services; nursing audiovisuals; paid internships; placement services for program completers; remedial services; resume preparation assistance; skills, simulation, or other laboratory; tutoring.
**Library Facilities** 476,656 volumes (14,285 in health, 1,804 in nursing); 54,115 periodical subscriptions (8,751 health-care related).

### BACCALAUREATE PROGRAMS

**Degree** BSN
**Available Programs** Generic Baccalaureate; RN Baccalaureate.
**Study Options** Full-time.
**Program Entrance Requirements** Minimum overall college GPA of 2.5, transcript of college record, CPR certification, written essay, health exam, immunizations, 2 letters of recommendation, minimum high school GPA of 2.5, minimum GPA in nursing prerequisites of 2.5, prerequisite course work. Transfer students are accepted. *Application deadline:* 6/1 (fall). *Application fee:* $25.
**Advanced Placement** Credit given for nursing courses completed elsewhere dependent upon specific evaluations.
**Expenses (2013–14)** *Tuition, state resident:* full-time $6000. *Tuition, nonresident:* full-time $14,000. *Room and board:* $6872; room only: $4532 per academic year.
**Financial Aid** 85% of baccalaureate students in nursing programs received some form of financial aid in 2012–13. *Gift aid (need-based):* Federal Pell, FSEOG, state, college/university gift aid from institutional funds, Federal Nursing. *Loans:* Federal Direct (Subsidized and Unsubsidized Stafford PLUS), state, college/university, Hinson-Hazelwood Loan Program. *Work-study:* Federal Work-Study, part-time campus jobs. *Financial aid application deadline:* 8/1(priority: 3/15).
**Contact** Dr. Glenda C. Walker, Dean, Canseco School of Nursing, Texas A&M International University, College of Nursing and Health Sciences, 5201 University Boulevard, Laredo, TX 78041-1900. *Telephone:* 956-326-2450. *Fax:* 956-326-2449. *E-mail:* glenda.walker@tamiu.edu.

### GRADUATE PROGRAMS

**Expenses (2013–14)** *Tuition, state resident:* full-time $3500. *Tuition, nonresident:* full-time $7790. *Room and board:* $6872; room only: $4532 per academic year.
**Financial Aid** 85% of graduate students in nursing programs received some form of financial aid in 2012–13.
**Contact** Dr. Glenda C. Walker, Dean, Canseco School of Nursing, Texas A&M International University, College of Nursing and Health Sciences, 5201 University Boulevard, Laredo, TX 78041-1900. *Telephone:* 956-326-2450. *Fax:* 956-326-2449. *E-mail:* glenda.walker@tamiu.edu.

#### MASTER'S DEGREE PROGRAM

**Degree** MSN
**Available Programs** Master's.
**Concentrations Available** Nursing administration. *Nurse practitioner programs in:* family health.
**Study Options** Full-time and part-time.
**Program Entrance Requirements** Clinical experience, minimum overall college GPA of 3.0, transcript of college record, CPR certification, written essay, immunizations, interview, 2 letters of recommendation, nursing research course. *Application deadline:* 6/1 (fall). *Application fee:* $25.
**Advanced Placement** Credit given for nursing courses completed elsewhere dependent upon specific evaluations.
**Degree Requirements** 45 total credit hours.

# Texas A&M University–Corpus Christi

## College of Nursing and Health Sciences
## Corpus Christi, Texas

*http://conhs.tamucc.edu/index.html*
Founded in 1947

### DEGREES • BSN • MSN

**Nursing Program Faculty** 64 (45% with doctorates).
**Baccalaureate Enrollment** 520 **Women** 79% **Men** 21% **Minority** 58% **International** .01% **Part-time** 13%
**Graduate Enrollment** 350 **Women** 84% **Men** 16% **Minority** 44% **Part-time** 99%
**Distance Learning Courses** Available.
**Nursing Student Activities** Nursing Honor Society, Sigma Theta Tau, Student Nurses' Association.
**Nursing Student Resources** Academic advising; academic or career counseling; assistance for students with disabilities; bookstore; campus computer network; career placement assistance; computer lab; computer-assisted instruction; e-mail services; employment services for current students; housing assistance; interactive nursing skills videos; Internet; learning resource lab; library services; nursing audiovisuals; placement

services for program completers; remedial services; resume preparation assistance; skills, simulation, or other laboratory; tutoring.
**Library Facilities** 731,586 volumes (500 in health, 350 in nursing); 1,901 periodical subscriptions (100 health-care related).

## BACCALAUREATE PROGRAMS

**Degree** BSN
**Available Programs** ADN to Baccalaureate; Accelerated Baccalaureate for Second Degree; Baccalaureate for Second Degree; Generic Baccalaureate; RN Baccalaureate.
**Study Options** Full-time and part-time.
**Online Degree Options** Yes.
**Program Entrance Requirements** Minimum overall college GPA of 3.0, transcript of college record, CPR certification, immunizations, professional liability insurance/malpractice insurance, prerequisite course work. Transfer students are accepted. *Application deadline:* 2/15 (fall), 7/31 (spring), 12/15 (summer). *Application fee:* $45.
**Advanced Placement** Credit by examination available. Credit given for nursing courses completed elsewhere dependent upon specific evaluations.
**Expenses (2013–14)** *Tuition, state resident:* full-time $7191; part-time $168 per credit hour. *Tuition, nonresident:* full-time $23,121; part-time $522 per credit hour. *International tuition:* $23,121 full-time. *Required fees:* full-time $4477; part-time $303 per credit; part-time $1492 per term.
**Financial Aid** 78% of baccalaureate students in nursing programs received some form of financial aid in 2012–13. *Gift aid (need-based):* Federal Pell, FSEOG, state, college/university gift aid from institutional funds. *Loans:* Perkins, state, college/university. *Work-study:* Federal Work-Study, part-time campus jobs. *Financial aid application deadline (priority):* 3/31.
**Contact** Dr. Cynthia O'Neal, Undergraduate Chair, College of Nursing and Health Sciences, Texas A&M University–Corpus Christi, 6300 Ocean Drive, Unit 5805, Corpus Christi, TX 78412-5503. *Telephone:* 361-825-2244. *Fax:* 361-825-2484. *E-mail:* Cynthia.O'Neal@tamucc.edu.

## GRADUATE PROGRAMS

**Expenses (2013–14)** *Tuition, area resident:* full-time $3522; part-time $196 per credit hour. *Tuition, state resident:* full-time $3122; part-time $196 per credit hour. *Tuition, nonresident:* full-time $9894; part-time $550 per credit hour. *International tuition:* $9894 full-time. *Required fees:* full-time $2880; part-time $263 per credit; part-time $891 per term.
**Financial Aid** 20% of graduate students in nursing programs received some form of financial aid in 2012–13.
**Contact** Dr. Chris Bray, Graduate Department Chair, College of Nursing and Health Sciences, Texas A&M University–Corpus Christi, 6300 Ocean Drive, Unit 5805, Corpus Christi, TX 78412. *Telephone:* 361-825-2798. *Fax:* 361-825-2484. *E-mail:* chris.bray@tamucc.edu.

### MASTER'S DEGREE PROGRAM

**Degree** MSN
**Available Programs** Master's; RN to Master's.
**Concentrations Available** Nursing administration; nursing education. *Nurse practitioner programs in:* family health.
**Study Options** Part-time.
**Online Degree Options** Yes (online only).
**Program Entrance Requirements** Minimum overall college GPA of 3.0, transcript of college record, CPR certification, written essay, immunizations, 3 letters of recommendation, resume, statistics course. *Application deadline:* 4/15 (fall), 11/15 (spring), 4/15 (summer). *Application fee:* $40.
**Advanced Placement** Credit given for nursing courses completed elsewhere dependent upon specific evaluations.
**Degree Requirements** 49 total credit hours, thesis or project.

### POST-MASTER'S PROGRAM

**Areas of Study** Nursing administration; nursing education. *Nurse practitioner programs in:* family health.

## CONTINUING EDUCATION PROGRAM

**Contact** Ms. Yvonne Serna, Chair of Continuing Education Committee, College of Nursing and Health Sciences, Texas A&M University–Corpus Christi, 6300 Ocean Drive, Island Hall Rm 342, Corpus Christi, TX 78412-5503. *Telephone:* 361-825-3790. *Fax:* 361-825-2484. *E-mail:* Yvonne.serna@tamucc.edu.

# Texas A&M University–Texarkana

### Nursing Department
### Texarkana, Texas

*http://www.tamut.edu/Academics/STEM/index.php*
Founded in 1971

**DEGREES • BSN • MSN**
**Nursing Program Faculty** 5 (60% with doctorates).
**Baccalaureate Enrollment** 31 **Women** 87% **Men** 13% **Minority** 23% **Part-time** 94%
**Graduate Enrollment** 26 **Women** 96% **Men** 4% **Minority** 15% **Part-time** 100%
**Nursing Student Activities** Nursing club.
**Nursing Student Resources** Academic advising; academic or career counseling; assistance for students with disabilities; bookstore; campus computer network; career placement assistance; computer lab; computer-assisted instruction; e-mail services; Internet; library services; nursing audiovisuals; resume preparation assistance.
**Library Facilities** 8,743 volumes in health, 2,558 volumes in nursing; 80 periodical subscriptions health-care related.

## BACCALAUREATE PROGRAMS

**Degree** BSN
**Available Programs** ADN to Baccalaureate.
**Study Options** Full-time and part-time.
**Program Entrance Requirements** Minimum overall college GPA of 2.0, transcript of college record, CPR certification, health exam, health insurance, immunizations, letters of recommendation, professional liability insurance/malpractice insurance, prerequisite course work, RN licensure. Transfer students are accepted. *Application deadline:* 7/15 (fall), 12/1 (spring), 4/1 (summer).
**Advanced Placement** Credit given for nursing courses completed elsewhere dependent upon specific evaluations.
**Contact** *Telephone:* 903-223-3175. *Fax:* 903-223-3107.

## GRADUATE PROGRAMS

**Contact** *Telephone:* 903-223-3175.

### MASTER'S DEGREE PROGRAM

**Degree** MSN
**Available Programs** Master's.
**Concentrations Available** Nursing administration; nursing education.
**Study Options** Full-time and part-time.
**Program Entrance Requirements** Minimum overall college GPA of 3.0, transcript of college record, written essay, 3 letters of recommendation, resume. *Application deadline:* 7/15 (fall), 12/1 (spring), 4/1 (summer).
**Degree Requirements** 36 total credit hours.

# Texas Christian University

### Harris College of Nursing
### Fort Worth, Texas

*http://www.nursing.tcu.edu/*
Founded in 1873

**DEGREES • BSN • DNP • MSN**
**Nursing Program Faculty** 52 (67% with doctorates).
**Baccalaureate Enrollment** 712 **Women** 92% **Men** 8% **Minority** 21%
**Graduate Enrollment** 259 **Women** 68% **Men** 32% **Minority** 24% **Part-time** 8%
**Distance Learning Courses** Available.
**Nursing Student Activities** Sigma Theta Tau, Student Nurses' Association.
**Nursing Student Resources** Academic advising; academic or career counseling; assistance for students with disabilities; bookstore; campus computer network; career placement assistance; computer lab; computer-assisted instruction; e-mail services; employment services for current students; externships; interactive nursing skills videos; Internet; learning resource lab; library services; nursing audiovisuals; other; placement services for program completers; remedial services; resume preparation assistance; skills, simulation, or other laboratory; tutoring; unpaid internships.
**Library Facilities** 1.4 million volumes (27,000 in health, 2,320 in nursing); 87,509 periodical subscriptions (298 health-care related).

## BACCALAUREATE PROGRAMS

**Degree** BSN
**Available Programs** Accelerated Baccalaureate for Second Degree; Generic Baccalaureate.
**Study Options** Full-time and part-time.
**Program Entrance Requirements** Minimum overall college GPA of 2.5, transcript of college record, CPR certification, written essay, health insurance, high school foreign language, 2 years high school math, 4 years high school science, high school transcript, immunizations, minimum high school GPA of 3.0, minimum GPA in nursing prerequisites of 2.5, prerequisite course work. Transfer students are accepted. *Application deadline:* 2/1 (fall), 10/1 (spring), 2/1 (summer). *Application fee:* $40.
**Advanced Placement** Credit by examination available. Credit given for nursing courses completed elsewhere dependent upon specific evaluations.
**Expenses (2013–14)** *Tuition:* full-time $36,500; part-time $1800 per credit hour. *International tuition:* $36,500 full-time. *Room and board:* $11,980; room only: $6700 per academic year. *Required fees:* full-time $460.
**Financial Aid** 70% of baccalaureate students in nursing programs received some form of financial aid in 2012–13. *Gift aid (need-based):* Federal Pell, FSEOG, state, private, college/university gift aid from institutional funds. *Loans:* Federal Nursing Student Loans, Federal Direct (Subsidized and Unsubsidized Stafford PLUS), Perkins, state. *Work-study:* Federal Work-Study, part-time campus jobs. *Financial aid application deadline:* 5/1(priority: 5/1).
**Contact** Ms. Marinda Allender, Director of Nursing Undergraduate Programs, Harris College of Nursing, Texas Christian University, TCU Box 298620, Fort Worth, TX 76129. *Telephone:* 817-257-7650. *Fax:* 817-257-7944. *E-mail:* m.allender@tcu.edu.

## GRADUATE PROGRAMS

**Expenses (2013–14)** *Tuition:* full-time $11,430; part-time $1270 per credit hour. *International tuition:* $11,430 full-time. *Required fees:* full-time $336.
**Financial Aid** 100% of graduate students in nursing programs received some form of financial aid in 2012–13.
**Contact** Ms. Mary Jane Allred, Administrative Program Specialist, Harris College of Nursing, Texas Christian University, TCU Box 298627, Fort Worth, TX 76129. *Telephone:* 817-257-6726. *Fax:* 817-257-8383. *E-mail:* m.allred@tcu.edu.

### MASTER'S DEGREE PROGRAM

**Degree** MSN
**Available Programs** Master's.
**Concentrations Available** Clinical nurse leader; nursing education. *Clinical nurse specialist programs in:* adult health, gerontology, pediatric.
**Study Options** Full-time and part-time.
**Online Degree Options** Yes (online only).
**Program Entrance Requirements** Clinical experience, computer literacy, minimum overall college GPA of 3.0, transcript of college record, CPR certification, written essay, immunizations, 3 letters of recommendation, professional liability insurance/malpractice insurance, prerequisite course work, resume. *Application deadline:* 11/15 (summer). *Application fee:* $60.
**Advanced Placement** Credit given for nursing courses completed elsewhere dependent upon specific evaluations.
**Degree Requirements** 40 total credit hours, thesis or project.

### POST-MASTER'S PROGRAM

**Areas of Study** Clinical nurse leader; nursing education. *Clinical nurse specialist programs in:* adult health, gerontology, pediatric.

### DOCTORAL DEGREE PROGRAM

**Degree** DNP
**Available Programs** Doctorate.
**Areas of Study** Advanced practice nursing, nurse anesthesia, nursing administration.
**Program Entrance Requirements** Minimum overall college GPA of 3.0, clinical experience, interview, 3 letters of recommendation, BSN or equivalent, vita, writing sample. *Application deadline:* 7/1 (summer). *Application fee:* $50.
**Degree Requirements** 30 total credit hours, oral exam, written exam.

## CONTINUING EDUCATION PROGRAM

**Contact** Ms. Barbara Patten, Program Planning and Continuing Nursing Education Coordinator, Harris College of Nursing, Texas Christian University, TCU Box 298620, Fort Worth, TX 76129. *Telephone:* 817-257-7368. *Fax:* 817-257-7944. *E-mail:* b.a.patten@tcu.edu.

# Texas State University–San Marcos

### St. David's School of Nursing
### San Marcos, Texas

***http://www.nursing.txstate.edu***
Founded in 1899

**DEGREES • BSN • MSN**
**Nursing Program Faculty** 36 (25% with doctorates).
**Baccalaureate Enrollment** 191 **Women** 88% **Men** 12% **Minority** 24%
**Graduate Enrollment** 33 **Women** 99% **Men** 1% **Minority** 29%
**Distance Learning Courses** Available.
**Nursing Student Activities** Nursing Honor Society, Student Nurses' Association, nursing club.
**Nursing Student Resources** Academic advising; academic or career counseling; assistance for students with disabilities; bookstore; campus computer network; computer lab; computer-assisted instruction; e-mail services; interactive nursing skills videos; Internet; library services; nursing audiovisuals; remedial services; resume preparation assistance; skills, simulation, or other laboratory; tutoring.
**Library Facilities** 1.6 million volumes (39,615 in health, 917 in nursing); 14,762 periodical subscriptions (11,734 health-care related).

## BACCALAUREATE PROGRAMS

**Degree** BSN
**Available Programs** Generic Baccalaureate.
**Site Options** Round Rock, TX.
**Study Options** Full-time.
**Program Entrance Requirements** Minimum overall college GPA of 2.9, transcript of college record, CPR certification, written essay, health exam, health insurance, high school foreign language, immunizations, 2 letters of recommendation, minimum GPA in nursing prerequisites of 3.0, professional liability insurance/malpractice insurance, prerequisite course work. *Application deadline:* 1/15 (fall). *Application fee:* $25.
**Expenses (2013–14)** *Tuition, state resident:* part-time $678 per credit hour. *Tuition, nonresident:* part-time $1032 per credit hour. *International tuition:* $1032 full-time.
**Financial Aid** 50% of baccalaureate students in nursing programs received some form of financial aid in 2012–13. *Gift aid (need-based):* Federal Pell, FSEOG, state, private, college/university gift aid from institutional funds. *Loans:* Federal Direct (Subsidized and Unsubsidized Stafford PLUS), Perkins, state, college/university, short-term emergency loans. *Work-study:* Federal Work-Study, part-time campus jobs. *Financial aid application deadline (priority):* 4/1.
**Contact** School of Nursing, St. David's School of Nursing, Texas State University–San Marcos, 1555 University Drive, Round Rock, TX 78665. *Telephone:* 512-716-2900. *Fax:* 512-716-2949.

## GRADUATE PROGRAMS

**Expenses (2013–14)** *Tuition, state resident:* part-time $638 per credit hour. *Tuition, nonresident:* part-time $992 per credit hour.
**Financial Aid** 67% of graduate students in nursing programs received some form of financial aid in 2012–13.
**Contact** Dr. Shirley A. Levenson, School of Nursing, St. David's School of Nursing, Texas State University–San Marcos, 1555 University Drive, Round Rock, TX 78665. *Telephone:* 512-716-2900. *Fax:* 512-716-2911. *E-mail:* sal11@txstate.edu.

### MASTER'S DEGREE PROGRAM

**Degree** MSN
**Available Programs** Master's.
**Concentrations Available** *Nurse practitioner programs in:* family health.
**Site Options** Round Rock, TX.
**Study Options** Full-time.
**Online Degree Options** Yes (online only).
**Program Entrance Requirements** Clinical experience, computer literacy, minimum overall college GPA of 3.0, transcript of college record, CPR certification, written essay, immunizations, 3 letters of recommen-

dation, nursing research course, professional liability insurance/malpractice insurance, resume, statistics course. *Application deadline:* 4/15 (fall). *Application fee:* $40.
**Advanced Placement** Credit given for nursing courses completed elsewhere dependent upon specific evaluations.
**Degree Requirements** 48 total credit hours, thesis or project.

# Texas Tech University Health Sciences Center

## School of Nursing
## Lubbock, Texas

*http://www.ttuhsc.edu/son*
Founded in 1969

**DEGREES • BSN • DNP • MSN**

**Nursing Program Faculty** 88 (48% with doctorates).
**Baccalaureate Enrollment** 878 **Women** 80% **Men** 20% **Minority** 45% **International** 20% **Part-time** 2%
**Graduate Enrollment** 489 **Women** 85% **Men** 15% **Minority** 34% **Part-time** 86%
**Distance Learning Courses** Available.
**Nursing Student Activities** Sigma Theta Tau, Student Nurses' Association.
**Nursing Student Resources** Academic advising; academic or career counseling; assistance for students with disabilities; bookstore; campus computer network; career placement assistance; computer lab; e-mail services; Internet; learning resource lab; library services; nursing audiovisuals; other; skills, simulation, or other laboratory; tutoring.
**Library Facilities** 320,818 volumes in health, 6,583 volumes in nursing; 28,960 periodical subscriptions health-care related.

### BACCALAUREATE PROGRAMS

**Degree** BSN
**Available Programs** Accelerated Baccalaureate for Second Degree; Generic Baccalaureate; RN Baccalaureate.
**Site Options** Odessa, TX; Abilene, TX.
**Study Options** Full-time.
**Online Degree Options** Yes (online only).
**Program Entrance Requirements** Transcript of college record, written essay, immunizations, minimum GPA in nursing prerequisites of 2.5, prerequisite course work, RN licensure. *Application deadline:* 12/15 (fall). *Application fee:* $40.
**Advanced Placement** Credit given for nursing courses completed elsewhere dependent upon specific evaluations.
**Expenses (2012–13)** *Tuition, state resident:* full-time $2625. *Tuition, nonresident:* full-time $7890. *International tuition:* $7890 full-time.
**Financial Aid** 86% of baccalaureate students in nursing programs received some form of financial aid in 2011–12.
**Contact** Dr. Kathy Sridaromont, Department Chair of Traditional Undergraduate Studies, School of Nursing, Texas Tech University Health Sciences Center, 3601 4th Street, MS 6264, Lubbock, TX 79430. *Telephone:* 806-743-2730. *Fax:* 806-743-1648. *E-mail:* kathy.sridaromont@ttuhsc.edu.

### GRADUATE PROGRAMS

**Expenses (2012–13)** *Tuition, state resident:* full-time $2025; part-time $1350 per semester. *Tuition, nonresident:* full-time $5184; part-time $3456 per semester. *International tuition:* $5184 full-time. *Required fees:* part-time $2016 per term.
**Financial Aid** 80% of graduate students in nursing programs received some form of financial aid in 2011–12. Institutionally sponsored loans, scholarships, and traineeships available. Aid available to part-time students. *Financial aid application deadline:* 12/1.
**Contact** Ms. Georgina Barrera, Graduate Program Student Affairs Coordinator, School of Nursing, Texas Tech University Health Sciences Center, 3601 4th Street, MS 6264, Lubbock, TX 79430. *Telephone:* 806-743-2762. *Fax:* 806-743-2324. *E-mail:* georgina.barrera@ttuhsc.edu.

### MASTER'S DEGREE PROGRAM

**Degree** MSN
**Available Programs** Master's.
**Concentrations Available** Nurse-midwifery; nursing administration; nursing education. *Nurse practitioner programs in:* acute care, family health, gerontology, pediatric.
**Study Options** Full-time and part-time.
**Online Degree Options** Yes (online only).
**Program Entrance Requirements** Clinical experience, computer literacy, minimum overall college GPA of 3.0, transcript of college record, CPR certification, written essay, immunizations, 3 letters of recommendation, nursing research course, statistics course. *Application deadline:* 5/1 (fall), 9/1 (spring). *Application fee:* $40.
**Advanced Placement** Credit given for nursing courses completed elsewhere dependent upon specific evaluations.
**Degree Requirements** 48 total credit hours, thesis or project, comprehensive exam.

### POST-MASTER'S PROGRAM

**Areas of Study** *Nurse practitioner programs in:* acute care, family health, gerontology, pediatric.

### DOCTORAL DEGREE PROGRAM

**Degree** DNP
**Available Programs** Doctorate.
**Areas of Study** Nursing administration, nursing education.
**Program Entrance Requirements** Clinical experience, minimum overall college GPA of 3.0, interview by faculty committee, interview, 3 letters of recommendation, MSN or equivalent, statistics course, vita, writing sample. *Application deadline:* 9/1 (summer).
**Degree Requirements** 48 total credit hours.

# Texas Tech University Health Sciences Center-El Paso

## Texas Tech University Health Sciences Center-El Paso
## El Paso, Texas

**DEGREE • BSN**

### BACCALAUREATE PROGRAMS

**Degree** BSN
**Available Programs** Accelerated Baccalaureate for Second Degree; Generic Baccalaureate.
**Online Degree Options** Yes.
**Contact** Jeanne Novotny, Founding Dean and Professor, Texas Tech University Health Sciences Center-El Paso, 415 East Yandell, El Paso, TX 79902. *Telephone:* 915-215-6106. *E-mail:* jeanne.novotny@ttuhsc.edu.

# Texas Woman's University

## College of Nursing
## Denton, Texas

*http://www.twu.edu/nursing*
Founded in 1901

**DEGREES • BS • MS • MS/MHA • PHD**

**Nursing Program Faculty** 250 (40% with doctorates).
**Baccalaureate Enrollment** 900 **Women** 90% **Men** 10% **Minority** 51% **International** 4% **Part-time** 14%
**Graduate Enrollment** 1,000 **Women** 94% **Men** 6% **Minority** 40% **International** 1% **Part-time** 85%
**Distance Learning Courses** Available.
**Nursing Student Activities** Nursing Honor Society, Sigma Theta Tau, Student Nurses' Association, nursing club.
**Nursing Student Resources** Academic advising; academic or career counseling; assistance for students with disabilities; bookstore; campus computer network; career placement assistance; computer lab; computer-assisted instruction; e-mail services; employment services for current students; interactive nursing skills videos; Internet; learning resource lab; library services; nursing audiovisuals; placement services for program completers; remedial services; resume preparation assistance; skills, simulation, or other laboratory; tutoring; unpaid internships.
**Library Facilities** 580,832 volumes (250,000 in health, 26,463 in nursing); 55,756 periodical subscriptions (2,644 health-care related).

### BACCALAUREATE PROGRAMS

**Degree** BS
**Available Programs** Baccalaureate for Second Degree; Generic Baccalaureate; RN Baccalaureate.

**Site Options** Houston, TX; Dallas, TX.

**Study Options** Full-time and part-time.

**Online Degree Options** Yes.

**Program Entrance Requirements** Transcript of college record, CPR certification, high school transcript, immunizations, minimum GPA in nursing prerequisites of 3.0, professional liability insurance/malpractice insurance, prerequisite course work. Transfer students are accepted. *Application deadline:* 2/1 (fall), 9/1 (spring). *Application fee:* $30.

**Advanced Placement** Credit given for nursing courses completed elsewhere dependent upon specific evaluations.

**Expenses (2013–14)** *Tuition, state resident:* full-time $5482; part-time $456 per credit hour. *Tuition, nonresident:* full-time $11,800; part-time $807 per credit hour. *Required fees:* full-time $2500.

**Financial Aid** ***Gift aid (need-based):*** Federal Pell, FSEOG, state, private, college/university gift aid from institutional funds, United Negro College Fund. *Loans:* Federal Nursing Student Loans, Federal Direct (Subsidized and Unsubsidized Stafford PLUS), Perkins, state, college/university, alternative loans. *Work-study:* Federal Work-Study, part-time campus jobs. *Financial aid application deadline (priority):* 4/1.

**Contact** Heather Close, Nursing Admissions Coordinator, College of Nursing, Texas Woman's University, PO Box 425498, Denton, TX 76204. *Telephone:* 940-898-2401. *Fax:* 940-898-2437. *E-mail:* nursing@twu.edu.

## GRADUATE PROGRAMS

**Financial Aid** 30% of graduate students in nursing programs received some form of financial aid in 2012–13. 10 research assistantships (averaging $12,942 per year), 1 teaching assistantship (averaging $12,942 per year) were awarded; career-related internships or fieldwork, Federal Work-Study, institutionally sponsored loans, scholarships, traineeships, and unspecified assistantships also available. Aid available to part-time students. *Financial aid application deadline:* 3/1.

**Contact** Dr. Ruth Johnson, Associate Dean of the Graduate School, College of Nursing, Texas Woman's University, PO Box 425649, Denton, TX 76204. *Telephone:* 940-898-3415. *E-mail:* rjohnson@twu.edu.

### MASTER'S DEGREE PROGRAM

**Degrees** MS; MS/MHA

**Available Programs** Master's; RN to Master's.

**Concentrations Available** Clinical nurse leader; health-care administration; nursing administration; nursing education. *Nurse practitioner programs in:* acute care, adult health, family health, pediatric,women's health.

**Site Options** Houston, TX; Dallas, TX.

**Study Options** Full-time and part-time.

**Online Degree Options** Yes.

**Program Entrance Requirements** Clinical experience, minimum overall college GPA of 3.0, transcript of college record, CPR certification, immunizations, professional liability insurance/malpractice insurance, statistics course, GRE or MAT. *Application deadline:* 2/1 (fall), 9/1 (spring).

**Advanced Placement** Credit given for nursing courses completed elsewhere dependent upon specific evaluations.

**Degree Requirements** 48 total credit hours, thesis or project.

### POST-MASTER'S PROGRAM

**Areas of Study** *Nurse practitioner programs in:* acute care, adult health, family health, pediatric,women's health.

### DOCTORAL DEGREE PROGRAM

**Degree** PhD

**Available Programs** Doctorate.

**Areas of Study** Nursing research, nursing science,women's health.

**Site Options** Houston, TX; Dallas, TX.

**Program Entrance Requirements** Minimum overall college GPA of 3.5, 2 letters of recommendation, MSN or equivalent, statistics course, vita, GRE (preferred minimum score 153 [500 old version] Verbal, 144 [500 old version] Quantitative, 4 Analytical).

**Degree Requirements** 60 total credit hours, dissertation, oral exam, written exam.

# University of Houston–Victoria
## School of Nursing
## Victoria, Texas

Founded in 1973

**DEGREES • BSN • MSN**

## BACCALAUREATE PROGRAMS

**Degree** BSN
**Available Programs** Accelerated Baccalaureate for Second Degree; RN Baccalaureate.
**Contact** *Telephone:* 361-570-4848.

## GRADUATE PROGRAMS

**Contact** *Telephone:* 361-570-4848.

### MASTER'S DEGREE PROGRAM

**Degree** MSN
**Available Programs** Master's; RN to Master's.
**Concentrations Available** Nursing administration; nursing education.
**Program Entrance Requirements** GRE or MAT.

# University of Mary Hardin-Baylor
## College of Nursing
## Belton, Texas

*http://www.umhb.edu/*
Founded in 1845

**DEGREES • BSN • MSN**

**Nursing Program Faculty** 48 (22% with doctorates).
**Baccalaureate Enrollment** 494 **Women** 90% **Men** 10% **Minority** 33% **International** 3%
**Graduate Enrollment** 42 **Women** 97% **Men** 3% **Minority** 22% **Part-time** 5%
**Distance Learning Courses** Available.
**Nursing Student Activities** Nursing Honor Society, Sigma Theta Tau, Student Nurses' Association.
**Nursing Student Resources** Academic advising; academic or career counseling; assistance for students with disabilities; bookstore; campus computer network; career placement assistance; computer lab; e-mail services; employment services for current students; housing assistance; Internet; learning resource lab; library services; nursing audiovisuals; placement services for program completers; remedial services; resume preparation assistance; skills, simulation, or other laboratory; tutoring.
**Library Facilities** 197,638 volumes (8,116 in health, 6,924 in nursing); 670 periodical subscriptions (132 health-care related).

## BACCALAUREATE PROGRAMS

**Degree** BSN
**Available Programs** ADN to Baccalaureate; Generic Baccalaureate.
**Study Options** Full-time and part-time.
**Program Entrance Requirements** Minimum overall college GPA of 3.0, transcript of college record, CPR certification, written essay, health exam, health insurance, high school transcript, immunizations, minimum GPA in nursing prerequisites of 3.0, prerequisite course work. Transfer students are accepted. *Application deadline:* 3/1 (fall), 10/1 (spring). Applications may be processed on a rolling basis for some programs.
**Advanced Placement** Credit given for nursing courses completed elsewhere dependent upon specific evaluations.
**Expenses (2013–14)** *Tuition:* full-time $18,360; part-time $765 per credit hour. *International tuition:* $18,360 full-time. *Room and board:* $6230; room only: $5250 per academic year. *Required fees:* full-time $2000; part-time $1000 per term.
**Financial Aid** 95% of baccalaureate students in nursing programs received some form of financial aid in 2012–13. *Gift aid (need-based):* Federal Pell, FSEOG, state, private, college/university gift aid from institutional funds. *Loans:* Federal Direct (Subsidized and Unsubsidized Stafford PLUS), Perkins, state. *Work-study:* Federal Work-Study, part-time campus jobs. *Financial aid application deadline (priority):* 3/1.
**Contact** Dr. Sharon Souter, Dean and Professor, College of Nursing, University of Mary Hardin-Baylor, Box 8015, 900 College Street, Belton, TX 76513-2599. *Telephone:* 254-295-4665. *Fax:* 254-295-4141. *E-mail:* lpehl@umhb.edu.

## GRADUATE PROGRAMS

**Expenses (2013–14)** *Tuition:* full-time $14,130; part-time $785 per contact hour. *International tuition:* $14,130 full-time. *Required fees:* full-time $1170; part-time $750 per term.
**Financial Aid** 40% of graduate students in nursing programs received some form of financial aid in 2012–13.
**Contact** Dr. Carrie Johnson, Director and Associate Professor, College of Nursing, University of Mary Hardin-Baylor, Box 8015, 900 College Street, Belton, TX 76513-2599. *Telephone:* 254-295-4178. *Fax:* 254-295-4141. *E-mail:* cjohnson@umhb.edu.

### MASTER'S DEGREE PROGRAM

**Degree** MSN
**Available Programs** Master's.
**Concentrations Available** Clinical nurse leader; nursing education. *Nurse practitioner programs in:* family health.
**Study Options** Full-time and part-time.
**Program Entrance Requirements** Clinical experience, computer literacy, minimum overall college GPA of 3.0, transcript of college record, CPR certification, written essay, immunizations, interview, 2 letters of recommendation, nursing research course, physical assessment course, professional liability insurance/malpractice insurance, prerequisite course work, statistics course. *Application deadline:* 4/1 (fall). Applications may be processed on a rolling basis for some programs. *Application fee:* $50.
**Advanced Placement** Credit given for nursing courses completed elsewhere dependent upon specific evaluations.
**Degree Requirements** 36 total credit hours, comprehensive exam.

### POST-MASTER'S PROGRAM

**Areas of Study** Clinical nurse leader; nursing education. *Nurse practitioner programs in:* family health.

# The University of Texas at Arlington
## College of Nursing
## Arlington, Texas

***http://www.uta.edu/nursing***
Founded in 1895

**DEGREES • BSN • MSN • MSN/MBA • MSN/MHA • MSN/MPH • PHD**
**Nursing Program Faculty** 126 (34% with doctorates).
**Baccalaureate Enrollment** 2,243 **Women** 89% **Men** 11% **Minority** 40% **International** 10% **Part-time** 8%
**Graduate Enrollment** 542 **Women** 91% **Men** 9% **Minority** 22% **Part-time** 70%
**Distance Learning Courses** Available.
**Nursing Student Activities** Nursing Honor Society, Sigma Theta Tau, Student Nurses' Association, nursing club.
**Nursing Student Resources** Academic advising; campus computer network; computer lab; e-mail services; externships; interactive nursing skills videos; Internet; learning resource lab; nursing audiovisuals; skills, simulation, or other laboratory; tutoring.
**Library Facilities** 1.6 million volumes (36,000 in health, 23,300 in nursing); 37,479 periodical subscriptions (530 health-care related).

## BACCALAUREATE PROGRAMS

**Degree** BSN
**Available Programs** Accelerated Baccalaureate; Accelerated Baccalaureate for Second Degree; Accelerated RN Baccalaureate; Baccalaureate for Second Degree; Generic Baccalaureate; RN Baccalaureate.
**Site Options** Fort Worth, TX; Dallas, TX; Waco, Grayson, Paris, Kaufman, TX.
**Study Options** Full-time and part-time.
**Program Entrance Requirements** Minimum overall college GPA of 2.5, transcript of college record, CPR certification, health insurance, immunizations, minimum high school GPA of 2.5, minimum GPA in nursing prerequisites of 2.5, professional liability insurance/malpractice insurance, prerequisite course work. Transfer students are accepted. *Application deadline:* 1/5 (fall), 6/1 (spring).
**Advanced Placement** Credit given for nursing courses completed elsewhere dependent upon specific evaluations.
**Contact** *Telephone:* 817-272-2776. *Fax:* 817-272-5006.

## GRADUATE PROGRAMS

**Contact** *Telephone:* 817-272-2776. *Fax:* 817-272-5006.

### MASTER'S DEGREE PROGRAM

**Degrees** MSN; MSN/MBA; MSN/MHA; MSN/MPH
**Available Programs** Master's.
**Concentrations Available** Health-care administration; nursing administration; nursing education. *Nurse practitioner programs in:* acute care, adult health, family health, gerontology, neonatal health, pediatric, psychiatric/mental health.
**Site Options** Fort Worth, TX; Dallas, TX.
**Study Options** Full-time and part-time.
**Online Degree Options** Yes.
**Program Entrance Requirements** Clinical experience, computer literacy, minimum overall college GPA of 3.0, transcript of college record, CPR certification, written essay, immunizations, physical assessment course, statistics course, GRE General Test if GPA less than 3.0. *Application deadline:* 6/1 (fall), 10/15 (spring). *Application fee:* $70.
**Advanced Placement** Credit given for nursing courses completed elsewhere dependent upon specific evaluations.
**Degree Requirements** 48 total credit hours.

### POST-MASTER'S PROGRAM

**Areas of Study** *Nurse practitioner programs in:* acute care, adult health, family health, gerontology, neonatal health, pediatric, psychiatric/mental health.

### DOCTORAL DEGREE PROGRAM

**Degree** PhD
**Available Programs** Doctorate; Post-Baccalaureate Doctorate.
**Areas of Study** Faculty preparation, nursing education, nursing research.
**Program Entrance Requirements** Clinical experience, minimum overall college GPA of 3.0, interview by faculty committee, interview, 3 letters of recommendation, statistics course, GRE General Test (waived for MSN-to-PhD applicants). *Application deadline:* 4/2 (fall). *Application fee:* $70.
**Degree Requirements** 54 total credit hours, dissertation, residency.

## CONTINUING EDUCATION PROGRAM

**Contact** *Telephone:* 817-272-0720. *Fax:* 817-272-5371.

# The University of Texas at Austin
## School of Nursing
## Austin, Texas

***http://www.utexas.edu/nursing***
Founded in 1883

**DEGREES • BSN • MSN • MSN/MBA • PHD**
**Nursing Program Faculty** 73 (62% with doctorates).
**Baccalaureate Enrollment** 791 **Women** 90.5% **Men** 9.5% **Minority** 33% **International** 1% **Part-time** 13%
**Graduate Enrollment** 300 **Women** 88% **Men** 12% **Minority** 27% **International** 9% **Part-time** 24%
**Distance Learning Courses** Available.
**Nursing Student Activities** Nursing Honor Society, Sigma Theta Tau, Student Nurses' Association, nursing club.
**Nursing Student Resources** Academic advising; academic or career counseling; assistance for students with disabilities; bookstore; campus computer network; career placement assistance; computer lab; computer-assisted instruction; e-mail services; externships; interactive nursing skills videos; Internet; learning resource lab; library services; nursing audiovisuals; other; remedial services; resume preparation assistance; skills, simulation, or other laboratory; tutoring; unpaid internships.
**Library Facilities** 10.9 million volumes (100,000 in health, 80,000 in nursing); 103,589 periodical subscriptions (504 health-care related).

## BACCALAUREATE PROGRAMS

**Degree** BSN
**Available Programs** Generic Baccalaureate; RN Baccalaureate.
**Study Options** Full-time.
**Program Entrance Requirements** Minimum overall college GPA of 2.75, transcript of college record, CPR certification, written essay, 3 years high school math, 2 years high school science, high school transcript, 3 letters of recommendation, minimum GPA in nursing prerequisites of 2.75, professional liability insurance/malpractice insurance, prerequisite

course work. Transfer students are accepted. *Application deadline:* 9/15 (fall), 2/15 (spring). *Application fee:* $50.
**Advanced Placement** Credit by examination available. Credit given for nursing courses completed elsewhere dependent upon specific evaluations.
**Expenses (2013–14)** *Tuition, state resident:* full-time $5181; part-time $1558 per hour. *Tuition, nonresident:* full-time $18,227; part-time $5473 per hour. *International tuition:* $18,227 full-time. *Room and board:* $9272; room only: $7272 per academic year.
**Financial Aid** 54% of baccalaureate students in nursing programs received some form of financial aid in 2012–13. *Gift aid (need-based):* Federal Pell, FSEOG, state, private, college/university gift aid from institutional funds. *Loans:* Federal Direct (Subsidized and Unsubsidized Stafford PLUS), Perkins, state. *Work-study:* Federal Work-Study, part-time campus jobs. *Financial aid application deadline:* Continuous.
**Contact** Christina Jarvis, Student Affairs Office, School of Nursing, The University of Texas at Austin, 1710 Red River Street, Austin, TX 78701-1412. *Telephone:* 512-232-4780. *Fax:* 512-232-4777. *E-mail:* sar@mail.nur.utexas.edu.

## GRADUATE PROGRAMS

**Expenses (2013–14)** *Tuition, state resident:* full-time $9482; part-time $3461 per semester. *Tuition, nonresident:* full-time $17,520; part-time $6221 per semester. *International tuition:* $17,520 full-time. *Room and board:* $9521 per academic year.
**Financial Aid** 35% of graduate students in nursing programs received some form of financial aid in 2012–13. Fellowships, research assistantships, teaching assistantships, scholarships and traineeships available. *Financial aid application deadline:* 2/1.
**Contact** Mr. Rudy Ortiz, Graduate Student Affairs, School of Nursing, The University of Texas at Austin, 1700 Red River Street, Graduate Student Affairs, Austin, TX 78701-1499. *Telephone:* 512-232-4701. *Fax:* 512-232-4777. *E-mail:* nugrad@uts.cc.utexas.edu.

### MASTER'S DEGREE PROGRAM

**Degrees** MSN; MSN/MBA
**Available Programs** Master's; Master's for Non-Nursing College Graduates; Master's for Nurses with Non-Nursing Degrees.
**Concentrations Available** Nursing administration. *Clinical nurse specialist programs in:* adult health. *Nurse practitioner programs in:* family health, pediatric, psychiatric/mental health.
**Study Options** Full-time and part-time.
**Program Entrance Requirements** Minimum overall college GPA of 3.0, transcript of college record, written essay, interview, 3 letters of recommendation, prerequisite course work, resume, statistics course, GRE General Test. *Application deadline:* 12/1 (fall), 11/1 (summer). *Application fee:* $65.
**Advanced Placement** Credit given for nursing courses completed elsewhere dependent upon specific evaluations.
**Degree Requirements** 39 total credit hours.

### POST-MASTER'S PROGRAM

**Areas of Study** *Clinical nurse specialist programs in:* adult health. *Nurse practitioner programs in:* family health, pediatric, psychiatric/mental health.

### DOCTORAL DEGREE PROGRAM

**Degree** PhD
**Available Programs** Doctorate; Doctorate for Nurses with Non-Nursing Degrees; Post-Baccalaureate Doctorate.
**Areas of Study** Addiction/substance abuse, aging, bio-behavioral research, clinical practice, community health, ethics, family health, gerontology, health promotion/disease prevention, health-care systems, human health and illness, illness and transition, individualized study, information systems, maternity-newborn, nursing administration, nursing research, nursing science, oncology,women's health.
**Program Entrance Requirements** Minimum overall college GPA of 3.0, interview, 3 letters of recommendation, MSN or equivalent, statistics course, vita, writing sample, GRE General Test. *Application deadline:* 12/1 (fall), 11/1 (summer). *Application fee:* $65.
**Degree Requirements** 57 total credit hours, dissertation, oral exam.

### POSTDOCTORAL PROGRAM

**Postdoctoral Program Contact** Dr. Lorraine Walker, Professor, School of Nursing, The University of Texas at Austin, 1700 Red River Street, Austin, TX 78701. *Telephone:* 512-232-4751. *Fax:* 512-232-4777. *E-mail:* lwalker@mail.nur.utexas.edu.

# The University of Texas at Brownsville

**Department of Nursing**
**Brownsville, Texas**

***http://www.utb.edu/vpaa/nursing/pages/default.aspx***
Founded in 1973

**DEGREES • BSN • MSN**
**Nursing Program Faculty** 13 (62% with doctorates).
**Baccalaureate Enrollment** 91 **Women** 74% **Men** 26% **Minority** 90% **International** 2% **Part-time** 82%
**Graduate Enrollment** 53 **Women** 77% **Men** 23% **Minority** 87% **International** 4% **Part-time** 47%
**Distance Learning Courses** Available.
**Nursing Student Activities** Nursing club.
**Nursing Student Resources** Academic advising; academic or career counseling; assistance for students with disabilities; bookstore; campus computer network; career placement assistance; computer lab; computer-assisted instruction; daycare for children of students; e-mail services; employment services for current students; housing assistance; interactive nursing skills videos; Internet; learning resource lab; library services; nursing audiovisuals; remedial services; resume preparation assistance; skills, simulation, or other laboratory; tutoring.

## BACCALAUREATE PROGRAMS

**Degree** BSN
**Available Programs** ADN to Baccalaureate.
**Study Options** Full-time and part-time.
**Online Degree Options** Yes (online only).
**Program Entrance Requirements** Minimum overall college GPA of 2.5, transcript of college record, CPR certification, immunizations, minimum GPA in nursing prerequisites of 2.5, professional liability insurance/malpractice insurance, prerequisite course work, RN licensure. Transfer students are accepted. *Application deadline:* 3/1 (fall), 11/1 (spring).
**Advanced Placement** Credit by examination available.
**Financial Aid** ***Gift aid (need-based):*** Federal Pell, FSEOG, state, private, college/university gift aid from institutional funds. *Loans:* Federal Direct (Subsidized and Unsubsidized Stafford PLUS), state, college/university. *Work-study:* Federal Work-Study, part-time campus jobs. *Financial aid application deadline (priority):* 3/1.
**Contact** Dr. Anne R. Rentfro, Associate Dean, College of Nursing, Department of Nursing, The University of Texas at Brownsville, 80 Fort Brown, Brownsville, TX 78520. *Telephone:* 956-882-5071. *Fax:* 956-882-5100. *E-mail:* anne.rentfro@utb.edu.

## GRADUATE PROGRAMS

**Contact** Dr. Eloisa G. Tamez, Director of Masters Program, Department of Nursing, The University of Texas at Brownsville, 80 Fort Brown, Brownsville, TX 78520. *Telephone:* 956-882-5079. *Fax:* 956-882-5100. *E-mail:* eloisa.tamez@utb.edu.

### MASTER'S DEGREE PROGRAM

**Degree** MSN
**Available Programs** Master's; Master's for Nurses with Non-Nursing Degrees.
**Concentrations Available** Nursing administration; nursing education. *Clinical nurse specialist programs in:* public health.
**Study Options** Full-time and part-time.
**Online Degree Options** Yes (online only).
**Program Entrance Requirements** Computer literacy, minimum overall college GPA of 3.0, transcript of college record, CPR certification, written essay, immunizations, interview, professional liability insurance/malpractice insurance, resume, statistics course. *Application deadline:* 4/1 (fall), 10/1 (spring). *Application fee:* $25.
**Advanced Placement** Credit given for nursing courses completed elsewhere dependent upon specific evaluations.
**Degree Requirements** 37 total credit hours, thesis or project.

## CONTINUING EDUCATION PROGRAM

**Contact** Dr. Anne Rentfro, Interim Associate Dean College of Nursing, Department of Nursing, The University of Texas at Brownsville, 80 Fort Brown, Brownsville, TX 78520. *Telephone:* 956-882-5084. *Fax:* 956-882-5100. *E-mail:* anne.rentfro@utb.edu.

## The University of Texas at El Paso
### School of Nursing
### El Paso, Texas

*http://www.utep.edu/*
Founded in 1913

**DEGREES • BSN • MSN**

**Nursing Program Faculty** 64 (27% with doctorates).
**Baccalaureate Enrollment** 514 **Women** 76.5% **Men** 23.5% **Minority** 80.4% **International** 2.7% **Part-time** 58.8%
**Graduate Enrollment** 153 **Women** 81% **Men** 19% **Minority** 61.4% **International** 3.3% **Part-time** 78.4%
**Distance Learning Courses** Available.
**Nursing Student Activities** Nursing Honor Society, Sigma Theta Tau, Student Nurses' Association.
**Nursing Student Resources** Academic advising; academic or career counseling; assistance for students with disabilities; bookstore; campus computer network; career placement assistance; computer lab; computer-assisted instruction; e-mail services; employment services for current students; interactive nursing skills videos; Internet; learning resource lab; library services; nursing audiovisuals; remedial services; skills, simulation, or other laboratory; tutoring.
**Library Facilities** 1.3 million volumes (71,389 in health, 13,043 in nursing); 3,065 periodical subscriptions (314 health-care related).

#### BACCALAUREATE PROGRAMS

**Degree** BSN
**Available Programs** Accelerated Baccalaureate; Generic Baccalaureate; RN Baccalaureate.
**Site Options** El Paso, TX.
**Study Options** Full-time and part-time.
**Program Entrance Requirements** Minimum overall college GPA of 2.0, transcript of college record, CPR certification, health exam, high school biology, high school math, high school science, high school transcript, immunizations, minimum GPA in nursing prerequisites of 2.5, professional liability insurance/malpractice insurance, prerequisite course work. Transfer students are accepted. *Application deadline:* 2/28 (fall), 9/30 (spring), 2/28 (summer).
**Advanced Placement** Credit by examination available. Credit given for nursing courses completed elsewhere dependent upon specific evaluations.
**Contact** *Telephone:* 915-747-7267. *Fax:* 915-747-8266.

#### GRADUATE PROGRAMS

**Contact** *Telephone:* 915-747-7226. *Fax:* 915-747-8266.

##### MASTER'S DEGREE PROGRAM

**Degree** MSN
**Available Programs** Master's; RN to Master's.
**Concentrations Available** Nursing administration; nursing education. *Nurse practitioner programs in:* family health.
**Site Options** El Paso, TX.
**Study Options** Full-time and part-time.
**Online Degree Options** Yes (online only).
**Program Entrance Requirements** Clinical experience, minimum overall college GPA of 3.0, transcript of college record, CPR certification, written essay, immunizations, interview, nursing research course, professional liability insurance/malpractice insurance, resume, statistics course. *Application deadline:* 9/1 (fall), 2/1 (spring). Applications may be processed on a rolling basis for some programs. *Application fee:* $45.
**Advanced Placement** Credit given for nursing courses completed elsewhere dependent upon specific evaluations.
**Degree Requirements** 33 total credit hours, thesis or project, comprehensive exam.

##### POST-MASTER'S PROGRAM

**Areas of Study** Nursing administration; nursing education. *Nurse practitioner programs in:* family health.

##### DOCTORAL DEGREE PROGRAM

**Program Entrance Requirements** GRE.

## The University of Texas at Tyler
### Program in Nursing
### Tyler, Texas

*http://www.uttyler.edu/nursing*
Founded in 1971

**DEGREES • BSN • MSN • MSN/MBA • PHD**

**Nursing Program Faculty** 65 (25% with doctorates).
**Baccalaureate Enrollment** 650 **Women** 70% **Men** 30% **Minority** 10% **International** 1% **Part-time** 15%
**Graduate Enrollment** 175 **Women** 88% **Men** 12% **Minority** 11% **Part-time** 88%
**Nursing Student Activities** Nursing Honor Society, Sigma Theta Tau, Student Nurses' Association, nursing club.
**Nursing Student Resources** Academic advising; academic or career counseling; assistance for students with disabilities; bookstore; campus computer network; career placement assistance; computer lab; computer-assisted instruction; e-mail services; employment services for current students; externships; interactive nursing skills videos; Internet; learning resource lab; library services; nursing audiovisuals; resume preparation assistance; skills, simulation, or other laboratory; tutoring.
**Library Facilities** 11,000 volumes in health, 5,500 volumes in nursing; 150 periodical subscriptions health-care related.

#### BACCALAUREATE PROGRAMS

**Degree** BSN
**Available Programs** ADN to Baccalaureate; Accelerated RN Baccalaureate; Generic Baccalaureate; International Nurse to Baccalaureate; LPN to Baccalaureate; LPN to RN Baccalaureate; RN Baccalaureate.
**Site Options** Longview, TX; Palestine, TX.
**Study Options** Full-time and part-time.
**Online Degree Options** Yes (online only).
**Program Entrance Requirements** Minimum overall college GPA of 2.75, transcript of college record, CPR certification, immunizations, minimum GPA in nursing prerequisites of 2.75, professional liability insurance/malpractice insurance, prerequisite course work. Transfer students are accepted. *Application deadline:* 2/15 (fall), 9/15 (spring).
**Advanced Placement** Credit given for nursing courses completed elsewhere dependent upon specific evaluations.
**Expenses (2012–13)** *Tuition, state resident:* full-time $7300. *Tuition, nonresident:* full-time $18,000.
**Financial Aid** 70% of baccalaureate students in nursing programs received some form of financial aid in 2011–12.
**Contact** Ms. Renee Lampkin, Director of Marketing/Advising, Program in Nursing, The University of Texas at Tyler, 3900 University Boulevard, Tyler, TX 75799. *Telephone:* 903-565-5534. *Fax:* 903-565-5533. *E-mail:* rlampkin@uttyler.edu.

#### GRADUATE PROGRAMS

**Financial Aid** 60% of graduate students in nursing programs received some form of financial aid in 2011–12. 1 fellowship (averaging $10,000 per year), 3 research assistantships (averaging $2,200 per year) were awarded; institutionally sponsored loans and scholarships also available. *Financial aid application deadline:* 7/1.
**Contact** Ms. RaeJean Griffin, Administrative Assistant II, Program in Nursing, The University of Texas at Tyler, 3900 University Boulevard, Tyler, TX 75799. *Telephone:* 903-566-7128. *Fax:* 903-565-5901. *E-mail:* rgriffin@uttyler.edu.

##### MASTER'S DEGREE PROGRAM

**Degrees** MSN; MSN/MBA
**Available Programs** Accelerated AD/RN to Master's; Accelerated RN to Master's; Master's; RN to Master's.
**Concentrations Available** Nursing administration; nursing education. *Nurse practitioner programs in:* family health, pediatric.
**Study Options** Full-time and part-time.
**Online Degree Options** Yes (online only).
**Program Entrance Requirements** Computer literacy, minimum overall college GPA of 3.0, transcript of college record, CPR certification, written essay, immunizations, 4 letters of recommendation, nursing research course, prerequisite course work, resume, statistics course, GRE General Test or MAT, GMAT. *Application deadline:* 3/15 (fall), 10/15 (spring).
**Advanced Placement** Credit given for nursing courses completed elsewhere dependent upon specific evaluations.
**Degree Requirements** 36 total credit hours, thesis or project, comprehensive exam.

**POST-MASTER'S PROGRAM**
**Areas of Study** Nursing administration; nursing education. *Nurse practitioner programs in:* family health, pediatric.

**DOCTORAL DEGREE PROGRAM**
**Degree** PhD
**Available Programs** Doctorate.
**Areas of Study** Nursing science.
**Program Entrance Requirements** Minimum overall college GPA of 3.0, interview by faculty committee, 3 letters of recommendation, MSN or equivalent, scholarly papers, statistics course, vita, writing sample.
**Degree Requirements** 65 total credit hours, dissertation, written exam.

# The University of Texas Health Science Center at Houston

## School of Nursing
## Houston, Texas

*http://www.son.uth.tmc.edu/*
Founded in 1972

**DEGREES • BSN • MSN • MSN/MPH • PHD**
**Nursing Program Faculty** 112 (54% with doctorates).
**Baccalaureate Enrollment** 497 **Women** 86% **Men** 14% **Minority** 45% **International** 1% **Part-time** 20%
**Graduate Enrollment** 350 **Women** 87% **Men** 13% **Minority** 35% **International** 12% **Part-time** 60%
**Distance Learning Courses** Available.
**Nursing Student Activities** Sigma Theta Tau, Student Nurses' Association.
**Nursing Student Resources** Academic advising; academic or career counseling; assistance for students with disabilities; bookstore; campus computer network; computer lab; computer-assisted instruction; e-mail services; employment services for current students; housing assistance; interactive nursing skills videos; Internet; learning resource lab; library services; nursing audiovisuals; paid internships; remedial services; skills, simulation, or other laboratory; tutoring.

### BACCALAUREATE PROGRAMS

**Degree** BSN
**Available Programs** ADN to Baccalaureate; Accelerated Baccalaureate for Second Degree; Generic Baccalaureate.
**Site Options** Houston, TX.
**Study Options** Full-time.
**Program Entrance Requirements** Transcript of college record, CPR certification, written essay, health exam, immunizations, interview, minimum GPA in nursing prerequisites of 2.75, prerequisite course work. Transfer students are accepted. *Application deadline:* 1/15 (fall), 9/1 (spring), 12/1 (summer). *Application fee:* $30.
**Advanced Placement** Credit given for nursing courses completed elsewhere dependent upon specific evaluations.
**Contact** *Telephone:* 713-500-2101. *Fax:* 713-500-2107.

### GRADUATE PROGRAMS

**Contact** *Telephone:* 713-500-2101. *Fax:* 713-500-2107.

**MASTER'S DEGREE PROGRAM**
**Degrees** MSN; MSN/MPH
**Available Programs** Master's.
**Concentrations Available** Nurse anesthesia; nursing administration; nursing education. *Clinical nurse specialist programs in:* acute care, adult health, critical care, gerontology. *Nurse practitioner programs in:* acute care, adult health, family health, gerontology, pediatric, psychiatric/mental health,women's health.
**Study Options** Full-time and part-time.
**Program Entrance Requirements** Clinical experience, minimum overall college GPA of 3.0, transcript of college record, CPR certification, immunizations, interview, 3 letters of recommendation, prerequisite course work, resume, statistics course, GRE or MAT. *Application deadline:* 4/15 (fall), 2/15 (summer). *Application fee:* $30.
**Advanced Placement** Credit given for nursing courses completed elsewhere dependent upon specific evaluations.
**Degree Requirements** 48 total credit hours, thesis or project.

**POST-MASTER'S PROGRAM**
**Areas of Study** Nursing administration; nursing education. *Clinical nurse specialist programs in:* acute care, adult health, critical care, gerontology, oncology. *Nurse practitioner programs in:* acute care, adult health, family health, gerontology, oncology, pediatric, psychiatric/mental health,women's health.

**DOCTORAL DEGREE PROGRAM**
**Degree** PhD
**Available Programs** Doctorate.
**Areas of Study** Addiction/substance abuse, advanced practice nursing, aging, bio-behavioral research, biology of health and illness, clinical practice, community health, critical care, ethics, faculty preparation, family health, gerontology, health policy, health promotion/disease prevention, health-care systems, human health and illness, illness and transition, individualized study, information systems, maternity-newborn, neuro-behavior, nurse case management, nursing administration, nursing education, nursing policy, nursing research, nursing science, oncology, urban health,women's health.
**Program Entrance Requirements** Minimum overall college GPA of 3.0, interview by faculty committee, 3 letters of recommendation, MSN or equivalent, vita, writing sample, GRE. *Application deadline:* 4/1 (fall). *Application fee:* $30.
**Degree Requirements** 66 total credit hours, dissertation.

### CONTINUING EDUCATION PROGRAM

**Contact** *Telephone:* 713-500-2116. *Fax:* 713-500-2026.

# The University of Texas Health Science Center at San Antonio

## School of Nursing
## San Antonio, Texas

*http://www.nursing.uthscsa.edu/*
Founded in 1976

**DEGREES • BSN • MSN • PHD**
**Nursing Program Faculty** 122 (63% with doctorates).
**Baccalaureate Enrollment** 558 **Women** 84.59% **Men** 15.41% **Minority** 53.23% **International** 1.79% **Part-time** 2.15%
**Graduate Enrollment** 258 **Women** 16% **Men** 84% **Minority** 54% **International** 2% **Part-time** 41%
**Distance Learning Courses** Available.
**Nursing Student Activities** Nursing Honor Society, Sigma Theta Tau, Student Nurses' Association, nursing club.
**Nursing Student Resources** Academic advising; academic or career counseling; assistance for students with disabilities; bookstore; campus computer network; career placement assistance; computer lab; computer-assisted instruction; e-mail services; employment services for current students; housing assistance; interactive nursing skills videos; Internet; learning resource lab; library services; nursing audiovisuals; placement services for program completers; remedial services; resume preparation assistance; skills, simulation, or other laboratory; tutoring.
**Library Facilities** 4,793 volumes in health, 4,091 volumes in nursing; 4,367 periodical subscriptions health-care related.

### BACCALAUREATE PROGRAMS

**Degree** BSN
**Available Programs** Accelerated Baccalaureate for Second Degree; Generic Baccalaureate.
**Study Options** Full-time.
**Program Entrance Requirements** Minimum overall college GPA of 2.5, transcript of college record, CPR certification, written essay, health insurance, immunizations, minimum GPA in nursing prerequisites of 3.0, professional liability insurance/malpractice insurance, prerequisite course work. Transfer students are accepted. *Application deadline:* 2/1 (fall), 8/1 (spring), 12/15 (summer). *Application fee:* $45.
**Advanced Placement** Credit given for nursing courses completed elsewhere dependent upon specific evaluations.
**Financial Aid** 84% of baccalaureate students in nursing programs received some form of financial aid in 2012–13.
**Contact** Dr. Ilene M. Decker, Associate Dean for Undergraduate Studies, School of Nursing, The University of Texas Health Science Center at San Antonio, 7703 Floyd Curl Drive, MC 7945, San Antonio, TX 78229-3900. *Telephone:* 210-567-5810. *Fax:* 210-567-3813. *E-mail:* deckerI@uthscsa.edu.

## GRADUATE PROGRAMS

**Financial Aid** 76% of graduate students in nursing programs received some form of financial aid in 2012–13. 3 fellowships with full tuition reimbursements available (averaging $30,000 per year) were awarded; research assistantships, teaching assistantships, institutionally sponsored loans and scholarships also available. *Financial aid application deadline:* 6/30.

**Contact** Dr. Ilene M. Decker, Associate Dean, School of Nursing, The University of Texas Health Science Center at San Antonio, 7703 Floyd Curl Drive, MC 7945, San Antonio, TX 78229-3900. *Telephone:* 210-567-5810. *Fax:* 210-567-3813. *E-mail:* DeckerI@uthscsa.edu.

### MASTER'S DEGREE PROGRAM

**Degree** MSN
**Available Programs** Master's; RN to Master's.
**Concentrations Available** Clinical nurse leader; nursing administration; nursing education. *Nurse practitioner programs in:* family health, gerontology, pediatric, psychiatric/mental health.
**Study Options** Full-time and part-time.
**Program Entrance Requirements** Computer literacy, minimum overall college GPA of 3.0, transcript of college record, CPR certification, written essay, immunizations, 3 letters of recommendation, professional liability insurance/malpractice insurance, statistics course. *Application deadline:* 2/1 (fall). *Application fee:* $45.
**Advanced Placement** Credit given for nursing courses completed elsewhere dependent upon specific evaluations.
**Degree Requirements** 50 total credit hours, thesis or project.

### POST-MASTER'S PROGRAM

**Areas of Study** *Nurse practitioner programs in:* family health, pediatric, psychiatric/mental health.

### DOCTORAL DEGREE PROGRAM

**Degree** PhD
**Available Programs** Doctorate; Post-Baccalaureate Doctorate.
**Areas of Study** Nursing research.
**Program Entrance Requirements** Clinical experience, minimum overall college GPA of 3.0, interview, 3 letters of recommendation, statistics course, vita, writing sample, GRE, MAT. *Application deadline:* 2/1 (fall). *Application fee:* $45.
**Degree Requirements** 80 total credit hours, dissertation.

## CONTINUING EDUCATION PROGRAM

**Contact** Laura Alvarado, Director of Lifelong Learning, School of Nursing, The University of Texas Health Science Center at San Antonio, 7703 Floyd Curl Drive, San Antonio, TX 78229-3900. *Telephone:* 210-567-0170. *Fax:* 210-567-5909. *E-mail:* AlvaradoLV@uthsca.edu.

# The University of Texas Medical Branch

**School of Nursing**
**Galveston, Texas**

*http://www.son.utmb.edu/*
Founded in 1891

## DEGREES • BSN • DNP • MSN

**Nursing Program Faculty** 58 (57% with doctorates).
**Baccalaureate Enrollment** 480 **Women** 84% **Men** 16% **Minority** 30% **International** 1% **Part-time** 8%
**Graduate Enrollment** 457 **Women** 86% **Men** 14% **Minority** 28% **International** .5% **Part-time** 79%
**Distance Learning Courses** Available.
**Nursing Student Activities** Nursing Honor Society, Sigma Theta Tau, Student Nurses' Association.
**Nursing Student Resources** Academic advising; academic or career counseling; assistance for students with disabilities; bookstore; campus computer network; career placement assistance; computer lab; computer-assisted instruction; e-mail services; employment services for current students; housing assistance; interactive nursing skills videos; Internet; learning resource lab; library services; nursing audiovisuals; resume preparation assistance; skills, simulation, or other laboratory; tutoring.
**Library Facilities** 287,643 volumes in health, 7,403 volumes in nursing; 11,327 periodical subscriptions health-care related.

## BACCALAUREATE PROGRAMS

**Degree** BSN
**Available Programs** Accelerated Baccalaureate for Second Degree; Generic Baccalaureate; RN Baccalaureate.
**Study Options** Full-time.
**Program Entrance Requirements** Minimum overall college GPA of 2.75, transcript of college record, CPR certification, written essay, health insurance, immunizations, interview, minimum GPA in nursing prerequisites of 2.75, professional liability insurance/malpractice insurance, prerequisite course work. Transfer students are accepted. *Application deadline:* 1/15 (fall), 6/15 (spring). *Application fee:* $25.
**Advanced Placement** Credit by examination available. Credit given for nursing courses completed elsewhere dependent upon specific evaluations.
**Expenses (2013–14)** *Tuition, state resident:* full-time $8622; part-time $192 per credit hour. *Tuition, nonresident:* full-time $24,652; part-time $548 per credit hour. *International tuition:* $24,652 full-time. *Room and board:* $14,424; room only: $10,332 per academic year. *Required fees:* full-time $5197.
**Financial Aid** 95% of baccalaureate students in nursing programs received some form of financial aid in 2012–13.
**Contact** Dr. Charlotte Wisnewski, Associate Professor and Director of Baccalaureate Programs, School of Nursing, The University of Texas Medical Branch, 301 University Boulevard, Galveston, TX 77555-1132. *Telephone:* 409-772-8235. *Fax:* 409-772-3770. *E-mail:* cwisnews@utmb.edu.

## GRADUATE PROGRAMS

**Expenses (2013–14)** *Tuition, state resident:* full-time $8681; part-time $235 per credit hour. *Tuition, nonresident:* full-time $21,778; part-time $589 per credit hour. *International tuition:* $21,778 full-time. *Room and board:* $14,424; room only: $10,332 per academic year. *Required fees:* full-time $5664.
**Financial Aid** 42% of graduate students in nursing programs received some form of financial aid in 2012–13.
**Contact** Dr. Maureer Wilder, Associate Professor and Masters Program Director, School of Nursing, The University of Texas Medical Branch, 301 University Boulevard, Galveston, TX 77555-1029. *Telephone:* 409-772-8241. *Fax:* 409-772-8323. *E-mail:* mwilder@utmb.edu.

### MASTER'S DEGREE PROGRAM

**Degree** MSN
**Available Programs** Master's.
**Concentrations Available** Clinical nurse leader; nursing administration; nursing education. *Nurse practitioner programs in:* family health, gerontology, neonatal health.
**Study Options** Full-time and part-time.
**Online Degree Options** Yes (online only).
**Program Entrance Requirements** Clinical experience, computer literacy, minimum overall college GPA of 3.0, transcript of college record, CPR certification, immunizations, interview, 3 letters of recommendation, professional liability insurance/malpractice insurance, prerequisite course work, statistics course. *Application deadline:* 3/1 (fall). *Application fee:* $60.
**Advanced Placement** Credit given for nursing courses completed elsewhere dependent upon specific evaluations.
**Degree Requirements** 46 total credit hours.

### POST-MASTER'S PROGRAM

**Areas of Study** Clinical nurse leader; nursing administration; nursing education. *Nurse practitioner programs in:* family health, gerontology, neonatal health.

### DOCTORAL DEGREE PROGRAM

**Degree** DNP
**Available Programs** Doctorate; Post-Baccalaureate Doctorate.
**Areas of Study** Health promotion/disease prevention.
**Online Degree Options** Yes (online only).
**Program Entrance Requirements** Clinical experience, minimum overall college GPA of 3.5, interview by faculty committee, interview, 3 letters of recommendation, MSN or equivalent, statistics course, vita, writing sample. *Application deadline:* 3/1 (fall). *Application fee:* $50.
**Degree Requirements** 63 total credit hours, residency.

# The University of Texas–Pan American

## Department of Nursing
## Edinburg, Texas

***http://www.utpa.edu/***
Founded in 1927

### DEGREES • BSN • MSN

**Nursing Program Faculty** 23 (45% with doctorates).
**Baccalaureate Enrollment** 170 **Women** 78% **Men** 22% **Minority** 90%
**Graduate Enrollment** 65 **Women** 88% **Men** 12% **Minority** 88% **Part-time** 75%
**Nursing Student Activities** Sigma Theta Tau, Student Nurses' Association.
**Nursing Student Resources** Academic advising; academic or career counseling; assistance for students with disabilities; bookstore; campus computer network; career placement assistance; computer lab; computer-assisted instruction; daycare for children of students; e-mail services; employment services for current students; housing assistance; interactive nursing skills videos; Internet; learning resource lab; library services; nursing audiovisuals; remedial services; skills, simulation, or other laboratory; tutoring.
**Library Facilities** 230 volumes in health, 200 volumes in nursing; 300 periodical subscriptions health-care related.

### BACCALAUREATE PROGRAMS

**Degree** BSN
**Available Programs** ADN to Baccalaureate; Generic Baccalaureate; RN Baccalaureate.
**Study Options** Full-time.
**Program Entrance Requirements** Transcript of college record, CPR certification, immunizations, minimum GPA in nursing prerequisites of 2.5, professional liability insurance/malpractice insurance, prerequisite course work. Transfer students are accepted. *Application deadline:* 10/1 (fall), 10/1 (spring).
**Contact** *Telephone:* 956-381-3491. *Fax:* 956-381-2875.

### GRADUATE PROGRAMS

**Contact** *Telephone:* 956-381-3491. *Fax:* 956-381-2875.

#### MASTER'S DEGREE PROGRAM

**Degree** MSN
**Available Programs** Master's.
**Concentrations Available** *Clinical nurse specialist programs in:* adult health. *Nurse practitioner programs in:* family health, pediatric.
**Study Options** Full-time and part-time.
**Program Entrance Requirements** Minimum overall college GPA of 2.75, transcript of college record, written essay, immunizations, 3 letters of recommendation, resume, statistics course. *Application deadline:* 7/1 (fall), 10/1 (winter), 4/1 (spring), 4/1 (summer).
**Advanced Placement** Credit given for nursing courses completed elsewhere dependent upon specific evaluations.
**Degree Requirements** 48 total credit hours, thesis or project.

#### POST-MASTER'S PROGRAM

**Areas of Study** *Clinical nurse specialist programs in:* adult health. *Nurse practitioner programs in:* family health, pediatric.

# University of the Incarnate Word

## Program in Nursing
## San Antonio, Texas

***http://www.uiw.edu/snhp***
Founded in 1881

### DEGREES • BSN • DNP • MSN

**Nursing Program Faculty** 39 (41% with doctorates).
**Baccalaureate Enrollment** 251 **Women** 87% **Men** 13% **Minority** 70% **International** 2%
**Graduate Enrollment** 66 **Women** 76% **Men** 24% **Minority** 39% **International** 10% **Part-time** 91%
**Distance Learning Courses** Available.
**Nursing Student Activities** Sigma Theta Tau, Student Nurses' Association.
**Nursing Student Resources** Academic advising; academic or career counseling; assistance for students with disabilities; bookstore; campus computer network; career placement assistance; computer lab; computer-assisted instruction; e-mail services; employment services for current students; externships; housing assistance; interactive nursing skills videos; Internet; learning resource lab; library services; nursing audiovisuals; paid internships; placement services for program completers; remedial services; resume preparation assistance; skills, simulation, or other laboratory; tutoring; unpaid internships.
**Library Facilities** 273,468 volumes (6,000 in health, 6,000 in nursing); 70,017 periodical subscriptions (3,048 health-care related).

### BACCALAUREATE PROGRAMS

**Degree** BSN
**Available Programs** ADN to Baccalaureate; Baccalaureate for Second Degree; Generic Baccalaureate.
**Study Options** Full-time.
**Online Degree Options** Yes.
**Program Entrance Requirements** Minimum overall college GPA of 2.5, transcript of college record, CPR certification, health exam, health insurance, immunizations, minimum GPA in nursing prerequisites of 2.5, professional liability insurance/malpractice insurance, prerequisite course work. Transfer students are accepted. *Application deadline:* 2/1 (fall), 9/1 (spring). *Application fee:* $20.
**Advanced Placement** Credit given for nursing courses completed elsewhere dependent upon specific evaluations.
**Expenses (2012–13)** *Tuition:* full-time $22,800; part-time $755 per credit hour. *Room and board:* $10,094 per academic year. *Required fees:* full-time $1990.
**Financial Aid** 90% of baccalaureate students in nursing programs received some form of financial aid in 2011–12.
**Contact** Ms. Heather Rodriguez, Office of Admissions, Program in Nursing, University of the Incarnate Word, 4301 Broadway, San Antonio, TX 78209. *Telephone:* 210-829-6005. *E-mail:* admis@uiwtx.edu.

### GRADUATE PROGRAMS

**Expenses (2012–13)** *Tuition:* full-time $18,840; part-time $785 per credit. *International tuition:* $18,840 full-time. *Required fees:* full-time $2352; part-time $98 per credit.
**Financial Aid** 75% of graduate students in nursing programs received some form of financial aid in 2011–12. Federal Work-Study, scholarships, and traineeships available. Aid available to part-time students.
**Contact** Dr. Holly B. Cassells, Director of Graduate Nursing Programs, Program in Nursing, University of the Incarnate Word, 4301 Broadway, San Antonio, TX 78209. *Telephone:* 210-829-3977. *Fax:* 210-829-3174. *E-mail:* cassells@uiwtx.edu.

#### MASTER'S DEGREE PROGRAM

**Degree** MSN
**Available Programs** Accelerated AD/RN to Master's; Master's.
**Concentrations Available** Clinical nurse leader. *Clinical nurse specialist programs in:* adult health.
**Study Options** Full-time and part-time.
**Program Entrance Requirements** Clinical experience, minimum overall college GPA of 3.0, transcript of college record, CPR certification, immunizations, 3 letters of recommendation, physical assessment course, professional liability insurance/malpractice insurance, statistics course. *Application deadline:* Applications may be processed on a rolling basis for some programs. *Application fee:* $20.
**Advanced Placement** Credit given for nursing courses completed elsewhere dependent upon specific evaluations.
**Degree Requirements** 42 total credit hours.

#### POST-MASTER'S PROGRAM

**Areas of Study** Clinical nurse leader. *Clinical nurse specialist programs in:* adult health.

#### DOCTORAL DEGREE PROGRAM

**Degree** DNP
**Available Programs** Doctorate.
**Areas of Study** Advanced practice nursing.
**Online Degree Options** Yes (online only).
**Program Entrance Requirements** Minimum overall college GPA of 3.0, interview, 3 letters of recommendation, MSN or equivalent, statistics course. *Application deadline:* Applications may be processed on a rolling basis for some programs. *Application fee:* $20.
**Degree Requirements** 33 total credit hours.

## Wayland Baptist University

### Bachelor of Science in Nursing Program
### Plainview, Texas

Founded in 1908

**DEGREE • BSN**

**Library Facilities** 131,163 volumes; 2,661 periodical subscriptions.

#### BACCALAUREATE PROGRAMS

**Degree** BSN
**Available Programs** RN Baccalaureate.
**Contact** *Telephone:* 210-826-7595 Ext. 228.

## West Texas A&M University

### Department of Nursing
### Canyon, Texas

***http://www.wtamu.edu/nursing***
Founded in 1909

**DEGREES • BSN • MSN**

**Nursing Program Faculty** 30 (23% with doctorates).
**Baccalaureate Enrollment** 380 **Women** 84% **Men** 16% **Minority** 27% **International** 1% **Part-time** 35%
**Graduate Enrollment** 54 **Women** 85% **Men** 15% **Minority** 9% **Part-time** 52%
**Nursing Student Activities** Sigma Theta Tau, Student Nurses' Association.
**Nursing Student Resources** Academic advising; academic or career counseling; assistance for students with disabilities; bookstore; campus computer network; career placement assistance; computer lab; computer-assisted instruction; daycare for children of students; e-mail services; employment services for current students; housing assistance; interactive nursing skills videos; Internet; learning resource lab; library services; nursing audiovisuals; placement services for program completers; remedial services; resume preparation assistance; skills, simulation, or other laboratory; tutoring.
**Library Facilities** 1.2 million volumes (17,000 in health, 10,000 in nursing); 19,264 periodical subscriptions (75 health-care related).

#### BACCALAUREATE PROGRAMS

**Degree** BSN
**Available Programs** ADN to Baccalaureate; Generic Baccalaureate; LPN to Baccalaureate.
**Study Options** Full-time and part-time.
**Program Entrance Requirements** Minimum overall college GPA of 2.5, transcript of college record, CPR certification, immunizations, minimum GPA in nursing prerequisites of 2.0, prerequisite course work. Transfer students are accepted.
**Advanced Placement** Credit given for nursing courses completed elsewhere dependent upon specific evaluations.
**Contact** *Telephone:* 806-651-2661. *Fax:* 806-651-2632.

#### GRADUATE PROGRAMS

**Contact** *Telephone:* 806-651-2637. *Fax:* 806-651-2632.

#### MASTER'S DEGREE PROGRAM

**Degree** MSN
**Available Programs** Master's; RN to Master's.
**Concentrations Available** Nursing administration; nursing education. *Nurse practitioner programs in:* family health.
**Study Options** Full-time and part-time.
**Program Entrance Requirements** Clinical experience, computer literacy, minimum overall college GPA of 3.0, transcript of college record, CPR certification, immunizations, nursing research course, prerequisite course work, statistics course, GRE General Test.
**Advanced Placement** Credit given for nursing courses completed elsewhere dependent upon specific evaluations.
**Degree Requirements** 39 total credit hours, thesis or project.

#### POST-MASTER'S PROGRAM

**Areas of Study** *Nurse practitioner programs in:* family health.

# UTAH

## Brigham Young University

### College of Nursing
### Provo, Utah

***http://nursing.byu.edu/***
Founded in 1875

**DEGREES • BS • MS**

**Nursing Program Faculty** 46 (43% with doctorates).
**Baccalaureate Enrollment** 370 **Women** 93.5% **Men** 6.5% **Minority** 5.4% **International** 2%
**Graduate Enrollment** 26 **Women** 69% **Men** 31% **Minority** 3%
**Nursing Student Activities** Nursing Honor Society, Sigma Theta Tau, Student Nurses' Association.
**Nursing Student Resources** Academic advising; academic or career counseling; assistance for students with disabilities; bookstore; campus computer network; career placement assistance; computer lab; computer-assisted instruction; e-mail services; employment services for current students; housing assistance; interactive nursing skills videos; Internet; learning resource lab; library services; nursing audiovisuals; other; paid internships; resume preparation assistance; skills, simulation, or other laboratory; tutoring.
**Library Facilities** 72,332 volumes in health, 5,217 volumes in nursing; 10,500 periodical subscriptions health-care related.

#### BACCALAUREATE PROGRAMS

**Degree** BS
**Available Programs** RN Baccalaureate.
**Study Options** Full-time.
**Program Entrance Requirements** Minimum overall college GPA, transcript of college record, CPR certification, written essay, 2 letters of recommendation, minimum GPA in nursing prerequisites of 3.0, prerequisite course work. Transfer students are accepted. *Application deadline:* 5/31 (fall), 9/30 (winter).
**Advanced Placement** Credit given for nursing courses completed elsewhere dependent upon specific evaluations.
**Financial Aid** 30% of baccalaureate students in nursing programs received some form of financial aid in 2012–13.
**Contact** Dr. Mark E. White, Advisement Center Supervisor, College of Nursing, Brigham Young University, 550 SWKT, Provo, UT 84602-5532. *Telephone:* 801-422-7211. *Fax:* 801-422-0536. *E-mail:* mark_white@byu.edu.

#### GRADUATE PROGRAMS

**Expenses (2013–14)** *Tuition:* full-time $12,260. *Room and board:* $7250; room only: $3350 per academic year.
**Financial Aid** 100% of graduate students in nursing programs received some form of financial aid in 2012–13. 2 research assistantships with full and partial tuition reimbursements available (averaging $10,000 per year), 3 teaching assistantships with full and partial tuition reimbursements available (averaging $10,000 per year) were awarded; institutionally sponsored loans, scholarships, tuition waivers (full), and unspecified assistantships also available. Aid available to part-time students. *Financial aid application deadline:* 2/1.
**Contact** Mrs. Lynete Jakins, Research Center and Graduate Program Secretary, College of Nursing, Brigham Young University, 400 SWKT, Provo, UT 84602-5532. *Telephone:* 801-422-4142. *Fax:* 801-422-0536. *E-mail:* nursing_graduate@byu.edu.

#### MASTER'S DEGREE PROGRAM

**Degree** MS
**Available Programs** Master's.
**Concentrations Available** *Nurse practitioner programs in:* family health.
**Study Options** Full-time and part-time.
**Program Entrance Requirements** Clinical experience, minimum overall college GPA of 3.0, transcript of college record, CPR certification, written essay, immunizations, interview, 3 letters of recommendation, prerequisite course work, resume, statistics course, GRE. *Application deadline:* 12/1 (spring). *Application fee:* $50.
**Advanced Placement** Credit given for nursing courses completed elsewhere dependent upon specific evaluations.
**Degree Requirements** 59 total credit hours, thesis or project.

**POST-MASTER'S PROGRAM**
**Areas of Study** *Nurse practitioner programs in:* family health.

## Dixie State University
### Nursing Department
### St. George, Utah

Founded in 1911
**DEGREE • BSN**
**Library Facilities** 166,120 volumes; 190 periodical subscriptions.

#### BACCALAUREATE PROGRAMS

**Degree** BSN
**Available Programs** RN Baccalaureate.
**Program Entrance Requirements** Written essay, immunizations, RN licensure. *Application deadline:* 3/15 (fall), 9/15 (spring).
**Contact** *Telephone:* 435-879-4802.

## Southern Utah University
### Department of Nursing
### Cedar City, Utah

*http://www.suu.edu/cose/nursing/*
Founded in 1897
**DEGREE • BSN**
**Nursing Program Faculty** 9 (2% with doctorates).
**Baccalaureate Enrollment** 96 **Women** 70% **Men** 30% **Minority** 5% **International** 1%
**Nursing Student Activities** Nursing Honor Society, Student Nurses' Association, nursing club.
**Nursing Student Resources** Academic advising; academic or career counseling; assistance for students with disabilities; bookstore; campus computer network; career placement assistance; computer lab; computer-assisted instruction; daycare for children of students; e-mail services; employment services for current students; externships; housing assistance; interactive nursing skills videos; Internet; learning resource lab; library services; nursing audiovisuals; remedial services; resume preparation assistance; skills, simulation, or other laboratory; tutoring.
**Library Facilities** 235,062 volumes (1,000 in health, 1,000 in nursing); 711 periodical subscriptions (5,000 health-care related).

#### BACCALAUREATE PROGRAMS

**Degree** BSN
**Available Programs** Generic Baccalaureate; RN Baccalaureate.
**Study Options** Full-time.
**Program Entrance Requirements** Minimum overall college GPA of 3.0, transcript of college record, written essay, health insurance, immunizations, 3 letters of recommendation, minimum GPA in nursing prerequisites of 3.0, prerequisite course work. Transfer students are accepted. *Application deadline:* 2/8 (fall), 9/12 (spring). *Application fee:* $20.
**Advanced Placement** Credit given for nursing courses completed elsewhere dependent upon specific evaluations.
**Expenses (2012–13)** *Tuition, state resident:* full-time $4100. *Tuition, nonresident:* full-time $14,500. *Room and board:* $7100; room only: $3600 per academic year. *Required fees:* full-time $540.
**Financial Aid** 80% of baccalaureate students in nursing programs received some form of financial aid in 2011–12.
**Contact** Vikki Robertson, Department Secretary, Department of Nursing, Southern Utah University, 351 West University Boulevard, GC 005, Cedar City, UT 84720. *Telephone:* 435-586-1906. *Fax:* 435-586-1984. *E-mail:* robertsonv@suu.edu.

## University of Phoenix–Utah Campus
### College of Health and Human Services
### Salt Lake City, Utah

Founded in 1984
**Nursing Program Faculty** 2
**Nursing Student Activities** Sigma Theta Tau.
**Nursing Student Resources** Academic advising; academic or career counseling; assistance for students with disabilities; bookstore; campus computer network; computer lab; computer-assisted instruction; e-mail services; interactive nursing skills videos; Internet; learning resource lab; library services; nursing audiovisuals; remedial services; skills, simulation, or other laboratory; tutoring.
**Library Facilities** 16,871 periodical subscriptions (1,300 health-care related).

## University of Utah
### College of Nursing
### Salt Lake City, Utah

*http://www.nursing.utah.edu/*
Founded in 1850
**DEGREES • BS • MS • PHD**
**Nursing Program Faculty** 105 (59% with doctorates).
**Baccalaureate Enrollment** 294 **Women** 82% **Men** 18% **Minority** 13% **International** 2% **Part-time** 35%
**Graduate Enrollment** 313 **Women** 80% **Men** 20% **Minority** 12% **International** 4% **Part-time** 24%
**Distance Learning Courses** Available.
**Nursing Student Activities** Sigma Theta Tau, Student Nurses' Association.
**Nursing Student Resources** Academic advising; academic or career counseling; assistance for students with disabilities; bookstore; campus computer network; career placement assistance; computer lab; computer-assisted instruction; e-mail services; employment services for current students; interactive nursing skills videos; Internet; learning resource lab; library services; nursing audiovisuals; remedial services; resume preparation assistance; skills, simulation, or other laboratory.
**Library Facilities** 4.2 million volumes (212,579 in health, 6,603 in nursing); 86,266 periodical subscriptions (5,201 health-care related).

#### BACCALAUREATE PROGRAMS

**Degree** BS
**Available Programs** ADN to Baccalaureate; Accelerated Baccalaureate; Baccalaureate for Second Degree; Generic Baccalaureate; RN Baccalaureate.
**Study Options** Full-time.
**Online Degree Options** Yes.
**Program Entrance Requirements** Minimum overall college GPA of 2.8, transcript of college record, CPR certification, written essay, health exam, immunizations, interview, 3 letters of recommendation, minimum GPA in nursing prerequisites of 3.0, prerequisite course work. Transfer students are accepted. *Application deadline:* 1/15 (fall), 1/15 (summer). *Application fee:* $55.
**Advanced Placement** Credit by examination available. Credit given for nursing courses completed elsewhere dependent upon specific evaluations.
**Expenses (2013–14)** *Tuition, state resident:* full-time $3841; part-time $2535 per semester. *Tuition, nonresident:* full-time $11,135; part-time $7349 per semester. *International tuition:* $11,135 full-time. *Room and board:* $10,602; room only: $9216 per academic year. *Required fees:* full-time $1000.
**Financial Aid** 65% of baccalaureate students in nursing programs received some form of financial aid in 2012–13. *Gift aid (need-based):* Federal Pell, FSEOG, state, private, college/university gift aid from institutional funds, Federal Nursing, TEACH Grants. *Loans:* Federal Nursing Student Loans, Federal Direct (Subsidized and Unsubsidized Stafford PLUS), Perkins, college/university, private loans. *Work-study:* Federal Work-Study. *Financial aid application deadline (priority):* 4/1.
**Contact** Ms. Jennifer Van Cott, Director, Student Services, College of Nursing, University of Utah, 10 South 2000 East, Salt Lake City, UT 84112-5880. *Telephone:* 801-585-6658. *Fax:* 801-581-3414. *E-mail:* jennifer.vancott@nurs.utah.edu.

#### GRADUATE PROGRAMS

**Financial Aid** 50% of graduate students in nursing programs received some form of financial aid in 2012–13. 78 fellowships with full and partial tuition reimbursements available, 4 research assistantships with full and partial tuition reimbursements available, 13 teaching assistantships with partial tuition reimbursements available were awarded; scholarships, traineeships, and unspecified assistantships also available. Aid available to part-time students. *Financial aid application deadline:* 3/15.

**Contact** Jennifer Van Cott, Director, Student Services, College of Nursing, University of Utah, 10 South 2000 East, Salt Lake City, UT 84112-5880. *Telephone:* 801-585-6658. *Fax:* 801-581-3414. *E-mail:* jennifer.vancott@nurs.utah.edu.

### MASTER'S DEGREE PROGRAM

**Degree** MS
**Available Programs** Master's; RN to Master's.
**Concentrations Available** Nursing education; nursing informatics. *Nurse practitioner programs in:* gerontology.
**Study Options** Full-time.
**Online Degree Options** Yes.
**Program Entrance Requirements** Clinical experience, minimum overall college GPA of 3.0, transcript of college record, CPR certification, written essay, immunizations, interview, 2 letters of recommendation, resume, statistics course. *Application deadline:* 1/15 (fall). *Application fee:* $60.
**Advanced Placement** Credit given for nursing courses completed elsewhere dependent upon specific evaluations.
**Degree Requirements** 38 total credit hours, thesis or project, comprehensive exam.

### POST-MASTER'S PROGRAM

**Areas of Study** Nurse-midwifery; nursing education; nursing informatics. *Nurse practitioner programs in:* acute care, adult health, family health, gerontology, neonatal health, pediatric, primary care, psychiatric/mental health,women's health.

### DOCTORAL DEGREE PROGRAM

**Degree** PhD
**Available Programs** Doctorate; Doctorate for Nurses with Non-Nursing Degrees; Post-Baccalaureate Doctorate.
**Areas of Study** Aging, bio-behavioral research, community health, critical care, ethics, faculty preparation, family health, gerontology, health policy, health promotion/disease prevention, health-care systems, human health and illness, illness and transition, individualized study, information systems, maternity-newborn, nursing administration, nursing education, nursing policy, nursing research, nursing science, oncology,women's health.
**Program Entrance Requirements** Clinical experience, minimum overall college GPA of 3.3, interview by faculty committee, interview, 3 letters of recommendation, statistics course, vita, writing sample. *Application deadline:* 1/15 (fall).
**Degree Requirements** 62 total credit hours, dissertation, oral exam, written exam, residency.

### POSTDOCTORAL PROGRAM

**Areas of Study** Aging, cancer care, chronic illness, gerontology, information systems, nursing informatics, nursing interventions, nursing research, nursing science,women's health.
**Postdoctoral Program Contact** Dr. Ginette A. Pepper, Associate Dean for Research and PhD Programs, College of Nursing, University of Utah, 10 South 2000 East, Salt Lake City, UT 84112-5880. *Telephone:* 801-585-7872. *Fax:* 801-581-4642. *E-mail:* ginny.pepper@nurs.utah.edu.

# Utah Valley University

## Department of Nursing
## Orem, Utah

*http://www.uvu.edu/*
Founded in 1941

### DEGREE • BSN

**Nursing Program Faculty** 22 (25% with doctorates).
**Baccalaureate Enrollment** 100 **Women** 60% **Men** 40% **Part-time** 99%
**Nursing Student Activities** Student Nurses' Association.
**Nursing Student Resources** Academic advising; academic or career counseling; assistance for students with disabilities; bookstore; campus computer network; career placement assistance; computer lab; computer-assisted instruction; daycare for children of students; e-mail services; employment services for current students; interactive nursing skills videos; Internet; learning resource lab; library services; nursing audiovisuals; resume preparation assistance; skills, simulation, or other laboratory; tutoring; unpaid internships.
**Library Facilities** 228,000 volumes (4,640 in health, 361 in nursing); 568 periodical subscriptions (200 health-care related).

### BACCALAUREATE PROGRAMS

**Degree** BSN
**Available Programs** ADN to Baccalaureate.
**Study Options** Part-time.
**Program Entrance Requirements** CPR certification, health exam, health insurance, immunizations, minimum GPA in nursing prerequisites of 2.5, prerequisite course work, RN licensure. Transfer students are accepted.
**Advanced Placement** Credit by examination available.
**Contact** *Telephone:* 801-863-8199. *Fax:* 801-863-6093.

# Weber State University

## Program in Nursing
## Ogden, Utah

*http://www.weber.edu/nursing*
Founded in 1889

### DEGREES • BSN • MSN

**Nursing Program Faculty** 42 (5% with doctorates).
**Baccalaureate Enrollment** 400 **Women** 86% **Men** 14% **Minority** 4% **International** 1% **Part-time** 3%
**Graduate Enrollment** 42 **Women** 86% **Men** 14% **Minority** 1%
**Distance Learning Courses** Available.
**Nursing Student Activities** Sigma Theta Tau, Student Nurses' Association.
**Nursing Student Resources** Academic advising; academic or career counseling; assistance for students with disabilities; bookstore; campus computer network; career placement assistance; computer lab; computer-assisted instruction; daycare for children of students; e-mail services; employment services for current students; housing assistance; interactive nursing skills videos; Internet; learning resource lab; library services; nursing audiovisuals; placement services for program completers; resume preparation assistance; skills, simulation, or other laboratory; tutoring; unpaid internships.
**Library Facilities** 721,422 volumes (800 in health, 800 in nursing); 718 periodical subscriptions (120 health-care related).

### BACCALAUREATE PROGRAMS

**Degree** BSN
**Available Programs** ADN to Baccalaureate.
**Site Options** Layton, UT.
**Study Options** Full-time and part-time.
**Program Entrance Requirements** Minimum overall college GPA of 3.0, transcript of college record, CPR certification, health insurance, minimum GPA in nursing prerequisites of 3.0, prerequisite course work, RN licensure. Transfer students are accepted. *Application deadline:* 3/10 (fall), 10/10 (spring). *Application fee:* $25.
**Financial Aid** 35% of baccalaureate students in nursing programs received some form of financial aid in 2012–13.
**Contact** Mr. Robert Holt, Enrollment Director, School of Nursing, Program in Nursing, Weber State University, 3903 University Circle, Ogden, UT 84408-3903. *Telephone:* 801-626-7774. *Fax:* 801-626-6397. *E-mail:* rholt@weber.edu.

### GRADUATE PROGRAMS

**Financial Aid** 20% of graduate students in nursing programs received some form of financial aid in 2012–13.
**Contact** Mr. Robert W. Holt, Enrollment Director, Program in Nursing, Weber State University, 3903 University Circle, Ogden, UT 84408-3903. *Telephone:* 801-626-7774. *Fax:* 801-626-6397. *E-mail:* rholt@weber.edu.

### MASTER'S DEGREE PROGRAM

**Degree** MSN
**Available Programs** Master's.
**Concentrations Available** Nursing administration; nursing education.
**Study Options** Full-time.
**Program Entrance Requirements** Clinical experience, minimum overall college GPA of 3.0, transcript of college record, CPR certification, written essay, immunizations, interview, 2 letters of recommendation, nursing research course, professional liability insurance/malpractice insurance, prerequisite course work, resume, statistics course. *Application deadline:* 3/1 (fall). *Application fee:* $100.
**Degree Requirements** 40 total credit hours, thesis or project.

## Western Governors University
### Online College of Health Professions
### Salt Lake City, Utah

Founded in 1998

**DEGREES • BS • MS**

**Baccalaureate Enrollment** 3,962
**Graduate Enrollment** 2,982
**Distance Learning Courses** Available.
**Nursing Student Resources** Academic advising; academic or career counseling; assistance for students with disabilities; campus computer network; computer lab; computer-assisted instruction; e-mail services; employment services for current students; interactive nursing skills videos; Internet; learning resource lab; library services; nursing audiovisuals; resume preparation assistance; skills, simulation, or other laboratory; tutoring.

#### BACCALAUREATE PROGRAMS

**Degree** BS
**Available Programs** Accelerated Baccalaureate; Accelerated RN Baccalaureate; Generic Baccalaureate; LPN to RN Baccalaureate; RN Baccalaureate.
**Site Options** Houston, TX; Indianapolis, IN; Los Angeles, CA.
**Study Options** Full-time.
**Online Degree Options** Yes (online only).
**Program Entrance Requirements** Transfer students are accepted. *Application deadline:* Applications may be processed on a rolling basis for some programs. *Application fee:* $65.
**Advanced Placement** Credit by examination available.
**Contact** Admissions, Online College of Health Professions, Western Governors University, 4001 South 700 East, Suite 700, Salt Lake City, UT 84107-2533. *Telephone:* 801-274-3280. *Fax:* 801-274-3305.

#### GRADUATE PROGRAMS

**Contact** Admissions, Online College of Health Professions, Western Governors University, 4001 South 700 East, Suite 700, Salt Lake City, UT 84107-2533. *Telephone:* 801-274-3280. *Fax:* 801-274-3305.

**MASTER'S DEGREE PROGRAM**
**Degree** MS
**Available Programs** Accelerated Master's; Accelerated RN to Master's; Master's; RN to Master's.
**Concentrations Available** Clinical nurse leader; health-care administration; nursing administration; nursing education.
**Study Options** Full-time.
**Online Degree Options** Yes (online only).
**Program Entrance Requirements** Computer literacy, transcript of college record, interview. *Application deadline:* Applications may be processed on a rolling basis for some programs. *Application fee:* $65.
**Advanced Placement** Credit by examination available.
**Degree Requirements** 30 total credit hours, thesis or project.

## Westminster College
### School of Nursing and Health Sciences
### Salt Lake City, Utah

***http://www.westminstercollege.edu/nursing/***
Founded in 1875

**DEGREES • BSN • MSN**

**Nursing Student Activities** Sigma Theta Tau, Student Nurses' Association, nursing club.
**Nursing Student Resources** Academic advising; academic or career counseling; assistance for students with disabilities; bookstore; campus computer network; career placement assistance; computer lab; computer-assisted instruction; e-mail services; employment services for current students; housing assistance; interactive nursing skills videos; Internet; learning resource lab; library services; nursing audiovisuals; placement services for program completers; remedial services; resume preparation assistance; skills, simulation, or other laboratory; tutoring.
**Library Facilities** 218,288 volumes; 22,033 periodical subscriptions.

#### BACCALAUREATE PROGRAMS

**Degree** BSN
**Available Programs** Baccalaureate for Second Degree; Generic Baccalaureate; RN Baccalaureate.
**Study Options** Full-time.
**Program Entrance Requirements** Transcript of college record, written essay, 3 letters of recommendation, minimum GPA in nursing prerequisites of 2.5, prerequisite course work. Transfer students are accepted.
**Contact** *Telephone:* 801-832-2150. *Fax:* 801-832-3110.

#### GRADUATE PROGRAMS

**Contact** *Telephone:* 801-832-2150. *Fax:* 801-832-3110.

**MASTER'S DEGREE PROGRAM**
**Degree** MSN
**Available Programs** Master's.
**Concentrations Available** Nursing education. *Nurse practitioner programs in:* family health.
**Program Entrance Requirements** Transcript of college record, written essay, 3 letters of recommendation, resume, GRE.
**Advanced Placement** Credit given for nursing courses completed elsewhere dependent upon specific evaluations.
**Degree Requirements** 42 total credit hours, thesis or project.

**POST-MASTER'S PROGRAM**
**Areas of Study** *Nurse practitioner programs in:* family health.

# VERMONT

## Norwich University
### Department of Nursing
### Northfield, Vermont

***http://profschools.norwich.edu/nursing/***
Founded in 1819

**DEGREE • BSN**

**Nursing Program Faculty** 8 (10% with doctorates).
**Baccalaureate Enrollment** 90 **Women** 90% **Men** 10% **Minority** 10% **Part-time** 20%
**Nursing Student Activities** Student Nurses' Association, nursing club.
**Nursing Student Resources** Academic advising; academic or career counseling; assistance for students with disabilities; bookstore; campus computer network; career placement assistance; computer lab; e-mail services; employment services for current students; externships; housing assistance; interactive nursing skills videos; Internet; learning resource lab; library services; nursing audiovisuals; placement services for program completers; remedial services; resume preparation assistance; skills, simulation, or other laboratory; tutoring; unpaid internships.
**Library Facilities** 280,000 volumes; 904 periodical subscriptions.

#### BACCALAUREATE PROGRAMS

**Degree** BSN
**Available Programs** ADN to Baccalaureate; Generic Baccalaureate; RN Baccalaureate.
**Site Options** Rutland, VT.
**Study Options** Full-time and part-time.
**Program Entrance Requirements** Minimum overall college GPA of 2.5, transcript of college record, CPR certification, written essay, health exam, health insurance, high school biology, high school chemistry, 2 years high school math, 2 years high school science, high school transcript, immunizations, interview, 2 letters of recommendation, minimum GPA in nursing prerequisites of 2.5. Transfer students are accepted.
**Advanced Placement** Credit given for nursing courses completed elsewhere dependent upon specific evaluations.
**Contact** *Telephone:* 802-485-2008. *Fax:* 802-485-2032.

## Southern Vermont College
### Department of Nursing
### Bennington, Vermont

*http://www.svc.edu/academics/divisions/nursing.html*
Founded in 1926

**DEGREE • BSN**
**Nursing Program Faculty** 12 (3% with doctorates).
**Baccalaureate Enrollment** 50 **Women** 85% **Men** 15% **Part-time** 10%
**Distance Learning Courses** Available.
**Nursing Student Activities** Student Nurses' Association.
**Nursing Student Resources** Academic advising; academic or career counseling; assistance for students with disabilities; bookstore; career placement assistance; computer lab; e-mail services; employment services for current students; Internet; learning resource lab; library services; nursing audiovisuals; resume preparation assistance; skills, simulation, or other laboratory; tutoring.
**Library Facilities** 20,270 volumes; 33,000 periodical subscriptions.

#### BACCALAUREATE PROGRAMS
**Degree** BSN
**Available Programs** ADN to Baccalaureate; Generic Baccalaureate.
**Study Options** Full-time and part-time.
**Program Entrance Requirements** CPR certification, written essay, health exam, high school chemistry, high school math, high school transcript, immunizations, interview, 2 letters of recommendation, minimum high school GPA of 2.8. Transfer students are accepted. *Application deadline:* Applications may be processed on a rolling basis for some programs. *Application fee:* $30.
**Advanced Placement** Credit by examination available.
**Contact** Dr. Mary Botter, Chair, Division of Nursing, Department of Nursing, Southern Vermont College, 982 Mansion Drive, Bennington, VT 05201. *Telephone:* 802-447-6347. *E-mail:* mbotter@svc.edu.

## University of Vermont
### Department of Nursing
### Burlington, Vermont

*http://www.uvm.edu/~cnhs/nursing*
Founded in 1791

**DEGREES • BS • MS**
**Nursing Program Faculty** 37 (14% with doctorates).
**Baccalaureate Enrollment** 282 **Women** 95% **Men** 5% **Minority** 9%
**Graduate Enrollment** 78 **Women** 90% **Men** 10% **Minority** 9% **Part-time** 23%
**Distance Learning Courses** Available.
**Nursing Student Activities** Nursing Honor Society, Sigma Theta Tau, Student Nurses' Association.
**Nursing Student Resources** Academic advising; academic or career counseling; assistance for students with disabilities; bookstore; campus computer network; career placement assistance; computer lab; computer-assisted instruction; e-mail services; employment services for current students; interactive nursing skills videos; Internet; learning resource lab; library services; nursing audiovisuals; remedial services; resume preparation assistance; skills, simulation, or other laboratory; tutoring.
**Library Facilities** 2.6 million volumes (126,689 in health, 1,437 in nursing); 30,000 periodical subscriptions (5,084 health-care related).

#### BACCALAUREATE PROGRAMS
**Degree** BS
**Available Programs** ADN to Baccalaureate; Generic Baccalaureate.
**Study Options** Full-time and part-time.
**Program Entrance Requirements** Minimum overall college GPA of 3.0, transcript of college record, written essay, health insurance, high school biology, high school chemistry, high school foreign language, 3 years high school math, 2 years high school science, high school transcript, immunizations, letters of recommendation, minimum GPA in nursing prerequisites of 2.0. Transfer students are accepted. *Application deadline:* 1/15 (fall). *Application fee:* $55.
**Advanced Placement** Credit by examination available. Credit given for nursing courses completed elsewhere dependent upon specific evaluations.
**Contact** *Telephone:* 802-656-0968.

#### GRADUATE PROGRAMS
**Contact** *Telephone:* 802-656-2018. *Fax:* 802-656-8306.

**MASTER'S DEGREE PROGRAM**
**Degree** MS
**Available Programs** Master's; Master's for Non-Nursing College Graduates; Master's for Nurses with Non-Nursing Degrees; RN to Master's.
**Concentrations Available** Nursing administration. *Nurse practitioner programs in:* adult health, family health, psychiatric/mental health.
**Study Options** Full-time and part-time.
**Program Entrance Requirements** Minimum overall college GPA of 3.0, transcript of college record, written essay, 3 letters of recommendation, physical assessment course, statistics course, GRE General Test. *Application deadline:* Applications may be processed on a rolling basis for some programs. *Application fee:* $40.
**Advanced Placement** Credit by examination available. Credit given for nursing courses completed elsewhere dependent upon specific evaluations.
**Degree Requirements** 57 total credit hours, thesis or project, comprehensive exam.

**POST-MASTER'S PROGRAM**
**Areas of Study** *Nurse practitioner programs in:* adult health, family health, psychiatric/mental health.

# VIRGIN ISLANDS

## University of the Virgin Islands
### Division of Nursing
### Saint Thomas, Virgin Islands

*http://www.uvi.edu/*
Founded in 1962

**DEGREE • BSN**
**Nursing Program Faculty** 8 (15% with doctorates).
**Baccalaureate Enrollment** 51 **Women** 98% **Men** 2% **Minority** 11% **International** 12% **Part-time** 20%
**Nursing Student Activities** Student Nurses' Association.
**Nursing Student Resources** Academic advising; academic or career counseling; assistance for students with disabilities; bookstore; campus computer network; career placement assistance; computer lab; computer-assisted instruction; e-mail services; employment services for current students; externships; housing assistance; interactive nursing skills videos; Internet; learning resource lab; library services; nursing audiovisuals; paid internships; remedial services; resume preparation assistance; skills, simulation, or other laboratory; tutoring.
**Library Facilities** 104,062 volumes (95,000 in health, 600 in nursing); 370 periodical subscriptions (15 health-care related).

#### BACCALAUREATE PROGRAMS
**Degree** BSN
**Available Programs** ADN to Baccalaureate; Generic Baccalaureate; LPN to Baccalaureate; RN Baccalaureate.
**Site Options** St. Croix, VI.
**Study Options** Full-time and part-time.
**Program Entrance Requirements** Minimum overall college GPA of 2.5, transcript of college record, CPR certification, health exam, 2 years high school math, high school transcript, immunizations, minimum GPA in nursing prerequisites of 2.5, professional liability insurance/malpractice insurance, prerequisite course work. Transfer students are accepted. *Application deadline:* 10/15 (fall). Applications may be processed on a rolling basis for some programs. *Application fee:* $25.
**Advanced Placement** Credit by examination available. Credit given for nursing courses completed elsewhere dependent upon specific evaluations.
**Expenses (2012–13)** *Tuition, state resident:* full-time $1995; part-time $133 per credit. *Tuition, nonresident:* full-time $5985; part-time $400 per credit. *International tuition:* $5985 full-time. *Room and board:* $5690; room only: $2800 per academic year. *Required fees:* full-time $484; part-time $373 per term.
**Financial Aid** 99% of baccalaureate students in nursing programs received some form of financial aid in 2011–12.

**Contact** Dr. Cheryl P. Franklin, Dean, Division of Nursing, University of the Virgin Islands, RR1, Box 10000, Kingshill, St. Croix, VI 00850-9781. *Telephone:* 340-778-1620 Ext. 4117. *Fax:* 340-693-1285. *E-mail:* cfrankl@uvi.edu.

# VIRGINIA

## Bon Secours Memorial College of Nursing

### Bon Secours Memorial College of Nursing
### Richmond, Virginia

**DEGREE • BSN**

#### BACCALAUREATE PROGRAMS

**Degree** BSN
**Available Programs** Generic Baccalaureate; RN Baccalaureate.
**Online Degree Options** Yes.
**Program Entrance Requirements** Minimum overall college GPA of 2.5, prerequisite course work.
**Contact** College of Nursing, Bon Secours Memorial College of Nursing, 8550 Magellan Parkway, Suite 1100, Richmond, VA 23227. *Telephone:* 804-627-5300.

## Eastern Mennonite University

### Department of Nursing
### Harrisonburg, Virginia

Founded in 1917

**DEGREES • BSN • MSN**
**Nursing Program Faculty** 12 (25% with doctorates).
**Baccalaureate Enrollment** 146 **Women** 92.5% **Men** 7.5% **Minority** 8.2%
**Graduate Enrollment** 13 **Women** 84.6% **Men** 15.4% **Minority** 8% **Part-time** 8%
**Distance Learning Courses** Available.
**Nursing Student Activities** Sigma Theta Tau, Student Nurses' Association.
**Nursing Student Resources** Academic advising; academic or career counseling; assistance for students with disabilities; bookstore; campus computer network; career placement assistance; computer lab; computer-assisted instruction; e-mail services; employment services for current students; externships; housing assistance; interactive nursing skills videos; Internet; learning resource lab; library services; nursing audiovisuals; placement services for program completers; remedial services; resume preparation assistance; skills, simulation, or other laboratory; tutoring.
**Library Facilities** 168,896 volumes (1,256 in health, 926 in nursing); 781 periodical subscriptions (33 health-care related).

#### BACCALAUREATE PROGRAMS

**Degree** BSN
**Available Programs** ADN to Baccalaureate; Baccalaureate for Second Degree; Generic Baccalaureate; LPN to Baccalaureate; RN Baccalaureate.
**Site Options** Lancaster , PA.
**Study Options** Full-time and part-time.
**Program Entrance Requirements** Minimum overall college GPA of 2.8, transcript of college record, CPR certification, written essay, health exam, health insurance, high school chemistry, high school transcript, immunizations, 3 letters of recommendation, minimum high school GPA of 2.0, minimum GPA in nursing prerequisites of 2.8, professional liability insurance/malpractice insurance, prerequisite course work. Transfer students are accepted. *Application deadline:* 2/2 (fall), 6/1 (spring). Applications may be processed on a rolling basis for some programs.
**Advanced Placement** Credit by examination available. Credit given for nursing courses completed elsewhere dependent upon specific evaluations.
**Contact** *Telephone:* 800-368-2665. *Fax:* 540-432-4118.

#### GRADUATE PROGRAMS

**Contact** *Telephone:* 540-432-4000 Ext. 4192. *Fax:* 540-432-4000 Ext. 4444.

**MASTER'S DEGREE PROGRAM**
**Degree** MSN
**Available Programs** Master's; Master's for Nurses with Non-Nursing Degrees.
**Concentrations Available** Nursing administration.
**Online Degree Options** Yes (online only).
**Program Entrance Requirements** Clinical experience, computer literacy, minimum overall college GPA of 3.0, transcript of college record, written essay, 2 letters of recommendation, nursing research course. *Application deadline:* 4/1 (fall). Applications may be processed on a rolling basis for some programs. *Application fee:* $25.
**Degree Requirements** 37 total credit hours, thesis or project.

## ECPI University

### BSN Program
### Virginia Beach, Virginia

***http://www.ecpi.edu/medical/program/nursing-bachelor-degree/***
Founded in 1966

**DEGREE • BSN**
**Nursing Program Faculty** 5 (60% with doctorates).
**Baccalaureate Enrollment** 30
**Distance Learning Courses** Available.
**Nursing Student Resources** Academic advising; academic or career counseling; assistance for students with disabilities; campus computer network; computer lab; e-mail services; Internet; library services; placement services for program completers; resume preparation assistance; tutoring.
**Library Facilities** 111,114 volumes; 293 periodical subscriptions.

#### BACCALAUREATE PROGRAMS

**Degree** BSN
**Available Programs** RN Baccalaureate.
**Study Options** Full-time and part-time.
**Online Degree Options** Yes.
**Program Entrance Requirements** CPR certification, health exam, immunizations, interview, minimum GPA in nursing prerequisites of 2.5, prerequisite course work, RN licensure. Transfer students are accepted. *Application deadline:* Applications may be processed on a rolling basis for some programs.
**Advanced Placement** Credit given for nursing courses completed elsewhere dependent upon specific evaluations.
**Contact** *Telephone:* 757-497-8400.

## George Mason University

### College of Health and Human Services
### Fairfax, Virginia

***http://chhs.gmu.edu/***
Founded in 1957

**DEGREES • BSN • MSN • PHD**
**Nursing Program Faculty** 72 (41% with doctorates).
**Baccalaureate Enrollment** 367 **Women** 91% **Men** 9% **Minority** 51% **International** 3% **Part-time** 22%
**Graduate Enrollment** 150 **Women** 95% **Men** 5% **Minority** 33% **International** 2% **Part-time** 80%
**Distance Learning Courses** Available.
**Nursing Student Activities** Nursing Honor Society, Sigma Theta Tau, Student Nurses' Association.
**Nursing Student Resources** Academic advising; academic or career counseling; assistance for students with disabilities; bookstore; campus computer network; career placement assistance; computer lab; computer-assisted instruction; e-mail services; employment services for current students; housing assistance; interactive nursing skills videos; Internet; library services; nursing audiovisuals; remedial services; resume preparation assistance; skills, simulation, or other laboratory; tutoring.
**Library Facilities** 2.5 million volumes (16,200 in nursing); 11,200 periodical subscriptions (700 health-care related).

## BACCALAUREATE PROGRAMS

**Degree** BSN
**Available Programs** Accelerated Baccalaureate for Second Degree; Generic Baccalaureate; RN Baccalaureate.
**Site Options** Prince William County, VA.
**Study Options** Full-time.
**Online Degree Options** Yes.
**Program Entrance Requirements** Minimum overall college GPA of 2.0, CPR certification, written essay, health exam, health insurance, immunizations, minimum high school GPA of 2.0, minimum GPA in nursing prerequisites of 3.0, professional liability insurance/malpractice insurance, prerequisite course work. Transfer students are accepted. *Application deadline:* 1/15 (fall). *Application fee:* $50.
**Contact** Office of Student Affairs, BSN Programs, School of Nursing, College of Health and Human Services, George Mason University, Mailstop 3C4, 4400 University Drive, Fairfax, VA 22030-4444. *Telephone:* 703-993-8896. *Fax:* 703-993-3606. *E-mail:* bsnapps@gmu.edu.

## GRADUATE PROGRAMS

**Financial Aid** 9 fellowships (averaging $26,347 per year), 27 research assistantships (averaging $19,716 per year), 4 teaching assistantships (averaging $19,500 per year) were awarded; career-related internships or fieldwork, Federal Work-Study, scholarships, unspecified assistantships, and health care benefits (for full-time research or teaching assistantship recipients) also available.
**Contact** Ms. Janice Lee-Beverly, Administrative Assistant, MSN Programs, School of Nursing, College of Health and Human Services, George Mason University, Mailstop 3C4, 4400 University Drive, Fairfax, VA 22030-4444. *Telephone:* 703-993-1947. *Fax:* 703-993-1949. *E-mail:* jleebev1@gmu.edu.

### MASTER'S DEGREE PROGRAM

**Degree** MSN
**Available Programs** Master's.
**Concentrations Available** Nursing administration; nursing education. *Clinical nurse specialist programs in:* adult health. *Nurse practitioner programs in:* adult health, family health, gerontology, psychiatric/mental health.
**Site Options** Prince William County, VA.
**Study Options** Full-time and part-time.
**Online Degree Options** Yes.
**Program Entrance Requirements** Clinical experience, computer literacy, minimum overall college GPA of 3.0, CPR certification, written essay, immunizations, 2 letters of recommendation, physical assessment course, professional liability insurance/malpractice insurance, statistics course. *Application deadline:* 4/1 (fall), 11/1 (spring). *Application fee:* $50.

### POST-MASTER'S PROGRAM

**Areas of Study** Nursing administration; nursing education.

### DOCTORAL DEGREE PROGRAM

**Degree** PhD
**Available Programs** Doctorate.
**Areas of Study** Individualized study.
**Site Options** Prince William County, VA.
**Program Entrance Requirements** Clinical experience, minimum overall college GPA of 3.5, interview, 3 letters of recommendation, MSN or equivalent, statistics course, writing sample, MAT. *Application deadline:* 3/1 (spring). *Application fee:* $60.
**Degree Requirements** 48 total credit hours, dissertation, written exam.

### POSTDOCTORAL PROGRAM

**Postdoctoral Program Contact** Jean Sorrell, Coordinator, College of Health and Human Services, George Mason University, Mailstop 3C4, 4400 University Drive, Fairfax, VA 22030-4444. *Telephone:* 703-993-1944. *Fax:* 703-993-1942. *E-mail:* jsorrell@gmu.edu.

## CONTINUING EDUCATION PROGRAM

**Contact** Ms. Sandy Kellerhals, Administrative Assistant for Academic Outreach, College of Health and Human Services, George Mason University, Mailstop 1B8, 4400 University Drive, Fairfax, VA 22030-4444. *Telephone:* 703-993-2120. *Fax:* 703-993-1622. *E-mail:* skellerh@gmu.edu.

# Hampton University
## School of Nursing
## Hampton, Virginia

*http://nursing.hamptonu.edu/*
Founded in 1868

## DEGREES • BS • MS • PHD

**Nursing Program Faculty** 26 (51% with doctorates).
**Baccalaureate Enrollment** 470 **Women** 93% **Men** 7% **Minority** 90% **International** 4% **Part-time** 4%
**Graduate Enrollment** 66 **Women** 100% **Minority** 80% **Part-time** 25%
**Distance Learning Courses** Available.
**Nursing Student Activities** Sigma Theta Tau, Student Nurses' Association.
**Nursing Student Resources** Academic advising; bookstore; computer lab; e-mail services; interactive nursing skills videos; Internet; library services; skills, simulation, or other laboratory; tutoring.
**Library Facilities** 526,154 volumes (4,000 in health, 2,000 in nursing); 32,187 periodical subscriptions (500 health-care related).

## BACCALAUREATE PROGRAMS

**Degree** BS
**Available Programs** Accelerated Baccalaureate; Generic Baccalaureate; LPN to Baccalaureate; LPN to RN Baccalaureate; RN Baccalaureate.
**Site Options** Virginia Beach, VA.
**Study Options** Full-time and part-time.
**Program Entrance Requirements** Minimum overall college GPA of 2.3, transcript of college record, CPR certification, written essay, health exam, health insurance, high school biology, high school chemistry, 3 years high school math, 2 years high school science, high school transcript, immunizations, 2 letters of recommendation, minimum high school GPA of 2.0, minimum high school rank 50%, minimum GPA in nursing prerequisites of 2.0, professional liability insurance/malpractice insurance. Transfer students are accepted. *Application deadline:* 3/1 (fall), 12/1 (spring).
**Advanced Placement** Credit by examination available. Credit given for nursing courses completed elsewhere dependent upon specific evaluations.
**Contact** *Telephone:* 757-727-5251.

## GRADUATE PROGRAMS

**Contact** *Telephone:* 757-727-5251. *Fax:* 757-727-5423.

### MASTER'S DEGREE PROGRAM

**Degree** MS
**Available Programs** Master's; RN to Master's.
**Concentrations Available** Health-care administration; nursing administration; nursing education. *Nurse practitioner programs in:* family health, gerontology, pediatric, primary care,women's health.
**Study Options** Full-time and part-time.
**Online Degree Options** Yes.
**Program Entrance Requirements** Clinical experience, computer literacy, minimum overall college GPA of 2.5, transcript of college record, written essay, interview, 2 letters of recommendation, nursing research course, physical assessment course, resume, statistics course, GRE General Test. *Application deadline:* 3/30 (fall), 11/1 (spring).
**Advanced Placement** Credit given for nursing courses completed elsewhere dependent upon specific evaluations.
**Degree Requirements** 46 total credit hours, thesis or project, comprehensive exam.

### DOCTORAL DEGREE PROGRAM

**Degree** PhD
**Available Programs** Doctorate.
**Areas of Study** Family health.
**Online Degree Options** Yes (online only).
**Program Entrance Requirements** Minimum overall college GPA of 3.5, interview by faculty committee, interview, 3 letters of recommendation, MSN or equivalent, statistics course, vita, writing sample. *Application deadline:* 3/30 (fall).
**Degree Requirements** 44 total credit hours, dissertation, oral exam, written exam, residency.

# James Madison University

## Department of Nursing
## Harrisonburg, Virginia

*http://www.nursing.jmu.edu/*
Founded in 1908

**DEGREES • BSN • DNP • MSN**

**Nursing Program Faculty** 45 (40% with doctorates).
**Baccalaureate Enrollment** 298 **Women** 96% **Men** 4% **Minority** 7%
**Graduate Enrollment** 72 **Women** 79% **Men** 21% **Minority** 4% **Part-time** 75%
**Distance Learning Courses** Available.
**Nursing Student Activities** Sigma Theta Tau, Student Nurses' Association.
**Nursing Student Resources** Academic advising; academic or career counseling; assistance for students with disabilities; bookstore; campus computer network; career placement assistance; computer lab; computer-assisted instruction; e-mail services; employment services for current students; externships; housing assistance; interactive nursing skills videos; Internet; learning resource lab; library services; nursing audiovisuals; paid internships; remedial services; resume preparation assistance; skills, simulation, or other laboratory; tutoring; unpaid internships.
**Library Facilities** 761,026 volumes (26,702 in health, 2,041 in nursing); 15,464 periodical subscriptions (8,814 health-care related).

### BACCALAUREATE PROGRAMS

**Degree** BSN
**Available Programs** Generic Baccalaureate; RN Baccalaureate.
**Study Options** Full-time.
**Program Entrance Requirements** Minimum overall college GPA of 3.0, transcript of college record, CPR certification, health exam, health insurance, immunizations, minimum GPA in nursing prerequisites of 2.0, prerequisite course work. Transfer students are accepted. *Application deadline:* 12/1 (fall), 7/1 (spring).
**Advanced Placement** Credit given for nursing courses completed elsewhere dependent upon specific evaluations.
**Expenses (2013–14)** *Tuition, state resident:* full-time $9176. *Tuition, nonresident:* full-time $23,654. *Room and board:* $4259 per academic year.
**Financial Aid** 50% of baccalaureate students in nursing programs received some form of financial aid in 2012–13. *Gift aid (need-based):* Federal Pell, FSEOG, state, private, college/university gift aid from institutional funds. *Loans:* Federal Direct (Subsidized and Unsubsidized Stafford PLUS), Perkins. *Work-study:* Federal Work-Study, part-time campus jobs. *Financial aid application deadline (priority):* 3/1.
**Contact** Ms. Becky Meadows, Administrative Assistant, Department of Nursing, James Madison University, 820 Madison Drive, Burruss Hall, MSC 4305, Harrisonburg, VA 22807. *Telephone:* 540-568-6314. *Fax:* 540-568-5613. *E-mail:* meadowra@jmu.edu.

### GRADUATE PROGRAMS

**Expenses (2013–14)** *Tuition, state resident:* part-time $410 per credit hour. *Tuition, nonresident:* part-time $1095 per credit hour.
**Contact** Dr. Patty Hale, Program Director, Department of Nursing, James Madison University, 820 Madison Drive, Burruss Hall, MSC 4305, Harrisonburg, VA 22807. *Telephone:* 540-568-6314. *Fax:* 540-568-7896. *E-mail:* halepj@jmu.edu.

#### MASTER'S DEGREE PROGRAM

**Degree** MSN
**Available Programs** Master's.
**Concentrations Available** Clinical nurse leader; nurse-midwifery; nursing administration. *Nurse practitioner programs in:* adult health, family health, gerontology.
**Study Options** Full-time and part-time.
**Program Entrance Requirements** Clinical experience, computer literacy, minimum overall college GPA of 2.8, transcript of college record, CPR certification, written essay, immunizations, 2 letters of recommendation, physical assessment course, prerequisite course work, resume, statistics course. *Application deadline:* 4/1 (fall), 10/1 (spring). Applications may be processed on a rolling basis for some programs. *Application fee:* $55.
**Advanced Placement** Credit given for nursing courses completed elsewhere dependent upon specific evaluations.
**Degree Requirements** 32 total credit hours.

#### DOCTORAL DEGREE PROGRAM

**Degree** DNP
**Available Programs** Doctorate.
**Areas of Study** Advanced practice nursing, clinical practice, clinical research, ethics, health policy, health promotion/disease prevention, health-care systems, individualized study, information systems, nursing administration, nursing policy, nursing research.
**Online Degree Options** Yes (online only).
**Program Entrance Requirements** Clinical experience, minimum overall college GPA of 3.2, interview, 3 letters of recommendation, MSN or equivalent, statistics course, vita, writing sample. *Application deadline:* Applications may be processed on a rolling basis for some programs.
**Degree Requirements** Oral exam, residency.

# Jefferson College of Health Sciences

## Nursing Education Program
## Roanoke, Virginia

*http://www.jchs.edu/*
Founded in 1982

**DEGREES • BSN • MSN**

**Nursing Program Faculty** 24 (17% with doctorates).
**Baccalaureate Enrollment** 260 **Women** 93% **Men** 7% **Minority** 15% **Part-time** 47%
**Graduate Enrollment** 32 **Women** 91% **Men** 9% **Minority** 9% **Part-time** 3%
**Distance Learning Courses** Available.
**Nursing Student Activities** Nursing Honor Society, Sigma Theta Tau, Student Nurses' Association.
**Nursing Student Resources** Academic advising; academic or career counseling; assistance for students with disabilities; bookstore; campus computer network; computer lab; computer-assisted instruction; e-mail services; externships; housing assistance; interactive nursing skills videos; Internet; learning resource lab; library services; nursing audiovisuals; skills, simulation, or other laboratory; tutoring.
**Library Facilities** 6,042 volumes (4,403 in health, 1,422 in nursing); 233 periodical subscriptions (277 health-care related).

### BACCALAUREATE PROGRAMS

**Degree** BSN
**Available Programs** ADN to Baccalaureate; Generic Baccalaureate; RN Baccalaureate.
**Site Options** Roanoke, VA.
**Study Options** Full-time and part-time.
**Program Entrance Requirements** Minimum overall college GPA of 2.0, transcript of college record, CPR certification, health exam, health insurance, high school biology, high school chemistry, 2 years high school math, 2 years high school science, high school transcript, immunizations, minimum high school GPA of 2.0, prerequisite course work. Transfer students are accepted.
**Advanced Placement** Credit by examination available. Credit given for nursing courses completed elsewhere dependent upon specific evaluations.
**Contact** *Telephone:* 540-985-9083. *Fax:* 540-224-6703.

### GRADUATE PROGRAMS

**Contact** *Telephone:* 540-985-9083. *Fax:* 540-224-6703.

#### MASTER'S DEGREE PROGRAM

**Degree** MSN
**Available Programs** Master's; Master's for Nurses with Non-Nursing Degrees.
**Concentrations Available** Nursing administration; nursing education.
**Site Options** Roanoke, VA.
**Study Options** Full-time.
**Program Entrance Requirements** Clinical experience, computer literacy, transcript of college record, 2 letters of recommendation, nursing research course, resume, statistics course.
**Degree Requirements** 37 total credit hours, thesis or project.

### CONTINUING EDUCATION PROGRAM

**Contact** *Telephone:* 540-767-6072.

## Liberty University
### Department of Nursing
### Lynchburg, Virginia

*http://www.liberty.edu/*
Founded in 1971

**DEGREES • BSN • MSN**
**Nursing Program Faculty** 25 (25% with doctorates).
**Baccalaureate Enrollment** 358 **Women** 93% **Men** 7% **Minority** 7% **International** 8%
**Graduate Enrollment** 280 **Women** 89% **Men** 11% **Minority** 29% **International** 3% **Part-time** 99%
**Distance Learning Courses** Available.
**Nursing Student Activities** Student Nurses' Association.
**Nursing Student Resources** Academic advising; academic or career counseling; assistance for students with disabilities; bookstore; campus computer network; career placement assistance; computer lab; e-mail services; externships; interactive nursing skills videos; Internet; learning resource lab; library services; nursing audiovisuals; resume preparation assistance; skills, simulation, or other laboratory; tutoring.
**Library Facilities** 402,115 volumes (3,632 in health, 3,000 in nursing); 75,441 periodical subscriptions (46 health-care related).

### BACCALAUREATE PROGRAMS

**Degree** BSN
**Available Programs** Generic Baccalaureate; RN Baccalaureate.
**Site Options** Lynchburg, VA.
**Study Options** Full-time and part-time.
**Program Entrance Requirements** Minimum overall college GPA of 3.0, transcript of college record, CPR certification, written essay, immunizations, 2 letters of recommendation, minimum GPA in nursing prerequisites of 3.0, professional liability insurance/malpractice insurance, prerequisite course work. Transfer students are accepted. *Application deadline:* 2/11 (spring).
**Advanced Placement** Credit given for nursing courses completed elsewhere dependent upon specific evaluations.
**Contact** *Telephone:* 804-582-2519. *Fax:* 804-582-7035.

### GRADUATE PROGRAMS

**Contact** *Telephone:* 804-582-2519.

**MASTER'S DEGREE PROGRAM**
**Degree** MSN
**Available Programs** Master's.
**Concentrations Available** Nursing education. *Clinical nurse specialist programs in:* acute care.
**Site Options** Lynchburg, VA.
**Study Options** Full-time and part-time.
**Online Degree Options** Yes (online only).
**Program Entrance Requirements** Clinical experience, computer literacy, minimum overall college GPA of 3.0, transcript of college record, CPR certification, written essay, immunizations, interview, 3 letters of recommendation, nursing research course, physical assessment course, prerequisite course work, resume, statistics course. *Application deadline:* Applications may be processed on a rolling basis for some programs. *Application fee:* $50.
**Degree Requirements** 36 total credit hours, thesis or project.

## Longwood University
### Nursing Program
### Farmville, Virginia

Founded in 1839

**DEGREE • BSN**
**Library Facilities** 478,036 volumes; 64,000 periodical subscriptions.

### BACCALAUREATE PROGRAMS

**Degree** BSN
**Available Programs** RN Baccalaureate.
**Contact** Dr. Melody Eaton, Nursing Program Director and Department Chair, Nursing Program, Longwood University, Stevens Hall, Suite 200, 201 High Street, Farmville, VA 23909. *Telephone:* 434-395-2936. *Fax:* 434-395-2006. *E-mail:* eatonmk@longwood.edu.

## Lynchburg College
### School of Health Sciences and Human Performance
### Lynchburg, Virginia

Founded in 1903

**DEGREES • BS • MSN**
**Nursing Program Faculty** 14 (38% with doctorates).
**Baccalaureate Enrollment** 95 **Women** 95% **Men** 5% **Minority** 8%
**Graduate Enrollment** 16 **Women** 87.5% **Men** 12.5% **Minority** 18.75% **International** 12.5% **Part-time** 100%
**Distance Learning Courses** Available.
**Nursing Student Activities** Nursing Honor Society, Sigma Theta Tau, Student Nurses' Association.
**Nursing Student Resources** Academic advising; academic or career counseling; assistance for students with disabilities; bookstore; campus computer network; career placement assistance; computer lab; computer-assisted instruction; e-mail services; employment services for current students; externships; housing assistance; interactive nursing skills videos; Internet; learning resource lab; library services; nursing audiovisuals; remedial services; resume preparation assistance; skills, simulation, or other laboratory; tutoring; unpaid internships.
**Library Facilities** 322,751 volumes (6,300 in health, 2,000 in nursing); 261 periodical subscriptions (100 health-care related).

### BACCALAUREATE PROGRAMS

**Degree** BS
**Available Programs** Accelerated Baccalaureate; Baccalaureate for Second Degree; Generic Baccalaureate.
**Study Options** Full-time and part-time.
**Program Entrance Requirements** Transcript of college record, high school biology, high school chemistry, 3 years high school math, high school science, high school transcript, minimum GPA in nursing prerequisites of 3.0, prerequisite course work. Transfer students are accepted. *Application deadline:* 4/1 (fall), 4/1 (summer). *Application fee:* $30.
**Advanced Placement** Credit given for nursing courses completed elsewhere dependent upon specific evaluations.
**Expenses (2013–14)** *Tuition:* full-time $32,620; part-time $900 per semester. *International tuition:* $32,620 full-time. *Room and board:* $34,470; room only: $4580 per academic year. *Required fees:* full-time $533.
**Financial Aid** 97% of baccalaureate students in nursing programs received some form of financial aid in 2012–13. *Gift aid (need-based):* Federal Pell, FSEOG, state, private, college/university gift aid from institutional funds. *Loans:* Federal Direct (Subsidized and Unsubsidized Stafford PLUS), Perkins. *Work-study:* Federal Work-Study, part-time campus jobs. *Financial aid application deadline (priority):* 3/5.
**Contact** Dr. Linda L. Andrews, EdD, Director of Nursing Program and Professor of Nursing, School of Health Sciences and Human Performance, Lynchburg College, 1501 Lakeside Drive, McMillan Nursing Building, Lynchburg, VA 24501-3199. *Telephone:* 434-544-8846. *Fax:* 434-544-8323. *E-mail:* andrews@lynchburg.edu.

### GRADUATE PROGRAMS

**Expenses (2013–14)** *Tuition:* full-time $8100; part-time $450 per credit hour. *International tuition:* $8100 full-time. *Room and board:* $9950; room only: $6980 per academic year.
**Financial Aid** 50% of graduate students in nursing programs received some form of financial aid in 2012–13.
**Contact** Dr. Nancy Overstreet, Director of Nursing Graduate Programs, School of Health Sciences and Human Performance, Lynchburg College, 1501 Lakeside Drive, Lynchburg, VA 24501. *Telephone:* 434-544-8340. *Fax:* 434-544-8323. *E-mail:* overstreet.n@lynchburg.edu.

**MASTER'S DEGREE PROGRAM**
**Degree** MSN
**Available Programs** Master's; RN to Master's.
**Concentrations Available** Clinical nurse leader; nursing education.
**Study Options** Full-time and part-time.
**Online Degree Options** Yes (online only).
**Program Entrance Requirements** Clinical experience, minimum overall college GPA of 3.0, transcript of college record, 3 letters of recommendation, physical assessment course, statistics course. *Application deadline:* 4/1 (fall), 10/1 (winter), 12/1 (spring), 4/1 (summer). Applications may be processed on a rolling basis for some programs. *Application fee:* $30.

**Advanced Placement** Credit given for nursing courses completed elsewhere dependent upon specific evaluations.
**Degree Requirements** 37 total credit hours, thesis or project.

# Marymount University
## School of Health Professions
## Arlington, Virginia

*http://www.marymount.edu/academics/schools/shp*
Founded in 1950

**DEGREES • BSN • DNP • MSN**
**Nursing Program Faculty** 20 (65% with doctorates).
**Baccalaureate Enrollment** 389 **Women** 90% **Men** 10% **Minority** 32% **International** 4% **Part-time** 17%
**Graduate Enrollment** 70 **Women** 91% **Men** 9% **Minority** 48% **International** 5% **Part-time** 84%
**Distance Learning Courses** Available.
**Nursing Student Activities** Sigma Theta Tau, Student Nurses' Association.
**Nursing Student Resources** Academic advising; academic or career counseling; assistance for students with disabilities; bookstore; campus computer network; career placement assistance; computer lab; computer-assisted instruction; e-mail services; externships; housing assistance; interactive nursing skills videos; Internet; learning resource lab; library services; nursing audiovisuals; paid internships; remedial services; resume preparation assistance; skills, simulation, or other laboratory; tutoring; unpaid internships.
**Library Facilities** 241,177 volumes (12,204 in health, 1,623 in nursing); 57,490 periodical subscriptions (2,906 health-care related).

### BACCALAUREATE PROGRAMS

**Degree** BSN
**Available Programs** ADN to Baccalaureate; Accelerated Baccalaureate for Second Degree; Generic Baccalaureate; RN Baccalaureate.
**Site Options** Arlington, VA.
**Study Options** Full-time and part-time.
**Program Entrance Requirements** Minimum overall college GPA of 2.5, health exam, health insurance, high school transcript, 2 letters of recommendation, minimum high school GPA of 2.5. Transfer students are accepted. *Application deadline:* Applications may be processed on a rolling basis for some programs. *Application fee:* $40.
**Advanced Placement** Credit by examination available. Credit given for nursing courses completed elsewhere dependent upon specific evaluations.
**Financial Aid** 84% of baccalaureate students in nursing programs received some form of financial aid in 2011–12. *Gift aid (need-based):* Federal Pell, FSEOG, state, private, college/university gift aid from institutional funds. *Loans:* Federal Direct (Subsidized and Unsubsidized Stafford PLUS), Perkins. *Work-study:* Federal Work-Study. *Financial aid application deadline (priority):* 3/1.
**Contact** Admissions Counselor, Undergraduate Admissions, School of Health Professions, Marymount University, 2807 North Glebe Road, Arlington, VA 22207-4299. *Telephone:* 800-548-7638. *Fax:* 703-522-0349. *E-mail:* admissions@marymount.edu.

### GRADUATE PROGRAMS

**Financial Aid** 57% of graduate students in nursing programs received some form of financial aid in 2011–12. Research assistantships with full and partial tuition reimbursements available, career-related internships or fieldwork, Federal Work-Study, scholarships, and unspecified assistantships available. Aid available to part-time students.
**Contact** Ms. Francesca Reed, Coordinator, Graduate Admissions, School of Health Professions, Marymount University, 2807 North Glebe Road, Arlington, VA 22207-4299. *Telephone:* 703-284-5906. *E-mail:* francesca.reed@marymount.edu.

#### MASTER'S DEGREE PROGRAM

**Degree** MSN
**Available Programs** Master's.
**Concentrations Available** *Nurse practitioner programs in:* family health.
**Site Options** Arlington, VA.
**Study Options** Full-time and part-time.
**Program Entrance Requirements** Minimum overall college GPA of 3.0, transcript of college record, CPR certification, immunizations, interview, 2 letters of recommendation, professional liability insurance/malpractice insurance, resume, statistics course, GRE, MAT. *Application deadline:* 9/15 (fall), 4/1 (spring). Applications may be processed on a rolling basis for some programs. *Application fee:* $40.
**Advanced Placement** Credit given for nursing courses completed elsewhere dependent upon specific evaluations.
**Degree Requirements** 42 total credit hours, comprehensive exam.

#### POST-MASTER'S PROGRAM

**Areas of Study** *Nurse practitioner programs in:* family health.

#### DOCTORAL DEGREE PROGRAM

**Degree** DNP
**Available Programs** Doctorate; Post-Baccalaureate Doctorate.
**Areas of Study** Advanced practice nursing.
**Site Options** Arlington, VA.
**Program Entrance Requirements** Clinical experience, minimum overall college GPA of 3.3, interview by faculty committee, interview, 2 letters of recommendation, MSN or equivalent, vita, writing sample, GRE. *Application deadline:* 4/1 (fall). *Application fee:* $40.
**Degree Requirements** 32 total credit hours, residency.

# Norfolk State University
## Department of Nursing
## Norfolk, Virginia

*http://cset.nsu.edu/nursing/*
Founded in 1935

**DEGREE • BSN**
**Nursing Program Faculty** 26 (40% with doctorates).
**Baccalaureate Enrollment** 133 **Women** 90% **Men** 10% **Minority** 85% **International** 15% **Part-time** 45%
**Distance Learning Courses** Available.
**Nursing Student Activities** Nursing Honor Society, Student Nurses' Association, nursing club.
**Nursing Student Resources** Academic advising; academic or career counseling; assistance for students with disabilities; bookstore; campus computer network; career placement assistance; computer lab; computer-assisted instruction; daycare for children of students; e-mail services; employment services for current students; externships; housing assistance; interactive nursing skills videos; Internet; learning resource lab; library services; nursing audiovisuals; paid internships; remedial services; resume preparation assistance; skills, simulation, or other laboratory; tutoring; unpaid internships.
**Library Facilities** 600 volumes in health, 300 volumes in nursing; 125 periodical subscriptions health-care related.

### BACCALAUREATE PROGRAMS

**Degree** BSN
**Available Programs** Accelerated Baccalaureate for Second Degree; Accelerated LPN to Baccalaureate; RN Baccalaureate.
**Site Options** Virginia Beach , VA.
**Study Options** Full-time and part-time.
**Program Entrance Requirements** Minimum overall college GPA of 2.5, transcript of college record, CPR certification, health exam, health insurance, high school biology, high school chemistry, 2 years high school math, high school transcript, immunizations, minimum high school GPA of 2.5, minimum GPA in nursing prerequisites of 2.5, professional liability insurance/malpractice insurance, prerequisite course work. Transfer students are accepted. *Application deadline:* 8/1 (fall), 12/1 (winter), 2/1 (spring), 8/1 (summer).
**Advanced Placement** Credit by examination available. Credit given for nursing courses completed elsewhere dependent upon specific evaluations.
**Contact** *Telephone:* 757-823-9015. *Fax:* 757-823-2131.

# Old Dominion University
## Department of Nursing
## Norfolk, Virginia

*http://www.odu.edu/nursing*
Founded in 1930

**DEGREES • BSN • DNP • MSN**
**Nursing Program Faculty** 27 (33% with doctorates).

**Baccalaureate Enrollment** 399 **Women** 91% **Men** 9% **Minority** 40% **Part-time** 46%

**Graduate Enrollment** 219 **Women** 92% **Men** 8% **Minority** 23% **Part-time** 47%

**Distance Learning Courses** Available.

**Nursing Student Activities** Sigma Theta Tau, Student Nurses' Association.

**Nursing Student Resources** Academic advising; academic or career counseling; assistance for students with disabilities; bookstore; campus computer network; career placement assistance; computer lab; computer-assisted instruction; e-mail services; externships; interactive nursing skills videos; Internet; learning resource lab; library services; nursing audiovisuals; paid internships; remedial services; resume preparation assistance; skills, simulation, or other laboratory; tutoring; unpaid internships.

**Library Facilities** 2.5 million volumes (44,144 in health, 3,622 in nursing); 10,754 periodical subscriptions (3,035 health-care related).

## BACCALAUREATE PROGRAMS

**Degree** BSN

**Available Programs** Accelerated Baccalaureate; Generic Baccalaureate; RN Baccalaureate.

**Site Options** Olympia, WA; Yavapai, AZ.

**Study Options** Full-time.

**Program Entrance Requirements** Transcript of college record, CPR certification, immunizations, minimum GPA in nursing prerequisites of 2.5, prerequisite course work. Transfer students are accepted. *Application deadline:* 2/1 (fall). *Application fee:* $40.

**Contact** *Telephone:* 757-683-5245. *Fax:* 757-683-5253.

## GRADUATE PROGRAMS

**Contact** *Telephone:* 757-683-4298. *Fax:* 757-683-5253.

### MASTER'S DEGREE PROGRAM

**Degree** MSN

**Available Programs** Master's; RN to Master's.

**Concentrations Available** Nurse anesthesia; nurse-midwifery; nursing administration; nursing education. *Nurse practitioner programs in:* family health,women's health.

**Site Options** Athens, GA; Olympia, WA; Yavapai, AZ.

**Study Options** Full-time and part-time.

**Online Degree Options** Yes (online only).

**Program Entrance Requirements** Clinical experience, computer literacy, minimum overall college GPA of 3.0, transcript of college record, CPR certification, written essay, immunizations, interview, 3 letters of recommendation, physical assessment course, statistics course. *Application deadline:* 6/1 (fall), 12/1 (winter). *Application fee:* $40.

**Advanced Placement** Credit given for nursing courses completed elsewhere dependent upon specific evaluations.

**Degree Requirements** 47 total credit hours, comprehensive exam.

### POST-MASTER'S PROGRAM

**Areas of Study** Nurse anesthesia; nurse-midwifery; nursing administration; nursing education. *Nurse practitioner programs in:* family health,women's health.

### DOCTORAL DEGREE PROGRAM

**Degree** DNP

**Available Programs** Doctorate.

**Areas of Study** Advanced practice nursing.

**Online Degree Options** Yes (online only).

**Program Entrance Requirements** Clinical experience, minimum overall college GPA of 3.0, 3 letters of recommendation, MSN or equivalent, statistics course, vita, writing sample. *Application deadline:* 11/15 (fall), 11/15 (winter), 11/15 (spring).

**Degree Requirements** 36 total credit hours.

## CONTINUING EDUCATION PROGRAM

**Contact** *Telephone:* 757-683-5261. *Fax:* 757-683-5253.

# Radford University

## School of Nursing
## Radford, Virginia

***http://www.radford.edu/nurs-web***
Founded in 1910

**DEGREES • BSN • DNP • MSN**

**Nursing Program Faculty** 42 (31% with doctorates).

**Baccalaureate Enrollment** 227

**Graduate Enrollment** 58

**Distance Learning Courses** Available.

**Nursing Student Activities** Nursing Honor Society, Sigma Theta Tau, Student Nurses' Association.

**Nursing Student Resources** Academic advising; academic or career counseling; assistance for students with disabilities; bookstore; campus computer network; career placement assistance; computer lab; computer-assisted instruction; e-mail services; employment services for current students; externships; housing assistance; interactive nursing skills videos; Internet; learning resource lab; library services; nursing audiovisuals; resume preparation assistance; skills, simulation, or other laboratory; tutoring; unpaid internships.

**Library Facilities** 680,679 volumes; 11,661 periodical subscriptions.

## BACCALAUREATE PROGRAMS

**Degree** BSN

**Available Programs** Baccalaureate for Second Degree; Generic Baccalaureate; RN Baccalaureate.

**Site Options** Roanoke, VA.

**Study Options** Full-time.

**Online Degree Options** Yes.

**Program Entrance Requirements** Minimum overall college GPA of 2.8, transcript of college record, CPR certification, written essay, health exam, health insurance, immunizations, prerequisite course work. Transfer students are accepted. *Application deadline:* 11/15 (fall), 8/1 (spring).

**Advanced Placement** Credit given for nursing courses completed elsewhere dependent upon specific evaluations.

**Contact** Dr. Anthony Ray Ramsey, Director, School of Nursing, Radford University, PO Box 6964, Radford, VA 24142. *Telephone:* 540-831-7700. *Fax:* 540-831-7716. *E-mail:* nurs-web@radford.edu.

## GRADUATE PROGRAMS

**Financial Aid** 1 fellowship, 2 teaching assistantships (averaging $10,000 per year) were awarded; career-related internships or fieldwork, Federal Work-Study, institutionally sponsored loans, scholarships, and unspecified assistantships also available.

**Contact** Dr. Virginia Burggraf, Graduate Program Coordinator, School of Nursing, Radford University, PO Box 6964, Radford, VA 24142. *Telephone:* 540-831-7714. *Fax:* 540-831-7716. *E-mail:* nurs-web@radford.edu.

### MASTER'S DEGREE PROGRAM

**Degree** MSN

**Available Programs** Master's.

**Concentrations Available** Nurse-midwifery. *Nurse practitioner programs in:* family health.

**Study Options** Full-time and part-time.

**Program Entrance Requirements** Clinical experience, computer literacy, transcript of college record, CPR certification, written essay, immunizations, interview, letters of recommendation, nursing research course, physical assessment course, professional liability insurance/malpractice insurance, resume, statistics course. *Application deadline:* Applications may be processed on a rolling basis for some programs.

**Degree Requirements** Thesis or project.

### POST-MASTER'S PROGRAM

**Areas of Study** Nurse-midwifery. *Nurse practitioner programs in:* family health.

### DOCTORAL DEGREE PROGRAM

**Degree** DNP

**Available Programs** Doctorate; Post-Baccalaureate Doctorate.

**Areas of Study** Advanced practice nursing, clinical practice, faculty preparation, family health, gerontology, maternity-newborn.

**Online Degree Options** Yes (online only).

**Program Entrance Requirements** Clinical experience, minimum overall college GPA of 3.0, interview by faculty committee, interview, 3

letters of recommendation, statistics course, vita, writing sample, GRE. *Application deadline:* Applications may be processed on a rolling basis for some programs.
**Degree Requirements** Residency.

# Sentara College of Health Sciences

## Bachelor of Science in Nursing Program
## Chesapeake, Virginia

**DEGREE • BSN**

### BACCALAUREATE PROGRAMS

**Degree** BSN
**Available Programs** Generic Baccalaureate; LPN to Baccalaureate; RN Baccalaureate.
**Study Options** Full-time and part-time.
**Online Degree Options** Yes.
**Program Entrance Requirements** Prerequisite course work.
**Contact** Admission Recruiter, Bachelor of Science in Nursing Program, Sentara College of Health Sciences, Suite 105, 1441 Crossways Boulevard, Chesapeake, VA 23320. *Telephone:* 757-388-2862. *E-mail:* salamb@sentara.com.

# Shenandoah University

## Division of Nursing
## Winchester, Virginia

***http://www.nursing.su.edu/***
Founded in 1875

**DEGREES • BSN • DNP • MSN • MSN/MBA**
**Nursing Program Faculty** 44 (30% with doctorates).
**Baccalaureate Enrollment** 350 **Women** 97% **Men** 3% **Minority** 10% **International** 3% **Part-time** 15%
**Graduate Enrollment** 120 **Women** 97% **Men** 3% **Minority** 10% **Part-time** 25%
**Nursing Student Activities** Nursing Honor Society, Sigma Theta Tau, Student Nurses' Association.
**Nursing Student Resources** Academic advising; academic or career counseling; assistance for students with disabilities; bookstore; campus computer network; computer lab; daycare for children of students; e-mail services; interactive nursing skills videos; Internet; learning resource lab; library services; nursing audiovisuals; resume preparation assistance; skills, simulation, or other laboratory; tutoring.
**Library Facilities** 211,976 volumes (500 in health, 200 in nursing); 76,250 periodical subscriptions (250 health-care related).

### BACCALAUREATE PROGRAMS

**Degree** BSN
**Available Programs** ADN to Baccalaureate; Accelerated Baccalaureate for Second Degree; Generic Baccalaureate; RN Baccalaureate.
**Site Options** Leesburg, VA.
**Study Options** Full-time and part-time.
**Program Entrance Requirements** Minimum overall college GPA of 3.0, transcript of college record, CPR certification, health exam, health insurance, high school biology, high school chemistry, 2 years high school math, high school transcript, immunizations, minimum high school GPA of 3.0, minimum GPA in nursing prerequisites of 3.0, prerequisite course work. Transfer students are accepted. *Application deadline:* Applications may be processed on a rolling basis for some programs.
**Advanced Placement** Credit by examination available. Credit given for nursing courses completed elsewhere dependent upon specific evaluations.
**Contact** *Telephone:* 540-678-4381. *Fax:* 540-665-5519.

### GRADUATE PROGRAMS

**Contact** *Telephone:* 540-665-5512. *Fax:* 540-665-5519.

**MASTER'S DEGREE PROGRAM**
**Degrees** MSN; MSN/MBA
**Available Programs** Master's; RN to Master's.
**Concentrations Available** Nurse case management; nurse-midwifery. *Clinical nurse specialist programs in:* psychiatric/mental health. *Nurse practitioner programs in:* family health, psychiatric/mental health.
**Study Options** Full-time and part-time.
**Program Entrance Requirements** Clinical experience, computer literacy, minimum overall college GPA of 3.0, transcript of college record, CPR certification, immunizations, interview, 3 letters of recommendation, nursing research course, physical assessment course, professional liability insurance/malpractice insurance, prerequisite course work, resume, statistics course, GRE General Test. *Application deadline:* Applications may be processed on a rolling basis for some programs.
**Advanced Placement** Credit given for nursing courses completed elsewhere dependent upon specific evaluations.
**Degree Requirements** 48 total credit hours, thesis or project.

**POST-MASTER'S PROGRAM**
**Areas of Study** Nurse-midwifery. *Nurse practitioner programs in:* family health, psychiatric/mental health.

**DOCTORAL DEGREE PROGRAM**
**Degree** DNP
**Available Programs** Doctorate; Post-Baccalaureate Doctorate.
**Program Entrance Requirements** Clinical experience, minimum overall college GPA of 3.0, interview by faculty committee, letters of recommendation, MSN or equivalent, statistics course, vita. *Application deadline:* Applications may be processed on a rolling basis for some programs.
**Degree Requirements** 30 total credit hours.

### CONTINUING EDUCATION PROGRAM

**Contact** *Telephone:* 540-678-4374.

# Stratford University

## School of Nursing
## Falls Church, Virginia

***http://www.stratford.edu/***
Founded in 1976

**DEGREE • BSN**
**Nursing Program Faculty** 3 (33% with doctorates).
**Baccalaureate Enrollment** 14 **Women** 64% **Men** 36% **Minority** 79% **International** 7% **Part-time** 80%
**Nursing Student Activities** Student Nurses' Association.
**Nursing Student Resources** Academic advising; campus computer network; career placement assistance; computer lab; computer-assisted instruction; e-mail services; employment services for current students; interactive nursing skills videos; Internet; learning resource lab; library services; nursing audiovisuals; placement services for program completers; resume preparation assistance; skills, simulation, or other laboratory; tutoring; unpaid internships.
**Library Facilities** 7,649 volumes (120 in health, 110 in nursing); 75 periodical subscriptions (600 health-care related).

### BACCALAUREATE PROGRAMS

**Degree** BSN
**Available Programs** Generic Baccalaureate.
**Study Options** Full-time and part-time.
**Program Entrance Requirements** Transcript of college record, written essay, high school transcript, 2 letters of recommendation. Transfer students are accepted. *Application deadline:* 9/30 (fall), 11/30 (winter), 2/28 (spring), 6/15 (summer). *Application fee:* $50.
**Advanced Placement** Credit by examination available.
**Contact** *Telephone:* 703-821-8570.

# University of Virginia

## School of Nursing
## Charlottesville, Virginia

***http://www.nursing.virginia.edu/***
Founded in 1819

**DEGREES • BSN • MSN • MSN/MBA • MSN/PHD • PHD**
**Nursing Program Faculty** 99 (65% with doctorates).

**Baccalaureate Enrollment** 370 **Women** 95% **Men** 5% **Minority** 30% **International** 2% **Part-time** 5%

**Graduate Enrollment** 350 **Women** 88% **Men** 12% **Minority** 25% **International** 2% **Part-time** 50%

**Distance Learning Courses** Available.

**Nursing Student Activities** Nursing Honor Society, Sigma Theta Tau, Student Nurses' Association, nursing club.

**Nursing Student Resources** Academic advising; academic or career counseling; assistance for students with disabilities; bookstore; campus computer network; career placement assistance; computer-assisted instruction; e-mail services; employment services for current students; housing assistance; interactive nursing skills videos; Internet; learning resource lab; library services; nursing audiovisuals; placement services for program completers; remedial services; resume preparation assistance; skills, simulation, or other laboratory; tutoring.

**Library Facilities** 5.7 million volumes (200,000 in health); 124,721 periodical subscriptions (1,000 health-care related).

## BACCALAUREATE PROGRAMS

**Degree** BSN

**Available Programs** ADN to Baccalaureate; Generic Baccalaureate; RN Baccalaureate.

**Study Options** Full-time.

**Program Entrance Requirements** Transcript of college record, written essay, high school biology, 3 years high school math, 2 years high school science, high school transcript, 1 letter of recommendation, minimum high school GPA. Transfer students are accepted. *Application deadline:* 1/1 (fall). *Application fee:* $75.

**Advanced Placement** Credit by examination available.

**Expenses (2013–14)** *Tuition, state resident:* full-time $10,016; part-time $334 per credit hour. *Tuition, nonresident:* full-time $36,720; part-time $1194 per credit hour. *International tuition:* $36,720 full-time. *Room and board:* $9730; room only: $5350 per academic year. *Required fees:* full-time $2656.

**Financial Aid** 60% of baccalaureate students in nursing programs received some form of financial aid in 2012–13.

**Contact** Mr. Clay Hysell, Assistant Dean for Admissions and Financial Aid, School of Nursing, University of Virginia, Claude Moore Nursing Education Building, PO Box 800826, Charlottesville, VA 22908. *Telephone:* 888-283-8703. *Fax:* 434-924-0528. *E-mail:* nursing-admissions@virginia.edu.

## GRADUATE PROGRAMS

**Expenses (2013–14)** *Tuition, state resident:* full-time $13,818; part-time $746 per credit hour. *Tuition, nonresident:* full-time $23,142; part-time $1264 per credit hour. *International tuition:* $23,142 full-time. *Required fees:* full-time $2466.

**Financial Aid** 80% of graduate students in nursing programs received some form of financial aid in 2012–13. Fellowships, research assistantships, teaching assistantships, Federal Work-Study and scholarships available.

**Contact** Mr. Clay D. Hysell, Assistant Dean for Admissions and Financial Aid, School of Nursing, University of Virginia, Claude Moore Nursing Education Building, PO Box 800826, Charlottesville, VA 22908. *Telephone:* 888-283-8703. *Fax:* 434-924-0528. *E-mail:* nursing-admissions@virginia.edu.

### MASTER'S DEGREE PROGRAM

**Degrees** MSN; MSN/MBA; MSN/PhD

**Available Programs** Master's; Master's for Non-Nursing College Graduates; Master's for Nurses with Non-Nursing Degrees; RN to Master's.

**Concentrations Available** Clinical nurse leader; nursing administration. *Clinical nurse specialist programs in:* acute care, medical-surgical. *Nurse practitioner programs in:* acute care, community health, family health, pediatric, primary care, psychiatric/mental health.

**Study Options** Full-time and part-time.

**Program Entrance Requirements** Clinical experience, minimum overall college GPA of 3.0, transcript of college record, written essay, interview, 3 letters of recommendation, prerequisite course work, resume, statistics course, GRE General Test, MAT. *Application deadline:* 11/1 (fall). *Application fee:* $75.

**Advanced Placement** Credit given for nursing courses completed elsewhere dependent upon specific evaluations.

**Degree Requirements** 34 total credit hours.

### POST-MASTER'S PROGRAM

**Areas of Study** Nursing administration. *Clinical nurse specialist programs in:* acute care, medical-surgical. *Nurse practitioner programs in:* acute care, family health, pediatric, primary care, psychiatric/mental health.

### DOCTORAL DEGREE PROGRAM

**Degree** PhD

**Available Programs** Doctorate; Post-Baccalaureate Doctorate.

**Areas of Study** Advanced practice nursing, aging, bio-behavioral research, clinical practice, clinical research, community health, critical care, ethics, faculty preparation, family health, forensic nursing, gerontology, health policy, health promotion/disease prevention, health-care systems, human health and illness, information systems, maternity-newborn, nursing administration, nursing education, nursing policy, nursing research, nursing science, oncology, palliative care, urban health,women's health.

**Program Entrance Requirements** Minimum overall college GPA of 3.0, interview by faculty committee, interview, 3 letters of recommendation, statistics course, vita, GRE General Test. *Application deadline:* 12/15 (fall). Applications may be processed on a rolling basis for some programs. *Application fee:* $75.

**Degree Requirements** 46 total credit hours, dissertation, written exam, residency.

### POSTDOCTORAL PROGRAM

**Areas of Study** Nursing research, nursing science.

**Postdoctoral Program Contact** Mr. Clay D. Hysell, Assistant Dean for Admissions and Financial Aid, School of Nursing, University of Virginia, McLeod Hall, PO Box 800826, Charlottesville, VA 22908. *Telephone:* 434-924-0141. *Fax:* 434-924-0528. *E-mail:* cdh6n@virginia.edu.

# The University of Virginia's College at Wise

## Department of Nursing
## Wise, Virginia

***http://www.uvawise.edu/***

Founded in 1954

## DEGREE • BSN

**Nursing Program Faculty** 10 (30% with doctorates).

**Baccalaureate Enrollment** 47 **Women** 79% **Men** 21% **Minority** 15% **Part-time** 5%

**Nursing Student Activities** Sigma Theta Tau, Student Nurses' Association.

**Nursing Student Resources** Academic advising; academic or career counseling; assistance for students with disabilities; bookstore; campus computer network; career placement assistance; computer lab; computer-assisted instruction; e-mail services; employment services for current students; externships; housing assistance; interactive nursing skills videos; Internet; learning resource lab; library services; nursing audiovisuals; resume preparation assistance; skills, simulation, or other laboratory; tutoring.

**Library Facilities** 159,245 volumes (4,654 in health, 2,761 in nursing); 3,634 periodical subscriptions (40 health-care related).

## BACCALAUREATE PROGRAMS

**Degree** BSN

**Available Programs** ADN to Baccalaureate; Generic Baccalaureate; RN Baccalaureate.

**Study Options** Full-time.

**Program Entrance Requirements** Minimum overall college GPA of 2.75, transcript of college record, CPR certification, written essay, health exam, health insurance, immunizations, minimum GPA in nursing prerequisites of 2.75, professional liability insurance/malpractice insurance, prerequisite course work. Transfer students are accepted. *Application deadline:* 11/1 (spring). *Application fee:* $25.

**Advanced Placement** Credit given for nursing courses completed elsewhere dependent upon specific evaluations.

**Contact** *Telephone:* 276-328-0275. *Fax:* 276-376-4589.

## Virginia Commonwealth University
### School of Nursing
### Richmond, Virginia

***http://www.nursing.vcu.edu/***
Founded in 1838

**DEGREES • BS • MS • PHD**
**Nursing Program Faculty** 129 (30% with doctorates).
**Baccalaureate Enrollment** 624 **Women** 90% **Men** 10% **Minority** 30% **Part-time** 43%
**Graduate Enrollment** 285 **Women** 94% **Men** 6% **Minority** 26% **Part-time** 67%
**Distance Learning Courses** Available.
**Nursing Student Activities** Sigma Theta Tau, Student Nurses' Association, nursing club.
**Nursing Student Resources** Academic advising; academic or career counseling; assistance for students with disabilities; bookstore; campus computer network; career placement assistance; computer lab; computer-assisted instruction; daycare for children of students; e-mail services; employment services for current students; externships; housing assistance; interactive nursing skills videos; Internet; learning resource lab; library services; nursing audiovisuals; paid internships; placement services for program completers; remedial services; resume preparation assistance; skills, simulation, or other laboratory; tutoring.
**Library Facilities** 2.5 million volumes (492,674 in health, 13,071 in nursing); 61,000 periodical subscriptions (14,256 health-care related).

#### BACCALAUREATE PROGRAMS

**Degree** BS
**Available Programs** ADN to Baccalaureate; Accelerated Baccalaureate for Second Degree; Generic Baccalaureate.
**Study Options** Full-time.
**Program Entrance Requirements** Minimum overall college GPA of 2.5, transcript of college record, CPR certification, written essay, immunizations, 3 letters of recommendation, minimum GPA in nursing prerequisites of 2.5, prerequisite course work. Transfer students are accepted. *Application deadline:* 2/1 (fall). *Application fee:* $40.
**Advanced Placement** Credit by examination available. Credit given for nursing courses completed elsewhere dependent upon specific evaluations.
**Expenses (2013–14)** *Tuition, state resident:* full-time $9536; part-time $425 per credit hour. *Tuition, nonresident:* full-time $25,814; part-time $922 per credit hour. *International tuition:* $25,814 full-time. *Room and board:* $8543; room only: $5215 per academic year. *Required fees:* full-time $2071; part-time $85 per credit.
**Financial Aid** 82% of baccalaureate students in nursing programs received some form of financial aid in 2012–13.
**Contact** Mrs. Susan L. Lipp, Assistant Dean of Enrollment and Student Services, School of Nursing, Virginia Commonwealth University, 1100 East Leigh Street, PO Box 980567, Richmond, VA 23298-0567. *Telephone:* 804-828-5171. *Fax:* 804-828-7743. *E-mail:* slipp@vcu.edu.

#### GRADUATE PROGRAMS

**Expenses (2013–14)** *Tuition, state resident:* full-time $9911; part-time $551 per credit hour. *Tuition, nonresident:* full-time $20,378; part-time $1132 per credit hour. *International tuition:* $20,378 full-time. *Room and board:* $8543; room only: $5215 per academic year. *Required fees:* full-time $1036; part-time $85 per credit.
**Financial Aid** 80% of graduate students in nursing programs received some form of financial aid in 2012–13. Fellowships, research assistantships, teaching assistantships, career-related internships or fieldwork and institutionally sponsored loans available.
**Contact** Mrs. Susan L. Lipp, Assistant Dean of Enrollment and Student Services, School of Nursing, Virginia Commonwealth University, 1100 East Leigh Street, PO Box 980567, Richmond, VA 23298-0567. *Telephone:* 804-828-5171. *Fax:* 804-828-7743. *E-mail:* slipp@vcu.edu.

#### MASTER'S DEGREE PROGRAM

**Degree** MS
**Available Programs** Master's; RN to Master's.
**Concentrations Available** Nursing administration. *Nurse practitioner programs in:* acute care, family health, psychiatric/mental health.
**Study Options** Full-time and part-time.
**Program Entrance Requirements** Computer literacy, minimum overall college GPA of 3.0, transcript of college record, CPR certification, written essay, immunizations, 3 letters of recommendation, prerequisite course work, resume, statistics course, GRE General Test. *Application deadline:* 3/15 (fall), 9/15 (spring). *Application fee:* $65.
**Advanced Placement** Credit given for nursing courses completed elsewhere dependent upon specific evaluations.
**Degree Requirements** 55 total credit hours.

#### POST-MASTER'S PROGRAM

**Areas of Study** Nursing administration. *Nurse practitioner programs in:* acute care, family health, psychiatric/mental health.

#### DOCTORAL DEGREE PROGRAM

**Degree** PhD
**Available Programs** Doctorate.
**Areas of Study** Bio-behavioral research.
**Online Degree Options** Yes (online only).
**Program Entrance Requirements** Minimum overall college GPA of 3.0, interview by faculty committee, interview, 3 letters of recommendation, MSN or equivalent, statistics course, vita, writing sample, GRE General Test. *Application deadline:* 2/1 (fall). *Application fee:* $65.
**Degree Requirements** 61 total credit hours, dissertation, written exam.

#### POSTDOCTORAL PROGRAM

**Postdoctoral Program Contact** Ms. Susan L. Lipp, Assistant Dean of Enrollment and Student Services, School of Nursing, Virginia Commonwealth University, 1100 East Leigh Street, PO Box 980567, Richmond, VA 23298-0567. *Telephone:* 804-828-5171. *Fax:* 804-828-7743. *E-mail:* slipp@vcu.edu.

# WASHINGTON

## Eastern Washington University
### Intercollegiate College of Nursing/Washington State University
### Cheney, Washington

***See description of programs under Intercollegiate College of Nursing/Washington State University (Spokane, Washington).***

## Gonzaga University
### Department of Nursing
### Spokane, Washington

***https://www.gonzaga.edu/***
Founded in 1887

**DEGREES • BSN • MSN**
**Nursing Program Faculty** 15 (73% with doctorates).
**Baccalaureate Enrollment** 233 **Women** 93% **Men** 7%
**Graduate Enrollment** 337 **Women** 94% **Men** 6% **Part-time** 14%
**Distance Learning Courses** Available.
**Nursing Student Activities** Sigma Theta Tau, Student Nurses' Association.
**Nursing Student Resources** Academic advising; academic or career counseling; assistance for students with disabilities; bookstore; campus computer network; computer lab; computer-assisted instruction; e-mail services; housing assistance; interactive nursing skills videos; Internet; learning resource lab; library services; nursing audiovisuals; resume preparation assistance; skills, simulation, or other laboratory; tutoring.
**Library Facilities** 286,482 volumes (35,000 in health, 950 in nursing); 58,763 periodical subscriptions (206 health-care related).

#### BACCALAUREATE PROGRAMS

**Degree** BSN
**Available Programs** Generic Baccalaureate.
**Study Options** Full-time and part-time.
**Program Entrance Requirements** Minimum overall college GPA of 2.9, transcript of college record, written essay, high school biology, high school chemistry, 4 years high school math, 4 years high school science,

high school transcript, 2 letters of recommendation, minimum high school GPA of 2.9, minimum GPA in nursing prerequisites of 2.0, prerequisite course work. Transfer students are accepted. *Application deadline:* 1/15 (fall), 9/15 (spring). *Application fee:* $50.

**Advanced Placement** Credit given for nursing courses completed elsewhere dependent upon specific evaluations.

**Contact** *Telephone:* 509-313-3580. *Fax:* 509-313-5827.

## GRADUATE PROGRAMS

**Contact** *Telephone:* 509-313-6640. *Fax:* 509-323-5827.

### MASTER'S DEGREE PROGRAM

**Degree** MSN

**Available Programs** Accelerated RN to Master's; Master's; Master's for Nurses with Non-Nursing Degrees.

**Concentrations Available** Health-care administration; nursing administration; nursing education. *Clinical nurse specialist programs in:* psychiatric/mental health. *Nurse practitioner programs in:* family health, primary care, psychiatric/mental health.

**Study Options** Full-time and part-time.

**Online Degree Options** Yes (online only).

**Program Entrance Requirements** Computer literacy, minimum overall college GPA of 3.0, transcript of college record, written essay, 2 letters of recommendation, resume, statistics course, MAT. *Application deadline:* Applications may be processed on a rolling basis for some programs.

**Advanced Placement** Credit given for nursing courses completed elsewhere dependent upon specific evaluations.

**Degree Requirements** 36 total credit hours.

### POST-MASTER'S PROGRAM

**Areas of Study** Health-care administration; nursing administration; nursing education. *Clinical nurse specialist programs in:* psychiatric/mental health. *Nurse practitioner programs in:* family health, primary care, psychiatric/mental health.

### DOCTORAL DEGREE PROGRAM

**Program Entrance Requirements** MAT or GRE within the last 5 years.

# Northwest University

**The Mark and Huldah Buntain School of Nursing**
**Kirkland, Washington**

*http://www.northwestu.edu/schools/nursing/*
Founded in 1934

**DEGREE • BS**

**Nursing Program Faculty** 24 (16% with doctorates).

**Baccalaureate Enrollment** 50 **Women** 87% **Men** 13% **Minority** 11%

**Nursing Student Resources** Academic advising; academic or career counseling; assistance for students with disabilities; bookstore; campus computer network; computer lab; computer-assisted instruction; e-mail services; employment services for current students; housing assistance; interactive nursing skills videos; Internet; learning resource lab; library services; nursing audiovisuals; other; remedial services; resume preparation assistance; skills, simulation, or other laboratory; tutoring; unpaid internships.

**Library Facilities** 100,356 volumes (1,922 in health, 387 in nursing); 13,443 periodical subscriptions (815 health-care related).

## BACCALAUREATE PROGRAMS

**Degree** BS

**Available Programs** Generic Baccalaureate.

**Study Options** Full-time.

**Program Entrance Requirements** Minimum overall college GPA of 3.0, transcript of college record, CPR certification, written essay, health exam, health insurance, high school transcript, immunizations, 2 letters of recommendation, minimum GPA in nursing prerequisites of 3.0, prerequisite course work. Transfer students are accepted. *Application deadline:* 1/30 (fall). *Application fee:* $35.

**Contact** *Telephone:* 800-669-3781 Ext. 7822. *Fax:* 425-889-7822.

# Olympic College

**Nursing Programs**
**Bremerton, Washington**

Founded in 1946

**DEGREE • BSN**

## BACCALAUREATE PROGRAMS

**Degree** BSN

**Available Programs** RN Baccalaureate.

**Study Options** Full-time and part-time.

**Program Entrance Requirements** Minimum overall college GPA of 2.5, minimum GPA in nursing prerequisites of 2.0, RN licensure.

**Contact** *Telephone:* 360-475-7748. *Fax:* 360-475-7628.

# Pacific Lutheran University

**School of Nursing**
**Tacoma, Washington**

*http://www.plu.edu/nursing/*
Founded in 1890

**DEGREES • BSN • MSN • MSN/MBA**

**Nursing Program Faculty** 30 (40% with doctorates).

**Baccalaureate Enrollment** 233 **Women** 89% **Men** 11% **Minority** 15% **International** 2%

**Graduate Enrollment** 56 **Women** 82% **Men** 18% **Minority** 6% **International** 2%

**Nursing Student Activities** Nursing Honor Society, Sigma Theta Tau, Student Nurses' Association, nursing club.

**Nursing Student Resources** Academic advising; academic or career counseling; assistance for students with disabilities; bookstore; campus computer network; career placement assistance; computer lab; computer-assisted instruction; e-mail services; employment services for current students; housing assistance; interactive nursing skills videos; Internet; learning resource lab; library services; nursing audiovisuals; other; resume preparation assistance; skills, simulation, or other laboratory; tutoring; unpaid internships.

**Library Facilities** 337,167 volumes (15,000 in health, 6,500 in nursing); 5,808 periodical subscriptions (150 health-care related).

## BACCALAUREATE PROGRAMS

**Degree** BSN

**Available Programs** Generic Baccalaureate; LPN to Baccalaureate.

**Study Options** Full-time.

**Program Entrance Requirements** Minimum overall college GPA of 3.0, transcript of college record, CPR certification, written essay, health exam, health insurance, high school foreign language, 2 years high school math, high school transcript, immunizations, 2 letters of recommendation, minimum GPA in nursing prerequisites of 2.75, professional liability insurance/malpractice insurance, prerequisite course work. Transfer students are accepted. *Application deadline:* 2/1 (fall), 2/1 (spring). Applications may be processed on a rolling basis for some programs.

**Advanced Placement** Credit by examination available. Credit given for nursing courses completed elsewhere dependent upon specific evaluations.

**Expenses (2013–14)** *Tuition:* full-time $34,440; part-time $1080 per credit hour. *International tuition:* $34,440 full-time.

**Financial Aid** 90% of baccalaureate students in nursing programs received some form of financial aid in 2012–13. *Gift aid (need-based):* Federal Pell, FSEOG, state, private, college/university gift aid from institutional funds, Federal Nursing. *Loans:* Federal Nursing Student Loans, Federal Direct (Subsidized and Unsubsidized Stafford PLUS), Perkins, state. *Work-study:* Federal Work-Study, part-time campus jobs. *Financial aid application deadline (priority):* 1/31.

**Contact** Admissions Coordinator, School of Nursing, Pacific Lutheran University, 12180 Park Avenue South, Tacoma, WA 98447-0029. *Telephone:* 253-535-7672. *Fax:* 253-535-7590.

## GRADUATE PROGRAMS

**Expenses (2013–14)** *Tuition:* part-time $1080 per credit hour.

**Financial Aid** 90% of graduate students in nursing programs received some form of financial aid in 2012–13. Fellowships, Federal Work-Study and scholarships available. *Financial aid application deadline:* 3/1.

**Contact** Dr. Teri M. Woo, Associate Dean for Graduate Nursing Programs, School of Nursing, Pacific Lutheran University, 12180 Park Avenue South, Tacoma, WA 98447-0029. *Telephone:* 253-535-7672. *Fax:* 253-535-7590. *E-mail:* gradnurs@plu.edu.

### MASTER'S DEGREE PROGRAM

**Degrees** MSN; MSN/MBA
**Available Programs** Accelerated Master's for Non-Nursing College Graduates; Master's; Master's for Nurses with Non-Nursing Degrees.
**Concentrations Available** Clinical nurse leader; health-care administration; nurse case management; nursing administration; nursing education. *Nurse practitioner programs in:* family health.
**Study Options** Full-time.
**Program Entrance Requirements** Clinical experience, computer literacy, minimum overall college GPA of 3.0, transcript of college record, CPR certification, written essay, immunizations, interview, 2 letters of recommendation, professional liability insurance/malpractice insurance, prerequisite course work, resume, statistics course, GRE General Test. *Application deadline:* 11/15 (summer). Applications may be processed on a rolling basis for some programs. *Application fee:* $40.
**Advanced Placement** Credit given for nursing courses completed elsewhere dependent upon specific evaluations.
**Degree Requirements** 33 total credit hours, thesis or project.

### CONTINUING EDUCATION PROGRAM

**Contact** Ms. Jessica J. Immerman, Coordinator, Continuing Nursing Education and Clinical Placements, School of Nursing, Pacific Lutheran University, 12180 Park Avenue South, Tacoma, WA 98447-0029. *Telephone:* 253-535-7683. *Fax:* 253-535-7590. *E-mail:* immermjJ@plu.edu.

## Seattle Pacific University

### School of Health Sciences
### Seattle, Washington

***http://www.spu.edu/depts/hsc***
Founded in 1891

**DEGREES • BS • MSN**
**Nursing Program Faculty** 23 (39% with doctorates).
**Baccalaureate Enrollment** 98 **Women** 91% **Men** 9% **Minority** 21% **International** 2%
**Graduate Enrollment** 61 **Women** 89% **Men** 11% **Minority** 39% **Part-time** 49%
**Nursing Student Activities** Nursing Honor Society, Sigma Theta Tau, Student Nurses' Association, nursing club.
**Nursing Student Resources** Academic advising; academic or career counseling; assistance for students with disabilities; bookstore; campus computer network; career placement assistance; computer lab; computer-assisted instruction; e-mail services; employment services for current students; housing assistance; Internet; learning resource lab; library services; nursing audiovisuals; placement services for program completers; remedial services; resume preparation assistance; skills, simulation, or other laboratory; tutoring; unpaid internships.
**Library Facilities** 217,369 volumes (11,539 in health, 1,791 in nursing); 2,729 periodical subscriptions (274 health-care related).

### BACCALAUREATE PROGRAMS

**Degree** BS
**Available Programs** Generic Baccalaureate; RN Baccalaureate.
**Study Options** Full-time.
**Program Entrance Requirements** Minimum overall college GPA of 2.75, transcript of college record, CPR certification, written essay, health exam, health insurance, high school transcript, immunizations, 1 letter of recommendation, minimum GPA in nursing prerequisites of 2.75, prerequisite course work. Transfer students are accepted. *Application deadline:* 1/15 (fall).
**Advanced Placement** Credit given for nursing courses completed elsewhere dependent upon specific evaluations.
**Contact** *Telephone:* 206-281-2612. *Fax:* 206-281-2767.

### GRADUATE PROGRAMS

**Contact** *Telephone:* 206-281-2888. *Fax:* 206-378-5480.

### MASTER'S DEGREE PROGRAM

**Degree** MSN
**Available Programs** Master's; Master's for Nurses with Non-Nursing Degrees.
**Concentrations Available** Nursing administration; nursing education. *Clinical nurse specialist programs in:* acute care, adult health, community health, critical care, gerontology, medical-surgical, oncology, palliative care, parent-child, pediatric,women's health. *Nurse practitioner programs in:* adult health, family health.
**Study Options** Full-time and part-time.
**Program Entrance Requirements** Clinical experience, computer literacy, minimum overall college GPA of 3.0, transcript of college record, CPR certification, written essay, immunizations, interview, 3 letters of recommendation, nursing research course, professional liability insurance/malpractice insurance, prerequisite course work, resume, statistics course, GRE General Test. *Application deadline:* 5/1 (fall). *Application fee:* $50.
**Advanced Placement** Credit given for nursing courses completed elsewhere dependent upon specific evaluations.
**Degree Requirements** 59 total credit hours, thesis or project, comprehensive exam.

### POST-MASTER'S PROGRAM

**Areas of Study** Nursing education. *Nurse practitioner programs in:* adult health, family health.

## Seattle University

### College of Nursing
### Seattle, Washington

***http://www.seattleu.edu/nursing***
Founded in 1891

**DEGREES • BSN • DNP • MSN**
**Nursing Program Faculty** 79 (42% with doctorates).
**Baccalaureate Enrollment** 464 **Women** 90% **Men** 10% **Minority** 37% **International** 1%
**Graduate Enrollment** 110 **Women** 89% **Men** 11% **Minority** 18% **International** 1%
**Distance Learning Courses** Available.
**Nursing Student Activities** Sigma Theta Tau, Student Nurses' Association.
**Nursing Student Resources** Academic advising; academic or career counseling; assistance for students with disabilities; bookstore; campus computer network; career placement assistance; computer lab; computer-assisted instruction; e-mail services; employment services for current students; housing assistance; interactive nursing skills videos; Internet; learning resource lab; library services; nursing audiovisuals; paid internships; remedial services; resume preparation assistance; skills, simulation, or other laboratory; tutoring.
**Library Facilities** 293,806 volumes; 1,569 periodical subscriptions.

### BACCALAUREATE PROGRAMS

**Degree** BSN
**Available Programs** Baccalaureate for Second Degree; Generic Baccalaureate.
**Study Options** Full-time.
**Program Entrance Requirements** Minimum overall college GPA of 2.75, transcript of college record, written essay, health insurance, high school biology, high school chemistry, high school foreign language, 3 years high school math, 2 years high school science, high school transcript, minimum GPA in nursing prerequisites of 3.0, prerequisite course work. Transfer students are accepted. *Application deadline:* 1/5 (winter). *Application fee:* $50.
**Financial Aid** 80% of baccalaureate students in nursing programs received some form of financial aid in 2012–13. *Gift aid (need-based):* Federal Pell, FSEOG, state, private, college/university gift aid from institutional funds, Federal Nursing. *Loans:* Federal Nursing Student Loans, Federal Direct (Subsidized and Unsubsidized Stafford PLUS), Perkins. *Work-study:* Federal Work-Study, part-time campus jobs. *Financial aid application deadline (priority):* 2/1.
**Contact** Rita Tower, Pre-Major Advisor, College of Nursing, Seattle University, 901 12th Avenue, PO Box 222000, Seattle, WA 98122-1090. *Telephone:* 206-296-2242. *Fax:* 206-296-5544. *E-mail:* rstower@seattleu.edu.

### GRADUATE PROGRAMS

**Financial Aid** 81% of graduate students in nursing programs received some form of financial aid in 2012–13. Fellowships, research assistant-

ships, career-related internships or fieldwork, Federal Work-Study, and scholarships available. Aid available to part-time students.
**Contact** Dr. Anne Hirsch, Associate Dean for Graduate Education, College of Nursing, Seattle University, 901 12th Avenue, PO Box 222000, Seattle, WA 98122-1090. *Telephone:* 206-296-5660. *Fax:* 206-296-5544. *E-mail:* nurse@seattleu.edu.

### MASTER'S DEGREE PROGRAM
**Degree** MSN
**Available Programs** Accelerated Master's for Nurses with Non-Nursing Degrees; Master's.
**Concentrations Available** *Clinical nurse specialist programs in:* community health. *Nurse practitioner programs in:* family health, gerontology, psychiatric/mental health.
**Study Options** Full-time.
**Program Entrance Requirements** Clinical experience, computer literacy, minimum overall college GPA of 3.0, transcript of college record, CPR certification, written essay, immunizations, interview, 2 letters of recommendation, professional liability insurance/malpractice insurance, prerequisite course work, resume, statistics course, GRE General Test. *Application deadline:* 12/1 (fall). *Application fee:* $55.
**Advanced Placement** Credit given for nursing courses completed elsewhere dependent upon specific evaluations.
**Degree Requirements** 110 total credit hours, thesis or project.

### POST-MASTER'S PROGRAM
**Areas of Study** *Clinical nurse specialist programs in:* community health. *Nurse practitioner programs in:* family health, gerontology, psychiatric/mental health.

### DOCTORAL DEGREE PROGRAM
**Degree** DNP
**Available Programs** Doctorate.
**Areas of Study** Advanced practice nursing, clinical practice, community health, critical care, family health, health policy, individualized study, information systems, nursing education, nursing policy, nursing research.
**Program Entrance Requirements** Clinical experience, minimum overall college GPA of 3.25, interview by faculty committee, 2 letters of recommendation, MSN or equivalent, writing sample. *Application deadline:* 5/1 (fall). Applications may be processed on a rolling basis for some programs. *Application fee:* $55.
**Degree Requirements** 40 total credit hours.

# University of Washington
## School of Nursing
## Seattle, Washington

***http://www.nursing.uw.edu/***
Founded in 1861

**DEGREES • BSN • DNP • MN • MN/MPH • PHD**
**Nursing Program Faculty** 246 (78% with doctorates).
**Baccalaureate Enrollment** 559 **Women** 84% **Men** 16% **Minority** 26% **International** 2% **Part-time** 13%
**Graduate Enrollment** 565 **Women** 87% **Men** 13% **Minority** 25% **International** 5% **Part-time** 59%
**Distance Learning Courses** Available.
**Nursing Student Activities** Sigma Theta Tau, Student Nurses' Association.
**Nursing Student Resources** Academic advising; academic or career counseling; assistance for students with disabilities; bookstore; campus computer network; computer lab; computer-assisted instruction; e-mail services; employment services for current students; interactive nursing skills videos; Internet; learning resource lab; library services; nursing audiovisuals; skills, simulation, or other laboratory.
**Library Facilities** 350,000 volumes in health; 2,400 periodical subscriptions health-care related.

### BACCALAUREATE PROGRAMS
**Degree** BSN
**Available Programs** ADN to Baccalaureate; Accelerated Baccalaureate; Generic Baccalaureate.
**Site Options** Bothell, WA; Tacoma, WA.
**Study Options** Full-time.
**Program Entrance Requirements** Minimum overall college GPA of 2.0, transcript of college record, written essay, 1 letter of recommendation, minimum GPA in nursing prerequisites of 2.0, prerequisite course work. *Application deadline:* 1/15 (fall).
**Expenses (2013–14)** *Tuition, state resident:* full-time $11,307; part-time $376 per credit. *Tuition, nonresident:* full-time $30,882; part-time $1030 per credit. *International tuition:* $30,882 full-time. *Room and board:* $9948; room only: $5550 per academic year. *Required fees:* full-time $1232.
**Financial Aid** ***Gift aid (need-based):*** Federal Pell, FSEOG, state, private, college/university gift aid from institutional funds. *Loans:* Federal Nursing Student Loans, Federal Direct (Subsidized and Unsubsidized Stafford PLUS), Perkins, college/university. *Work-study:* Federal Work-Study, part-time campus jobs. *Financial aid application deadline (priority):* 2/28.
**Contact** Academic Services, School of Nursing, University of Washington, Box 357260, Health Sciences Building, Room T310, Seattle, WA 98195. *Telephone:* 206-543-8736. *Fax:* 206-543-3624. *E-mail:* sonas@u.washington.edu.

### GRADUATE PROGRAMS
**Financial Aid** Fellowships, research assistantships, teaching assistantships, Federal Work-Study, institutionally sponsored loans, scholarships, and traineeships available.
**Contact** Academic Services, School of Nursing, University of Washington, Box 357260, Health Sciences Building, Room T310, Seattle, WA 98195. *Telephone:* 206-543-8736. *Fax:* 206-543-3624. *E-mail:* sonas@u.washington.edu.

### MASTER'S DEGREE PROGRAM
**Degrees** MN; MN/MPH
**Available Programs** Master's; Master's for Nurses with Non-Nursing Degrees.
**Concentrations Available** *Clinical nurse specialist programs in:* community health.
**Site Options** Bothell, WA; Tacoma, WA.
**Study Options** Full-time and part-time.
**Program Entrance Requirements** Minimum overall college GPA of 3.0, transcript of college record, written essay, 3 letters of recommendation, resume, statistics course, GRE. *Application deadline:* 1/15 (fall). *Application fee:* $85.
**Advanced Placement** Credit given for nursing courses completed elsewhere dependent upon specific evaluations.
**Degree Requirements** 38 total credit hours, thesis or project.

**Degree** MS
**Available Programs** Master's; Master's for Nurses with Non-Nursing Degrees; Master's for Non-Nursing College Graduates.
**Concentrations Available** Nursing informatics.
**Study Options** Full-time and part-time.
**Online Degree Options** Yes (online only).
**Program Entrance Requirements** Minimum overall college GPA of 3.0, transcript of college record, written essay, 3 letters of recommendation, resume, statistics course. *Application deadline:* 5/1 (fall). *Application fee:* $85.
**Advanced Placement** Credit given for nursing courses completed elsewhere dependent upon specific evaluations.
**Degree Requirements** 46 total credit hours, thesis or project.

### POST-MASTER'S PROGRAM
**Areas of Study** Nurse-midwifery. *Clinical nurse specialist programs in:* pediatric, perinatal, psychiatric/mental health. *Nurse practitioner programs in:* neonatal health, pediatric, psychiatric/mental health.

### DOCTORAL DEGREE PROGRAM
**Degree** DNP
**Available Programs** Doctorate; Doctorate for Nurses with Non-Nursing Degrees; Post-Baccalaureate Doctorate.
**Areas of Study** Advanced practice nursing.
**Program Entrance Requirements** Minimum overall college GPA of 3.0, 3 letters of recommendation, statistics course, vita, writing sample, GRE. *Application deadline:* 1/15 (fall). *Application fee:* $85.
**Degree Requirements** 93 total credit hours, oral exam.

**Degree** PhD
**Available Programs** Doctorate, Doctorate for Nurses with Non-Nursing Degrees, Post-Baccalaureate Doctorate.
**Areas of Study** Clinical research, health policy, nursing education, nursing research, nursing science.

**Program Entrance Requirements** Minimum overall college GPA of 3.0, 3 letters of recommendation, statistics course, vita, writing sample. *Application deadline:* 1/15 (fall). *Application fee:* $85.
**Degree Requirements** 93 total credit hours, dissertation, oral exam, written exam.

**POSTDOCTORAL PROGRAM**
**Postdoctoral Program Contact** Academic Services, School of Nursing, University of Washington, Box 357260, Health Sciences Building, Room T310, Seattle, WA 98195. *Telephone:* 206-543-8736. *Fax:* 206-685-1613. *E-mail:* sonas@u.washington.edu.

### CONTINUING EDUCATION PROGRAM

**Contact** Martha Duhamel, Assistant Dean for Continuing Nursing Education, School of Nursing, University of Washington, Box 359440, Seattle, WA 98195-9440. *Telephone:* 206-543-1047. *Fax:* 206-543-6953. *E-mail:* marthadu@u.washington.edu.

## Walla Walla University
### School of Nursing
### College Place, Washington

***http://www.wallawalla.edu/nursing***
Founded in 1892

**DEGREE • BS**
**Nursing Program Faculty** 25 (12% with doctorates).
**Baccalaureate Enrollment** 190 **Women** 82% **Men** 18% **Minority** 21% **International** 1% **Part-time** 2%
**Nursing Student Activities** Nursing Honor Society, nursing club.
**Nursing Student Resources** Academic advising; academic or career counseling; assistance for students with disabilities; bookstore; campus computer network; computer lab; e-mail services; Internet; learning resource lab; library services; nursing audiovisuals; skills, simulation, or other laboratory; tutoring.
**Library Facilities** 10,000 volumes in health, 7,000 volumes in nursing; 450 periodical subscriptions health-care related.

### BACCALAUREATE PROGRAMS

**Degree** BS
**Available Programs** ADN to Baccalaureate; Generic Baccalaureate; LPN to Baccalaureate; RN Baccalaureate.
**Site Options** Portland, OR.
**Study Options** Full-time.
**Program Entrance Requirements** Minimum overall college GPA of 2.75, transcript of college record, CPR certification, written essay, health exam, health insurance, high school biology, 3 years high school math, 2 years high school science, high school transcript, immunizations, 3 letters of recommendation, minimum high school GPA of 2.75, minimum GPA in nursing prerequisites of 2.75, prerequisite course work. Transfer students are accepted. *Application deadline:* 4/15 (fall), 2/1 (summer). *Application fee:* $40.
**Advanced Placement** Credit given for nursing courses completed elsewhere dependent upon specific evaluations.
**Expenses (2013–14)** *Tuition:* full-time $24,822; part-time $648 per credit. *International tuition:* $24,822 full-time. *Room and board:* $5970; room only: $3360 per academic year. *Required fees:* full-time $1155; part-time $20 per credit.
**Financial Aid** 95% of baccalaureate students in nursing programs received some form of financial aid in 2012–13.
**Contact** Jan Thurnhofer, Student Program Advisor, School of Nursing, Walla Walla University, 10345 SE Market Street, Portland, OR 97216. *Telephone:* 503-251-6115 Ext. 7304. *Fax:* 503-251-6249. *E-mail:* jant@wallawalla.edu.

## Washington State University
### Intercollegiate College of Nursing/Washington State University
### Pullman, Washington

***See description of programs under Intercollegiate College of Nursing/Washington State University (Spokane, Washington).***

## Washington State University College of Nursing
### Washington State University College of Nursing
### Spokane, Washington

***http://www.nursing.wsu.edu/***

**DEGREES • BSN • MN • PHD**
**Nursing Program Faculty** 114 (39% with doctorates).
**Baccalaureate Enrollment** 759 **Women** 84% **Men** 16% **Minority** 22% **Part-time** 29%
**Graduate Enrollment** 274 **Women** 89% **Men** 11% **Minority** 12% **International** 1% **Part-time** 83%
**Distance Learning Courses** Available.
**Nursing Student Activities** Nursing Honor Society, Sigma Theta Tau, Student Nurses' Association, nursing club.
**Nursing Student Resources** Academic advising; academic or career counseling; assistance for students with disabilities; bookstore; campus computer network; computer lab; computer-assisted instruction; e-mail services; interactive nursing skills videos; Internet; learning resource lab; library services; nursing audiovisuals; other; remedial services; resume preparation assistance; skills, simulation, or other laboratory; tutoring; unpaid internships.
**Library Facilities** 15,000 volumes in health, 7,000 volumes in nursing; 2,000 periodical subscriptions health-care related.

### BACCALAUREATE PROGRAMS

**Degree** BSN
**Available Programs** Generic Baccalaureate; RN Baccalaureate.
**Site Options** Richland, WA; Yakima, WA; Vancouver, WA.
**Study Options** Full-time.
**Program Entrance Requirements** Minimum overall college GPA of 2.8, transcript of college record, CPR certification, health insurance, immunizations, interview, minimum GPA in nursing prerequisites of 2.8, professional liability insurance/malpractice insurance, prerequisite course work. Transfer students are accepted. *Application deadline:* 1/15 (fall), 8/5 (spring). *Application fee:* $45.
**Advanced Placement** Credit given for nursing courses completed elsewhere dependent upon specific evaluations.
**Contact** *Telephone:* 509-324-7337. *Fax:* 509-324-7336.

### GRADUATE PROGRAMS

**Contact** *Telephone:* 509-324-7334. *Fax:* 509-324-7336.

**MASTER'S DEGREE PROGRAM**
**Degree** MN
**Available Programs** Accelerated Master's for Nurses with Non-Nursing Degrees; Accelerated RN to Master's; Master's.
**Concentrations Available** Nurse case management; nursing administration; nursing education. *Clinical nurse specialist programs in:* community health. *Nurse practitioner programs in:* family health, psychiatric/mental health.
**Site Options** Richland, WA; Yakima, WA; Vancouver, WA.
**Study Options** Full-time and part-time.
**Program Entrance Requirements** Computer literacy, minimum overall college GPA of 3.0, transcript of college record, CPR certification, written essay, immunizations, interview, 3 letters of recommendation, physical assessment course, professional liability insurance/malpractice insurance, prerequisite course work, statistics course. *Application deadline:* 2/1 (fall), 10/1 (spring).
**Advanced Placement** Credit given for nursing courses completed elsewhere dependent upon specific evaluations.
**Degree Requirements** 45 total credit hours, thesis or project.

**POST-MASTER'S PROGRAM**
**Areas of Study** *Nurse practitioner programs in:* family health, psychiatric/mental health.

**DOCTORAL DEGREE PROGRAM**
**Degree** PhD
**Available Programs** Doctorate.
**Areas of Study** Nursing education, nursing research.
**Program Entrance Requirements** Minimum overall college GPA of 3.5, interview by faculty committee, 3 letters of recommendation, MSN or equivalent, scholarly papers, statistics course, vita. *Application deadline:* 1/10 (summer).
**Degree Requirements** 72 total credit hours, dissertation.

### CONTINUING EDUCATION PROGRAM

**Contact** *Telephone:* 509-324-7354. *Fax:* 509-324-7341.

## Whitworth College

### Intercollegiate College of Nursing/Washington State University
### Spokane, Washington

*See description of programs under Intercollegiate College of Nursing/Washington State University (Spokane, Washington).*

# WEST VIRGINIA

## Alderson Broaddus University

### Department of Nursing
### Philippi, West Virginia

*http://www.ab.edu/*
Founded in 1871

### DEGREE • BSN

**Nursing Program Faculty** 13 (1% with doctorates).
**Baccalaureate Enrollment** 96 **Women** 94% **Men** 6% **Minority** 2% **International** 1% **Part-time** 2%
**Nursing Student Activities** Student Nurses' Association.
**Nursing Student Resources** Academic advising; academic or career counseling; assistance for students with disabilities; bookstore; campus computer network; career placement assistance; computer lab; computer-assisted instruction; e-mail services; employment services for current students; Internet; learning resource lab; library services; nursing audiovisuals; remedial services; resume preparation assistance; skills, simulation, or other laboratory; tutoring.
**Library Facilities** 50,000 volumes (6,000 in health, 1,000 in nursing); 11,000 periodical subscriptions (172 health-care related).

### BACCALAUREATE PROGRAMS

**Degree** BSN
**Available Programs** Generic Baccalaureate; LPN to RN Baccalaureate; RN Baccalaureate.
**Study Options** Full-time.
**Program Entrance Requirements** Minimum overall college GPA of 2.0, transcript of college record, CPR certification, health exam, high school chemistry, high school transcript, immunizations, minimum GPA in nursing prerequisites of 2.25, professional liability insurance/malpractice insurance, prerequisite course work. Transfer students are accepted. *Application deadline:* 7/30 (fall), 1/5 (winter). Applications may be processed on a rolling basis for some programs. *Application fee:* $25.
**Advanced Placement** Credit by examination available. Credit given for nursing courses completed elsewhere dependent upon specific evaluations.
**Contact** *Telephone:* 304-457-6384. *Fax:* 304-457-6293.

## American Public University System

### Bachelor of Science in Nursing
### Charles Town, West Virginia

Founded in 1991

### DEGREE • BSN

**Library Facilities** 150,000 volumes; 35,000 periodical subscriptions.

### BACCALAUREATE PROGRAMS

**Degree** BSN
**Available Programs** RN Baccalaureate.
**Online Degree Options** Yes (online only).
**Contact** Nursing Program Information, Bachelor of Science in Nursing, American Public University System, 111 West Congress Street, Charles Town, WV 25414. *Telephone:* 304-724-3700.

## Bluefield State College

### Program in Nursing
### Bluefield, West Virginia

*http://www.bluefieldstate.edu/*
Founded in 1895

### DEGREE • BSN

**Nursing Program Faculty** 15
**Baccalaureate Enrollment** 4 **Women** 93% **Men** 7% **Part-time** 20%
**Distance Learning Courses** Available.
**Nursing Student Activities** Nursing Honor Society, Sigma Theta Tau, Student Nurses' Association.
**Nursing Student Resources** Academic advising; academic or career counseling; assistance for students with disabilities; bookstore; campus computer network; career placement assistance; computer lab; computer-assisted instruction; e-mail services; housing assistance; interactive nursing skills videos; Internet; learning resource lab; library services; nursing audiovisuals; resume preparation assistance; skills, simulation, or other laboratory; tutoring.
**Library Facilities** 5,649 volumes in health, 1,250 volumes in nursing; 200 periodical subscriptions health-care related.

### BACCALAUREATE PROGRAMS

**Degree** BSN
**Available Programs** ADN to Baccalaureate; RN Baccalaureate.
**Site Options** Beckley, WV; Bluefield, WV.
**Study Options** Full-time and part-time.
**Online Degree Options** Yes (online only).
**Program Entrance Requirements** Minimum overall college GPA of 2.5, transcript of college record, CPR certification, health exam, health insurance, high school chemistry, immunizations, minimum high school GPA of 2.8, minimum GPA in nursing prerequisites of 2.5, prerequisite course work, RN licensure. Transfer students are accepted. *Application deadline:* 3/1 (fall), 4/15 (spring).
**Financial Aid** 35% of baccalaureate students in nursing programs received some form of financial aid in 2012–13. *Gift aid (need-based):* Federal Pell, FSEOG, state. *Loans:* Federal Direct (Subsidized and Unsubsidized Stafford PLUS), Perkins. *Work-study:* Federal Work-Study, part-time campus jobs. *Financial aid application deadline (priority):* 3/1.
**Contact** Ms. Beth Pritchett, Director, Program in Nursing, Bluefield State College, 219 Rock Street, Bluefield, WV 24701. *Telephone:* 304-327-4139. *Fax:* 304-327-4219. *E-mail:* bpritchett@bluefieldstate.edu.

## Fairmont State University

### School of Nursing and Allied Health Administration
### Fairmont, West Virginia

*http://www.fairmontstate.edu/*
Founded in 1865

### DEGREE • BSN

**Nursing Program Faculty** 4 (75% with doctorates).
**Baccalaureate Enrollment** 150 **Women** 96% **Men** 4% **International** 1% **Part-time** 40%
**Distance Learning Courses** Available.
**Nursing Student Activities** Sigma Theta Tau, Student Nurses' Association.
**Nursing Student Resources** Academic advising; academic or career counseling; assistance for students with disabilities; bookstore; campus computer network; career placement assistance; computer lab; computer-assisted instruction; e-mail services; housing assistance; interactive nursing skills videos; Internet; learning resource lab; library services; nursing audiovisuals; placement services for program completers; remedial services; resume preparation assistance; skills, simulation, or other laboratory; tutoring.
**Library Facilities** 280,000 volumes (9,000 in health, 1,100 in nursing); 895 periodical subscriptions (50 health-care related).

## BACCALAUREATE PROGRAMS

**Degree** BSN
**Available Programs** ADN to Baccalaureate; Accelerated RN Baccalaureate; RN Baccalaureate.
**Study Options** Full-time and part-time.
**Program Entrance Requirements** Minimum overall college GPA of 2.0, transcript of college record, CPR certification, health exam, high school transcript, immunizations, minimum high school GPA of 2.0, RN licensure. Transfer students are accepted. *Application deadline:* 8/15 (fall), 8/15 (winter), 1/2 (spring), 5/15 (summer). Applications may be processed on a rolling basis for some programs.
**Advanced Placement** Credit by examination available. Credit given for nursing courses completed elsewhere dependent upon specific evaluations.
**Contact** *Telephone:* 304-367-4074. *Fax:* 304-367-4268.

## CONTINUING EDUCATION PROGRAM

**Contact** *Telephone:* 304-367-4074. *Fax:* 304-367-4268.

# Marshall University

### College of Health Professions
### Huntington, West Virginia

***http://www.marshall.edu/cohp***
Founded in 1837

**DEGREES • BSN • MSN**
**Nursing Program Faculty** 35 (23% with doctorates).
**Baccalaureate Enrollment** 345 **Women** 80% **Men** 20% **Minority** 5% **Part-time** 35%
**Graduate Enrollment** 100 **Women** 90% **Men** 10% **Part-time** 60%
**Nursing Student Activities** Sigma Theta Tau, Student Nurses' Association, nursing club.
**Nursing Student Resources** Academic advising; academic or career counseling; assistance for students with disabilities; bookstore; campus computer network; career placement assistance; computer lab; computer-assisted instruction; daycare for children of students; e-mail services; employment services for current students; externships; housing assistance; interactive nursing skills videos; Internet; learning resource lab; library services; nursing audiovisuals; placement services for program completers; remedial services; resume preparation assistance; skills, simulation, or other laboratory; tutoring.
**Library Facilities** 1.9 million volumes (20,200 in health, 6,400 in nursing); 33,622 periodical subscriptions (500 health-care related).

## BACCALAUREATE PROGRAMS

**Degree** BSN
**Available Programs** Accelerated RN Baccalaureate; Generic Baccalaureate.
**Study Options** Full-time and part-time.
**Program Entrance Requirements** Minimum overall college GPA of 2.5, transcript of college record, high school transcript, minimum high school GPA of 2.5. Transfer students are accepted.
**Advanced Placement** Credit given for nursing courses completed elsewhere dependent upon specific evaluations.
**Contact** *Telephone:* 304-696-2639. *Fax:* 304-696-6739.

## GRADUATE PROGRAMS

**Contact** *Telephone:* 304-696-2639. *Fax:* 304-696-6739.

### MASTER'S DEGREE PROGRAM

**Degree** MSN
**Available Programs** Master's.
**Concentrations Available** Nursing administration; nursing education. *Nurse practitioner programs in:* family health.
**Study Options** Full-time and part-time.
**Program Entrance Requirements** Minimum overall college GPA of 3.0, transcript of college record, nursing research course, resume, statistics course, GRE General Test.
**Advanced Placement** Credit given for nursing courses completed elsewhere dependent upon specific evaluations.
**Degree Requirements** 36 total credit hours, thesis or project.

### POST-MASTER'S PROGRAM

**Areas of Study** Nursing administration; nursing education. *Nurse practitioner programs in:* family health.

# Shepherd University

### Department of Nursing Education
### Shepherdstown, West Virginia

***http://www.shepherd.edu/nurseweb/***
Founded in 1871

**DEGREE • BSN**
**Nursing Program Faculty** 8 (50% with doctorates).
**Baccalaureate Enrollment** 144 **Women** 92% **Men** 8% **Minority** 18% **International** 4%
**Nursing Student Activities** Nursing Honor Society, Student Nurses' Association.
**Nursing Student Resources** Academic advising; academic or career counseling; assistance for students with disabilities; bookstore; campus computer network; career placement assistance; computer lab; computer-assisted instruction; e-mail services; interactive nursing skills videos; Internet; learning resource lab; library services; nursing audiovisuals; remedial services; resume preparation assistance; skills, simulation, or other laboratory; tutoring.
**Library Facilities** 285,494 volumes (4,997 in health, 462 in nursing); 45,260 periodical subscriptions (1,956 health-care related).

## BACCALAUREATE PROGRAMS

**Degree** BSN
**Available Programs** ADN to Baccalaureate; Generic Baccalaureate; RN Baccalaureate.
**Study Options** Full-time.
**Program Entrance Requirements** Minimum overall college GPA of 2.5, transcript of college record, CPR certification, written essay, health exam, health insurance, immunizations, interview, minimum GPA in nursing prerequisites of 2.0, professional liability insurance/malpractice insurance, prerequisite course work. Transfer students are accepted. *Application deadline:* 3/1 (fall), 10/1 (spring).
**Advanced Placement** Credit by examination available. Credit given for nursing courses completed elsewhere dependent upon specific evaluations.
**Contact** *Telephone:* 304-876-5341. *Fax:* 304-876-5169.

## CONTINUING EDUCATION PROGRAM

**Contact** *Telephone:* 304-876-5341. *Fax:* 304-876-5169.

# University of Charleston

### Department of Nursing
### Charleston, West Virginia

***http://www.ucwv.edu/majors/nursing/***
Founded in 1888

**DEGREE • BSN**
**Nursing Program Faculty** 6 (33% with doctorates).
**Baccalaureate Enrollment** 65 **Women** 97% **Men** 3% **Minority** 3% **International** 1% **Part-time** 1%
**Nursing Student Activities** Nursing Honor Society, Sigma Theta Tau, Student Nurses' Association, nursing club.
**Nursing Student Resources** Academic advising; academic or career counseling; assistance for students with disabilities; bookstore; campus computer network; career placement assistance; computer lab; computer-assisted instruction; e-mail services; employment services for current students; externships; housing assistance; interactive nursing skills videos; Internet; learning resource lab; library services; nursing audiovisuals; paid internships; placement services for program completers; remedial services; resume preparation assistance; skills, simulation, or other laboratory; tutoring; unpaid internships.
**Library Facilities** 94,267 volumes (3,900 in health, 1,550 in nursing); 150 periodical subscriptions (75 health-care related).

## BACCALAUREATE PROGRAMS

**Degree** BSN
**Available Programs** Generic Baccalaureate.
**Study Options** Full-time and part-time.
**Program Entrance Requirements** Minimum overall college GPA of 2.75, transcript of college record, CPR certification, health exam, high school biology, 1 year of high school math, high school transcript, immunizations, minimum high school GPA of 2.25, minimum GPA in nursing prerequisites of 2.75, professional liability insurance/malpractice

insurance, prerequisite course work. Transfer students are accepted. *Application deadline:* Applications may be processed on a rolling basis for some programs.
**Advanced Placement** Credit given for nursing courses completed elsewhere dependent upon specific evaluations.
**Contact** *Telephone:* 304-357-4750. *Fax:* 304-357-4781.

# West Liberty University
## Department of Health Sciences
## West Liberty, West Virginia

***http://www.westliberty.edu/nursing/index.htm***
Founded in 1837

### DEGREE • BSN
**Nursing Program Faculty** 12 (33% with doctorates).
**Baccalaureate Enrollment** 123 **Women** 88% **Men** 12% **Minority** 3% **International** 1%
**Distance Learning Courses** Available.
**Nursing Student Activities** Student Nurses' Association.
**Nursing Student Resources** Academic advising; academic or career counseling; assistance for students with disabilities; bookstore; campus computer network; career placement assistance; computer lab; computer-assisted instruction; e-mail services; externships; housing assistance; interactive nursing skills videos; Internet; learning resource lab; library services; nursing audiovisuals; placement services for program completers; remedial services; resume preparation assistance; skills, simulation, or other laboratory; tutoring; unpaid internships.
**Library Facilities** 2,500 volumes in health, 750 volumes in nursing; 350 periodical subscriptions health-care related.

### BACCALAUREATE PROGRAMS
**Degree** BSN
**Available Programs** Accelerated RN Baccalaureate; Generic Baccalaureate.
**Site Options** Triadelphia, WV.
**Study Options** Full-time and part-time.
**Program Entrance Requirements** Minimum overall college GPA of 3.0, transcript of college record, health exam, immunizations, minimum high school GPA of 3.0, minimum GPA in nursing prerequisites of 2.0, prerequisite course work. Transfer students are accepted. *Application deadline:* 3/31 (spring).
**Advanced Placement** Credit by examination available. Credit given for nursing courses completed elsewhere dependent upon specific evaluations.
**Expenses (2012–13)** *Tuition, state resident:* full-time $6422. *Tuition, nonresident:* full-time $13,990. *Room and board:* $8200 per academic year. *Required fees:* full-time $275.
**Financial Aid** 90% of baccalaureate students in nursing programs received some form of financial aid in 2011–12.
**Contact** Dr. Rose Kutlenios, Interim Program Director, Nursing, Department of Health Sciences, West Liberty University, 208 University Drive, College Union Box 140, West Liberty, WV 26074. *Telephone:* 304-336-8911. *Fax:* 304-336-5104. *E-mail:* rose.kutlenios@westliberty.edu.

# West Virginia University
## School of Nursing
## Morgantown, West Virginia

***http://www.nursing.hsc.wvu.edu/***
Founded in 1867

### DEGREES • BSN • DNP • MSN • PHD
**Nursing Program Faculty** 88 (52% with doctorates).
**Baccalaureate Enrollment** 680 **Women** 90% **Men** 10% **Minority** 6.5% **International** 1.3% **Part-time** 17.5%
**Graduate Enrollment** 202 **Women** 94% **Men** 6% **Minority** 9.4% **International** .5% **Part-time** 66.8%
**Distance Learning Courses** Available.
**Nursing Student Activities** Nursing Honor Society, Sigma Theta Tau, Student Nurses' Association.
**Nursing Student Resources** Academic advising; academic or career counseling; assistance for students with disabilities; bookstore; campus computer network; career placement assistance; computer lab; computer-assisted instruction; daycare for children of students; e-mail services; employment services for current students; externships; housing assistance; interactive nursing skills videos; Internet; learning resource lab; library services; nursing audiovisuals; other; paid internships; remedial services; resume preparation assistance; skills, simulation, or other laboratory; tutoring.
**Library Facilities** 1.9 million volumes (78,811 in health, 4,496 in nursing); 59,860 periodical subscriptions (73,528 health-care related).

### BACCALAUREATE PROGRAMS
**Degree** BSN
**Available Programs** ADN to Baccalaureate; Accelerated Baccalaureate; Accelerated Baccalaureate for Second Degree; Generic Baccalaureate; RN Baccalaureate.
**Site Options** Montgomery, WV; Glenville, WV.
**Study Options** Full-time.
**Program Entrance Requirements** Minimum overall college GPA of 3.0, transcript of college record, CPR certification, health insurance, high school biology, high school chemistry, 3 years high school math, 3 years high school science, high school transcript, immunizations, interview, minimum high school GPA of 3.0, minimum GPA in nursing prerequisites of 3.0, prerequisite course work. Transfer students are accepted. *Application deadline:* 1/15 (fall), 5/15 (spring). *Application fee:* $30.
**Advanced Placement** Credit by examination available. Credit given for nursing courses completed elsewhere dependent upon specific evaluations.
**Expenses (2013–14)** *Tuition, state resident:* full-time $8688; part-time $362 per credit hour. *Tuition, nonresident:* full-time $21,912; part-time $913 per credit hour. *Room and board:* $8848 per academic year.
**Financial Aid** 93% of baccalaureate students in nursing programs received some form of financial aid in 2012–13. *Gift aid (need-based):* Federal Pell, FSEOG, state, private, college/university gift aid from institutional funds. *Loans:* Federal Nursing Student Loans, Federal Direct (Subsidized and Unsubsidized Stafford PLUS), Perkins, college/university. *Work-study:* Federal Work-Study, part-time campus jobs. *Financial aid application deadline:* 3/1.
**Contact** Mrs. Kim McCourt, Recruiting and Outreach Coordinator, School of Nursing, West Virginia University, PO Box 9640, 6400 Health Sciences Center South, Morgantown, WV 26506-9600. *Telephone:* 304-293-1386. *Fax:* 304-293-2546. *E-mail:* kmccourt@hsc.wvu.edu.

### GRADUATE PROGRAMS
**Expenses (2013–14)** *Tuition, state resident:* part-time $495 per credit hour. *Tuition, nonresident:* part-time $1216 per credit hour.
**Financial Aid** 88% of graduate students in nursing programs received some form of financial aid in 2012–13. 1 teaching assistantship with tuition reimbursement available (averaging $10,000 per year) was awarded; institutionally sponsored loans, tuition waivers (partial), and graduate administrative assistantships also available. *Financial aid application deadline:* 2/1.
**Contact** Mrs. Kim McCourt, Recruiting and Outreach Coordinator, School of Nursing, West Virginia University, PO Box 9640, 6400 RCB Health Sciences Center South, Morgantown, WV 26506-9600. *Telephone:* 304-293-1386. *Fax:* 304-293-2546. *E-mail:* kmccourt@hsc.wvu.edu.

#### MASTER'S DEGREE PROGRAM
**Degree** MSN
**Available Programs** Accelerated AD/RN to Master's; Accelerated Master's; Accelerated RN to Master's; Master's; RN to Master's.
**Concentrations Available** Nursing administration. *Nurse practitioner programs in:* family health, neonatal health, pediatric,women's health.
**Site Options** Charleston, WV.
**Study Options** Full-time and part-time.
**Online Degree Options** Yes (online only).
**Program Entrance Requirements** Computer literacy, minimum overall college GPA of 3.0, transcript of college record, CPR certification, written essay, immunizations, 3 letters of recommendation, nursing research course, physical assessment course, resume, statistics course. *Application deadline:* 2/1 (fall). *Application fee:* $60.
**Advanced Placement** Credit by examination available. Credit given for nursing courses completed elsewhere dependent upon specific evaluations.
**Degree Requirements** 44 total credit hours.

#### POST-MASTER'S PROGRAM
**Areas of Study** Nursing administration. *Nurse practitioner programs in:* family health, neonatal health, pediatric,women's health.

**DOCTORAL DEGREE PROGRAM**
**Degree** DNP
**Available Programs** Doctorate.
**Areas of Study** Addiction/substance abuse, advanced practice nursing, aging, bio-behavioral research, clinical practice, community health, ethics, family health, gerontology, health promotion/disease prevention, human health and illness, individualized study, maternity-newborn, neuro-behavior, nursing administration, oncology,women's health.
**Online Degree Options** Yes (online only).
**Program Entrance Requirements** Minimum overall college GPA of 3.0, 3 letters of recommendation, MSN or equivalent, statistics course, vita, writing sample. *Application deadline:* 3/1 (summer). *Application fee:* $50.
**Degree Requirements** 44 total credit hours, Capstone project, oral exam.

**Degree** PhD
**Available Programs** Doctorate.
**Areas of Study** Addiction/substance abuse, aging, bio-behavioral research, community health, ethics, gerontology, health promotion/disease prevention, individualized study, nursing research, oncology,women's health.
**Site Options** Charleston, WV.
**Program Entrance Requirements** Minimum overall college GPA of 3.0, interview by faculty committee, 3 letters of recommendation, MSN or equivalent, statistics course, vita, writing sample, GRE General Test (PhD). *Application deadline:* 3/1 (summer). *Application fee:* $60.
**Degree Requirements** 55 total credit hours, dissertation, oral exam, written exam, residency.

## CONTINUING EDUCATION PROGRAM

**Contact** Office of Extended Learning, School of Nursing, West Virginia University, PO Box 6800, 150 Clay Street, Morgantown, WV 26506-6800. *Telephone:* 800-253-2762. *Fax:* 304-293-4899. *E-mail:* elearn@mail.wvu.edu.

# West Virginia Wesleyan College

**School of Nursing**
**Buckhannon, West Virginia**

***http://www.wvwc.edu/***
Founded in 1890

**DEGREES • BSN • MSN**
**Nursing Program Faculty** 11 (36% with doctorates).
**Baccalaureate Enrollment** 140 **Women** 94% **Men** 6% **Minority** 2%
**Graduate Enrollment** 20 **Women** 97% **Men** 3%
**Nursing Student Activities** Nursing Honor Society, Sigma Theta Tau, Student Nurses' Association.
**Nursing Student Resources** Academic advising; academic or career counseling; assistance for students with disabilities; bookstore; campus computer network; career placement assistance; computer-assisted instruction; e-mail services; employment services for current students; externships; interactive nursing skills videos; Internet; learning resource lab; library services; nursing audiovisuals; placement services for program completers; remedial services; resume preparation assistance; skills, simulation, or other laboratory; tutoring.
**Library Facilities** 130,000 volumes (4,000 in health, 600 in nursing); 14,500 periodical subscriptions (90 health-care related).

## BACCALAUREATE PROGRAMS

**Degree** BSN
**Available Programs** Generic Baccalaureate.
**Study Options** Full-time and part-time.
**Program Entrance Requirements** Minimum overall college GPA of 3.0, transcript of college record, CPR certification, health exam, health insurance, high school transcript, immunizations, interview, minimum high school GPA of 2.5, minimum GPA in nursing prerequisites of 2.0, prerequisite course work. Transfer students are accepted. *Application deadline:* 6/15 (fall), 12/15 (spring). Applications may be processed on a rolling basis for some programs.
**Advanced Placement** Credit by examination available. Credit given for nursing courses completed elsewhere dependent upon specific evaluations.
**Expenses (2012–13)** *Tuition:* full-time $12,390; part-time $1040 per credit hour. *International tuition:* $12,390 full-time. *Room and board:* $7510; room only: $3840 per academic year. *Required fees:* full-time $1024; part-time $512 per term.
**Financial Aid** 95% of baccalaureate students in nursing programs received some form of financial aid in 2011–12. *Gift aid (need-based):* Federal Pell, FSEOG, state, private, college/university gift aid from institutional funds, Federal Nursing. *Loans:* Federal Nursing Student Loans, Federal Direct (Subsidized and Unsubsidized Stafford PLUS), Perkins. *Work-study:* Federal Work-Study, part-time campus jobs. *Financial aid application deadline (priority):* 2/15.
**Contact** Dr. Judith McKinney, Professor and Director, School of Nursing, West Virginia Wesleyan College, 59 College Avenue, Buckhannon, WV 26201-2995. *Telephone:* 304-473-8224. *Fax:* 304-473-8435. *E-mail:* mckinney@wvwc.edu.

## GRADUATE PROGRAMS

**Expenses (2012–13)** *Tuition:* full-time $10,200; part-time $425 per credit hour. *International tuition:* $10,200 full-time. *Required fees:* full-time $780; part-time $195 per term.
**Financial Aid** 50% of graduate students in nursing programs received some form of financial aid in 2011–12.
**Contact** Dr. Sue Leight, Associate Professor and Director of MSN Program, School of Nursing, West Virginia Wesleyan College, 59 College Avenue, Buckhannon, WV 26201. *Telephone:* 304-473-8228. *E-mail:* leight@wvwc.edu.

**MASTER'S DEGREE PROGRAM**
**Degree** MSN
**Available Programs** Master's.
**Concentrations Available** Nurse-midwifery; nursing administration; nursing education. *Nurse practitioner programs in:* psychiatric/mental health.
**Study Options** Full-time and part-time.
**Program Entrance Requirements** Minimum overall college GPA of 3.0, transcript of college record, CPR certification, immunizations, interview, letters of recommendation, physical assessment course, professional liability insurance/malpractice insurance, resume, statistics course. *Application deadline:* 8/1 (fall), 12/10 (spring), 5/1 (summer). Applications may be processed on a rolling basis for some programs. *Application fee:* $50.
**Degree Requirements** 36 total credit hours, thesis or project.

# Wheeling Jesuit University

**Department of Nursing**
**Wheeling, West Virginia**

***http://www.wju.edu/***
Founded in 1954

**DEGREES • BSN • MSN**
**Nursing Program Faculty** 26 (35% with doctorates).
**Baccalaureate Enrollment** 133 **Women** 93% **Men** 7% **Minority** 1% **International** 1% **Part-time** 52%
**Graduate Enrollment** 177 **Women** 94% **Men** 6% **Minority** 3% **Part-time** 88%
**Distance Learning Courses** Available.
**Nursing Student Activities** Sigma Theta Tau, Student Nurses' Association.
**Nursing Student Resources** Academic advising; academic or career counseling; assistance for students with disabilities; bookstore; campus computer network; career placement assistance; computer lab; computer-assisted instruction; e-mail services; employment services for current students; externships; housing assistance; Internet; learning resource lab; library services; nursing audiovisuals; placement services for program completers; remedial services; resume preparation assistance; skills, simulation, or other laboratory; tutoring.
**Library Facilities** 282,379 volumes (5,065 in nursing); 232 periodical subscriptions (90 health-care related).

## BACCALAUREATE PROGRAMS

**Degree** BSN
**Available Programs** Accelerated Baccalaureate for Second Degree; Generic Baccalaureate; RN Baccalaureate.
**Study Options** Full-time and part-time.
**Online Degree Options** Yes.
**Program Entrance Requirements** Minimum overall college GPA of 2.75, transcript of college record, CPR certification, health exam, health insurance, high school transcript, immunizations, minimum GPA in nursing prerequisites of 2.0, prerequisite course work. Transfer students

are accepted. *Application deadline:* Applications may be processed on a rolling basis for some programs.
**Advanced Placement** Credit by examination available. Credit given for nursing courses completed elsewhere dependent upon specific evaluations.
**Financial Aid** 97% of baccalaureate students in nursing programs received some form of financial aid in 2012–13. *Gift aid (need-based):* Federal Pell, FSEOG, state, private, college/university gift aid from institutional funds, Federal Nursing. *Loans:* Federal Nursing Student Loans, Federal Direct (Subsidized and Unsubsidized Stafford PLUS), Perkins, alternative loans. *Work-study:* Federal Work-Study, part-time campus jobs. *Financial aid application deadline (priority):* 3/1.
**Contact** Admissions Office, Department of Nursing, Wheeling Jesuit University, 316 Washington Avenue, Wheeling, WV 26003-6233. *Telephone:* 304-243-2359. *Fax:* 304-243-2397.

## GRADUATE PROGRAMS

**Financial Aid** 95% of graduate students in nursing programs received some form of financial aid in 2012–13. Scholarships and unspecified assistantships available. *Financial aid application deadline:* 8/1.
**Contact** Mrs. Carol Carroll, Program Contact, Department of Nursing, Wheeling Jesuit University, 316 Washington Avenue, Wheeling, WV 26003-6233. *Telephone:* 304-243-2344. *Fax:* 304-243-2608. *E-mail:* ccarroll@wju.edu.

### MASTER'S DEGREE PROGRAM

**Degree** MSN
**Available Programs** Master's; RN to Master's.
**Concentrations Available** Nursing administration; nursing education. *Nurse practitioner programs in:* family health.
**Site Options** Charleston, WV.
**Study Options** Full-time and part-time.
**Online Degree Options** Yes (online only).
**Program Entrance Requirements** Computer literacy, minimum overall college GPA of 3.0, 3 letters of recommendation, statistics course, GRE General Test or MAT. *Application deadline:* Applications may be processed on a rolling basis for some programs.
**Advanced Placement** Credit given for nursing courses completed elsewhere dependent upon specific evaluations.
**Degree Requirements** 42 total credit hours, thesis or project, comprehensive exam.

### POST-MASTER'S PROGRAM

**Areas of Study** Nursing administration; nursing education. *Nurse practitioner programs in:* family health.

# WISCONSIN

## Alverno College
### Division of Nursing
### Milwaukee, Wisconsin

*http://www.alverno.edu/*
Founded in 1887

### DEGREES • BSN • MSN

**Nursing Program Faculty** 39 (5% with doctorates).
**Baccalaureate Enrollment** 763 **Women** 100% **Minority** 24% **Part-time** 22%
**Graduate Enrollment** 43 **Women** 96% **Men** 4% **Minority** 9% **Part-time** 62%
**Nursing Student Activities** Student Nurses' Association.
**Nursing Student Resources** Academic advising; academic or career counseling; assistance for students with disabilities; bookstore; campus computer network; career placement assistance; computer lab; computer-assisted instruction; daycare for children of students; e-mail services; employment services for current students; externships; housing assistance; interactive nursing skills videos; Internet; learning resource lab; library services; nursing audiovisuals; remedial services; resume preparation assistance; skills, simulation, or other laboratory; tutoring; unpaid internships.
**Library Facilities** 177,846 volumes; 46,569 periodical subscriptions.

## BACCALAUREATE PROGRAMS

**Degree** BSN
**Available Programs** ADN to Baccalaureate; Baccalaureate for Second Degree; Generic Baccalaureate; LPN to Baccalaureate; RN Baccalaureate.
**Study Options** Full-time and part-time.
**Program Entrance Requirements** Minimum overall college GPA of 2.5, transcript of college record, written essay, high school biology, high school chemistry, 3 years high school math, 2 years high school science, high school transcript, minimum high school GPA of 2.0, prerequisite course work. Transfer students are accepted.
**Advanced Placement** Credit by examination available. Credit given for nursing courses completed elsewhere dependent upon specific evaluations.
**Contact** *Telephone:* 414-382-6276. *Fax:* 414-382-6279.

## GRADUATE PROGRAMS

**Contact** *Telephone:* 414-382-6278. *Fax:* 414-382-6279.

### MASTER'S DEGREE PROGRAM

**Degree** MSN
**Available Programs** Master's.
**Concentrations Available** Nursing education. *Clinical nurse specialist programs in:* adult health, gerontology, medical-surgical.
**Study Options** Full-time and part-time.
**Program Entrance Requirements** Clinical experience, transcript of college record, CPR certification, written essay, immunizations, 3 letters of recommendation, physical assessment course, statistics course.
**Advanced Placement** Credit given for nursing courses completed elsewhere dependent upon specific evaluations.
**Degree Requirements** 39 total credit hours, thesis or project.

## CONTINUING EDUCATION PROGRAM

**Contact** *Telephone:* 414-382-6177. *Fax:* 414-382-6354.

## Bellin College
### Nursing Program
### Green Bay, Wisconsin

*http://www.bellincollege.edu/*
Founded in 1909

### DEGREES • BSN • MSN

**Nursing Program Faculty** 20 (21% with doctorates).
**Baccalaureate Enrollment** 274 **Women** 92% **Men** 8% **Minority** 5% **International** 1% **Part-time** 9%
**Graduate Enrollment** 32 **Women** 93% **Men** 7% **Minority** 2% **Part-time** 81%
**Distance Learning Courses** Available.
**Nursing Student Activities** Sigma Theta Tau, Student Nurses' Association.
**Nursing Student Resources** Academic advising; academic or career counseling; assistance for students with disabilities; career placement assistance; computer lab; computer-assisted instruction; e-mail services; interactive nursing skills videos; Internet; learning resource lab; library services; nursing audiovisuals; resume preparation assistance; skills, simulation, or other laboratory; tutoring.
**Library Facilities** 7,000 volumes (7,000 in health, 4,000 in nursing); 225 periodical subscriptions (190 health-care related).

## BACCALAUREATE PROGRAMS

**Degree** BSN
**Available Programs** Accelerated Baccalaureate; Accelerated Baccalaureate for Second Degree; Baccalaureate for Second Degree; Generic Baccalaureate.
**Study Options** Full-time and part-time.
**Program Entrance Requirements** Minimum overall college GPA of 2.7, transcript of college record, CPR certification, health exam, health insurance, high school biology, high school chemistry, 3 years high school math, 3 years high school science, high school transcript, immunizations, interview, 3 letters of recommendation, minimum high school GPA of 3.25, minimum GPA in nursing prerequisites of 2.7. Transfer students are accepted. *Application deadline:* Applications may be processed on a rolling basis for some programs. *Application fee:* $30.

**Advanced Placement** Credit by examination available. Credit given for nursing courses completed elsewhere dependent upon specific evaluations.
**Contact** *Telephone:* 920-433-6651. *Fax:* 920-433-1922.

## GRADUATE PROGRAMS

**Contact** *Telephone:* 920-433-3624. *Fax:* 920-433-1922.

### MASTER'S DEGREE PROGRAM

**Degree** MSN
**Available Programs** Master's.
**Concentrations Available** Nursing administration; nursing education.
**Study Options** Full-time and part-time.
**Online Degree Options** Yes.
**Program Entrance Requirements** Computer literacy, minimum overall college GPA of 3.0, transcript of college record, written essay, interview, 3 letters of recommendation, nursing research course, resume, statistics course. *Application deadline:* Applications may be processed on a rolling basis for some programs. *Application fee:* $50.
**Advanced Placement** Credit given for nursing courses completed elsewhere dependent upon specific evaluations.
**Degree Requirements** 38 total credit hours, thesis or project.

# Cardinal Stritch University

**Ruth S. Coleman College of Nursing**
**Milwaukee, Wisconsin**

*http://www.stritch.edu/nursing*
Founded in 1937

**DEGREES • BSN • MSN**
**Nursing Program Faculty** 36 (11% with doctorates).
**Baccalaureate Enrollment** 98 **Women** 90% **Men** 10% **Minority** 17% **International** 6%
**Graduate Enrollment** 15 **Women** 100% **Minority** 13%
**Nursing Student Activities** Student Nurses' Association.
**Nursing Student Resources** Academic advising; academic or career counseling; assistance for students with disabilities; bookstore; campus computer network; career placement assistance; computer lab; e-mail services; employment services for current students; interactive nursing skills videos; Internet; learning resource lab; library services; nursing audiovisuals; remedial services; resume preparation assistance; skills, simulation, or other laboratory; tutoring.
**Library Facilities** 124,897 volumes (4,500 in health, 600 in nursing); 667 periodical subscriptions (1,500 health-care related).

## BACCALAUREATE PROGRAMS

**Degree** BSN
**Available Programs** ADN to Baccalaureate.
**Site Options** Menomonee Falls, WI; Milwaukee, WI.
**Study Options** Full-time and part-time.
**Program Entrance Requirements** Minimum overall college GPA of 2.33, transcript of college record, RN licensure. Transfer students are accepted. *Application deadline:* Applications may be processed on a rolling basis for some programs.
**Advanced Placement** Credit by examination available. Credit given for nursing courses completed elsewhere dependent upon specific evaluations.
**Contact** *Telephone:* 414-410-4966. *Fax:* 414-410-4049.

## GRADUATE PROGRAMS

**Contact** *Telephone:* 414-410-4966. *Fax:* 414-410-4049.

### MASTER'S DEGREE PROGRAM

**Degree** MSN
**Available Programs** Accelerated Master's.
**Concentrations Available** Nursing education.
**Study Options** Full-time.
**Program Entrance Requirements** Computer literacy, minimum overall college GPA of 3.0, transcript of college record, CPR certification, written essay, immunizations, interview, 3 letters of recommendation, nursing research course, resume. *Application deadline:* Applications may be processed on a rolling basis for some programs.
**Advanced Placement** Credit given for nursing courses completed elsewhere dependent upon specific evaluations.
**Degree Requirements** 36 total credit hours, thesis or project.

# Carroll University

**Nursing Program**
**Waukesha, Wisconsin**

*http://www.carrollu.edu/programs/nursing/*
Founded in 1846

**DEGREE • BSN**
**Nursing Program Faculty** 18
**Baccalaureate Enrollment** 331 **Women** 91.5% **Men** 8.5% **Minority** 8.8% **International** .3% **Part-time** 5.4%
**Nursing Student Activities** Sigma Theta Tau, Student Nurses' Association.
**Nursing Student Resources** Academic advising; academic or career counseling; assistance for students with disabilities; bookstore; campus computer network; computer lab; computer-assisted instruction; e-mail services; housing assistance; interactive nursing skills videos; Internet; learning resource lab; library services; nursing audiovisuals; resume preparation assistance; skills, simulation, or other laboratory; tutoring.
**Library Facilities** 150,000 volumes; 65,200 periodical subscriptions.

## BACCALAUREATE PROGRAMS

**Degree** BSN
**Available Programs** ADN to Baccalaureate; Generic Baccalaureate.
**Study Options** Full-time.
**Program Entrance Requirements** Minimum overall college GPA of 2.75, transcript of college record, written essay, health exam, health insurance, high school biology, high school chemistry, 3 years high school math, high school transcript, minimum high school GPA of 2.75, minimum GPA in nursing prerequisites of 2.75, prerequisite course work. Transfer students are accepted. *Application deadline:* Applications may be processed on a rolling basis for some programs.
**Expenses (2013–14)** *Tuition:* full-time $27,039; part-time $440 per credit. *International tuition:* $27,039 full-time. *Room and board:* $8513; room only: $4535 per academic year. *Required fees:* full-time $525; part-time $263 per term.
**Financial Aid** 98% of baccalaureate students in nursing programs received some form of financial aid in 2012–13.
**Contact** Ms. Angela Rose Brindowski, Chair, Department of Nursing, Nursing Program, Carroll University, 100 North East Avenue, Waukesha, WI 53186. *Telephone:* 262-524-4927. *E-mail:* abrindow@carrollu.edu.

# Columbia College of Nursing

**Columbia College of Nursing/Mount Mary College Nursing Program**
**Milwaukee, Wisconsin**

***See description of programs under Columbia College of Nursing/Mount Mary College Nursing Program (Milwaukee, Wisconsin).***

# Columbia College of Nursing/Mount Mary College Nursing Program

**Columbia College of Nursing/Mount Mary College Nursing Program**
**Milwaukee, Wisconsin**

*http://www.mtmary.edu/*
Founded in 2002

**DEGREE • BSN**
**Nursing Program Faculty** 20 (7% with doctorates).
**Baccalaureate Enrollment** 250 **Women** 95% **Men** 5% **Minority** 15% **Part-time** 20%
**Nursing Student Activities** Sigma Theta Tau, Student Nurses' Association.
**Nursing Student Resources** Academic advising; academic or career counseling; bookstore; campus computer network; career placement assistance; computer lab; computer-assisted instruction; daycare for children of students; e-mail services; employment services for current

students; housing assistance; interactive nursing skills videos; Internet; learning resource lab; library services; nursing audiovisuals; resume preparation assistance; skills, simulation, or other laboratory; tutoring.

### BACCALAUREATE PROGRAMS

**Degree** BSN
**Available Programs** Baccalaureate for Second Degree; Generic Baccalaureate; RN Baccalaureate.
**Site Options** Milwaukee, WI.
**Study Options** Full-time and part-time.
**Program Entrance Requirements** Minimum overall college GPA of 2.8, transcript of college record, health exam, health insurance, high school biology, high school chemistry, 2 years high school math, 2 years high school science, high school transcript, minimum high school GPA of 2.5, minimum high school rank 40%, minimum GPA in nursing prerequisites of 2.8, prerequisite course work. Transfer students are accepted.
**Advanced Placement** Credit by examination available. Credit given for nursing courses completed elsewhere dependent upon specific evaluations.
**Contact** *Telephone:* 414-256-1219 Ext. 193. *Fax:* 414-256-0180.

## Concordia University Wisconsin
### Program in Nursing
### Mequon, Wisconsin

*http://www.cuw.edu/*
Founded in 1881

**DEGREES • BSN • DNP • MSN**
**Nursing Program Faculty** 12 (3% with doctorates).
**Baccalaureate Enrollment** 420 **Women** 92% **Men** 8% **Minority** 10% **International** 1% **Part-time** 32%
**Graduate Enrollment** 611 **Women** 95% **Men** 5% **Minority** 8% **International** 1% **Part-time** 44%
**Distance Learning Courses** Available.
**Nursing Student Activities** Nursing Honor Society, Sigma Theta Tau, Student Nurses' Association.
**Nursing Student Resources** Academic advising; academic or career counseling; assistance for students with disabilities; bookstore; campus computer network; career placement assistance; computer lab; computer-assisted instruction; e-mail services; employment services for current students; externships; interactive nursing skills videos; Internet; learning resource lab; library services; nursing audiovisuals; paid internships; placement services for program completers; resume preparation assistance; skills, simulation, or other laboratory; tutoring.
**Library Facilities** 3,893 volumes in health, 1,011 volumes in nursing; 922 periodical subscriptions health-care related.

### BACCALAUREATE PROGRAMS

**Degree** BSN
**Available Programs** ADN to Baccalaureate; Generic Baccalaureate; LPN to RN Baccalaureate; RN Baccalaureate.
**Site Options** Mequon, WI; Milwaukee, WI.
**Study Options** Full-time.
**Program Entrance Requirements** Transcript of college record, CPR certification, health exam, health insurance, high school transcript, immunizations, minimum high school GPA of 2.75, minimum GPA in nursing prerequisites of 2.75, RN licensure. Transfer students are accepted. *Application deadline:* 7/15 (fall), 7/15 (winter), 10/15 (spring), 3/15 (summer). *Application fee:* $50.
**Advanced Placement** Credit given for nursing courses completed elsewhere dependent upon specific evaluations.
**Contact** *Telephone:* 262-243-4374. *Fax:* 262-243-4466.

### GRADUATE PROGRAMS

**Contact** *Telephone:* 262-243-4538. *Fax:* 262-243-4506.

#### MASTER'S DEGREE PROGRAM

**Degree** MSN
**Available Programs** Master's.
**Concentrations Available** Nursing education. *Nurse practitioner programs in:* adult health, family health, gerontology.
**Site Options** multiple cities and states; Mequon, WI; Milwaukee, WI.
**Study Options** Full-time and part-time.
**Program Entrance Requirements** Clinical experience, computer literacy, minimum overall college GPA of 3.0, transcript of college record, CPR certification, written essay, immunizations, interview, 2 letters of recommendation, physical assessment course, professional liability insurance/malpractice insurance, resume, statistics course. *Application deadline:* 6/1 (fall), 10/15 (spring). *Application fee:* $50.
**Advanced Placement** Credit given for nursing courses completed elsewhere dependent upon specific evaluations.
**Degree Requirements** 44 total credit hours, thesis or project.

#### POST-MASTER'S PROGRAM

**Areas of Study** *Nurse practitioner programs in:* family health.

#### DOCTORAL DEGREE PROGRAM

**Degree** DNP
**Available Programs** Doctorate.
**Areas of Study** Family health, gerontology.
**Site Options** multiple cities and states; Mequon, WI; Milwaukee, WI.
**Online Degree Options** Yes (online only).
**Program Entrance Requirements** Clinical experience, minimum overall college GPA of 3.0, 2 letters of recommendation, MSN or equivalent, vita, writing sample. *Application deadline:* 4/1 (spring). *Application fee:* $50.
**Degree Requirements** 35 total credit hours, dissertation.

## Edgewood College
### Program in Nursing
### Madison, Wisconsin

*http://www.edgewood.edu/*
Founded in 1927

**DEGREES • BS • MS • MSN/MBA**
**Nursing Program Faculty** 36 (25% with doctorates).
**Baccalaureate Enrollment** 220 **Women** 90% **Men** 10% **Minority** 2% **International** 1% **Part-time** 35%
**Graduate Enrollment** 45 **Women** 86% **Men** 14% **Minority** 2% **Part-time** 100%
**Distance Learning Courses** Available.
**Nursing Student Activities** Sigma Theta Tau, Student Nurses' Association.
**Nursing Student Resources** Academic advising; academic or career counseling; assistance for students with disabilities; bookstore; campus computer network; career placement assistance; computer lab; computer-assisted instruction; e-mail services; employment services for current students; externships; housing assistance; interactive nursing skills videos; Internet; learning resource lab; library services; nursing audiovisuals; paid internships; remedial services; resume preparation assistance; skills, simulation, or other laboratory; tutoring; unpaid internships.
**Library Facilities** 92,054 volumes (4,500 in health, 1,000 in nursing); 26,700 periodical subscriptions (45 health-care related).

### BACCALAUREATE PROGRAMS

**Degree** BS
**Available Programs** Accelerated Baccalaureate for Second Degree; Baccalaureate for Second Degree; Generic Baccalaureate.
**Site Options** Madison, WI.
**Study Options** Full-time and part-time.
**Program Entrance Requirements** Minimum overall college GPA of 2.75, transcript of college record, CPR certification, written essay, health exam, high school biology, high school chemistry, high school foreign language, high school math, high school transcript, immunizations, interview, minimum high school GPA of 2.75, minimum GPA in nursing prerequisites of 2.75, prerequisite course work. Transfer students are accepted. *Application deadline:* 1/15 (fall), 9/15 (spring). *Application fee:* $40.
**Advanced Placement** Credit given for nursing courses completed elsewhere dependent upon specific evaluations.
**Contact** *Telephone:* 608-663-2280. *Fax:* 608-663-2863.

### GRADUATE PROGRAMS

**Contact** *Telephone:* 608-663-2280. *Fax:* 608-663-2863.

#### MASTER'S DEGREE PROGRAM

**Degrees** MS; MSN/MBA
**Available Programs** Master's.
**Concentrations Available** Nursing administration; nursing education.
**Site Options** Madison, WI.
**Study Options** Full-time and part-time.

**Program Entrance Requirements** Clinical experience, computer literacy, minimum overall college GPA of 3.0, transcript of college record, CPR certification, written essay, immunizations, interview, 2 letters of recommendation, nursing research course, prerequisite course work, resume, statistics course. *Application deadline:* Applications may be processed on a rolling basis for some programs.
**Advanced Placement** Credit given for nursing courses completed elsewhere dependent upon specific evaluations.
**Degree Requirements** 36 total credit hours, thesis or project.

# Herzing University Online

## Program in Nursing
## Milwaukee, Wisconsin

### DEGREES • BSN • MSN

**Nursing Program Faculty** 24 (95% with doctorates).
**Baccalaureate Enrollment** 45
**Distance Learning Courses** Available.
**Nursing Student Resources** Academic advising; academic or career counseling; assistance for students with disabilities; bookstore; campus computer network; career placement assistance; computer-assisted instruction; e-mail services; interactive nursing skills videos; learning resource lab; library services; other; skills, simulation, or other laboratory; tutoring.

### BACCALAUREATE PROGRAMS

**Degree** BSN
**Available Programs** RN Baccalaureate.
**Online Degree Options** Yes (online only).
**Contact** Nursing Information, Program in Nursing, Herzing University Online, Administrative Offices, W140 N8917 Lilly Road, Menomonee Falls, WI 53051. *Telephone:* 866-508-0748. *Fax:* 414-727-7090. *E-mail:* admissions@onl.herzing.edu.

### GRADUATE PROGRAMS

**Contact** Mr. Usama Saleh, PhD, Department Chair of Nursing, Program in Nursing, Herzing University Online, W140 N8917 Lilly Road, Menomonee Falls, WI 53051. *Telephone:* 866-508-0748 Ext. 598. *E-mail:* usaleh@herzing.edu.

#### MASTER'S DEGREE PROGRAM

**Degree** MSN
**Available Programs** Master's.
**Concentrations Available** Nursing administration; nursing education. *Nurse practitioner programs in:* family health.
**Study Options** Full-time and part-time.
**Online Degree Options** Yes (online only).
**Program Entrance Requirements** Minimum overall college GPA of 2.75. *Application deadline:* Applications may be processed on a rolling basis for some programs.
**Degree Requirements** 36 total credit hours, comprehensive exam.

# Maranatha Baptist Bible College

## Nursing Department
## Watertown, Wisconsin

***http://www.mbbc.edu***
Founded in 1968

### DEGREE • BSN

**Baccalaureate Enrollment** 58
**Nursing Student Activities** Student Nurses' Association.
**Nursing Student Resources** Academic advising; academic or career counseling; assistance for students with disabilities; bookstore; campus computer network; career placement assistance; computer lab; computer-assisted instruction; e-mail services; employment services for current students; housing assistance; interactive nursing skills videos; Internet; learning resource lab; library services; nursing audiovisuals; skills, simulation, or other laboratory; tutoring.

### BACCALAUREATE PROGRAMS

**Degree** BSN
**Available Programs** RN Baccalaureate.
**Program Entrance Requirements** Minimum overall college GPA of 2.5, CPR certification, written essay, health exam, immunizations, interview, minimum high school GPA, minimum GPA in nursing prerequisites of 2.5, prerequisite course work. Transfer students are accepted. *Application deadline:* Applications may be processed on a rolling basis for some programs.
**Contact** *Telephone:* 920-206-4050.

# Marian University

## School of Nursing
## Fond du Lac, Wisconsin

***http://www.mariancollege.edu/***
Founded in 1936

### DEGREES • BSN • MSN

**Baccalaureate Enrollment** 221 **Women** 95% **Men** 5% **Minority** 1% **Part-time** 7%
**Graduate Enrollment** 39 **Women** 97% **Men** 3% **Part-time** 15%
**Nursing Student Activities** Student Nurses' Association.
**Nursing Student Resources** Academic advising; academic or career counseling; assistance for students with disabilities; bookstore; career placement assistance; computer lab; daycare for children of students; e-mail services; externships; interactive nursing skills videos; Internet; learning resource lab; library services; nursing audiovisuals.
**Library Facilities** 161,589 volumes (3,000 in health, 2,500 in nursing); 1,381 periodical subscriptions (91 health-care related).

### BACCALAUREATE PROGRAMS

**Degree** BSN
**Available Programs** ADN to Baccalaureate; Generic Baccalaureate.
**Site Options** Appleton, WI; Beaver Dam, WI.
**Study Options** Full-time and part-time.
**Program Entrance Requirements** Transcript of college record, high school biology, high school chemistry, 3 years high school math, high school science, high school transcript, minimum high school GPA of 2.5. Transfer students are accepted.
**Advanced Placement** Credit given for nursing courses completed elsewhere dependent upon specific evaluations.
**Contact** *Telephone:* 920-923-8732. *Fax:* 920-923-8770.

### GRADUATE PROGRAMS

**Contact** *Telephone:* 920-923-8094. *Fax:* 920-923-8094.

#### MASTER'S DEGREE PROGRAM

**Degree** MSN
**Available Programs** Master's.
**Concentrations Available** Nursing education. *Nurse practitioner programs in:* adult health.
**Study Options** Full-time and part-time.
**Program Entrance Requirements** Clinical experience, minimum overall college GPA of 3.0, transcript of college record, CPR certification, written essay, immunizations, 3 letters of recommendation, nursing research course, professional liability insurance/malpractice insurance, resume, statistics course.
**Advanced Placement** Credit given for nursing courses completed elsewhere dependent upon specific evaluations.
**Degree Requirements** 39 total credit hours, thesis or project.

#### POST-MASTER'S PROGRAM

**Areas of Study** Nursing education.

# Marquette University

## College of Nursing
## Milwaukee, Wisconsin

***http://www.marquette.edu/nursing***
Founded in 1881

### DEGREES • BSN • DNP • MSN • MSN/MBA • PHD

**Nursing Program Faculty** 65 (58% with doctorates).
**Baccalaureate Enrollment** 490 **Women** 94% **Men** 6% **Minority** 15% **International** .2% **Part-time** .6%
**Graduate Enrollment** 388 **Women** 92% **Men** 8% **Minority** 9% **International** .5% **Part-time** 73%

**Distance Learning Courses** Available.
**Nursing Student Activities** Nursing Honor Society, Sigma Theta Tau, Student Nurses' Association.
**Nursing Student Resources** Academic advising; academic or career counseling; assistance for students with disabilities; bookstore; campus computer network; career placement assistance; computer lab; computer-assisted instruction; daycare for children of students; e-mail services; employment services for current students; housing assistance; interactive nursing skills videos; Internet; learning resource lab; library services; nursing audiovisuals; remedial services; resume preparation assistance; skills, simulation, or other laboratory; tutoring.
**Library Facilities** 1.7 million volumes (58,852 in health, 10,818 in nursing); 45,200 periodical subscriptions (6,100 health-care related).

## BACCALAUREATE PROGRAMS

**Degree** BSN
**Available Programs** Generic Baccalaureate.
**Study Options** Full-time and part-time.
**Program Entrance Requirements** Minimum overall college GPA of 3.0, transcript of college record, written essay, high school biology, high school chemistry, 3 years high school math, high school transcript, 1 letter of recommendation, minimum high school GPA of 2.5, minimum high school rank 25%. *Application deadline:* 12/1 (fall).
**Advanced Placement** Credit given for nursing courses completed elsewhere dependent upon specific evaluations.
**Expenses (2013–14)** *Tuition:* full-time $34,200; part-time $995 per credit hour. *Room and board:* $10,730; room only: $5500 per academic year. *Required fees:* full-time $934.
**Financial Aid** 100% of baccalaureate students in nursing programs received some form of financial aid in 2012–13. *Gift aid (need-based):* Federal Pell, FSEOG, state, private, college/university gift aid from institutional funds. *Loans:* Federal Nursing Student Loans, Federal Direct (Subsidized and Unsubsidized Stafford PLUS), Perkins, state, college/university. *Work-study:* Federal Work-Study, part-time campus jobs. *Financial aid application deadline:* Continuous.
**Contact** Dr. Kerry Kosmoski-Goepfert, Associate Dean for Undergraduate Programs, College of Nursing, Marquette University, Clark Hall, PO Box 1881, Milwaukee, WI 53201-1881. *Telephone:* 414-288-3809. *Fax:* 414-288-1597. *E-mail:* kerry.goepfert@marquette.edu.

## GRADUATE PROGRAMS

**Expenses (2013–14)** *Tuition:* part-time $1025 per credit.
**Financial Aid** 81% of graduate students in nursing programs received some form of financial aid in 2012–13. 1 fellowship with partial tuition reimbursement available (averaging $17,500 per year), 2 research assistantships with full tuition reimbursements available (averaging $13,285 per year), 8 teaching assistantships with full tuition reimbursements available (averaging $13,912 per year) were awarded; career-related internships or fieldwork, Federal Work-Study, scholarships, tuition waivers (partial), and unspecified assistantships also available. Aid available to part-time students. *Financial aid application deadline:* 2/15.
**Contact** Dr. Maureen O'Brien, Associate Dean for Graduate Programs, College of Nursing, Marquette University, Clark Hall, PO Box 1881, Milwaukee, WI 53201-1881. *Telephone:* 414-288-3869. *Fax:* 414-288-1597. *E-mail:* maureen.obrien@marquette.edu.

### MASTER'S DEGREE PROGRAM

**Degrees** MSN; MSN/MBA
**Available Programs** Accelerated Master's for Non-Nursing College Graduates; Master's; Master's for Non-Nursing College Graduates; Master's for Nurses with Non-Nursing Degrees.
**Concentrations Available** Clinical nurse leader; nurse-midwifery; nursing administration. *Clinical nurse specialist programs in:* adult health, pediatric. *Nurse practitioner programs in:* acute care, adult health, pediatric.
**Study Options** Full-time and part-time.
**Program Entrance Requirements** Minimum overall college GPA of 3.0, transcript of college record, CPR certification, written essay, immunizations, 3 letters of recommendation, nursing research course, physical assessment course, prerequisite course work, resume, statistics course, GRE General Test. *Application deadline:* 2/15 (fall), 11/15 (spring). Applications may be processed on a rolling basis for some programs. *Application fee:* $50.
**Advanced Placement** Credit given for nursing courses completed elsewhere dependent upon specific evaluations.
**Degree Requirements** 42 total credit hours, comprehensive exam.

### POST-MASTER'S PROGRAM

**Areas of Study** Nurse-midwifery; nursing administration. *Clinical nurse specialist programs in:* adult health. *Nurse practitioner programs in:* acute care, adult health, family health, pediatric.

### DOCTORAL DEGREE PROGRAM

**Degree** DNP
**Available Programs** Doctorate, Post-Baccalaureate Doctorate.
**Areas of Study** Advanced practice nursing, health-care systems, nursing administration.
**Program Entrance Requirements** Minimum overall college GPA of 3.0, 3 letters of recommendation, statistics course, vita. *Application deadline:* 2/15 (fall).
**Degree Requirements** 69 total credit hours, residency.

**Degree** PhD
**Available Programs** Doctorate; Post-Baccalaureate Doctorate.
**Areas of Study** Aging, faculty preparation, health promotion/disease prevention, health-care systems, human health and illness, illness and transition, nursing administration, nursing education, nursing research, nursing science.
**Program Entrance Requirements** Minimum overall college GPA of 3.2, interview, 3 letters of recommendation, MSN or equivalent, statistics course, vita, writing sample, GRE General Test. *Application deadline:* 2/15 (fall), 11/15 (spring). Applications may be processed on a rolling basis for some programs. *Application fee:* $50.
**Degree Requirements** 51 total credit hours, dissertation, oral exam, written exam, residency.

***See display on next page and full description on page 480.***

# Milwaukee School of Engineering
## School of Nursing
## Milwaukee, Wisconsin

***http://www.msoe.edu/nursing***
Founded in 1903

**DEGREE • BSN**
**Nursing Program Faculty** 27 (26% with doctorates).
**Baccalaureate Enrollment** 239 **Women** 86% **Men** 14% **Minority** 22% **International** .01% **Part-time** 2.3%
**Nursing Student Activities** Nursing Honor Society, Student Nurses' Association.
**Nursing Student Resources** Academic advising; academic or career counseling; assistance for students with disabilities; bookstore; campus computer network; career placement assistance; computer lab; computer-assisted instruction; e-mail services; employment services for current students; externships; housing assistance; interactive nursing skills videos; Internet; learning resource lab; library services; nursing audiovisuals; placement services for program completers; remedial services; resume preparation assistance; skills, simulation, or other laboratory; tutoring.
**Library Facilities** 168,488 volumes (2,528 in health, 2,528 in nursing); 3,436 periodical subscriptions (8,625 health-care related).

## BACCALAUREATE PROGRAMS

**Degree** BSN
**Available Programs** Accelerated Baccalaureate; Accelerated Baccalaureate for Second Degree; Accelerated RN Baccalaureate; Baccalaureate for Second Degree; Generic Baccalaureate; RN Baccalaureate.
**Study Options** Full-time and part-time.
**Program Entrance Requirements** Minimum overall college GPA of 3.0, transcript of college record, CPR certification, health exam, health insurance, high school biology, high school chemistry, 4 years high school math, 2 years high school science, high school transcript, immunizations, minimum high school GPA of 2.75. Transfer students are accepted. *Application deadline:* 9/1 (fall), 12/1 (winter), 3/1 (spring). Applications may be processed on a rolling basis for some programs.
**Advanced Placement** Credit by examination available. Credit given for nursing courses completed elsewhere dependent upon specific evaluations.
**Expenses (2013–14)** *Tuition:* full-time $32,880; part-time $570 per credit. *International tuition:* $32,880 full-time. *Room and board:* $8271; room only: $5280 per academic year. *Required fees:* full-time $1590.
**Financial Aid** 99% of baccalaureate students in nursing programs received some form of financial aid in 2012–13. *Gift aid (need-based):* Federal Pell, FSEOG, state, private, college/university gift aid from insti-

tutional funds. *Loans:* Federal Direct (Subsidized and Unsubsidized Stafford PLUS), Perkins, state, college/university. *Work-study:* Federal Work-Study. *Financial aid application deadline (priority):* 3/15.

**Contact** Dr. Debra L. Jenks, Chair, School of Nursing, Milwaukee School of Engineering, 1025 North Broadway Street, Milwaukee, WI 53202-3109. *Telephone:* 414-277-4516. *Fax:* 414-277-4540. *E-mail:* jenks@msoe.edu.

### CONTINUING EDUCATION PROGRAM

**Contact** Dr. Debra L. Jenks, Department Chair, School of Nursing, Milwaukee School of Engineering, 1025 N Broadway, Milwaukee, WI 53202. *Telephone:* 414-277-4516. *Fax:* 414-277-4540. *E-mail:* jenks@msoe.edu.

## Mount Mary College

### Columbia College of Nursing/Mount Mary College Nursing Program
### Milwaukee, Wisconsin

***See description of programs under Columbia College of Nursing/Mount Mary College Nursing Program (Milwaukee, Wisconsin).***

## Silver Lake College of the Holy Family

### Nursing Program
### Manitowoc, Wisconsin

Founded in 1869

**DEGREE • BSN**

**Nursing Program Faculty** 5

**Baccalaureate Enrollment** 13 **Women** 93% **Men** 7% **Part-time** 100%

**Distance Learning Courses** Available.

**Nursing Student Resources** Academic advising; assistance for students with disabilities; bookstore; campus computer network; computer lab; computer-assisted instruction; e-mail services; interactive nursing skills videos; Internet; library services; nursing audiovisuals; tutoring.

**Library Facilities** 62,418 volumes; 259 periodical subscriptions.

### BACCALAUREATE PROGRAMS

**Degree** BSN

**Available Programs** ADN to Baccalaureate.

**Study Options** Part-time.

**Online Degree Options** Yes.

**Program Entrance Requirements** Minimum overall college GPA of 2.0, transcript of college record, health insurance, immunizations, 1 letter of recommendation, minimum GPA in nursing prerequisites, prerequisite course work, RN licensure. Transfer students are accepted. *Application deadline:* Applications may be processed on a rolling basis for some programs.

**Advanced Placement** Credit given for nursing courses completed elsewhere dependent upon specific evaluations.

**Expenses (2013–14)** *Tuition:* part-time $430 per credit.

**Financial Aid** 93% of baccalaureate students in nursing programs received some form of financial aid in 2012–13.

**Contact** Brianna Neuser, BSN Completion Program Director, Nursing Program, Silver Lake College of the Holy Family, 2406 South Alverno Road, Manitowoc, WI 54220. *Telephone:* 920-686-6213. *E-mail:* brianna.neuser@sl.edu.

# University of Phoenix–Milwaukee Campus

## College of Health and Human Services
## Milwaukee, Wisconsin

***http://www.phoenix.edu/campus-locations/wi/milwaukee-campus/milwaukee-campus.html***

**DEGREES • BSN • MSN • PHD**

### BACCALAUREATE PROGRAMS

**Degree** BSN
**Available Programs** RN Baccalaureate.
**Contact** *Telephone:* 262-785-0608.

### GRADUATE PROGRAMS

**Contact** *Telephone:* 262-785-0608.

**MASTER'S DEGREE PROGRAM**
**Degree** MSN
**Available Programs** Master's.

**DOCTORAL DEGREE PROGRAM**
**Degree** PhD
**Available Programs** Doctorate.

# University of Wisconsin–Eau Claire

## College of Nursing and Health Sciences
## Eau Claire, Wisconsin

***http://www.uwec.edu/conhs/index.htm***
Founded in 1916

**DEGREES • BSN • DNP • MSN**

**Nursing Program Faculty** 47 (28% with doctorates).
**Baccalaureate Enrollment** 401 **Women** 91% **Men** 9% **Minority** 4% **Part-time** 20%
**Graduate Enrollment** 102 **Women** 96% **Men** 4% **Minority** 1% **Part-time** 61%
**Distance Learning Courses** Available.
**Nursing Student Activities** Sigma Theta Tau, Student Nurses' Association.
**Nursing Student Resources** Academic advising; academic or career counseling; assistance for students with disabilities; bookstore; campus computer network; career placement assistance; computer lab; computer-assisted instruction; daycare for children of students; e-mail services; employment services for current students; housing assistance; interactive nursing skills videos; Internet; learning resource lab; library services; nursing audiovisuals; other; placement services for program completers; remedial services; resume preparation assistance; skills, simulation, or other laboratory; tutoring.
**Library Facilities** 666,340 volumes (17,256 in health, 1,984 in nursing); 63,825 periodical subscriptions (3,893 health-care related).

### BACCALAUREATE PROGRAMS

**Degree** BSN
**Available Programs** ADN to Baccalaureate; Accelerated Baccalaureate for Second Degree; Generic Baccalaureate; RN Baccalaureate.
**Site Options** Marshfield, WI.
**Study Options** Full-time.
**Program Entrance Requirements** Minimum overall college GPA of 3.0, transcript of college record, CPR certification, written essay, health exam, high school biology, high school chemistry, high school foreign language, 3 years high school math, 3 years high school science, high school transcript, immunizations, minimum GPA in nursing prerequisites of 2.5, prerequisite course work. Transfer students are accepted. *Application deadline:* 5/1 (fall), 12/1 (spring). *Application fee:* $86.
**Advanced Placement** Credit given for nursing courses completed elsewhere dependent upon specific evaluations.
**Contact** *Telephone:* 715-836-5287. *Fax:* 715-836-5925.

### GRADUATE PROGRAMS

**Contact** *Telephone:* 715-836-5287. *Fax:* 715-836-5925.

**MASTER'S DEGREE PROGRAM**
**Degree** MSN
**Available Programs** Master's; RN to Master's.
**Concentrations Available** Nursing administration; nursing education. *Clinical nurse specialist programs in:* adult health. *Nurse practitioner programs in:* adult health, family health, gerontology.
**Site Options** Marshfield, WI.
**Study Options** Full-time and part-time.
**Program Entrance Requirements** Clinical experience, minimum overall college GPA of 3.0, transcript of college record, CPR certification, written essay, immunizations, 3 letters of recommendation, physical assessment course, professional liability insurance/malpractice insurance, statistics course. *Application deadline:* 1/15 (summer). Applications may be processed on a rolling basis for some programs. *Application fee:* $86.
**Advanced Placement** Credit given for nursing courses completed elsewhere dependent upon specific evaluations.
**Degree Requirements** 42 total credit hours, thesis or project.

**POST-MASTER'S PROGRAM**
**Areas of Study** Nursing administration; nursing education. *Clinical nurse specialist programs in:* adult health. *Nurse practitioner programs in:* adult health, family health, gerontology.

**DOCTORAL DEGREE PROGRAM**
**Degree** DNP
**Available Programs** Doctorate; Post-Baccalaureate Doctorate.
**Areas of Study** Family health, gerontology, nursing administration.
**Program Entrance Requirements** Clinical experience, minimum overall college GPA of 3.00, 3 letters of recommendation, statistics course, vita, writing sample. *Application deadline:* 1/4 (summer). Applications may be processed on a rolling basis for some programs. *Application fee:* $86.
**Degree Requirements** 72 total credit hours.

### CONTINUING EDUCATION PROGRAM

**Contact** *Telephone:* 715-836-5645. *Fax:* 715-836-5263.

# University of Wisconsin–Green Bay

## BSN–LINC Online RN–BSN Program
## Green Bay, Wisconsin

***http://www.uwgb.edu/nursing/***
Founded in 1968

**DEGREES • BSN • MSN**

**Nursing Program Faculty** 12 (67% with doctorates).
**Baccalaureate Enrollment** 441 **Women** 91% **Men** 9% **Minority** 7% **International** 1% **Part-time** 97%
**Graduate Enrollment** 18
**Distance Learning Courses** Available.
**Nursing Student Activities** Sigma Theta Tau, Student Nurses' Association.
**Nursing Student Resources** Academic advising; academic or career counseling; assistance for students with disabilities; bookstore; campus computer network; career placement assistance; computer lab; computer-assisted instruction; e-mail services; employment services for current students; Internet; learning resource lab; library services; nursing audiovisuals; resume preparation assistance; skills, simulation, or other laboratory; tutoring.
**Library Facilities** 360,795 volumes (1,000 in health, 675 in nursing); 4,452 periodical subscriptions (100 health-care related).

### BACCALAUREATE PROGRAMS

**Degree** BSN
**Available Programs** ADN to Baccalaureate; RN Baccalaureate.
**Site Options** Marinette, WI; Rhinelander, WI.
**Study Options** Full-time and part-time.
**Online Degree Options** Yes.
**Program Entrance Requirements** Minimum overall college GPA of 2.5, transcript of college record, RN licensure. Transfer students are accepted. *Application fee:* $44.
**Expenses (2013–14)** *Tuition, area resident:* part-time $319 per credit. *Tuition, state resident:* part-time $452 per credit. *Tuition, nonresident:* part-time $415 per credit.

**Financial Aid** 45% of baccalaureate students in nursing programs received some form of financial aid in 2012–13.
**Contact** Ms. Sharon Gajeski, Advisor, BSN–LINC Online RN–BSN Program, University of Wisconsin–Green Bay, 2420 Nicolet Drive, Green Bay, WI 54311-7001. *Telephone:* 920-465-2570. *Fax:* 920-465-2854. *E-mail:* gajeskis@uwgb.edu.

## GRADUATE PROGRAMS

**Expenses (2013–14)** *Tuition, state resident:* part-time $571 per credit. *Tuition, nonresident:* part-time $571 per credit.
**Contact** Dr. Janet Reilly, Director of MSN-LINC, BSN–LINC Online RN–BSN Program, University of Wisconsin–Green Bay, Nursing, 2420 Nicolet Drive, RH 325, Green Bay, WI 54311-7001. *Telephone:* 920-465-2365. *Fax:* 920-465-2854. *E-mail:* reillyj@uwgb.edu.

### MASTER'S DEGREE PROGRAM

**Degree** MSN
**Available Programs** Master's.
**Concentrations Available** Health-care administration; nursing administration.
**Study Options** Part-time.
**Online Degree Options** Yes (online only).
**Program Entrance Requirements** Minimum overall college GPA of 3.0, written essay, 3 letters of recommendation, resume, statistics course. *Application fee:* $54.
**Advanced Placement** Credit given for nursing courses completed elsewhere dependent upon specific evaluations.
**Degree Requirements** 34 total credit hours.

# University of Wisconsin–Madison

## School of Nursing
## Madison, Wisconsin

***http://www.son.wisc.edu/***
Founded in 1848

## DEGREES • BS • PHD

**Nursing Program Faculty** 52 (35% with doctorates).
**Baccalaureate Enrollment** 384 **Women** 86% **Men** 14% **Minority** 11% **International** 2% **Part-time** 25%
**Graduate Enrollment** 164 **Women** 95% **Men** 5% **Minority** 7% **International** 4% **Part-time** 60%
**Distance Learning Courses** Available.
**Nursing Student Activities** Nursing Honor Society, Sigma Theta Tau, Student Nurses' Association, nursing club.
**Nursing Student Resources** Academic advising; academic or career counseling; assistance for students with disabilities; bookstore; campus computer network; career placement assistance; computer lab; computer-assisted instruction; e-mail services; externships; interactive nursing skills videos; Internet; learning resource lab; library services; nursing audiovisuals; resume preparation assistance; skills, simulation, or other laboratory; tutoring.
**Library Facilities** 334,000 volumes in health, 8,300 volumes in nursing; 1,500 periodical subscriptions health-care related.

## BACCALAUREATE PROGRAMS

**Degree** BS
**Available Programs** ADN to Baccalaureate; Generic Baccalaureate; RN Baccalaureate.
**Study Options** Full-time.
**Program Entrance Requirements** Minimum overall college GPA of 2.75, transcript of college record, CPR certification, written essay, high school chemistry, high school foreign language, 3 years high school math, 3 years high school science, high school transcript, immunizations, minimum GPA in nursing prerequisites of 2.75, prerequisite course work. Transfer students are accepted. *Application deadline:* 2/1 (fall). *Application fee:* $50.
**Advanced Placement** Credit by examination available. Credit given for nursing courses completed elsewhere dependent upon specific evaluations.
**Expenses (2013–14)** *Tuition, state resident:* full-time $10,402. *Tuition, nonresident:* full-time $26,652. *Room and board:* $8354 per academic year.
**Financial Aid** 65% of baccalaureate students in nursing programs received some form of financial aid in 2012–13. *Gift aid (need-based):* Federal Pell, FSEOG, state, private, college/university gift aid from institutional funds. *Loans:* Federal Direct (Subsidized and Unsubsidized Stafford PLUS), Perkins. *Work-study:* Federal Work-Study, part-time campus jobs. *Financial aid application deadline:* Continuous.
**Contact** Nursing Admissions, School of Nursing, University of Wisconsin–Madison, 600 Highland Avenue, Room K6/146, Madison, WI 53792-2455. *Telephone:* 608-263-5202. *Fax:* 608-263-5296. *E-mail:* ugadmit@son.wisc.edu.

## GRADUATE PROGRAMS

**Expenses (2013–14)** *Tuition, state resident:* full-time $12,068. *Tuition, nonresident:* full-time $25,188. *Room and board:* $8980 per academic year.
**Financial Aid** 55% of graduate students in nursing programs received some form of financial aid in 2012–13. 8 fellowships with full tuition reimbursements available (averaging $26,900 per year), 8 research assistantships with full tuition reimbursements available (averaging $18,000 per year), 5 teaching assistantships with full tuition reimbursements available (averaging $11,000 per year) were awarded; career-related internships or fieldwork, Federal Work-Study, institutionally sponsored loans, scholarships, traineeships, and unspecified assistantships also available. Aid available to part-time students. *Financial aid application deadline:* 3/1.
**Contact** Caroline Luscombe, Graduate Program Coordinator, School of Nursing, University of Wisconsin–Madison, 600 Highland Avenue, Room K6/140, Clinical Science Center, Madison, WI 53792-2455. *Telephone:* 608-263-5258. *Fax:* 608-263-5296. *E-mail:* luscombe@wisc.edu.

### DOCTORAL DEGREE PROGRAM

**Degree** PhD
**Available Programs** Doctorate; Post-Baccalaureate Doctorate.
**Areas of Study** Aging, bio-behavioral research, biology of health and illness, community health, faculty preparation, family health, gerontology, health policy, health promotion/disease prevention, human health and illness, information systems, nursing education, nursing research, oncology,women's health.
**Program Entrance Requirements** Minimum overall college GPA of 3.0, interview, 3 letters of recommendation, scholarly papers, vita, writing sample, GRE General Test. *Application deadline:* 1/15 (fall), 9/15 (spring). *Application fee:* $56.
**Degree Requirements** 60 total credit hours, dissertation, written exam, residency.

### POSTDOCTORAL PROGRAM

**Areas of Study** Adolescent health, aging, cancer care, chronic illness, community health, family health, gerontology, health promotion/disease prevention, individualized study, nursing informatics, nursing interventions, nursing research, vulnerable population,women's health.
**Postdoctoral Program Contact** Carol Aspinwall, Student Services Coordinator, School of Nursing, University of Wisconsin–Madison, 600 Highland Avenue, Room K6/133, Madison, WI 53792-2455. *Telephone:* 608-263-9109. *Fax:* 608-263-5296. *E-mail:* caaspinwall@wisc.edu.

## CONTINUING EDUCATION PROGRAM

**Contact** Ms. Marilyn Haynes Brokopp, Clinical Associate Professor, School of Nursing, University of Wisconsin–Madison, 600 Highland Avenue, Room H6/158, Clinical Science Center, Madison, WI 53792-2455. *Telephone:* 608-262-1179. *Fax:* 608-263-5332. *E-mail:* haynesbrokop@wisc.edu.

# University of Wisconsin–Milwaukee

## College of Nursing
## Milwaukee, Wisconsin

***http://www.nursing.uwm.edu/***
Founded in 1956

## DEGREES • BSN • DNP • MN • PHD

**Nursing Program Faculty** 29 (100% with doctorates).
**Baccalaureate Enrollment** 1,154 **Women** 85% **Men** 15% **Minority** 25% **International** .75% **Part-time** 23%
**Graduate Enrollment** 255 **Women** 90% **Men** 10% **Minority** 15% **International** 3% **Part-time** 54%
**Distance Learning Courses** Available.
**Nursing Student Activities** Sigma Theta Tau, Student Nurses' Association.

**Nursing Student Resources** Academic advising; academic or career counseling; assistance for students with disabilities; bookstore; campus computer network; career placement assistance; computer lab; computer-assisted instruction; e-mail services; interactive nursing skills videos; Internet; learning resource lab; library services; nursing audiovisuals; remedial services; skills, simulation, or other laboratory; tutoring.
**Library Facilities** 2.3 million volumes (330,089 in health, 179,089 in nursing); 73,211 periodical subscriptions (926 health-care related).

## BACCALAUREATE PROGRAMS

**Degree** BSN
**Available Programs** ADN to Baccalaureate; Generic Baccalaureate; RN Baccalaureate.
**Site Options** Kenosha, WI; West Bend, WI.
**Study Options** Full-time and part-time.
**Program Entrance Requirements** Minimum overall college GPA of 2.75, transcript of college record, written essay, high school biology, high school chemistry, high school foreign language, 3 years high school math, 3 years high school science; high school transcript, minimum high school GPA of 2.0, minimum GPA in nursing prerequisites of 2.75, prerequisite course work. Transfer students are accepted. *Application deadline:* 1/15 (fall), 8/15 (spring). *Application fee:* $44.
**Advanced Placement** Credit given for nursing courses completed elsewhere dependent upon specific evaluations.
**Expenses (2013–14)** *Tuition, state resident:* full-time $8090; part-time $337 per credit. *Tuition, nonresident:* full-time $17,820; part-time $506 per credit. *International tuition:* $17,820 full-time. *Room and board:* $10,086; room only: $6420 per academic year. *Required fees:* full-time $1210; part-time $605 per term.
**Financial Aid** 89% of baccalaureate students in nursing programs received some form of financial aid in 2012–13. *Gift aid (need-based):* Federal Pell, FSEOG, state, private, college/university gift aid from institutional funds, Federal Nursing. *Loans:* Federal Nursing Student Loans, Federal Direct (Subsidized and Unsubsidized Stafford PLUS), Perkins, state, alternative loans. *Work-study:* Federal Work-Study. *Financial aid application deadline (priority):* 3/1.
**Contact** Ms. Donna Wier, Senior Advisor, College of Nursing, University of Wisconsin–Milwaukee, PO Box 413, Student Affairs, Milwaukee, WI 53201. *Telephone:* 414-229-5481. *Fax:* 414-229-5554. *E-mail:* ddw@uwm.edu.

## GRADUATE PROGRAMS

**Expenses (2013–14)** *Tuition, state resident:* full-time $10,386; part-time $649 per credit. *Tuition, nonresident:* full-time $22,852; part-time $1428 per credit. *International tuition:* $22,852 full-time. *Room and board:* $12,846; room only: $3666 per academic year. *Required fees:* full-time $1210; part-time $605 per term.
**Financial Aid** 65% of graduate students in nursing programs received some form of financial aid in 2012–13. 3 fellowships, 1 research assistantship, 9 teaching assistantships were awarded; career-related internships or fieldwork, Federal Work-Study, unspecified assistantships, and project assistantships also available. Aid available to part-time students. *Financial aid application deadline:* 4/15.
**Contact** Ms. Robin Jens, Director, Student Services, College of Nursing, University of Wisconsin–Milwaukee, PO Box 413, Student Affairs, Milwaukee, WI 53201. *Telephone:* 414-229-2494. *Fax:* 414-229-5554. *E-mail:* rjens@uwm.edu.

### MASTER'S DEGREE PROGRAM

**Degree** MN
**Available Programs** Master's; Master's for Non-Nursing College Graduates.
**Concentrations Available** Clinical nurse leader.
**Study Options** Full-time and part-time.
**Program Entrance Requirements** Minimum overall college GPA of 3.0, transcript of college record, written essay, 3 letters of recommendation, prerequisite course work, resume, statistics course, GRE General Test or MAT. *Application deadline:* 1/1 (fall), 9/1 (spring). *Application fee:* $56.
**Advanced Placement** Credit given for nursing courses completed elsewhere dependent upon specific evaluations.
**Degree Requirements** 33 total credit hours.

### DOCTORAL DEGREE PROGRAM

**Degree** DNP
**Available Programs** Doctorate, Post-Baccalaureate Doctorate.
**Areas of Study** Advanced practice nursing, clinical practice, community health, family health, gerontology, health-care systems, human health and illness, individualized study, maternity-newborn, neurobehavior,women's health.
**Online Degree Options** Yes.
**Program Entrance Requirements** Minimum overall college GPA of 3.2, interview, 3 letters of recommendation, scholarly papers, statistics course, vita, writing sample. *Application deadline:* 1/1 (fall), 9/1 (spring), 11/1 (summer). Applications may be processed on a rolling basis for some programs. *Application fee:* $56.
**Degree Requirements** 64 total credit hours, residency.

**Degrees** DNP; PhD
**Available Programs** Doctorate; Post-Baccalaureate Doctorate.
**Areas of Study** Health-care systems, individualized study, neurobehavior, nursing research,women's health.
**Online Degree Options** Yes (online only).
**Program Entrance Requirements** Minimum overall college GPA of 3.2, interview, 3 letters of recommendation, scholarly papers, statistics course, vita, writing sample, GRE. *Application deadline:* 1/1 (fall), 9/1 (spring), 11/1 (summer). Applications may be processed on a rolling basis for some programs. *Application fee:* $56.
**Degree Requirements** 64 total credit hours, dissertation, oral exam, written exam.

***See display on next page and full description on page 492.***

# University of Wisconsin–Oshkosh
## College of Nursing
## Oshkosh, Wisconsin

*http://www.uwosh.edu/con*
Founded in 1871

**DEGREES • BSN • DNP • MSN**
**Nursing Program Faculty** 92 (13% with doctorates).
**Baccalaureate Enrollment** 635 **Women** 88% **Men** 12% **Minority** 6% **Part-time** 35%
**Graduate Enrollment** 136 **Women** 95% **Men** 5% **Minority** 7% **International** 1% **Part-time** 76%
**Distance Learning Courses** Available.
**Nursing Student Activities** Sigma Theta Tau, Student Nurses' Association.
**Nursing Student Resources** Academic advising; academic or career counseling; assistance for students with disabilities; bookstore; campus computer network; career placement assistance; computer lab; computer-assisted instruction; daycare for children of students; e-mail services; employment services for current students; externships; housing assistance; interactive nursing skills videos; Internet; learning resource lab; library services; nursing audiovisuals; other; paid internships; placement services for program completers; remedial services; resume preparation assistance; skills, simulation, or other laboratory; tutoring; unpaid internships.
**Library Facilities** 446,774 volumes; 5,219 periodical subscriptions.

## BACCALAUREATE PROGRAMS

**Degree** BSN
**Available Programs** ADN to Baccalaureate; Accelerated Baccalaureate; Accelerated Baccalaureate for Second Degree; Baccalaureate for Second Degree; Generic Baccalaureate; RN Baccalaureate.
**Site Options** Wausau, WI; Sheboygan/Manitowoc, WI; Janesville, WI.
**Study Options** Full-time and part-time.
**Online Degree Options** Yes.
**Program Entrance Requirements** Minimum overall college GPA of 2.75, transcript of college record, CPR certification, written essay, 3 years high school math, 3 years high school science, immunizations, interview, minimum high school rank 50%, minimum GPA in nursing prerequisites of 2.75, prerequisite course work. Transfer students are accepted. *Application deadline:* 1/30 (fall), 8/30 (spring).
**Advanced Placement** Credit by examination available. Credit given for nursing courses completed elsewhere dependent upon specific evaluations.
**Expenses (2013–14)** *Tuition, state resident:* full-time $6422; part-time $273 per credit. *Tuition, nonresident:* full-time $13,995; part-time $583 per credit. *International tuition:* $13,995 full-time. *Room and board:* $6872; room only: $3864 per academic year. *Required fees:* full-time $979; part-time $41 per credit.
**Financial Aid** 68% of baccalaureate students in nursing programs received some form of financial aid in 2012–13.

**Contact** Ms. Molly Gottfried, Undergraduate Program Assistant, College of Nursing, University of Wisconsin–Oshkosh, 800 Algoma Boulevard, Oshkosh, WI 54901-8660. *Telephone:* 920-424-1077. *Fax:* 920-424-0123. *E-mail:* gottfrim@uwosh.edu.

## GRADUATE PROGRAMS

**Expenses (2013–14)** *Tuition, state resident:* full-time $7640; part-time $424 per credit. *Tuition, nonresident:* full-time $16,771; part-time $932 per credit. *International tuition:* $16,771 full-time. *Room and board:* $6872; room only: $3864 per academic year. *Required fees:* full-time $979; part-time $54 per credit.

**Financial Aid** 48% of graduate students in nursing programs received some form of financial aid in 2012–13. Fellowships, research assistantships with partial tuition reimbursements available, institutionally sponsored loans, scholarships, traineeships, tuition waivers (partial), and unspecified assistantships available. *Financial aid application deadline:* 3/15.

**Contact** Ms. Katrina Helmer, Graduate Program Assistant, College of Nursing, University of Wisconsin–Oshkosh, College of Nursing, 800 Algoma Boulevard, Oshkosh, WI 54901-8660. *Telephone:* 920-424-2106. *Fax:* 920-424-0123. *E-mail:* congrad@uwosh.edu.

### MASTER'S DEGREE PROGRAM

**Degree** MSN
**Available Programs** Master's; RN to Master's.
**Concentrations Available** Clinical nurse leader; nursing education.
**Study Options** Full-time and part-time.
**Online Degree Options** Yes (online only).
**Program Entrance Requirements** Computer literacy, minimum overall college GPA of 3.0, transcript of college record, CPR certification, written essay, immunizations, interview, 3 letters of recommendation, resume, statistics course. *Application deadline:* 1/31 (fall). *Application fee:* $56.
**Advanced Placement** Credit given for nursing courses completed elsewhere dependent upon specific evaluations.
**Degree Requirements** 37 total credit hours, thesis or project.

### POST-MASTER'S PROGRAM

**Areas of Study** Clinical nurse leader; nursing education; nursing informatics.

### DOCTORAL DEGREE PROGRAM

**Degree** DNP
**Available Programs** Doctorate; Post-Baccalaureate Doctorate.
**Areas of Study** Advanced practice nursing.
**Program Entrance Requirements** Minimum overall college GPA of 3.0, interview, 3 letters of recommendation, MSN or equivalent, statistics course, vita, writing sample. *Application deadline:* 1/31 (fall). *Application fee:* $56.
**Degree Requirements** 74 total credit hours, residency.

## CONTINUING EDUCATION PROGRAM

**Contact** Dr. Karen Heikel, Assistant Vice Chancellor, College of Nursing, University of Wisconsin–Oshkosh, 800 Algoma Boulevard, Oshkosh, WI 54901-8660. *Telephone:* 920-424-1463. *Fax:* 920-424-1803. *E-mail:* heikelk@uwosh.edu.

# University of Wisconsin–Waukesha

**Columbia College of Nursing/Mount Mary College Nursing Program**
**Waukesha, Wisconsin**

***See description of programs under Columbia College of Nursing/Mount Mary College Nursing Program (Milwaukee, Wisconsin).***

# Viterbo University

**School of Nursing**
**La Crosse, Wisconsin**

***http://www.viterbo.edu/***
Founded in 1890

**DEGREES • BSN • DNP • MSN**

**Nursing Program Faculty** 32 (8% with doctorates).

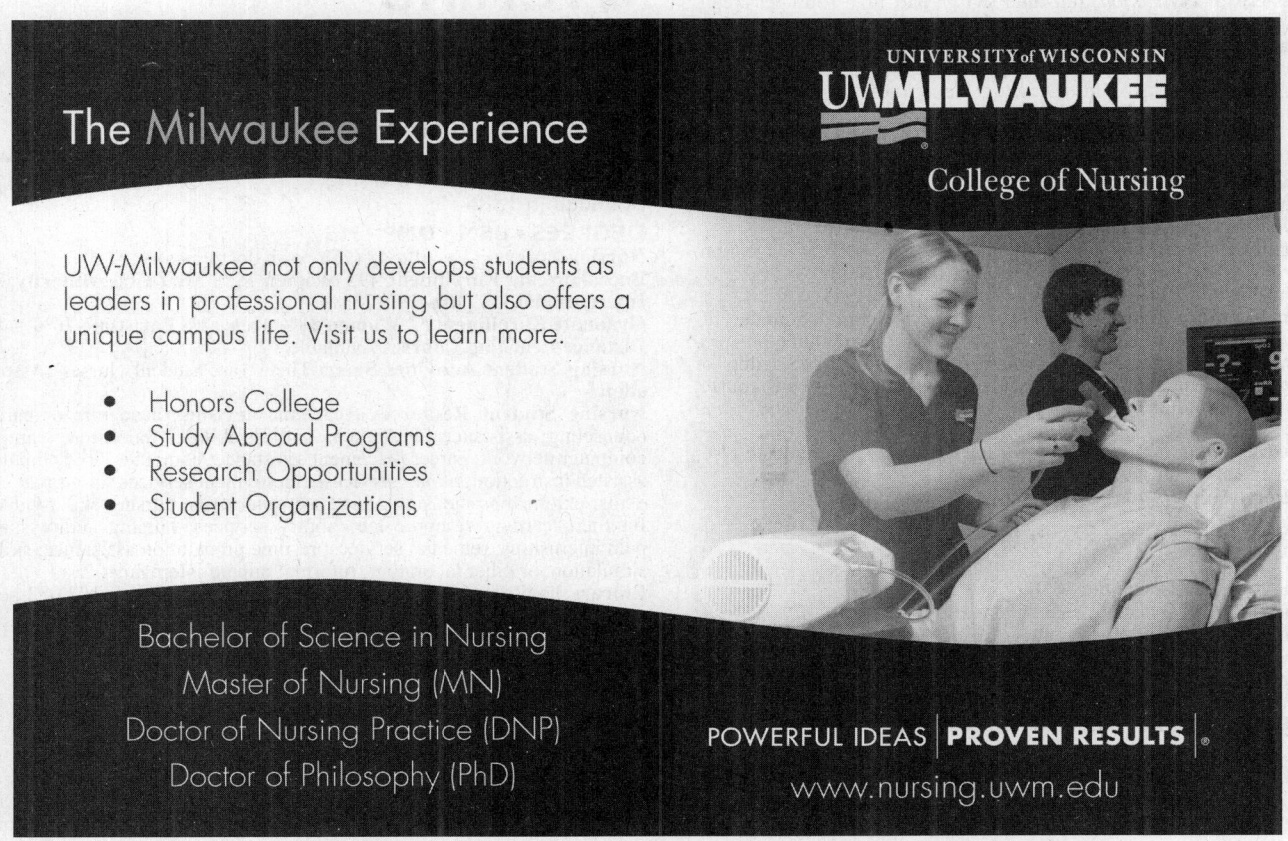

**Baccalaureate Enrollment** 688 **Women** 94% **Men** 6% **Minority** 3% **International** 1% **Part-time** 5%
**Graduate Enrollment** 60 **Women** 99% **Men** 1% **Minority** 1% **Part-time** 15%
**Nursing Student Activities** Sigma Theta Tau, Student Nurses' Association.
**Nursing Student Resources** Academic advising; academic or career counseling; assistance for students with disabilities; bookstore; campus computer network; career placement assistance; computer lab; computer-assisted instruction; e-mail services; interactive nursing skills videos; Internet; learning resource lab; library services; nursing audiovisuals; remedial services; resume preparation assistance; skills, simulation, or other laboratory; tutoring.
**Library Facilities** 92,300 volumes (5,200 in health, 3,398 in nursing); 229 periodical subscriptions (312 health-care related).

### BACCALAUREATE PROGRAMS

**Degree** BSN
**Available Programs** Generic Baccalaureate; RN Baccalaureate.
**Site Options** Madison, WI; Rochester, MN; Janesville, WI.
**Study Options** Full-time and part-time.
**Program Entrance Requirements** Minimum overall college GPA of 2.75, transcript of college record, CPR certification, health exam, high school chemistry, 2 years high school math, 2 years high school science, high school transcript, immunizations, minimum high school GPA of 3.0, minimum high school rank 55%, minimum GPA in nursing prerequisites of 2.75, prerequisite course work. Transfer students are accepted. *Application deadline:* Applications may be processed on a rolling basis for some programs.
**Advanced Placement** Credit given for nursing courses completed elsewhere dependent upon specific evaluations.
**Expenses (2013–14)** *Tuition:* full-time $22,740; part-time $670 per credit. *Room and board:* $3800 per academic year. *Required fees:* full-time $2670; part-time $260 per credit; part-time $295 per term.
**Financial Aid** 98% of baccalaureate students in nursing programs received some form of financial aid in 2012–13.
**Contact** Mr. Robert Forget, Dean of Admission, School of Nursing, Viterbo University, 900 Viterbo Drive, La Crosse, WI 54601. *Telephone:* 608-796-3012. *Fax:* 608-796-3050. *E-mail:* rlforget@viterbo.edu.

### GRADUATE PROGRAMS

**Expenses (2013–14)** *Tuition:* full-time $8400; part-time $700 per credit. *Required fees:* full-time $120; part-time $10 per credit.
**Financial Aid** 33% of graduate students in nursing programs received some form of financial aid in 2012–13.
**Contact** Dr. Bonnie Nesbitt, Director, School of Nursing, Viterbo University, 900 Viterbo Drive, La Crosse, WI 54601. *Telephone:* 608-796-3688. *Fax:* 608-796-3668. *E-mail:* bjnesbitt@viterbo.edu.

#### MASTER'S DEGREE PROGRAM

**Degree** MSN
**Available Programs** Master's.
**Concentrations Available** Clinical nurse leader; nursing education. *Nurse practitioner programs in:* adult health, family health.
**Study Options** Full-time and part-time.
**Program Entrance Requirements** Clinical experience, computer literacy, minimum overall college GPA of 3.0, transcript of college record, CPR certification, written essay, immunizations, interview, 3 letters of recommendation, nursing research course, physical assessment course, resume, statistics course. *Application deadline:* 2/15 (fall). *Application fee:* $50.
**Advanced Placement** Credit given for nursing courses completed elsewhere dependent upon specific evaluations.
**Degree Requirements** 40 total credit hours, thesis or project.

#### DOCTORAL DEGREE PROGRAM

**Degree** DNP
**Available Programs** Doctorate.
**Areas of Study** Advanced practice nursing.
**Program Entrance Requirements** Clinical experience, minimum overall college GPA of 3.0, interview by faculty committee, 2 letters of recommendation, statistics course, vita, writing sample. *Application deadline:* 2/15 (fall). *Application fee:* $50.
**Degree Requirements** 66 total credit hours, residency.

### CONTINUING EDUCATION PROGRAM

**Contact** Ms. Delayne Vogel, Continuing Education Coordinator, School of Nursing, Viterbo University, 900 Viterbo Drive, La Crosse, WI 54601. *Telephone:* 608-796-3692. *Fax:* 608-796-3668. *E-mail:* dgvogel@viterbo.edu.

## Wisconsin Lutheran College
**Nursing Program**
**Milwaukee, Wisconsin**

Founded in 1973

**DEGREE • BSN**
**Nursing Program Faculty** 2
**Baccalaureate Enrollment** 14
**Nursing Student Activities** Student Nurses' Association.
**Nursing Student Resources** Academic advising; academic or career counseling; assistance for students with disabilities; bookstore; campus computer network; career placement assistance; computer lab; computer-assisted instruction; e-mail services; externships; housing assistance; interactive nursing skills videos; Internet; learning resource lab; library services; nursing audiovisuals; skills, simulation, or other laboratory; tutoring.
**Library Facilities** 78,107 volumes; 310 periodical subscriptions.

### BACCALAUREATE PROGRAMS

**Degree** BSN
**Available Programs** Generic Baccalaureate.
**Study Options** Full-time.
**Program Entrance Requirements** Minimum overall college GPA of 2.75, transcript of college record, written essay, high school foreign language, interview, 3 letters of recommendation, minimum GPA in nursing prerequisites of 2.0, prerequisite course work. Transfer students are accepted. *Application deadline:* 3/15 (spring).
**Contact** *Telephone:* 414-443-8800.

### CONTINUING EDUCATION PROGRAM

**Contact** *Telephone:* 414-443-8800.

# WYOMING

## University of Wyoming
**Fay W. Whitney School of Nursing**
**Laramie, Wyoming**

***http://www.uwyo.edu/nursing***
Founded in 1886

**DEGREES • BSN • DNP • MS**
**Nursing Program Faculty** 48 (25% with doctorates).
**Baccalaureate Enrollment** 492 **Women** 87% **Men** 13% **Minority** 7% **International** 1% **Part-time** 73%
**Graduate Enrollment** 52 **Women** 88% **Men** 12% **Part-time** 46%
**Distance Learning Courses** Available.
**Nursing Student Activities** Sigma Theta Tau, Student Nurses' Association.
**Nursing Student Resources** Academic advising; academic or career counseling; assistance for students with disabilities; bookstore; campus computer network; career placement assistance; computer lab; computer-assisted instruction; e-mail services; employment services for current students; externships; housing assistance; interactive nursing skills videos; Internet; learning resource lab; library services; nursing audiovisuals; paid internships; remedial services; resume preparation assistance; skills, simulation, or other laboratory; tutoring; unpaid internships.
**Library Facilities** 3.9 million volumes (56,231 in health); 103,083 periodical subscriptions (1,689 health-care related).

### BACCALAUREATE PROGRAMS

**Degree** BSN
**Available Programs** ADN to Baccalaureate; Accelerated Baccalaureate for Second Degree; Generic Baccalaureate.
**Study Options** Full-time.
**Online Degree Options** Yes.
**Program Entrance Requirements** Transcript of college record, CPR certification, written essay, immunizations, interview, 2 letters of recom-

mendation, minimum GPA in nursing prerequisites of 2.75, professional liability insurance/malpractice insurance, prerequisite course work. Transfer students are accepted. *Application deadline:* 2/1 (fall). *Application fee:* $30.
**Advanced Placement** Credit given for nursing courses completed elsewhere dependent upon specific evaluations.
**Expenses (2013–14)** *Tuition, area resident:* part-time $108 per credit hour. *Tuition, state resident:* part-time $108. *Tuition, nonresident:* part-time $432 per credit hour.
**Contact** Ms. Debbie A. Shoefelt, Credentials Analyst/Academic Advisor, Fay W. Whitney School of Nursing, University of Wyoming, Department 3065, 1000 East University Avenue, Laramie, WY 82071. *Telephone:* 307-766-4292. *Fax:* 307-766-4294. *E-mail:* basicbsn@uwyo.edu.

### GRADUATE PROGRAMS

**Expenses (2013–14)** *Tuition, area resident:* part-time $304 per credit hour. *Tuition, state resident:* part-time $307. *Tuition, nonresident:* part-time $643 per credit hour.
**Financial Aid** Research assistantships (averaging $10,062 per year), teaching assistantships (averaging $10,062 per year) were awarded; career-related internships or fieldwork, institutionally sponsored loans, scholarships, traineeships, and unspecified assistantships also available.
**Contact** Ms. Crystal McFadden, Office Associate, Fay W. Whitney School of Nursing, University of Wyoming, Department 3065, 1000 East University Avenue, Laramie, WY 82071. *Telephone:* 307-766-6568. *Fax:* 307-766-4294. *E-mail:* gradnurse@uwyo.edu.

#### MASTER'S DEGREE PROGRAM

**Degree** MS
**Available Programs** Master's; Master's for Nurses with Non-Nursing Degrees.
**Concentrations Available** Nursing education.
**Study Options** Part-time.
**Online Degree Options** Yes (online only).
**Program Entrance Requirements** Clinical experience, minimum overall college GPA of 3.0, transcript of college record, CPR certification, written essay, immunizations, 3 letters of recommendation, professional liability insurance/malpractice insurance, resume, statistics course, GRE General Test. *Application deadline:* 2/1 (fall). *Application fee:* $50.
**Degree Requirements** 36 total credit hours.

#### POST-MASTER'S PROGRAM

**Areas of Study** Nursing education.

#### DOCTORAL DEGREE PROGRAM

**Degree** DNP
**Available Programs** Doctorate.
**Areas of Study** Advanced practice nursing, clinical practice, ethics, family health, health policy, health promotion/disease prevention, human health and illness, individualized study, information systems, nursing policy,women's health.
**Program Entrance Requirements** Clinical experience, minimum overall college GPA of 3.5, interview by faculty committee, 3 letters of recommendation, vita, writing sample. *Application deadline:* 2/1 (fall). *Application fee:* $50.
**Degree Requirements** 84 total credit hours.

# CANADA

## ALBERTA

## Athabasca University

### Centre for Nursing and Health Studies
### Athabasca, Alberta

***http://www.athabascau.ca/cnhs/***
Founded in 1970

**DEGREES • BN • MN • MN/MHSA**

**Nursing Program Faculty** 130 (45% with doctorates).
**Baccalaureate Enrollment** 3,647
**Graduate Enrollment** 1,382
**Distance Learning Courses** Available.
**Nursing Student Activities** Student Nurses' Association.
**Nursing Student Resources** Academic advising; academic or career counseling; assistance for students with disabilities; bookstore; campus computer network; computer lab; computer-assisted instruction; e-mail services; interactive nursing skills videos; Internet; library services; nursing audiovisuals; remedial services; skills, simulation, or other laboratory; tutoring.
**Library Facilities** 178,808 volumes; 32,619 periodical subscriptions.

### BACCALAUREATE PROGRAMS

**Degree** BN
**Available Programs** Generic Baccalaureate; LPN to RN Baccalaureate; RN Baccalaureate.
**Study Options** Full-time and part-time.
**Program Entrance Requirements** CPR certification, immunizations, RN licensure. Transfer students are accepted. *Application deadline:* Applications may be processed on a rolling basis for some programs.
**Advanced Placement** Credit by examination available. Credit given for nursing courses completed elsewhere dependent upon specific evaluations.
**Expenses (2013–14)** *Tuition, state resident:* part-time CAN$663 per course. *Tuition, nonresident:* part-time CAN$777 per course. *International tuition:* CAN$1249 full-time.
**Contact** Gayle Deren-Purdy, Undergraduate Student Advisor, Centre for Nursing and Health Studies, Athabasca University, 1 University Drive, Athabasca, AB T9S 3A3. *Telephone:* 800-788-9041 Ext. 6446. *Fax:* 780-675-6468. *E-mail:* gayled@athabascau.ca.

### GRADUATE PROGRAMS

**Expenses (2013–14)** *Tuition:* part-time CAN$1395 per course. *International tuition:* CAN$1595 full-time.
**Contact** Ms. Donna Dunn Hart, Graduate Student Advisor, Centre for Nursing and Health Studies, Athabasca University, 1 University Drive, Athabasca, AB T9S 3A3. *Telephone:* 800-788-9041 Ext. 6300. *Fax:* 780-675-6468. *E-mail:* donnad@athabascau.ca.

#### MASTER'S DEGREE PROGRAM

**Degrees** MN; MN/MHSA
**Available Programs** Master's; Master's for Nurses with Non-Nursing Degrees.
**Concentrations Available** Nursing administration; nursing education. *Nurse practitioner programs in:* community health, family health, primary care.
**Study Options** Full-time and part-time.
**Online Degree Options** Yes.
**Program Entrance Requirements** Clinical experience, computer literacy, minimum overall college GPA of 3.0, transcript of college record, written essay, 3 letters of recommendation, resume. *Application deadline:* 3/1 (fall), 12/1 (spring). *Application fee:* CAN$150.
**Advanced Placement** Credit given for nursing courses completed elsewhere dependent upon specific evaluations.
**Degree Requirements** 33 total credit hours, thesis or project, comprehensive exam.

**POST-MASTER'S PROGRAM**
**Areas of Study** *Nurse practitioner programs in:* community health, family health.

# University of Alberta
## Faculty of Nursing
## Edmonton, Alberta

***http://www.nursing.ualberta.ca/***
Founded in 1906

**DEGREES • BSCN • MN • PHD**
**Nursing Program Faculty** 106 (50% with doctorates).
**Baccalaureate Enrollment** 1,615 **Women** 93% **Men** 7% **International** 1% **Part-time** 7%
**Graduate Enrollment** 173 **Women** 90% **Men** 10% **International** 7% **Part-time** 60%
**Distance Learning Courses** Available.
**Nursing Student Activities** Nursing Honor Society, Sigma Theta Tau, Student Nurses' Association.
**Nursing Student Resources** Academic advising; academic or career counseling; assistance for students with disabilities; bookstore; campus computer network; career placement assistance; computer lab; computer-assisted instruction; daycare for children of students; e-mail services; employment services for current students; housing assistance; interactive nursing skills videos; Internet; learning resource lab; library services; nursing audiovisuals; other; paid internships; remedial services; resume preparation assistance; skills, simulation, or other laboratory; tutoring; unpaid internships.
**Library Facilities** 9.7 million volumes (115,000 in health, 19,000 in nursing); 2,400 periodical subscriptions health-care related.

### BACCALAUREATE PROGRAMS

**Degree** BScN
**Available Programs** Accelerated Baccalaureate for Second Degree; Baccalaureate for Second Degree; Generic Baccalaureate; RN Baccalaureate; RPN to Baccalaureate.
**Site Options** Grande Prairie, AB; Fort McMurray, AB; Red Deer, AB.
**Study Options** Full-time.
**Program Entrance Requirements** Minimum overall college GPA of 3.5, transcript of college record, CPR certification, health exam, high school biology, high school chemistry, 3 years high school math, 3 years high school science, high school transcript, immunizations, minimum high school rank 85%. Transfer students are accepted. *Application deadline:* 5/1 (fall). Applications may be processed on a rolling basis for some programs. *Application fee:* CAN$115.
**Advanced Placement** Credit given for nursing courses completed elsewhere dependent upon specific evaluations.
**Contact** Help Desk, Faculty of Nursing, University of Alberta, 3 Edmonton Clinic Health Authority, Edmonton, AB T6G 1C9. *Telephone:* 780-492-5300. *Fax:* 780-492-2551. *E-mail:* undergraduate@nurs.ualberta.ca.

### GRADUATE PROGRAMS

**Financial Aid** 47% of graduate students in nursing programs received some form of financial aid in 2012–13. 12 fellowships with partial tuition reimbursements available (averaging $23,868 per year), 27 research assistantships with partial tuition reimbursements available (averaging $6,186 per year), 12 teaching assistantships with partial tuition reimbursements available (averaging $2,365 per year) were awarded; institutionally sponsored loans and scholarships also available.
**Contact** Yvette Labiuk, Graduate Services Administrator, Faculty of Nursing, University of Alberta, 4-171 Edmonton Clinic Health Academy, 11405 87 Avenue, Edmonton, AB T6G 1C9. *Telephone:* 780-492-9546. *Fax:* 780-492-2551. *E-mail:* nursing.graduate@ualberta.ca.

**MASTER'S DEGREE PROGRAM**
**Degree** MN
**Available Programs** Master's.
**Concentrations Available** *Nurse practitioner programs in:* adult health, gerontology.
**Study Options** Full-time and part-time.
**Program Entrance Requirements** Clinical experience, computer literacy, minimum overall college GPA of 3.0, transcript of college record, CPR certification, 3 letters of recommendation, nursing research course, physical assessment course, resume, statistics course. *Application deadline:* 2/1 (fall). *Application fee:* CAN$100.
**Advanced Placement** Credit given for nursing courses completed elsewhere dependent upon specific evaluations.
**Degree Requirements** 39 total credit hours, thesis or project.

**POST-MASTER'S PROGRAM**
**Areas of Study** *Nurse practitioner programs in:* adult health, gerontology.

**DOCTORAL DEGREE PROGRAM**
**Degree** PhD
**Available Programs** Doctorate.
**Areas of Study** Aging, community health, ethics, family health, gerontology, health policy, health promotion/disease prevention, health-care systems, nursing education, nursing policy, nursing research.
**Program Entrance Requirements** Clinical experience, minimum overall college GPA of 3.0, 3 letters of recommendation, MSN or equivalent, scholarly papers, statistics course, vita, writing sample. *Application deadline:* 2/1 (fall). *Application fee:* CAN$100.
**Degree Requirements** 36 total credit hours, dissertation, oral exam, written exam, residency.

**POSTDOCTORAL PROGRAM**
**Postdoctoral Program Contact** Dr. Phyllis Giovannetti, Associate Dean, Graduate Education, Faculty of Nursing, University of Alberta, Clinical Sciences Building, 3rd Floor, Edmonton, AB T6G 2G3. *Telephone:* 780-492-6764. *Fax:* 780-492-2551. *E-mail:* phyllis.giovannetti@ualberta.ca.

# University of Calgary
## Faculty of Nursing
## Calgary, Alberta

***http://www.ucalgary.ca/nu***
Founded in 1945

**DEGREES • BN • MN • PHD**
**Nursing Program Faculty** 50 (85% with doctorates).
**Baccalaureate Enrollment** 930 **Women** 90% **Men** 10% **Minority** 5% **International** 1%
**Graduate Enrollment** 110 **Women** 95% **Men** 5% **Minority** 1% **International** 1% **Part-time** 21%
**Nursing Student Activities** Student Nurses' Association.
**Nursing Student Resources** Academic advising; academic or career counseling; assistance for students with disabilities; bookstore; campus computer network; career placement assistance; computer lab; computer-assisted instruction; daycare for children of students; e-mail services; externships; housing assistance; interactive nursing skills videos; Internet; learning resource lab; library services; nursing audiovisuals; remedial services; resume preparation assistance; skills, simulation, or other laboratory; tutoring.
**Library Facilities** 3.3 million volumes; 37,285 periodical subscriptions.

### BACCALAUREATE PROGRAMS

**Degree** BN
**Available Programs** Accelerated Baccalaureate; Accelerated Baccalaureate for Second Degree; Baccalaureate for Second Degree; Generic Baccalaureate; RN Baccalaureate.
**Site Options** Medicine Hat, AB.
**Study Options** Full-time.
**Program Entrance Requirements** Minimum overall college GPA of 3.3, transcript of college record, CPR certification, health exam, high school biology, high school chemistry, 3 years high school math, high school transcript, immunizations, minimum high school rank 78%. Transfer students are accepted.
**Advanced Placement** Credit by examination available. Credit given for nursing courses completed elsewhere dependent upon specific evaluations.
**Contact** *Telephone:* 403-220-4636. *Fax:* 403-284-4803.

### GRADUATE PROGRAMS

**Contact** *Telephone:* 403-220-6241. *Fax:* 403-284-4803.

**MASTER'S DEGREE PROGRAM**
**Degree** MN
**Available Programs** Master's; RN to Master's.
**Concentrations Available** *Clinical nurse specialist programs in:* acute care, adult health, cardiovascular, community health, critical care, family

health, gerontology, maternity-newborn, medical-surgical, parent-child, pediatric, perinatal, psychiatric/mental health, public health, rehabilitation,women's health. *Nurse practitioner programs in:* acute care, adult health, neonatal health.
**Study Options** Full-time and part-time.
**Program Entrance Requirements** Clinical experience, computer literacy, minimum overall college GPA of 3.0, transcript of college record, CPR certification, written essay, 3 letters of recommendation, nursing research course, statistics course.
**Advanced Placement** Credit given for nursing courses completed elsewhere dependent upon specific evaluations.
**Degree Requirements** 30 total credit hours, thesis or project, comprehensive exam.

### POST-MASTER'S PROGRAM

**Areas of Study** *Nurse practitioner programs in:* acute care, adult health, neonatal health.

### DOCTORAL DEGREE PROGRAM

**Degree** PhD
**Available Programs** Doctorate; Doctorate for Nurses with Non-Nursing Degrees.
**Areas of Study** Advanced practice nursing, aging, clinical practice, community health, critical care, ethics, family health, gerontology, health promotion/disease prevention, health-care systems, human health and illness, illness and transition, individualized study, maternity-newborn, neuro-behavior, nursing research,women's health.
**Program Entrance Requirements** Clinical experience, minimum overall college GPA of 3.0, 3 letters of recommendation, MSN or equivalent, scholarly papers, statistics course, vita, writing sample.
**Degree Requirements** Dissertation, oral exam, written exam.

## University of Lethbridge

### Faculty of Health Sciences
### Lethbridge, Alberta

***http://www.uleth.ca/healthsciences***
Founded in 1967

### DEGREES • BN • M SC

**Nursing Program Faculty** 40 (18% with doctorates).
**Baccalaureate Enrollment** 688 **Women** 87% **Men** 13%
**Graduate Enrollment** 9 **Women** 67% **Men** 33%
**Nursing Student Activities** Nursing club.
**Nursing Student Resources** Academic advising; academic or career counseling; assistance for students with disabilities; bookstore; campus computer network; career placement assistance; computer lab; computer-assisted instruction; daycare for children of students; e-mail services; employment services for current students; housing assistance; interactive nursing skills videos; Internet; learning resource lab; library services; nursing audiovisuals; other; remedial services; resume preparation assistance; skills, simulation, or other laboratory; tutoring; unpaid internships.
**Library Facilities** 602,148 volumes (14,743 in health, 2,554 in nursing); 6,533 periodical subscriptions (11,168 health-care related).

### BACCALAUREATE PROGRAMS

**Degree** BN
**Available Programs** Accelerated Baccalaureate; Baccalaureate for Second Degree; Generic Baccalaureate.
**Site Options** Lethbridge, AB.
**Study Options** Full-time.
**Program Entrance Requirements** CPR certification, high school biology, high school chemistry, 3 years high school math, 3 years high school science, high school transcript, immunizations, minimum high school rank 70%. Transfer students are accepted. *Application deadline:* 3/1 (fall). *Application fee:* CAN$100.
**Advanced Placement** Credit given for nursing courses completed elsewhere dependent upon specific evaluations.
**Financial Aid** ***Gift aid (need-based):*** private, college/university gift aid from institutional funds. *Financial aid application deadline:* Continuous.
**Contact** Sherry Hogeweide, Academic Advisor, Faculty of Health Sciences, University of Lethbridge, 4401 University Drive, Lethbridge, AB T1K 3M4. *Telephone:* 403-329-2220. *Fax:* 403-329-2668. *E-mail:* nursing@uleth.ca.

### GRADUATE PROGRAMS

**Contact** Dr. Brad Hagen, Graduate Studies Coordinator, Faculty of Health Sciences, University of Lethbridge, 4401 University Drive, Lethbridge, AB T1K 3M4. *Telephone:* 403-329-2299. *Fax:* 403-329-2668. *E-mail:* brad.hagen@uleth.ca.

### MASTER'S DEGREE PROGRAM

**Degree** M Sc
**Available Programs** Master's.
**Study Options** Full-time and part-time.
**Program Entrance Requirements** Clinical experience, computer literacy, minimum overall college GPA of 3.0, transcript of college record, CPR certification, immunizations, interview, 3 letters of recommendation. *Application deadline:* 3/1 (fall).
**Degree Requirements** Thesis or project, comprehensive exam.

# BRITISH COLUMBIA

## British Columbia Institute of Technology

### School of Health Sciences
### Burnaby, British Columbia

***http://www.bcit.ca/health/***
Founded in 1964

### DEGREE • BSN

**Nursing Program Faculty** 96
**Baccalaureate Enrollment** 546 **Women** 90% **Men** 10%
**Distance Learning Courses** Available.
**Nursing Student Activities** Student Nurses' Association.
**Nursing Student Resources** Academic advising; academic or career counseling; assistance for students with disabilities; bookstore; campus computer network; computer lab; computer-assisted instruction; e-mail services; housing assistance; interactive nursing skills videos; Internet; learning resource lab; library services; nursing audiovisuals; paid internships; resume preparation assistance; skills, simulation, or other laboratory; tutoring; unpaid internships.
**Library Facilities** 169,404 volumes (10,000 in health, 2,600 in nursing); 1,080 periodical subscriptions (110 health-care related).

### BACCALAUREATE PROGRAMS

**Degree** BSN
**Available Programs** RN Baccalaureate; RPN to Baccalaureate.
**Study Options** Full-time.
**Program Entrance Requirements** Transcript of college record, CPR certification, high school chemistry, 11 years high school math, high school transcript, immunizations, prerequisite course work. Transfer students are accepted. *Application deadline:* 4/1 (fall), 10/1 (winter). *Application fee:* CAN$62.
**Advanced Placement** Credit given for nursing courses completed elsewhere dependent upon specific evaluations.
**Expenses (2013–14)** *Tuition, area resident:* full-time CAN$5846.
**Financial Aid** 70% of baccalaureate students in nursing programs received some form of financial aid in 2012–13. *Financial aid application deadline:* Continuous.
**Contact** Ms. Loreen Martin, Administrative Coordinator, School of Health Sciences, British Columbia Institute of Technology, 3700 Willingdon Avenue, SE12, Room 418, Burnaby, BC V5G 3H2. *Telephone:* 604-432-8884. *Fax:* 604-436-9590. *E-mail:* loreen_martin@bcit.ca.

### CONTINUING EDUCATION PROGRAM

**Contact** Ms. Pauline O'Reilly, Program Head, School of Health Sciences, British Columbia Institute of Technology, 3700 Willingdon Avenue, SE12, Room 328, Burnaby, BC V5G 3H2. *Telephone:* 604-451-7115. *E-mail:* pauline_o'reilly@bcit.ca.

# Kwantlen Polytechnic University

## Faculty of Community and Health Sciences
## Surrey, British Columbia

*http://www.kwantlen.ca/*
Founded in 1981

**DEGREE • BSN**

**Nursing Program Faculty** 60 (13% with doctorates).

**Baccalaureate Enrollment** 360 **Women** 90% **Men** 10% **Part-time** 13%

**Nursing Student Activities** Student Nurses' Association.

**Nursing Student Resources** Academic advising; academic or career counseling; assistance for students with disabilities; bookstore; campus computer network; career placement assistance; computer lab; computer-assisted instruction; e-mail services; employment services for current students; interactive nursing skills videos; Internet; learning resource lab; library services; nursing audiovisuals; remedial services; resume preparation assistance; skills, simulation, or other laboratory.

### BACCALAUREATE PROGRAMS

**Degree** BSN

**Available Programs** Accelerated Baccalaureate for Second Degree; Generic Baccalaureate; RN Baccalaureate.

**Study Options** Full-time.

**Program Entrance Requirements** CPR certification, health insurance, high school biology, high school chemistry, high school math, 2 years high school science, high school transcript, immunizations. Transfer students are accepted.

**Advanced Placement** Credit given for nursing courses completed elsewhere dependent upon specific evaluations.

**Expenses (2012–13)** *Tuition, area resident:* full-time CAN$4000. *Required fees:* full-time CAN$200.

**Financial Aid** 40% of baccalaureate students in nursing programs received some form of financial aid in 2011–12.

**Contact** Ms. Pam Kubossek, Admissions Assistant, Faculty of Community and Health Sciences, Kwantlen Polytechnic University, 12666 72nd Avenue, Surrey, BC V3W 2M8. *Telephone:* 604-599-2141. *E-mail:* Pam.Kubossek@kwantlen.ca.

# Thompson Rivers University

## School of Nursing
## Kamloops, British Columbia

*http://www.tru.ca/nursing.html*
Founded in 1970

**DEGREE • BSN**

**Nursing Program Faculty** 56

**Library Facilities** 285,426 volumes (7,326 in health, 2,275 in nursing); 9,585 periodical subscriptions (89 health-care related).

### BACCALAUREATE PROGRAMS

**Degree** BSN

**Study Options** Full-time and part-time.

**Program Entrance Requirements** Minimum overall college GPA of 2.7, transcript of college record, CPR certification, health exam, high school biology, high school chemistry, high school foreign language, high school math, high school science, high school transcript, immunizations, interview, 2 letters of recommendation, minimum high school GPA of 2.3, minimum GPA in nursing prerequisites of 2.3. Transfer students are accepted.

**Advanced Placement** Credit given for nursing courses completed elsewhere dependent upon specific evaluations.

**Contact** *Telephone:* 250-828-5435. *Fax:* 250-828-5450.

### CONTINUING EDUCATION PROGRAM

**Contact** *Telephone:* 250-828-5210. *Fax:* 250-371-5510.

# Trinity Western University

## Department of Nursing
## Langley, British Columbia

*http://www.twu.ca/*
Founded in 1962

**DEGREES • BSCN • MSN**

**Nursing Program Faculty** 13 (23% with doctorates).

**Baccalaureate Enrollment** 187 **Women** 91.5% **Men** 8.5% **Minority** 14% **International** 10%

**Graduate Enrollment** 63 **Women** 100% **Minority** 32% **International** .5% **Part-time** 6%

**Nursing Student Activities** Student Nurses' Association, nursing club.

**Nursing Student Resources** Academic advising; academic or career counseling; assistance for students with disabilities; bookstore; campus computer network; career placement assistance; computer lab; computer-assisted instruction; e-mail services; employment services for current students; housing assistance; interactive nursing skills videos; Internet; learning resource lab; library services; nursing audiovisuals; remedial services; resume preparation assistance; skills, simulation, or other laboratory; tutoring.

**Library Facilities** 2,500 volumes in health, 800 volumes in nursing; 369 periodical subscriptions health-care related.

### BACCALAUREATE PROGRAMS

**Degree** BScN

**Available Programs** Generic Baccalaureate.

**Study Options** Full-time.

**Program Entrance Requirements** Minimum overall college GPA of 2.0, CPR certification, health insurance, high school biology, high school chemistry, 1 year of high school math, 2 years high school science, high school transcript, immunizations, 2 letters of recommendation, minimum high school GPA of 2.7, minimum GPA in nursing prerequisites of 2.3. Transfer students are accepted. *Application deadline:* 2/28 (fall).

**Advanced Placement** Credit given for nursing courses completed elsewhere dependent upon specific evaluations.

**Expenses (2013–14)** *Room and board:* CAN$7550 per academic year.

**Financial Aid** 99% of baccalaureate students in nursing programs received some form of financial aid in 2012–13. *Gift aid (need-based):* private, college/university gift aid from institutional funds. *Loans:* federal and provincial loans. *Financial aid application deadline (priority):* 2/28.

**Contact** Dr. Sonya Grypma, Dean, Department of Nursing, Trinity Western University, 7600 Glover Road, Langley, BC V2Y 1Y1. *Telephone:* 604-888-7511 Ext. 3283. *Fax:* 604-513-2012. *E-mail:* sonya.grypma@twu.ca.

### GRADUATE PROGRAMS

**Expenses (2013–14)** *Tuition:* part-time CAN$670 per credit hour.

**Financial Aid** 20% of graduate students in nursing programs received some form of financial aid in 2012–13.

**Contact** Ms. Guelda Redman, MSN Administrative Assistant, Department of Nursing, Trinity Western University, 7600 Glover Road, Langley, BC V2Y 1Y1. *Telephone:* 604-888-7511 Ext. 3270. *Fax:* 604-513-2012. *E-mail:* guelda.redman@twu.ca.

#### MASTER'S DEGREE PROGRAM

**Degree** MSN

**Available Programs** Master's.

**Study Options** Part-time.

**Program Entrance Requirements** Minimum overall college GPA of 3.0, transcript of college record, 2 letters of recommendation, statistics course. *Application deadline:* 5/1 (summer).

**Advanced Placement** Credit given for nursing courses completed elsewhere dependent upon specific evaluations.

**Degree Requirements** 30 total credit hours, thesis or project.

# The University of British Columbia

## Program in Nursing
## Vancouver, British Columbia

*http://www.nursing.ubc.ca/*
Founded in 1915

**DEGREES • BSN • MSN • MSN/MPH • PHD**

**Nursing Program Faculty** 55 (51% with doctorates).
**Baccalaureate Enrollment** 239 **Women** 83.8% **Men** 16.2% **International** 12%
**Graduate Enrollment** 210 **Women** 91.4% **Men** 8.6% **International** 8.6% **Part-time** 25.7%
**Nursing Student Activities** Sigma Theta Tau, Student Nurses' Association, nursing club.
**Nursing Student Resources** Academic advising; academic or career counseling; assistance for students with disabilities; bookstore; campus computer network; career placement assistance; computer lab; computer-assisted instruction; e-mail services; employment services for current students; housing assistance; interactive nursing skills videos; Internet; learning resource lab; library services; nursing audiovisuals; remedial services; resume preparation assistance; skills, simulation, or other laboratory.
**Library Facilities** 6.4 million volumes (160,000 in health, 11,000 in nursing); 875,000 periodical subscriptions (17,000 health-care related).

### BACCALAUREATE PROGRAMS

**Degree** BSN
**Available Programs** Accelerated Baccalaureate; Accelerated Baccalaureate for Second Degree.
**Study Options** Full-time.
**Program Entrance Requirements** Minimum overall college GPA of 2.8, transcript of college record, CPR certification, written essay, health insurance, immunizations, interview, 2 letters of recommendation, professional liability insurance/malpractice insurance, prerequisite course work. *Application deadline:* 12/1 (winter). *Application fee:* CAN$219.
**Expenses (2013–14)** *Tuition, state resident:* full-time CAN$7671. *Tuition, nonresident:* full-time CAN$7671. *International tuition:* CAN$37,280 full-time. *Room and board:* CAN$8824; room only: CAN$4738 per academic year. *Required fees:* full-time CAN$886.
**Financial Aid** 68% of baccalaureate students in nursing programs received some form of financial aid in 2012–13. *Gift aid (need-based):* state, private, college/university gift aid from institutional funds, Canadian Federal and Provincial Grants. *Loans:* college/university, Canadian federal and provincial loans. *Work-study:* part-time campus jobs. *Financial aid application deadline:* 9/15(priority: 4/15).
**Contact** Ruxandra Vasiljevic, Undergraduate Admissions Assistant, Program in Nursing, The University of British Columbia, T201-2211 Wesbrook Mall, Vancouver, BC V6T 2B5. *Telephone:* 604-822-9754. *Fax:* 604-822-7466. *E-mail:* information@nursing.ubc.ca.

### GRADUATE PROGRAMS

**Expenses (2013–14)** *Tuition, area resident:* full-time CAN$4436; part-time CAN$845 per semester. *Tuition, state resident:* full-time CAN$4436. *Tuition, nonresident:* full-time CAN$4436. *International tuition:* CAN$7794 full-time. *Room and board:* CAN$8824; room only: CAN$4738 per academic year. *Required fees:* full-time CAN$797.
**Financial Aid** 63% of graduate students in nursing programs received some form of financial aid in 2012–13. 4 fellowships (averaging $8,000 per year), 14 research assistantships (averaging $800 per year), 3 teaching assistantships were awarded.
**Contact** Mr. Drew St. Laurent, Recruitment and Graduate Admissions Officer, Program in Nursing, The University of British Columbia, T201-2211 Wesbrook Mall, Vancouver, BC V6T 2B5. *Telephone:* 604-822-7446. *E-mail:* student.services@nursing.ubc.ca.

#### MASTER'S DEGREE PROGRAM

**Degrees** MSN; MSN/MPH
**Available Programs** Master's.
**Concentrations Available** Nursing administration; nursing education. *Clinical nurse specialist programs in:* adult health, cardiovascular, community health, family health, gerontology, maternity-newborn, oncology, parent-child, pediatric, perinatal, psychiatric/mental health, public health,women's health. *Nurse practitioner programs in:* community health, family health, primary care.
**Study Options** Full-time and part-time.
**Program Entrance Requirements** Computer literacy, minimum overall college GPA of 3.3, transcript of college record, 3 letters of recommendation, resume, GRE. *Application deadline:* 12/1 (fall). *Application fee:* CAN$93.
**Advanced Placement** Credit given for nursing courses completed elsewhere dependent upon specific evaluations.
**Degree Requirements** 33 total credit hours, thesis or project.

#### DOCTORAL DEGREE PROGRAM

**Degree** PhD
**Available Programs** Doctorate.
**Areas of Study** Addiction/substance abuse, advanced practice nursing, aging, clinical practice, clinical research, community health, ethics, faculty preparation, family health, gerontology, health policy, health promotion/disease prevention, health-care systems, human health and illness, illness and transition, individualized study, information systems, maternity-newborn, nursing administration, nursing education, nursing policy, nursing research, nursing science, oncology, palliative care, urban health,women's health.
**Program Entrance Requirements** Interview, 3 letters of recommendation, MSN or equivalent, vita, writing sample, GRE. *Application deadline:* 12/1 (fall). Applications may be processed on a rolling basis for some programs. *Application fee:* CAN$153.
**Degree Requirements** 18 total credit hours, dissertation, oral exam.

#### POSTDOCTORAL PROGRAM

**Areas of Study** Addiction/substance abuse, adolescent health, aging, cancer care, chronic illness, community health, family health, gerontology, health promotion/disease prevention, individualized study, infection prevention/skin care, information systems, neuro-behavior, nursing informatics, nursing interventions, nursing research, nursing science, outcomes, self-care, vulnerable population,women's health.
**Postdoctoral Program Contact** Dr. Lynda Balneaves, Associate Director, Research, Program in Nursing, The University of British Columbia, T201-2211 Wesbrook Mall, Vancouver, BC V6T 2B5. *Telephone:* 604-822-7679. *Fax:* 604-822-7466. *E-mail:* Lynda.Balneaves@nursing.ubc.ca.

# University of Northern British Columbia

## Nursing Programme
## Prince George, British Columbia

*http://www.unbc.ca/nursing/*
Founded in 1994

**DEGREES • BSCN • M SC N**

**Nursing Program Faculty** 40 (18% with doctorates).
**Baccalaureate Enrollment** 600
**Graduate Enrollment** 60
**Distance Learning Courses** Available.
**Nursing Student Activities** Student Nurses' Association.
**Nursing Student Resources** Academic advising; academic or career counseling; assistance for students with disabilities; bookstore; campus computer network; computer lab; computer-assisted instruction; e-mail services; employment services for current students; externships; Internet; learning resource lab; library services; nursing audiovisuals; skills, simulation, or other laboratory.
**Library Facilities** 310,433 volumes (4,000 in health, 2,000 in nursing); 19,570 periodical subscriptions (300 health-care related).

### BACCALAUREATE PROGRAMS

**Degree** BScN
**Available Programs** Generic Baccalaureate; RN Baccalaureate.
**Site Options** Prince George, BC; Quesnel, BC; Terrace, BC.
**Study Options** Full-time.
**Program Entrance Requirements** Minimum overall college GPA of 2.33, transcript of college record, CPR certification, health exam, high school biology, high school chemistry, 1 year of high school math, 4 years high school science, high school transcript, immunizations, minimum high school GPA of 2.3, minimum high school rank 65%, minimum GPA in nursing prerequisites of 2.0, professional liability insurance/malpractice insurance. Transfer students are accepted. *Application deadline:* 3/31 (fall). *Application fee:* CAN$35.
**Advanced Placement** Credit given for nursing courses completed elsewhere dependent upon specific evaluations.
**Contact** *Telephone:* 250-960-5645.

## GRADUATE PROGRAMS

**Contact** *Telephone:* 250-960-5848. *Fax:* 250-960-6410.

### MASTER'S DEGREE PROGRAM

**Degree** M Sc N
**Available Programs** Master's.
**Concentrations Available** *Nurse practitioner programs in:* family health.
**Study Options** Full-time and part-time.
**Program Entrance Requirements** Clinical experience, minimum overall college GPA of 3.0, transcript of college record, CPR certification, written essay, 3 letters of recommendation, nursing research course, professional liability insurance/malpractice insurance, prerequisite course work. *Application deadline:* 2/15 (fall). *Application fee:* CAN$75.
**Advanced Placement** Credit given for nursing courses completed elsewhere dependent upon specific evaluations.
**Degree Requirements** 51 total credit hours, thesis or project.

### POSTDOCTORAL PROGRAM

**Areas of Study** Chronic illness, community health, family health, health promotion/disease prevention, individualized study, nursing interventions, nursing research, nursing science, outcomes, vulnerable population.
**Postdoctoral Program Contact***Telephone:* 250-960-6507. *Fax:* 250-960-6410.

# University of Victoria

## School of Nursing
## Victoria, British Columbia

***http://www.web.uvic.ca/nurs/***
Founded in 1963

## DEGREES • BSN • MN • PHD

**Nursing Program Faculty** 21 (95% with doctorates).
**Baccalaureate Enrollment** 1,100 **Women** 95% **Men** 5% **Part-time** 50%
**Nursing Student Activities** Student Nurses' Association.
**Nursing Student Resources** Academic advising; assistance for students with disabilities; bookstore; campus computer network; computer lab; e-mail services; employment services for current students; interactive nursing skills videos; Internet; library services; nursing audiovisuals; remedial services; resume preparation assistance; unpaid internships.
**Library Facilities** 1.8 million volumes; 14,000 periodical subscriptions.

## BACCALAUREATE PROGRAMS

**Degree** BSN
**Site Options** Vancouver, BC.
**Program Entrance Requirements** Minimum overall college GPA of 3.5, transcript of college record, CPR certification, high school transcript, immunizations, prerequisite course work. Transfer students are accepted.
**Contact** *Telephone:* 250-721-7961. *Fax:* 250-721-6231.

## GRADUATE PROGRAMS

**Contact** *Telephone:* 250-721-7961. *Fax:* 250-721-6231.

### MASTER'S DEGREE PROGRAM

**Degree** MN
**Available Programs** Master's.
**Site Options** Victoria.
**Study Options** Full-time and part-time.
**Program Entrance Requirements** Clinical experience, transcript of college record, letters of recommendation.
**Advanced Placement** Credit given for nursing courses completed elsewhere dependent upon specific evaluations.
**Degree Requirements** 18 total credit hours, thesis or project.

### DOCTORAL DEGREE PROGRAM

**Degree** PhD
**Program Entrance Requirements** Clinical experience, MSN or equivalent.
**Degree Requirements** Dissertation.

# Vancouver Island University

## Department of Nursing
## Nanaimo, British Columbia

***http://www.viu.ca/calendar/Health/bscnursing.asp***
Founded in 1969

## DEGREE • BSCN

**Nursing Program Faculty** 36 (2% with doctorates).
**Baccalaureate Enrollment** 279 **Women** 92% **Men** 8% **Minority** 6%
**Distance Learning Courses** Available.
**Nursing Student Activities** Student Nurses' Association.
**Nursing Student Resources** Academic advising; academic or career counseling; assistance for students with disabilities; bookstore; campus computer network; computer lab; computer-assisted instruction; e-mail services; employment services for current students; housing assistance; interactive nursing skills videos; Internet; learning resource lab; library services; nursing audiovisuals; remedial services; resume preparation assistance; skills, simulation, or other laboratory; tutoring; unpaid internships.
**Library Facilities** 9,475 volumes in health, 1,299 volumes in nursing; 800 periodical subscriptions health-care related.

## BACCALAUREATE PROGRAMS

**Degree** BScN
**Available Programs** Generic Baccalaureate; LPN to RN Baccalaureate.
**Study Options** Full-time.
**Program Entrance Requirements** CPR certification, health insurance, high school biology, high school chemistry, 11 years high school math, high school transcript, immunizations, minimum GPA in nursing prerequisites of 3.0, prerequisite course work. Transfer students are accepted. *Application deadline:* 2/28 (fall). *Application fee:* CAN$35.
**Advanced Placement** Credit given for nursing courses completed elsewhere dependent upon specific evaluations.
**Expenses (2013–14)** *Tuition, area resident:* full-time CAN$4000.
**Financial Aid** 53% of baccalaureate students in nursing programs received some form of financial aid in 2012–13. *Gift aid (need-based):* private, college/university gift aid from institutional funds. *Loans:* government student loans.
**Contact** Dr. Sherry Dahlke, Chair of Bachelor of Science in Nursing Programs, Department of Nursing, Vancouver Island University, 900 Fifth Street, Nanaimo, BC V9R 5S5. *Telephone:* 250-740-6260. *Fax:* 250-740-6468. *E-mail:* Sherry.Dahlke@viu.ca.

## CONTINUING EDUCATION PROGRAM

**Contact** Ms. Cheryl Dill, Program Coordinator, Department of Nursing, Vancouver Island University, 900 Fifth Street, Nanaimo, BC V9R 5S5. *Telephone:* 250-740-6327. *E-mail:* Cheryl.Dill@viu.ca.

# MANITOBA

# Brandon University

## School of Health Studies
## Brandon, Manitoba

***http://www.brandonu.ca/health-studies/***
Founded in 1899

## DEGREE • BN

**Nursing Program Faculty** 20 (40% with doctorates).
**Baccalaureate Enrollment** 480 **Women** 95% **Men** 5% **Minority** 10% **Part-time** 25%
**Distance Learning Courses** Available.
**Nursing Student Activities** Nursing Honor Society, Sigma Theta Tau, Student Nurses' Association.
**Nursing Student Resources** Academic advising; academic or career counseling; assistance for students with disabilities; bookstore; campus computer network; career placement assistance; computer lab; computer-assisted instruction; e-mail services; employment services for current students; housing assistance; interactive nursing skills videos; Internet; library services; resume preparation assistance; skills, simulation, or other laboratory; tutoring.
**Library Facilities** 238,816 volumes; 1,699 periodical subscriptions.

## BACCALAUREATE PROGRAMS

**Degree** BN
**Available Programs** Baccalaureate for Second Degree; Generic Baccalaureate; LPN to Baccalaureate; RN Baccalaureate.
**Site Options** Winnipeg, MB.
**Study Options** Full-time and part-time.
**Program Entrance Requirements** Minimum overall college GPA of 2.0, CPR certification, immunizations, minimum GPA in nursing prerequisites of 2.0, prerequisite course work. Transfer students are accepted. *Application deadline:* 5/1 (fall).
**Advanced Placement** Credit given for nursing courses completed elsewhere dependent upon specific evaluations.
**Contact** *Telephone:* 204-571-8567. *Fax:* 204-571-8568.

# University of Manitoba

## Faculty of Nursing
## Winnipeg, Manitoba

***http://www.umanitoba.ca/faculties/nursing/***
Founded in 1877

**DEGREES • BN • MN • PHD**
**Nursing Program Faculty** 54 (53% with doctorates).
**Baccalaureate Enrollment** 965 **Women** 87% **Men** 13% **Part-time** 25%
**Graduate Enrollment** 84 **Women** 85% **Men** 15% **Part-time** 38%
**Distance Learning Courses** Available.
**Nursing Student Activities** Nursing Honor Society, Sigma Theta Tau, Student Nurses' Association.
**Nursing Student Resources** Academic advising; academic or career counseling; assistance for students with disabilities; bookstore; campus computer network; computer lab; computer-assisted instruction; daycare for children of students; e-mail services; employment services for current students; housing assistance; interactive nursing skills videos; Internet; learning resource lab; library services; skills, simulation, or other laboratory; unpaid internships.
**Library Facilities** 2 million volumes (137,100 in health, 5,000 in nursing); 47,299 periodical subscriptions (2,208 health-care related).

## BACCALAUREATE PROGRAMS

**Degree** BN
**Available Programs** Baccalaureate for Second Degree; Generic Baccalaureate; RN Baccalaureate.
**Site Options** Thompson, MB; The Pas, MB.
**Study Options** Full-time and part-time.
**Program Entrance Requirements** Minimum overall college GPA of 2.5, transcript of college record, CPR certification, high school chemistry, high school math, high school science, high school transcript, immunizations, minimum high school GPA of 2.5, prerequisite course work. Transfer students are accepted. *Application deadline:* 4/1 (fall).
**Advanced Placement** Credit given for nursing courses completed elsewhere dependent upon specific evaluations.
**Contact** Dr. Terri Ashcroft, Associate Dean, Undergraduate Program, Faculty of Nursing, University of Manitoba, 277 Helen Glass Centre for Nursing, Winnipeg, MB R3T 2N2. *Telephone:* 204-474-6220. *Fax:* 204-474-7682. *E-mail:* terri.ashcroft@umanitoba.ca.

## GRADUATE PROGRAMS

**Contact** Dr. Jo-Ann Sawatzky, Associate Dean, Graduate Programs, Faculty of Nursing, University of Manitoba, 281-89 Curry Place, Winnipeg, MB R3T 2N2. *Telephone:* 204-474-9317. *Fax:* 204-474-7682. *E-mail:* joann.sawatzky@ad.umanitoba.ca.

### MASTER'S DEGREE PROGRAM

**Degree** MN
**Available Programs** Master's.
**Concentrations Available** Nursing administration. *Clinical nurse specialist programs in:* acute care, family health, gerontology, perinatal,women's health. *Nurse practitioner programs in:* primary care.
**Study Options** Full-time and part-time.
**Program Entrance Requirements** Clinical experience, minimum overall college GPA of 3.0, transcript of college record, written essay, 3 letters of recommendation, nursing research course, resume, statistics course. *Application deadline:* 4/1 (fall).
**Advanced Placement** Credit given for nursing courses completed elsewhere dependent upon specific evaluations.
**Degree Requirements** 27 total credit hours, thesis or project, comprehensive exam.

### DOCTORAL DEGREE PROGRAM

**Degree** PhD
**Available Programs** Doctorate.
**Areas of Study** Nursing science.
**Program Entrance Requirements** Clinical experience, letters of recommendation, MSN or equivalent. *Application deadline:* 4/1 (fall).
**Degree Requirements** 21 total credit hours, dissertation.

## CONTINUING EDUCATION PROGRAM

**Contact** Dr. Beverly O'Connell, Professor, Faculty of Nursing, University of Manitoba, 293 Helen Glass Centre for Nursing, Winnipeg, MB R3T 2N2. *Telephone:* 204-474-9201. *Fax:* 204-474-7500. *E-mail:* beverly.oconnell@umanitoba.ca.

# NEW BRUNSWICK

# Université de Moncton

## School of Nursing
## Moncton, New Brunswick

***http://www.umoncton.ca/umcm-fsssc-scienceinfirmiere***
Founded in 1963

**DEGREES • BSCN • M SC N**
**Nursing Program Faculty** 64 (17% with doctorates).
**Baccalaureate Enrollment** 548 **Women** 86% **Men** 14% **Minority** 4% **International** 6% **Part-time** 1%
**Graduate Enrollment** 56 **Women** 89% **Men** 11% **Minority** 2% **International** 2% **Part-time** 100%
**Distance Learning Courses** Available.
**Nursing Student Activities** Student Nurses' Association.
**Nursing Student Resources** Academic or career counseling; assistance for students with disabilities; bookstore; campus computer network; career placement assistance; computer lab; computer-assisted instruction; daycare for children of students; e-mail services; employment services for current students; externships; housing assistance; Internet; library services; nursing audiovisuals; placement services for program completers; resume preparation assistance; skills, simulation, or other laboratory; tutoring; unpaid internships.
**Library Facilities** 789,046 volumes (10,757 in health, 3,807 in nursing); 2,059 periodical subscriptions (210 health-care related).

## BACCALAUREATE PROGRAMS

**Degree** BScN
**Available Programs** RN Baccalaureate.
**Site Options** Edmundston, NB; Bathurst, NB; Moncton, NB.
**Study Options** Full-time.
**Program Entrance Requirements** Transcript of college record, CPR certification, high school biology, high school chemistry, 30411 years high school math, high school science, high school transcript, immunizations, minimum high school rank 65%. Transfer students are accepted. *Application deadline:* 4/1 (winter). *Application fee:* CAN$50.
**Advanced Placement** Credit given for nursing courses completed elsewhere dependent upon specific evaluations.
**Expenses (2012–13)** *Tuition, state resident:* full-time CAN$5292; part-time CAN$178 per credit. *Tuition, nonresident:* full-time CAN$5292; part-time CAN$178 per credit. *International tuition:* CAN$8972 full-time. *Room and board:* CAN$5162; room only: CAN$3937 per academic year. *Required fees:* full-time CAN$338.
**Financial Aid** 50% of baccalaureate students in nursing programs received some form of financial aid in 2011–12.
**Contact** Yoland Bordeleau, Bureau de recrutement, School of Nursing, Université de Moncton, Pavillon Leopold Taillon, Moncton, NB E1A 3E9. *Telephone:* 506-858-4443. *Fax:* 506-858-4538. *E-mail:* yoland.bordeleau@umoncton.ca.

## GRADUATE PROGRAMS

**Expenses (2012–13)** *Tuition:* part-time CAN$206 per credit. *Room and board:* CAN$5162; room only: CAN$3937 per academic year.
**Financial Aid** 4% of graduate students in nursing programs received some form of financial aid in 2011–12.
**Contact** Yoland Bordeleau, Bureau de recrutement, School of Nursing, Université de Moncton, Pavillon Leopold Taillon, Moncton, NB E1A

3E9. *Telephone:* 506-858-4443. *Fax:* 506-858-4538. *E-mail:* yoland.bordeleau@umoncton.ca.

**MASTER'S DEGREE PROGRAM**
**Degree** M Sc N
**Available Programs** Master's; RN to Master's.
**Concentrations Available** Health-care administration; nurse case management; nursing administration; nursing education. *Clinical nurse specialist programs in:* community health, family health, home health care, occupational health, pediatric, psychiatric/mental health, public health, school health. *Nurse practitioner programs in:* adult health, community health, family health, oncology, primary care.
**Site Options** Moncton, NB.
**Study Options** Full-time and part-time.
**Program Entrance Requirements** Minimum overall college GPA of 3.0, transcript of college record, CPR certification, written essay, immunizations, 2 letters of recommendation, resume, statistics course. *Application deadline:* 6/1 (summer). *Application fee:* CAN$50.
**Advanced Placement** Credit given for nursing courses completed elsewhere dependent upon specific evaluations.
**Degree Requirements** 45 total credit hours, thesis or project.

## CONTINUING EDUCATION PROGRAM

**Contact** Mrs. Denise Savoie, Directrice du service la clientle, School of Nursing, Université de Moncton, ducation permanente, 18 avenue Antonine-Maillet, Moncton, NB E1A 3E9. *Telephone:* 506-858-4621. *Fax:* 506-858-4480. *E-mail:* denise.savoie@umoncton.ca.

# University of New Brunswick Fredericton

### Faculty of Nursing
### Fredericton, New Brunswick

***http://www.unbf.ca/nursing/***
Founded in 1785

### DEGREES • BN • MN

**Nursing Program Faculty** 75 (17% with doctorates).
**Baccalaureate Enrollment** 706 **Women** 94% **Men** 6% **International** 1%
**Graduate Enrollment** 53 **Women** 96% **Men** 4% **Part-time** 30%
**Distance Learning Courses** Available.
**Nursing Student Activities** Student Nurses' Association, nursing club.
**Nursing Student Resources** Academic advising; academic or career counseling; assistance for students with disabilities; bookstore; campus computer network; computer lab; computer-assisted instruction; daycare for children of students; e-mail services; employment services for current students; interactive nursing skills videos; Internet; learning resource lab; library services; nursing audiovisuals; resume preparation assistance; skills, simulation, or other laboratory; tutoring.
**Library Facilities** 1.3 million volumes (12,547 in health, 1,910 in nursing); 47,249 periodical subscriptions (250 health-care related).

## BACCALAUREATE PROGRAMS

**Degree** BN
**Available Programs** Accelerated Baccalaureate; Generic Baccalaureate.
**Site Options** Bathurst, NB; Moncton, NB; Fredericton, NB.
**Study Options** Full-time.
**Program Entrance Requirements** Minimum overall college GPA of 3.0, transcript of college record, CPR certification, written essay, health exam, high school biology, high school chemistry, 60 years high school math, high school transcript, immunizations, interview, minimum high school rank 70%, prerequisite course work. Transfer students are accepted. *Application deadline:* 3/31 (fall). *Application fee:* CAN$55.
**Advanced Placement** Credit given for nursing courses completed elsewhere dependent upon specific evaluations.
**Contact** Ms. Pam Wiebe, Administrative Assistant, Faculty of Nursing, University of New Brunswick Fredericton, PO Box 4400, Fredericton, NB E3B 5A3. *Telephone:* 506-458-7670. *Fax:* 506-453-3512. *E-mail:* pwiebe@unb.ca.

## GRADUATE PROGRAMS

**Contact** Mr. Francis Perry, Graduate Assistant, Faculty of Nursing, University of New Brunswick Fredericton, PO Box 4400, Fredericton, NB E3B 5A3. *Telephone:* 506-451-6844. *Fax:* 506-447-3374. *E-mail:* fperry@unb.ca.

**MASTER'S DEGREE PROGRAM**
**Degree** MN
**Available Programs** Master's.
**Concentrations Available** Nurse case management; nursing administration; nursing education; nursing informatics. *Clinical nurse specialist programs in:* acute care, adult health, cardiovascular, community health, critical care, family health, gerontology, maternity-newborn, medical-surgical, oncology, parent-child, pediatric, psychiatric/mental health, public health, school health,women's health. *Nurse practitioner programs in:* acute care, adult health, community health, family health, gerontology, neonatal health, pediatric, primary care, psychiatric/mental health,women's health.
**Site Options** Fredericton, NB.
**Study Options** Full-time and part-time.
**Program Entrance Requirements** Clinical experience, computer literacy, minimum overall college GPA of 3.3, transcript of college record, CPR certification, written essay, immunizations, 3 letters of recommendation, nursing research course, physical assessment course, prerequisite course work, statistics course. *Application deadline:* 1/2 (winter). *Application fee:* CAN$50.
**Advanced Placement** Credit given for nursing courses completed elsewhere dependent upon specific evaluations.
**Degree Requirements** 27 total credit hours, thesis or project.

## CONTINUING EDUCATION PROGRAM

**Contact** Mr. Lee Heenan, Administrative Assistant, Faculty of Nursing, University of New Brunswick Fredericton, PO Box 4400, Fredericton, NB E3B 5A3. *Telephone:* 506-458-7625. *Fax:* 506-447-3057. *E-mail:* nursing@unb.ca.

# NEWFOUNDLAND AND LABRADOR

# Memorial University of Newfoundland

### School of Nursing
### St. John's, Newfoundland and Labrador

***http://www.nurs.mun.ca/***
Founded in 1925

### DEGREES • BN • MN

**Nursing Program Faculty** 42 (30% with doctorates).
**Baccalaureate Enrollment** 642 **Women** 92% **Men** 8% **International** 2% **Part-time** 50%
**Graduate Enrollment** 100 **Women** 91% **Men** 9% **International** 1% **Part-time** 82%
**Distance Learning Courses** Available.
**Nursing Student Activities** Student Nurses' Association.
**Nursing Student Resources** Academic advising; academic or career counseling; assistance for students with disabilities; bookstore; campus computer network; computer lab; computer-assisted instruction; daycare for children of students; e-mail services; employment services for current students; externships; interactive nursing skills videos; Internet; learning resource lab; library services; nursing audiovisuals; remedial services; skills, simulation, or other laboratory; tutoring.
**Library Facilities** 1.9 million volumes (40,000 in health, 5,000 in nursing); 17,170 periodical subscriptions (3,800 health-care related).

## BACCALAUREATE PROGRAMS

**Degree** BN
**Available Programs** Accelerated Baccalaureate; Generic Baccalaureate; LPN to Baccalaureate; RN Baccalaureate.
**Study Options** Full-time.
**Program Entrance Requirements** Minimum overall college GPA of 3.0, transcript of college record, written essay, high school biology, high school chemistry, high school foreign language, high school math, high school science, high school transcript, 2 letters of recommendation, minimum high school rank 80%. Transfer students are accepted. *Application deadline:* 3/1 (fall).
**Contact** *Telephone:* 709-737-6871. *Fax:* 709-737-3890.

## GRADUATE PROGRAMS

**Contact** *Telephone:* 709-777-6679. *Fax:* 709-777-7037.

**MASTER'S DEGREE PROGRAM**
**Degree** MN
**Available Programs** Master's.
**Concentrations Available** Nursing education. *Nurse practitioner programs in:* acute care.
**Study Options** Full-time and part-time.
**Online Degree Options** Yes (online only).
**Program Entrance Requirements** Clinical experience, minimum overall college GPA of 3.0, transcript of college record, written essay, 2 letters of recommendation, nursing research course, professional liability insurance/malpractice insurance, prerequisite course work, resume, statistics course. *Application deadline:* 2/15 (fall). *Application fee:* CAN$40.
**Advanced Placement** Credit given for nursing courses completed elsewhere dependent upon specific evaluations.
**Degree Requirements** 28 total credit hours, thesis or project.

**POST-MASTER'S PROGRAM**
**Areas of Study** *Nurse practitioner programs in:* acute care.

# NOVA SCOTIA

## St. Francis Xavier University

### Department of Nursing
### Antigonish, Nova Scotia

*http://www.stfx.ca/*
Founded in 1853

**DEGREE • BSCN**
**Nursing Program Faculty** 67 (10% with doctorates).
**Baccalaureate Enrollment** 1,067 **Women** 90% **Men** 10% **Minority** 5% **International** 1% **Part-time** 40%
**Nursing Student Activities** Student Nurses' Association, nursing club.
**Nursing Student Resources** Academic advising; academic or career counseling; assistance for students with disabilities; bookstore; campus computer network; career placement assistance; computer lab; computer-assisted instruction; daycare for children of students; e-mail services; employment services for current students; externships; housing assistance; interactive nursing skills videos; Internet; learning resource lab; library services; nursing audiovisuals; other; paid internships; placement services for program completers; remedial services; resume preparation assistance; skills, simulation, or other laboratory; tutoring; unpaid internships.
**Library Facilities** 320,317 volumes (4,000 in health, 4,000 in nursing); 24,293 periodical subscriptions (1,015 health-care related).

### BACCALAUREATE PROGRAMS

**Degree** BScN
**Available Programs** Accelerated Baccalaureate; Accelerated Baccalaureate for Second Degree; Accelerated LPN to Baccalaureate; Generic Baccalaureate; RN Baccalaureate.
**Site Options** Sydney, NS.
**Study Options** Full-time.
**Program Entrance Requirements** Transcript of college record, CPR certification, health exam, high school biology, high school chemistry, 2 years high school math, 2 years high school science, high school transcript, immunizations, minimum high school GPA, prerequisite course work. Transfer students are accepted.
**Advanced Placement** Credit given for nursing courses completed elsewhere dependent upon specific evaluations.
**Contact** *Telephone:* 902-867-5386. *Fax:* 902-867-2329.

### CONTINUING EDUCATION PROGRAM

**Contact** *Telephone:* 902-867-5186. *Fax:* 902-867-5154.

# ONTARIO

## Brock University

### Department of Nursing
### St. Catharines, Ontario

*http://www.brocku.ca/nursing/*
Founded in 1964

**DEGREE • BSCN**
**Nursing Program Faculty** 27
**Nursing Student Activities** Student Nurses' Association, nursing club.
**Nursing Student Resources** Academic advising; academic or career counseling; assistance for students with disabilities; bookstore; campus computer network; computer lab; computer-assisted instruction; daycare for children of students; e-mail services; employment services for current students; housing assistance; interactive nursing skills videos; Internet; learning resource lab; library services; nursing audiovisuals; other; resume preparation assistance; skills, simulation, or other laboratory; tutoring.
**Library Facilities** 769,873 volumes.

### BACCALAUREATE PROGRAMS

**Degree** BScN
**Available Programs** Generic Baccalaureate; RN Baccalaureate.
**Study Options** Full-time.
**Program Entrance Requirements** High school biology, high school chemistry.
**Contact** *Telephone:* 905-688-5550 Ext. 4660.

## Lakehead University

### School of Nursing
### Thunder Bay, Ontario

*http://www.lakeheadu.ca/*
Founded in 1965

**DEGREE • BSCN**
**Nursing Program Faculty** 15 (20% with doctorates).
**Baccalaureate Enrollment** 575 **Women** 82% **Men** 18%
**Distance Learning Courses** Available.
**Nursing Student Activities** Student Nurses' Association.
**Nursing Student Resources** Academic advising; academic or career counseling; assistance for students with disabilities; bookstore; campus computer network; career placement assistance; computer lab; daycare for children of students; e-mail services; employment services for current students; externships; housing assistance; interactive nursing skills videos; Internet; library services; nursing audiovisuals; resume preparation assistance; skills, simulation, or other laboratory; tutoring; unpaid internships.
**Library Facilities** 715,276 volumes; 44,533 periodical subscriptions.

### BACCALAUREATE PROGRAMS

**Degree** BScN
**Available Programs** Accelerated Baccalaureate; Generic Baccalaureate; RN Baccalaureate.
**Study Options** Full-time and part-time.
**Online Degree Options** Yes.
**Program Entrance Requirements** Transcript of college record, CPR certification, health insurance, high school biology, high school chemistry, 4 years high school math, high school transcript, immunizations, minimum high school GPA. Transfer students are accepted. *Application deadline:* 1/12 (winter). Applications may be processed on a rolling basis for some programs.
**Advanced Placement** Credit given for nursing courses completed elsewhere dependent upon specific evaluations.
**Contact** *Telephone:* 807-343-8439. *Fax:* 807-343-8246.

# Laurentian University
## School of Nursing
## Sudbury, Ontario

*http://www.laurentian.ca/content/program/nursing/overview*
Founded in 1960

### DEGREES • BSCN • M SC N

**Nursing Program Faculty** 15 (10% with doctorates).
**Baccalaureate Enrollment** 260 **Women** 90% **Men** 10%
**Distance Learning Courses** Available.
**Nursing Student Activities** Student Nurses' Association.
**Nursing Student Resources** Academic advising; academic or career counseling; assistance for students with disabilities; bookstore; campus computer network; career placement assistance; computer lab; computer-assisted instruction; daycare for children of students; e-mail services; employment services for current students; externships; housing assistance; interactive nursing skills videos; Internet; learning resource lab; library services; nursing audiovisuals; placement services for program completers; remedial services; resume preparation assistance; skills, simulation, or other laboratory; tutoring; unpaid internships.

### BACCALAUREATE PROGRAMS

**Degree** BScN
**Available Programs** Generic Baccalaureate; RN Baccalaureate.
**Study Options** Full-time.
**Program Entrance Requirements** CPR certification, high school biology, high school chemistry, high school transcript, immunizations. Transfer students are accepted. *Application deadline:* Applications may be processed on a rolling basis for some programs.
**Financial Aid** ***Gift aid (need-based):*** state, private, college/university gift aid from institutional funds. *Loans:* college/university. *Work-study:* part-time campus jobs. *Financial aid application deadline:* Continuous.
**Contact** Ms. Fran Guilbeault, Administrative Assistant, School of Nursing, Laurentian University, 935 Ramsey Lake Road, Sudbury, ON P3E 2C6. *Telephone:* 705-675-1151 Ext. 3800. *Fax:* 705-675-4861. *E-mail:* fguilbeault@laurentian.ca.

### GRADUATE PROGRAMS

**Contact** Fran Guilbeault, Administrative Assistant, School of Nursing, Laurentian University, 935 Ramsey Lake Road, Sudbury, ON P3E 2C6. *Telephone:* 705-675-1151 Ext. 3800. *Fax:* 705-675-4861. *E-mail:* fguilbeault@laurentian.ca.

#### MASTER'S DEGREE PROGRAM

**Degree** M Sc N
**Available Programs** Master's.
**Study Options** Full-time and part-time.
**Program Entrance Requirements** Clinical experience, written essay, letters of recommendation, resume.
**Degree Requirements** Thesis or project.

### CONTINUING EDUCATION PROGRAM

**Contact** Mrs. Fran Guilbeault, Administrative Assistant, School of Nursing, Laurentian University, 935 Ramsey Lake Road, Sudbury, ON P3E 2C6. *Telephone:* 705-675-1151 Ext. 3800. *Fax:* 705-675-4861. *E-mail:* fguilbeault@laurentian.ca.

# McMaster University
## School of Nursing
## Hamilton, Ontario

*http://www.fhs.mcmaster.ca/nursing*
Founded in 1887

### DEGREES • BSCN • M SC • MSN/PHD • PHD

**Nursing Program Faculty** 53 (47% with doctorates).
**Baccalaureate Enrollment** 548 **Women** 90% **Men** 10% **Part-time** 20%
**Nursing Student Activities** Student Nurses' Association.
**Nursing Student Resources** Academic advising; academic or career counseling; assistance for students with disabilities; bookstore; campus computer network; career placement assistance; computer lab; daycare for children of students; e-mail services; employment services for current students; housing assistance; Internet; learning resource lab; library services; nursing audiovisuals; placement services for program completers; remedial services; resume preparation assistance; skills, simulation, or other laboratory; tutoring.
**Library Facilities** 1.7 million volumes (150,446 in health); 57,487 periodical subscriptions (89,267 health-care related).

### BACCALAUREATE PROGRAMS

**Degree** BScN
**Available Programs** Baccalaureate for Second Degree; Generic Baccalaureate; RN Baccalaureate.
**Site Options** Kitchener, ON.
**Study Options** Full-time and part-time.
**Program Entrance Requirements** CPR certification, health exam, high school biology, high school chemistry, 4 years high school math, 4 years high school science, high school transcript, immunizations, minimum high school GPA of 3.0, minimum high school rank 75%. Transfer students are accepted.
**Advanced Placement** Credit by examination available. Credit given for nursing courses completed elsewhere dependent upon specific evaluations.
**Contact** *Telephone:* 905-525-9140 Ext. 22232. *Fax:* 905-528-4727.

### GRADUATE PROGRAMS

**Contact** *Telephone:* 905-525-9140 Ext. 22982. *Fax:* 905-546-1129.

#### MASTER'S DEGREE PROGRAM

**Degrees** M Sc; MSN/PhD
**Available Programs** Master's.
**Concentrations Available** *Clinical nurse specialist programs in:* perinatal. *Nurse practitioner programs in:* neonatal health.
**Study Options** Full-time and part-time.
**Program Entrance Requirements** Transcript of college record, written essay, 2 letters of recommendation.
**Advanced Placement** Credit given for nursing courses completed elsewhere dependent upon specific evaluations.
**Degree Requirements** Thesis or project.

#### DOCTORAL DEGREE PROGRAM

**Degree** PhD
**Available Programs** Doctorate.
**Program Entrance Requirements** 2 letters of recommendation, MSN or equivalent, vita.
**Degree Requirements** Dissertation, oral exam.

# Nipissing University
## Nursing Department
## North Bay, Ontario

*http://www.nipissingu.ca/nursing/*
Founded in 1992

### DEGREE • BSCN

**Nursing Program Faculty** 12 (3% with doctorates).
**Baccalaureate Enrollment** 378 **Women** 91% **Men** 9%
**Distance Learning Courses** Available.
**Nursing Student Activities** Student Nurses' Association.
**Nursing Student Resources** Academic advising; academic or career counseling; assistance for students with disabilities; bookstore; campus computer network; career placement assistance; computer lab; computer-assisted instruction; e-mail services; employment services for current students; housing assistance; interactive nursing skills videos; Internet; learning resource lab; library services; nursing audiovisuals; placement services for program completers; remedial services; resume preparation assistance; skills, simulation, or other laboratory; tutoring; unpaid internships.
**Library Facilities** 715,494 volumes (2,800 in health, 1,820 in nursing); 19,115 periodical subscriptions (2,430 health-care related).

### BACCALAUREATE PROGRAMS

**Degree** BScN
**Available Programs** RN Baccalaureate; RPN to Baccalaureate.
**Study Options** Full-time.
**Online Degree Options** Yes.
**Program Entrance Requirements** Minimum overall college GPA of 3.0, transcript of college record, CPR certification, high school biology, high school chemistry, high school transcript, immunizations, minimum high school rank 70%. Transfer students are accepted. *Application*

*deadline:* 4/1 (fall). Applications may be processed on a rolling basis for some programs. *Application fee:* CAN$130.
**Advanced Placement** Credit given for nursing courses completed elsewhere dependent upon specific evaluations.
**Financial Aid** 44% of baccalaureate students in nursing programs received some form of financial aid in 2012–13.
**Contact** Registrar's Office, Nursing Department, Nipissing University, 100 College Drive, PO Box 5002, North Bay, ON P1B 8L7. *Telephone:* 705-474-3450 Ext. 4521. *E-mail:* registrar@nipssingu.ca.

# Queen's University at Kingston

## School of Nursing
## Kingston, Ontario

***http://www.nursing.queensu.ca/***
Founded in 1841

**DEGREES • BNSC • M SC • PHD**
**Nursing Program Faculty** 20 (80% with doctorates).
**Baccalaureate Enrollment** 440 **Women** 90% **Men** 10% **Minority** 4% **International** 2%
**Graduate Enrollment** 110 **Women** 87% **Men** 13% **Minority** 4% **International** 4%
**Distance Learning Courses** Available.
**Nursing Student Activities** Student Nurses' Association.
**Nursing Student Resources** Academic advising; academic or career counseling; assistance for students with disabilities; bookstore; campus computer network; career placement assistance; computer lab; computer-assisted instruction; e-mail services; employment services for current students; housing assistance; interactive nursing skills videos; Internet; learning resource lab; library services; nursing audiovisuals; resume preparation assistance; skills, simulation, or other laboratory; tutoring; unpaid internships.
**Library Facilities** 3.5 million volumes (5,209 in health, 3,652 in nursing); 16,109 periodical subscriptions (1,054 health-care related).

### BACCALAUREATE PROGRAMS

**Degree** BNSc
**Available Programs** Accelerated Baccalaureate; Generic Baccalaureate.
**Site Options** Napanee, ON.
**Study Options** Full-time.
**Program Entrance Requirements** CPR certification, high school biology, high school chemistry, high school math, high school science, high school transcript, immunizations, minimum high school GPA, minimum high school rank. Transfer students are accepted. *Application deadline:* 2/1 (fall). *Application fee:* CAN$130.
**Advanced Placement** Credit given for nursing courses completed elsewhere dependent upon specific evaluations.
**Expenses (2013–14)** *Tuition, area resident:* full-time CAN$5877. *International tuition:* CAN$24,696 full-time. *Required fees:* full-time CAN$1032.
**Financial Aid** 41% of baccalaureate students in nursing programs received some form of financial aid in 2012–13.
**Contact** Dr. Christina Godfrey, Chair, Admissions Committee, School of Nursing, Queen's University at Kingston, Cataraqui Building, 92 Barrie Street, Kingston, ON K7L 3N6. *Telephone:* 613-533-2668 Ext. 78760. *Fax:* 613-533-6770. *E-mail:* christina.godfrey@queensu.ca.

### GRADUATE PROGRAMS

**Expenses (2013–14)** *Tuition, area resident:* full-time CAN$6258. *International tuition:* CAN$12,366 full-time. *Required fees:* full-time CAN$1065.
**Financial Aid** 100% of graduate students in nursing programs received some form of financial aid in 2012–13. 25 fellowships (averaging $6,636 per year), 4 research assistantships, 9 teaching assistantships (averaging $2,592 per year) were awarded; institutionally sponsored loans and scholarships also available. *Financial aid application deadline:* 2/1.
**Contact** Dr. Diane Buchanan, Graduate Coordinator, School of Nursing, Queen's University at Kingston, Cataraqui Building, 92 Barrie Street, Kingston, ON K7L 3N6. *Telephone:* 613-533-6000 Ext. 78907. *Fax:* 613-533-6770. *E-mail:* buchan@queensu.ca.

#### MASTER'S DEGREE PROGRAM

**Degree** M Sc
**Available Programs** Master's.
**Concentrations Available** *Nurse practitioner programs in:* primary care.
**Study Options** Full-time.
**Program Entrance Requirements** Minimum overall college GPA of 3.0, transcript of college record, 2 letters of recommendation, nursing research course, prerequisite course work, resume, statistics course. *Application deadline:* 2/1 (fall). *Application fee:* CAN$105.
**Degree Requirements** 15 total credit hours, thesis or project.

#### DOCTORAL DEGREE PROGRAM

**Degree** PhD
**Available Programs** Doctorate.
**Areas of Study** Illness and transition, nursing science.
**Program Entrance Requirements** Minimum overall college GPA of 3.2, 2 letters of recommendation, MSN or equivalent, statistics course, vita. *Application deadline:* 2/1 (fall). *Application fee:* CAN$105.
**Degree Requirements** 15 total credit hours, dissertation, oral exam, written exam, residency.

# Ryerson University

## Program in Nursing
## Toronto, Ontario

***http://www.ryerson.ca/nursing***
Founded in 1948

**DEGREES • BSCN • MN**
**Nursing Program Faculty** 83 (94% with doctorates).
**Baccalaureate Enrollment** 1,953 **Women** 89% **Men** 11% **International** 1% **Part-time** 25.75%
**Graduate Enrollment** 168 **Women** 89% **Men** 11% **Part-time** 28%
**Distance Learning Courses** Available.
**Nursing Student Activities** Sigma Theta Tau, Student Nurses' Association, nursing club.
**Nursing Student Resources** Academic advising; academic or career counseling; assistance for students with disabilities; bookstore; campus computer network; career placement assistance; computer lab; computer-assisted instruction; daycare for children of students; e-mail services; employment services for current students; housing assistance; interactive nursing skills videos; Internet; learning resource lab; library services; nursing audiovisuals; remedial services; resume preparation assistance; skills, simulation, or other laboratory; tutoring.
**Library Facilities** 487,361 volumes (29,163 in health, 4,963 in nursing); 28,075 periodical subscriptions (5,567 health-care related).

### BACCALAUREATE PROGRAMS

**Degree** BScN
**Available Programs** International Nurse to Baccalaureate; RN Baccalaureate; RPN to Baccalaureate.
**Study Options** Full-time.
**Online Degree Options** Yes.
**Program Entrance Requirements** Transcript of college record, CPR certification, health exam, health insurance, high school biology, high school chemistry, 3 years high school math, 4 years high school science, high school transcript, immunizations, minimum high school rank, minimum GPA in nursing prerequisites of 3.0. *Application deadline:* 3/1 (fall). *Application fee:* CAN$215.
**Expenses (2013–14)** *International tuition:* CAN$21,000 full-time.
**Financial Aid** ***Gift aid (need-based):*** college/university gift aid from institutional funds. *Loans:* Federal Direct (Subsidized and Unsubsidized Stafford). *Financial aid application deadline:* 1/15.
**Contact** Heather Palmer, Senior Admission Officer, Program in Nursing, Ryerson University, 350 Victoria Street, Toronto, ON M5B 2K3. *Telephone:* 416-979-5000 Ext. 4122. *Fax:* 416-979-5221. *E-mail:* hpalmer@ryerson.ca.

### GRADUATE PROGRAMS

**Financial Aid** 11% of graduate students in nursing programs received some form of financial aid in 2012–13.
**Contact** Mr. Gerry Warner, Program Administrator, Program in Nursing, Ryerson University, 350 Victoria Street, Toronto, ON M5B 2K3. *Telephone:* 416-979-5000 Ext. 7852. *Fax:* 416-979-5332. *E-mail:* gerry.warner@ryerson.ca.

#### MASTER'S DEGREE PROGRAM

**Degree** MN
**Available Programs** Master's.

**Concentrations Available** *Clinical nurse specialist programs in:* adult health, community health, family health, public health. *Nurse practitioner programs in:* primary care.
**Study Options** Full-time and part-time.
**Program Entrance Requirements** Minimum overall college GPA of 3.33, transcript of college record, written essay, immunizations, 2 letters of recommendation, nursing research course, physical assessment course, resume. *Application deadline:* 1/31 (fall). Applications may be processed on a rolling basis for some programs. *Application fee:* CAN$110.
**Advanced Placement** Credit given for nursing courses completed elsewhere dependent upon specific evaluations.
**Degree Requirements** 10 total credit hours, thesis or project.

## CONTINUING EDUCATION PROGRAM

**Contact** Paula Mastrilli, Program Manager, Program in Nursing, Ryerson University, 297 Victoria Street, POD 481-D, Toronto, ON M5B 2K3. *Telephone:* 416-979-0000 Ext. 5178. *Fax:* 416-542-5878. *E-mail:* pmastril@gwemail.ryerson.ca.

# Trent University

## Nursing Program
## Peterborough, Ontario

***http://www.trentu.ca/nursing/***
Founded in 1963

### DEGREE • BSCN

**Nursing Program Faculty** 45 (10% with doctorates).
**Baccalaureate Enrollment** 694 **Part-time** 11%
**Distance Learning Courses** Available.
**Nursing Student Activities** Student Nurses' Association.
**Nursing Student Resources** Academic advising; academic or career counseling; assistance for students with disabilities; bookstore; campus computer network; career placement assistance; computer lab; computer-assisted instruction; e-mail services; employment services for current students; housing assistance; interactive nursing skills videos; Internet; learning resource lab; library services; nursing audiovisuals; remedial services; resume preparation assistance; skills, simulation, or other laboratory; tutoring.
**Library Facilities** 6,393 volumes in health, 1,281 volumes in nursing; 360 periodical subscriptions health-care related.

### BACCALAUREATE PROGRAMS

**Degree** BScN
**Available Programs** Accelerated Baccalaureate; Generic Baccalaureate.
**Site Options** Peterborough, ON; Toronto, ON.
**Study Options** Full-time.
**Program Entrance Requirements** CPR certification, health exam, high school biology, high school chemistry, 4 years high school math, 4 years high school science, high school transcript, immunizations, minimum high school rank 70%. Transfer students are accepted.
**Advanced Placement** Credit given for nursing courses completed elsewhere dependent upon specific evaluations.
**Financial Aid** ***Loans:*** Sallie Mae Smart Option Loans.
**Contact** Nursing Enrolment Advisor, Nursing Program, Trent University, 1600 West Bank Drive, Peterborough, ON K9J 7B8. *Telephone:* 705-748-1011 Ext. 7809. *Fax:* 705-748-1629. *E-mail:* nursingadmissions@trentu.ca.

# University of Ottawa

## School of Nursing
## Ottawa, Ontario

***http://www.health.uottawa.ca/sn/***
Founded in 1848

### DEGREES • BSCN • M SC N • PHD

**Nursing Program Faculty** 125 (33% with doctorates).
**Baccalaureate Enrollment** 1,542 **Women** 87.94% **Men** 12.06% **Part-time** 15.82%
**Graduate Enrollment** 224 **Women** 90.18% **Men** 9.82% **Part-time** 60.71%
**Distance Learning Courses** Available.
**Nursing Student Activities** Sigma Theta Tau, Student Nurses' Association.
**Nursing Student Resources** Academic advising; academic or career counseling; assistance for students with disabilities; bookstore; campus computer network; career placement assistance; computer lab; computer-assisted instruction; e-mail services; employment services for current students; housing assistance; interactive nursing skills videos; Internet; learning resource lab; library services; nursing audiovisuals; remedial services; resume preparation assistance; skills, simulation, or other laboratory; tutoring.
**Library Facilities** 3.8 million volumes (46,081 in health, 8,911 in nursing); 90,710 periodical subscriptions (8,304 health-care related).

### BACCALAUREATÈ PROGRAMS

**Degree** BScN
**Available Programs** Accelerated Baccalaureate for Second Degree; Accelerated RN Baccalaureate; Generic Baccalaureate; International Nurse to Baccalaureate; RN Baccalaureate; RPN to Baccalaureate.
**Site Options** Hawkesbury, ON; Pembroke, ON; Hawkesbury, ON.
**Study Options** Full-time.
**Program Entrance Requirements** Transcript of college record, high school biology, high school chemistry, high school math, high school transcript, minimum high school GPA. Transfer students are accepted. *Application deadline:* 3/30 (fall). *Application fee:* CAN$130.
**Advanced Placement** Credit given for nursing courses completed elsewhere dependent upon specific evaluations.
**Expenses (2013–14)** *Tuition, area resident:* full-time CAN$5835; part-time CAN$231 per credit. *Room and board:* room only: CAN$5545 per academic year. *Required fees:* full-time CAN$677; part-time CAN$117 per term.
**Financial Aid** ***Gift aid (need-based):*** state, private, college/university gift aid from institutional funds. *Loans:* Federal Direct (Subsidized and Unsubsidized Stafford PLUS). *Work-study:* part-time campus jobs. *Financial aid application deadline:* 1/31.
**Contact** Ms. Julie Monette, Undergraduate Studies Office, School of Nursing, University of Ottawa, 125 Universit, Ottawa, ON K1N 6N5. *Telephone:* 613-562-5853. *Fax:* 613-562-5149. *E-mail:* esecr@uottawa.ca.

### GRADUATE PROGRAMS

**Expenses (2013–14)** *Tuition, area resident:* full-time CAN$3258; part-time CAN$392 per credit. *International tuition:* CAN$5301 full-time. *Room and board:* room only: CAN$5545 per academic year. *Required fees:* full-time CAN$662; part-time CAN$111 per credit.
**Financial Aid** Fellowships, research assistantships, teaching assistantships, career-related internships or fieldwork, Federal Work-Study, scholarships, traineeships, tuition waivers (full and partial), and unspecified assistantships available.
**Contact** Dr. Jocelyne Tourigny, Assistant Director of Graduate Program, School of Nursing, University of Ottawa, 451 Smyth Road, Ottawa, ON K1H 8M5. *Telephone:* 613-562-5800 Ext. 8422. *Fax:* 613-562-5443. *E-mail:* jtourign@uottawa.ca.

### MASTER'S DEGREE PROGRAM

**Degree** M Sc N
**Available Programs** Master's.
**Concentrations Available** *Clinical nurse specialist programs in:* acute care, adult health, cardiovascular, community health, critical care, family health, forensic nursing, gerontology, home health care, maternity-newborn, medical-surgical, occupational health, oncology, palliative care, parent-child, pediatric, perinatal, psychiatric/mental health, public health, rehabilitation, school health,women's health. *Nurse practitioner programs in:* primary care.
**Study Options** Full-time and part-time.
**Program Entrance Requirements** Clinical experience, minimum overall college GPA of 3.0, transcript of college record, written essay, immunizations, 3 letters of recommendation, nursing research course, physical assessment course, prerequisite course work, resume, statistics course. *Application deadline:* 2/15 (winter).
**Advanced Placement** Credit given for nursing courses completed elsewhere dependent upon specific evaluations.
**Degree Requirements** 24 total credit hours, thesis or project.

### DOCTORAL DEGREE PROGRAM

**Degree** PhD
**Available Programs** Doctorate; Doctorate for Nurses with Non-Nursing Degrees.
**Areas of Study** Aging, community health, critical care, ethics, forensic nursing, gerontology, health policy, health promotion/disease prevention, health-care systems, human health and illness, illness and transition,

maternity-newborn, nursing education, nursing policy, nursing research, nursing science, oncology,women's health.
**Program Entrance Requirements** Minimum overall college GPA of 3.5, 3 letters of recommendation, MSN or equivalent, statistics course, vita, writing sample. *Application deadline:* 9/11 (fall). *Application fee:* CAN$100.
**Degree Requirements** 18 total credit hours, dissertation, oral exam, written exam, residency.

### POSTDOCTORAL PROGRAM

**Areas of Study** Addiction/substance abuse, aging, cancer care, chronic illness, community health, health promotion/disease prevention, information systems, nursing interventions, nursing research, nursing science, outcomes, vulnerable population,women's health.
**Postdoctoral Program Contact** Dr. Jocelyne Tourigny, Assistant Director of Graduate Program, School of Nursing, University of Ottawa, 451 Smyth Road, Ottawa, ON K1H 8M5. *Telephone:* 613-562-5800 Ext. 8422. *Fax:* 613-562-5443. *E-mail:* jtourign@uottawa.ca.

# University of Toronto

## Faculty of Nursing
## Toronto, Ontario

***http://www.bloomberg.nursing.utoronto.ca/***
Founded in 1827

**DEGREES • BSCN • MN • PHD**
**Nursing Program Faculty** 250 (50% with doctorates).
**Baccalaureate Enrollment** 340 **Women** 87% **Men** 13% **International** 5%
**Graduate Enrollment** 360
**Distance Learning Courses** Available.
**Nursing Student Activities** Sigma Theta Tau, Student Nurses' Association, nursing club.
**Nursing Student Resources** Academic advising; academic or career counseling; assistance for students with disabilities; bookstore; campus computer network; career placement assistance; computer lab; computer-assisted instruction; daycare for children of students; e-mail services; employment services for current students; externships; housing assistance; interactive nursing skills videos; Internet; learning resource lab; library services; nursing audiovisuals; paid internships; remedial services; resume preparation assistance; skills, simulation, or other laboratory; tutoring.
**Library Facilities** 14.5 million volumes; 97,753 periodical subscriptions.

### BACCALAUREATE PROGRAMS

**Degree** BScN
**Available Programs** Accelerated Baccalaureate; Accelerated Baccalaureate for Second Degree; Accelerated RN Baccalaureate; Baccalaureate for Second Degree.
**Study Options** Full-time.
**Program Entrance Requirements** Minimum overall college GPA of 3.0, CPR certification, written essay, immunizations, 2 letters of recommendation, minimum GPA in nursing prerequisites of 3.0, prerequisite course work. *Application deadline:* 2/1 (fall).
**Contact** *Telephone:* 416-978-2392. *Fax:* 416-978-8222.

### GRADUATE PROGRAMS

**Contact** *Telephone:* 416-978-2392. *Fax:* 416-978-8222.

### MASTER'S DEGREE PROGRAM

**Degree** MN
**Available Programs** Master's.
**Concentrations Available** Clinical nurse leader; health-care administration; nurse anesthesia; nursing administration; nursing education; nursing informatics. *Clinical nurse specialist programs in:* acute care, adult health, cardiovascular, community health, critical care, family health, gerontology, maternity-newborn, medical-surgical, occupational health, oncology, palliative care, parent-child, pediatric, perinatal, psychiatric/mental health, public health, rehabilitation, school health,women's health. *Nurse practitioner programs in:* acute care, adult health, family health, gerontology, neonatal health, oncology, pediatric, primary care.
**Study Options** Full-time.
**Online Degree Options** Yes.
**Program Entrance Requirements** Clinical experience, minimum overall college GPA of 3.0, transcript of college record, CPR certification, written essay, 2 letters of recommendation, prerequisite course work, resume, statistics course. *Application deadline:* 3/15 (fall).
**Degree Requirements** 9 total credit hours.

### POST-MASTER'S PROGRAM

**Areas of Study** Nurse anesthesia. *Clinical nurse specialist programs in:* acute care, adult health, gerontology, maternity-newborn, pediatric. *Nurse practitioner programs in:* acute care, adult health, pediatric, primary care.

### DOCTORAL DEGREE PROGRAM

**Degree** PhD
**Available Programs** Doctorate; Doctorate for Nurses with Non-Nursing Degrees; Post-Baccalaureate Doctorate.
**Areas of Study** Addiction/substance abuse, advanced practice nursing, aging, bio-behavioral research, biology of health and illness, community health, critical care, ethics, faculty preparation, family health, gerontology, health policy, health promotion/disease prevention, health-care systems, human health and illness, individualized study, information systems, maternity-newborn, neuro-behavior, nurse case management, nursing administration, nursing education, nursing policy, nursing research, nursing science, oncology, urban health,women's health.
**Program Entrance Requirements** Minimum overall college GPA of 3.3, interview by faculty committee, 2 letters of recommendation, MSN or equivalent, scholarly papers, statistics course, vita, writing sample. *Application deadline:* 2/1 (fall).
**Degree Requirements** 6 total credit hours, dissertation, oral exam.

### POSTDOCTORAL PROGRAM

**Postdoctoral Program Contact***Telephone:* 416-978-8069.

# The University of Western Ontario

## School of Nursing
## London, Ontario

***http://www.uwo.ca/fhs/nursing***
Founded in 1878

**DEGREES • BSCN • M SC N • PHD**
**Nursing Program Faculty** 101 (18% with doctorates).
**Baccalaureate Enrollment** 1,153 **Women** 93.24% **Men** 6.76% **Part-time** 13.53%
**Graduate Enrollment** 54 **Women** 89% **Men** 11% **Part-time** 28%
**Nursing Student Activities** Nursing Honor Society, Sigma Theta Tau, Student Nurses' Association.
**Nursing Student Resources** Academic advising; academic or career counseling; assistance for students with disabilities; bookstore; campus computer network; computer lab; computer-assisted instruction; daycare for children of students; e-mail services; employment services for current students; housing assistance; interactive nursing skills videos; Internet; learning resource lab; library services; nursing audiovisuals; resume preparation assistance; unpaid internships.
**Library Facilities** 4.7 million volumes (357,263 in health, 40 in nursing); 108,417 periodical subscriptions (250 health-care related).

### BACCALAUREATE PROGRAMS

**Degree** BScN
**Available Programs** Accelerated Baccalaureate; Generic Baccalaureate; RN Baccalaureate.
**Study Options** Full-time.
**Program Entrance Requirements** CPR certification, high school biology, high school chemistry, 4 years high school math, high school science, high school transcript, immunizations, minimum high school rank 80%. Transfer students are accepted.
**Advanced Placement** Credit given for nursing courses completed elsewhere dependent upon specific evaluations.
**Contact** *Telephone:* 519-661-2111 Ext. 86564. *Fax:* 519-661-3928.

### GRADUATE PROGRAMS

**Contact** *Telephone:* 519-661-3409. *Fax:* 519-661-3928.

### MASTER'S DEGREE PROGRAM

**Degree** M Sc N

**Available Programs** Master's.
**Concentrations Available** Health-care administration; nursing administration; nursing education. *Clinical nurse specialist programs in:* acute care, adult health, community health, psychiatric/mental health, public health,women's health. *Nurse practitioner programs in:* community health.
**Study Options** Full-time and part-time.
**Program Entrance Requirements** Minimum overall college GPA of 3.5, transcript of college record, written essay, interview, 2 letters of recommendation, nursing research course, prerequisite course work, resume, statistics course.
**Advanced Placement** Credit given for nursing courses completed elsewhere dependent upon specific evaluations.
**Degree Requirements** 7 total credit hours, thesis or project.

### DOCTORAL DEGREE PROGRAM

**Degree** PhD
**Available Programs** Doctorate.
**Areas of Study** Addiction/substance abuse, advanced practice nursing, aging, clinical practice, community health, faculty preparation, health policy, health promotion/disease prevention, health-care systems, human health and illness, individualized study, nurse case management, nursing administration, nursing education, nursing research, nursing science,women's health.
**Program Entrance Requirements** Clinical experience, minimum overall college GPA of 3.5, interview by faculty committee, interview, 2 letters of recommendation, MSN or equivalent, scholarly papers, statistics course, vita, writing sample.
**Degree Requirements** 4 total credit hours, dissertation, written exam.

### POSTDOCTORAL PROGRAM

**Areas of Study** Addiction/substance abuse, community health, health promotion/disease prevention, vulnerable population,women's health.
**Postdoctoral Program Contact***Telephone:* 519-661-2111 Ext. 86573.

## University of Windsor

**Faculty of Nursing**
**Windsor, Ontario**

***http://www.uwindsor.ca/nursing***
Founded in 1857

**DEGREES • BSCN • M SC N**

**Nursing Program Faculty** 192 (8% with doctorates).
**Baccalaureate Enrollment** 880 **Women** 81% **Men** 19% **International** .3% **Part-time** 3.75%
**Graduate Enrollment** 66 **Women** 85% **Men** 15% **Part-time** 36%
**Distance Learning Courses** Available.
**Nursing Student Activities** Nursing Honor Society, Sigma Theta Tau, Student Nurses' Association, nursing club.
**Nursing Student Resources** Academic advising; academic or career counseling; assistance for students with disabilities; bookstore; campus computer network; career placement assistance; computer lab; computer-assisted instruction; e-mail services; employment services for current students; interactive nursing skills videos; Internet; learning resource lab; library services; nursing audiovisuals; placement services for program completers; remedial services; resume preparation assistance; skills, simulation, or other laboratory; tutoring.
**Library Facilities** 8 million volumes (65,328 in nursing); 83,605 periodical subscriptions.

### BACCALAUREATE PROGRAMS

**Degree** BScN
**Available Programs** Generic Baccalaureate.
**Study Options** Full-time.
**Program Entrance Requirements** CPR certification, health exam, health insurance, high school biology, high school chemistry, high school math, 4 years high school science, high school transcript, immunizations, minimum high school rank 80%. Transfer students are accepted. *Application deadline:* 1/14 (fall). *Application fee:* CAN$130.
**Advanced Placement** Credit given for nursing courses completed elsewhere dependent upon specific evaluations.
**Expenses (2013–14)** *Tuition, area resident:* full-time CAN$5724; part-time CAN$572 per course. *International tuition:* CAN$20,170 full-time. *Room and board:* CAN$10,485; room only: CAN$5055 per academic year. *Required fees:* full-time CAN$1014; part-time CAN$17 per credit; part-time CAN$395 per term.
**Financial Aid** 33% of baccalaureate students in nursing programs received some form of financial aid in 2012–13.
**Contact** Nursing Contact, Faculty of Nursing, University of Windsor, 401 Sunset Avenue, Windsor, ON N9B 3P4. *Telephone:* 519-253-3000 Ext. 2258. *Fax:* 519-973-7084. *E-mail:* nurse@uwindsor.ca.

### GRADUATE PROGRAMS

**Expenses (2013–14)** *Tuition, area resident:* full-time CAN$5111; part-time CAN$1278 per term. *International tuition:* CAN$12,010 full-time. *Room and board:* CAN$10,485; room only: CAN$5055 per academic year. *Required fees:* full-time CAN$1009; part-time CAN$13 per credit; part-time CAN$88 per term.
**Financial Aid** 33% of graduate students in nursing programs received some form of financial aid in 2012–13.
**Contact** Dr. Debbie Kane, Graduate Coordinator, Faculty of Nursing, University of Windsor, 401 Sunset Avenue, Windsor, ON N9B 3P4. *Telephone:* 519-253-3000 Ext. 2268. *Fax:* 519-973-7084. *E-mail:* dkane@uwindsor.ca.

### MASTER'S DEGREE PROGRAM

**Degree** M Sc N
**Available Programs** Master's.
**Concentrations Available** Clinical nurse leader; nursing administration. *Nurse practitioner programs in:* primary care.
**Study Options** Full-time and part-time.
**Program Entrance Requirements** Minimum overall college GPA of 3.0, transcript of college record, written essay, 3 letters of recommendation, nursing research course, physical assessment course, prerequisite course work, statistics course. *Application deadline:* 2/15 (fall). *Application fee:* CAN$105.
**Advanced Placement** Credit given for nursing courses completed elsewhere dependent upon specific evaluations.
**Degree Requirements** 6 total credit hours, thesis or project.

### CONTINUING EDUCATION PROGRAM

**Contact** Nursing Main Office, Faculty of Nursing, University of Windsor, 401 Sunset Avenue, Windsor, ON N9B 3P4. *Telephone:* 519-253-3000 Ext. 2258. *Fax:* 519-973-7084. *E-mail:* nurse@uwindsor.ca.

## York University

**School of Nursing**
**Toronto, Ontario**

Founded in 1959

**DEGREE • BSCN**

**Nursing Program Faculty** 19 (79% with doctorates).
**Baccalaureate Enrollment** 850 **Women** 96% **Men** 4% **Minority** 30% **International** 1% **Part-time** 15%
**Nursing Student Resources** Academic advising; academic or career counseling; assistance for students with disabilities; bookstore; campus computer network; career placement assistance; computer lab; computer-assisted instruction; daycare for children of students; e-mail services; employment services for current students; housing assistance; interactive nursing skills videos; Internet; learning resource lab; library services; nursing audiovisuals; skills, simulation, or other laboratory; unpaid internships.
**Library Facilities** 6.5 million volumes; 540,000 periodical subscriptions.

### BACCALAUREATE PROGRAMS

**Degree** BScN
**Available Programs** Generic Baccalaureate; RN Baccalaureate.
**Site Options** King City, ON; Barrie, ON; Oshawa, ON.
**Study Options** Full-time and part-time.
**Program Entrance Requirements** CPR certification, written essay, health exam, high school biology, high school chemistry, high school math, high school science, high school transcript, immunizations, 1 letter of recommendation, minimum high school GPA, minimum GPA in nursing prerequisites. Transfer students are accepted.
**Advanced Placement** Credit by examination available. Credit given for nursing courses completed elsewhere dependent upon specific evaluations.
**Contact** *Telephone:* 416-736-5271 Ext. 66351. *Fax:* 416-736-5714.

### CONTINUING EDUCATION PROGRAM

**Contact** *Telephone:* 416-736-5271. *Fax:* 416-736-5714.

# PRINCE EDWARD ISLAND

## University of Prince Edward Island

### School of Nursing
### Charlottetown, Prince Edward Island

Founded in 1834

**DEGREE • BSCN**

**Nursing Program Faculty** 10 (2% with doctorates).
**Baccalaureate Enrollment** 211 **Women** 97% **Men** 3% **International** 1%
**Nursing Student Activities** Nursing Honor Society, Student Nurses' Association, nursing club.
**Nursing Student Resources** Academic advising; academic or career counseling; assistance for students with disabilities; bookstore; campus computer network; career placement assistance; computer lab; computer-assisted instruction; daycare for children of students; e-mail services; employment services for current students; housing assistance; interactive nursing skills videos; Internet; learning resource lab; library services; nursing audiovisuals; placement services for program completers; remedial services; resume preparation assistance; skills, simulation, or other laboratory; tutoring.
**Library Facilities** 402,808 volumes; 26,196 periodical subscriptions.

### BACCALAUREATE PROGRAMS

**Degree** BScN
**Available Programs** Generic Baccalaureate.
**Study Options** Full-time and part-time.
**Program Entrance Requirements** Transcript of college record, CPR certification, high school chemistry, high school math, high school science, high school transcript, immunizations, minimum high school GPA of 3.0, minimum high school rank 75%, minimum GPA in nursing prerequisites of 3.0, prerequisite course work. Transfer students are accepted.
**Advanced Placement** Credit given for nursing courses completed elsewhere dependent upon specific evaluations.
**Contact** *Telephone:* 902-566-0733. *Fax:* 902-566-0777.

# QUEBEC

## McGill University

### School of Nursing
### Montréal, Quebec

***http://www.mcgill.ca/***
Founded in 1821

**DEGREES • BSCN • M SC • PHD**

**Nursing Program Faculty** 163 (13% with doctorates).
**Baccalaureate Enrollment** 438 **Women** 90% **Men** 10% **International** 2% **Part-time** 25%
**Graduate Enrollment** 93 **Women** 90% **Men** 10% **International** 5% **Part-time** 26%
**Nursing Student Activities** Student Nurses' Association.
**Nursing Student Resources** Academic advising; academic or career counseling; assistance for students with disabilities; bookstore; campus computer network; career placement assistance; computer lab; e-mail services; Internet; learning resource lab; library services; nursing audiovisuals; skills, simulation, or other laboratory; tutoring; unpaid internships.
**Library Facilities** 4.2 million volumes; 49,433 periodical subscriptions.

### BACCALAUREATE PROGRAMS

**Degree** BScN
**Available Programs** Accelerated RN Baccalaureate; Generic Baccalaureate; RN Baccalaureate.
**Study Options** Full-time.
**Program Entrance Requirements** Minimum overall college GPA of 3.0, transcript of college record, high school chemistry, 4 years high school math, 4 years high school science, high school transcript, minimum high school GPA of 3.3, minimum high school rank 25%. Transfer students are accepted. *Application deadline:* 1/15 (fall), 11/1 (winter). *Application fee:* CAN$85.
**Advanced Placement** Credit given for nursing courses completed elsewhere dependent upon specific evaluations.
**Contact** *Telephone:* 514-398-3784. *Fax:* 514-398-8455.

### GRADUATE PROGRAMS

**Contact** *Telephone:* 514-398-4151. *Fax:* 514-398-8455.

#### MASTER'S DEGREE PROGRAM

**Degree** M Sc
**Available Programs** Master's; Master's for Non-Nursing College Graduates.
**Concentrations Available** Nursing administration. *Clinical nurse specialist programs in:* acute care, adult health, cardiovascular, community health, critical care, family health, gerontology, home health care, maternity-newborn, medical-surgical, oncology, parent-child, pediatric, perinatal, psychiatric/mental health, public health, rehabilitation,women's health. *Nurse practitioner programs in:* neonatal health, primary care.
**Study Options** Full-time.
**Program Entrance Requirements** Clinical experience, minimum overall college GPA of 3.0, transcript of college record, CPR certification, written essay, immunizations, interview, 3 letters of recommendation, resume, statistics course. *Application deadline:* 1/15 (fall). *Application fee:* CAN$85.
**Degree Requirements** 53 total credit hours, thesis or project.

#### DOCTORAL DEGREE PROGRAM

**Degree** PhD
**Available Programs** Doctorate; Post-Baccalaureate Doctorate.
**Areas of Study** Family health, health-care systems, human health and illness, nursing administration, nursing research, oncology.
**Program Entrance Requirements** Minimum overall college GPA of 3.3, interview, 2 letters of recommendation, MSN or equivalent, statistics course, vita, writing sample. *Application deadline:* 1/15 (fall). *Application fee:* CAN$85.
**Degree Requirements** 90 total credit hours, dissertation, oral exam, written exam, residency.

#### POSTDOCTORAL PROGRAM

**Areas of Study** Cancer care, chronic illness.
**Postdoctoral Program Contact***Telephone:* 514-398-4157. *Fax:* 514-398-8455.

## Université de Montréal

### Faculty of Nursing
### Montréal, Quebec

***http://www.scinf.umontreal.ca/***
Founded in 1920

**DEGREES • BSCN • M SC • PHD**

**Nursing Program Faculty** 43 (92% with doctorates).
**Baccalaureate Enrollment** 1,300 **Women** 80% **Men** 20% **Minority** 30% **International** 10% **Part-time** 10%
**Graduate Enrollment** 300 **Women** 75% **Men** 25% **Minority** 20% **International** 3% **Part-time** 60%
**Distance Learning Courses** Available.
**Nursing Student Activities** Student Nurses' Association.
**Nursing Student Resources** Academic advising; academic or career counseling; assistance for students with disabilities; bookstore; campus computer network; career placement assistance; computer lab; computer-assisted instruction; daycare for children of students; e-mail services; employment services for current students; externships; housing assistance; interactive nursing skills videos; Internet; learning resource lab; library services; nursing audiovisuals; other; placement services for program completers; remedial services; resume preparation assistance; skills, simulation, or other laboratory; tutoring.

**Library Facilities** 4 million volumes (32,536 in health, 32,536 in nursing); 18,330 periodical subscriptions (1,319 health-care related).

## BACCALAUREATE PROGRAMS

**Degree** BScN
**Available Programs** RN Baccalaureate.
**Site Options** Laval, QC.
**Study Options** Full-time.
**Program Entrance Requirements** Transcript of college record, CPR certification, high school biology, high school chemistry, immunizations, minimum high school GPA. Transfer students are accepted. *Application deadline:* 3/1 (fall), 10/3 (winter). *Application fee:* CAN$85.
**Advanced Placement** Credit given for nursing courses completed elsewhere dependent upon specific evaluations.
**Contact** Catherine Sarrazin, Assistant to Vice Dean, Faculty of Nursing, Université de Montréal, Pav. Marg. d'Youville, CP 6128 Succursale Centre-Ville, Montreal, QC H3C 3J7. *Telephone:* 514-343-6439. *Fax:* 514-343-2306. *E-mail:* catherine.sarrazin@umontreal.ca.

## GRADUATE PROGRAMS

**Expenses (2013–14)** *Tuition, state resident:* full-time CAN$3336. *Tuition, nonresident:* full-time CAN$9352. *International tuition:* CAN$22,423 full-time. *Room and board:* room only: CAN$3700 per academic year. *Required fees:* full-time CAN$1112.
**Financial Aid** 30% of graduate students in nursing programs received some form of financial aid in 2012–13. Fellowships, research assistantships, teaching assistantships, career-related internships or fieldwork, Federal Work-Study, and institutionally sponsored loans available.
**Contact** Suzanne Pinel, Assistant to the Vice Dean of Studies, Faculty of Nursing, Université de Montréal, Pav. Marg. d'Youville, CP 6128 Succursale Centre-Ville, Montreal, QC H3C 3J7. *Telephone:* 514-343-6111 Ext. 7098. *Fax:* 514-343-6111 Ext. 2705. *E-mail:* suzanne.pinel@umontreal.ca.

### MASTER'S DEGREE PROGRAM

**Degree** M Sc
**Available Programs** Master's; RN to Master's.
**Concentrations Available** Clinical nurse leader; nursing administration; nursing education. *Clinical nurse specialist programs in:* acute care, adult health, cardiovascular, community health, family health, gerontology, maternity-newborn, medical-surgical, occupational health, oncology, palliative care, parent-child, psychiatric/mental health, public health, rehabilitation,women's health. *Nurse practitioner programs in:* acute care, family health, primary care.
**Study Options** Full-time and part-time.
**Program Entrance Requirements** Minimum overall college GPA of 3.0, transcript of college record, CPR certification, written essay, immunizations, nursing research course, resume, statistics course. *Application deadline:* 3/1 (fall). *Application fee:* CAN$90.
**Degree Requirements** 45 total credit hours, thesis or project.

### POST-MASTER'S PROGRAM

**Areas of Study** *Nurse practitioner programs in:* acute care, family health, primary care.

### DOCTORAL DEGREE PROGRAM

**Degree** PhD
**Available Programs** Doctorate.
**Areas of Study** Addiction/substance abuse, aging, bio-behavioral research, clinical practice, community health, critical care, family health, gerontology, health policy, health promotion/disease prevention, health-care systems, human health and illness, illness and transition, maternity-newborn, neuro-behavior, nursing administration, nursing education, nursing policy, nursing research, nursing science, oncology, urban health,women's health.
**Program Entrance Requirements** Minimum overall college GPA of 3.4, interview by faculty committee, 2 letters of recommendation, MSN or equivalent, statistics course, vita, writing sample. *Application deadline:* 3/1 (fall). *Application fee:* CAN$90.
**Degree Requirements** 90 total credit hours, dissertation, oral exam.

### POSTDOCTORAL PROGRAM

**Areas of Study** Adolescent health, aging, cancer care, chronic illness, community health, family health, gerontology, health promotion/disease prevention, individualized study, neuro-behavior, nursing informatics, nursing interventions, nursing research, nursing science, outcomes, self-care, vulnerable population,women's health.
**Postdoctoral Program Contact** Ms. Chantal Cara, Vice Dean, Research, Faculty of Nursing, Université de Montréal, Pav. Marg. d'Youville, CP 6128 Succursale Centre-Ville, Montreal, QC H3C 3J7. *Telephone:* 514-343-5835. *Fax:* 514-343-2306. *E-mail:* chantal.cara@umontreal.ca.

## CONTINUING EDUCATION PROGRAM

**Contact** Ms. Camille Sasseville, Program Coordinator, Faculty of Nursing, Université de Montréal, Pav. Marg. d'Youville, CP 6128 Succursale Centre-Ville, Montreal, QC H3C 3J7. *Telephone:* 514-343-6111 Ext. 84164. *E-mail:* camille.sasseville@umontreal.ca.

# Université de Sherbrooke
## Department of Nursing
## Sherbrooke, Quebec

***http://www.usherbrooke.ca/scinf/***
Founded in 1954

**DEGREES • BSCN • M SC • PHD**
**Nursing Program Faculty** 17 (76% with doctorates).
**Baccalaureate Enrollment** 482 **Women** 90% **Men** 10% **Minority** .5% **Part-time** 30%
**Graduate Enrollment** 61 **Women** 95% **Men** 5% **Part-time** 50%
**Nursing Student Activities** Student Nurses' Association.
**Nursing Student Resources** Academic advising; academic or career counseling; assistance for students with disabilities; bookstore; computer lab; computer-assisted instruction; e-mail services; externships; housing assistance; Internet; learning resource lab; library services; nursing audiovisuals; tutoring.
**Library Facilities** 1.2 million volumes (40,000 in health, 4,000 in nursing); 43,478 periodical subscriptions (3,000 health-care related).

## BACCALAUREATE PROGRAMS

**Degree** BScN
**Available Programs** RN Baccalaureate.
**Site Options** Longueuil, QC.
**Study Options** Full-time and part-time.
**Program Entrance Requirements** Transcript of college record, high school chemistry, 4 years high school math, immunizations, professional liability insurance/malpractice insurance, RN licensure. Transfer students are accepted.
**Advanced Placement** Credit given for nursing courses completed elsewhere dependent upon specific evaluations.
**Contact** *Telephone:* 819-563-5355. *Fax:* 819-820-6816.

## GRADUATE PROGRAMS

**Contact** *Telephone:* 819-564-5354. *Fax:* 819-820-6816.

### MASTER'S DEGREE PROGRAM

**Degree** M Sc
**Available Programs** Master's.
**Concentrations Available** *Clinical nurse specialist programs in:* acute care, community health, family health, gerontology.
**Site Options** Longueuil, QC.
**Study Options** Full-time and part-time.
**Program Entrance Requirements** Transcript of college record, interview, 3 letters of recommendation, nursing research course, professional liability insurance/malpractice insurance, resume.
**Degree Requirements** 45 total credit hours, thesis or project.

### DOCTORAL DEGREE PROGRAM

**Degree** PhD
**Available Programs** Doctorate.
**Areas of Study** Advanced practice nursing, aging, biology of health and illness, clinical practice, community health, critical care, family health, gerontology, health promotion/disease prevention, human health and illness, illness and transition, information systems, maternity-newborn, neuro-behavior, nurse case management, nursing administration, nursing education, nursing policy, nursing research, nursing science, oncology,women's health.
**Site Options** Longueuil, QC.
**Program Entrance Requirements** Clinical experience, interview, 3 letters of recommendation, MSN or equivalent, statistics course, vita, writing sample.
**Degree Requirements** 90 total credit hours, dissertation, oral exam, written exam.

POSTDOCTORAL PROGRAM
**Postdoctoral Program Contact** *Telephone:* 819-564-5355. *Fax:* 819-820-6816.

# Université du Québec à Chicoutimi

## Program in Nursing
## Chicoutimi, Quebec

Founded in 1969

**DEGREES • BNSC • MS/MPH • MSN**

**Nursing Program Faculty** 12 (30% with doctorates).
**Baccalaureate Enrollment** 600 **Women** 90% **Men** 10% **Minority** 5% **Part-time** 75%
**Graduate Enrollment** 30 **Women** 90% **Men** 10% **Minority** 2% **Part-time** 80%
**Distance Learning Courses** Available.
**Nursing Student Activities** Nursing Honor Society, Student Nurses' Association.
**Nursing Student Resources** Academic advising; academic or career counseling; assistance for students with disabilities; bookstore; campus computer network; computer lab; computer-assisted instruction; e-mail services; employment services for current students; externships; housing assistance; interactive nursing skills videos; Internet; learning resource lab; library services; nursing audiovisuals; resume preparation assistance; skills, simulation, or other laboratory; tutoring; unpaid internships.
**Library Facilities** 689,214 volumes (8,000 in health, 6,300 in nursing); 5,092 periodical subscriptions (5,250 health-care related).

### BACCALAUREATE PROGRAMS

**Degree** BNSc
**Available Programs** Accelerated RN Baccalaureate; Generic Baccalaureate; RN Baccalaureate.
**Site Options** St. Felicien, QC; Sept-Iles, QC; Alma, QC.
**Study Options** Full-time and part-time.
**Program Entrance Requirements** Transcript of college record, health exam, high school biology, high school chemistry, high school math, immunizations, interview. Transfer students are accepted. *Application deadline:* 3/1 (fall), 3/1 (winter). *Application fee:* CAN$50.
**Advanced Placement** Credit given for nursing courses completed elsewhere dependent upon specific evaluations.
**Financial Aid** 5% of baccalaureate students in nursing programs received some form of financial aid in 2012–13. *Gift aid (need-based):* private, college/university gift aid from institutional funds. *Loans:* college/university. *Work-study:* part-time campus jobs.
**Contact** Mme. Anna Gauthier, Secretary, Program in Nursing, Université du Québec à Chicoutimi, 555 Boulevard de l'Universite, Chicoutimi, QC G7H 2B1. *Telephone:* 418-545-5011 Ext. 5315. *Fax:* 418-615-1205. *E-mail:* anna_gauthier@uqac.ca.

### GRADUATE PROGRAMS

**Financial Aid** 2% of graduate students in nursing programs received some form of financial aid in 2012–13.
**Contact** Mrs. Marie Tremblay, RN, Director of Master Degree Program, Program in Nursing, Université du Québec à Chicoutimi, 555 Boulevard de l'Universit, Saguenay, QC G7H 2B1. *Telephone:* 418-545-5011 Ext. 5331. *Fax:* 418-615-1205. *E-mail:* Marie_Tremblay@uqac.ca.

MASTER'S DEGREE PROGRAM
**Degrees** MS/MPH; MSN
**Available Programs** Accelerated RN to Master's; Master's; RN to Master's.
**Concentrations Available** *Clinical nurse specialist programs in:* acute care, adult health, cardiovascular, community health, critical care, family health, gerontology, home health care, maternity-newborn, medical-surgical, occupational health, oncology, parent-child, pediatric, perinatal, psychiatric/mental health, public health, rehabilitation, school health,women's health. *Nurse practitioner programs in:* primary care.
**Site Options** St. Felicien, QC; Sept-Iles, QC; Alma, QC.
**Study Options** Full-time and part-time.
**Program Entrance Requirements** Clinical experience, minimum overall college GPA of 3.2, transcript of college record, written essay, interview, 3 letters of recommendation, nursing research course, professional liability insurance/malpractice insurance, resume, statistics course. *Application deadline:* 3/1 (fall), 11/1 (winter). *Application fee:* CAN$50.
**Advanced Placement** Credit given for nursing courses completed elsewhere dependent upon specific evaluations.
**Degree Requirements** 45 total credit hours, thesis or project, comprehensive exam.

POST-MASTER'S PROGRAM
**Areas of Study** *Nurse practitioner programs in:* primary care.

# Université du Québec à Rimouski

## Program in Nursing
## Rimouski, Quebec

*http://www.uquebec.ca/mscinf/*
Founded in 1973

**DEGREES • BSCN • M SC N**

**Nursing Program Faculty** 17 (53% with doctorates).
**Baccalaureate Enrollment** 750 **Women** 90% **Men** 10% **Part-time** 74%
**Graduate Enrollment** 24 **Women** 96% **Men** 4% **Part-time** 92%
**Distance Learning Courses** Available.
**Nursing Student Activities** Student Nurses' Association.
**Nursing Student Resources** Academic advising; academic or career counseling; assistance for students with disabilities; bookstore; campus computer network; career placement assistance; computer lab; daycare for children of students; e-mail services; employment services for current students; housing assistance; Internet; learning resource lab; library services; nursing audiovisuals; other; placement services for program completers; resume preparation assistance; skills, simulation, or other laboratory; tutoring.
**Library Facilities** 263,142 volumes (5,200 in health, 1,100 in nursing); 3,951 periodical subscriptions (1,300 health-care related).

### BACCALAUREATE PROGRAMS

**Degree** BScN
**Available Programs** RN Baccalaureate.
**Site Options** Rimouski, QC; Lvis, QC.
**Study Options** Full-time and part-time.
**Program Entrance Requirements** Transcript of college record, professional liability insurance/malpractice insurance, prerequisite course work. Transfer students are accepted.
**Advanced Placement** Credit by examination available.
**Contact** *Telephone:* 418-723-1986 Ext. 1568. *Fax:* 418-724-1450.

### GRADUATE PROGRAMS

**Contact** *Telephone:* 418-723-1986 Ext. 1345. *Fax:* 418-724-1450.

MASTER'S DEGREE PROGRAM
**Degree** M Sc N
**Available Programs** Master's.
**Concentrations Available** *Clinical nurse specialist programs in:* community health, critical care, gerontology, psychiatric/mental health.
**Site Options** Rimouski, QC; Lvis, QC.
**Study Options** Full-time and part-time.
**Program Entrance Requirements** Clinical experience, transcript of college record, interview, 3 letters of recommendation, nursing research course, prerequisite course work, statistics course.
**Advanced Placement** Credit given for nursing courses completed elsewhere dependent upon specific evaluations.
**Degree Requirements** 45 total credit hours, thesis or project.

### CONTINUING EDUCATION PROGRAM

**Contact** *Telephone:* 418-723-1986 Ext. 1818. *Fax:* 418-724-1525.

# Université du Québec à Trois-Rivières

## Program in Nursing
## Trois-Rivières, Quebec

*http://www.uqtr.ca/*
Founded in 1969

**DEGREES • BSN • MSN**

**Nursing Program Faculty** 28 (30% with doctorates).

**Baccalaureate Enrollment** 180 **Women** 95% **Men** 5% **Minority** 5% **International** 1% **Part-time** 75%
**Graduate Enrollment** 50 **Women** 97% **Men** 3% **Minority** 1% **Part-time** 90%
**Distance Learning Courses** Available.
**Nursing Student Activities** Student Nurses' Association.
**Nursing Student Resources** Academic advising; academic or career counseling; assistance for students with disabilities; bookstore; campus computer network; career placement assistance; computer lab; computer-assisted instruction; daycare for children of students; e-mail services; employment services for current students; externships; interactive nursing skills videos; Internet; learning resource lab; library services; nursing audiovisuals; placement services for program completers; resume preparation assistance; skills, simulation, or other laboratory; tutoring; unpaid internships.
**Library Facilities** 464,338 volumes (2,000 in health, 500 in nursing); 2,000 periodical subscriptions health-care related.

## BACCALAUREATE PROGRAMS

**Degree** BSN
**Available Programs** Generic Baccalaureate; RN Baccalaureate.
**Study Options** Full-time and part-time.
**Program Entrance Requirements** Transcript of college record, CPR certification, high school biology, high school chemistry, prerequisite course work, RN licensure. Transfer students are accepted. *Application deadline:* 3/1 (fall). Applications may be processed on a rolling basis for some programs. *Application fee:* CAN$30.
**Advanced Placement** Credit given for nursing courses completed elsewhere dependent upon specific evaluations.
**Contact** *Telephone:* 819-376-5011 Ext. 3471. *Fax:* 819-376-5048.

## GRADUATE PROGRAMS

**Contact** *Telephone:* 819-376-5011 Ext. 3460.

### MASTER'S DEGREE PROGRAM

**Degree** MSN
**Available Programs** Master's.
**Concentrations Available** *Clinical nurse specialist programs in:* acute care, adult health, community health, critical care, family health, home health care, maternity-newborn, medical-surgical, pediatric, perinatal, psychiatric/mental health, public health. *Nurse practitioner programs in:* primary care.
**Study Options** Full-time and part-time.
**Program Entrance Requirements** Minimum overall college GPA of 3, transcript of college record, CPR certification, immunizations, 3 letters of recommendation, nursing research course, physical assessment course, prerequisite course work, statistics course. *Application deadline:* 8/29 (fall), 11/29 (winter), 4/29 (spring). Applications may be processed on a rolling basis for some programs. *Application fee:* CAN$30.
**Advanced Placement** Credit by examination available.
**Degree Requirements** 45 total credit hours, thesis or project.

# Université du Québec en Abitibi-Témiscamingue

## Département des sciences sociales et de la santé
## Rouyn-Noranda, Quebec

*http://www.uqat.ca/en/*
Founded in 1983

## DEGREE • BN

**Nursing Program Faculty** 12
**Baccalaureate Enrollment** 78 **Women** 95% **Men** 5% **Part-time** 64%
**Nursing Student Resources** Academic advising; assistance for students with disabilities; bookstore; campus computer network; computer lab; computer-assisted instruction; housing assistance; Internet; library services; resume preparation assistance; skills, simulation, or other laboratory.
**Library Facilities** 135,882 volumes (3,239 in health, 715 in nursing); 302 periodical subscriptions (17 health-care related).

## BACCALAUREATE PROGRAMS

**Degree** BN
**Program Entrance Requirements** Transfer students are accepted.
**Contact** *Telephone:* 819-762-0971 Ext. 2370. *Fax:* 819-797-4727.

# Université du Québec en Outaouais

## Département des Sciences Infirmières
## Gatineau, Quebec

*http://www.uqo.ca/*
Founded in 1981

## DEGREES • BSCN • M SC N

**Nursing Program Faculty** 21 (71% with doctorates).
**Baccalaureate Enrollment** 900 **Women** 90% **Men** 10% **Minority** 20% **Part-time** 40%
**Graduate Enrollment** 40 **Women** 99% **Men** 1% **Minority** 6% **Part-time** 100%
**Nursing Student Activities** Student Nurses' Association.
**Nursing Student Resources** Academic advising; academic or career counseling; assistance for students with disabilities; bookstore; campus computer network; computer lab; daycare for children of students; e-mail services; employment services for current students; externships; housing assistance; Internet; learning resource lab; library services; nursing audiovisuals; placement services for program completers; skills, simulation, or other laboratory.
**Library Facilities** 230,910 volumes; 12,351 periodical subscriptions.

## BACCALAUREATE PROGRAMS

**Degree** BScN
**Available Programs** Generic Baccalaureate; RN Baccalaureate.
**Site Options** St. Jerome, QC.
**Study Options** Full-time and part-time.
**Program Entrance Requirements** CPR certification, high school chemistry, immunizations, RN licensure. Transfer students are accepted. *Application deadline:* 3/1 (fall). *Application fee:* CAN$30.
**Advanced Placement** Credit by examination available. Credit given for nursing courses completed elsewhere dependent upon specific evaluations.
**Financial Aid** ***Loans:*** college/university.
**Contact** Prof. Robert Bilterys, Directeur, Département des Sciences Infirmières, Université du Québec en Outaouais, 5, rue Saint-Joseph, Succursale Hull, Hull, QC J8X 3X7. *Telephone:* 819-595-3900 Ext. 4102. *Fax:* 819-595-3801. *E-mail:* robert.bilterys@uqo.ca.

## GRADUATE PROGRAMS

**Contact** Prof. Robert Bilterys, Director, Département des Sciences Infirmières, Université du Québec en Outaouais, CP 1250, Succursale Hull, Gatineau, QC J8X 3X7. *Telephone:* 819-595-3900 Ext. 4102. *Fax:* 819-595-2202. *E-mail:* robert.bilterys@uqo.ca.

### MASTER'S DEGREE PROGRAM

**Degree** M Sc N
**Available Programs** Master's.
**Concentrations Available** Health-care administration. *Clinical nurse specialist programs in:* community health, critical care, psychiatric/mental health, rehabilitation. *Nurse practitioner programs in:* primary care.
**Site Options** St. Jerome, QC.
**Study Options** Full-time and part-time.
**Program Entrance Requirements** Computer literacy, minimum overall college GPA of 3.2, 3 letters of recommendation, nursing research course, resume, statistics course. *Application deadline:* 5/1 (fall), 11/1 (winter), 3/1 (spring). *Application fee:* CAN$30.
**Advanced Placement** Credit given for nursing courses completed elsewhere dependent upon specific evaluations.
**Degree Requirements** 45 total credit hours, thesis or project.

## CONTINUING EDUCATION PROGRAM

**Contact** Ms. Monique Fecteau, Commis senior au soutien la pdagogie, Département des Sciences Infirmières, Université du Québec en Outaouais, Dcanat de la formation continue et des partenariats (DFCP), UQO - Gatineau, Gatineau, QC J8X 3X7. *E-mail:* monique.fecteau@uqo.ca.

## Université Laval

### Faculty of Nursing
### Québec, Quebec

*http://www.fsi.ulaval.ca/*
Founded in 1852

**DEGREES • BSCN • MSN • PHD**
**Nursing Program Faculty** 25 (64% with doctorates).
**Baccalaureate Enrollment** 798 **Women** 94% **Men** 6% **Minority** 18% **International** 12% **Part-time** 32%
**Graduate Enrollment** 116 **Women** 72% **Men** 28% **Minority** 32% **International** 24% **Part-time** 22%
**Distance Learning Courses** Available.
**Nursing Student Activities** Student Nurses' Association, nursing club.
**Nursing Student Resources** Academic advising; academic or career counseling; assistance for students with disabilities; bookstore; campus computer network; career placement assistance; computer lab; computer-assisted instruction; daycare for children of students; e-mail services; employment services for current students; externships; housing assistance; interactive nursing skills videos; Internet; learning resource lab; library services; nursing audiovisuals; placement services for program completers; resume preparation assistance; skills, simulation, or other laboratory; tutoring.
**Library Facilities** 3 million volumes (118,994 in health, 3,781 in nursing); 13,928 periodical subscriptions (624 health-care related).

#### BACCALAUREATE PROGRAMS

**Degree** BScN
**Available Programs** Accelerated Baccalaureate; Accelerated RN Baccalaureate; Generic Baccalaureate; RN Baccalaureate.
**Study Options** Full-time and part-time.
**Program Entrance Requirements** Transcript of college record, high school biology, high school chemistry, 5 years high school math, high school transcript, immunizations, minimum high school GPA. Transfer students are accepted.
**Advanced Placement** Credit given for nursing courses completed elsewhere dependent upon specific evaluations.
**Contact** *Telephone:* 418-656-2131 Ext. 7930. *Fax:* 418-656-7747.

#### GRADUATE PROGRAMS

**Contact** *Telephone:* 418-656-3356. *Fax:* 418-656-7304.

**MASTER'S DEGREE PROGRAM**
**Degree** MSN
**Available Programs** Accelerated Master's; Master's.
**Concentrations Available** Clinical nurse leader; health-care administration; nursing administration. *Clinical nurse specialist programs in:* acute care, adult health, cardiovascular, community health, critical care, family health, gerontology, oncology, palliative care, parent-child, pediatric, perinatal, psychiatric/mental health, public health, rehabilitation. *Nurse practitioner programs in:* adult health, primary care.
**Study Options** Full-time and part-time.
**Program Entrance Requirements** Clinical experience, transcript of college record, 2 letters of recommendation, nursing research course, resume, statistics course, French exam.
**Advanced Placement** Credit given for nursing courses completed elsewhere dependent upon specific evaluations.
**Degree Requirements** 45 total credit hours, thesis or project.

**POST-MASTER'S PROGRAM**
**Areas of Study** *Clinical nurse specialist programs in:* acute care, adult health, cardiovascular, community health, critical care, family health, gerontology, oncology, palliative care, parent-child, pediatric, perinatal, psychiatric/mental health, public health, rehabilitation. *Nurse practitioner programs in:* adult health, primary care.

**DOCTORAL DEGREE PROGRAM**
**Degree** PhD
**Available Programs** Doctorate.
**Areas of Study** Community health, nursing science.
**Program Entrance Requirements** Clinical experience, interview, 2 letters of recommendation, MSN or equivalent, scholarly papers, statistics course, vita, writing sample.
**Degree Requirements** 96 total credit hours, dissertation, oral exam, written exam.

**POSTDOCTORAL PROGRAM**
**Areas of Study** Aging, cancer care, community health, gerontology, health promotion/disease prevention, nursing interventions, nursing research, nursing science, outcomes.
**Postdoctoral Program Contact***Telephone:* 418-656-3356. *Fax:* 418-656-7747.

#### CONTINUING EDUCATION PROGRAM

**Contact** *Telephone:* 418-656-2131 Ext. 6712. *Fax:* 418-656-7747.

# SASKATCHEWAN

## University of Saskatchewan

### College of Nursing
### Saskatoon, Saskatchewan

*http://www.usask.ca/nursing/*
Founded in 1907

**DEGREES • BSN • MN • PHD**
**Nursing Program Faculty** 134 (20% with doctorates).
**Baccalaureate Enrollment** 1,678 **Women** 93% **Men** 7% **Minority** 5% **Part-time** 17%
**Graduate Enrollment** 50 **Women** 94% **Men** 6% **Minority** 2% **Part-time** 62%
**Distance Learning Courses** Available.
**Nursing Student Activities** Student Nurses' Association.
**Nursing Student Resources** Academic advising; academic or career counseling; assistance for students with disabilities; bookstore; campus computer network; computer lab; computer-assisted instruction; daycare for children of students; e-mail services; employment services for current students; interactive nursing skills videos; Internet; learning resource lab; library services; nursing audiovisuals; other; remedial services; resume preparation assistance; skills, simulation, or other laboratory; tutoring.
**Library Facilities** 2.5 million volumes (92,505 in health, 3,932 in nursing); 47,055 periodical subscriptions (3,069 health-care related).

#### BACCALAUREATE PROGRAMS

**Degree** BSN
**Available Programs** Accelerated Baccalaureate; Accelerated RN Baccalaureate; Baccalaureate for Second Degree; Generic Baccalaureate; RN Baccalaureate.
**Site Options** Regina , SK; Prince Albert, SK; Saskatoon , SK.
**Study Options** Full-time and part-time.
**Program Entrance Requirements** Transcript of college record, CPR certification, high school biology, high school chemistry, 4 years high school math, 4 years high school science, high school transcript, immunizations, minimum high school GPA of 2.0. Transfer students are accepted. *Application deadline:* 1/15 (fall). *Application fee:* CAN$90.
**Advanced Placement** Credit given for nursing courses completed elsewhere dependent upon specific evaluations.
**Contact** *Telephone:* 306-966-6231. *Fax:* 306-966-6621.

#### GRADUATE PROGRAMS

**Contact** *Telephone:* 306-966-1477. *Fax:* 306-966-6703.

**MASTER'S DEGREE PROGRAM**
**Degree** MN
**Available Programs** Master's.
**Concentrations Available** Nursing education. *Nurse practitioner programs in:* primary care.
**Site Options** Saskatoon , SK.
**Study Options** Full-time and part-time.
**Program Entrance Requirements** Minimum overall college GPA of 2.5, transcript of college record, 3 letters of recommendation, nursing research course, statistics course. *Application deadline:* 11/15 (fall). *Application fee:* CAN$75.
**Advanced Placement** Credit given for nursing courses completed elsewhere dependent upon specific evaluations.
**Degree Requirements** 24 total credit hours, thesis or project.

**POST-MASTER'S PROGRAM**
**Areas of Study** *Nurse practitioner programs in:* primary care.

**DOCTORAL DEGREE PROGRAM**
**Degree** PhD
**Available Programs** Doctorate.
**Areas of Study** Individualized study.
**Site Options** Saskatoon , SK.
**Program Entrance Requirements** Minimum overall college GPA of 4, 3 letters of recommendation, MSN or equivalent, statistics course, vita. *Application deadline:* 11/15 (fall). *Application fee:* CAN$75.
**Degree Requirements** 18 total credit hours, dissertation, oral exam, written exam.

## CONTINUING EDUCATION PROGRAM

**Contact** *Telephone:* 306-966-6261. *Fax:* 306-966-7673.

# TWO-PAGE DESCRIPTIONS

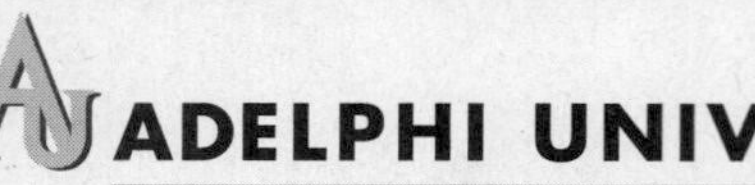

COLLEGE OF NURSING AND PUBLIC HEALTH

*Leading to New Horizons in Nursing*

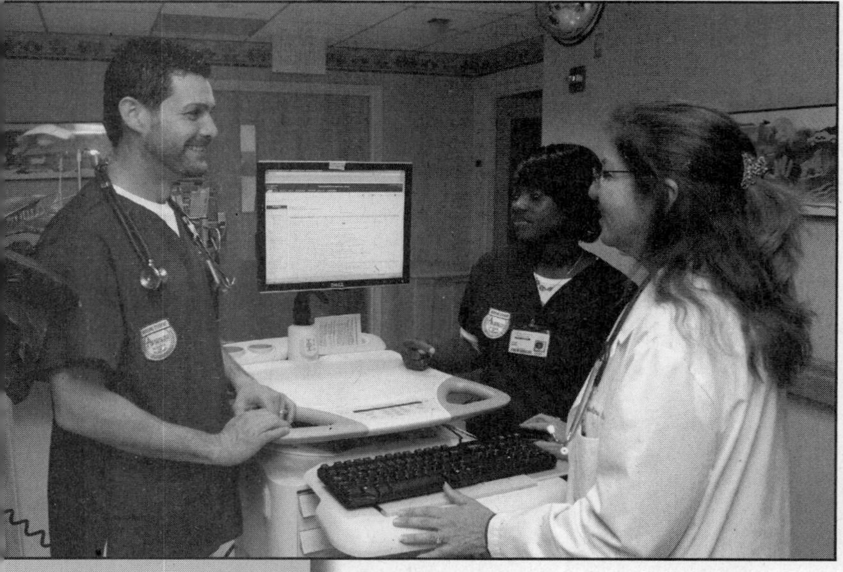

*Adelphi College of Nursing and Public Health students benefit from a progressive curriculum, unique partnerships, and hands-on clinical training.*

With a strong foundation built on seventy years of nursing education and a new vision for the future, the College of Nursing and Public Health focuses on issues within population health and has combined hallmark nursing programs with relevant healthcare programs to tackle today's health issues and those in the future. College of Nursing and Public Health students benefit from a holistic approach that focuses on community intervention, health maintenance and management, wellness, and environmental health.

The College offers three basic undergraduate programs leading to a Bachelor of Science in Nursing. The basic curriculum is for those seeking a B.S. in Nursing and to meet the New York State licensing requirements as a registered professional nurse (R.N.). A second curriculum (ASCEND) is for current registered nurses continuing their education to receive a B.S. in Nursing. This one-day-a-week R.N. to B.S. program includes not only classroom, but some online courses as well.

The third program, the Professional Acceleration to Healthcare (PATH) program, is a 14-month intensive program for those who have a bachelor's degree in another discipline and are now seeking a degree in nursing. Candidates for the accelerated PATH program must have all of their prerequisites completed with a grade of C+ or better at the time of application submission.

Adelphi's nursing programs combine theory, clinical practice, and community service. The College's students partner with community healthcare providers and receive innovative clinical education with esteemed faculty members who have a passion for teaching and the profession of nursing. Adelphi maintains an extensive network of partnerships in more than 100 healthcare settings, from acute care to community environments.

Adelphi has clinical affiliations with all the major health systems, hospitals, and community agencies in the metropolitan New York area.

On Adelphi's Garden City campus and at the Manhattan Center, students have access to the Nursing Resource Center, which features learning labs designed to simulate hospital settings and simulation labs for real-time problem scenario learning.

Candidates seeking admission as freshmen must meet the general admission requirements of Adelphi University. Those who have college credits or an associate degree may apply as transfer students. A minimum cumulative GPA of 3.0 is required for admission to the ASCEND program. A maximum of 64 credits may be transferred from a regionally accredited community college, and a maximum of 90 credits may be transferred from a regionally accredited university.

Successful completion of the Test of Essential Academic Skills (TEAS), Version V, is an admission prerequisite for transfer students to the College of Nursing and Public Health B.S. program.

At the graduate level, the emphasis is on the development of scholarly critical thinkers with a focus on a specialty practice area and the ability to translate knowledge into practice. In Adelphi's nurse practitioner program, through the process of critical thinking, students learn to understand the nature of complex human and environmental systems and to develop strategies for effective intervention. In addition, the core of the master's curriculum provides the knowledge base and experience needed to develop specific specialty skills, evaluate research designs and methodologies, and to utilize findings providing evidence-based practice.

Graduate programs include the following: M.S. in Adult/Geriatric Nurse Practitioner; M.S. in Nursing Administration; M.S. in Nursing Education; M.S. in Nutrition (fully online); Master of Public Health; Ph.D. in Nursing; and M.S. in Healthcare Informatics (traditional and online). Post-master's certificates are available in most of the above.

Graduate applicants must submit a completed application, an essay, letters of reference, and a $50 nonrefundable application fee. In addition, they must have official copies of standardized test scores forwarded to Adelphi, as well as official transcripts from all colleges and universities previously attended.

---

- *2013–14 UNDERGRADUATE TUITION & FEES FOR FULL-TIME (12–17 CREDITS PER SEMESTER) NURSING UPPER DIVISION STUDENTS:*

  *Resident (living on campus): $43,130*

  *Nonresident: $30,800*

- *2013–14 GRADUATE TUITION & FEES FOR PART-TIME (6 CREDITS PER SEMESTER) STUDENTS:*

  *Nonresident: $1,115 per credit hour (Graduate nursing students do not live on campus)*

- *APPLICATION DEADLINES:*

  *Ph.D. program (fall admission only): January 15*

  *Accelerated RN program (PATH) has a May start; January 15.*

  *All other programs: rolling admission*

- *FACULTY INFORMATION:*

  *nursing.adelphi.edu/faculty*

- *MULTIMEDIA:*

  *http://nursing.adelphi.edu/about*

**CONTACT INFORMATION**

**Adelphi University College of Nursing and Public Health**
**One South Avenue**
**Garden City, NY 11530**
**800-ADELPHI (toll-free)**
**E-mail: nursing@adelphi.edu**
**Website: http://nursing.adelphi.edu**

**UNDERGRADUATE NURSING PROGRAM:**
**Phone: 516-877-3050**
**E-mail: admissions@adelphi.edu**

**GRADUATE NURSING PROGRAM:**
**Phone: 516-877-3050**
**E-mail: graduateadmissions@adelphi.edu**
**Find us on Facebook®:** facebook.com/AdelphiU
**Follow us on Twitter™:** twitter.com/adelphiu

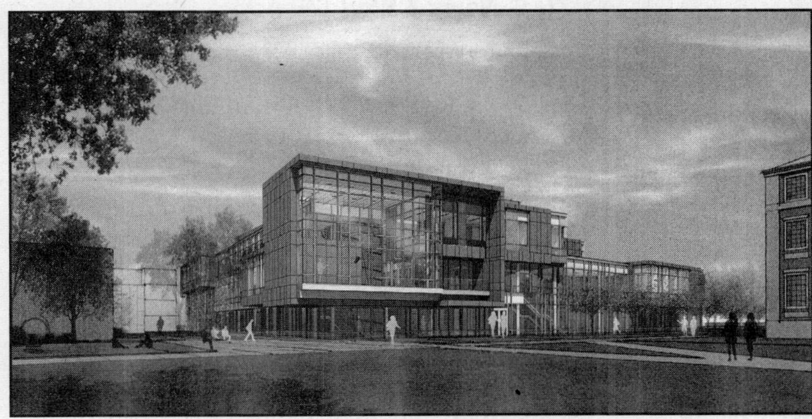

*In Fall 2013, Adelphi broke ground on the Nexus Building and Welcome Center—the future home of the College of Nursing and Public Health. The new building will feature classrooms and at least 10 examination rooms, including an intensive care room, a delivery room, and a home-care lab. The exam rooms will have closed-circuit TV to observe student performance.*

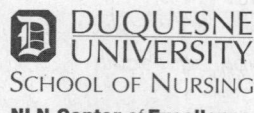

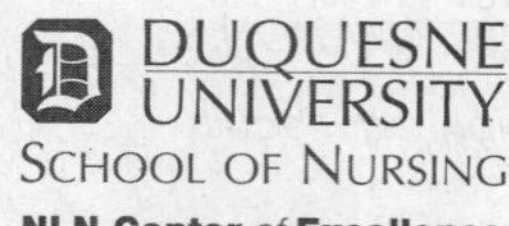


The Duquesne University School of Nursing was the first nursing school in Pennsylvania to offer a Bachelor of Science in Nursing degree and the first in the nation with an entirely online doctorate in nursing program.

Undergraduate nursing students use e-textbooks for both classroom and clinical learning.

Twice recognized as a National League for Nursing Center of Excellence, the School of Nursing is accredited by the Commission on Collegiate Nursing Education and approved by the Pennsylvania State Board of Nursing.

Since its founding in 1878, Duquesne University has earned a reputation for academic excellence and having a faculty that is committed to teaching and to helping students succeed. Today, Duquesne is experiencing an exciting period of growth and increased recognition:

**U.S. News & World Report:**

- Duquesne University School of Nursing's online Graduate Program has been ranked No. 6 in the nation among the 2014 Best Online Graduate Nursing Programs.
- A top-tier university among the 1,800 American institutions considered for 2014.
- The only private university in Pennsylvania listed among the 20 most financially efficient top-ranked schools.
- Among the nation's top 100 popular schools. For the third time, Duquesne is described as having a "top reputation and students are highly motivated to go there."
- Offering high academic quality at a good price, Duquesne appears as number 44 on the 2013 Great Schools at Great Prices list.

**Princeton Review**

- Among The Best 378 Colleges for 2014, which profiles only 15 percent of American four-year colleges.
- One of the Best in the Northeast, Duquesne was one of only 220 institutions chosen for 2012.
- Named for the second year in the *Guide to 311 Green Colleges* as one of America's most environmentally responsible schools.

In addition, Duquesne University is 16th in the nation among small research universities, according to a Chronicle of Higher Education index that measured faculty productivity among more than 7,300 doctoral programs

From the beginning, Duquesne has worked diligently to improve the quality of life for the people of Pittsburgh. To that end, the School of Nursing operates a Nurse-Managed Wellness Center for underserved communities, where nurses and other health-care providers promote health and wellness and monitor chronic medical conditions. These clinics offer students an invaluable learning experience as well as an opportunity for community service. The School of Nursing is also home to the Center for Nursing Research, which supports qualitative and quantitative inquiry in areas related to health disparities, cultural competence, and chronic deviations from health.

Duquesne's green, self-contained, 49-acre campus—centrally located in a city with an international reputation for leadership in medicine and technology—has superb recreational facilities and student services and is only minutes away from Pittsburgh's rich cultural, sports, and entertainment offerings.

## Bachelor of Science in Nursing (B.S.N.) Program

Clinical experiences, which begin in the sophomore year, create a strong foundation for nursing practice, and Duquesne's students complete over 810 clinical hours in hospitals and community health facilities. The clinical faculty-to-student ratio is 1:8.

Duquesne's nursing labs have the latest nursing simulators for helping students gain patient-care skills in a controlled environment designed to improve decision making and develop teamwork, communications, and leadership skills.

Nursing students can add international perspectives by participating in faculty-led, summertime study-abroad programs or for-credit learning experiences in Nicaragua during spring break. The University offers semester-long programs at a satellite campus in Italy and at an International Study Center in Ireland.

## Second Degree B.S.N. Program

The Second Degree Bachelor of Science in Nursing (B.S.N.) program enables the non-nurse with a baccalaureate degree to obtain a B.S.N. in twelve months. The program includes three semesters of course work and over 630 hours of clinical experience.

## RN–B.S.N. Program

This new and completely online program, beginning fall 2014, enables the registered nurse with an ADN or diploma degree in nursing to obtain the B.S.N. degree. The courses are 7½ weeks in length and are innovative, relevant, and student-friendly. Students may also choose 6 credits from the following: ethics, quality and safety, forensics, veterans' health, global health and human rights, and professional development.

## Graduate Programs

All graduate nursing programs are offered exclusively online in a user-friendly, asynchronous format. Online learning provides flexibility for professional nurses with busy schedules and permits students to earn degrees in a reasonable length of time. Course work is highly interactive, so students communicate often with instructors and classmates. Online flexibility plus academic rigor make the Duquesne University School of Nursing the ideal choice for graduate nursing education.

### Master of Science in Nursing (M.S.N.)

Family (Individual Across the Lifespan) Nurse Practitioner
Forensic Nursing
Nursing Education

### Post-Master's Certificates

Family (Individual Across the Lifespan) Nurse Practitioner
Forensic Nursing

### Ph.D. in Nursing

### Doctor of Nursing Practice (D.N.P.)

Visit www.duq.edu/nursing for complete admission requirements and application instructions, or call 412-396-4945 or e-mail nursing@duq.edu.

---

- *2013–14 FULL-TIME UNDERGRADUATE TUITION & FEES: $31,385 ($1,039 per credit)*
- *2013–14 FULL-TIME GRADUATE TUITION & FEES: $1,132 per credit*
- *APPLICATION DEADLINES:*

  *B.S.N.: May 1*

  *B.S.N. (transfer students): April 1 (fall admission); November 1 (spring admission)*

  *Second Degree B.S.N.: March 1*

  *RN–B.S.N.: June 13*

  *M.S.N.: March 1*

  *Ph.D.: January 15*

  *D.N.P.: February 1*

  *Visit www.duq.edu/nursing for complete admission requirements and application instructions.*
- *FACULTY INFORMATION: www.duq.edu/nursing*

**CONTACT INFORMATION**

**Susan Hardner, Nurse Recruiter**
**545-A Fisher Hall**
**Duquesne University**
**600 Forbes Avenue**
**Pittsburgh, Pennsylvania 15282**
**Phone: 412-396-4945**
**Fax: 412-396-6346**
**E-mail: nursing@duq.edu**
**Web site: http://www.duq.edu/academics/schools/nursing**
**Facebook: https://www.facebook.com/DUNursing**
**Twitter: https://twitter.com/dunursing**
**YouTube: http://www.youtube.com/dunursing**
**LinkedIn: http://www.linkedin.com/groups/Duquesne-University-School-Nursing-4803465**
**GooglePlus: https://plus.google.com/118445490080314869545/posts**
**Pinterest: https://www.pinterest.com/dunursing/**
**Instagram: http://instagram.com/dunursing#**
**NursesLounge: http://community.nurseslounge.com/groups/b93d6a735c/summary**

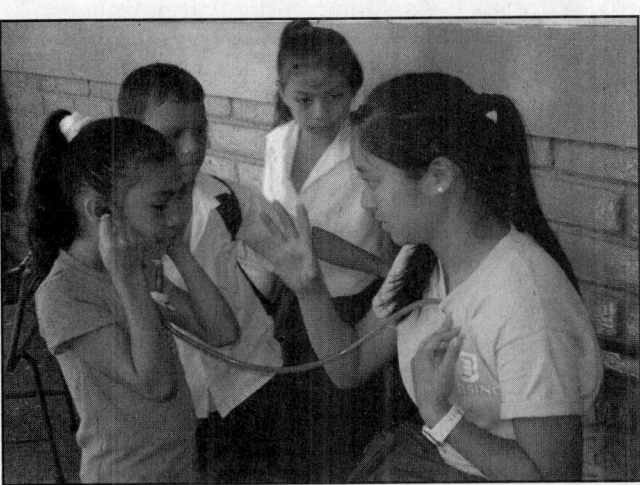

*The School of Nursing encourages students to engage in international travel and study to explore global health issues. Since 1995, students and faculty have traveled to many locations, such as Nicaragua, in a spirit of service, learning, and international collaboration.*

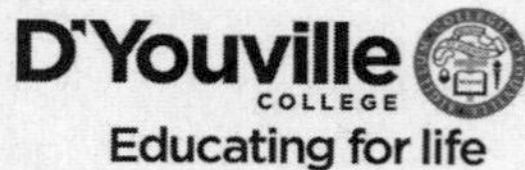

## School of Nursing

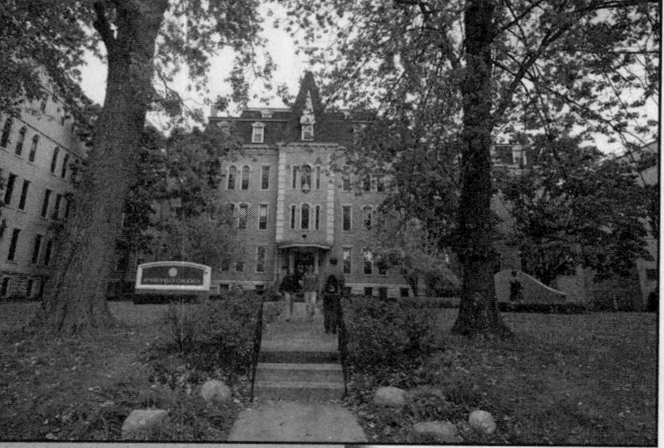

The Koessler Administration Building dates back to 1872 when it was the home of Holy Angels Academy, a private boarding school for young ladies in elementary and secondary grades. In 1908, a charter established D'Youville College and the Academy of the Holy Angels. As the College grew, the Academy moved to another location in Buffalo in 1930. Today, the landmark building houses the President's suite and other administrative offices.

*Educating competent, compassionate, knowledgeable, professional nurses.*

D'Youville College is a private, co-educational liberal arts and professional college offering students a high-quality education in more than thirty undergraduate and graduate degree programs. Founded in 1908 by the Grey Nuns as the first college for women in western New York to offer baccalaureate degrees to women, it was named for their founder, Saint Marguerite D'Youville. The current enrollment is 3,100 men and women; the student-faculty ratio is 12:1, allowing for individual attention and student support by faculty. The College is committed to helping its students grow academically, socially, and personally throughout their college experience. The Learning Center and other college-wide support services are available to enhance students' opportunity for success. Many student organizations, including pre-professional student associations, expand the learning environment.

D'Youville College has been growing and attracting students from all over the world since 1908, particularly in the areas of professional health-related programs. D'Youville College has been educating and preparing professional nurses for careers since 1942; the first Bachelor of Science in Nursing (B.S.N.) class graduated in 1946. Since then, nursing education programs at D'Youville have continued to grow, and the school of nursing is now the largest single education entity on campus. D'Youville offers a four-year Bachelor of Science in Nursing. The B.S.N. program combines a liberal arts foundation with professional nursing classroom and clinical instruction. An active Student Nurses Association orients students to the role that professional organizations play in life-long professional practice and promotion of health for populations.

Classroom instruction concentrates on preparing students for critical thinking and clinical decision making required for clinical practice. Students begin their clinical experiences at area hospitals, long-term care facilities, community agencies, and other health-related facilities and services. On-campus nursing laboratory instruction and practice with low-, mid-, and high-fidelity simulators; standardized patients; and inter-professional learning opportunities help to prepare students for actual clinical practice. Clinical practice begins in the sophomore year. Areas of clinical experience include geriatrics, pediatrics, obstetrics/gynecology, behavioral health, community health, and medical/surgical nursing. Some area hospital systems provide paid competitive internship opportunities for students between their junior and senior years. D'Youville enjoys partnerships and active affiliations with area health-care facilities and agencies where students develop their clinical competencies. Within a narrow geographic area surrounding the college campus and its nearby suburbs are several institutions of the Catholic Health System; Erie County Medical Center (including WNY's Level 1 Trauma and Burn Center); Buffalo Psychiatric Center, Kaleida Health Care System (including Women and Children's Hospital of Buffalo and the Gates Vascular Institute); the Visiting Nurses Association of Western New York; the world-renowned Roswell Park Cancer Institute; Buffalo's VA hospital; and numerous community health agencies and services that provide for primary care and population health. Opportunity is available for service-learning locally and in third-world locations.

In 1957, the RN to B.S.N. program was initiated, offering a specialized curriculum for licensed professional nurses with nursing diplomas and associate degrees. Professional nurses can complete a two-year RN to B.S.N. online program.

Graduate programs offer several options for baccalaureate–prepared nurses to continue their professional development: the Master of Science (M.S.) in community health nursing, with concentrations in advanced clinical nursing, nursing management, or nursing education; the M.S. in family nurse practitioner studies; and a post-master's certificate in family nurse practitioner studies. Begun in fall 2012, D'Youville now offers a Doctor of Nursing Practice (DNP). The DNP can be taken as a post-baccalaureate degree or as a post-master's degree. Admission and progression in the program is individualized to the student's prior preparation.

All baccalaureate and masters programs offered by the School of Nursing are fully accredited by the Commission on Collegiate Nursing Education (CCNE) and approved by the New York State Education Department. The DNP program is approved by the New York State Education Department; the application for accreditation by CCNE will be made one year prior to the graduation of the first class, which is the standard procedure for new programs.

The nursing faculty members are committed, dedicated educators who pride themselves on providing individual attention to students. Faculty members represent diverse educational and clinical preparation and expertise. Their active practice in a variety of specialty practice areas, their research and other scholarly work, and their participation in professional organizations enrich the teaching/learning opportunities provided at D'Youville.

D'Youville College admits students on a rolling admissions basis but recommends students submit applications well before the start of the semester. Applications are reviewed as they are received by the Admissions Office. Freshman applicants must submit a completed application; official high school transcripts, and SAT or ACT scores. Transfer students must also submit official transcripts from all colleges previously attended. Graduate and doctorate applicants present evidence of their undergraduate education from an accredited college or university and their current unrestricted license to practice as a professional registered nurse and/or nurse practitioner.

- *2013–14 UNDERGRADUATE TUITION & FEES:*
  *Full-time: $23,092*
  *Room and Board: $10,800 per year*
- *2013–14 GRADUATE TUITION & FEES:*
  *$850 per credit*
- *APPLICATION DEADLINES: Rolling admissions*
- *FACULTY: http://www.dyc.edu/academics/nursing/faculty.asp*

**CONTACT INFORMATION**

**Dr. Judith Lewis**
**School of Nursing**
**D'Youville College**
**320 Porter Avenue**
**Buffalo, New York 14201**
**Phone: 716-829-7600**
**800-777-3921 (toll-free)**
**Fax: 716-829-7900**
**E-mail: admissions@dyc.edu**
**Web site: http://www.dyc.edu/academics/nursing/**

**UNDERGRADUATE NURSING PROGRAM**

**Dr. Steve Smith, Director of Admissions**
**Phone: 716-829-7600**
**E-mail: admissions@dyc.edu**

**GRADUATE NURSING PROGRAM**

**Mark Pavone, Director of Graduate Admissions**
**Phone: 716-829-8400**
**E-mail: graduateadmissions@dyc.edu**

**Find us on Facebook®:** http://www.dyc.edu/facebook
**Follow us on Twitter™:** http://twitter.com/uanursing

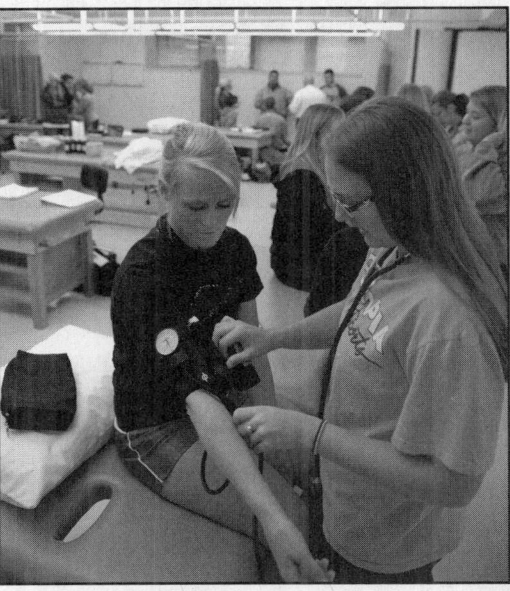

*D'Youville College is internationally known for its wide array of health-care academic offerings. Majors include nursing, physician assistant, occupational and physical therapy, pharmacy, chiropractic, and dietetics. All majors include a strong liberal arts component.*

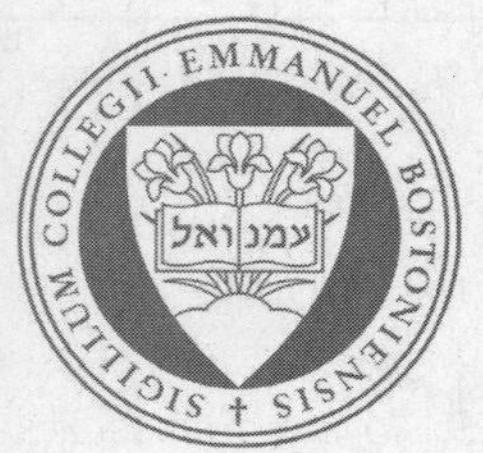


# EMMANUEL COLLEGE

## Graduate Studies + Nursing

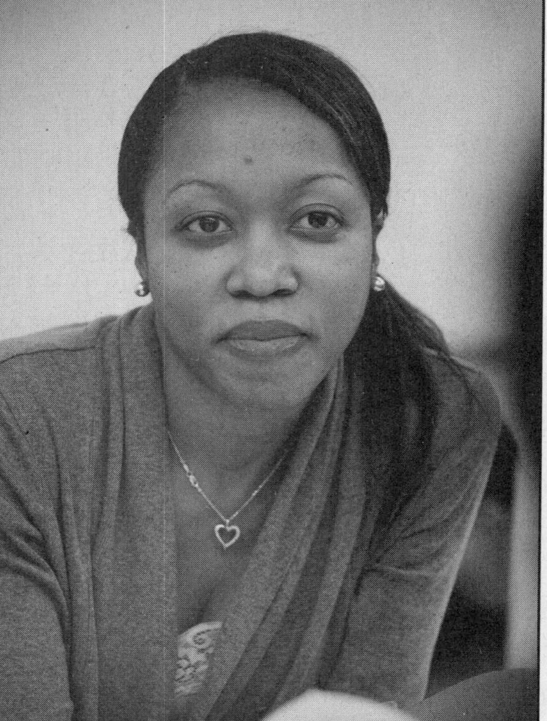

*Students benefit from small, interactive classes.*

### UNDERGRADUATE AND GRADUATE PROGRAMS IN NURSING FOR RNS

Emmanuel College, located in the heart of the Longwood Medical and Academic Area (LMA) of Boston, offers a Bachelor of Science in Nursing (BSN), a Master of Science in Nursing (MSN), and Certificates of Graduate Study in nursing education and nursing management. The curriculum has been tailored to meet students' learning needs and career goals in an ever-changing environment. Faculty and advisors work one-on-one with students to develop individualized plans for nursing study and professional development.

The Bachelor of Science in Nursing (RN to BSN) program prepares students to think critically, appreciate diverse human experience, and use personal and professional values in everyday life. Emmanuel College's program is health promotion–based, enabling students to meet career goals in a constantly changing healthcare environment. Teaching and learning strategies throughout Emmanuel College's nursing courses prepare graduates with the knowledge, skills, and attitudes necessary to continuously improve the quality and safety of the healthcare systems in which they work. The BSN and MSN programs are fully accredited by the Commission on Collegiate Nursing Education (CCNE).

The Master of Science in Nursing program prepares students for an advanced role as a nurse educator or nurse manager/administrator. These distinctive tracks offer students the knowledge and expertise to thrive in a wide variety of clinical settings and to work with diverse populations. Students who choose the education concentration are qualified to pursue roles in clinical education, staff development, and as nursing faculty members; graduates of the management track are prepared for management/administration positions such as nurse executive, administrator, manager, director, coordinator, and case manager.

The newly launched Certificates in Graduate Study in Nursing at Emmanuel offer the opportunity for nurses who have completed a Master of Science in Nursing to further develop their skills in the nursing education and nursing management tracks. These certificate programs enable students to strengthen and broaden the advanced skills and knowledge needed to explore new professional directions.

As respected professionals with years of experience in nursing, Emmanuel College faculty members maintain a strong and up-to-date command in their areas of expertise in research and teaching. As understanding nurse educators, they cultivate lively dialogue so that students share first-hand perspectives on patient care, healthcare issues, and other key subjects. Emmanuel College professors are clinicians, researchers and teachers who serve as true advocates. Each student works directly with a full-time member of the nursing faculty as a dedicated advisor. This provides students with the individual attention necessary to get the most from their plan of study.

With an average class size of 15 students, students have the ability to engage in lively classroom discussions, to share their unique experiences as RNs, and to exchange views and clinical knowledge. Classes meet evenings or Saturday mornings every other week, enabling students to fit academics into their professional and personal schedules. All modified accelerated courses include independent study, and students can set their own pace with flexible program scheduling. Graduate nursing classes meet seven times during the semester and undergraduate nursing classes meet six times. All courses are offered at Emmanuel College's easy-to-reach Boston campus in the Longwood Medical and Academic Area. Emmanuel offers on-campus parking for visitors, as well as parking passes for purchase by Graduate Studies + Nursing students.

The BSN program has enrollment and application opportunities multiple times per year and is also available by request at employer sites. The MSN and graduate certificate programs have new cohorts beginning each fall semester, and the preferred application deadline for the MSN is April 30. More information is available on the website at www.emmanuel.edu/nursing.

- *2013–14 TUITION & FEES*

  *Bachelor of Science in Nursing (BSN):*

  *$1,816 per 4-credit course*

  *Master of Science (MSN) and Certificates in Graduate Study in Nursing:*

  *$2,581 per 3-credit course*

  *There are no additional fees associated with these programs.*

- *APPLICATION DEADLINES*

  *Bachelor of Science in Nursing (BSN):*

  *There are enrollment opportunities multiple times per year. An application form must be submitted prior to enrollment.*

  *Master of Science in Nursing (MSN) and Certificates in Graduate Study in Nursing:*

  *The preferred application deadline is April 30th for enrollment in the fall semester.*
  *There is no application fee.*

- *FACULTY INFORMATION*

  *emmanuel.edu/nursing*

**CONTACT INFORMATION**

**Helen Muterperl, Assistant Director**
**Graduate Admissions /Nursing Programs**
**Emmanuel College**
**Graduate Studies + Nursing**
**400 The Fenway**
**Boston, Massachusetts 02115**
**Phone: 617-735-9700**
**E-mail: graduatestudies@emmanuel.edu**
**Website: www.emmanuel.edu/nursing**

**Find us on Facebook®:** http://www.facebook.com/emmanuelgpp

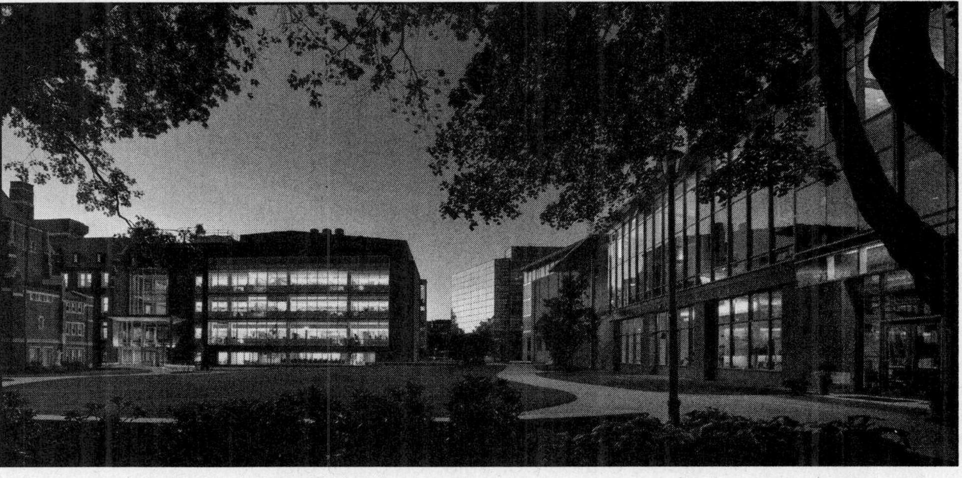

*Emmanuel's Boston campus is located in the world-renowned Longwood Medical and Academic Area.*

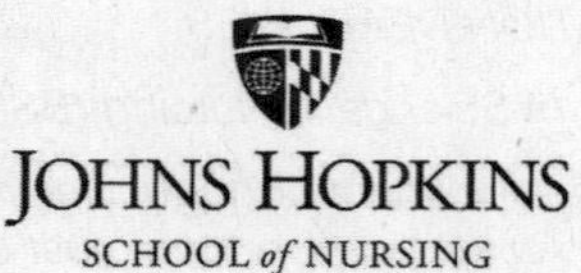


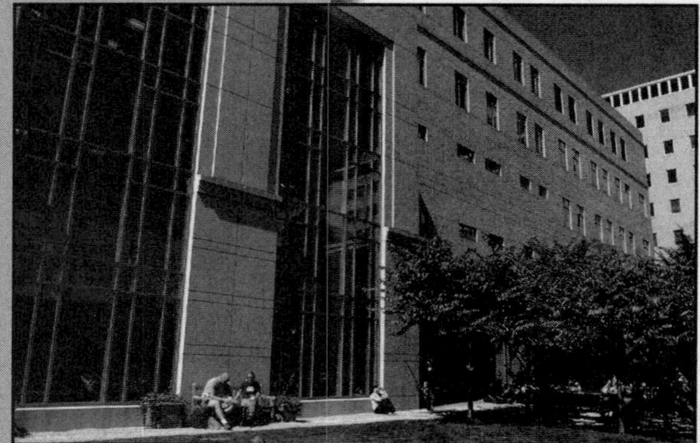

The Johns Hopkins University School of Nursing is a place where exceptional people discover possibilities that forever change their lives and the world. With more than a century of established excellence in connection with The Johns Hopkins Hospital and the University, the School of Nursing is both connected to the past and focused on the future. It attracts students and faculty from around the world to collaborate, research, and learn the best practices to advance the science and art of nursing. Hopkins students enjoy the advantages of an education at an institution with a worldwide reputation and an outstanding network of alumni who are willing to serve as guides and mentors. A rigorous academic curriculum, which includes a strong scientific orientation, gives students the background to understand the healthcare decisions they will make as professionals.

Recognized as a leader by its peers, the School of Nursing ranked first in the nation for Community Health Nursing Programs and first overall for Graduate Programs in the 2012 edition of *U.S. News & World Report.* The School is ranked first among nursing schools in the United States in the National Institutes of Health (NIH) research funding. Named a Center of Excellence in Nursing Education in 2010 by the National League for Nursing, the School is located adjacent to the top-ranked Johns Hopkins University schools of Medicine and Public Health and The Johns Hopkins Hospital.

Johns Hopkins University is accredited by Middle States Commission on Higher Education. The bachelor's and master's programs of the School of Nursing are fully accredited by the National League for Nursing Accrediting Commission (NLNAC) and the Commission on Collegiate Nursing Education (CCNE). In addition, the bachelor's and master's programs are approved by the Maryland State Board of Examiners of Nurses. The bachelor's, master's, and doctoral programs are endorsed by the Maryland State Board for Higher Education. The School's Doctor of Nursing Practice (DNP) program went through the accreditation process with the Commission on Collegiate Nursing Education (CCNE) in fall 2009 and received full accreditation until 2015. The School is also proud to be the only Paul D. Coverdell Fellows Program in nursing.

A complete bachelor's and master's application consists of an application form and a nonrefundable $75 application fee. Doctoral applicants pay an application fee of $100. Applicants to the bachelor's program are required to submit three letters of recommendation and official college- or university-level transcripts. A grade point average (GPA) above 3.0 (on a 4.0 scale) is recommended. Personal interviews may be requested.

Applicants to the master's program are required to have graduated from a bachelor's or master's degree program in nursing with a GPA above 3.0 (on a 4.0 scale), a current Maryland state nursing license, academic and professional references, written expression of goals, and official transcripts from all previous colleges/universities attended. Personal interviews may be requested.

---

- *2014–15 UNDERGRADUATE TUITION & FEES:*

  **Summer-Entry Accelerated Bachelor's Program:**
  *Tuition: $67,344 (for entire 13-month program)*
  *Housing, food, books, fees, and other costs: $29,632*

  **Fall-Entry Accelerated Bachelor's Program:**
  *Tuition: $67,765 (for entire 17-month program)*
  *Housing, food, books, fees, and other costs: $33,412*

**Accelerated BS-MSN with Paid Clinical Residency Program:** *Bachelor's tuition: $67,765 (full-time—12 credit hours/semester). Housing, food, books, fees, and other costs: $33,412. Master's tuition dependent on track.*

- *2014–15 GRADUATE TUITION & FEES:*

**MSN Program:**
*Tuition: $33,984 (full-time—12 credit hours/semester); $1,416 per credit (part-time). Housing, food, books, fees, and other costs: $18,866*

**MSN/MPH Program:**
*Tuition: $54,376 (full-time—16 credit hours/semester); $1,431 per credit (part-time). Housing, food, books, fees, and other costs: $23,110*

**PhD Program:**
*Tuition: $40,626 (full-time—9 credit hours/semester); $2,257 per credit (part-time). Housing, food, books, fees, and other costs: $18,866*

**DNP Program:**
*Tuition: $33,816 (for entire 40 credit program); $1,409 per credit (part-time). Housing, food, books, fees, and other costs: $18,866*

- *APPLICATION DEADLINES:*

**Bachelor's Program:** *November 1 (early decision); December 1 (summer entry); January 15 (fall entry)*

**Accelerated BS-MSN with Paid Clinical Residency Program:** *November 1 (early decision); January 15 (regular decision)*

**Master's Program:** *March 15 (fall entry); September 1 (spring entry); January 15 (summer entry)*

*Special Deadlines:*

*MSN/MPH and MSN/MPH Nurse Practitioner: December 1 (summer entry)*

*MSN in Public Health Nursing/Nurse-Midwifery Track: December 1 (fall entry)*

*MSN Primary Care Nurse Practitioner (Adult-Geriatric, Family, Pediatric): December 1 (fall entry)*

*Note: BS to MSN students who are enrolled in the Bachelor's degree portion of the program must confirm their planned fall enrollment in the MSN program by February 1.*

- **Post-Degree Options**

*Family Primary Care Nurse Practitioner: December 1 (fall entry)*

*Applied Health Informatics: June 1 (fall entry)*

*Forensic Nursing:*
*November 1 (spring entry); June 1 (fall entry)*

*Nurse Educator: July 15 (fall entry); December 1 (spring entry); May 1 (summer entry)*

*Adult-Gerontology Acute Care, Pediatric Primary Care, and Adult-Geriatric Nurse Practitioner: January 15 (fall entry)*

*Accelerated Acute Care Nurse Practitioner: September 1 (spring entry)*

**PhD Program:**
*March 1 (fall entry); January 15 (for full eligibility for scholarship opportunities).*

**DNP Program:**
*January 1 (summer entry)*

- *FACULTY INFORMATION:* *http://nursing.jhu.edu/faculty*
- *MULTIMEDIA:* *http://youtube.com/hopkinsnursing*

**CONTACT INFORMATION**

**Office of Admissions and Student Services**
**Johns Hopkins University School of Nursing**
**525 North Wolfe Street**
**Baltimore, Maryland 21205**
**Phone: 410-955-7548**
**Fax: 410-614-7086**
**E-mail: jhuson@jhu.edu**
**Web site: www.nursing.jhu.edu**

**Find us on Facebook®:** www.facebook.com/jhunursing
**Follow us on Twitter™:** twitter.com/JHUNursing

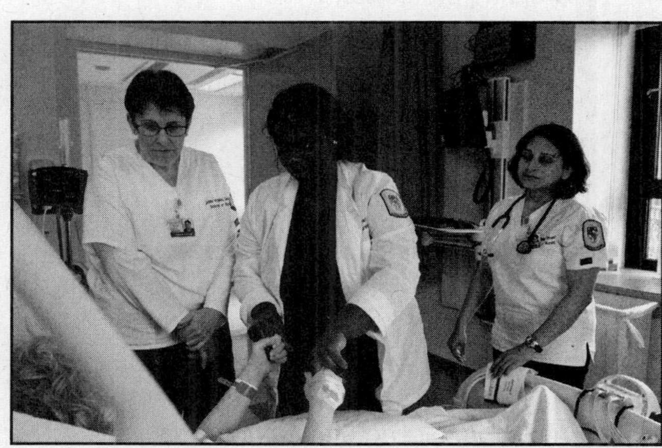

*Students work closely with clinical instructors at The Johns Hopkins Hospital.*

# LUTHER COLLEGE

## Department of Nursing

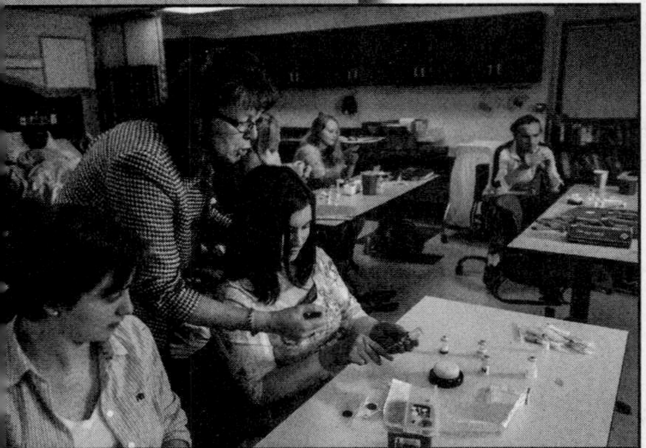

*The nursing major at Luther College offers an integrated program of liberal arts and 14 professional nursing courses, giving students a broad approach to nursing and providing a base for graduate study or immediate entry into the profession. Students gain clinical experience at healthcare sites such as St. Marys Hospital, an affiliate of Mayo Clinic in Rochester, Minnesota.*

The goal of Luther's nursing faculty is to prepare nurses to function autonomously and interdependently with individuals, families, groups, and communities to promote, maintain, and restore optimal health in a variety of health-care settings. The nursing major, therefore, offers an integrated program of liberal arts and 14 professional nursing courses. The program gives students a broad approach to nursing, providing a base for graduate study or immediate entry into the nursing profession.

Following graduation, Luther nursing students may take the National Council Licensure Examination for Registered Nurses (NCLEX-RN). More information is available upon request.

The first year at Luther provides a foundation in the liberal arts and sciences. All nursing majors are assigned a faculty adviser to help each student decide whether to pursue a nursing curriculum plan. All students interested in nursing are invited to participate in the Luther Student Nurses Association (LSNA).

Clinical nursing courses begin in the fall of the sophomore year. Nursing courses at this level emphasize health assessment, health promotion, clinical reasoning, and fundamental skills throughout the life span in a variety of settings. These learning experiences develop new communication and interpersonal skills.

Third-year students experience a concentrated study of nursing concepts by caring for children, childbearing families, and adults with physical and emotional problems. The sites for this clinical experience are inpatient and ambulatory care areas at Mayo Clinic; the Federal Medical Center; and a variety of community-based agencies in Rochester, Minnesota.

The senior year provides final preparation for entry into the practice of professional nursing. Courses focus on promoting health and preventing illness in childbearing families and in community groups. Students further develop leadership management and research skills through selected areas of nursing.

Minimum academic requirements must be met to be considered for enrollment in nursing courses. However, meeting the minimum requirements does not guarantee placement in the courses. Decisions affecting progression in the major are made at the end of each semester.

The study of nursing at Luther incorporates academic classroom learning, based in the newly renovated Valders Hall of Science, and clinical experience in several community facilities. These include Winneshiek Medical Center; the Decorah Free Clinic; Mayo Clinic: Methodist Hospital and Mayo Clinic: Saint Marys Hospital; the Federal Medical Center; and a variety of community-based health-care agencies in Decorah, Iowa and Rochester, Minnesota.

Nursing scholarships are available to incoming students on a competitive basis upon admission. Selection of recipients is based on academic information submitted on the application and the high school transcript. Scholarship renewal is based on satisfactory academic and clinical performance in the major.

All nursing students benefit from the Bernice Fischer Cross and Bert S. Cross Perpetual Endowment for the Luther College Mayo Nursing Program and Health Sciences Program. This is used for equal-share assistance for the Luther College nursing students enrolled in the curriculum provided at Mayo Clinic in Rochester, Minnesota. The endowment is not a need-based scholarship.

Located in the northeast Iowa town of Decorah (resident population: 8,100), Luther College is an undergraduate liberal arts institution of about 2,500 students that is affiliated with the Lutheran church (ELCA). The Upper Iowa River—the only waterway in the state designated as wild and scenic—flows through the lower portion of Luther's 200-acre central campus and borders Decorah's business district. Decorah is known nationwide for its recreational opportunities, numerous cultural heritage events and festivals, pedestrian-friendly village center, and its conscious efforts to thrive as a small town. Public transportation includes commercial airports in Rochester (Minnesota), Waterloo (Iowa), and La Crosse (Wisconsin); a municipal airport in Decorah; and train and bus depots in La Crosse, Wisconsin.

- *2014–15 UNDERGRADUATE TUITION & FEES:*

  *The comprehensive fee is $45,260 ($38,170 tuition, $3,140 room, $3,950 board).*

- *APPLICATION DEADLINES:*

  *Luther College operates on rolling admission. There is no application deadline.*

- *FACULTY INFORMATION:*

  *http://www.luther.edu/nursing/faculty/*

- *MULTIMEDIA:*

  *http://www.luther.edu/video/*

**CONTACT INFORMATION**

**LaDonna McGohan, Head**
**Department of Nursing**
**Luther College**
**700 College Drive**
**Decorah, Iowa 52101**
**Phone: 563-387-1057**
**800-458-8437 (toll-free)**
**E-mail: mcgola01@luther.edu**
**Web site: http://www.luther.edu/nursing/**

**Find us on Facebook®:** www.facebook.com/luthercollege1861
**Follow us on Twitter™:** www.twitter.com/luthercollege

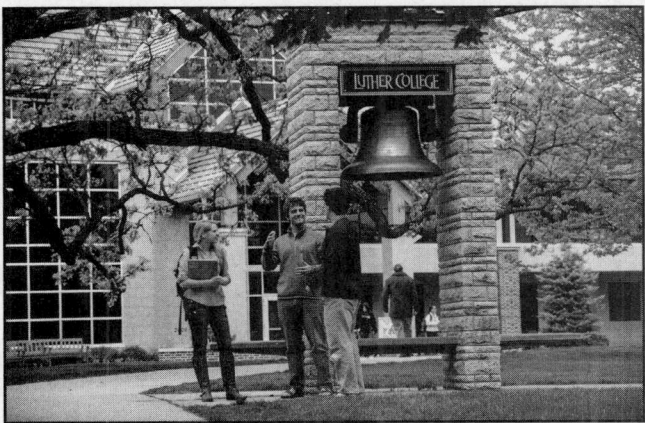


*Luther College students learn in a community that emphasizes rigorous academics, a world-class music program, champion athletics, and opportunities to put their classroom learning to the test through internships, independent research, and study abroad. Typically, 98 percent of Luther graduates are employed, attending graduate school, or engaged in an internship or volunteer work within eight months of graduation.*

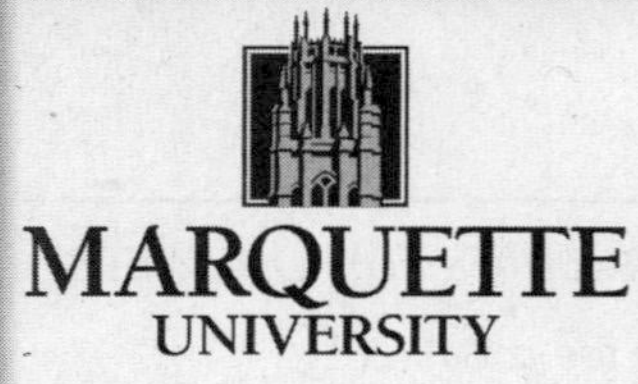


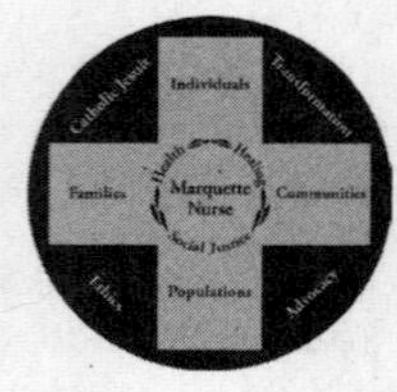

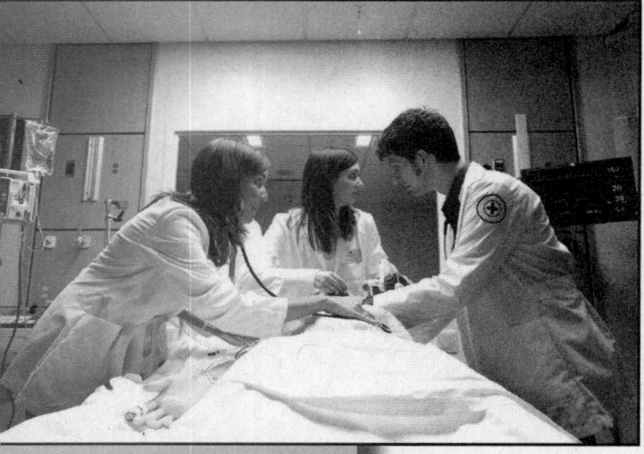

*Simulated Cardiac Arrest Resuscitation*

The four-year Bachelor of Science in Nursing (B.S.N.) degree program at Marquette University provides a strong academic foundation in nursing, natural and social science, and humanities. Preparation for a professional nursing role is emphasized through the development of clinical, cognitive, and leadership skills and personal and professional values. Students are **admitted directly as freshmen** into the College of Nursing, which **assures placement in clinical nursing courses.** Nursing courses begin on the first day of enrollment. Clinical reasoning, introduced in the first year through course assignments and simulation experiences, is further developed through five clinical rotations in health-care agencies across the sophomore, junior, and senior years. A low student-teacher ratio (8:1) affords personal attention in all clinical rotations, including maternity, community health, nursing care for children and adults with chronic and acute conditions, and transition into professional practice.

The 128-credit B.S.N. program includes courses in the humanities, physical-biological sciences, and social-behavioral sciences as well as electives and courses in the nursing major. A University Core of Common Studies is foundational for all majors at Marquette University. Lower-division nursing courses are Dimensions of Professional Nursing in the Jesuit Tradition, Nursing and Health in the Jesuit Tradition, Health Assessment and Fundamentals I and II, Pathophysiology I and II, and Concepts and Interventions for the Promotion of Mental Health. Upper-division courses include Pharmacology, Evidence-Based Practice and Nursing Research, Maternity Nursing and Women's Health, Family and Community-Centered Nursing*, Community and Population Health Nursing, Nursing Concepts and Interventions for the Care of Adults—Older Adults I and II, Nursing Care for Persons with Chronic and Acute Conditions*, Family Centered Nursing of Children, Quality and Safety in Nursing, Leadership in Professional Nursing Practice, Transition into Professional Nursing*, and Palliative Care. [The asterisk (*) denotes clinical practice courses.]

Marquette University College of Nursing offers the Master of Science in Nursing (M.S.N.) degree and post-master's certificates that prepare graduates for advanced practice roles or leadership roles within health-care systems. Individuals may enter through three pathways: post-B.S.N.; Direct Entry (DE), a combined RN and generalist M.S.N. for those with non-nursing bachelor's degrees; and ADN-prepared nurses with bachelor's degrees in other disciplines. Graduates are academically eligible to seek formal professional certification as nurse practitioners, clinical nurse specialists, nurse midwives, nurse administrators, or clinical nurse leaders, depending on the specialty option completed. Seven specialty options are available: systems leadership and health care quality, clinical nurse leader, and advanced practice programs in nurse midwifery, adult-older adult primary or acute care, adult-older adult clinical nurse specialist, and pediatric primary or acute care. Full-time students complete the 39–49 credit programs in four to six semesters.

At the Ph.D. program level, a 69-credit B.S.N. to Ph.D. program and a 51-credit post-M.S.N./Ph.D. program to prepare nurse scientists as teachers/scholars who focus on knowledge generation related to vulnerable populations.

At the Doctor of Nursing Practice (D.N.P.) level, a 63–69 credit B.S.N. to D.N.P. program or a 33-credit post-M.S.N. program, is another route to leadership in advanced practice nursing. The program emphasizes translational research, epidemiology, informatics, health policy, statistics, and professional issues. All students complete a two-semester capstone clinical project. A residency course is also required.

The College is affiliated with more than ninety health-care agencies in Wisconsin and the surrounding states. These agencies include hospitals, clinics, home care facilities, public health departments, schools, parishes, long-term-care facilities, and hospice. Many of these agencies offer excellent student employment opportunities as well as financial aid and loan forgiveness programs once students graduate from the program.

Marquette is located on an 80-acre campus with excellent facilities. The College of Nursing has many technology-enhanced classrooms and a well-equipped Wheaton Franciscan Health Care Center for Clinical Simulation, including SIM-MAN G, a birthing simulator, and many other advanced simulation technology models for student learning. The Simulation Center provides media resources and practice labs supplied with state-of-the-art models and equipment necessary to develop a solid foundation for clinical practice. Students participate in simulation exercises that are videotaped for maximal learning before entering into complex health-care systems.

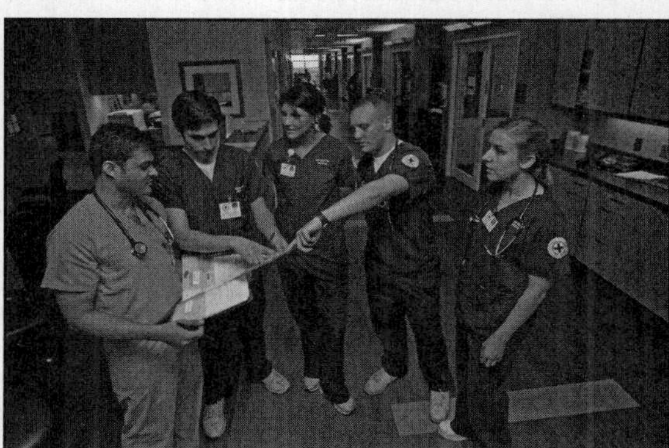

*Intensive Care Unit Patient Consultation.*

- *2013–14 UNDERGRADUATE TUITION & FEES:*

  *Full-time tuition: $34,200*

  *Typical room and board: $10,730; Fees: $440*

- *2013–14 GRADUATE TUITION & FEES:*

  *$1,025 per credit hour*

  *15-Month Direct Entry Pre-MSN Program: $52,480 paid in four payments (summer, fall, spring, and summer)*

- *APPLICATION DEADLINES:*

  *Undergraduate: December 1*

  *Graduate and Post-Grad: August 1 for fall; November 1 for spring*

  *D.N.P.: February 15*

  *Direct Entry (DE) Master's: December 31 for May start*

- *FACULTY INFORMATION:*

  *http://www.mu.edu/facstaff*

- *MULTIMEDIA: http://www.mu.edu/nursing*

**CONTACT INFORMATION**

**Undergraduate Nursing Program:**

**Mary Grant**
**Undergraduate Program Assistant**
**Phone: 414-288-3809**
**E-mail: mary.grant@mu.edu**

**Graduate Nursing Program:**

**Karen Nest**
**Graduate Program Coordinator**
**Phone: 414-288-3810**
**E-mail: Karen.nest@mu.edu**

**Graduate Program & Communication Coordinator**
**College of Nursing**
**Marquette University**
**P.O. Box 1881**
**Milwaukee, Wisconsin 53233**
**Phone: 414-288-3869**
**Fax: 414-288-1939**
**Web site: http://www.mu.edu/nursing**

**Find us on Facebook®**: http://www.facebook.com/MarquetteU
**Follow us on Twitter™**: http://www.twitter.com/marquetteu

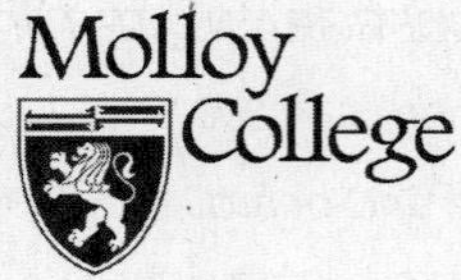

## Division of Nursing

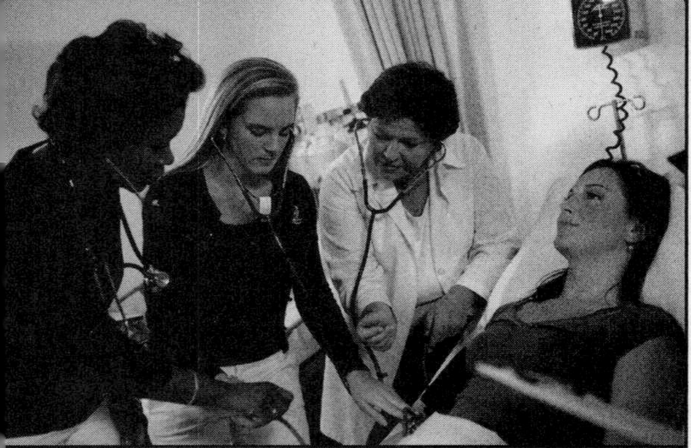

*Molloy's undergraduate nursing program is one of the largest in the United States, and the College also offers multiple graduate programs, including a Ph.D. in Nursing.*

*An Emphasis on Human Compassion, Dignity, and Respect*

At Molloy, nursing is both art and science. One of the country's largest and most respected programs, Molloy's Nursing Division curriculum immerses students in clinical practice with an emphasis on human compassion, dignity, and respect for the patient. Molloy's programs proactively respond to the changing needs of today's health-care environment, providing students with individualized attention from an expert faculty that is easily accessible and always committed to students' success.

From Molloy's fully equipped, state-of-the-art learning laboratory to its innovative clinical practice opportunities, at Molloy students can find all the resources and support they need to become an effective, humanistic health-care provider—whether students are just beginning their nursing education or are professionals who are ready to take their career to the next level. At Molloy, students benefit from a comprehensive array of:

- Undergraduate programs. Offering a wealth of hands-on clinical experiences beginning in a student's sophomore year, Molloy's bachelor's degree program prepares students for a vital role in health care. Already working in health care or in another career? Consider one of Molloy's dual-degree programs, the degree completion program for registered nurses, the LPN to B.S./RN career mobility program, or the accelerated dual-degree program for second degree students holding a non-nursing baccalaureate or higher degree.
- Graduate programs. Focused on advanced theory and its application in a selected area of nursing, Molloy offers seven distinct tracks leading to master's degrees and nine master's certificates concentrating on advanced clinical practice, administrative and informatics expertise, and specialty training in education. Nurse Practitioner tracks are available in Pediatrics, Adult, Family or Psychiatry, Clinical Nurse Specialist (CNS): Adult Health, Nursing Education, or Nursing Administration with Informatics.
- Doctoral program. Molloy's first doctoral program is designed to prepare doctoral students to become leaders, advancing the profession of nursing through research, education, administration, and health policy.

Molloy College launched its first doctoral program, a Ph.D. in Nursing, in fall 2010. According to Veronica Feeg, Ph.D., RN, FAAN, Associate Dean and Director of the Doctoral Program, "Doctoral education is important for our profession and the Ph.D. at Molloy will produce the researchers and scholars who will lead the discipline."

"We expect that our Ph.D. graduates will leave Molloy prepared to serve our communities, develop the next generation of nursing leaders and have a strong voice in health policy decisions that affect us all," said Jeannine D. Muldoon, Ph.D., RN, Dean of the Division of Nursing.

"Molloy's Ph.D. in Nursing further demonstrates the College's commitment to academic excellence," said Valerie H. Collins, Ph.D., Vice President of Academic Affairs and Dean of Faculty. "Molloy's Nursing programs have always been among the finest in the country—the undergraduate program is among the largest in the United States—so we are pleased that the College's first doctoral program comes from this Division."

A Ph.D. from Molloy prepares nurses for leadership roles in academia, health policy formulation, health-care administration, and clinical practice. The curriculum focuses on theory, research, the humanities, and methodology. Essential elements of the curriculum feature leadership through caring, both in educational and organizational/policy settings, as well as theory and research in the nursing profession. Students are required to complete 45 credits of course work and a dissertation.

- *2013–14 UNDERGRADUATE TUITION & FEES:*

  *Tuition: $24,700*

  *Fees: $1,010*

- *2013–14 GRADUATE TUITION & FEES:*

  *Master's program:*
  *Tuition: $895 per credit*

  *Fees: $720 (if taking 1–4 credits); $880 (if taking 5 or more credits)*

  *Ph.D. program: $1,000/credit; fees same as for Master's program*

- *APPLICATION DEADLINES:*

  *Undergraduate: Rolling admissions*

  *Master's program: Rolling admissions*

  *Ph.D. program: February 1*

**CONTACT INFORMATION**

**Molloy College**
**1000 Hempstead Avenue**
**Rockville Centre, New York 11571**
**Phone: 888-4-MOLLOY (toll-free)**
**Website: http://www.molloy.edu**

**Undergraduate Admissions**
**Phone: 516-323-4000**
**E-mail: admissions@molloy.edu**

**Graduate and Ph.D. Admissions**
**Alina Haitz**
**Phone: 516-323-4008**
**E-mail: ahaitz@molloy.edu**

**Find us on Facebook®: http://www.facebook.com/GoMolloy**
**Follow us on Twitter™: http://www.twitter.com/MolloyCollege**

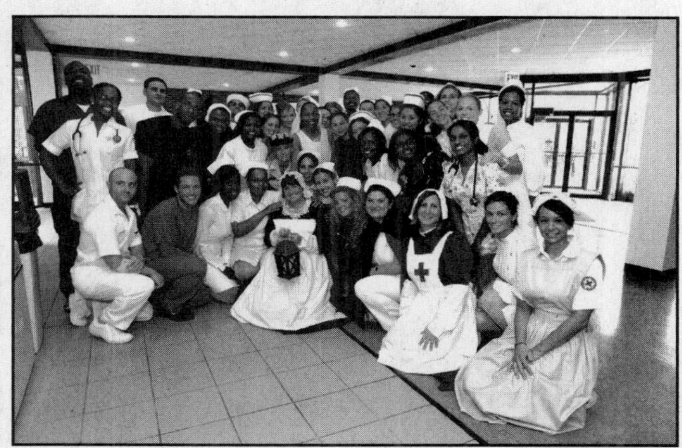

*Molloy College recently celebrated the launch of its new Ph.D. program with a series of lectures and a "nursing fashion show" that featured students wearing uniforms from various decades.*

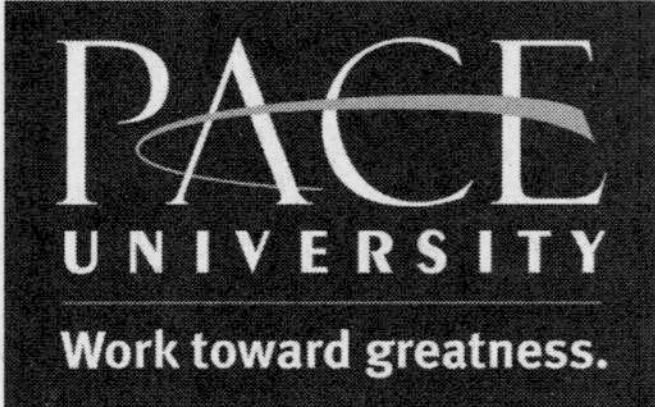


*Discover unlimited opportunities in the health professions at Pace!*

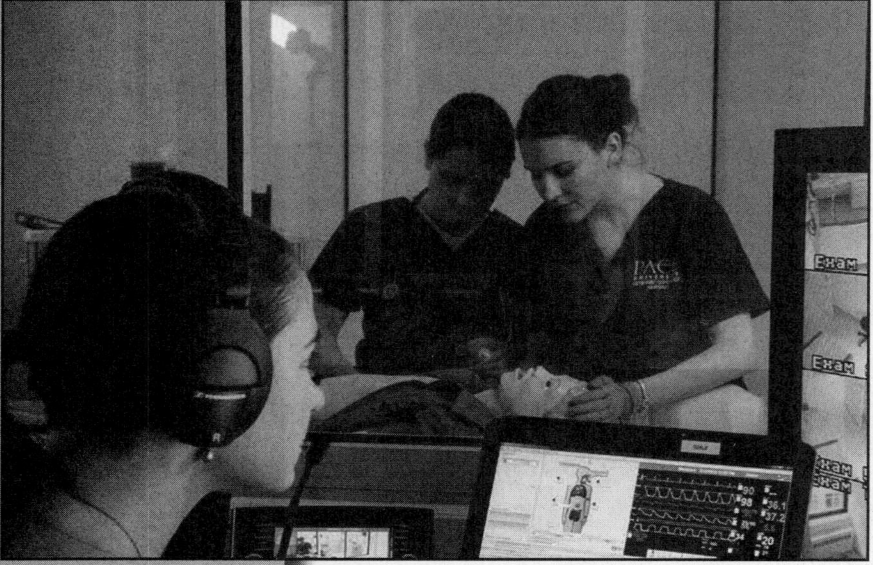

*The Clinical Education Labs (CEL) offer state-of-the-art resources on both Pleasantville (PLV) and New York City (NYC) campuses.*

## The College of Health Professions

The Lienhard School of Nursing is part of Pace University's College of Health Professions, which was established in 2010 in an effort to showcase and expand health profession majors at Pace University. The College is made up of the Lienhard School of Nursing and the Pace University–Lenox Hill Hospital Physician Assistant Studies Program. The College's vision is innovative leadership in education, practice, and scholarship for the health professions. Its mission is to educate and challenge students for the health professions to be innovators and leaders who will positively impact global health care.

## The Lienhard School of Nursing

Set within urban and suburban settings, the Lienhard School of Nursing (LSN) partners with many well-known primary, acute, and tertiary care facilities and community agencies to foster human growth and dignity and provide primary health care. The School is committed to helping individuals, families, and communities at local, national, and international levels that strive to meet health-care demands now and in the future. Lienhard's vision is to be a leader in innovation and excellence in education, research, and practice in primary health care.

The Lienhard School of Nursing considers teaching and learning its highest priorities and is committed to the integration of scholarship and practice. Graduates have the competitive edge through the School's focus on highly developed clinical skills and critical thinking, evidence-based practice, cultural competence, and leadership. LSN's primary health-care focus is intended to promote improved health outcomes for clients.

For more than 48 years, The Lienhard School of Nursing has been educating practitioners to deliver health care to individuals and families. Its master's program is nationally ranked by *U.S. News & World Report*. In addition, its DNP program prepares nurses for the most advanced level of clinical practice.

Lienhard School of Nursing graduates are prepared to be leaders in both academic and health-care settings.

The Lienhard School of Nursing has many distinguished programs, faculty members, and services that give students a great start to nursing practice. The following programs are available:

- 4-year B.S. (Pleasantville campus only)
- Bridge Program to Advanced Degree (for RNs with a bachelor's degree in a field other than nursing)
- Accelerated BS in Nursing for non-nurse college graduates
- iPace RN/BS Completion Program for RNs with an associate degree or diploma in nursing

- MS/Family Nurse Practitioner (FNP)—Certificates of Advanced Graduate Studies (CAGS) also offered
- MA in Nursing Education (offered in a blended online and in-class format)—Certificates of Advanced Graduate Studies (CAGS) also offered
- Acute Care Adult NP: Certificate of Advanced Graduate Study
- FNP–DNP (Family Nurse Practitioner–Doctor of Nursing Practice)
- Doctor of Nursing Practice (DNP) (New York City campus only)

## What makes Lienhard School of Nursing programs unique?

- NCLEX pass rates are excellent and consistently exceed state and national averages.
- Students in the RN-4 program start nursing classes in their freshman year and clinicals in their sophomore year—earlier than many other programs, giving them an edge.
- The faculty is composed of excellent teachers/clinicians who partner with New York's premier hospitals and health-care organizations to share their expertise while creating unparalleled clinical experiences for Lienhard students. Graduates are prepared to be leaders in both academic and health-care settings.

Pace University's motto is *Opportunitas,* and it is the foundation of the LSN philosophy—offering students the *opportunity* to discover and fulfill their potential and offering a distinguished faculty and an outstanding staff the *opportunity* to achieve excellence.

Based on Lienhard School of Nursing's long and rich history of educating nurses, students can be confident that they will be prepared for positions of responsibility in all areas of health care and nursing education.

---

- *2014–15 UNDERGRADUATE TUITION & FEES:*

  *For up-to-date, detailed information, visit:*

  *www.pace.edu/tuition*
- *2014–15 GRADUATE TUITION & FEES:*

  *For up-to-date, detailed information, visit:*

  *www.pace.edu/tuition-grad*
- *APPLICATION DEADLINES (domestic students):*

  *RN-4 Program—February 15*
  *ABSN 1-Year FT Program*
  *(Fall-New York City Campus)—March 1*
  *ABSN 1-Year FT Program*
  *(Spring–Westchester Campus)—September 1*
  *ABSN 2-Year Program*
  *(Fall–New York City Campus)—March 1*
  *ABSN 2-Year Program*
  *(Spring–Westchester Campus)—September 1*
  *FNP Program (Fall)—March 1*
  *Nursing Education (Fall)—March 1*
  *Acute Care Adult NP (Fall)—March 1*
  *DNP Program (Fall 2014 Cohort)—March 1*
- *FACULTY INFORMATION:*

  *www.pace.edu/lienhard/faculty*
- *MULTIMEDIA:*

  *www.pace.edu/lienhard*

**CONTACT INFORMATION**

**Sally Hay, Staff Assistant**
**Lienhard School of Nursing, College of Health Professions**
**Pace University**
**861 Bedford Road**
**Pleasantville, New York 10570**
**Phone: 914-773-3552**
**866-722-3338 (general info; toll-free)**
**E-mail: nursing@pace.edu**
**Web site: www.pace.edu/lienhard**

**Find Lienhard on Facebook®:**
https://www.facebook.com/lienhardnursing
**Follow Pace University on Twitter™:** http://twitter.com/paceuniversity

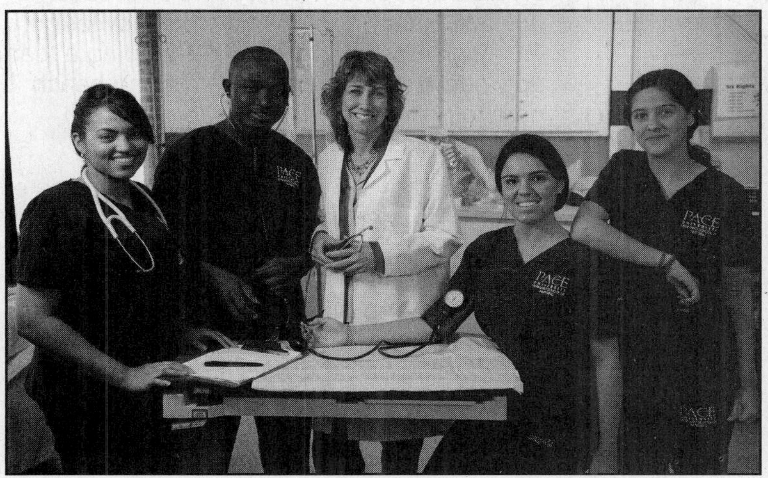

*Professor Andrea Sonenberg, DNSc, RN, with Lienhard School of Nursing students.*

# QUINNIPIAC UNIVERSITY

## School of Nursing

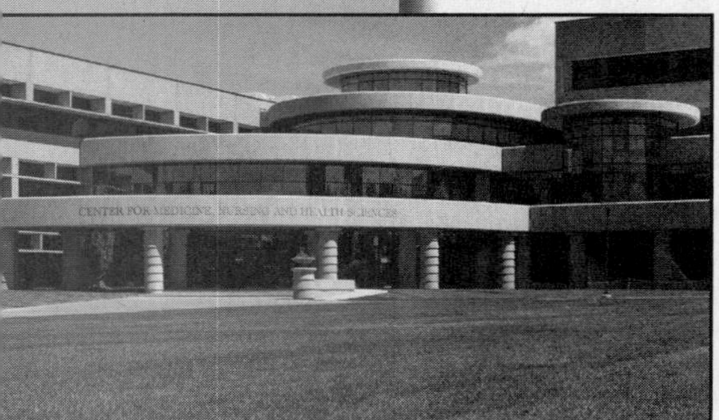

*Education with a Personal Touch.*

*Professional nursing courses take place in the Center for Medicine, Nursing and Health Sciences on Quinnipiac's 104-acre North Haven campus.*

Quinnipiac University (QU), located in Hamden, Connecticut, just 8 miles from New Haven and midway between New York City and Boston, has 6,400 undergraduate and 2,200 graduate students. QU offers the B.S. in Nursing, an Accelerated B.S.N. for those who hold a non-nursing college degree, an RN to B.S.N Completion Track, a Master's of Science in Nursing (M.S.N. in Nursing), and the Doctorate of Nursing Practice (D.N.P.) for postbaccalaureate and post-master's students. The School of Nursing is located on the North Haven campus along with the Schools of Medicine, Health Sciences, Education, and Law.

Quinnipiac views nursing as a research-based profession that is goal-directed as well as creative and concerned with the health and dignity of the whole person. The art of delivering high-quality nursing care depends on the successful mastery and application of intellectually rigorous nursing knowledge. Quinnipiac goes further by developing a team approach to health care in providing health care to patients of all ages, abilities, and backgrounds.

Accredited by the Commission on Collegiate Nursing Education (CCNE) Quinnipiac's bachelor's degree program in nursing offers the theoretical and clinical education students need to enter professional nursing practice. Graduates of the traditional and accelerated second degree programs are eligible to take the NCLEX-RN exam and are well prepared for graduate study in nursing. The nursing curriculum fosters professional socialization for future roles and responsibilities within the profession. Graduates of the program are prepared as generalists to begin the practice of holistic professional nursing, with sound theoretical foundations and nearly 700 hours of diverse clinical practice and laboratory experiences. In addition to the traditional four-year program, and the accelerated second degree option, an online RN to BSN completion program provides Associate Degree and Diploma trained nurses with an opportunity to develop competencies in research, community and public health, quality, safety, and leadership.

The graduate nursing program, also accredited by CCNE, prepares professional nurses at an advanced theoretical and clinical practice level in order to address present and potential societal health needs. Two available post-B.S.N. tracks are Adult-Gerontology Nurse Practitioner and Family Nurse Practitioner. Two post-master's tracks, The Care of Populations and Nursing Leadership, are also available. All tracks in the graduate nursing program lead to the Doctorate of Nursing Practice (D.N.P.) degree. Proposed options for post-B.S.N. and post-M.S.N. tracks in nurse anesthesia are in requisite approval processes from national and state authorities. Proposed options for post-B.S.N. and post-M.S.N. tracks in nurse anesthesia are in requisite approval processes from national and state authorities and are expected to open in Summer 2014. The graduate nursing program broadens the scope of practice and provides for the acquisition of expertise in an area of certified specialization (Adult-Gerontology Nurse Practitioner or Family Nurse Practitioner), as well as leadership roles in advanced specialty practice, population health and health-care systems. The graduate nursing program includes core courses that cover bioethics, Evidence-based practice, organizational systems, epidemiology, and health-care policy.

Quinnipiac's strong affiliates with health-care providers in the area allow students to complete clinical work within institutions such as Yale-New Haven Health system, St. Vincent's Medical Center, Connecticut Children's Medical Center, Mid-State Medical Center, Middlesex Hospital, the Hartford Healthcare system as well as in private practices, clinics, schools, and other community-based settings.

Quinnipiac's Mount Carmel Campus is the primary location for housing, recreation, and course work for undergraduates in their first two years. Starting in the junior year, the professional courses in nursing take place on the nearby 104-acre North Haven campus in the Center for Medicine, Nursing & Health Sciences, a remarkable facility with state-of-the-art technologies to prepare health-care professionals in a variety of fields. The Clinical Simulation Labs house "patients" that are lifelike simulation mannequins. Cameras capture the simulation for student assessment. The variety of labs and technology provide an educational setting for nursing students to learn across the lifespan, across the continuum of care, and across the disciplines. The Physical Diagnosis Lab, Physical Exam Suite, Health Assessment Lab, and the Standardized Patient center duplicate care in an outpatient primary care setting, such as an emergency room or doctor's office.

For more on the North Haven campus, see www.quinnipiac.edu/resources-facilities/.

Students applying as freshmen into the nursing program should file their application for admission by November 15. Information regarding admission requirements can be found at http://www.quinnipiac.edu/apply.

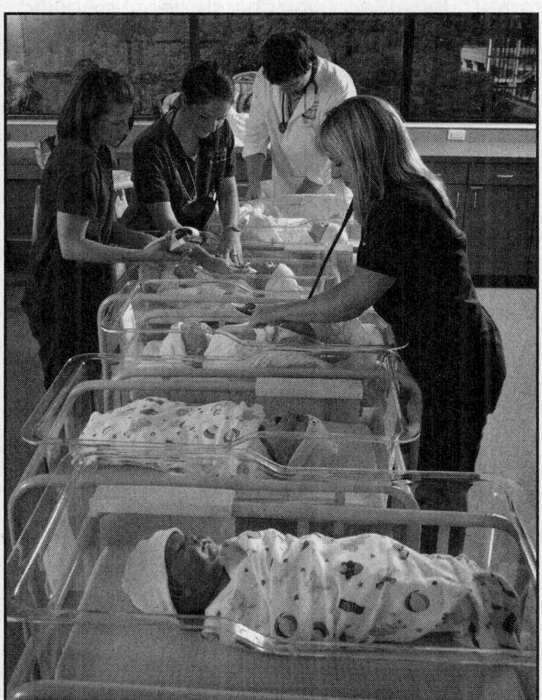

*In the pediatrics maternity lab, students learn about fetal development and birthing. Students are taught to bathe and swaddle infants as well as how to educate new mothers about infant care.*

Transfer students must have a minimum 3.0 GPA and are considered on a space-available basis.

The accelerated (second degree) nursing program begins in August. The complete application and all supporting documents must be filed by January 1.
See www.quinnipiac.edu/accelerated for details.

Graduate admission information for the M.S., D.N.P., and the various tracks can be found at www.quinnipiac.edu/gradnursing.

---

- *2014–15 UNDERGRADUATE TUITION & FEES:*

  *Full-time: $40,670 (tuition and fees); $14,490 (room and board)*

  *Part-time: $930 per credit*
- *2014–15 GRADUATE TUITION: $930 per credit plus $37 per credit student fee.*
- *APPLICATION DEADLINES:*

  *Undergraduate applicants should apply by Nov. 15 for fall admission*

  *Graduate students should ideally apply by June 1 for the fall semester; the program has rolling admissions.*
- *FACULTY INFORMATION:*

  *http://www.quinnipiac.edu/nursing*
- *MULTIMEDIA:*

  *http://www.quinnipiac.edu/tour*

**CONTACT INFORMATION**

**Joan Isaac Mohr**
**VP for Admissions & Financial Aid**
**Admissions Office**
**Quinnipiac University**
**275 Mt. Carmel Avenue**
**Hamden, Connecticut 06518**
**Phone: 203-582-8600**
**800-462-1944 (toll-free)**
**Fax: 203-582-8906**
**E-mail: admissions@quinnipiac.edu**
**Web site: http://www.quinnipiac.edu**

**Undergraduate Nursing Program:**
**Office of Undergraduate Admissions**
**Phone: 203-582-8600**
**E-mail: admissions@quinnipiac.edu**

**Graduate Nursing Program:**
**Office of Graduate Admissions**
**Phone: 203-582-8672**
**E-mail: graduate@quinnipiac.edu**

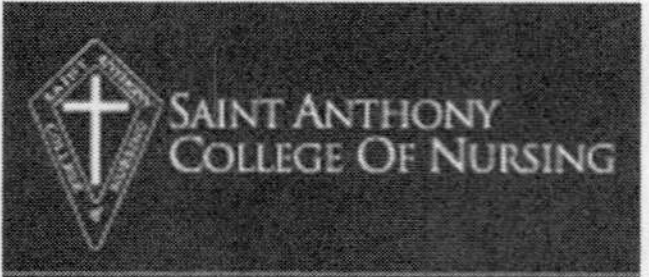


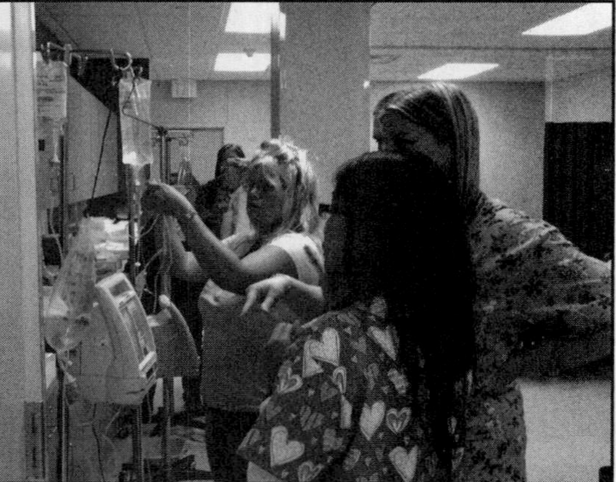

*Personal, individualized attention in a caring environment.*

*SACN students attain a broad spectrum of scientific, critical thinking, humanistic, communication, and leadership concepts and experiences expected of today's medical professionals.*

Saint Anthony College of Nursing (SACN) is a specialized college granting the Bachelor of Science in Nursing (B.S.N.) and Master of Science in Nursing (M.S.N.) degrees. The College is located in Rockford, Illinois, in the north-central part of the state. The surrounding area provides much to see and do. Students receive excellent academic instruction along with abundant clinical experience.

Striving for excellence in nursing education, SACN's upper-division baccalaureate nursing program integrates Christian ideals, values, and practices, while building on a broad foundation of general education courses in the humanities and sciences.

SACN students are admitted as juniors, entering with the prerequisite credits from another regionally accredited college or university. They complete the last two years of a four-year Bachelor of Science in Nursing (B.S.N.) degree, which provides a broad spectrum of scientific, critical thinking, humanistic, communication, and leadership concepts and experiences expected of today's medical professionals. These last two years build on the broad base of two academic years (64 semester hours) transferred from another regionally accredited college or university. To this end, cooperative agreements have been reached with several of the community colleges in the area. Prospective students are encouraged to work with the SACN admissions office at the beginning of their college career to ensure transfer of credits.

Clinical sites for B.S.N. students include Carrie Lynn Children's Center, Walter Lawson's Children's Home, Rosecrance Treatment Centers, Northern Illinois Hospice, Rockford Memorial Hospital, Rockford Public Schools, OSF Saint Anthony Medical Center, Visiting Nurses Association, Winnebago County Health Department, Winnebago County Housing Authority, and many other institutions.

Registered Nurses with an associate degree or diploma in nursing may apply for admission to the RN-to-BSN program. This program is designed with the working nurse in mind. Courses are held one night per week with a hybrid format (partially online and partially face-to-face), allowing the student flexibility and convenience. The RN-to-BSN program is offered on the main campus as well as in Freeport, Illinois, on Highland Community College's campus.

Graduate students enroll in a program designed for the part-time student to complete within three or four years, leading to a Master of Science in Nursing degree for nurse educators, clinical nurse leaders, clinical nurse specialists in adult health concepts, and family nurse practitioners. The faculty and staff members are well known for their ability to provide personal, individualized attention in a caring environment. Classes are generally held one night per week, with additional work done online.

Students entering the master's program must enter with a bachelor's degree. Students may present with a baccalaureate degree in nursing (B.S.N.) or a baccalaureate in a field other than nursing. Licensure as a registered nurse is required for the state in which they will partake of their clinical practicum. If the student's baccalaureate degree is not in nursing, he or she must successfully complete an undergraduate nursing concepts course and nursing research course from a regionally accredited college or university prior to enrolling in the master's-level nursing concepts course or nursing research course.

A post-master's certificate is available for those who already have earned an M.S.N. degree but would like to take courses toward eligibility for the Nurse Educator Certificate. Student-at-Large status is available for graduate students. Interested students should contact the Graduate Affairs Office for details.

The student-to-faculty ratio at SACN is less than 8:1. The NCLEX-RN pass rate for 2013 was 97 percent, considerably higher than the state average of 85 percent or the national average of 83 percent. In addition, 85 percent of all undergraduate students applied for and received financial aid. Because SACN is a nonresidential facility, students commute from their homes or find a residence in the Rockford area.

Saint Anthony College of Nursing is accredited by the Higher Learning Commission, member of the North Central Association of Colleges and Schools (NCA). The B.S.N. and M.S.N. programs are accredited by the Commission on Collegiate Nursing Education.

---

- *FACULTY INFORMATION: http://www.sacn.edu/contact/*
- *MULTIMEDIA: http://www.sacn.edu*

- *2013–14 UNDERGRADUATE TUITION & FEES*

  *Full-time: $10,544 per semester*

  *Part-time: $659 per credit*

  *Testing fees vary from $93–$120*

  *Supplies fee: $60 (first semester)*

  *Graduation fee: $200*
- *2013–14 GRADUATE TUITION & FEES: $803 per credit*
- *APPLICATION DEADLINES:*

  *Undergraduate students: September 15 (spring admission); February 15 (fall admission)*

  *Graduate students: February 1*

**CONTACT INFORMATION**

**Nancy Sanders, Associate Dean**
**Saint Anthony College of Nursing**
**5658 E. State Street**
**Rockford, Illinois 61108-2468**
**Phone: 815-395-5100**
**Fax: 815-395-2275**
**E-mail: admissions@sacn.edu**
**Web site: http://www.sacn.edu**

**UNDERGRADUATE NURSING PROGRAM:**
**April Lipnitzky**
**Supervisor of Enrollment Management**
**Phone: 815-227-2141**
**E-mail: admissions@sacn.edu**

**GRADUATE NURSING PROGRAM:**
**Melissa Wrolstad**
**Graduate Affairs Specialist**
**Phone: 815-395-5476**
**E-mail: melissawrolstad@sacn.edu**

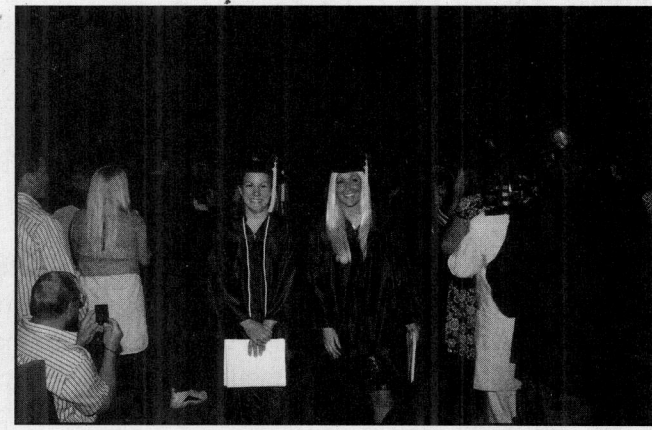

*Saint Anthony College of Nursing students have a high graduation rate—92 percent of all students who attend the first day of class (full-time and part-time) will graduate.*

# ST. FRANCIS COLLEGE

THE SMALL COLLEGE OF BIG DREAMS

St. Francis College has been recognized by "U.S. News & World Report" among the best regional colleges in the north and by "Assisted Living Today" as a Top 20 College Course for Geriatrics and Senior Care. The College was also named by Forbes.com to its America's Best Colleges List.

## NURSING PROGRAM

*Building a foundation of knowledge that will contribute to the development of the nursing profession and society as a whole.*

### Quality Private Education

Graduates of the St. Francis College Nursing Program go on to a wide variety of nursing careers at many of the best hospitals and health-care institutions in New York and nationally. St. Francis students are accepted into top graduate programs in nursing that include Columbia University Teacher's College, Long Island University, New York University, Pace University, and SUNY Downstate, among others. The College's well-rounded nursing program is excellent preparation for graduate school admission and careers such as nurse practitioners, clinical specialists, administrators and nurse educators.

### Academic Excellence

St. Francis College consistently makes the grade when it comes to college rankings. *U.S. News & World Report* classifies St. Francis as one of the "best regional colleges in the North," while Forbes.com places St. Francis on its America's Top Colleges list for the fourth year in a row. St. Francis was also recognized by *Assisted Living Today* as a Top 20 College Course for Geriatrics and Senior Care.

### Prepare Yourself for the Future of Nursing

The Nursing Program at St. Francis College offers a Bachelor of Science degree with a major in nursing to qualified high school graduates and transfer students interested in preparing for the NCLEX Exam (BSN Pre-Licensure Nursing Program), as well as to qualified students with a valid New York State RN license (RN to BS Program). St. Francis is registered with the New York State Education Department and accredited by the Commission on Collegiate Nursing Education (CCNE), the accrediting arm of the American Association of Colleges of Nursing (AACN). In addition to a nursing curriculum, students gain valuable knowledge and skills in liberal arts and sciences through courses focused on mathematics, natural sciences, social sciences, advanced writing, and oral communication.

The Pre-Licensure Nursing Program is open to students interested in full-time study only. For those students who are already registered nurses (RN to BS), flexible scheduling allows for full- or part-time study. In fact, the RN to BS program is designed for nurses who wish to keep working while continuing their education. All students are required to complete the program within a maximum five-year period.

### Department Mission

The mission of the Department of Nursing is consistent with the overall mission of the College—to promote the development of the whole person by integrating a liberal arts education with pre-professional programs designed to prepare nurses for the rigors of an increasingly technological and globalized marketplace and society. The department's mission encompasses the Franciscan and Catholic traditions that underpin its commitment to academic excellence, spiritual and moral values, physical fitness, social responsibility, and lifelong learning. These traditions include the Franciscan tradition of service, equality, aesthetics, freedom, honor, dignity, justice, and truth that are demonstrated within the context of professional nursing standards at the baccalaureate level (AACN Baccalaureate Essentials; ANA Standards of Clinical Nursing Practice). This nursing program builds a foundation of knowledge that will contribute to the development of the nursing profession as well as society as a whole.

Students who successfully complete the St. Francis Nursing program are able to:

- Integrate knowledge from bio/psycho/social/spiritual dimensions in caring for individuals, families, groups, and communities.
- Apply the nursing process in the delivery of culturally competent nursing care.
- Apply principles of leadership and management in caring for individuals, families, groups, and communities.
- Demonstrate accountability and responsibility for individual nursing actions.
- Collaborate as a member of a multidisciplinary healthcare team.
- Analyze research findings and technological advances for their applicability to clinical practice.
- Analyze national and international health policy initiatives for their impact on service, equality, aesthetics, freedom, human dignity, justice, and health of populations.
- Critically analyze the rationale for the nursing care provided.
- Incorporate the Franciscan tradition of service, equality, aesthetics, freedom, honor, dignity, justice, and truth into daily nursing practice.
- Recognize the legal and ethical health policy ramifications central to the delivery of health care.
- Demonstrate proficiency in the use of technology in the delivery of nursing care.
- Be prepared to sit for the Registered Nurse Licensing Exam (NCLEX).
- Be prepared for entrance into graduate schools that prepare nurses for advanced nursing roles including nurse practitioner, clinical specialist, and other specialties in the nursing profession that require advanced practice in nursing.

For details on tuition and fees, application deadlines, and more information, please visit the College's Web site at www.sfc.edu.

- *FACULTY:*
  www.sfc.edu/nursing
- *APPLICATION INFORMATION:*
  *Students are encouraged to apply through the St. Francis College website. Apply online at www.sfc.edu.*

**CONTACT INFORMATION**

**Office of Admissions**
**St. Francis College**
**180 Remsen Street**
**Brooklyn Heights, NY 11201**
**Phone: 718-489-5200**
**Web sites: www.sfc.edu**
**www.sfc.edu/nursing**

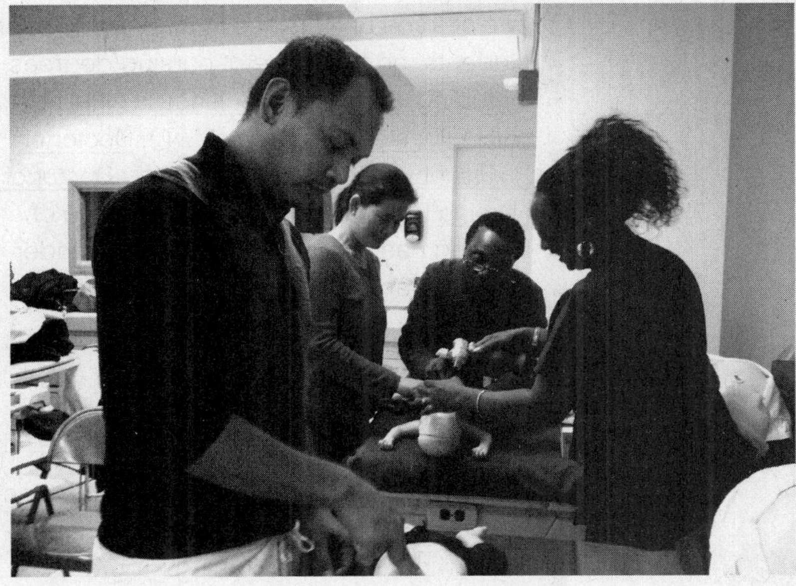

*Hands-on work with Sim Baby exposes St. Francis Nursing students to real-world medical scenarios.*

UNIVERSITY of WISCONSIN
UWMILWAUKEE

College of Nursing

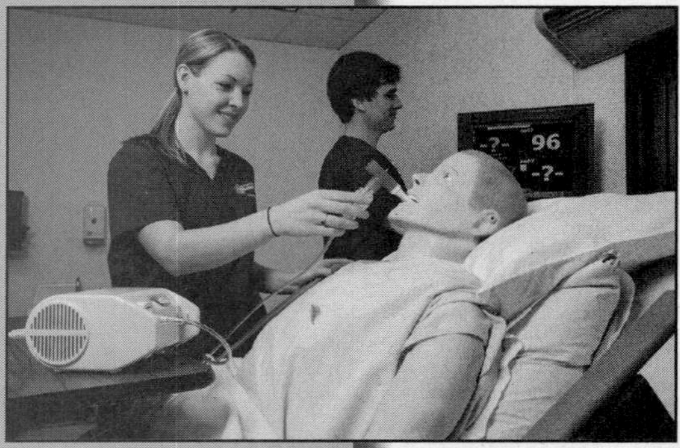

Students at UW-Milwaukee engage in experiential learning, clinical training, and high-level critical thinking.

## *IDEAS: Innovation, Discovery, Engagement, Access, Solutions.*

As Wisconsin's largest nursing program, the University of Wisconsin–Milwaukee College of Nursing has made its home in the commercial, cultural, and economic capital of Wisconsin for over 45 years. Across Southeastern Wisconsin, UW-Milwaukee's competitive, collaborative nursing program is valued for its ability to prepare science-based, compassionate nurse leaders through innovative, superior educational programs. The College is a vibrant, innovative environment for teaching, research, practice, and service to the community and the profession. The College is one of three universities in the state to offer students the full range of nursing degrees including: Bachelor of Science in Nursing (B.S.), Master of Nursing (M.N.), Doctor of Philosophy in Nursing (Ph.D.) and Doctor of Nursing Practice (D.N.P.). The College of Nursing has an enrollment of 1,154 undergraduate and 255 graduate students.

The College of Nursing's faculty creates innovative classroom environments and provide the latest technological teaching tools. The College is consistently ranked in the top 10 percent for academic excellence by the *U.S. News and World Report* of colleges with Graduate Nursing Programs. Faculty members embrace practice by engaging regional and global communities in the development of solutions to improve health care.

The College enjoys clinical practice and research partnerships with over 130 clinical facilities throughout Southeast Wisconsin and beyond. The College's Community Nursing Centers address the health needs of at-risk urban populations, engaging with community members to provide health-care solutions aligned with their needs. Nationally recognized initiatives include the Collaborative for Intelligent Health Information Systems Initiative (CIHISI), a research center dedicated to creating health information technology solutions that improve the access, quality, and costs of health care. The Pediatric Nursing Research Consortium, a partnership with Children's Hospital of Wisconsin, the Medical College of Wisconsin, and Marquette University, combines the resources of clinical and academic researchers to create translational research in the care of children and families. The Self Management Science Center, a continuation of NIH Funded P20, expands research aimed at enhancing the science of the self-management in individuals and families. Faculty members have also extended the scope of international research to health care in rural Malawi, Thailand and Kenya. The College also maintains a 15-year partnership with two sister nursing schools in South Korea. The baccalaureate, master, and doctorate programs are accredited by the Commission on Collegiate Nursing Education. The College of Nursing is also affiliated with Sigma Theta Tau International, Eta Nu Chapter, and the Nursing Centers Research Network.

The undergraduate nursing program is built upon a rigorous science-based curriculum and requires a dedication to scholarship and a passion for health care. Students master nursing theory and practice through hands-on learning and technology. With focused clinical cohorts, teachers are key in student success providing mentorship, career preparation, and support. The College of Nursing continues to expand and enhance its graduate program opportunities. The College offers the Master in Nursing (M.N.) with two entry options. Entry to the Master of Nursing degree is for nurses and non-nurses who hold a bachelor's degree. The program provides the framework for practice as a clinical nurse leader, public health nurse, clinical research manager, health informatics specialist or nurse manager. In addition to the Master of Nursing, the College offers two doctoral programs: Doctor of Nursing Practice (D.N.P.) and Doctor of Philosophy in Nursing (Ph.D.) in face-to-face and online formats.

Graduate program application deadlines depend on the program of interest. Generally, applications are due to UWM by February 1 for fall enrollment and October 1 for spring semester enrollment. Prospective students are encouraged to visit the College website at www.nursing.uwm.edu for more detailed information about admission requirements.

- *2013–14 UNDERGRADUATE TUITION & FEES:*
  *Annual Full-time: $9,300 (residents)*
  *$19,028 (nonresidents)*

  *Additional tuition differential fee of $32 per credit is due upon admission to the clinical major.*
- *2013–14 GRADUATE TUITION & FEES:*
  *Annual Full-time: $11,596 (residents)*
  *$24,061 (nonresidents)*
- *APPLICATION DEADLINES:*
  *Undergraduate: December 2 for spring admission; March 1 for fall admission*

  *Graduate: February 1 for fall admission; October 1 for spring admission*

**CONTACT INFORMATION**

**Office of Student Affairs**
**University of Wisconsin–Milwaukee College of Nursing**
**1921 East Hartford Avenue**
**Milwaukee, Wisconsin 53201**
**Phone: 414-229-5047**
**Fax: 414-229-5554**
**E-mail: asknursing@uwm.edu**
**Web site: www.nursing.uwm.edu**

**Find us on Facebook®:** https://www.facebook.com/UWMNursing

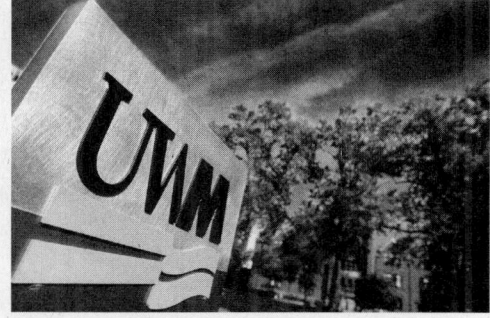


*Connect with businesses, corporations and recreational hotspots that make Milwaukee the economic/cultural/entertainment capital of Wisconsin.*

# INDEXES

# Baccalaureate Programs

## ACCELERATED BACCALAUREATE

### U.S. AND U.S. TERRITORIES

#### Alabama

University of South Alabama, College of Nursing, *Mobile (BSN)*

#### Arizona

Arizona State University at the Downtown Phoenix Campus, College of Nursing, *Phoenix (BSN)*

Chamberlain College of Nursing, *Phoenix (BSN)*

University of Phoenix–Online Campus, Online Campus, *Phoenix (BSN)*

University of Phoenix–Phoenix Campus, College of Nursing, *Tempe (BSN)*

University of Phoenix–Southern Arizona Campus, College of Social Sciences, *Tucson (BSN)*

#### California

American University of Health Sciences, School of Nursing, *Signal Hill (BSN)*

Azusa Pacific University, School of Nursing, *Azusa (BSN)*

California State University, Long Beach, School of Nursing, *Long Beach (BSN)*

California State University, Northridge, Nursing Program, *Northridge (BSN)*

California State University, San Marcos, School of Nursing, *San Marcos (BSN)*

Mount St. Mary's College, Department of Nursing, *Los Angeles (BSN, BSc PN)*

Samuel Merritt University, School of Nursing, *Oakland (BSN)*

University of Phoenix–Bay Area Campus, College of Nursing, *San Jose (BSN)*

University of Phoenix–Sacramento Valley Campus, College of Nursing, *Sacramento (BSN)*

University of Phoenix–San Diego Campus, College of Nursing, *San Diego (BSN)*

University of Phoenix–Southern California Campus, College of Nursing, *Costa Mesa (BSN)*

#### Colorado

Denver School of Nursing, *Denver (BSN)*

Platt College, School of Nursing, *Aurora (BSN)*

Regis University, School of Nursing, *Denver (BSN)*

University of Colorado Denver, College of Nursing, *Aurora (BS)*

University of Northern Colorado, School of Nursing, *Greeley (BS)*

#### Connecticut

St. Vincent's College, Nursing Program, *Bridgeport (BSN)*

Southern Connecticut State University, Department of Nursing, *New Haven (BS)*

#### District of Columbia

The Catholic University of America, School of Nursing, *Washington (BSN)*

#### Florida

Barry University, Division of Nursing, *Miami Shores (BSN)*

Florida Southern College, School of Nursing & Health Sciences, *Lakeland (BSN)*

Florida State University, College of Nursing, *Tallahassee (BSN)*

Jacksonville University, School of Nursing, *Jacksonville (BSN)*

University of Phoenix–North Florida Campus, College of Nursing, *Jacksonville (BSN)*

University of Phoenix–West Florida Campus, College of Nursing, *Temple Terrace (BSN)*

#### Georgia

Kennesaw State University, School of Nursing, *Kennesaw (BSN)*

#### Hawaii

University of Phoenix–Hawaii Campus, College of Nursing, *Honolulu (BSN)*

#### Illinois

Olivet Nazarene University, Division of Nursing, *Bourbonnais (BSN)*

Resurrection University, *Chicago (BSN)*

Southern Illinois University Edwardsville, School of Nursing, *Edwardsville (BS)*

Trinity College of Nursing and Health Sciences, *Rock Island (BSN)*

#### Indiana

Ball State University, School of Nursing, *Muncie (BS)*

Marian University, School of Nursing, *Indianapolis (BSN)*

Purdue University North Central, Department of Nursing, *Westville (BS)*

Valparaiso University, College of Nursing, *Valparaiso (BSN)*

#### Iowa

Allen College, Program in Nursing, *Waterloo (BSN)*

#### Kansas

MidAmerica Nazarene University, Division of Nursing, *Olathe (BSN)*

Wichita State University, School of Nursing, *Wichita (BSN)*

#### Louisiana

University of Phoenix–Louisiana Campus, College of Nursing, *Metairie (BSN)*

#### Maine

University of Maine at Fort Kent, Department of Nursing, *Fort Kent (BSN)*

#### Maryland

Bowie State University, Department of Nursing, *Bowie (BSN)*

The Johns Hopkins University, School of Nursing, *Baltimore (BS)*

#### Massachusetts

MCPHS University, School of Nursing, *Boston (BSN)*

MGH Institute of Health Professions, School of Nursing, *Boston (BSN)*

Regis College, School of Nursing, Science and Health Professions, *Weston (BSN)*

Simmons College, School of Nursing and Health Sciences, *Boston (BS)*

#### Michigan

Northern Michigan University, College of Nursing and Allied Health Science, *Marquette (BSN)*

#### Missouri

Cox College, Department of Nursing, *Springfield (BSN)*

Goldfarb School of Nursing at Barnes-Jewish College, *St. Louis (BSN)*

Graceland University, School of Nursing, *Independence (BSN)*

Maryville University of Saint Louis, Nursing Program, School of Health Professions, *St. Louis (BSN)*

Research College of Nursing, College of Nursing, *Kansas City (BSN)*

Saint Louis University, School of Nursing, *St. Louis (BSN)*

University of Missouri, Sinclair School of Nursing, *Columbia (BSN)*

University of Missouri–Kansas City, School of Nursing and Health Studies, *Kansas City (BSN)*

University of Missouri–St. Louis, College of Nursing, *St. Louis (BSN)*

William Jewell College, Department of Nursing, *Liberty (BS)*

#### Nebraska

University of Nebraska Medical Center, College of Nursing, *Omaha (BSN)*

#### Nevada

Roseman University of Health Sciences, College of Nursing, *Henderson (BSN)*

University of Nevada, Las Vegas, School of Nursing, *Las Vegas (BSN)*

University of Nevada, Reno, Orvis School of Nursing, *Reno (BSN)*

#### New Jersey

Caldwell College, Nursing Programs, *Caldwell (BSN)*

#### New Mexico

University of Phoenix–New Mexico Campus, College of Nursing, *Albuquerque (BSN)*

#### New York

Columbia University, School of Nursing, *New York (BS)*

Hartwick College, Department of Nursing, *Oneonta (BS)*

Hunter College of the City University of New York, Hunter-Bellevue School of Nursing, *New York (BSN)*

Mount Saint Mary College, Division of Nursing, *Newburgh (BSN)*

The Sage Colleges, Department of Nursing, *Troy (BS)*

State University of New York Institute of Technology, School of Nursing and Health Systems, *Utica (BS)*

Stony Brook University, State University of New York, School of Nursing, *Stony Brook (BS)*

### North Carolina

Queens University of Charlotte, Presbyterian School of Nursing, *Charlotte (BSN)*

The University of North Carolina at Chapel Hill, School of Nursing, *Chapel Hill (BSN)*

Western Carolina University, School of Nursing, *Cullowhee (BSN)*

### Ohio

Ashland University, Dwight Schar College of Nursing and Health Sciences, *Ashland (BSN)*

Chamberlain College of Nursing, *Columbus (BSN)*

Franklin University, Nursing Program, *Columbus (BSN)*

Kent State University, College of Nursing, *Kent (BSN)*

University of Phoenix–Cleveland Campus, College of Nursing, *Independence (BSN)*

Ursuline College, The Breen School of Nursing, *Pepper Pike (BSN)*

Walsh University, Department of Nursing, *North Canton (BSN)*

### Oklahoma

Northwestern Oklahoma State University, Division of Nursing, *Alva (BSN)*

Oklahoma City University, Kramer School of Nursing, *Oklahoma City (BSN)*

### Oregon

Oregon Health & Science University, School of Nursing, *Portland (BS)*

### Pennsylvania

DeSales University, Department of Nursing and Health, *Center Valley (BSN)*

Drexel University, College of Nursing and Health Professions, *Philadelphia (BSN)*

Edinboro University of Pennsylvania, Department of Nursing, *Edinboro (BSN)*

Lock Haven University of Pennsylvania, Nursing Program, *Lock Haven (BSN)*

Moravian College, Department of Nursing, *Bethlehem (BS)*

Thomas Jefferson University, Department of Nursing, *Philadelphia (BSN)*

University of Pennsylvania, School of Nursing, *Philadelphia (BSN)*

Waynesburg University, Department of Nursing, *Waynesburg (BSN)*

### Puerto Rico

Inter American University of Puerto Rico, Metropolitan Campus, Carmen Torres de Tiburcio School of Nursing, *San Juan (BSN)*

### South Carolina

Clemson University, School of Nursing, *Clemson (BS)*

Lander University, School of Nursing, *Greenwood (BSN)*

Medical University of South Carolina, College of Nursing, *Charleston (BSN)*

### South Dakota

South Dakota State University, College of Nursing, *Brookings (BS)*

University of Sioux Falls, School of Nursing, *Sioux Falls (BSN)*

### Tennessee

Belmont University, School of Nursing, *Nashville (BSN)*

Carson-Newman University, Department of Nursing, *Jefferson City (BSN)*

Cumberland University, Rudy School of Nursing and Health Professions, *Lebanon (BSN)*

Lincoln Memorial University, Caylor School of Nursing, *Harrogate (BSN)*

University of Memphis, Loewenberg School of Nursing, *Memphis (BSN)*

The University of Tennessee, College of Nursing, *Knoxville (BSN)*

The University of Tennessee Health Science Center, College of Nursing, *Memphis (BSN)*

### Texas

The University of Texas at Arlington, College of Nursing, *Arlington (BSN)*

The University of Texas at El Paso, School of Nursing, *El Paso (BSN)*

### Utah

University of Utah, College of Nursing, *Salt Lake City (BS)*

Western Governors University, Online College of Health Professions, *Salt Lake City (BS)*

### Virginia

Hampton University, School of Nursing, *Hampton (BS)*

Lynchburg College, School of Health Sciences and Human Performance, *Lynchburg (BS)*

Old Dominion University, Department of Nursing, *Norfolk (BSN)*

### Washington

University of Washington, School of Nursing, *Seattle (BSN)*

### West Virginia

West Virginia University, School of Nursing, *Morgantown (BSN)*

### Wisconsin

Bellin College, Nursing Program, *Green Bay (BSN)*

Milwaukee School of Engineering, School of Nursing, *Milwaukee (BSN)*

University of Wisconsin–Oshkosh, College of Nursing, *Oshkosh (BSN)*

## CANADA

### Alberta

University of Calgary, Faculty of Nursing, *Calgary (BN)*

University of Lethbridge, Faculty of Health Sciences, *Lethbridge (BN)*

### British Columbia

The University of British Columbia, Program in Nursing, *Vancouver (BSN)*

### New Brunswick

University of New Brunswick Fredericton, Faculty of Nursing, *Fredericton (BN)*

### Newfoundland and Labrador

Memorial University of Newfoundland, School of Nursing, *St. John's (BN)*

### Nova Scotia

St. Francis Xavier University, Department of Nursing, *Antigonish (BScN)*

### Ontario

Lakehead University, School of Nursing, *Thunder Bay (BScN)*

Queen's University at Kingston, School of Nursing, *Kingston (BNSc)*

Trent University, Nursing Program, *Peterborough (BScN)*

University of Toronto, Faculty of Nursing, *Toronto (BScN)*

The University of Western Ontario, School of Nursing, *London (BScN)*

### Quebec

Université Laval, Faculty of Nursing, *Québec (BScN)*

### Saskatchewan

University of Saskatchewan, College of Nursing, *Saskatoon (BSN)*

# ACCELERATED BACCALAUREATE FOR SECOND DEGREE

## U.S. AND U.S. TERRITORIES

### Alabama

Samford University, Ida V. Moffett School of Nursing, *Birmingham (BSN)*

### Arizona

Arizona State University at the Downtown Phoenix Campus, College of Nursing, *Phoenix (BSN)*

Brookline College, Baccalaureate Nursing Program, *Phoenix (BSN)*

Chamberlain College of Nursing, *Phoenix (BSN)*

Northern Arizona University, School of Nursing, *Flagstaff (BSN)*

### Arkansas

Arkansas State University, Department of Nursing, *State University (BSN)*

### California

Concordia University, Bachelor of Science in Nursing Program, *Irvine (BSN)*

Loma Linda University, School of Nursing, *Loma Linda (BS)*

### Colorado

Colorado State University–Pueblo, Department of Nursing, *Pueblo (BSN)*

Denver School of Nursing, *Denver (BSN)*

Metropolitan State University of Denver, Department of Health Professions, *Denver (BSN)*

University of Colorado Colorado Springs, Beth-El College of Nursing and Health Sciences, *Colorado Springs (BSN)*

### Connecticut

Fairfield University, School of Nursing, *Fairfield (BSN)*

Quinnipiac University, School of Nursing, *Hamden (BSN)*

University of Connecticut, School of Nursing, *Storrs (BS)*

### Delaware

University of Delaware, School of Nursing, *Newark (BSN)*

### District of Columbia

The Catholic University of America, School of Nursing, *Washington (BSN)*

Georgetown University, School of Nursing and Health Studies, *Washington (BSN)*
The George Washington University, School of Nursing, *Washington (BSN)*

### Florida

Barry University, Division of Nursing, *Miami Shores (BSN)*
Florida Atlantic University, Christine E. Lynn College of Nursing, *Boca Raton (BSN)*
Florida International University, Nursing Program, *Miami (BSN)*
Florida Southern College, School of Nursing & Health Sciences, *Lakeland (BSN)*
Jacksonville University, School of Nursing, *Jacksonville (BSN)*
Remington College of Nursing, *Lake Mary (BSN)*
University of Central Florida, College of Nursing, *Orlando (BSN)*
University of Florida, College of Nursing, *Gainesville (BSN)*
University of Miami, School of Nursing and Health Studies, *Coral Gables (BSN)*
University of North Florida, School of Nursing, *Jacksonville (BSN)*
University of South Florida, College of Nursing, *Tampa (BS)*

### Georgia

Albany State University, College of Sciences and Health Professions, *Albany (BSN)*
Armstrong Atlantic State University, Program in Nursing, *Savannah (BSN)*
Emory University, Nell Hodgson Woodruff School of Nursing, *Atlanta (BSN)*
Kennesaw State University, School of Nursing, *Kennesaw (BSN)*

### Idaho

Idaho State University, Department of Nursing, *Pocatello (BS)*

### Illinois

Blessing–Rieman College of Nursing, *Quincy (BSN)*
Bradley University, Department of Nursing, *Peoria (BSN, BSc PN)*
Illinois State University, Mennonite College of Nursing, *Normal (BSN)*
Lewis University, Program in Nursing, *Romeoville (BSN)*
Loyola University Chicago, Marcella Niehoff School of Nursing, *Maywood (BSN)*
Methodist College, *Peoria (BSN)*
Resurrection University, *Chicago (BSN)*
Saint Xavier University, School of Nursing, *Chicago (BSN)*
Trinity College of Nursing and Health Sciences, *Rock Island (BSN)*

### Indiana

Ball State University, School of Nursing, *Muncie (BS)*
Indiana State University, Department of Nursing, *Terre Haute (BS)*
Indiana University Northwest, School of Nursing, *Gary (BSN)*
Indiana University–Purdue University Indianapolis, School of Nursing, *Indianapolis (BSN)*
Indiana University South Bend, College of Health Sciences, *South Bend (BSN)*
Indiana Wesleyan University, School of Nursing, *Marion (BSN)*
Marian University, School of Nursing, *Indianapolis (BSN)*
Purdue University, School of Nursing, *West Lafayette (BS)*
Purdue University Calumet, School of Nursing, *Hammond (BS)*
Purdue University North Central, Department of Nursing, *Westville (BS)*
Saint Joseph's College, St. Elizabeth School of Nursing, *Rensselaer (BSN)*
University of Indianapolis, School of Nursing, *Indianapolis (BSN)*

### Iowa

Allen College, Program in Nursing, *Waterloo (BSN)*

### Kansas

Wichita State University, School of Nursing, *Wichita (BSN)*

### Kentucky

Bellarmine University, Donna and Allan Lansing School of Nursing and Health Sciences, *Louisville (BSN, MSCE)*
Northern Kentucky University, Department of Nursing, *Highland Heights (BSN)*
Spalding University, School of Nursing, *Louisville (BSN)*
University of Louisville, School of Nursing, *Louisville (BSN)*

### Louisiana

Louisiana State University Health Sciences Center, School of Nursing, *New Orleans (BSN)*
Our Lady of the Lake College, Division of Nursing, *Baton Rouge (BSN)*
Southeastern Louisiana University, School of Nursing, *Hammond (BS)*
University of Louisiana at Lafayette, College of Nursing, *Lafayette (BSN)*

### Maine

University of Southern Maine, School of Nursing, *Portland (BS)*

### Maryland

The Johns Hopkins University, School of Nursing, *Baltimore (BS)*
Salisbury University, Nursing DNP Program, *Salisbury (BS)*

### Massachusetts

Curry College, Division of Nursing, *Milton (BS)*
MCPHS University, School of Nursing, *Boston (BSN)*
Regis College, School of Nursing, Science and Health Professions, *Weston (BSN)*
Salem State University, Program in Nursing, *Salem (BSN)*
Simmons College, School of Nursing and Health Sciences, *Boston (BS)*
University of Massachusetts Amherst, School of Nursing, *Amherst (BS)*
University of Massachusetts Boston, College of Nursing and Health Sciences, *Boston (BS)*

### Michigan

Ferris State University, School of Nursing, *Big Rapids (BSN)*
Grand Valley State University, Kirkhof College of Nursing, *Allendale (BSN)*
Michigan State University, College of Nursing, *East Lansing (BSN)*
Saginaw Valley State University, College of Health and Human Services, *University Center (BSN)*
University of Detroit Mercy, McAuley School of Nursing, *Detroit (BSN)*
University of Michigan, School of Nursing, *Ann Arbor (BSN)*
University of Michigan–Flint, Department of Nursing, *Flint (BSN)*
Wayne State University, College of Nursing, *Detroit (BSN)*

### Minnesota

The College of St. Scholastica, Department of Nursing, *Duluth (BS)*
Concordia College, Department of Nursing, *Moorhead (BA)*
Minnesota State University Mankato, School of Nursing, *Mankato (BS)*

### Mississippi

University of Mississippi Medical Center, School of Nursing, *Jackson (BSN)*

### Missouri

Central Methodist University, College of Liberal Arts and Sciences, *Fayette (BSN)*
Cox College, Department of Nursing, *Springfield (BSN)*
Goldfarb School of Nursing at Barnes-Jewish College, *St. Louis (BSN)*
Research College of Nursing, College of Nursing, *Kansas City (BSN)*
Saint Louis University, School of Nursing, *St. Louis (BSN)*
University of Missouri, Sinclair School of Nursing, *Columbia (BSN)*

### Montana

Montana State University, College of Nursing, *Bozeman (BSN)*

### Nebraska

Creighton University, School of Nursing, *Omaha (BSN)*
Nebraska Methodist College, Department of Nursing, *Omaha (BSN)*
University of Nebraska Medical Center, College of Nursing, *Omaha (BSN)*

### Nevada

Nevada State College at Henderson, Nursing Program, *Henderson (BSN)*
Roseman University of Health Sciences, College of Nursing, *Henderson (BSN)*

### New Jersey

Fairleigh Dickinson University, Metropolitan Campus, Henry P. Becton School of Nursing and Allied Health, *Teaneck (BSN)*
Felician College, Division of Nursing and Health Management, *Lodi (BSN)*
New Jersey City University, Department of Nursing, *Jersey City (BSN)*
Rutgers, The State University of New Jersey, Newark, Rutgers School of Nursing, *Newark (BSN)*
Seton Hall University, College of Nursing, *South Orange (BSN)*

William Paterson University of New Jersey, Department of Nursing, *Wayne (BSN)*

**New York**

Adelphi University, College of Nursing and Public Health, *Garden City (BS)*

The College of New Rochelle, School of Nursing, *New Rochelle (BSN)*

Columbia University, School of Nursing, *New York (BS)*

Concordia College–New York, Nursing Program, *Bronxville (BS)*

Dominican College, Department of Nursing, *Orangeburg (BSN)*

Hartwick College, Department of Nursing, *Oneonta (BS)*

Lehman College of the City University of New York, Department of Nursing, *Bronx (BS)*

Le Moyne College, Nursing Programs, *Syracuse (BS)*

Long Island University–LIU Brooklyn, School of Nursing, *Brooklyn (BS)*

Molloy College, Division of Nursing, *Rockville Centre (BS)*

New York University, College of Nursing, *New York (BS)*

Niagara University, Department of Nursing, *Niagara University (BS)*

Pace University, Lienhard School of Nursing, *New York (BS)*

The Sage Colleges, Department of Nursing, *Troy (BS)*

State University of New York Downstate Medical Center, College of Nursing, *Brooklyn (BS)*

University at Buffalo, the State University of New York, School of Nursing, *Buffalo (BS)*

University of Rochester, School of Nursing, *Rochester (BS)*

Utica College, Department of Nursing, *Utica (BS)*

**North Carolina**

Duke University, School of Nursing, *Durham (BSN)*

North Carolina Agricultural and Technical State University, School of Nursing, *Greensboro (BSN)*

Queens University of Charlotte, Presbyterian School of Nursing, *Charlotte (BSN)*

The University of North Carolina at Chapel Hill, School of Nursing, *Chapel Hill (BSN)*

**North Dakota**

University of North Dakota, College of Nursing, *Grand Forks (BSN)*

**Ohio**

Ashland University, Dwight Schar College of Nursing and Health Sciences, *Ashland (BSN)*

Capital University, School of Nursing, *Columbus (BSN)*

Chamberlain College of Nursing, *Columbus (BSN)*

Cleveland State University, School of Nursing, *Cleveland (BSN)*

Kent State University, College of Nursing, *Kent (BSN)*

Mount Carmel College of Nursing, Nursing Programs, *Columbus (BSN)*

The University of Akron, School of Nursing, *Akron (BSN)*

University of Cincinnati, College of Nursing, *Cincinnati (BSN)*

Ursuline College, The Breen School of Nursing, *Pepper Pike (BSN)*

Walsh University, Department of Nursing, *North Canton (BSN)*

Wright State University, College of Nursing and Health, *Dayton (BSN)*

**Oklahoma**

Oklahoma City University, Kramer School of Nursing, *Oklahoma City (BSN)*

University of Oklahoma Health Sciences Center, College of Nursing, *Oklahoma City (BSN)*

**Oregon**

Linfield College, School of Nursing, *McMinnville (BSN)*

**Pennsylvania**

Drexel University, College of Nursing and Health Professions, *Philadelphia (BSN)*

Duquesne University, School of Nursing, *Pittsburgh (BSN)*

Edinboro University of Pennsylvania, Department of Nursing, *Edinboro (BSN)*

Holy Family University, School of Nursing and Allied Health Professions, *Philadelphia (BSN)*

Thomas Jefferson University, Department of Nursing, *Philadelphia (BSN)*

University of Pennsylvania, School of Nursing, *Philadelphia (BSN)*

University of Pittsburgh, School of Nursing, *Pittsburgh (BSN)*

Villanova University, College of Nursing, *Villanova (BSN)*

Waynesburg University, Department of Nursing, *Waynesburg (BSN)*

West Chester University of Pennsylvania, Department of Nursing, *West Chester (BSN)*

Wilkes University, Department of Nursing, *Wilkes-Barre (BS)*

**South Carolina**

Lander University, School of Nursing, *Greenwood (BSN)*

Medical University of South Carolina, College of Nursing, *Charleston (BSN)*

**Tennessee**

Belmont University, School of Nursing, *Nashville (BSN)*

Cumberland University, Rudy School of Nursing and Health Professions, *Lebanon (BSN)*

East Tennessee State University, College of Nursing, *Johnson City (BSN)*

Union University, School of Nursing, *Jackson (BSN)*

University of Memphis, Loewenberg School of Nursing, *Memphis (BSN)*

The University of Tennessee Health Science Center, College of Nursing, *Memphis (BSN)*

**Texas**

Baylor University, Louise Herrington School of Nursing, *Dallas (BSN)*

Texas A&M Health Science Center, College of Nursing, *College Station (BSN)*

Texas A&M University–Corpus Christi, College of Nursing and Health Sciences, *Corpus Christi (BSN)*

Texas Christian University, Harris College of Nursing, *Fort Worth (BSN)*

Texas Tech University Health Sciences Center, School of Nursing, *Lubbock (BSN)*

Texas Tech University Health Sciences Center-El Paso, *El Paso (BSN)*

University of Houston–Victoria, School of Nursing, *Victoria (BSN)*

The University of Texas at Arlington, College of Nursing, *Arlington (BSN)*

The University of Texas Health Science Center at Houston, School of Nursing, *Houston (BSN)*

The University of Texas Health Science Center at San Antonio, School of Nursing, *San Antonio (BSN)*

The University of Texas Medical Branch, School of Nursing, *Galveston (BSN)*

**Virginia**

George Mason University, College of Health and Human Services, *Fairfax (BSN)*

Marymount University, School of Health Professions, *Arlington (BSN)*

Norfolk State University, Department of Nursing, *Norfolk (BSN)*

Shenandoah University, Division of Nursing, *Winchester (BSN)*

Virginia Commonwealth University, School of Nursing, *Richmond (BS)*

**West Virginia**

West Virginia University, School of Nursing, *Morgantown (BSN)*

Wheeling Jesuit University, Department of Nursing, *Wheeling (BSN)*

**Wisconsin**

Bellin College, Nursing Program, *Green Bay (BSN)*

Edgewood College, Program in Nursing, *Madison (BS)*

Milwaukee School of Engineering, School of Nursing, *Milwaukee (BSN)*

University of Wisconsin–Eau Claire, College of Nursing and Health Sciences, *Eau Claire (BSN)*

University of Wisconsin–Oshkosh, College of Nursing, *Oshkosh (BSN)*

**Wyoming**

University of Wyoming, Fay W. Whitney School of Nursing, *Laramie (BSN)*

**CANADA**

**Alberta**

University of Alberta, Faculty of Nursing, *Edmonton (BScN)*

University of Calgary, Faculty of Nursing, *Calgary (BN)*

**British Columbia**

Kwantlen Polytechnic University, Faculty of Community and Health Sciences, *Surrey (BSN)*

The University of British Columbia, Program in Nursing, *Vancouver (BSN)*

**Nova Scotia**

St. Francis Xavier University, Department of Nursing, *Antigonish (BScN)*

**Ontario**

University of Ottawa, School of Nursing, *Ottawa (BScN)*

University of Toronto, Faculty of Nursing, *Toronto (BScN)*

## ACCELERATED LPN TO BACCALAUREATE

### U.S. AND U.S. TERRITORIES

**California**

San Francisco State University, School of Nursing, *San Francisco (BSN)*

**Massachusetts**

Fitchburg State University, Department of Nursing, *Fitchburg (BS)*

**New York**

Dominican College, Department of Nursing, *Orangeburg (BSN)*

**Oklahoma**

Northwestern Oklahoma State University, Division of Nursing, *Alva (BSN)*

Oklahoma Baptist University, School of Nursing, *Shawnee (BSN)*

**Pennsylvania**

Wilkes University, Department of Nursing, *Wilkes-Barre (BS)*

**South Dakota**

Mount Marty College, Nursing Program, *Yankton (BSN)*

**Virginia**

Norfolk State University, Department of Nursing, *Norfolk (BSN)*

### CANADA

**Nova Scotia**

St. Francis Xavier University, Department of Nursing, *Antigonish (BScN)*

## ACCELERATED RN BACCALAUREATE

### U.S. AND U.S. TERRITORIES

**Arizona**

Arizona State University at the Downtown Phoenix Campus, College of Nursing, *Phoenix (BSN)*

**Arkansas**

University of Arkansas for Medical Sciences, College of Nursing, *Little Rock (BSN)*

**California**

Azusa Pacific University, School of Nursing, *Azusa (BSN)*

Loma Linda University, School of Nursing, *Loma Linda (BS)*

West Coast University, Nursing Programs, *North Hollywood (BSN)*

**Colorado**

Colorado State University–Pueblo, Department of Nursing, *Pueblo (BSN)*

**Delaware**

Wilmington University, College of Health Professions, *New Castle (BSN)*

**Florida**

Northwest Florida State College, RN to BSN Degree Program, *Niceville (BSN)*

**Georgia**

Georgia State University, Byrdine F. Lewis School of Nursing and Health Professions, *Atlanta (BS)*

Thomas University, Division of Nursing, *Thomasville (BSN)*

University of West Georgia, School of Nursing, *Carrollton (BSN)*

**Idaho**

Boise State University, Department of Nursing, *Boise (BS)*

**Illinois**

Benedictine University, Department of Nursing, *Lisle (BSN)*

Lakeview College of Nursing, *Danville (BSN)*

Lewis University, Program in Nursing, *Romeoville (BSN)*

Resurrection University, *Chicago (BSN)*

University of St. Francis, Leach College of Nursing, *Joliet (BSN)*

**Indiana**

Indiana University Kokomo, Indiana University School of Nursing, *Kokomo (BSN)*

Marian University, School of Nursing, *Indianapolis (BSN)*

Purdue University Calumet, School of Nursing, *Hammond (BS)*

**Iowa**

Allen College, Program in Nursing, *Waterloo (BSN)*

Mount Mercy University, Department of Nursing, *Cedar Rapids (BSN)*

**Kansas**

MidAmerica Nazarene University, Division of Nursing, *Olathe (BSN)*

Tabor College, Department of Nursing, *Hillsboro (BSN)*

**Kentucky**

Eastern Kentucky University, Department of Baccalaureate and Graduate Nursing, *Richmond (BSN)*

Midway College, Program in Nursing (Baccalaureate), *Midway (BSN)*

Spalding University, School of Nursing, *Louisville (BSN)*

**Maine**

University of New England, Department of Nursing, *Biddeford (BSN)*

**Maryland**

Coppin State University, Helene Fuld School of Nursing, *Baltimore (BSN)*

Notre Dame of Maryland University, Department of Nursing, *Baltimore (BS)*

Stevenson University, Nursing Division, *Stevenson (BS)*

Washington Adventist University, Nursing Department, *Takoma Park (BS)*

**Massachusetts**

Regis College, School of Nursing, Science and Health Professions, *Weston (BSN)*

University of Massachusetts Amherst, School of Nursing, *Amherst (BS)*

**Michigan**

Ferris State University, School of Nursing, *Big Rapids (BSN)*

**Missouri**

Chamberlain College of Nursing, *St. Louis (BSN)*

Maryville University of Saint Louis, Nursing Program, School of Health Professions, *St. Louis (BSN)*

Missouri State University, Department of Nursing, *Springfield (BSN)*

**Nebraska**

Clarkson College, Master of Science in Nursing Program, *Omaha (BSN)*

Nebraska Methodist College, Department of Nursing, *Omaha (BSN)*

Nebraska Wesleyan University, Department of Nursing, *Lincoln (BSN)*

University of Nebraska Medical Center, College of Nursing, *Omaha (BSN)*

**New Jersey**

College of Saint Elizabeth, Department of Nursing, *Morristown (BSN)*

Rutgers, The State University of New Jersey, Camden, Rutgers School of Nursing–Camden, *Camden (BS)*

Seton Hall University, College of Nursing, *South Orange (BSN)*

**New York**

Binghamton University, State University of New York, Decker School of Nursing, *Vestal (BS)*

The College of New Rochelle, School of Nursing, *New Rochelle (BSN)*

Columbia University, School of Nursing, *New York (BS)*

Daemen College, Department of Nursing, *Amherst (BS)*

Dominican College, Department of Nursing, *Orangeburg (BSN)*

Keuka College, Division of Nursing, *Keuka Park (BS)*

Lehman College of the City University of New York, Department of Nursing, *Bronx (BS)*

Medgar Evers College of the City University of New York, Department of Nursing, *Brooklyn (BSN)*

Mercy College, Programs in Nursing, *Dobbs Ferry (BS)*

Molloy College, Division of Nursing, *Rockville Centre (BS)*

Mount Saint Mary College, Division of Nursing, *Newburgh (BSN)*

St. John Fisher College, Wegmans School of Nursing, *Rochester (BS)*

State University of New York Institute of Technology, School of Nursing and Health Systems, *Utica (BS)*

University of Rochester, School of Nursing, *Rochester (BS)*

**North Carolina**

Winston-Salem State University, Department of Nursing, *Winston-Salem (BSN)*

**Ohio**

College of Mount St. Joseph, Department of Nursing, *Cincinnati (BSN)*

Defiance College, Bachelor's Degree in Nursing, *Defiance (BSN)*

Ohio Northern University, Nursing Program, *Ada (BSN)*

Otterbein University, Department of Nursing, *Westerville (BSN)*

The University of Akron, School of Nursing, *Akron (BSN)*

Ursuline College, The Breen School of Nursing, *Pepper Pike (BSN)*

### Oklahoma

Bacone College, Department of Nursing, *Muskogee (BSN)*

Northeastern State University, Department of Nursing, *Tahlequah (BSN)*

Northwestern Oklahoma State University, Division of Nursing, *Alva (BSN)*

Oklahoma Wesleyan University, School of Nursing, *Bartlesville (BSN)*

### Pennsylvania

Carlow University, School of Nursing, *Pittsburgh (BSN)*

DeSales University, Department of Nursing and Health, *Center Valley (BSN)*

Eastern University, Program in Nursing, *St. Davids (BSN)*

Gwynedd Mercy University, School of Nursing, *Gwynedd Valley (BSN)*

Holy Family University, School of Nursing and Allied Health Professions, *Philadelphia (BSN)*

Immaculata University, Division of Nursing, *Immaculata (BSN)*

La Roche College, Department of Nursing and Nursing Management, *Pittsburgh (BSN)*

Misericordia University, Department of Nursing, *Dallas (BSN)*

Mount Aloysius College, Division of Nursing, *Cresson (BSN)*

Neumann University, Program in Nursing and Health Sciences, *Aston (BS)*

Thomas Jefferson University, Department of Nursing, *Philadelphia (BSN)*

University of Pennsylvania, School of Nursing, *Philadelphia (BSN)*

Wilkes University, Department of Nursing, *Wilkes-Barre (BS)*

### South Carolina

Lander University, School of Nursing, *Greenwood (BSN)*

### Tennessee

Aquinas College, School of Nursing, *Nashville (BSN)*

Cumberland University, Rudy School of Nursing and Health Professions, *Lebanon (BSN)*

East Tennessee State University, College of Nursing, *Johnson City (BSN)*

King College, School of Nursing, *Bristol (BSN)*

University of Memphis, Loewenberg School of Nursing, *Memphis (BSN)*

### Texas

The University of Texas at Arlington, College of Nursing, *Arlington (BSN)*

The University of Texas at Tyler, Program in Nursing, *Tyler (BSN)*

### Utah

Western Governors University, Online College of Health Professions, *Salt Lake City (BS)*

### West Virginia

Fairmont State University, School of Nursing and Allied Health Administration, *Fairmont (BSN)*

Marshall University, College of Health Professions, *Huntington (BSN)*

West Liberty University, Department of Health Sciences, *West Liberty (BSN)*

### Wisconsin

Milwaukee School of Engineering, School of Nursing, *Milwaukee (BSN)*

## CANADA

### Ontario

University of Ottawa, School of Nursing, *Ottawa (BScN)*

University of Toronto, Faculty of Nursing, *Toronto (BScN)*

### Quebec

McGill University, School of Nursing, *Montréal (BScN)*

Université du Québec à Chicoutimi, Program in Nursing, *Chicoutimi (BNSc)*

Université Laval, Faculty of Nursing, *Québec (BScN)*

### Saskatchewan

University of Saskatchewan, College of Nursing, *Saskatoon (BSN)*

# ADN TO BACCALAUREATE

## U.S. AND U.S. TERRITORIES

### Alabama

Tuskegee University, Program in Nursing, *Tuskegee (BSN)*

University of Mobile, School of Nursing, *Mobile (BSN)*

University of South Alabama, College of Nursing, *Mobile (BSN)*

### Arizona

Grand Canyon University, College of Nursing and Health Sciences, *Phoenix (BSN)*

Northern Arizona University, School of Nursing, *Flagstaff (BSN)*

### Arkansas

Arkansas Tech University, Program in Nursing, *Russellville (BSN)*

Harding University, College of Nursing, *Searcy (BSN)*

Henderson State University, Department of Nursing, *Arkadelphia (BSN)*

Southern Arkansas University–Magnolia, Department of Nursing, *Magnolia (BSN)*

University of Arkansas at Monticello, School of Nursing, *Monticello (BSN)*

University of Arkansas for Medical Sciences, College of Nursing, *Little Rock (BSN)*

University of Arkansas–Fort Smith, Carol McKelvey Moore School of Nursing, *Fort Smith (BSN)*

University of Central Arkansas, Department of Nursing, *Conway (BSN)*

### California

Azusa Pacific University, School of Nursing, *Azusa (BSN)*

Biola University, Department of Nursing, *La Mirada (BSN)*

California Baptist University, School of Nursing, *Riverside (BSN)*

California State University, Bakersfield, Program in Nursing, *Bakersfield (BSN)*

California State University, Chico, School of Nursing, *Chico (BSN)*

California State University, East Bay, Department of Nursing and Health Sciences, *Hayward (BS)*

California State University, Fresno, Department of Nursing, *Fresno (BSN)*

California State University, Fullerton, Department of Nursing, *Fullerton (BSN)*

California State University, Long Beach, School of Nursing, *Long Beach (BSN)*

California State University, Northridge, Nursing Program, *Northridge (BSN)*

California State University, Sacramento, School of Nursing, *Sacramento (BSN)*

California State University, Stanislaus, Department of Nursing, *Turlock (BSN)*

Loma Linda University, School of Nursing, *Loma Linda (BS)*

Mount St. Mary's College, Department of Nursing, *Los Angeles (BSN, BSc PN)*

Pacific Union College, Department of Nursing, *Angwin (BSN)*

Point Loma Nazarene University, School of Nursing, *San Diego (BSN)*

San Diego State University, School of Nursing, *San Diego (BSN)*

San Francisco State University, School of Nursing, *San Francisco (BSN)*

### Colorado

Colorado Mesa University, Department of Nursing and Radiologic Sciences, *Grand Junction (BSN)*

Colorado State University–Pueblo, Department of Nursing, *Pueblo (BSN)*

Denver School of Nursing, *Denver (BSN)*

Metropolitan State University of Denver, Department of Health Professions, *Denver (BSN)*

### Connecticut

Southern Connecticut State University, Department of Nursing, *New Haven (BS)*

University of Hartford, College of Education, Nursing, and Health Professions, *West Hartford (BSN)*

### Florida

Barry University, Division of Nursing, *Miami Shores (BSN)*

Jacksonville University, School of Nursing, *Jacksonville (BSN)*

Northwest Florida State College, RN to BSN Degree Program, *Niceville (BSN)*

St. Petersburg College, Department of Nursing, *St. Petersburg (BSN)*

University of Central Florida, College of Nursing, *Orlando (BSN)*

University of South Florida, College of Nursing, *Tampa (BS)*

The University of Tampa, Department of Nursing, *Tampa (BSN)*

University of West Florida, Department of Nursing, *Pensacola (BSN)*

### Georgia

Albany State University, College of Sciences and Health Professions, *Albany (BSN)*

Armstrong Atlantic State University, Program in Nursing, *Savannah (BSN)*
Brenau University, College of Health and Science, *Gainesville (BSN)*
Georgia Southern University, School of Nursing, *Statesboro (BSN)*
Kennesaw State University, School of Nursing, *Kennesaw (BSN)*
Middle Georgia State College, School of Nursing and Health Sciences, *Cochran (BSN)*
Thomas University, Division of Nursing, *Thomasville (BSN)*
University of North Georgia, Department of Nursing, *Dahlonega (BSN)*

### Guam
University of Guam, School of Nursing and Health Sciences, *Mangilao (BSN)*

### Hawaii
University of Hawaii at Hilo, Department in Nursing, *Hilo (BSN)*
University of Hawaii at Manoa, School of Nursing and Dental Hygiene, *Honolulu (BSN)*

### Idaho
Idaho State University, Department of Nursing, *Pocatello (BS)*
Lewis-Clark State College, Division of Nursing and Health Sciences, *Lewiston (BSN)*

### Illinois
Blessing–Rieman College of Nursing, *Quincy (BSN)*
Bradley University, Department of Nursing, *Peoria (BSN, BSc PN)*
Eastern Illinois University, Nursing Program, *Charleston (BSN)*
MacMurray College, Department of Nursing, *Jacksonville (BSN)*
McKendree University, Department of Nursing, *Lebanon (BSN)*
Northern Illinois University, School of Nursing and Health Studies, *De Kalb (BS)*
Resurrection University, *Chicago (BSN)*
Rockford University, Department of Nursing, *Rockford (BSN)*
Southern Illinois University Edwardsville, School of Nursing, *Edwardsville (BS)*
Trinity Christian College, Department of Nursing, *Palos Heights (BSN)*
Trinity College of Nursing and Health Sciences, *Rock Island (BSN)*
University of Illinois at Chicago, College of Nursing, *Chicago (BSN)*

### Indiana
Bethel College, School of Nursing, *Mishawaka (BSN)*
Huntington University, Department of Nursing, *Huntington (BSN)*
Indiana University East, School of Nursing, *Richmond (BSN)*
Indiana University–Purdue University Indianapolis, School of Nursing, *Indianapolis (BSN)*
Purdue University, School of Nursing, *West Lafayette (BS)*
Purdue University North Central, Department of Nursing, *Westville (BS)*
University of Indianapolis, School of Nursing, *Indianapolis (BSN)*
University of Saint Francis, Department of Nursing, *Fort Wayne (BSN)*

### Iowa
Allen College, Program in Nursing, *Waterloo (BSN)*
Briar Cliff University, Department of Nursing, *Sioux City (BSN)*
Iowa Wesleyan College, Division of Nursing, *Mount Pleasant (BSN)*
Mercy College of Health Sciences, Division of Nursing, *Des Moines (BSN)*
Mount Mercy University, Department of Nursing, *Cedar Rapids (BSN)*

### Kansas
Emporia State University, Newman Division of Nursing, *Emporia (BSN)*
Kansas Wesleyan University, Department of Nursing Education, *Salina (BSN)*
Tabor College, Department of Nursing, *Hillsboro (BSN)*
The University of Kansas, School of Nursing, *Kansas City (BSN)*
Washburn University, School of Nursing, *Topeka (BSN)*
Wichita State University, School of Nursing, *Wichita (BSN)*

### Kentucky
Kentucky State University, School of Nursing, *Frankfort (BSN)*
Midway College, Program in Nursing (Baccalaureate), *Midway (BSN)*
Morehead State University, Department of Nursing, *Morehead (BSN)*
Western Kentucky University, School of Nursing, *Bowling Green (BSN)*

### Louisiana
McNeese State University, College of Nursing, *Lake Charles (BSN)*
Northwestern State University of Louisiana, College of Nursing and Allied Health, *Shreveport (BSN)*
Our Lady of the Lake College, Division of Nursing, *Baton Rouge (BSN)*
University of Louisiana at Lafayette, College of Nursing, *Lafayette (BSN)*
University of Louisiana at Monroe, Nursing, *Monroe (BS)*

### Maine
University of Southern Maine, School of Nursing, *Portland (BS)*

### Maryland
Salisbury University, Nursing DNP Program, *Salisbury (BS)*
Stevenson University, Nursing Division, *Stevenson (BS)*

### Massachusetts
American International College, Division of Nursing, *Springfield (BSN)*
Anna Maria College, Department of Nursing, *Paxton (BSN)*
Framingham State University, Department of Nursing, *Framingham (BS)*
Regis College, School of Nursing, Science and Health Professions, *Weston (BSN)*
Salem State University, Program in Nursing, *Salem (BSN)*
Simmons College, School of Nursing and Health Sciences, *Boston (BS)*
Worcester State University, Department of Nursing, *Worcester (BS)*

### Michigan
Andrews University, Department of Nursing, *Berrien Springs (BS)*
Davenport University, Division of Nursing, *Grand Rapids (BSN)*
Eastern Michigan University, School of Nursing, *Ypsilanti (BSN)*
Grand Valley State University, Kirkhof College of Nursing, *Allendale (BSN)*
Lake Superior State University, Department of Nursing, *Sault Sainte Marie (BSN)*
Madonna University, College of Nursing and Health, *Livonia (BSN)*
Saginaw Valley State University, College of Health and Human Services, *University Center (BSN)*
Spring Arbor University, Program in Nursing, *Spring Arbor (BSN)*
Western Michigan University, College of Health and Human Services, *Kalamazoo (BSN)*

### Minnesota
Augsburg College, Program in Nursing, *Minneapolis (BS)*
The College of St. Scholastica, Department of Nursing, *Duluth (BS)*
Minnesota State University Moorhead, School of Nursing and Healthcare Leadership, *Moorhead (BSN)*
St. Catherine University, Department of Nursing, *St. Paul (BS)*

### Mississippi
Delta State University, School of Nursing, *Cleveland (BSN)*
Mississippi University for Women, College of Nursing and Speech Language Pathology, *Columbus (BSN)*
University of Mississippi Medical Center, School of Nursing, *Jackson (BSN)*
University of Southern Mississippi, School of Nursing, *Hattiesburg (BSN)*
William Carey University, School of Nursing, *Hattiesburg (BSN)*

### Missouri
Central Methodist University, College of Liberal Arts and Sciences, *Fayette (BSN)*
Chamberlain College of Nursing, *St. Louis (BSN)*
Cox College, Department of Nursing, *Springfield (BSN)*
Goldfarb School of Nursing at Barnes-Jewish College, *St. Louis (BSN)*
Graceland University, School of Nursing, *Independence (BSN)*
Missouri Southern State University, Department of Nursing, *Joplin (BSN)*
Missouri State University, Department of Nursing, *Springfield (BSN)*
Missouri Western State University, Department of Nursing, *St. Joseph (BSN)*
University of Central Missouri, Department of Nursing, *Warrensburg (BS)*
University of Missouri, Sinclair School of Nursing, *Columbia (BSN)*
Webster University, Department of Nursing, *St. Louis (BSN)*

### Montana
Montana State University–Northern, College of Nursing, *Havre (BSN)*

**Nebraska**

Clarkson College, Master of Science in Nursing Program, *Omaha (BSN)*

College of Saint Mary, Division of Health Care Professions, *Omaha (BSN)*

Midland University, Department of Nursing, *Fremont (BSN)*

Nebraska Wesleyan University, Department of Nursing, *Lincoln (BSN)*

Union College, Division of Health Sciences, *Lincoln (BSN)*

University of Nebraska Medical Center, College of Nursing, *Omaha (BSN)*

**Nevada**

Great Basin College, BSN Program, *Elko (BSN)*

Touro University, School of Nursing, *Henderson (BSN)*

University of Nevada, Reno, Orvis School of Nursing, *Reno (BSN)*

**New Hampshire**

Franklin Pierce University, Master of Science in Nursing, *Rindge (BS)*

Rivier University, Division of Nursing, *Nashua (BS)*

**New Jersey**

College of Saint Elizabeth, Department of Nursing, *Morristown (BSN)*

Kean University, Department of Nursing, *Union (BSN)*

Monmouth University, Marjorie K. Unterberg School of Nursing, *West Long Branch (BSN)*

Saint Peter's University, Nursing Program, *Jersey City (BSN)*

Seton Hall University, College of Nursing, *South Orange (BSN)*

William Paterson University of New Jersey, Department of Nursing, *Wayne (BSN)*

**New Mexico**

Eastern New Mexico University, Department of Allied Health–Nursing, *Portales (BSN)*

**New York**

The College at Brockport, State University of New York, Department of Nursing, *Brockport (BSN)*

Daemen College, Department of Nursing, *Amherst (BS)*

Elmira College, Program in Nursing Education, *Elmira (BS)*

Lehman College of the City University of New York, Department of Nursing, *Bronx (BS)*

Le Moyne College, Nursing Programs, *Syracuse (BS)*

Long Island University–LIU Brooklyn, School of Nursing, *Brooklyn (BS)*

Medgar Evers College of the City University of New York, Department of Nursing, *Brooklyn (BSN)*

Molloy College, Division of Nursing, *Rockville Centre (BS)*

The Sage Colleges, Department of Nursing, *Troy (BS)*

St. Francis College, Department of Nursing, *Brooklyn Heights (BS)*

St. John Fisher College, Wegmans School of Nursing, *Rochester (BS)*

State University of New York at Plattsburgh, Department of Nursing, *Plattsburgh (BS)*

State University of New York Institute of Technology, School of Nursing and Health Systems, *Utica (BS)*

State University of New York Upstate Medical University, College of Nursing, *Syracuse (BS)*

University of Rochester, School of Nursing, *Rochester (BS)*

York College of the City University of New York, Program in Nursing, *Jamaica (BS)*

**North Carolina**

Barton College, School of Nursing, *Wilson (BSN)*

East Carolina University, College of Nursing, *Greenville (BSN)*

Gardner-Webb University, School of Nursing, *Boiling Springs (BSN)*

Lees-McRae College, Nursing Program, *Banner Elk (BSN)*

Lenoir-Rhyne University, Program in Nursing, *Hickory (BS)*

Queens University of Charlotte, Presbyterian School of Nursing, *Charlotte (BSN)*

The University of North Carolina at Charlotte, School of Nursing, *Charlotte (BSN)*

The University of North Carolina at Greensboro, School of Nursing, *Greensboro (BSN)*

Winston-Salem State University, Department of Nursing, *Winston-Salem (BSN)*

**North Dakota**

Dickinson State University, Department of Nursing, *Dickinson (BSN)*

North Dakota State University, Department of Nursing, *Fargo (BSN)*

University of North Dakota, College of Nursing, *Grand Forks (BSN)*

**Ohio**

Ashland University, Dwight Schar College of Nursing and Health Sciences, *Ashland (BSN)*

Capital University, School of Nursing, *Columbus (BSN)*

Cedarville University, School of Nursing, *Cedarville (BSN)*

Defiance College, Bachelor's Degree in Nursing, *Defiance (BSN)*

Kent State University, College of Nursing, *Kent (BSN)*

Lourdes University, School of Nursing, *Sylvania (BSN)*

Malone University, School of Nursing, *Canton (BSN)*

Miami University, Department of Nursing, *Hamilton (BSN)*

Mount Vernon Nazarene University, School of Nursing and Health Sciences, *Mount Vernon (BS)*

Shawnee State University, Department of Nursing, *Portsmouth (BSN)*

The University of Akron, School of Nursing, *Akron (BSN)*

University of Cincinnati, College of Nursing, *Cincinnati (BSN)*

The University of Toledo, College of Nursing, *Toledo (BSN)*

Urbana University, College of Nursing and Allied Health, *Urbana (BSN)*

Ursuline College, The Breen School of Nursing, *Pepper Pike (BSN)*

**Oklahoma**

East Central University, Department of Nursing, *Ada (BS)*

Northwestern Oklahoma State University, Division of Nursing, *Alva (BSN)*

Oklahoma Baptist University, School of Nursing, *Shawnee (BSN)*

Oklahoma City University, Kramer School of Nursing, *Oklahoma City (BSN)*

Oklahoma Panhandle State University, Bachelor of Science in Nursing Program, *Goodwell (BSN)*

Oklahoma Wesleyan University, School of Nursing, *Bartlesville (BSN)*

Oral Roberts University, Anna Vaughn School of Nursing, *Tulsa (BSN)*

Rogers State University, Nursing Program, *Claremore (BSN)*

Southern Nazarene University, School of Nursing, *Bethany (BS)*

Southwestern Oklahoma State University, School of Nursing, *Weatherford (BSN)*

University of Oklahoma Health Sciences Center, College of Nursing, *Oklahoma City (BSN)*

**Oregon**

Linfield College, School of Nursing, *McMinnville (BSN)*

**Pennsylvania**

Bloomsburg University of Pennsylvania, Department of Nursing, *Bloomsburg (BSN)*

Clarion University of Pennsylvania, School of Nursing, *Oil City (BSN)*

DeSales University, Department of Nursing and Health, *Center Valley (BSN)*

Edinboro University of Pennsylvania, Department of Nursing, *Edinboro (BSN)*

Gannon University, Villa Maria School of Nursing, *Erie (BSN)*

Gwynedd Mercy University, School of Nursing, *Gwynedd Valley (BSN)*

Holy Family University, School of Nursing and Allied Health Professions, *Philadelphia (BSN)*

Marywood University, Department of Nursing, *Scranton (BSN)*

Mount Aloysius College, Division of Nursing, *Cresson (BSN)*

Neumann University, Program in Nursing and Health Sciences, *Aston (BS)*

Penn State University Park, School of Nursing, *University Park (BS)*

Slippery Rock University of Pennsylvania, Department of Nursing, *Slippery Rock (BSN)*

Thomas Jefferson University, Department of Nursing, *Philadelphia (BSN)*

University of Pennsylvania, School of Nursing, *Philadelphia (BSN)*

Villanova University, College of Nursing, *Villanova (BSN)*

Widener University, School of Nursing, *Chester (BSN)*

Wilkes University, Department of Nursing, *Wilkes-Barre (BS)*

York College of Pennsylvania, Department of Nursing, *York (BS)*

**Puerto Rico**

Inter American University of Puerto Rico, Metropolitan Campus, Carmen Torres de Tiburcio School of Nursing, *San Juan (BSN)*

University of Puerto Rico, Medical Sciences Campus, School of Nursing, *San Juan (BSN)*

### Rhode Island

University of Rhode Island, College of Nursing, *Kingston (BS)*

### South Carolina

Charleston Southern University, Wingo School of Nursing, *Charleston (BSN)*

Francis Marion University, Department of Nursing, *Florence (BSN)*

Newberry College, Department of Nursing, *Newberry (BSN)*

University of South Carolina Aiken, School of Nursing, *Aiken (BSN)*

### South Dakota

Mount Marty College, Nursing Program, *Yankton (BSN)*

Presentation College, Department of Nursing, *Aberdeen (BSN)*

### Tennessee

Austin Peay State University, School of Nursing, *Clarksville (BSN)*

Belmont University, School of Nursing, *Nashville (BSN)*

Bethel University, Nursing Program, *McKenzie (BSN)*

Cumberland University, Rudy School of Nursing and Health Professions, *Lebanon (BSN)*

East Tennessee State University, College of Nursing, *Johnson City (BSN)*

Lincoln Memorial University, Caylor School of Nursing, *Harrogate (BSN)*

Milligan College, Department of Nursing, *Milligan College (BSN)*

Southern Adventist University, School of Nursing, *Collegedale (BS)*

Tennessee Technological University, Whitson-Hester School of Nursing, *Cookeville (BSN)*

Tennessee Wesleyan College, Fort Sanders Nursing Department, *Knoxville (BSN)*

University of Memphis, Loewenberg School of Nursing, *Memphis (BSN)*

The University of Tennessee at Chattanooga, School of Nursing, *Chattanooga (BSN)*

The University of Tennessee at Martin, Department of Nursing, *Martin (BSN)*

The University of Tennessee Health Science Center, College of Nursing, *Memphis (BSN)*

### Texas

Lamar University, Department of Nursing, *Beaumont (BSN)*

Midwestern State University, Nursing Program, *Wichita Falls (BSN)*

Tarleton State University, Department of Nursing, *Stephenville (BSN)*

Texas A&M Health Science Center, College of Nursing, *College Station (BSN)*

Texas A&M University–Corpus Christi, College of Nursing and Health Sciences, *Corpus Christi (BSN)*

Texas A&M University–Texarkana, Nursing Department, *Texarkana (BSN)*

University of Mary Hardin-Baylor, College of Nursing, *Belton (BSN)*

The University of Texas at Brownsville, Department of Nursing, *Brownsville (BSN)*

The University of Texas at Tyler, Program in Nursing, *Tyler (BSN)*

The University of Texas Health Science Center at Houston, School of Nursing, *Houston (BSN)*

The University of Texas–Pan American, Department of Nursing, *Edinburg (BSN)*

University of the Incarnate Word, Program in Nursing, *San Antonio (BSN)*

West Texas A&M University, Department of Nursing, *Canyon (BSN)*

### Utah

University of Utah, College of Nursing, *Salt Lake City (BS)*

Utah Valley University, Department of Nursing, *Orem (BSN)*

Weber State University, Program in Nursing, *Ogden (BSN)*

### Vermont

Norwich University, Department of Nursing, *Northfield (BSN)*

Southern Vermont College, Department of Nursing, *Bennington (BSN)*

University of Vermont, Department of Nursing, *Burlington (BS)*

### Virgin Islands

University of the Virgin Islands, Division of Nursing, *Saint Thomas (BSN)*

### Virginia

Eastern Mennonite University, Department of Nursing, *Harrisonburg (BSN)*

Jefferson College of Health Sciences, Nursing Education Program, *Roanoke (BSN)*

Marymount University, School of Health Professions, *Arlington (BSN)*

Shenandoah University, Division of Nursing, *Winchester (BSN)*

University of Virginia, School of Nursing, *Charlottesville (BSN)*

The University of Virginia's College at Wise, Department of Nursing, *Wise (BSN)*

Virginia Commonwealth University, School of Nursing, *Richmond (BS)*

### Washington

University of Washington, School of Nursing, *Seattle (BSN)*

Walla Walla University, School of Nursing, *College Place (BS)*

### West Virginia

Bluefield State College, Program in Nursing, *Bluefield (BSN)*

Fairmont State University, School of Nursing and Allied Health Administration, *Fairmont (BSN)*

Shepherd University, Department of Nursing Education, *Shepherdstown (BSN)*

West Virginia University, School of Nursing, *Morgantown (BSN)*

### Wisconsin

Alverno College, Division of Nursing, *Milwaukee (BSN)*

Cardinal Stritch University, Ruth S. Coleman College of Nursing, *Milwaukee (BSN)*

Carroll University, Nursing Program, *Waukesha (BSN)*

Concordia University Wisconsin, Program in Nursing, *Mequon (BSN)*

Marian University, School of Nursing, *Fond du Lac (BSN)*

Silver Lake College of the Holy Family, Nursing Program, *Manitowoc (BSN)*

University of Wisconsin–Eau Claire, College of Nursing and Health Sciences, *Eau Claire (BSN)*

University of Wisconsin–Green Bay, BSN–LINC Online RN–BSN Program, *Green Bay (BSN)*

University of Wisconsin–Madison, School of Nursing, *Madison (BS)*

University of Wisconsin–Milwaukee, College of Nursing, *Milwaukee (BSN)*

University of Wisconsin–Oshkosh, College of Nursing, *Oshkosh (BSN)*

### Wyoming

University of Wyoming, Fay W. Whitney School of Nursing, *Laramie (BSN)*

## BACCALAUREATE FOR SECOND DEGREE

## U.S. AND U.S. TERRITORIES

### Alabama

Samford University, Ida V. Moffett School of Nursing, *Birmingham (BSN)*

Spring Hill College, Division of Nursing, *Mobile (BSN)*

The University of Alabama, Capstone College of Nursing, *Tuscaloosa (BSN)*

The University of Alabama at Birmingham, School of Nursing, *Birmingham (BSN)*

The University of Alabama in Huntsville, College of Nursing, *Huntsville (BSN)*

### Arizona

Arizona State University at the Downtown Phoenix Campus, College of Nursing, *Phoenix (BSN)*

### Arkansas

Arkansas Tech University, Program in Nursing, *Russellville (BSN)*

University of Arkansas for Medical Sciences, College of Nursing, *Little Rock (BSN)*

### California

California State University, Chico, School of Nursing, *Chico (BSN)*

California State University, Dominguez Hills, Program in Nursing, *Carson (BSN)*

California State University, Fullerton, Department of Nursing, *Fullerton (BSN)*

California State University, Long Beach, School of Nursing, *Long Beach (BSN)*

California State University, Sacramento, School of Nursing, *Sacramento (BSN)*

Dominican University of California, Program in Nursing, *San Rafael (BSN)*

Loma Linda University, School of Nursing, *Loma Linda (BS)*

National University, Department of Nursing, *La Jolla (BSN)*

University of California, Irvine, Program in Nursing Science, *Irvine (BS)*

### Colorado

Colorado State University–Pueblo, Department of Nursing, *Pueblo (BSN)*

### Connecticut

University of Saint Joseph, Department of Nursing, *West Hartford (BS)*

**Florida**

Barry University, Division of Nursing, *Miami Shores (BSN)*

Florida Southern College, School of Nursing & Health Sciences, *Lakeland (BSN)*

Jacksonville University, School of Nursing, *Jacksonville (BSN)*

**Georgia**

Emory University, Nell Hodgson Woodruff School of Nursing, *Atlanta (BSN)*

Georgia Southwestern State University, School of Nursing, *Americus (BSN)*

Kennesaw State University, School of Nursing, *Kennesaw (BSN)*

**Illinois**

Bradley University, Department of Nursing, *Peoria (BSN, BSc PN)*

Methodist College, *Peoria (BSN)*

Millikin University, School of Nursing, *Decatur (BSN)*

Resurrection University, *Chicago (BSN)*

Saint Anthony College of Nursing, *Rockford (BSN)*

University of Illinois at Chicago, College of Nursing, *Chicago (BSN)*

Western Illinois University, School of Nursing, *Macomb (BSN)*

**Indiana**

Ball State University, School of Nursing, *Muncie (BS)*

Indiana University Bloomington, Department of Nursing–Bloomington Division, *Bloomington (BSN)*

Marian University, School of Nursing, *Indianapolis (BSN)*

Purdue University, School of Nursing, *West Lafayette (BS)*

Purdue University North Central, Department of Nursing, *Westville (BS)*

**Iowa**

Allen College, Program in Nursing, *Waterloo (BSN)*

Clarke University, Department of Nursing and Health, *Dubuque (BS)*

Iowa Wesleyan College, Division of Nursing, *Mount Pleasant (BSN)*

Morningside College, Department of Nursing Education, *Sioux City (BSN)*

**Kansas**

Washburn University, School of Nursing, *Topeka (BSN)*

**Kentucky**

Eastern Kentucky University, Department of Baccalaureate and Graduate Nursing, *Richmond (BSN)*

University of Kentucky, College of Nursing, *Lexington (BSN)*

Western Kentucky University, School of Nursing, *Bowling Green (BSN)*

**Maryland**

Coppin State University, Helene Fuld School of Nursing, *Baltimore (BSN)*

Stevenson University, Nursing Division, *Stevenson (BS)*

**Massachusetts**

Regis College, School of Nursing, Science and Health Professions, *Weston (BSN)*

Simmons College, School of Nursing and Health Sciences, *Boston (BS)*

**Michigan**

Eastern Michigan University, School of Nursing, *Ypsilanti (BSN)*

Ferris State University, School of Nursing, *Big Rapids (BSN)*

Saginaw Valley State University, College of Health and Human Services, *University Center (BSN)*

**Minnesota**

St. Catherine University, Department of Nursing, *St. Paul (BS)*

**Missouri**

Cox College, Department of Nursing, *Springfield (BSN)*

Missouri Southern State University, Department of Nursing, *Joplin (BSN)*

Research College of Nursing, College of Nursing, *Kansas City (BSN)*

University of Missouri–St. Louis, College of Nursing, *St. Louis (BSN)*

**Montana**

Montana State University, College of Nursing, *Bozeman (BSN)*

**Nebraska**

Clarkson College, Master of Science in Nursing Program, *Omaha (BSN)*

University of Nebraska Medical Center, College of Nursing, *Omaha (BSN)*

**Nevada**

University of Nevada, Reno, Orvis School of Nursing, *Reno (BSN)*

**New Jersey**

Caldwell College, Nursing Programs, *Caldwell (BSN)*

Seton Hall University, College of Nursing, *South Orange (BSN)*

**New York**

College of Mount Saint Vincent, Department of Nursing, *Riverdale (BS)*

The College of New Rochelle, School of Nursing, *New Rochelle (BSN)*

Columbia University, School of Nursing, *New York (BS)*

Lehman College of the City University of New York, Department of Nursing, *Bronx (BS)*

Molloy College, Division of Nursing, *Rockville Centre (BS)*

The Sage Colleges, Department of Nursing, *Troy (BS)*

St. John Fisher College, Wegmans School of Nursing, *Rochester (BS)*

Wagner College, Department of Nursing, *Staten Island (BS)*

**North Carolina**

Queens University of Charlotte, Presbyterian School of Nursing, *Charlotte (BSN)*

The University of North Carolina at Chapel Hill, School of Nursing, *Chapel Hill (BSN)*

The University of North Carolina at Greensboro, School of Nursing, *Greensboro (BSN)*

Winston-Salem State University, Department of Nursing, *Winston-Salem (BSN)*

**North Dakota**

University of North Dakota, College of Nursing, *Grand Forks (BSN)*

**Ohio**

Ashland University, Dwight Schar College of Nursing and Health Sciences, *Ashland (BSN)*

Kent State University, College of Nursing, *Kent (BSN)*

Ursuline College, The Breen School of Nursing, *Pepper Pike (BSN)*

Wright State University, College of Nursing and Health, *Dayton (BSN)*

**Oklahoma**

Northwestern Oklahoma State University, Division of Nursing, *Alva (BSN)*

Oklahoma Baptist University, School of Nursing, *Shawnee (BSN)*

Oklahoma City University, Kramer School of Nursing, *Oklahoma City (BSN)*

Oklahoma Wesleyan University, School of Nursing, *Bartlesville (BSN)*

Southern Nazarene University, School of Nursing, *Bethany (BS)*

**Oregon**

Linfield College, School of Nursing, *McMinnville (BSN)*

**Pennsylvania**

Bloomsburg University of Pennsylvania, Department of Nursing, *Bloomsburg (BSN)*

Carlow University, School of Nursing, *Pittsburgh (BSN)*

Cedar Crest College, Department of Nursing, *Allentown (BS)*

DeSales University, Department of Nursing and Health, *Center Valley (BSN)*

Eastern University, Program in Nursing, *St. Davids (BSN)*

Edinboro University of Pennsylvania, Department of Nursing, *Edinboro (BSN)*

Gannon University, Villa Maria School of Nursing, *Erie (BSN)*

Indiana University of Pennsylvania, Department of Nursing and Allied Health, *Indiana (BSN)*

La Salle University, School of Nursing and Health Sciences, *Philadelphia (BSN)*

Misericordia University, Department of Nursing, *Dallas (BSN)*

Neumann University, Program in Nursing and Health Sciences, *Aston (BS)*

Robert Morris University, School of Nursing and Health Sciences, *Moon Township (BSN)*

Thomas Jefferson University, Department of Nursing, *Philadelphia (BSN)*

University of Pennsylvania, School of Nursing, *Philadelphia (BSN)*

The University of Scranton, Department of Nursing, *Scranton (BSN)*

Villanova University, College of Nursing, *Villanova (BSN)*

**Rhode Island**

Rhode Island College, Department of Nursing, *Providence (BSN)*

**South Carolina**

Lander University, School of Nursing, *Greenwood (BSN)*

**South Dakota**

Presentation College, Department of Nursing, *Aberdeen (BSN)*

**Tennessee**

Austin Peay State University, School of Nursing, *Clarksville (BSN)*

Belmont University, School of Nursing, *Nashville (BSN)*

Cumberland University, Rudy School of Nursing and Health Professions, *Lebanon (BSN)*

Milligan College, Department of Nursing, *Milligan College (BSN)*

Tennessee Technological University, Whitson-Hester School of Nursing, *Cookeville (BSN)*

University of Memphis, Loewenberg School of Nursing, *Memphis (BSN)*

The University of Tennessee at Chattanooga, School of Nursing, *Chattanooga (BSN)*

**Texas**

Texas A&M University–Corpus Christi, College of Nursing and Health Sciences, *Corpus Christi (BSN)*

Texas Woman's University, College of Nursing, *Denton (BS)*

The University of Texas at Arlington, College of Nursing, *Arlington (BSN)*

University of the Incarnate Word, Program in Nursing, *San Antonio (BSN)*

**Utah**

University of Utah, College of Nursing, *Salt Lake City (BS)*

Westminster College, School of Nursing and Health Sciences, *Salt Lake City (BSN)*

**Virginia**

Eastern Mennonite University, Department of Nursing, *Harrisonburg (BSN)*

Lynchburg College, School of Health Sciences and Human Performance, *Lynchburg (BS)*

Radford University, School of Nursing, *Radford (BSN)*

**Washington**

Seattle University, College of Nursing, *Seattle (BSN)*

**Wisconsin**

Alverno College, Division of Nursing, *Milwaukee (BSN)*

Bellin College, Nursing Program, *Green Bay (BSN)*

Columbia College of Nursing/Mount Mary College Nursing Program, *Milwaukee (BSN)*

Edgewood College, Program in Nursing, *Madison (BS)*

Milwaukee School of Engineering, School of Nursing, *Milwaukee (BSN)*

University of Wisconsin–Oshkosh, College of Nursing, *Oshkosh (BSN)*

## CANADA

**Alberta**

University of Alberta, Faculty of Nursing, *Edmonton (BScN)*

University of Calgary, Faculty of Nursing, *Calgary (BN)*

University of Lethbridge, Faculty of Health Sciences, *Lethbridge (BN)*

**Manitoba**

Brandon University, School of Health Studies, *Brandon (BN)*

University of Manitoba, Faculty of Nursing, *Winnipeg (BN)*

**Ontario**

McMaster University, School of Nursing, *Hamilton (BScN)*

University of Toronto, Faculty of Nursing, *Toronto (BScN)*

**Saskatchewan**

University of Saskatchewan, College of Nursing, *Saskatoon (BSN)*

# GENERIC BACCALAUREATE

## U.S. AND U.S. TERRITORIES

**Alabama**

Auburn University, School of Nursing, *Auburn University (BSN)*

Auburn University at Montgomery, School of Nursing, *Montgomery (BSN)*

Jacksonville State University, College of Nursing and Health Sciences, *Jacksonville (BSN)*

Oakwood University, Department of Nursing, *Huntsville (BS)*

Samford University, Ida V. Moffett School of Nursing, *Birmingham (BSN)*

Spring Hill College, Division of Nursing, *Mobile (BSN)*

Troy University, School of Nursing, *Troy (BSN)*

Tuskegee University, Program in Nursing, *Tuskegee (BSN)*

The University of Alabama, Capstone College of Nursing, *Tuscaloosa (BSN)*

The University of Alabama at Birmingham, School of Nursing, *Birmingham (BSN)*

The University of Alabama in Huntsville, College of Nursing, *Huntsville (BSN)*

University of Mobile, School of Nursing, *Mobile (BSN)*

University of North Alabama, College of Nursing and Allied Health, *Florence (BSN)*

University of South Alabama, College of Nursing, *Mobile (BSN)*

**Alaska**

University of Alaska Anchorage, School of Nursing, *Anchorage (BS)*

**Arizona**

Arizona State University at the Downtown Phoenix Campus, College of Nursing, *Phoenix (BSN)*

Brookline College, Baccalaureate Nursing Program, *Phoenix (BSN)*

Northern Arizona University, School of Nursing, *Flagstaff (BSN)*

The University of Arizona, College of Nursing, *Tucson (BSN)*

**Arkansas**

Arkansas State University, Department of Nursing, *State University (BSN)*

Arkansas Tech University, Program in Nursing, *Russellville (BSN)*

Harding University, College of Nursing, *Searcy (BSN)*

Henderson State University, Department of Nursing, *Arkadelphia (BSN)*

Southern Arkansas University–Magnolia, Department of Nursing, *Magnolia (BSN)*

University of Arkansas, Eleanor Mann School of Nursing, *Fayetteville (BSN)*

University of Arkansas at Monticello, School of Nursing, *Monticello (BSN)*

University of Arkansas at Pine Bluff, Department of Nursing, *Pine Bluff (BSN)*

University of Arkansas for Medical Sciences, College of Nursing, *Little Rock (BSN)*

University of Arkansas–Fort Smith, Carol McKelvey Moore School of Nursing, *Fort Smith (BSN)*

University of Central Arkansas, Department of Nursing, *Conway (BSN)*

**California**

American University of Health Sciences, School of Nursing, *Signal Hill (BSN)*

Azusa Pacific University, School of Nursing, *Azusa (BSN)*

Biola University, Department of Nursing, *La Mirada (BSN)*

California Baptist University, School of Nursing, *Riverside (BSN)*

California State University, Bakersfield, Program in Nursing, *Bakersfield (BSN)*

California State University Channel Islands, Nursing Program, *Camarillo (BSN)*

California State University, Chico, School of Nursing, *Chico (BSN)*

California State University, East Bay, Department of Nursing and Health Sciences, *Hayward (BS)*

California State University, Fresno, Department of Nursing, *Fresno (BSN)*

California State University, Fullerton, Department of Nursing, *Fullerton (BSN)*

California State University, Long Beach, School of Nursing, *Long Beach (BSN)*

California State University, Los Angeles, School of Nursing, *Los Angeles (BSN)*

California State University, Sacramento, School of Nursing, *Sacramento (BSN)*

California State University, San Bernardino, Department of Nursing, *San Bernardino (BSN)*

California State University, San Marcos, School of Nursing, *San Marcos (BSN)*

California State University, Stanislaus, Department of Nursing, *Turlock (BSN)*

Dominican University of California, Program in Nursing, *San Rafael (BSN)*

Loma Linda University, School of Nursing, *Loma Linda (BS)*

Mount St. Mary's College, Department of Nursing, *Los Angeles (BSN, BSc PN)*

National University, Department of Nursing, *La Jolla (BSN)*

Point Loma Nazarene University, School of Nursing, *San Diego (BSN)*

Samuel Merritt University, School of Nursing, *Oakland (BSN)*

San Diego State University, School of Nursing, *San Diego (BSN)*

San Francisco State University, School of Nursing, *San Francisco (BSN)*

San Jose State University, The Valley Foundation School of Nursing, *San Jose (BS)*

Sonoma State University, Department of Nursing, *Rohnert Park (BSN)*

University of California, Irvine, Program in Nursing Science, *Irvine (BS)*
University of California, Los Angeles, School of Nursing, *Los Angeles (BS)*
University of San Francisco, School of Nursing, *San Francisco (BSN)*

### Colorado

Adams State University, Nursing Program, *Alamosa (BSN)*
Colorado Christian University, Nursing Programs, *Lakewood (BSN)*
Colorado Mesa University, Department of Nursing and Radiologic Sciences, *Grand Junction (BSN)*
Colorado State University–Pueblo, Department of Nursing, *Pueblo (BSN)*
Denver School of Nursing, *Denver (BSN)*
Regis University, School of Nursing, *Denver (BSN)*
University of Colorado Colorado Springs, Beth-El College of Nursing and Health Sciences, *Colorado Springs (BSN)*
University of Colorado Denver, College of Nursing, *Aurora (BS)*
University of Northern Colorado, School of Nursing, *Greeley (BS)*

### Connecticut

Central Connecticut State University, Department of Nursing, *New Britain (BSN)*
Fairfield University, School of Nursing, *Fairfield (BSN)*
Quinnipiac University, School of Nursing, *Hamden (BSN)*
Sacred Heart University, Program in Nursing, *Fairfield (BSN)*
Southern Connecticut State University, Department of Nursing, *New Haven (BS)*
University of Connecticut, School of Nursing, *Storrs (BS)*
University of Saint Joseph, Department of Nursing, *West Hartford (BS)*
Western Connecticut State University, Department of Nursing, *Danbury (BS)*

### Delaware

Delaware State University, Department of Nursing, *Dover (BSN)*
University of Delaware, School of Nursing, *Newark (BSN)*
Wesley College, Nursing Program, *Dover (BSN)*

### District of Columbia

The Catholic University of America, School of Nursing, *Washington (BSN)*
Georgetown University, School of Nursing and Health Studies, *Washington (BSN)*
Howard University, Division of Nursing, *Washington (BSN)*
Trinity Washington University, Nursing Program, *Washington (BSN)*

### Florida

Adventist University of Health Sciences, Department of Nursing, *Orlando (BSN)*
Barry University, Division of Nursing, *Miami Shores (BSN)*
Bethune-Cookman University, School of Nursing, *Daytona Beach (BSN)*
Florida Agricultural and Mechanical University, School of Nursing, *Tallahassee (BSN)*
Florida Atlantic University, Christine E. Lynn College of Nursing, *Boca Raton (BSN)*
Florida Gulf Coast University, School of Nursing, *Fort Myers (BSN)*
Florida International University, Nursing Program, *Miami (BSN)*
Florida Southern College, School of Nursing & Health Sciences, *Lakeland (BSN)*
Florida State University, College of Nursing, *Tallahassee (BSN)*
Jacksonville University, School of Nursing, *Jacksonville (BSN)*
Kaplan University Online, The School of Nursing Online, *Fort Lauderdale (BSN)*
Nova Southeastern University, College of Health Care Sciences, *Fort Lauderdale (BSN)*
University of Central Florida, College of Nursing, *Orlando (BSN)*
University of Florida, College of Nursing, *Gainesville (BSN)*
University of Miami, School of Nursing and Health Studies, *Coral Gables (BSN)*
University of North Florida, School of Nursing, *Jacksonville (BSN)*
University of South Florida, College of Nursing, *Tampa (BS)*
The University of Tampa, Department of Nursing, *Tampa (BSN)*
University of West Florida, Department of Nursing, *Pensacola (BSN)*

### Georgia

Albany State University, College of Sciences and Health Professions, *Albany (BSN)*
Armstrong Atlantic State University, Program in Nursing, *Savannah (BSN)*
Brenau University, College of Health and Science, *Gainesville (BSN)*
Clayton State University, Department of Nursing, *Morrow (BSN)*
Columbus State University, Nursing Program, *Columbus (BSN)*
Emory University, Nell Hodgson Woodruff School of Nursing, *Atlanta (BSN)*
Georgia College & State University, College of Health Sciences, *Milledgeville (BSN)*
Georgia Regents University, School of Nursing, *Augusta (BSN)*
Georgia Southern University, School of Nursing, *Statesboro (BSN)*
Georgia Southwestern State University, School of Nursing, *Americus (BSN)*
Georgia State University, Byrdine F. Lewis School of Nursing and Health Professions, *Atlanta (BS)*
Kennesaw State University, School of Nursing, *Kennesaw (BSN)*
LaGrange College, Department of Nursing, *LaGrange (BSN)*
Georgia Baptist College of Nursing, *Atlanta (BSN)*
Middle Georgia State College, School of Nursing and Health Sciences, *Cochran (BSN)*
Piedmont College, School of Nursing, *Demorest (BSN)*
Shorter University, School of Nursing, *Rome (BSN)*
University of West Georgia, School of Nursing, *Carrollton (BSN)*
Valdosta State University, College of Nursing, *Valdosta (BSN)*

### Guam

University of Guam, School of Nursing and Health Sciences, *Mangilao (BSN)*

### Hawaii

Chaminade University of Honolulu, Nursing Program, *Honolulu (BSN)*
Hawai`i Pacific University, College of Nursing and Health Sciences, *Honolulu (BSN)*
University of Hawaii at Hilo, Department in Nursing, *Hilo (BSN)*
University of Hawaii at Manoa, School of Nursing and Dental Hygiene, *Honolulu (BSN)*

### Idaho

Boise State University, Department of Nursing, *Boise (BS)*
Idaho State University, Department of Nursing, *Pocatello (BS)*
Lewis-Clark State College, Division of Nursing and Health Sciences, *Lewiston (BSN)*
Northwest Nazarene University, School of Health and Science, *Nampa (BSN)*

### Illinois

Aurora University, School of Nursing, *Aurora (BSN)*
Blessing–Rieman College of Nursing, *Quincy (BSN)*
Bradley University, Department of Nursing, *Peoria (BSN, BSc PN)*
Chicago State University, Department of Nursing, *Chicago (BSN)*
Elmhurst College, Deicke Center for Nursing Education, *Elmhurst (BS)*
Illinois State University, Mennonite College of Nursing, *Normal (BSN)*
Illinois Wesleyan University, School of Nursing, *Bloomington (BSN)*
Lakeview College of Nursing, *Danville (BSN)*
Lewis University, Program in Nursing, *Romeoville (BSN)*
Loyola University Chicago, Marcella Niehoff School of Nursing, *Maywood (BSN)*
MacMurray College, Department of Nursing, *Jacksonville (BSN)*
Methodist College, *Peoria (BSN)*
Millikin University, School of Nursing, *Decatur (BSN)*
Northern Illinois University, School of Nursing and Health Studies, *De Kalb (BS)*
North Park University, School of Nursing, *Chicago (BS)*
Olivet Nazarene University, Division of Nursing, *Bourbonnais (BSN)*
Rockford University, Department of Nursing, *Rockford (BSN)*
Saint Anthony College of Nursing, *Rockford (BSN)*
Saint Francis Medical Center College of Nursing, Baccalaureate Nursing Program, *Peoria (BSN)*
St. John's College, Department of Nursing, *Springfield (BSN)*
Saint Xavier University, School of Nursing, *Chicago (BSN)*
Southern Illinois University Edwardsville, School of Nursing, *Edwardsville (BS)*
Trinity Christian College, Department of Nursing, *Palos Heights (BSN)*
Trinity College of Nursing and Health Sciences, *Rock Island (BSN)*

University of Illinois at Chicago, College of Nursing, *Chicago (BSN)*
University of St. Francis, Leach College of Nursing, *Joliet (BSN)*
Western Illinois University, School of Nursing, *Macomb (BSN)*

**Indiana**

Anderson University, School of Nursing, *Anderson (BSN)*
Ball State University, School of Nursing, *Muncie (BS)*
Bethel College, School of Nursing, *Mishawaka (BSN)*
Goshen College, Department of Nursing, *Goshen (BSN)*
Huntington University, Department of Nursing, *Huntington (BSN)*
Indiana State University, Department of Nursing, *Terre Haute (BS)*
Indiana University Bloomington, Department of Nursing–Bloomington Division, *Bloomington (BSN)*
Indiana University East, School of Nursing, *Richmond (BSN)*
Indiana University Kokomo, Indiana University School of Nursing, *Kokomo (BSN)*
Indiana University Northwest, School of Nursing, *Gary (BSN)*
Indiana University–Purdue University Fort Wayne, Department of Nursing, *Fort Wayne (BS)*
Indiana University–Purdue University Indianapolis, School of Nursing, *Indianapolis (BSN)*
Indiana University South Bend, College of Health Sciences, *South Bend (BSN)*
Indiana University Southeast, Division of Nursing, *New Albany (BSN)*
Indiana Wesleyan University, School of Nursing, *Marion (BSN)*
Marian University, School of Nursing, *Indianapolis (BSN)*
Purdue University, School of Nursing, *West Lafayette (BS)*
Purdue University Calumet, School of Nursing, *Hammond (BS)*
Saint Mary's College, Department of Nursing, *Notre Dame (BS)*
University of Evansville, Department of Nursing, *Evansville (BSN)*
University of Indianapolis, School of Nursing, *Indianapolis (BSN)*
University of Saint Francis, Department of Nursing, *Fort Wayne (BSN)*
University of Southern Indiana, College of Nursing and Health Professions, *Evansville (BSN)*
Valparaiso University, College of Nursing, *Valparaiso (BSN)*

**Iowa**

Allen College, Program in Nursing, *Waterloo (BSN)*
Briar Cliff University, Department of Nursing, *Sioux City (BSN)*
Clarke University, Department of Nursing and Health, *Dubuque (BS)*
Coe College, Department of Nursing, *Cedar Rapids (BSN)*
Dordt College, Nursing Program, *Sioux Center (BSN)*
Grand View University, Division of Nursing, *Des Moines (BSN)*
Iowa Wesleyan College, Division of Nursing, *Mount Pleasant (BSN)*
Luther College, Department of Nursing, *Decorah (BA)*
Morningside College, Department of Nursing Education, *Sioux City (BSN)*
Mount Mercy University, Department of Nursing, *Cedar Rapids (BSN)*
Northwestern College, Nursing Program, *Orange City (BSN)*
St. Ambrose University, Program in Nursing (BSN), *Davenport (BSN)*
The University of Iowa, College of Nursing, *Iowa City (BSN)*

**Kansas**

Baker University, School of Nursing, *Topeka (BSN)*
Benedictine College, Department of Nursing, *Atchison (BSN)*
Bethel College, Department of Nursing, *North Newton (BSN)*
Emporia State University, Newman Division of Nursing, *Emporia (BSN)*
Fort Hays State University, Department of Nursing, *Hays (BSN)*
Kansas Wesleyan University, Department of Nursing Education, *Salina (BSN)*
Newman University, Division of Nursing, *Wichita (BSN)*
Pittsburg State University, Department of Nursing, *Pittsburg (BSN)*
The University of Kansas, School of Nursing, *Kansas City (BSN)*
University of Saint Mary, Bachelor of Science in Nursing Program, *Leavenworth (BSN)*
Washburn University, School of Nursing, *Topeka (BSN)*
Wichita State University, School of Nursing, *Wichita (BSN)*

**Kentucky**

Bellarmine University, Donna and Allan Lansing School of Nursing and Health Sciences, *Louisville (BSN, MSCE)*
Berea College, Department of Nursing, *Berea (BSN)*
Eastern Kentucky University, Department of Baccalaureate and Graduate Nursing, *Richmond (BSN)*
Kentucky Christian University, School of Nursing, *Grayson (BSN)*
Morehead State University, Department of Nursing, *Morehead (BSN)*
Murray State University, Program in Nursing, *Murray (BSN)*
Northern Kentucky University, Department of Nursing, *Highland Heights (BSN)*
Spalding University, School of Nursing, *Louisville (BSN)*
Thomas More College, Program in Nursing, *Crestview Hills (BSN)*
Union College, School of Nursing & Health Sciences, *Barbourville (BSN)*
University of Kentucky, College of Nursing, *Lexington (BSN)*
University of Louisville, School of Nursing, *Louisville (BSN)*
Western Kentucky University, School of Nursing, *Bowling Green (BSN)*

**Louisiana**

Dillard University, Division of Nursing, *New Orleans (BSN)*
Grambling State University, School of Nursing, *Grambling (BSN)*
Louisiana College, Department of Nursing, *Pineville (BSN)*
Louisiana State University Health Sciences Center, School of Nursing, *New Orleans (BSN)*
McNeese State University, College of Nursing, *Lake Charles (BSN)*
Nicholls State University, Department of Nursing, *Thibodaux (BSN)*
Northwestern State University of Louisiana, College of Nursing and Allied Health, *Shreveport (BSN)*
Our Lady of Holy Cross College, Division of Nursing, *New Orleans (BSN)*
Our Lady of the Lake College, Division of Nursing, *Baton Rouge (BSN)*
Southeastern Louisiana University, School of Nursing, *Hammond (BS)*
Southern University and Agricultural and Mechanical College, School of Nursing, *Baton Rouge (BSN)*
University of Louisiana at Lafayette, College of Nursing, *Lafayette (BSN)*
University of Louisiana at Monroe, Nursing, *Monroe (BS)*

**Maine**

Husson University, School of Nursing, *Bangor (BSN)*
Saint Joseph's College of Maine, Master of Science in Nursing Program, *Standish (BSN)*
University of Maine, School of Nursing, *Orono (BSN)*
University of Maine at Fort Kent, Department of Nursing, *Fort Kent (BSN)*
University of New England, Department of Nursing, *Biddeford (BSN)*
University of Southern Maine, School of Nursing, *Portland (BS)*

**Maryland**

Bowie State University, Department of Nursing, *Bowie (BSN)*
Coppin State University, Helene Fuld School of Nursing, *Baltimore (BSN)*
Salisbury University, Nursing DNP Program, *Salisbury (BS)*
Stevenson University, Nursing Division, *Stevenson (BS)*
Towson University, Department of Nursing, *Towson (BS)*
University of Maryland, Baltimore, Master's Program in Nursing, *Baltimore (BSN)*
Washington Adventist University, Nursing Department, *Takoma Park (BS)*

**Massachusetts**

American International College, Division of Nursing, *Springfield (BSN)*
Becker College, Nursing Programs, *Worcester (BSN)*
Boston College, William F. Connell School of Nursing, *Chestnut Hill (BS)*
Curry College, Division of Nursing, *Milton (BS)*
Elms College, Division of Nursing, *Chicopee (BS)*

Endicott College, Major in Nursing, *Beverly (BS)*
Fitchburg State University, Department of Nursing, *Fitchburg (BS)*
Labouré College, Bachelor of Science in Nursing Program, *Boston (BSN)*
Northeastern University, School of Nursing, *Boston (BSN)*
Regis College, School of Nursing, Science and Health Professions, *Weston (BSN)*
Salem State University, Program in Nursing, *Salem (BSN)*
Simmons College, School of Nursing and Health Sciences, *Boston (BS)*
University of Massachusetts Amherst, School of Nursing, *Amherst (BS)*
University of Massachusetts Boston, College of Nursing and Health Sciences, *Boston (BS)*
University of Massachusetts Dartmouth, College of Nursing, *North Dartmouth (BSN)*
University of Massachusetts Lowell, School of Nursing, *Lowell (BS)*
Worcester State University, Department of Nursing, *Worcester (BS)*

### Michigan

Andrews University, Department of Nursing, *Berrien Springs (BS)*
Calvin College, Department of Nursing, *Grand Rapids (BSN)*
Davenport University, Division of Nursing, *Grand Rapids (BSN)*
Davenport University, Bachelor of Science in Nursing Program, *Kalamazoo (BSN)*
Eastern Michigan University, School of Nursing, *Ypsilanti (BSN)*
Finlandia University, College of Professional Studies, *Hancock (BSN)*
Grand Valley State University, Kirkhof College of Nursing, *Allendale (BSN)*
Hope College, Department of Nursing, *Holland (BSN)*
Lake Superior State University, Department of Nursing, *Sault Sainte Marie (BSN)*
Madonna University, College of Nursing and Health, *Livonia (BSN)*
Michigan State University, College of Nursing, *East Lansing (BSN)*
Northern Michigan University, College of Nursing and Allied Health Science, *Marquette (BSN)*
Oakland University, School of Nursing, *Rochester (BSN)*
Rochester College, School of Nursing, *Rochester Hills (BSN)*
Saginaw Valley State University, College of Health and Human Services, *University Center (BSN)*
Siena Heights University, Nursing Program, *Adrian (BSN)*
University of Detroit Mercy, McAuley School of Nursing, *Detroit (BSN)*
University of Michigan, School of Nursing, *Ann Arbor (BSN)*
Wayne State University, College of Nursing, *Detroit (BSN)*
Western Michigan University, College of Health and Human Services, *Kalamazoo (BSN)*

### Minnesota

Bemidji State University, Department of Nursing, *Bemidji (BS)*
Bethel University, Department of Nursing, *St. Paul (BSN)*
College of Saint Benedict, Department of Nursing, *Saint Joseph (BS)*
The College of St. Scholastica, Department of Nursing, *Duluth (BS)*
Concordia College, Department of Nursing, *Moorhead (BA)*
Crown College, Nursing Department, *St. Bonifacius (BSN)*
Globe University–Woodbury, Bachelor of Science in Nursing, *Woodbury (BS)*
Gustavus Adolphus College, Department of Nursing, *St. Peter (BA)*
Herzing University, Nursing Program, *Minneapolis (BSN)*
Metropolitan State University, College of Health, Community and Professional Studies, *St. Paul (BSN)*
Minnesota Intercollegiate Nursing Consortium, *Northfield (BA)*
Minnesota State University Mankato, School of Nursing, *Mankato (BS)*
St. Catherine University, Department of Nursing, *St. Paul (BS)*
St. Cloud State University, Department of Nursing Science, *St. Cloud (BS)*
St. Olaf College, Department of Nursing, *Northfield (BA)*
University of Minnesota, Twin Cities Campus, School of Nursing, *Minneapolis (BSN)*
Winona State University, College of Nursing and Health Sciences, *Winona (BS)*

### Mississippi

Alcorn State University, School of Nursing, *Natchez (BSN)*
Delta State University, School of Nursing, *Cleveland (BSN)*
Mississippi College, School of Nursing, *Clinton (BSN)*
Mississippi University for Women, College of Nursing and Speech Language Pathology, *Columbus (BSN)*
University of Mississippi Medical Center, School of Nursing, *Jackson (BSN)*
University of Southern Mississippi, School of Nursing, *Hattiesburg (BSN)*
William Carey University, School of Nursing, *Hattiesburg (BSN)*

### Missouri

Avila University, School of Nursing, *Kansas City (BSN)*
Central Methodist University, College of Liberal Arts and Sciences, *Fayette (BSN)*
Chamberlain College of Nursing, *St. Louis (BSN)*
College of the Ozarks, Armstrong McDonald School of Nursing, *Point Lookout (BSN)*
Cox College, Department of Nursing, *Springfield (BSN)*
Goldfarb School of Nursing at Barnes-Jewish College, *St. Louis (BSN)*
Graceland University, School of Nursing, *Independence (BSN)*
Maryville University of Saint Louis, Nursing Program, School of Health Professions, *St. Louis (BSN)*
Missouri Southern State University, Department of Nursing, *Joplin (BSN)*
Missouri State University, Department of Nursing, *Springfield (BSN)*
Missouri Western State University, Department of Nursing, *St. Joseph (BSN)*
Research College of Nursing, College of Nursing, *Kansas City (BSN)*
Saint Louis University, School of Nursing, *St. Louis (BSN)*
Saint Luke's College of Health Sciences, Nursing College, *Kansas City (BSN)*
Southeast Missouri State University, Department of Nursing, *Cape Girardeau (BSN)*
Truman State University, Program in Nursing, *Kirksville (BSN)*
University of Central Missouri, Department of Nursing, *Warrensburg (BS)*
University of Missouri, Sinclair School of Nursing, *Columbia (BSN)*
University of Missouri–Kansas City, School of Nursing and Health Studies, *Kansas City (BSN)*
University of Missouri–St. Louis, College of Nursing, *St. Louis (BSN)*
William Jewell College, Department of Nursing, *Liberty (BS)*

### Montana

Carroll College, Department of Nursing, *Helena (BS)*
Montana State University, College of Nursing, *Bozeman (BSN)*

### Nebraska

Bryan College of Health Sciences, School of Nursing, *Lincoln (BSN)*
Clarkson College, Master of Science in Nursing Program, *Omaha (BSN)*
College of Saint Mary, Division of Health Care Professions, *Omaha (BSN)*
Creighton University, School of Nursing, *Omaha (BSN)*
Midland University, Department of Nursing, *Fremont (BSN)*
Nebraska Methodist College, Department of Nursing, *Omaha (BSN)*
Union College, Division of Health Sciences, *Lincoln (BSN)*
University of Nebraska Medical Center, College of Nursing, *Omaha (BSN)*

### Nevada

Nevada State College at Henderson, Nursing Program, *Henderson (BSN)*
Roseman University of Health Sciences, College of Nursing, *Henderson (BSN)*
Touro University, School of Nursing, *Henderson (BSN)*
University of Nevada, Las Vegas, School of Nursing, *Las Vegas (BSN)*
University of Nevada, Reno, Orvis School of Nursing, *Reno (BSN)*

### New Hampshire

Colby-Sawyer College, Department of Nursing, *New London (BSN)*
Rivier University, Division of Nursing, *Nashua (BS)*
University of New Hampshire, Department of Nursing, *Durham (BS)*

### New Jersey

Bloomfield College, Division of Nursing, *Bloomfield (BS)*
Caldwell College, Nursing Programs, *Caldwell (BSN)*

The College of New Jersey, School of Nursing, Health and Exercise Science, *Ewing (BSN)*
Fairleigh Dickinson University, Metropolitan Campus, Henry P. Becton School of Nursing and Allied Health, *Teaneck (BSN)*
Felician College, Division of Nursing and Health Management, *Lodi (BSN)*
Georgian Court University, The Georgian Court-Meridian Health School of Nursing, *Lakewood (BSN)*
Ramapo College of New Jersey, Master of Science in Nursing Program, *Mahwah (BSN)*
Rutgers, The State University of New Jersey, Camden, Rutgers School of Nursing–Camden, *Camden (BS)*
Saint Peter's University, Nursing Program, *Jersey City (BSN)*
Seton Hall University, College of Nursing, *South Orange (BSN)*
Thomas Edison State College, School of Nursing, *Trenton (BSN)*
William Paterson University of New Jersey, Department of Nursing, *Wayne (BSN)*

### New Mexico

New Mexico State University, School of Nursing, *Las Cruces (BSN)*
University of New Mexico, College of Nursing, *Albuquerque (BSN)*

### New York

Adelphi University, College of Nursing and Public Health, *Garden City (BS)*
Binghamton University, State University of New York, Decker School of Nursing, *Vestal (BS)*
The College at Brockport, State University of New York, Department of Nursing, *Brockport (BSN)*
College of Mount Saint Vincent, Department of Nursing, *Riverdale (BS)*
The College of New Rochelle, School of Nursing, *New Rochelle (BSN)*
Concordia College–New York, Nursing Program, *Bronxville (BS)*
Dominican College, Department of Nursing, *Orangeburg (BSN)*
D'Youville College, School of Nursing, *Buffalo (BSN)*
Elmira College, Program in Nursing Education, *Elmira (BS)*
Farmingdale State College, Nursing Department, *Farmingdale (BS)*
Hartwick College, Department of Nursing, *Oneonta (BS)*
Hunter College of the City University of New York, Hunter-Bellevue School of Nursing, *New York (BSN)*
Lehman College of the City University of New York, Department of Nursing, *Bronx (BS)*
Long Island University–LIU Brooklyn, School of Nursing, *Brooklyn (BS)*
Molloy College, Division of Nursing, *Rockville Centre (BS)*
Mount Saint Mary College, Division of Nursing, *Newburgh (BSN)*
Nazareth College of Rochester, Department of Nursing, *Rochester (BS)*
New York Institute of Technology, Department of Nursing, *Old Westbury (BSN)*
New York University, College of Nursing, *New York (BS)*
Niagara University, Department of Nursing, *Niagara University (BS)*
Pace University, Lienhard School of Nursing, *New York (BS)*
Roberts Wesleyan College, Division of Nursing, *Rochester (BScN)*
The Sage Colleges, Department of Nursing, *Troy (BS)*
St. Francis College, Department of Nursing, *Brooklyn Heights (BS)*
St. John Fisher College, Wegmans School of Nursing, *Rochester (BS)*
State University of New York at Plattsburgh, Department of Nursing, *Plattsburgh (BS)*
State University of New York College of Technology at Alfred, Nursing Program, *Alfred (BSN)*
Stony Brook University, State University of New York, School of Nursing, *Stony Brook (BS)*
Trocaire College, Nursing Program, *Buffalo (BS)*
University at Buffalo, the State University of New York, School of Nursing, *Buffalo (BS)*
Utica College, Department of Nursing, *Utica (BS)*
Wagner College, Department of Nursing, *Staten Island (BS)*

### North Carolina

Appalachian State University, Department of Nursing, *Boone (BSN)*
Barton College, School of Nursing, *Wilson (BSN)*
East Carolina University, College of Nursing, *Greenville (BSN)*
Fayetteville State University, Program in Nursing, *Fayetteville (BSN)*
Gardner-Webb University, School of Nursing, *Boiling Springs (BSN)*
Lenoir-Rhyne University, Program in Nursing, *Hickory (BS)*
North Carolina Agricultural and Technical State University, School of Nursing, *Greensboro (BSN)*
North Carolina Central University, Department of Nursing, *Durham (BSN)*
Queens University of Charlotte, Presbyterian School of Nursing, *Charlotte (BSN)*
The University of North Carolina at Chapel Hill, School of Nursing, *Chapel Hill (BSN)*
The University of North Carolina at Charlotte, School of Nursing, *Charlotte (BSN)*
The University of North Carolina at Greensboro, School of Nursing, *Greensboro (BSN)*
The University of North Carolina at Pembroke, Nursing Program, *Pembroke (BSN)*
The University of North Carolina Wilmington, School of Nursing, *Wilmington (BS)*
Western Carolina University, School of Nursing, *Cullowhee (BSN)*
Winston-Salem State University, Department of Nursing, *Winston-Salem (BSN)*

### North Dakota

Minot State University, Department of Nursing, *Minot (BSN)*
North Dakota State University, Department of Nursing, *Fargo (BSN)*
University of Mary, Division of Nursing, *Bismarck (BSN)*
University of North Dakota, College of Nursing, *Grand Forks (BSN)*

### Ohio

Ashland University, Dwight Schar College of Nursing and Health Sciences, *Ashland (BSN)*
Capital University, School of Nursing, *Columbus (BSN)*
Case Western Reserve University, Frances Payne Bolton School of Nursing, *Cleveland (BSN)*
Cleveland State University, School of Nursing, *Cleveland (BSN)*
College of Mount St. Joseph, Department of Nursing, *Cincinnati (BSN)*
Franciscan University of Steubenville, Department of Nursing, *Steubenville (BSN)*
Franklin University, Nursing Program, *Columbus (BSN)*
Hiram College, Nursing Department, *Hiram (BSN)*
Hondros College, Nursing Programs, *Westerville (BSN)*
Kent State University, College of Nursing, *Kent (BSN)*
Kettering College, Division of Nursing, *Kettering (BSN)*
Lourdes University, School of Nursing, *Sylvania (BSN)*
Malone University, School of Nursing, *Canton (BSN)*
Mercy College of Ohio, Division of Nursing, *Toledo (BSN)*
Miami University, Department of Nursing, *Hamilton (BSN)*
Miami University Hamilton, Bachelor of Science in Nursing Program, *Hamilton (BSN)*
Mount Carmel College of Nursing, Nursing Programs, *Columbus (BSN)*
Mount Vernon Nazarene University, School of Nursing and Health Sciences, *Mount Vernon (BS)*
Muskingum University, Department of Nursing, *New Concord (BSN)*
Notre Dame College, Nursing Department, *South Euclid (BSN)*
The Ohio State University, College of Nursing, *Columbus (BSN)*
Ohio University, School of Nursing, *Athens (BSN)*
Otterbein University, Department of Nursing, *Westerville (BSN)*
The University of Akron, School of Nursing, *Akron (BSN)*
University of Cincinnati, College of Nursing, *Cincinnati (BSN)*
The University of Toledo, College of Nursing, *Toledo (BSN)*
Ursuline College, The Breen School of Nursing, *Pepper Pike (BSN)*
Walsh University, Department of Nursing, *North Canton (BSN)*
Wright State University, College of Nursing and Health, *Dayton (BSN)*
Xavier University, School of Nursing, *Cincinnati (BSN)*

### Oklahoma

East Central University, Department of Nursing, *Ada (BS)*
Langston University, School of Nursing and Health Professions, *Langston (BSN)*

Northwestern Oklahoma State University, Division of Nursing, *Alva (BSN)*
Oklahoma Baptist University, School of Nursing, *Shawnee (BSN)*
Oklahoma Christian University, Nursing Program, *Oklahoma City (BSN)*
Oklahoma City University, Kramer School of Nursing, *Oklahoma City (BSN)*
Oklahoma Wesleyan University, School of Nursing, *Bartlesville (BSN)*
Oral Roberts University, Anna Vaughn School of Nursing, *Tulsa (BSN)*
Southern Nazarene University, School of Nursing, *Bethany (BS)*
Southwestern Oklahoma State University, School of Nursing, *Weatherford (BSN)*
University of Central Oklahoma, Department of Nursing, *Edmond (BSN)*
University of Oklahoma Health Sciences Center, College of Nursing, *Oklahoma City (BSN)*
University of Tulsa, School of Nursing, *Tulsa (BSN)*

### Oregon

George Fox University, Nursing Department, *Newberg (BSN)*
Linfield College, School of Nursing, *McMinnville (BSN)*
Oregon Health & Science University, School of Nursing, *Portland (BS)*
University of Portland, School of Nursing, *Portland (BSN)*

### Pennsylvania

Alvernia University, Nursing, *Reading (BSN)*
Bloomsburg University of Pennsylvania, Department of Nursing, *Bloomsburg (BSN)*
Carlow University, School of Nursing, *Pittsburgh (BSN)*
Cedar Crest College, Department of Nursing, *Allentown (BS)*
DeSales University, Department of Nursing and Health, *Center Valley (BSN)*
Drexel University, College of Nursing and Health Professions, *Philadelphia (BSN)*
Duquesne University, School of Nursing, *Pittsburgh (BSN)*
Eastern University, Program in Nursing, *St. Davids (BSN)*
East Stroudsburg University of Pennsylvania, Department of Nursing, *East Stroudsburg (BS)*
Edinboro University of Pennsylvania, Department of Nursing, *Edinboro (BSN)*
Gannon University, Villa Maria School of Nursing, *Erie (BSN)*
Holy Family University, School of Nursing and Allied Health Professions, *Philadelphia (BSN)*
Immaculata University, Division of Nursing, *Immaculata (BSN)*
Indiana University of Pennsylvania, Department of Nursing and Allied Health, *Indiana (BSN)*
La Salle University, School of Nursing and Health Sciences, *Philadelphia (BSN)*
Mansfield University of Pennsylvania, Department of Health Sciences–Nursing, *Mansfield (BSN)*
Marywood University, Department of Nursing, *Scranton (BSN)*
Messiah College, Department of Nursing, *Mechanicsburg (BSN)*
Misericordia University, Department of Nursing, *Dallas (BSN)*
Moravian College, Department of Nursing, *Bethlehem (BS)*
Neumann University, Program in Nursing and Health Sciences, *Aston (BS)*
Penn State University Park, School of Nursing, *University Park (BS)*
Robert Morris University, School of Nursing and Health Sciences, *Moon Township (BSN)*
Saint Francis University, Department of Nursing, *Loretto (BSN)*
Temple University, Department of Nursing, *Philadelphia (BSN)*
Thomas Jefferson University, Department of Nursing, *Philadelphia (BSN)*
University of Pennsylvania, School of Nursing, *Philadelphia (BSN)*
University of Pittsburgh, School of Nursing, *Pittsburgh (BSN)*
University of Pittsburgh at Bradford, Department of Nursing, *Bradford (BSN)*
The University of Scranton, Department of Nursing, *Scranton (BSN)*
Villanova University, College of Nursing, *Villanova (BSN)*
Waynesburg University, Department of Nursing, *Waynesburg (BSN)*
West Chester University of Pennsylvania, Department of Nursing, *West Chester (BSN)*
Widener University, School of Nursing, *Chester (BSN)*
Wilkes University, Department of Nursing, *Wilkes-Barre (BS)*
York College of Pennsylvania, Department of Nursing, *York (BS)*

### Puerto Rico

Inter American University of Puerto Rico, Arecibo Campus, Nursing Program, *Arecibo (BS)*
Inter American University of Puerto Rico, Metropolitan Campus, Carmen Torres de Tiburcio School of Nursing, *San Juan (BSN)*
Pontifical Catholic University of Puerto Rico, Department of Nursing, *Ponce (BSN)*
Universidad Adventista de las Antillas, Department of Nursing, *Mayagüez (BSN)*
Universidad del Turabo, Nursing Program, *Gurabo (BS)*
University of Puerto Rico in Arecibo, Department of Nursing, *Arecibo (BSN)*
University of Puerto Rico in Humacao, Department of Nursing, *Humacao (BS)*
University of Puerto Rico, Mayagüez Campus, Department of Nursing, *Mayagüez (BSN)*
University of Puerto Rico, Medical Sciences Campus, School of Nursing, *San Juan (BSN)*
University of the Sacred Heart, Program in Nursing, *San Juan (BSN)*

### Rhode Island

Rhode Island College, Department of Nursing, *Providence (BSN)*
Salve Regina University, Department of Nursing, *Newport (BS)*
University of Rhode Island, College of Nursing, *Kingston (BS)*

### South Carolina

Charleston Southern University, Wingo School of Nursing, *Charleston (BSN)*
Clemson University, School of Nursing, *Clemson (BS)*
Francis Marion University, Department of Nursing, *Florence (BSN)*
Lander University, School of Nursing, *Greenwood (BSN)*
Newberry College, Department of Nursing, *Newberry (BSN)*
South Carolina State University, Department of Nursing, *Orangeburg (BSN)*
University of South Carolina, College of Nursing, *Columbia (BSN)*
University of South Carolina Aiken, School of Nursing, *Aiken (BSN)*
University of South Carolina Beaufort, Nursing Program, *Bluffton (BSN)*
University of South Carolina Upstate, Mary Black School of Nursing, *Spartanburg (BSN)*

### South Dakota

Augustana College, Department of Nursing, *Sioux Falls (BA)*
Mount Marty College, Nursing Program, *Yankton (BSN)*
National American University, School of Nursing, *Rapid City (BSN)*
Presentation College, Department of Nursing, *Aberdeen (BSN)*
South Dakota State University, College of Nursing, *Brookings (BS)*
University of Sioux Falls, School of Nursing, *Sioux Falls (BSN)*
The University of South Dakota, Department of Nursing, *Vermillion (BSN)*

### Tennessee

Austin Peay State University, School of Nursing, *Clarksville (BSN)*
Baptist College of Health Sciences, Nursing Division, *Memphis (BSN)*
Belmont University, School of Nursing, *Nashville (BSN)*
Bethel University, Nursing Program, *McKenzie (BSN)*
Carson-Newman University, Department of Nursing, *Jefferson City (BSN)*
Cumberland University, Rudy School of Nursing and Health Professions, *Lebanon (BSN)*
East Tennessee State University, College of Nursing, *Johnson City (BSN)*
King College, School of Nursing, *Bristol (BSN)*
Lincoln Memorial University, Caylor School of Nursing, *Harrogate (BSN)*
Lipscomb University, Department of Nursing, *Nashville (BSN)*
Martin Methodist College, Division of Nursing, *Pulaski (BSN)*
Middle Tennessee State University, School of Nursing, *Murfreesboro (BSN)*
Milligan College, Department of Nursing, *Milligan College (BSN)*
South College, Department of Nursing, *Knoxville (BSN)*
Tennessee State University, Division of Nursing, *Nashville (BSN)*
Tennessee Technological University, Whitson-Hester School of Nursing, *Cookeville (BSN)*
Tennessee Wesleyan College, Fort Sanders Nursing Department, *Knoxville (BSN)*

Union University, School of Nursing, *Jackson (BSN)*

University of Memphis, Loewenberg School of Nursing, *Memphis (BSN)*

The University of Tennessee, College of Nursing, *Knoxville (BSN)*

The University of Tennessee at Chattanooga, School of Nursing, *Chattanooga (BSN)*

The University of Tennessee at Martin, Department of Nursing, *Martin (BSN)*

## Texas

Angelo State University, Department of Nursing and Rehabilitation Sciences, *San Angelo (BSN)*

Baylor University, Louise Herrington School of Nursing, *Dallas (BSN)*

Concordia University Texas, School of Nursing, *Austin (BSN)*

East Texas Baptist University, Department of Nursing, *Marshall (BSN)*

Houston Baptist University, School of Nursing and Allied Health, *Houston (BSN)*

Lamar University, Department of Nursing, *Beaumont (BSN)*

Midwestern State University, Nursing Program, *Wichita Falls (BSN)*

Patty Hanks Shelton School of Nursing, *Abilene (BSN)*

Prairie View A&M University, College of Nursing, *Houston (BSN)*

Sam Houston State University, Nursing Program, *Huntsville (BSN)*

Southwestern Adventist University, Department of Nursing, *Keene (BS)*

Stephen F. Austin State University, Richard and Lucille Dewitt School of Nursing, *Nacogdoches (BSN)*

Tarleton State University, Department of Nursing, *Stephenville (BSN)*

Texas A&M Health Science Center, College of Nursing, *College Station (BSN)*

Texas A&M International University, Canseco School of Nursing, *Laredo (BSN)*

Texas A&M University–Corpus Christi, College of Nursing and Health Sciences, *Corpus Christi (BSN)*

Texas Christian University, Harris College of Nursing, *Fort Worth (BSN)*

Texas State University–San Marcos, St. David's School of Nursing, *San Marcos (BSN)*

Texas Tech University Health Sciences Center, School of Nursing, *Lubbock (BSN)*

Texas Tech University Health Sciences Center-El Paso, *El Paso (BSN)*

Texas Woman's University, College of Nursing, *Denton (BS)*

University of Mary Hardin-Baylor, College of Nursing, *Belton (BSN)*

The University of Texas at Arlington, College of Nursing, *Arlington (BSN)*

The University of Texas at Austin, School of Nursing, *Austin (BSN)*

The University of Texas at El Paso, School of Nursing, *El Paso (BSN)*

The University of Texas at Tyler, Program in Nursing, *Tyler (BSN)*

The University of Texas Health Science Center at Houston, School of Nursing, *Houston (BSN)*

The University of Texas Health Science Center at San Antonio, School of Nursing, *San Antonio (BSN)*

The University of Texas Medical Branch, School of Nursing, *Galveston (BSN)*

The University of Texas–Pan American, Department of Nursing, *Edinburg (BSN)*

University of the Incarnate Word, Program in Nursing, *San Antonio (BSN)*

West Texas A&M University, Department of Nursing, *Canyon (BSN)*

## Utah

Southern Utah University, Department of Nursing, *Cedar City (BSN)*

University of Utah, College of Nursing, *Salt Lake City (BS)*

Western Governors University, Online College of Health Professions, *Salt Lake City (BS)*

Westminster College, School of Nursing and Health Sciences, *Salt Lake City (BSN)*

## Vermont

Norwich University, Department of Nursing, *Northfield (BSN)*

Southern Vermont College, Department of Nursing, *Bennington (BSN)*

University of Vermont, Department of Nursing, *Burlington (BS)*

## Virgin Islands

University of the Virgin Islands, Division of Nursing, *Saint Thomas (BSN)*

## Virginia

Bon Secours Memorial College of Nursing, *Richmond (BSN)*

Eastern Mennonite University, Department of Nursing, *Harrisonburg (BSN)*

George Mason University, College of Health and Human Services, *Fairfax (BSN)*

Hampton University, School of Nursing, *Hampton (BS)*

James Madison University, Department of Nursing, *Harrisonburg (BSN)*

Jefferson College of Health Sciences, Nursing Education Program, *Roanoke (BSN)*

Liberty University, Department of Nursing, *Lynchburg (BSN)*

Lynchburg College, School of Health Sciences and Human Performance, *Lynchburg (BS)*

Marymount University, School of Health Professions, *Arlington (BSN)*

Old Dominion University, Department of Nursing, *Norfolk (BSN)*

Radford University, School of Nursing, *Radford (BSN)*

Sentara College of Health Sciences, Bachelor of Science in Nursing Program, *Chesapeake (BSN)*

Shenandoah University, Division of Nursing, *Winchester (BSN)*

Stratford University, School of Nursing, *Falls Church (BSN)*

University of Virginia, School of Nursing, *Charlottesville (BSN)*

The University of Virginia's College at Wise, Department of Nursing, *Wise (BSN)*

Virginia Commonwealth University, School of Nursing, *Richmond (BS)*

## Washington

Gonzaga University, Department of Nursing, *Spokane (BSN)*

Northwest University, The Mark and Huldah Buntain School of Nursing, *Kirkland (BS)*

Pacific Lutheran University, School of Nursing, *Tacoma (BSN)*

Seattle Pacific University, School of Health Sciences, *Seattle (BS)*

Seattle University, College of Nursing, *Seattle (BSN)*

University of Washington, School of Nursing, *Seattle (BSN)*

Walla Walla University, School of Nursing, *College Place (BS)*

Washington State University College of Nursing, *Spokane (BSN)*

## West Virginia

Alderson Broaddus University, Department of Nursing, *Philippi (BSN)*

Marshall University, College of Health Professions, *Huntington (BSN)*

Shepherd University, Department of Nursing Education, *Shepherdstown (BSN)*

University of Charleston, Department of Nursing, *Charleston (BSN)*

West Liberty University, Department of Health Sciences, *West Liberty (BSN)*

West Virginia University, School of Nursing, *Morgantown (BSN)*

West Virginia Wesleyan College, School of Nursing, *Buckhannon (BSN)*

Wheeling Jesuit University, Department of Nursing, *Wheeling (BSN)*

## Wisconsin

Alverno College, Division of Nursing, *Milwaukee (BSN)*

Bellin College, Nursing Program, *Green Bay (BSN)*

Carroll University, Nursing Program, *Waukesha (BSN)*

Columbia College of Nursing/Mount Mary College Nursing Program, *Milwaukee (BSN)*

Concordia University Wisconsin, Program in Nursing, *Mequon (BSN)*

Edgewood College, Program in Nursing, *Madison (BS)*

Marian University, School of Nursing, *Fond du Lac (BSN)*

Marquette University, College of Nursing, *Milwaukee (BSN)*

Milwaukee School of Engineering, School of Nursing, *Milwaukee (BSN)*

University of Wisconsin–Eau Claire, College of Nursing and Health Sciences, *Eau Claire (BSN)*

University of Wisconsin–Madison, School of Nursing, *Madison (BS)*

University of Wisconsin–Milwaukee, College of Nursing, *Milwaukee (BSN)*

University of Wisconsin–Oshkosh, College of Nursing, *Oshkosh (BSN)*

Viterbo University, School of Nursing, *La Crosse (BSN)*

Wisconsin Lutheran College, Nursing Program, *Milwaukee (BSN)*

## Wyoming

University of Wyoming, Fay W. Whitney School of Nursing, *Laramie (BSN)*

## CANADA

### Alberta

Athabasca University, Centre for Nursing and Health Studies, *Athabasca (BN)*
University of Alberta, Faculty of Nursing, *Edmonton (BScN)*
University of Calgary, Faculty of Nursing, *Calgary (BN)*
University of Lethbridge, Faculty of Health Sciences, *Lethbridge (BN)*

### British Columbia

Kwantlen Polytechnic University, Faculty of Community and Health Sciences, *Surrey (BSN)*
Trinity Western University, Department of Nursing, *Langley (BScN)*
University of Northern British Columbia, Nursing Programme, *Prince George (BScN)*
Vancouver Island University, Department of Nursing, *Nanaimo (BScN)*

### Manitoba

Brandon University, School of Health Studies, *Brandon (BN)*
University of Manitoba, Faculty of Nursing, *Winnipeg (BN)*

### New Brunswick

University of New Brunswick Fredericton, Faculty of Nursing, *Fredericton (BN)*

### Newfoundland and Labrador

Memorial University of Newfoundland, School of Nursing, *St. John's (BN)*

### Nova Scotia

St. Francis Xavier University, Department of Nursing, *Antigonish (BScN)*

### Ontario

Brock University, Department of Nursing, *St. Catharines (BScN)*
Lakehead University, School of Nursing, *Thunder Bay (BScN)*
Laurentian University, School of Nursing, *Sudbury (BScN)*
McMaster University, School of Nursing, *Hamilton (BScN)*
Queen's University at Kingston, School of Nursing, *Kingston (BNSc)*
Trent University, Nursing Program, *Peterborough (BScN)*
University of Ottawa, School of Nursing, *Ottawa (BScN)*
The University of Western Ontario, School of Nursing, *London (BScN)*
University of Windsor, Faculty of Nursing, *Windsor (BScN)*
York University, School of Nursing, *Toronto (BScN)*

### Prince Edward Island

University of Prince Edward Island, School of Nursing, *Charlottetown (BScN)*

### Quebec

McGill University, School of Nursing, *Montréal (BScN)*
Université du Québec à Chicoutimi, Program in Nursing, *Chicoutimi (BNSc)*
Université du Québec à Trois-Rivières, Program in Nursing, *Trois-Rivières (BSN)*
Université du Québec en Outaouais, Département des Sciences Infirmières, *Gatineau (BScN)*
Université Laval, Faculty of Nursing, *Québec (BScN)*

### Saskatchewan

University of Saskatchewan, College of Nursing, *Saskatoon (BSN)*

## INTERNATIONAL NURSE TO BACCALAUREATE

## U.S. AND U.S. TERRITORIES

### Delaware

Wesley College, Nursing Program, *Dover (BSN)*
Wilmington University, College of Health Professions, *New Castle (BSN)*

### Georgia

Thomas University, Division of Nursing, *Thomasville (BSN)*

### Hawaii

Hawai`i Pacific University, College of Nursing and Health Sciences, *Honolulu (BSN)*

### Iowa

Morningside College, Department of Nursing Education, *Sioux City (BSN)*

### Massachusetts

Salem State University, Program in Nursing, *Salem (BSN)*

### Nebraska

Nebraska Wesleyan University, Department of Nursing, *Lincoln (BSN)*
University of Nebraska Medical Center, College of Nursing, *Omaha (BSN)*

### New Jersey

College of Saint Elizabeth, Department of Nursing, *Morristown (BSN)*
Seton Hall University, College of Nursing, *South Orange (BSN)*

### New York

College of Mount Saint Vincent, Department of Nursing, *Riverdale (BS)*
Daemen College, Department of Nursing, *Amherst (BS)*
Lehman College of the City University of New York, Department of Nursing, *Bronx (BS)*
The Sage Colleges, Department of Nursing, *Troy (BS)*
St. Francis College, Department of Nursing, *Brooklyn Heights (BS)*

### Oklahoma

Oklahoma City University, Kramer School of Nursing, *Oklahoma City (BSN)*
Oklahoma Wesleyan University, School of Nursing, *Bartlesville (BSN)*

### Pennsylvania

Eastern University, Program in Nursing, *St. Davids (BSN)*
Edinboro University of Pennsylvania, Department of Nursing, *Edinboro (BSN)*
Gannon University, Villa Maria School of Nursing, *Erie (BSN)*
Holy Family University, School of Nursing and Allied Health Professions, *Philadelphia (BSN)*
Marywood University, Department of Nursing, *Scranton (BSN)*
Neumann University, Program in Nursing and Health Sciences, *Aston (BS)*
Villanova University, College of Nursing, *Villanova (BSN)*

### South Dakota

Mount Marty College, Nursing Program, *Yankton (BSN)*

### Texas

The University of Texas at Tyler, Program in Nursing, *Tyler (BSN)*

## CANADA

### Ontario

Ryerson University, Program in Nursing, *Toronto (BScN)*
University of Ottawa, School of Nursing, *Ottawa (BScN)*

## LPN TO BACCALAUREATE

## U.S. AND U.S. TERRITORIES

### Arizona

University of Phoenix–Phoenix Campus, College of Nursing, *Tempe (BSN)*
University of Phoenix–Southern Arizona Campus, College of Social Sciences, *Tucson (BSN)*

### Arkansas

Arkansas State University, Department of Nursing, *State University (BSN)*
Arkansas Tech University, Program in Nursing, *Russellville (BSN)*
Harding University, College of Nursing, *Searcy (BSN)*
Henderson State University, Department of Nursing, *Arkadelphia (BSN)*
University of Arkansas, Eleanor Mann School of Nursing, *Fayetteville (BSN)*
University of Arkansas at Monticello, School of Nursing, *Monticello (BSN)*
University of Arkansas for Medical Sciences, College of Nursing, *Little Rock (BSN)*
University of Central Arkansas, Department of Nursing, *Conway (BSN)*

### California

Biola University, Department of Nursing, *La Mirada (BSN)*
California State University, Fullerton, Department of Nursing, *Fullerton (BSN)*
California State University, Long Beach, School of Nursing, *Long Beach (BSN)*
California State University, San Bernardino, Department of Nursing, *San Bernardino (BSN)*
California State University, Stanislaus, Department of Nursing, *Turlock (BSN)*
Loma Linda University, School of Nursing, *Loma Linda (BS)*
National University, Department of Nursing, *La Jolla (BSN)*
University of Phoenix–Sacramento Valley Campus, College of Nursing, *Sacramento (BSN)*

**Colorado**

Colorado Mesa University, Department of Nursing and Radiologic Sciences, *Grand Junction (BSN)*

Colorado State University–Pueblo, Department of Nursing, *Pueblo (BSN)*

**Delaware**

Delaware State University, Department of Nursing, *Dover (BSN)*

Wesley College, Nursing Program, *Dover (BSN)*

**District of Columbia**

Howard University, Division of Nursing, *Washington (BSN)*

**Florida**

Barry University, Division of Nursing, *Miami Shores (BSN)*

**Georgia**

Armstrong Atlantic State University, Program in Nursing, *Savannah (BSN)*

Piedmont College, School of Nursing, *Demorest (BSN)*

**Hawaii**

Hawai`i Pacific University, College of Nursing and Health Sciences, *Honolulu (BSN)*

University of Phoenix–Hawaii Campus, College of Nursing, *Honolulu (BSN)*

**Idaho**

Boise State University, Department of Nursing, *Boise (BS)*

Lewis-Clark State College, Division of Nursing and Health Sciences, *Lewiston (BSN)*

**Illinois**

Bradley University, Department of Nursing, *Peoria (BSN, BSc PN)*

Chicago State University, Department of Nursing, *Chicago (BSN)*

**Indiana**

Ball State University, School of Nursing, *Muncie (BS)*

Indiana State University, Department of Nursing, *Terre Haute (BS)*

Purdue University Calumet, School of Nursing, *Hammond (BS)*

Purdue University North Central, Department of Nursing, *Westville (BS)*

**Iowa**

Allen College, Program in Nursing, *Waterloo (BSN)*

Briar Cliff University, Department of Nursing, *Sioux City (BSN)*

Iowa Wesleyan College, Division of Nursing, *Mount Pleasant (BSN)*

Morningside College, Department of Nursing Education, *Sioux City (BSN)*

**Kansas**

Bethel College, Department of Nursing, *North Newton (BSN)*

Emporia State University, Newman Division of Nursing, *Emporia (BSN)*

Newman University, Division of Nursing, *Wichita (BSN)*

Washburn University, School of Nursing, *Topeka (BSN)*

**Louisiana**

Dillard University, Division of Nursing, *New Orleans (BSN)*

McNeese State University, College of Nursing, *Lake Charles (BSN)*

Nicholls State University, Department of Nursing, *Thibodaux (BSN)*

Northwestern State University of Louisiana, College of Nursing and Allied Health, *Shreveport (BSN)*

Our Lady of the Lake College, Division of Nursing, *Baton Rouge (BSN)*

University of Louisiana at Lafayette, College of Nursing, *Lafayette (BSN)*

University of Louisiana at Monroe, Nursing, *Monroe (BS)*

University of Phoenix–Louisiana Campus, College of Nursing, *Metairie (BSN)*

**Massachusetts**

Salem State University, Program in Nursing, *Salem (BSN)*

Simmons College, School of Nursing and Health Sciences, *Boston (BS)*

**Michigan**

Lake Superior State University, Department of Nursing, *Sault Sainte Marie (BSN)*

Madonna University, College of Nursing and Health, *Livonia (BSN)*

Northern Michigan University, College of Nursing and Allied Health Science, *Marquette (BSN)*

**Missouri**

Cox College, Department of Nursing, *Springfield (BSN)*

Maryville University of Saint Louis, Nursing Program, School of Health Professions, *St. Louis (BSN)*

Missouri Southern State University, Department of Nursing, *Joplin (BSN)*

Missouri State University, Department of Nursing, *Springfield (BSN)*

**Montana**

Montana State University, College of Nursing, *Bozeman (BSN)*

**Nebraska**

Clarkson College, Master of Science in Nursing Program, *Omaha (BSN)*

College of Saint Mary, Division of Health Care Professions, *Omaha (BSN)*

Nebraska Methodist College, Department of Nursing, *Omaha (BSN)*

Union College, Division of Health Sciences, *Lincoln (BSN)*

University of Nebraska Medical Center, College of Nursing, *Omaha (BSN)*

**New Hampshire**

Rivier University, Division of Nursing, *Nashua (BS)*

**New Jersey**

William Paterson University of New Jersey, Department of Nursing, *Wayne (BSN)*

**New York**

College of Mount Saint Vincent, Department of Nursing, *Riverdale (BS)*

Dominican College, Department of Nursing, *Orangeburg (BSN)*

Molloy College, Division of Nursing, *Rockville Centre (BS)*

Nazareth College of Rochester, Department of Nursing, *Rochester (BS)*

The Sage Colleges, Department of Nursing, *Troy (BS)*

**North Carolina**

The University of North Carolina at Greensboro, School of Nursing, *Greensboro (BSN)*

Winston-Salem State University, Department of Nursing, *Winston-Salem (BSN)*

**North Dakota**

Dickinson State University, Department of Nursing, *Dickinson (BSN)*

North Dakota State University, Department of Nursing, *Fargo (BSN)*

University of Mary, Division of Nursing, *Bismarck (BSN)*

University of North Dakota, College of Nursing, *Grand Forks (BSN)*

**Ohio**

Lourdes University, School of Nursing, *Sylvania (BSN)*

Otterbein University, Department of Nursing, *Westerville (BSN)*

The University of Akron, School of Nursing, *Akron (BSN)*

**Oklahoma**

Langston University, School of Nursing and Health Professions, *Langston (BSN)*

Northwestern Oklahoma State University, Division of Nursing, *Alva (BSN)*

Oklahoma Baptist University, School of Nursing, *Shawnee (BSN)*

Oklahoma Wesleyan University, School of Nursing, *Bartlesville (BSN)*

Southern Nazarene University, School of Nursing, *Bethany (BS)*

University of Central Oklahoma, Department of Nursing, *Edmond (BSN)*

**Pennsylvania**

Alvernia University, Nursing, *Reading (BSN)*

Cedar Crest College, Department of Nursing, *Allentown (BS)*

Indiana University of Pennsylvania, Department of Nursing and Allied Health, *Indiana (BSN)*

La Salle University, School of Nursing and Health Sciences, *Philadelphia (BSN)*

Marywood University, Department of Nursing, *Scranton (BSN)*

Neumann University, Program in Nursing and Health Sciences, *Aston (BS)*

Waynesburg University, Department of Nursing, *Waynesburg (BSN)*

York College of Pennsylvania, Department of Nursing, *York (BS)*

**South Dakota**

Mount Marty College, Nursing Program, *Yankton (BSN)*

**Tennessee**

Baptist College of Health Sciences, Nursing Division, *Memphis (BSN)*

Carson-Newman University, Department of Nursing, *Jefferson City (BSN)*

East Tennessee State University, College of Nursing, *Johnson City (BSN)*

Milligan College, Department of Nursing, *Milligan College (BSN)*

Union University, School of Nursing, *Jackson (BSN)*

**Texas**

Prairie View A&M University, College of Nursing, *Houston (BSN)*

Tarleton State University, Department of Nursing, *Stephenville (BSN)*

The University of Texas at Tyler, Program in Nursing, *Tyler (BSN)*

West Texas A&M University, Department of Nursing, *Canyon (BSN)*

**Virgin Islands**

University of the Virgin Islands, Division of Nursing, *Saint Thomas (BSN)*

**Virginia**

Eastern Mennonite University, Department of Nursing, *Harrisonburg (BSN)*

Hampton University, School of Nursing, *Hampton (BS)*

Sentara College of Health Sciences, Bachelor of Science in Nursing Program, *Chesapeake (BSN)*

**Washington**

Pacific Lutheran University, School of Nursing, *Tacoma (BSN)*

Walla Walla University, School of Nursing, *College Place (BS)*

**Wisconsin**

Alverno College, Division of Nursing, *Milwaukee (BSN)*

### CANADA

**Manitoba**

Brandon University, School of Health Studies, *Brandon (BN)*

**Newfoundland and Labrador**

Memorial University of Newfoundland, School of Nursing, *St. John's (BN)*

## LPN TO RN BACCALAUREATE

### U.S. AND U.S. TERRITORIES

**Arkansas**

Harding University, College of Nursing, *Searcy (BSN)*

University of Arkansas, Eleanor Mann School of Nursing, *Fayetteville (BSN)*

University of Central Arkansas, Department of Nursing, *Conway (BSN)*

**California**

California State University, Chico, School of Nursing, *Chico (BSN)*

California State University, Los Angeles, School of Nursing, *Los Angeles (BSN)*

California State University, Sacramento, School of Nursing, *Sacramento (BSN)*

Holy Names University, Department of Nursing, *Oakland (BSN)*

Point Loma Nazarene University, School of Nursing, *San Diego (BSN)*

**Colorado**

Colorado Mesa University, Department of Nursing and Radiologic Sciences, *Grand Junction (BSN)*

Colorado State University–Pueblo, Department of Nursing, *Pueblo (BSN)*

Denver School of Nursing, *Denver (BSN)*

**Florida**

Barry University, Division of Nursing, *Miami Shores (BSN)*

**Georgia**

Georgia Southern University, School of Nursing, *Statesboro (BSN)*

Georgia Southwestern State University, School of Nursing, *Americus (BSN)*

**Idaho**

Idaho State University, Department of Nursing, *Pocatello (BS)*

Lewis-Clark State College, Division of Nursing and Health Sciences, *Lewiston (BSN)*

**Illinois**

MacMurray College, Department of Nursing, *Jacksonville (BSN)*

Saint Xavier University, School of Nursing, *Chicago (BSN)*

**Indiana**

Ball State University, School of Nursing, *Muncie (BS)*

Saint Joseph's College, St. Elizabeth School of Nursing, *Rensselaer (BSN)*

**Iowa**

Iowa Wesleyan College, Division of Nursing, *Mount Pleasant (BSN)*

**Kansas**

Wichita State University, School of Nursing, *Wichita (BSN)*

**Louisiana**

Dillard University, Division of Nursing, *New Orleans (BSN)*

Grambling State University, School of Nursing, *Grambling (BSN)*

McNeese State University, College of Nursing, *Lake Charles (BSN)*

Southeastern Louisiana University, School of Nursing, *Hammond (BS)*

**Massachusetts**

Salem State University, Program in Nursing, *Salem (BSN)*

Worcester State University, Department of Nursing, *Worcester (BS)*

**Michigan**

Lake Superior State University, Department of Nursing, *Sault Sainte Marie (BSN)*

**Mississippi**

Alcorn State University, School of Nursing, *Natchez (BSN)*

**Missouri**

Chamberlain College of Nursing, *St. Louis (BSN)*

Cox College, Department of Nursing, *Springfield (BSN)*

**Nebraska**

Clarkson College, Master of Science in Nursing Program, *Omaha (BSN)*

Midland University, Department of Nursing, *Fremont (BSN)*

Nebraska Methodist College, Department of Nursing, *Omaha (BSN)*

University of Nebraska Medical Center, College of Nursing, *Omaha (BSN)*

**New Hampshire**

Rivier University, Division of Nursing, *Nashua (BS)*

**New York**

College of Mount Saint Vincent, Department of Nursing, *Riverdale (BS)*

Molloy College, Division of Nursing, *Rockville Centre (BS)*

**North Dakota**

Dickinson State University, Department of Nursing, *Dickinson (BSN)*

**Ohio**

Lourdes University, School of Nursing, *Sylvania (BSN)*

The University of Akron, School of Nursing, *Akron (BSN)*

**Oklahoma**

Northwestern Oklahoma State University, Division of Nursing, *Alva (BSN)*

Oklahoma Baptist University, School of Nursing, *Shawnee (BSN)*

University of Oklahoma Health Sciences Center, College of Nursing, *Oklahoma City (BSN)*

University of Tulsa, School of Nursing, *Tulsa (BSN)*

**Pennsylvania**

Alvernia University, Nursing, *Reading (BSN)*

Bloomsburg University of Pennsylvania, Department of Nursing, *Bloomsburg (BSN)*

La Roche College, Department of Nursing and Nursing Management, *Pittsburgh (BSN)*

Neumann University, Program in Nursing and Health Sciences, *Aston (BS)*

The University of Scranton, Department of Nursing, *Scranton (BSN)*

Wilkes University, Department of Nursing, *Wilkes-Barre (BS)*

**South Dakota**

Mount Marty College, Nursing Program, *Yankton (BSN)*

Presentation College, Department of Nursing, *Aberdeen (BSN)*

**Tennessee**

Belmont University, School of Nursing, *Nashville (BSN)*

Middle Tennessee State University, School of Nursing, *Murfreesboro (BSN)*

Milligan College, Department of Nursing, *Milligan College (BSN)*

The University of Tennessee at Martin, Department of Nursing, *Martin (BSN)*

**Texas**

Southwestern Adventist University, Department of Nursing, *Keene (BS)*

The University of Texas at Tyler, Program in Nursing, *Tyler (BSN)*

### Utah

Western Governors University, Online College of Health Professions, *Salt Lake City (BS)*

### Virginia

Hampton University, School of Nursing, *Hampton (BS)*

### West Virginia

Alderson Broaddus University, Department of Nursing, *Philippi (BSN)*

### Wisconsin

Concordia University Wisconsin, Program in Nursing, *Mequon (BSN)*

## CANADA

### Alberta

Athabasca University, Centre for Nursing and Health Studies, *Athabasca (BN)*

### British Columbia

Vancouver Island University, Department of Nursing, *Nanaimo (BScN)*

# RN BACCALAUREATE

## U.S. AND U.S. TERRITORIES

### Alabama

Auburn University at Montgomery, School of Nursing, *Montgomery (BSN)*

Jacksonville State University, College of Nursing and Health Sciences, *Jacksonville (BSN)*

Oakwood University, Department of Nursing, *Huntsville (BS)*

Stillman College, Nursing Major, *Tuscaloosa (BSN)*

Troy University, School of Nursing, *Troy (BSN)*

Tuskegee University, Program in Nursing, *Tuskegee (BSN)*

The University of Alabama, Capstone College of Nursing, *Tuscaloosa (BSN)*

The University of Alabama at Birmingham, School of Nursing, *Birmingham (BSN)*

The University of Alabama in Huntsville, College of Nursing, *Huntsville (BSN)*

University of Mobile, School of Nursing, *Mobile (BSN)*

University of North Alabama, College of Nursing and Allied Health, *Florence (BSN)*

University of South Alabama, College of Nursing, *Mobile (BSN)*

### Alaska

University of Alaska Anchorage, School of Nursing, *Anchorage (BS)*

### Arizona

Arizona State University at the Downtown Phoenix Campus, College of Nursing, *Phoenix (BSN)*

Chamberlain College of Nursing, *Phoenix (BSN)*

Grand Canyon University, College of Nursing and Health Sciences, *Phoenix (BSN)*

Northern Arizona University, School of Nursing, *Flagstaff (BSN)*

### Arkansas

Arkansas State University, Department of Nursing, *State University (BSN)*

Arkansas Tech University, Program in Nursing, *Russellville (BSN)*

Harding University, College of Nursing, *Searcy (BSN)*

Southern Arkansas University–Magnolia, Department of Nursing, *Magnolia (BSN)*

University of Arkansas, Eleanor Mann School of Nursing, *Fayetteville (BSN)*

University of Arkansas at Little Rock, BSN Programs, *Little Rock (BSN)*

University of Arkansas at Monticello, School of Nursing, *Monticello (BSN)*

University of Arkansas for Medical Sciences, College of Nursing, *Little Rock (BSN)*

University of Central Arkansas, Department of Nursing, *Conway (BSN)*

### California

Biola University, Department of Nursing, *La Mirada (BSN)*

Brandman University, School of Nursing and Health Professions, *Irvine (BSN)*

California Baptist University, School of Nursing, *Riverside (BSN)*

California State University Channel Islands, Nursing Program, *Camarillo (BSN)*

California State University, Chico, School of Nursing, *Chico (BSN)*

California State University, Dominguez Hills, Program in Nursing, *Carson (BSN)*

California State University, Fullerton, Department of Nursing, *Fullerton (BSN)*

California State University, Los Angeles, School of Nursing, *Los Angeles (BSN)*

California State University, San Bernardino, Department of Nursing, *San Bernardino (BSN)*

Concordia University, Bachelor of Science in Nursing Program, *Irvine (BSN)*

Dominican University of California, Program in Nursing, *San Rafael (BSN)*

Fresno Pacific University, RN to BSN Program, *Fresno (BSN)*

Holy Names University, Department of Nursing, *Oakland (BSN)*

Loma Linda University, School of Nursing, *Loma Linda (BS)*

National University, Department of Nursing, *La Jolla (BSN)*

Point Loma Nazarene University, School of Nursing, *San Diego (BSN)*

San Diego State University, School of Nursing, *San Diego (BSN)*

San Francisco State University, School of Nursing, *San Francisco (BSN)*

University of Phoenix–Central Valley Campus, College of Health and Human Services, *Fresno (BSN)*

Vanguard University of Southern California, Nursing Program, *Costa Mesa (BSN)*

West Coast University, Nursing Programs, *North Hollywood (BSN)*

### Colorado

Adams State University, Nursing Program, *Alamosa (BSN)*

American Sentinel University, RN to Bachelor of Science Nursing, *Aurora (BSN)*

Colorado Christian University, Nursing Programs, *Lakewood (BSN)*

Colorado Mesa University, Department of Nursing and Radiologic Sciences, *Grand Junction (BSN)*

Colorado State University–Pueblo, Department of Nursing, *Pueblo (BSN)*

Denver School of Nursing, *Denver (BSN)*

Regis University, School of Nursing, *Denver (BSN)*

University of Colorado Colorado Springs, Beth-El College of Nursing and Health Sciences, *Colorado Springs (BSN)*

University of Colorado Denver, College of Nursing, *Aurora (BS)*

University of Northern Colorado, School of Nursing, *Greeley (BS)*

### Connecticut

Central Connecticut State University, Department of Nursing, *New Britain (BSN)*

Fairfield University, School of Nursing, *Fairfield (BSN)*

Quinnipiac University, School of Nursing, *Hamden (BSN)*

Sacred Heart University, Program in Nursing, *Fairfield (BSN)*

Southern Connecticut State University, Department of Nursing, *New Haven (BS)*

University of Hartford, College of Education, Nursing, and Health Professions, *West Hartford (BSN)*

University of Saint Joseph, Department of Nursing, *West Hartford (BS)*

Western Connecticut State University, Department of Nursing, *Danbury (BS)*

### Delaware

Delaware State University, Department of Nursing, *Dover (BSN)*

University of Delaware, School of Nursing, *Newark (BSN)*

Wilmington University, College of Health Professions, *New Castle (BSN)*

### District of Columbia

Howard University, Division of Nursing, *Washington (BSN)*

Trinity Washington University, Nursing Program, *Washington (BSN)*

University of the District of Columbia, Nursing Education Program, *Washington (BSN)*

### Florida

Adventist University of Health Sciences, Department of Nursing, *Orlando (BSN)*

Barry University, Division of Nursing, *Miami Shores (BSN)*

Bethune-Cookman University, School of Nursing, *Daytona Beach (BSN)*

Broward College, Nursing Program, *Fort Lauderdale (BSN)*

Edison State College, Bachelor of Science in Nursing Program, *Fort Myers (BSN)*

Florida Atlantic University, Christine E. Lynn College of Nursing, *Boca Raton (BSN)*

Florida International University, Nursing Program, *Miami (BSN)*

Florida Southern College, School of Nursing & Health Sciences, *Lakeland (BSN)*

Florida State College at Jacksonville, Nursing Department, *Jacksonville (BSN)*

Indian River State College, Bachelor of Science in Nursing Program, *Fort Pierce (BSN)*

Keiser University, Nursing Programs, *Fort Lauderdale (BSN)*

Keiser University, Nursing Programs, *Fort Myers (BSN)*

Keiser University, Nursing Programs, *Jacksonville (BSN)*
Keiser University, Nursing Programs, *Lakeland (BSN)*
Keiser University, Nursing Programs, *Melbourne (BSN)*
Keiser University, Nursing Programs, *Miami (BSN)*
Keiser University, Nursing Programs, *Orlando (BSN)*
Keiser University, Nursing Programs, *Port St. Lucie (BSN)*
Keiser University, Nursing Programs, *Sarasota (BSN)*
Keiser University, Nursing Programs, *Tallahassee (BSN)*
Keiser University, Nursing Programs, *Tampa (BSN)*
Miami Dade College, School of Nursing, *Miami (BSN)*
Northwest Florida State College, RN to BSN Degree Program, *Niceville (BSN)*
Nova Southeastern University, College of Health Care Sciences, *Fort Lauderdale (BSN)*
Palm Beach Atlantic University, School of Nursing, *West Palm Beach (BSN)*
Polk State College, RN to BSN Program, *Winter Haven (BSN)*
St. Petersburg College, Department of Nursing, *St. Petersburg (BSN)*
State College of Florida Manatee-Sarasota, Nursing Degree Program, *Bradenton (BSN)*
University of Central Florida, College of Nursing, *Orlando (BSN)*
University of Miami, School of Nursing and Health Studies, *Coral Gables (BSN)*
University of North Florida, School of Nursing, *Jacksonville (BSN)*
University of Phoenix–South Florida Campus, College of Nursing, *Miramar (BSN)*
The University of Tampa, Department of Nursing, *Tampa (BSN)*
University of West Florida, Department of Nursing, *Pensacola (BSN)*

## Georgia

Armstrong Atlantic State University, Program in Nursing, *Savannah (BSN)*
Brenau University, College of Health and Science, *Gainesville (BSN)*
Clayton State University, Department of Nursing, *Morrow (BSN)*
College of Coastal Georgia, Department of Nursing and Health Sciences, *Brunswick (BSN)*
Columbus State University, Nursing Program, *Columbus (BSN)*
Georgia College & State University, College of Health Sciences, *Milledgeville (BSN)*
Georgia Southwestern State University, School of Nursing, *Americus (BSN)*
Gordon State College, Division of Nursing and Health Sciences, *Barnesville (BSN)*
Kennesaw State University, School of Nursing, *Kennesaw (BSN)*
LaGrange College, Department of Nursing, *LaGrange (BSN)*
Georgia Baptist College of Nursing, *Atlanta (BSN)*
Piedmont College, School of Nursing, *Demorest (BSN)*
Thomas University, Division of Nursing, *Thomasville (BSN)*
Valdosta State University, College of Nursing, *Valdosta (BSN)*

## Guam

University of Guam, School of Nursing and Health Sciences, *Mangilao (BSN)*

## Hawaii

Hawai`i Pacific University, College of Nursing and Health Sciences, *Honolulu (BSN)*
University of Hawaii at Hilo, Department in Nursing, *Hilo (BSN)*
University of Hawaii at Manoa, School of Nursing and Dental Hygiene, *Honolulu (BSN)*

## Idaho

Boise State University, Department of Nursing, *Boise (BS)*
Brigham Young University–Idaho, Department of Nursing, *Rexburg (BSN)*

## Illinois

Aurora University, School of Nursing, *Aurora (BSN)*
Blessing–Rieman College of Nursing, *Quincy (BSN)*
Bradley University, Department of Nursing, *Peoria (BSN, BSc PN)*
Chicago State University, Department of Nursing, *Chicago (BSN)*
Elmhurst College, Deicke Center for Nursing Education, *Elmhurst (BS)*
Governors State University, College of Health and Human Services, *University Park (BS)*
Illinois State University, Mennonite College of Nursing, *Normal (BSN)*
Lakeview College of Nursing, *Danville (BSN)*
Loyola University Chicago, Marcella Niehoff School of Nursing, *Maywood (BSN)*
Methodist College, *Peoria (BSN)*
Millikin University, School of Nursing, *Decatur (BSN)*
Northern Illinois University, School of Nursing and Health Studies, *De Kalb (BS)*
North Park University, School of Nursing, *Chicago (BS)*
Olivet Nazarene University, Division of Nursing, *Bourbonnais (BSN)*
Resurrection University, *Chicago (BSN)*
Rockford University, Department of Nursing, *Rockford (BSN)*
Saint Anthony College of Nursing, *Rockford (BSN)*
Saint Francis Medical Center College of Nursing, Baccalaureate Nursing Program, *Peoria (BSN)*
Trinity College of Nursing and Health Sciences, *Rock Island (BSN)*
University of Illinois at Chicago, College of Nursing, *Chicago (BSN)*
Western Illinois University, School of Nursing, *Macomb (BSN)*

## Indiana

Anderson University, School of Nursing, *Anderson (BSN)*
Ball State University, School of Nursing, *Muncie (BS)*
Bethel College, School of Nursing, *Mishawaka (BSN)*
Goshen College, Department of Nursing, *Goshen (BSN)*
Huntington University, Department of Nursing, *Huntington (BSN)*
Indiana State University, Department of Nursing, *Terre Haute (BS)*
Indiana University Bloomington, Department of Nursing–Bloomington Division, *Bloomington (BSN)*
Indiana University East, School of Nursing, *Richmond (BSN)*
Indiana University Northwest, School of Nursing, *Gary (BSN)*
Indiana University–Purdue University Fort Wayne, Department of Nursing, *Fort Wayne (BS)*
Indiana University–Purdue University Indianapolis, School of Nursing, *Indianapolis (BSN)*
Indiana University South Bend, College of Health Sciences, *South Bend (BSN)*
Indiana University Southeast, Division of Nursing, *New Albany (BSN)*
Indiana Wesleyan University, School of Nursing, *Marion (BSN)*
Marian University, School of Nursing, *Indianapolis (BSN)*
Purdue University, School of Nursing, *West Lafayette (BS)*
Purdue University North Central, Department of Nursing, *Westville (BS)*
Saint Joseph's College, St. Elizabeth School of Nursing, *Rensselaer (BSN)*
University of Evansville, Department of Nursing, *Evansville (BSN)*
University of Indianapolis, School of Nursing, *Indianapolis (BSN)*
University of Saint Francis, Department of Nursing, *Fort Wayne (BSN)*
University of Southern Indiana, College of Nursing and Health Professions, *Evansville (BSN)*
Valparaiso University, College of Nursing, *Valparaiso (BSN)*
Vincennes University, Department of Nursing, *Vincennes (BSN)*

## Iowa

Allen College, Program in Nursing, *Waterloo (BSN)*
Briar Cliff University, Department of Nursing, *Sioux City (BSN)*
Clarke University, Department of Nursing and Health, *Dubuque (BS)*
Grand View University, Division of Nursing, *Des Moines (BSN)*
Iowa Wesleyan College, Division of Nursing, *Mount Pleasant (BSN)*
Morningside College, Department of Nursing Education, *Sioux City (BSN)*
St. Ambrose University, Program in Nursing (BSN), *Davenport (BSN)*
University of Dubuque, School of Professional Programs, *Dubuque (BSN)*
The University of Iowa, College of Nursing, *Iowa City (BSN)*
Upper Iowa University, RN-BSN Nursing Program, *Fayette (BSN)*

## Kansas

Baker University, School of Nursing, *Topeka (BSN)*
Bethel College, Department of Nursing, *North Newton (BSN)*

Emporia State University, Newman Division of Nursing, *Emporia (BSN)*
Fort Hays State University, Department of Nursing, *Hays (BSN)*
Kansas Wesleyan University, Department of Nursing Education, *Salina (BSN)*
MidAmerica Nazarene University, Division of Nursing, *Olathe (BSN)*
Newman University, Division of Nursing, *Wichita (BSN)*
Pittsburg State University, Department of Nursing, *Pittsburg (BSN)*
The University of Kansas, School of Nursing, *Kansas City (BSN)*
University of Saint Mary, Bachelor of Science in Nursing Program, *Leavenworth (BSN)*
Washburn University, School of Nursing, *Topeka (BSN)*
Wichita State University, School of Nursing, *Wichita (BSN)*

**Kentucky**

Bellarmine University, Donna and Allan Lansing School of Nursing and Health Sciences, *Louisville (BSN, MSCE)*
Eastern Kentucky University, Department of Baccalaureate and Graduate Nursing, *Richmond (BSN)*
Midway College, Program in Nursing (Baccalaureate), *Midway (BSN)*
Morehead State University, Department of Nursing, *Morehead (BSN)*
Murray State University, Program in Nursing, *Murray (BSN)*
Northern Kentucky University, Department of Nursing, *Highland Heights (BSN)*
University of Kentucky, College of Nursing, *Lexington (BSN)*
University of Louisville, School of Nursing, *Louisville (BSN)*
University of Pikeville, RN to BSN Completion Program, *Pikeville (BSN)*
Western Kentucky University, School of Nursing, *Bowling Green (BSN)*

**Louisiana**

Dillard University, Division of Nursing, *New Orleans (BSN)*
Grambling State University, School of Nursing, *Grambling (BSN)*
Louisiana State University at Alexandria, Nursing Program, *Alexandria (BSN)*
Louisiana State University Health Sciences Center, School of Nursing, *New Orleans (BSN)*
Loyola University New Orleans, School of Nursing, *New Orleans (BSN)*
Nicholls State University, Department of Nursing, *Thibodaux (BSN)*
Northwestern State University of Louisiana, College of Nursing and Allied Health, *Shreveport (BSN)*
Our Lady of the Lake College, Division of Nursing, *Baton Rouge (BSN)*
Southeastern Louisiana University, School of Nursing, *Hammond (BS)*
University of Louisiana at Monroe, Nursing, *Monroe (BS)*

**Maine**

Saint Joseph's College of Maine, Master of Science in Nursing Program, *Standish (BSN)*
University of Maine, School of Nursing, *Orono (BSN)*
University of Maine at Fort Kent, Department of Nursing, *Fort Kent (BSN)*
University of New England, Department of Nursing, *Biddeford (BSN)*
University of Southern Maine, School of Nursing, *Portland (BS)*

**Maryland**

Bowie State University, Department of Nursing, *Bowie (BSN)*
Coppin State University, Helene Fuld School of Nursing, *Baltimore (BSN)*
Frostburg State University, Nursing Department, *Frostburg (BSN)*
Notre Dame of Maryland University, Department of Nursing, *Baltimore (BS)*
Salisbury University, Nursing DNP Program, *Salisbury (BS)*
Stevenson University, Nursing Division, *Stevenson (BS)*
Towson University, Department of Nursing, *Towson (BS)*
University of Maryland, Baltimore, Master's Program in Nursing, *Baltimore (BSN)*

**Massachusetts**

American International College, Division of Nursing, *Springfield (BSN)*
Anna Maria College, Department of Nursing, *Paxton (BSN)*
Becker College, Nursing Programs, *Worcester (BSN)*
Curry College, Division of Nursing, *Milton (BS)*
Elms College, Division of Nursing, *Chicopee (BS)*
Emmanuel College, Department of Nursing, *Boston (BS)*
Endicott College, Major in Nursing, *Beverly (BS)*
Fitchburg State University, Department of Nursing, *Fitchburg (BS)*
Regis College, School of Nursing, Science and Health Professions, *Weston (BSN)*
Simmons College, School of Nursing and Health Sciences, *Boston (BS)*
University of Massachusetts Boston, College of Nursing and Health Sciences, *Boston (BS)*
University of Massachusetts Dartmouth, College of Nursing, *North Dartmouth (BSN)*
University of Massachusetts Lowell, School of Nursing, *Lowell (BS)*

**Michigan**

Davenport University, Division of Nursing, *Grand Rapids (BSN)*
Davenport University, Bachelor of Science in Nursing Program, *Kalamazoo (BSN)*
Eastern Michigan University, School of Nursing, *Ypsilanti (BSN)*
Ferris State University, School of Nursing, *Big Rapids (BSN)*
Finlandia University, College of Professional Studies, *Hancock (BSN)*
Grand Valley State University, Kirkhof College of Nursing, *Allendale (BSN)*
Lake Superior State University, Department of Nursing, *Sault Sainte Marie (BSN)*
Madonna University, College of Nursing and Health, *Livonia (BSN)*
Michigan State University, College of Nursing, *East Lansing (BSN)*
Northern Michigan University, College of Nursing and Allied Health Science, *Marquette (BSN)*
Oakland University, School of Nursing, *Rochester (BSN)*
The Robert B. Miller College, School of Nursing, *Battle Creek (BSN)*
Rochester College, School of Nursing, *Rochester Hills (BSN)*
Saginaw Valley State University, College of Health and Human Services, *University Center (BSN)*
Siena Heights University, Nursing Program, *Adrian (BSN)*
University of Detroit Mercy, McAuley School of Nursing, *Detroit (BSN)*
University of Michigan, School of Nursing, *Ann Arbor (BSN)*
University of Michigan–Flint, Department of Nursing, *Flint (BSN)*

**Minnesota**

Bemidji State University, Department of Nursing, *Bemidji (BS)*
Bethel University, Department of Nursing, *St. Paul (BSN)*
Capella University, Nursing Programs, *Minneapolis (BSN)*
Metropolitan State University, College of Health, Community and Professional Studies, *St. Paul (BSN)*
Minnesota State University Mankato, School of Nursing, *Mankato (BS)*
Minnesota State University Moorhead, School of Nursing and Healthcare Leadership, *Moorhead (BSN)*
St. Catherine University, Department of Nursing, *St. Paul (BS)*
Saint Mary's University of Minnesota, B.S. in Nursing, *Winona (BS)*
Walden University, Nursing Programs, *Minneapolis (BSN)*
Winona State University, College of Nursing and Health Sciences, *Winona (BS)*

**Mississippi**

Alcorn State University, School of Nursing, *Natchez (BSN)*
Mississippi College, School of Nursing, *Clinton (BSN)*

**Missouri**

Chamberlain College of Nursing, *St. Louis (BSN)*
Cox College, Department of Nursing, *Springfield (BSN)*
Goldfarb School of Nursing at Barnes-Jewish College, *St. Louis (BSN)*
Graceland University, School of Nursing, *Independence (BSN)*
Lincoln University, Department of Nursing, *Jefferson City (BSN)*
Maryville University of Saint Louis, Nursing Program, School of Health Professions, *St. Louis (BSN)*
Missouri Southern State University, Department of Nursing, *Joplin (BSN)*
Missouri State University, Department of Nursing, *Springfield (BSN)*
Saint Louis University, School of Nursing, *St. Louis (BSN)*

Southeast Missouri State University, Department of Nursing, *Cape Girardeau (BSN)*

Southwest Baptist University, College of Nursing, *Bolivar (BSN)*

University of Central Missouri, Department of Nursing, *Warrensburg (BS)*

University of Missouri, Sinclair School of Nursing, *Columbia (BSN)*

University of Missouri–Kansas City, School of Nursing and Health Studies, *Kansas City (BSN)*

University of Missouri–St. Louis, College of Nursing, *St. Louis (BSN)*

Webster University, Department of Nursing, *St. Louis (BSN)*

**Montana**

Montana State University–Northern, College of Nursing, *Havre (BSN)*

Salish Kootenai College, Nursing Department, *Pablo (BS)*

University of Great Falls, B.S. in Nursing Degree Completion Program, *Great Falls (BSN)*

**Nebraska**

Bryan College of Health Sciences, School of Nursing, *Lincoln (BSN)*

Clarkson College, Master of Science in Nursing Program, *Omaha (BSN)*

Creighton University, School of Nursing, *Omaha (BSN)*

Midland University, Department of Nursing, *Fremont (BSN)*

Nebraska Methodist College, Department of Nursing, *Omaha (BSN)*

Nebraska Wesleyan University, Department of Nursing, *Lincoln (BSN)*

University of Nebraska Medical Center, College of Nursing, *Omaha (BSN)*

**Nevada**

Great Basin College, BSN Program, *Elko (BSN)*

Nevada State College at Henderson, Nursing Program, *Henderson (BSN)*

Touro University, School of Nursing, *Henderson (BSN)*

University of Nevada, Reno, Orvis School of Nursing, *Reno (BSN)*

**New Hampshire**

Franklin Pierce University, Master of Science in Nursing, *Rindge (BS)*

Rivier University, Division of Nursing, *Nashua (BS)*

Saint Anselm College, Department of Nursing, *Manchester (BSN)*

University of New Hampshire, Department of Nursing, *Durham (BS)*

**New Jersey**

Bloomfield College, Division of Nursing, *Bloomfield (BS)*

Caldwell College, Nursing Programs, *Caldwell (BSN)*

The College of New Jersey, School of Nursing, Health and Exercise Science, *Ewing (BSN)*

College of Saint Elizabeth, Department of Nursing, *Morristown (BSN)*

Fairleigh Dickinson University, Metropolitan Campus, Henry P. Becton School of Nursing and Allied Health, *Teaneck (BSN)*

Kean University, Department of Nursing, *Union (BSN)*

Monmouth University, Marjorie K. Unterberg School of Nursing, *West Long Branch (BSN)*

New Jersey City University, Department of Nursing, *Jersey City (BSN)*

Ramapo College of New Jersey, Master of Science in Nursing Program, *Mahwah (BSN)*

The Richard Stockton College of New Jersey, Program in Nursing, *Galloway (BSN)*

Rowan University, RN to BSN Program, *Glassboro (BSN)*

Rutgers, The State University of New Jersey, Camden, Rutgers School of Nursing–Camden, *Camden (BS)*

Rutgers, The State University of New Jersey, Newark, Rutgers School of Nursing, *Newark (BSN)*

Saint Peter's University, Nursing Program, *Jersey City (BSN)*

Seton Hall University, College of Nursing, *South Orange (BSN)*

William Paterson University of New Jersey, Department of Nursing, *Wayne (BSN)*

**New Mexico**

New Mexico Highlands University, Department of Nursing, *Las Vegas (BSN)*

New Mexico State University, School of Nursing, *Las Cruces (BSN)*

Northern New Mexico College, College of Nursing and Health Sciences, *Espa&nnola (BSN)*

University of New Mexico, College of Nursing, *Albuquerque (BSN)*

Western New Mexico University, Nursing Department, *Silver City (BNSc)*

**New York**

Adelphi University, College of Nursing and Public Health, *Garden City (BS)*

The College of New Rochelle, School of Nursing, *New Rochelle (BSN)*

College of Staten Island of the City University of New York, Department of Nursing, *Staten Island (BS)*

Daemen College, Department of Nursing, *Amherst (BS)*

Dominican College, Department of Nursing, *Orangeburg (BSN)*

D'Youville College, School of Nursing, *Buffalo (BSN)*

Elmira College, Program in Nursing Education, *Elmira (BS)*

Excelsior College, School of Nursing, *Albany (BS)*

Farmingdale State College, Nursing Department, *Farmingdale (BS)*

Hartwick College, Department of Nursing, *Oneonta (BS)*

Hunter College of the City University of New York, Hunter-Bellevue School of Nursing, *New York (BSN)*

Lehman College of the City University of New York, Department of Nursing, *Bronx (BS)*

Le Moyne College, Nursing Programs, *Syracuse (BS)*

Long Island University–LIU Post, Department of Nursing, *Brookville (BS)*

Maria College, RN Baccalaureate Completion Program, *Albany (BSN)*

Mercy College, Programs in Nursing, *Dobbs Ferry (BS)*

Molloy College, Division of Nursing, *Rockville Centre (BS)*

Mount Saint Mary College, Division of Nursing, *Newburgh (BSN)*

Nazareth College of Rochester, Department of Nursing, *Rochester (BS)*

New York City College of Technology of the City University of New York, Department of Nursing, *Brooklyn (BS)*

New York University, College of Nursing, *New York (BS)*

Niagara University, Department of Nursing, *Niagara University (BS)*

Pace University, Lienhard School of Nursing, *New York (BS)*

Roberts Wesleyan College, Division of Nursing, *Rochester (BScN)*

The Sage Colleges, Department of Nursing, *Troy (BS)*

St. Francis College, Department of Nursing, *Brooklyn Heights (BS)*

St. John Fisher College, Wegmans School of Nursing, *Rochester (BS)*

St. Joseph's College, New York, Department of Nursing, *Brooklyn (BSN)*

State University of New York at Plattsburgh, Department of Nursing, *Plattsburgh (BS)*

State University of New York College of Technology at Delhi, Bachelor of Science in Nursing Program, *Delhi (BSN)*

State University of New York Downstate Medical Center, College of Nursing, *Brooklyn (BS)*

State University of New York Empire State College, Bachelor of Science in Nursing Program, *Saratoga Springs (BS)*

State University of New York Institute of Technology, School of Nursing and Health Systems, *Utica (BS)*

Stony Brook University, State University of New York, School of Nursing, *Stony Brook (BS)*

University at Buffalo, the State University of New York, School of Nursing, *Buffalo (BS)*

University of Rochester, School of Nursing, *Rochester (BS)*

Utica College, Department of Nursing, *Utica (BS)*

York College of the City University of New York, Program in Nursing, *Jamaica (BS)*

**North Carolina**

Appalachian State University, Department of Nursing, *Boone (BSN)*

Barton College, School of Nursing, *Wilson (BSN)*

Cabarrus College of Health Sciences, Louise Harkey School of Nursing, *Concord (BSN)*

Fayetteville State University, Program in Nursing, *Fayetteville (BSN)*

North Carolina Agricultural and Technical State University, School of Nursing, *Greensboro (BSN)*

Queens University of Charlotte, Presbyterian School of Nursing, *Charlotte (BSN)*

The University of North Carolina at Charlotte, School of Nursing, *Charlotte (BSN)*

The University of North Carolina at Greensboro, School of Nursing, *Greensboro (BSN)*

The University of North Carolina at Pembroke, Nursing Program, *Pembroke (BSN)*

The University of North Carolina Wilmington, School of Nursing, *Wilmington (BS)*

Western Carolina University, School of Nursing, *Cullowhee (BSN)*

Winston-Salem State University, Department of Nursing, *Winston-Salem (BSN)*

### North Dakota

Dickinson State University, Department of Nursing, *Dickinson (BSN)*

Minot State University, Department of Nursing, *Minot (BSN)*

Sanford College of Nursing, *Bismarck (BSN)*

University of Mary, Division of Nursing, *Bismarck (BSN)*

### Ohio

Ashland University, Dwight Schar College of Nursing and Health Sciences, *Ashland (BSN)*

Capital University, School of Nursing, *Columbus (BSN)*

Cedarville University, School of Nursing, *Cedarville (BSN)*

Chamberlain College of Nursing, *Columbus (BSN)*

Cleveland State University, School of Nursing, *Cleveland (BSN)*

Defiance College, Bachelor's Degree in Nursing, *Defiance (BSN)*

Franciscan University of Steubenville, Department of Nursing, *Steubenville (BSN)*

Kent State University, College of Nursing, *Kent (BSN)*

Kettering College, Division of Nursing, *Kettering (BSN)*

Lourdes University, School of Nursing, *Sylvania (BSN)*

Malone University, School of Nursing, *Canton (BSN)*

Mercy College of Ohio, Division of Nursing, *Toledo (BSN)*

Miami University, Department of Nursing, *Hamilton (BSN)*

Miami University Hamilton, Bachelor of Science in Nursing Program, *Hamilton (BSN)*

Mount Carmel College of Nursing, Nursing Programs, *Columbus (BSN)*

Notre Dame College, Nursing Department, *South Euclid (BSN)*

Ohio Northern University, Nursing Program, *Ada (BSN)*

The Ohio State University, College of Nursing, *Columbus (BSN)*

Ohio University, School of Nursing, *Athens (BSN)*

Otterbein University, Department of Nursing, *Westerville (BSN)*

Shawnee State University, Department of Nursing, *Portsmouth (BSN)*

University of Cincinnati, College of Nursing, *Cincinnati (BSN)*

University of Rio Grande, Holzer School of Nursing, *Rio Grande (BSN)*

The University of Toledo, College of Nursing, *Toledo (BSN)*

Ursuline College, The Breen School of Nursing, *Pepper Pike (BSN)*

Walsh University, Department of Nursing, *North Canton (BSN)*

Wright State University, College of Nursing and Health, *Dayton (BSN)*

### Oklahoma

Langston University, School of Nursing and Health Professions, *Langston (BSN)*

Northeastern State University, Department of Nursing, *Tahlequah (BSN)*

Northwestern Oklahoma State University, Division of Nursing, *Alva (BSN)*

Oklahoma Baptist University, School of Nursing, *Shawnee (BSN)*

Oklahoma City University, Kramer School of Nursing, *Oklahoma City (BSN)*

Oklahoma Wesleyan University, School of Nursing, *Bartlesville (BSN)*

Oral Roberts University, Anna Vaughn School of Nursing, *Tulsa (BSN)*

Southwestern Oklahoma State University, School of Nursing, *Weatherford (BSN)*

University of Central Oklahoma, Department of Nursing, *Edmond (BSN)*

University of Tulsa, School of Nursing, *Tulsa (BSN)*

### Oregon

Oregon Health & Science University, School of Nursing, *Portland (BS)*

### Pennsylvania

Alvernia University, Nursing, *Reading (BSN)*

California University of Pennsylvania, Department of Nursing, *California (BSN)*

Cedar Crest College, Department of Nursing, *Allentown (BS)*

Chatham University, Nursing Programs, *Pittsburgh (BSN)*

Clarion University of Pennsylvania, School of Nursing, *Oil City (BSN)*

DeSales University, Department of Nursing and Health, *Center Valley (BSN)*

Drexel University, College of Nursing and Health Professions, *Philadelphia (BSN)*

East Stroudsburg University of Pennsylvania, Department of Nursing, *East Stroudsburg (BS)*

Gannon University, Villa Maria School of Nursing, *Erie (BSN)*

Gwynedd Mercy University, School of Nursing, *Gwynedd Valley (BSN)*

Immaculata University, Division of Nursing, *Immaculata (BSN)*

La Roche College, Department of Nursing and Nursing Management, *Pittsburgh (BSN)*

La Salle University, School of Nursing and Health Sciences, *Philadelphia (BSN)*

Lock Haven University of Pennsylvania, Nursing Program, *Lock Haven (BSN)*

Mansfield University of Pennsylvania, Department of Health Sciences–Nursing, *Mansfield (BSN)*

Marywood University, Department of Nursing, *Scranton (BSN)*

Millersville University of Pennsylvania, Department of Nursing, *Millersville (BSN)*

Misericordia University, Department of Nursing, *Dallas (BSN)*

Moravian College, Department of Nursing, *Bethlehem (BS)*

Penn State University Park, School of Nursing, *University Park (BS)*

Pennsylvania College of Health Sciences, Bachelor of Science in Nursing Program, *Lancaster (BSN)*

Pennsylvania College of Technology, School of Health Sciences, *Williamsport (BSN)*

Robert Morris University, School of Nursing and Health Sciences, *Moon Township (BSN)*

Slippery Rock University of Pennsylvania, Department of Nursing, *Slippery Rock (BSN)*

Temple University, Department of Nursing, *Philadelphia (BSN)*

Thomas Jefferson University, Department of Nursing, *Philadelphia (BSN)*

University of Pennsylvania, School of Nursing, *Philadelphia (BSN)*

University of Pittsburgh, School of Nursing, *Pittsburgh (BSN)*

University of Pittsburgh at Bradford, Department of Nursing, *Bradford (BSN)*

The University of Scranton, Department of Nursing, *Scranton (BSN)*

Villanova University, College of Nursing, *Villanova (BSN)*

West Chester University of Pennsylvania, Department of Nursing, *West Chester (BSN)*

Widener University, School of Nursing, *Chester (BSN)*

Wilkes University, Department of Nursing, *Wilkes-Barre (BS)*

York College of Pennsylvania, Department of Nursing, *York (BS)*

### Puerto Rico

Inter American University of Puerto Rico, Aguadilla Campus, Nursing Program, *Aguadilla (BSN)*

Universidad Adventista de las Antillas, Department of Nursing, *Mayagüez (BSN)*

### Rhode Island

Rhode Island College, Department of Nursing, *Providence (BSN)*

Salve Regina University, Department of Nursing, *Newport (BS)*

University of Rhode Island, College of Nursing, *Kingston (BS)*

### South Carolina

Charleston Southern University, Wingo School of Nursing, *Charleston (BSN)*

Clemson University, School of Nursing, *Clemson (BS)*

Coastal Carolina University, Nursing Completion Program, *Conway (BSN)*

Lander University, School of Nursing, *Greenwood (BSN)*

South Carolina State University, Department of Nursing, *Orangeburg (BSN)*

University of South Carolina Aiken, School of Nursing, *Aiken (BSN)*

University of South Carolina Beaufort, Nursing Program, *Bluffton (BSN)*

University of South Carolina Upstate, Mary Black School of Nursing, *Spartanburg (BSN)*

### South Dakota

Mount Marty College, Nursing Program, *Yankton (BSN)*

Presentation College, Department of Nursing, *Aberdeen (BSN)*

South Dakota State University, College of Nursing, *Brookings (BS)*

University of Sioux Falls, School of Nursing, *Sioux Falls (BSN)*

The University of South Dakota, Department of Nursing, *Vermillion (BSN)*

### Tennessee

Austin Peay State University, School of Nursing, *Clarksville (BSN)*
Baptist College of Health Sciences, Nursing Division, *Memphis (BSN)*
Belmont University, School of Nursing, *Nashville (BSN)*
Carson-Newman University, Department of Nursing, *Jefferson City (BSN)*
Christian Brothers University, RN to BSN Program, *Memphis (BSN)*
Cumberland University, Rudy School of Nursing and Health Professions, *Lebanon (BSN)*
East Tennessee State University, College of Nursing, *Johnson City (BSN)*
Lincoln Memorial University, Caylor School of Nursing, *Harrogate (BSN)*
Middle Tennessee State University, School of Nursing, *Murfreesboro (BSN)*
Milligan College, Department of Nursing, *Milligan College (BSN)*
Tennessee State University, Division of Nursing, *Nashville (BSN)*
Tennessee Technological University, Whitson-Hester School of Nursing, *Cookeville (BSN)*
Tennessee Wesleyan College, Fort Sanders Nursing Department, *Knoxville (BSN)*
Union University, School of Nursing, *Jackson (BSN)*
University of Memphis, Loewenberg School of Nursing, *Memphis (BSN)*
The University of Tennessee, College of Nursing, *Knoxville (BSN)*
The University of Tennessee Health Science Center, College of Nursing, *Memphis (BSN)*

### Texas

Angelo State University, Department of Nursing and Rehabilitation Sciences, *San Angelo (BSN)*
Houston Baptist University, School of Nursing and Allied Health, *Houston (BSN)*
Lamar University, Department of Nursing, *Beaumont (BSN)*
Lubbock Christian University, Department of Nursing, *Lubbock (BSN)*
Patty Hanks Shelton School of Nursing, *Abilene (BSN)*
Prairie View A&M University, College of Nursing, *Houston (BSN)*
Southwestern Adventist University, Department of Nursing, *Keene (BS)*
Stephen F. Austin State University, Richard and Lucille Dewitt School of Nursing, *Nacogdoches (BSN)*
Texas A&M Health Science Center, College of Nursing, *College Station (BSN)*
Texas A&M International University, Canseco School of Nursing, *Laredo (BSN)*
Texas A&M University–Corpus Christi, College of Nursing and Health Sciences, *Corpus Christi (BSN)*
Texas Tech University Health Sciences Center, School of Nursing, *Lubbock (BSN)*
Texas Woman's University, College of Nursing, *Denton (BS)*
University of Houston–Victoria, School of Nursing, *Victoria (BSN)*
The University of Texas at Arlington, College of Nursing, *Arlington (BSN)*
The University of Texas at Austin, School of Nursing, *Austin (BSN)*
The University of Texas at El Paso, School of Nursing, *El Paso (BSN)*
The University of Texas at Tyler, Program in Nursing, *Tyler (BSN)*
The University of Texas Medical Branch, School of Nursing, *Galveston (BSN)*
The University of Texas–Pan American, Department of Nursing, *Edinburg (BSN)*
Wayland Baptist University, Bachelor of Science in Nursing Program, *Plainview (BSN)*

### Utah

Brigham Young University, College of Nursing, *Provo (BS)*
Dixie State University, Nursing Department, *St. George (BSN)*
Southern Utah University, Department of Nursing, *Cedar City (BSN)*
University of Utah, College of Nursing, *Salt Lake City (BS)*
Western Governors University, Online College of Health Professions, *Salt Lake City (BS)*
Westminster College, School of Nursing and Health Sciences, *Salt Lake City (BSN)*

### Vermont

Norwich University, Department of Nursing, *Northfield (BSN)*

### Virgin Islands

University of the Virgin Islands, Division of Nursing, *Saint Thomas (BSN)*

### Virginia

Bon Secours Memorial College of Nursing, *Richmond (BSN)*
Eastern Mennonite University, Department of Nursing, *Harrisonburg (BSN)*
ECPI University, BSN Program, *Virginia Beach (BSN)*
George Mason University, College of Health and Human Services, *Fairfax (BSN)*
Hampton University, School of Nursing, *Hampton (BS)*
James Madison University, Department of Nursing, *Harrisonburg (BSN)*
Jefferson College of Health Sciences, Nursing Education Program, *Roanoke (BSN)*
Liberty University, Department of Nursing, *Lynchburg (BSN)*
Longwood University, Nursing Program, *Farmville (BSN)*
Marymount University, School of Health Professions, *Arlington (BSN)*
Norfolk State University, Department of Nursing, *Norfolk (BSN)*
Old Dominion University, Department of Nursing, *Norfolk (BSN)*
Radford University, School of Nursing, *Radford (BSN)*
Sentara College of Health Sciences, Bachelor of Science in Nursing Program, *Chesapeake (BSN)*
Shenandoah University, Division of Nursing, *Winchester (BSN)*
University of Virginia, School of Nursing, *Charlottesville (BSN)*
The University of Virginia's College at Wise, Department of Nursing, *Wise (BSN)*

### Washington

Olympic College, Nursing Programs, *Bremerton (BSN)*
Seattle Pacific University, School of Health Sciences, *Seattle (BS)*
Walla Walla University, School of Nursing, *College Place (BS)*
Washington State University College of Nursing, *Spokane (BSN)*

### West Virginia

Alderson Broaddus University, Department of Nursing, *Philippi (BSN)*
American Public University System, Bachelor of Science in Nursing, *Charles Town (BSN)*
Bluefield State College, Program in Nursing, *Bluefield (BSN)*
Fairmont State University, School of Nursing and Allied Health Administration, *Fairmont (BSN)*
Shepherd University, Department of Nursing Education, *Shepherdstown (BSN)*
West Virginia University, School of Nursing, *Morgantown (BSN)*
Wheeling Jesuit University, Department of Nursing, *Wheeling (BSN)*

### Wisconsin

Alverno College, Division of Nursing, *Milwaukee (BSN)*
Columbia College of Nursing/Mount Mary College Nursing Program, *Milwaukee (BSN)*
Concordia University Wisconsin, Program in Nursing, *Mequon (BSN)*
Herzing University Online, Program in Nursing, *Milwaukee (BSN)*
Maranatha Baptist Bible College, Nursing Department, *Watertown (BSN)*
Milwaukee School of Engineering, School of Nursing, *Milwaukee (BSN)*
University of Phoenix–Milwaukee Campus, College of Health and Human Services, *Milwaukee (BSN)*
University of Wisconsin–Eau Claire, College of Nursing and Health Sciences, *Eau Claire (BSN)*
University of Wisconsin–Green Bay, BSN–LINC Online RN–BSN Program, *Green Bay (BSN)*
University of Wisconsin–Madison, School of Nursing, *Madison (BS)*
University of Wisconsin–Milwaukee, College of Nursing, *Milwaukee (BSN)*
University of Wisconsin–Oshkosh, College of Nursing, *Oshkosh (BSN)*
Viterbo University, School of Nursing, *La Crosse (BSN)*

## CANADA

### Alberta

Athabasca University, Centre for Nursing and Health Studies, *Athabasca (BN)*
University of Alberta, Faculty of Nursing, *Edmonton (BScN)*
University of Calgary, Faculty of Nursing, *Calgary (BN)*

### British Columbia

British Columbia Institute of Technology, School of Health Sciences, *Burnaby (BSN)*
Kwantlen Polytechnic University, Faculty of Community and Health Sciences, *Surrey (BSN)*

University of Northern British Columbia, Nursing Programme, *Prince George (BScN)*

### Manitoba

Brandon University, School of Health Studies, *Brandon (BN)*

University of Manitoba, Faculty of Nursing, *Winnipeg (BN)*

### New Brunswick

Université de Moncton, School of Nursing, *Moncton (BScN)*

### Newfoundland and Labrador

Memorial University of Newfoundland, School of Nursing, *St. John's (BN)*

### Nova Scotia

St. Francis Xavier University, Department of Nursing, *Antigonish (BScN)*

### Ontario

Brock University, Department of Nursing, *St. Catharines (BScN)*

Lakehead University, School of Nursing, *Thunder Bay (BScN)*

Laurentian University, School of Nursing, *Sudbury (BScN)*

McMaster University, School of Nursing, *Hamilton (BScN)*

Nipissing University, Nursing Department, *North Bay (BScN)*

Ryerson University, Program in Nursing, *Toronto (BScN)*

University of Ottawa, School of Nursing, *Ottawa (BScN)*

The University of Western Ontario, School of Nursing, *London (BScN)*

York University, School of Nursing, *Toronto (BScN)*

### Quebec

McGill University, School of Nursing, *Montréal (BScN)*

Université de Montréal, Faculty of Nursing, *Montréal (BScN)*

Université de Sherbrooke, Department of Nursing, *Sherbrooke (BScN)*

Université du Québec à Chicoutimi, Program in Nursing, *Chicoutimi (BNSc)*

Université du Québec à Rimouski, Program in Nursing, *Rimouski (BScN)*

Université du Québec à Trois-Rivières, Program in Nursing, *Trois-Rivières (BSN)*

Université du Québec en Outaouais, Département des Sciences Infirmières, *Gatineau (BScN)*

Université Laval, Faculty of Nursing, *Québec (BScN)*

### Saskatchewan

University of Saskatchewan, College of Nursing, *Saskatoon (BSN)*

## RPN TO BACCALAUREATE

## U.S. AND U.S. TERRITORIES

### California

San Jose State University, The Valley Foundation School of Nursing, *San Jose (BS)*

### Massachusetts

Curry College, Division of Nursing, *Milton (BS)*

### Michigan

Lake Superior State University, Department of Nursing, *Sault Sainte Marie (BSN)*

University of Michigan–Flint, Department of Nursing, *Flint (BSN)*

### Nebraska

University of Nebraska Medical Center, College of Nursing, *Omaha (BSN)*

### Ohio

Franciscan University of Steubenville, Department of Nursing, *Steubenville (BSN)*

### Pennsylvania

Chatham University, Nursing Programs, *Pittsburgh (BSN)*

## CANADA

### Alberta

University of Alberta, Faculty of Nursing, *Edmonton (BScN)*

### British Columbia

British Columbia Institute of Technology, School of Health Sciences, *Burnaby (BSN)*

### Ontario

Nipissing University, Nursing Department, *North Bay (BScN)*

Ryerson University, Program in Nursing, *Toronto (BScN)*

University of Ottawa, School of Nursing, *Ottawa (BScN)*

# Master's Degree Programs

## ACCELERATED AD/RN TO MASTER'S

### U.S. AND U.S. TERRITORIES

**Alabama**

Spring Hill College, Division of Nursing, *Mobile (MSN)*

The University of Alabama at Birmingham, School of Nursing, *Birmingham (MSN, MSN/MPH)*

**California**

University of San Francisco, School of Nursing, *San Francisco (MSN)*

Western University of Health Sciences, College of Graduate Nursing, *Pomona (MSN)*

**Delaware**

Wesley College, Nursing Program, *Dover (MSN)*

Wilmington University, College of Health Professions, *New Castle (MSN, MSN/MBA, MSN/MS)*

**Florida**

Florida International University, Nursing Program, *Miami (MSN)*

**Georgia**

Brenau University, College of Health and Science, *Gainesville (MSN)*

**Kentucky**

Frontier Nursing University, Nursing Degree Programs, *Hyden (MSN)*

**Massachusetts**

Regis College, School of Nursing, Science and Health Professions, *Weston (MSN)*

**Michigan**

Ferris State University, School of Nursing, *Big Rapids (MSN, MSN/MBA)*

Saginaw Valley State University, College of Health and Human Services, *University Center (MSN)*

University of Detroit Mercy, McAuley School of Nursing, *Detroit (MSN)*

**Missouri**

Missouri State University, Department of Nursing, *Springfield (MSN)*

**Nebraska**

Nebraska Wesleyan University, Department of Nursing, *Lincoln (MSN)*

**New York**

Daemen College, Department of Nursing, *Amherst (MS)*

State University of New York Institute of Technology, School of Nursing and Health Systems, *Utica (MS)*

**Ohio**

Case Western Reserve University, Frances Payne Bolton School of Nursing, *Cleveland (MSN, MSN/MA, MSN/MBA, MSN/PhD)*

Walsh University, Department of Nursing, *North Canton (MSN)*

**Oklahoma**

Oklahoma City University, Kramer School of Nursing, *Oklahoma City (MSN, MSN/MBA)*

**Pennsylvania**

DeSales University, Department of Nursing and Health, *Center Valley (MSN, MSN/MBA)*

Gannon University, Villa Maria School of Nursing, *Erie (MSN)*

The University of Scranton, Department of Nursing, *Scranton (MSN)*

Wilkes University, Department of Nursing, *Wilkes-Barre (MS)*

**Tennessee**

Carson-Newman University, Department of Nursing, *Jefferson City (MSN)*

Middle Tennessee State University, School of Nursing, *Murfreesboro (MSN)*

**Texas**

The University of Texas at Tyler, Program in Nursing, *Tyler (MSN, MSN/MBA)*

University of the Incarnate Word, Program in Nursing, *San Antonio (MSN)*

**West Virginia**

West Virginia University, School of Nursing, *Morgantown (MSN)*

## ACCELERATED MASTER'S

### U.S. AND U.S. TERRITORIES

**Alabama**

University of South Alabama, College of Nursing, *Mobile (MSN)*

**Arizona**

The University of Arizona, College of Nursing, *Tucson (MSN)*

**California**

California State University, Fresno, Department of Nursing, *Fresno (MSN)*

California State University, Long Beach, School of Nursing, *Long Beach (MSN, MSN/MHA)*

University of Phoenix–Sacramento Valley Campus, College of Nursing, *Sacramento (MSN, MSN/MHA)*

Western University of Health Sciences, College of Graduate Nursing, *Pomona (MSN)*

**Georgia**

Thomas University, Division of Nursing, *Thomasville (MSN, MSN/MBA)*

**Hawaii**

University of Hawaii at Manoa, School of Nursing and Dental Hygiene, *Honolulu (MS, MSN/MBA)*

**Illinois**

Benedictine University, Department of Nursing, *Lisle (MSN)*

Lewis University, Program in Nursing, *Romeoville (MSN, MSN/MBA)*

**Maryland**

Stevenson University, Nursing Division, *Stevenson (MS)*

**Massachusetts**

Boston College, William F. Connell School of Nursing, *Chestnut Hill (MS, MS/MA, MS/MBA, MSN/PhD)*

Regis College, School of Nursing, Science and Health Professions, *Weston (MSN)*

Simmons College, School of Nursing and Health Sciences, *Boston (MS)*

University of Massachusetts Lowell, School of Nursing, *Lowell (MS)*

**Nebraska**

Nebraska Wesleyan University, Department of Nursing, *Lincoln (MSN)*

**New York**

The Sage Colleges, Department of Nursing, *Troy (MS, MS/MBA)*

**Ohio**

Ursuline College, The Breen School of Nursing, *Pepper Pike (MSN, MSN/MBA)*

**Oklahoma**

Oklahoma City University, Kramer School of Nursing, *Oklahoma City (MSN, MSN/MBA)*

Southern Nazarene University, School of Nursing, *Bethany (MS)*

**Pennsylvania**

Carlow University, School of Nursing, *Pittsburgh (MSN)*

Thomas Jefferson University, Department of Nursing, *Philadelphia (MSN)*

Waynesburg University, Department of Nursing, *Waynesburg (MSN, MSN/MBA)*

**Utah**

Western Governors University, Online College of Health Professions, *Salt Lake City (MS)*

**West Virginia**

West Virginia University, School of Nursing, *Morgantown (MSN)*

**Wisconsin**

Cardinal Stritch University, Ruth S. Coleman College of Nursing, *Milwaukee (MSN)*

### CANADA

**Quebec**

Université Laval, Faculty of Nursing, *Québec (MSN)*

## ACCELERATED MASTER'S FOR NON-NURSING COLLEGE GRADUATES

### U.S. AND U.S. TERRITORIES

**Alabama**

The University of Alabama at Birmingham, School of Nursing, *Birmingham (MSN, MSN/MPH)*

**Arizona**

The University of Arizona, College of Nursing, *Tucson (MSN)*

**California**

Azusa Pacific University, School of Nursing, *Azusa (MSN)*

California Baptist University, School of Nursing, *Riverside (MSN)*
San Francisco State University, School of Nursing, *San Francisco (MSN)*
University of San Diego, Hahn School of Nursing and Health Science, *San Diego (MSN)*
University of San Francisco, School of Nursing, *San Francisco (MSN)*
Western University of Health Sciences, College of Graduate Nursing, *Pomona (MSN)*

### Georgia
Georgia Regents University, School of Nursing, *Augusta (MSN)*

### Illinois
Millikin University, School of Nursing, *Decatur (MSN)*

### Indiana
University of Indianapolis, School of Nursing, *Indianapolis (MSN)*

### Maryland
University of Maryland, Baltimore, Master's Program in Nursing, *Baltimore (MS, MSN/MBA, MSN/MPH)*

### Massachusetts
Boston College, William F. Connell School of Nursing, *Chestnut Hill (MS, MS/MA, MS/MBA, MSN/PhD)*
Regis College, School of Nursing, Science and Health Professions, *Weston (MSN)*
Salem State University, Program in Nursing, *Salem (MSN, MSN/MBA)*
Simmons College, School of Nursing and Health Sciences, *Boston (MS)*
University of Massachusetts Worcester, Graduate School of Nursing, *Worcester (MS)*

### Missouri
Saint Louis University, School of Nursing, *St. Louis (MSN)*

### New Jersey
Seton Hall University, College of Nursing, *South Orange (MSN, MSN/MA, MSN/MBA)*

### New York
Columbia University, School of Nursing, *New York (MS, MSN/MBA, MSN/MPH)*
Mercy College, Programs in Nursing, *Dobbs Ferry (MS)*

### North Carolina
East Carolina University, College of Nursing, *Greenville (MSN)*

### Ohio
College of Mount St. Joseph, Department of Nursing, *Cincinnati (MN)*
University of Cincinnati, College of Nursing, *Cincinnati (MSN, MSN/MBA, MSN/PhD)*
Xavier University, School of Nursing, *Cincinnati (MSN, MSN/MBA, MSN/Ed D)*

### Oregon
Oregon Health & Science University, School of Nursing, *Portland (MS, MN/MPH)*

### Pennsylvania
University of Pennsylvania, School of Nursing, *Philadelphia (MSN, MSN/MBA, MSN/MPH, MSN/PhD)*

### Washington
Pacific Lutheran University, School of Nursing, *Tacoma (MSN, MSN/MBA)*

### Wisconsin
Marquette University, College of Nursing, *Milwaukee (MSN, MSN/MBA)*

## ACCELERATED MASTER'S FOR NURSES WITH NON-NURSING DEGREES

## U.S. AND U.S. TERRITORIES

### California
Azusa Pacific University, School of Nursing, *Azusa (MSN)*
California State University, Los Angeles, School of Nursing, *Los Angeles (MSN)*
Charles Drew University of Medicine and Science, School of Nursing, *Los Angeles (MSN)*
San Francisco State University, School of Nursing, *San Francisco (MSN)*

### Delaware
Wilmington University, College of Health Professions, *New Castle (MSN, MSN/MBA, MSN/MS)*

### Illinois
Lewis University, Program in Nursing, *Romeoville (MSN, MSN/MBA)*
Resurrection University, *Chicago (MSN)*

### Kentucky
Western Kentucky University, School of Nursing, *Bowling Green (MSN)*

### Massachusetts
Regis College, School of Nursing, Science and Health Professions, *Weston (MSN)*

### New Jersey
Kean University, Department of Nursing, *Union (MSN, MSN/MPA)*
Seton Hall University, College of Nursing, *South Orange (MSN, MSN/MA, MSN/MBA)*

### New York
Columbia University, School of Nursing, *New York (MS, MSN/MBA, MSN/MPH)*
Mercy College, Programs in Nursing, *Dobbs Ferry (MS)*

### North Carolina
East Carolina University, College of Nursing, *Greenville (MSN)*

### Oklahoma
Oklahoma City University, Kramer School of Nursing, *Oklahoma City (MSN, MSN/MBA)*
Southern Nazarene University, School of Nursing, *Bethany (MS)*

### Pennsylvania
University of Pennsylvania, School of Nursing, *Philadelphia (MSN, MSN/MBA, MSN/MPH, MSN/PhD)*
Waynesburg University, Department of Nursing, *Waynesburg (MSN, MSN/MBA)*

### Tennessee
University of Memphis, Loewenberg School of Nursing, *Memphis (MSN)*

### Washington
Seattle University, College of Nursing, *Seattle (MSN)*
Washington State University College of Nursing, *Spokane (MN)*

## ACCELERATED RN TO MASTER'S

## U.S. AND U.S. TERRITORIES

### California
California State University, Los Angeles, School of Nursing, *Los Angeles (MSN)*

### Delaware
Wesley College, Nursing Program, *Dover (MSN)*

### Georgia
Brenau University, College of Health and Science, *Gainesville (MSN)*

### Illinois
Lewis University, Program in Nursing, *Romeoville (MSN, MSN/MBA)*
Saint Francis Medical Center College of Nursing, Baccalaureate Nursing Program, *Peoria (MSN)*

### Iowa
The University of Iowa, College of Nursing, *Iowa City (MSN, MSN/MBA, MSN/MPH)*

### Kentucky
Spalding University, School of Nursing, *Louisville (MSN)*

### Maryland
Stevenson University, Nursing Division, *Stevenson (MS)*

### Massachusetts
Regis College, School of Nursing, Science and Health Professions, *Weston (MSN)*
University of Massachusetts Lowell, School of Nursing, *Lowell (MS)*

### Michigan
Ferris State University, School of Nursing, *Big Rapids (MSN, MSN/MBA)*
University of Michigan, School of Nursing, *Ann Arbor (MS, MSN/MBA, MSN/MPH)*
University of Michigan–Flint, Department of Nursing, *Flint (MSN)*

### Minnesota
Capella University, Nursing Programs, *Minneapolis (MSN)*
Minnesota State University Mankato, School of Nursing, *Mankato (MSN, MSN/MS)*

### Missouri
Maryville University of Saint Louis, Nursing Program, School of Health Professions, *St. Louis (MSN)*

### Nebraska
Nebraska Wesleyan University, Department of Nursing, *Lincoln (MSN)*

### New Jersey
Fairleigh Dickinson University, Metropolitan Campus, Henry P. Becton School of Nursing and Allied Health, *Teaneck (MSN)*

Felician College, Division of Nursing and Health Management, *Lodi (MSN, MA/MSM)*

Seton Hall University, College of Nursing, *South Orange (MSN, MSN/MA, MSN/MBA)*

### New York

Daemen College, Department of Nursing, *Amherst (MS)*

Mercy College, Programs in Nursing, *Dobbs Ferry (MS)*

The Sage Colleges, Department of Nursing, *Troy (MS, MS/MBA)*

State University of New York Institute of Technology, School of Nursing and Health Systems, *Utica (MS)*

State University of New York Upstate Medical University, College of Nursing, *Syracuse (MS)*

### Ohio

Kent State University, College of Nursing, *Kent (MSN, MSN/MBA, MSN/MPA)*

### Oklahoma

Oklahoma City University, Kramer School of Nursing, *Oklahoma City (MSN, MSN/MBA)*

### Pennsylvania

Gannon University, Villa Maria School of Nursing, *Erie (MSN)*

Thomas Jefferson University, Department of Nursing, *Philadelphia (MSN)*

The University of Scranton, Department of Nursing, *Scranton (MSN)*

Waynesburg University, Department of Nursing, *Waynesburg (MSN, MSN/MBA)*

Wilkes University, Department of Nursing, *Wilkes-Barre (MS)*

### Tennessee

King College, School of Nursing, *Bristol (MSN, MSN/MBA)*

Southern Adventist University, School of Nursing, *Collegedale (MSN, MSN/MBA)*

### Texas

The University of Texas at Tyler, Program in Nursing, *Tyler (MSN, MSN/MBA)*

### Utah

Western Governors University, Online College of Health Professions, *Salt Lake City (MS)*

### Washington

Gonzaga University, Department of Nursing, *Spokane (MSN)*

Washington State University College of Nursing, *Spokane (MN)*

### West Virginia

West Virginia University, School of Nursing, *Morgantown (MSN)*

## CANADA

### Quebec

Université du Québec à Chicoutimi, Program in Nursing, *Chicoutimi (MSN, MS/MPH)*

# JOINT DEGREES

## U.S. AND U.S. TERRITORIES

### Alabama

The University of Alabama at Birmingham, School of Nursing, *Birmingham (MSN, MSN/MPH)*

### Arizona

Arizona State University at the Downtown Phoenix Campus, College of Nursing, *Phoenix (MS, MS/MPH)*

Grand Canyon University, College of Nursing and Health Sciences, *Phoenix (MS, MSN/MBA)*

University of Phoenix–Online Campus, Online Campus, *Phoenix (MSN, MSN/MBA, MSN/MHA)*

University of Phoenix–Phoenix Campus, College of Nursing, *Tempe (MSN, MSN/MBA, MSN/MHA)*

### California

California State University, Long Beach, School of Nursing, *Long Beach (MSN, MSN/MHA)*

Holy Names University, Department of Nursing, *Oakland (MSN, MSN/MBA)*

University of California, Davis, The Betty Irene Moore School of Nursing, *Davis (MS, MSN/MS)*

University of California, Los Angeles, School of Nursing, *Los Angeles (MSN, MSN/MBA)*

University of Phoenix–Bay Area Campus, College of Nursing, *San Jose (MSN, MSN/MBA, MSN/MHA)*

University of Phoenix–Sacramento Valley Campus, College of Nursing, *Sacramento (MSN, MSN/MHA)*

University of Phoenix–Southern California Campus, College of Nursing, *Costa Mesa (MSN, MSN/MBA, MSN/MHA)*

### Connecticut

Yale University, School of Nursing, *New Haven (MSN, MSN/MPH, MSN/MDIV)*

### Delaware

Wilmington University, College of Health Professions, *New Castle (MSN, MSN/MBA, MSN/MS)*

### District of Columbia

The Catholic University of America, School of Nursing, *Washington (MSN, MA/MSM)*

### Florida

Barry University, Division of Nursing, *Miami Shores (MSN, MSN/MBA)*

Florida Southern College, School of Nursing & Health Sciences, *Lakeland (MSN, MSN/MBA)*

Jacksonville University, School of Nursing, *Jacksonville (MSN, MSN/MBA)*

University of Florida, College of Nursing, *Gainesville (MSN, MSN/PhD)*

University of Phoenix–North Florida Campus, College of Nursing, *Jacksonville (MSN, MSN/MHA, MSN/Ed D)*

University of Phoenix–South Florida Campus, College of Nursing, *Miramar (MSN, MSN/MBA, MSN/MHA)*

University of South Florida, College of Nursing, *Tampa (MS, MS/MPH)*

### Georgia

Emory University, Nell Hodgson Woodruff School of Nursing, *Atlanta (MSN, MSN/MPH)*

Thomas University, Division of Nursing, *Thomasville (MSN, MSN/MBA)*

### Hawaii

Hawai`i Pacific University, College of Nursing and Health Sciences, *Honolulu (MSN, MSN/MBA)*

University of Hawaii at Manoa, School of Nursing and Dental Hygiene, *Honolulu (MS, MSN/MBA)*

### Idaho

Boise State University, Department of Nursing, *Boise (MSN, MSN/MS)*

### Illinois

Elmhurst College, Deicke Center for Nursing Education, *Elmhurst (MS, MSN/MBA)*

Lewis University, Program in Nursing, *Romeoville (MSN, MSN/MBA)*

Loyola University Chicago, Marcella Niehoff School of Nursing, *Maywood (MSN, MSN/MBA)*

McKendree University, Department of Nursing, *Lebanon (MSN, MSN/MBA)*

Northern Illinois University, School of Nursing and Health Studies, *De Kalb (MS, MSN/MPH)*

North Park University, School of Nursing, *Chicago (MS, MSN/MA, MSN/MBA, MSN/MM)*

Saint Xavier University, School of Nursing, *Chicago (MSN, MSN/MBA)*

University of Illinois at Chicago, College of Nursing, *Chicago (MS, MS/MBA, MS/MPH)*

### Indiana

Anderson University, School of Nursing, *Anderson (MSN, MSN/MBA)*

Valparaiso University, College of Nursing, *Valparaiso (MSN, MSN/MBA)*

### Iowa

The University of Iowa, College of Nursing, *Iowa City (MSN, MSN/MBA, MSN/MPH)*

### Kansas

The University of Kansas, School of Nursing, *Kansas City (MS, MS/MHSA, MS/MPH)*

### Kentucky

Bellarmine University, Donna and Allan Lansing School of Nursing and Health Sciences, *Louisville (Certificate of Completion, MSN, MSN/MBA)*

### Maine

Saint Joseph's College of Maine, Master of Science in Nursing Program, *Standish (MSN, MSN/MHA)*

University of Southern Maine, School of Nursing, *Portland (MS, MS/MBA)*

### Maryland

The Johns Hopkins University, School of Nursing, *Baltimore (MSN, MSN/MBA, MSN/MPH, MSN/PhD)*

University of Maryland, Baltimore, Master's Program in Nursing, *Baltimore (MS, MSN/MBA, MSN/MPH)*

### Massachusetts

Boston College, William F. Connell School of Nursing, *Chestnut Hill (MS, MS/MA, MS/MBA, MSN/PhD)*

Salem State University, Program in Nursing, *Salem (MSN, MSN/MBA)*

### Michigan

Ferris State University, School of Nursing, *Big Rapids (MSN, MSN/MBA)*

Madonna University, College of Nursing and Health, *Livonia (MSN, MSN/MBA)*

Spring Arbor University, Program in Nursing, *Spring Arbor (MSN, MSN/MBA)*

University of Michigan, School of Nursing, *Ann Arbor (MS, MSN/MBA, MSN/MPH)*

### Minnesota

Minnesota State University Mankato, School of Nursing, *Mankato (MSN, MSN/MS)*

### Missouri

University of Missouri, Sinclair School of Nursing, *Columbia (MSN, MSN/PhD)*

### Nevada

University of Nevada, Reno, Orvis School of Nursing, *Reno (MSN, MSN/MPH)*

### New Jersey

Felician College, Division of Nursing and Health Management, *Lodi (MSN, MA/MSM)*

Kean University, Department of Nursing, *Union (MSN, MSN/MPA)*

Rutgers, The State University of New Jersey, Newark, Rutgers School of Nursing, *Newark (MSN, MSN/MPH)*

Seton Hall University, College of Nursing, *South Orange (MSN, MSN/MA, MSN/MBA)*

### New York

Adelphi University, College of Nursing and Public Health, *Garden City (MS, MS/MBA)*

Columbia University, School of Nursing, *New York (MS, MSN/MBA, MSN/MPH)*

Hunter College of the City University of New York, Hunter-Bellevue School of Nursing, *New York (MS, MSN/MPA, MSN/MPH)*

Molloy College, Division of Nursing, *Rockville Centre (MS, MS/MBA)*

New York University, College of Nursing, *New York (MS, MS/MPH, MSN/MPA)*

The Sage Colleges, Department of Nursing, *Troy (MS, MS/MBA)*

State University of New York Downstate Medical Center, College of Nursing, *Brooklyn (MS, MS/MPH)*

### North Carolina

Duke University, School of Nursing, *Durham (MSN, MSN/MBA)*

Gardner-Webb University, School of Nursing, *Boiling Springs (MSN, MSN/MBA)*

Queens University of Charlotte, Presbyterian School of Nursing, *Charlotte (MSN, MSN/MBA)*

The University of North Carolina at Greensboro, School of Nursing, *Greensboro (MSN, MSN/MBA)*

### Ohio

Capital University, School of Nursing, *Columbus (MSN, MN/MBA, MSN/JD, MSN/MDIV)*

Case Western Reserve University, Frances Payne Bolton School of Nursing, *Cleveland (MSN, MSN/MA, MSN/MBA, MSN/PhD)*

Cleveland State University, School of Nursing, *Cleveland (MSN, MSN/MBA)*

Kent State University, College of Nursing, *Kent (MSN, MSN/MBA, MSN/MPA)*

The Ohio State University, College of Nursing, *Columbus (MS, MS/MPH)*

University of Cincinnati, College of Nursing, *Cincinnati (MSN, MSN/MBA, MSN/PhD)*

Ursuline College, The Breen School of Nursing, *Pepper Pike (MSN, MSN/MBA)*

Wright State University, College of Nursing and Health, *Dayton (MS, MS/MBA)*

Xavier University, School of Nursing, *Cincinnati (MSN, MSN/MBA, MSN/Ed D)*

### Oklahoma

Oklahoma City University, Kramer School of Nursing, *Oklahoma City (MSN, MSN/MBA)*

### Oregon

Oregon Health & Science University, School of Nursing, *Portland (MS, MN/MPH)*

### Pennsylvania

Bloomsburg University of Pennsylvania, Department of Nursing, *Bloomsburg (MSN, MSN/MBA)*

DeSales University, Department of Nursing and Health, *Center Valley (MSN, MSN/MBA)*

La Salle University, School of Nursing and Health Sciences, *Philadelphia (MSN, MSN/MBA)*

Marywood University, Department of Nursing, *Scranton (MSN, MSN/MPH)*

Penn State University Park, School of Nursing, *University Park (MS, MSN/PhD)*

University of Pennsylvania, School of Nursing, *Philadelphia (MSN, MSN/MBA, MSN/MPH, MSN/PhD)*

Waynesburg University, Department of Nursing, *Waynesburg (MSN, MSN/MBA)*

Widener University, School of Nursing, *Chester (MSN, MSN/PhD)*

### Tennessee

King College, School of Nursing, *Bristol (MSN, MSN/MBA)*

Southern Adventist University, School of Nursing, *Collegedale (MSN, MSN/MBA)*

The University of Tennessee, College of Nursing, *Knoxville (MSN, MSN/PhD)*

Vanderbilt University, Vanderbilt University School of Nursing, *Nashville (MSN, MSN/MDIV, MSN/MTS)*

### Texas

Lamar University, Department of Nursing, *Beaumont (MSN, MSN/MBA)*

Texas Woman's University, College of Nursing, *Denton (MS, MS/MHA)*

The University of Texas at Arlington, College of Nursing, *Arlington (MSN, MSN/MBA, MSN/MHA, MSN/MPH)*

The University of Texas at Austin, School of Nursing, *Austin (MSN, MSN/MBA)*

The University of Texas at Tyler, Program in Nursing, *Tyler (MSN, MSN/MBA)*

The University of Texas Health Science Center at Houston, School of Nursing, *Houston (MSN, MSN/MPH)*

### Virginia

Shenandoah University, Division of Nursing, *Winchester (MSN, MSN/MBA)*

University of Virginia, School of Nursing, *Charlottesville (MSN, MSN/MBA, MSN/PhD)*

### Washington

Pacific Lutheran University, School of Nursing, *Tacoma (MSN, MSN/MBA)*

University of Washington, School of Nursing, *Seattle (MN, MN/MPH)*

### Wisconsin

Edgewood College, Program in Nursing, *Madison (MS, MSN/MBA)*

Marquette University, College of Nursing, *Milwaukee (MSN, MSN/MBA)*

## CANADA

### Alberta

Athabasca University, Centre for Nursing and Health Studies, *Athabasca (MN, MN/MHSA)*

### British Columbia

The University of British Columbia, Program in Nursing, *Vancouver (MSN, MSN/MPH)*

### Ontario

McMaster University, School of Nursing, *Hamilton (M Sc, MSN/PhD)*

### Quebec

Université du Québec à Chicoutimi, Program in Nursing, *Chicoutimi (MSN, MS/MPH)*

# MASTER'S

## U.S. AND U.S. TERRITORIES

### Alabama

Auburn University, School of Nursing, *Auburn University (MSN)*

Auburn University at Montgomery, School of Nursing, *Montgomery (MSN)*

Jacksonville State University, College of Nursing and Health Sciences, *Jacksonville (MSN)*

Samford University, Ida V. Moffett School of Nursing, *Birmingham (MSN)*

Spring Hill College, Division of Nursing, *Mobile (MSN)*

Troy University, School of Nursing, *Troy (MSN)*

The University of Alabama, Capstone College of Nursing, *Tuscaloosa (MSN, MSN/Ed D)*

The University of Alabama at Birmingham, School of Nursing, *Birmingham (MSN, MSN/MPH)*

The University of Alabama in Huntsville, College of Nursing, *Huntsville (MSN)*

University of Mobile, School of Nursing, *Mobile (MSN)*

University of North Alabama, College of Nursing and Allied Health, *Florence (MSN)*

University of South Alabama, College of Nursing, *Mobile (MSN)*

### Alaska

University of Alaska Anchorage, School of Nursing, *Anchorage (MS)*

**Arizona**

Arizona State University at the Downtown Phoenix Campus, College of Nursing, *Phoenix (MS, MS/MPH)*

Chamberlain College of Nursing, *Phoenix (MSN)*

Grand Canyon University, College of Nursing and Health Sciences, *Phoenix (MS, MSN/MBA)*

Northern Arizona University, School of Nursing, *Flagstaff (MS)*

University of Phoenix–Online Campus, Online Campus, *Phoenix (MSN, MSN/MBA, MSN/MHA)*

University of Phoenix–Phoenix Campus, College of Nursing, *Tempe (MSN, MSN/MBA, MSN/MHA)*

University of Phoenix–Southern Arizona Campus, College of Social Sciences, *Tucson (MSN)*

**Arkansas**

Arkansas State University, Department of Nursing, *State University (MSN)*

Arkansas Tech University, Program in Nursing, *Russellville (MSN)*

University of Arkansas, Eleanor Mann School of Nursing, *Fayetteville (MSN)*

University of Arkansas for Medical Sciences, College of Nursing, *Little Rock (MN Sc)*

University of Central Arkansas, Department of Nursing, *Conway (MSN)*

**California**

Azusa Pacific University, School of Nursing, *Azusa (MSN)*

Brandman University, School of Nursing and Health Professions, *Irvine (MS)*

California Baptist University, School of Nursing, *Riverside (MSN)*

California State University, Chico, School of Nursing, *Chico (MSN)*

California State University, Dominguez Hills, Program in Nursing, *Carson (MSN)*

California State University, Fresno, Department of Nursing, *Fresno (MSN)*

California State University, Fullerton, Department of Nursing, *Fullerton (MSN)*

California State University, Long Beach, School of Nursing, *Long Beach (MSN, MSN/MHA)*

California State University, Los Angeles, School of Nursing, *Los Angeles (MSN)*

California State University, Sacramento, School of Nursing, *Sacramento (MS)*

California State University, San Bernardino, Department of Nursing, *San Bernardino (MSN)*

Charles Drew University of Medicine and Science, School of Nursing, *Los Angeles (MSN)*

Dominican University of California, Program in Nursing, *San Rafael (MSN)*

Holy Names University, Department of Nursing, *Oakland (MSN, MSN/MBA)*

Loma Linda University, School of Nursing, *Loma Linda (MS)*

Mount St. Mary's College, Department of Nursing, *Los Angeles (MSN)*

Point Loma Nazarene University, School of Nursing, *San Diego (MSN)*

Samuel Merritt University, School of Nursing, *Oakland (MSN)*

San Diego State University, School of Nursing, *San Diego (MSN)*

San Francisco State University, School of Nursing, *San Francisco (MSN)*

San Jose State University, The Valley Foundation School of Nursing, *San Jose (MS)*

University of California, Davis, The Betty Irene Moore School of Nursing, *Davis (MS, MSN/MS)*

University of California, Irvine, Program in Nursing Science, *Irvine (MS)*

University of California, Los Angeles, School of Nursing, *Los Angeles (MSN, MSN/MBA)*

University of California, San Francisco, School of Nursing, *San Francisco (MS)*

University of Phoenix–Bay Area Campus, College of Nursing, *San Jose (MSN, MSN/MBA, MSN/MHA)*

University of Phoenix–San Diego Campus, College of Nursing, *San Diego (MSN, MSN/Ed D)*

University of Phoenix–Southern California Campus, College of Nursing, *Costa Mesa (MSN, MSN/MBA, MSN/MHA)*

University of San Diego, Hahn School of Nursing and Health Science, *San Diego (MSN)*

Western University of Health Sciences, College of Graduate Nursing, *Pomona (MSN)*

**Colorado**

American Sentinel University, RN to Bachelor of Science Nursing, *Aurora (MSN)*

Aspen University, Graduate School of Health Professions and Studies, *Denver (MSN)*

Colorado State University–Pueblo, Department of Nursing, *Pueblo (MS)*

Regis University, School of Nursing, *Denver (MS)*

University of Colorado Colorado Springs, Beth-El College of Nursing and Health Sciences, *Colorado Springs (MSN)*

University of Colorado Denver, College of Nursing, *Aurora (MS)*

University of Northern Colorado, School of Nursing, *Greeley (MS)*

**Connecticut**

Fairfield University, School of Nursing, *Fairfield (MSN)*

Quinnipiac University, School of Nursing, *Hamden (MSN)*

Sacred Heart University, Program in Nursing, *Fairfield (MSN)*

Southern Connecticut State University, Department of Nursing, *New Haven (MSN)*

University of Connecticut, School of Nursing, *Storrs (MS)*

University of Hartford, College of Education, Nursing, and Health Professions, *West Hartford (MSN)*

University of Saint Joseph, Department of Nursing, *West Hartford (MS)*

Western Connecticut State University, Department of Nursing, *Danbury (MS)*

Yale University, School of Nursing, *New Haven (MSN, MSN/MPH, MSN/MDIV)*

**Delaware**

Delaware State University, Department of Nursing, *Dover (MS)*

University of Delaware, School of Nursing, *Newark (MSN)*

Wesley College, Nursing Program, *Dover (MSN)*

Wilmington University, College of Health Professions, *New Castle (MSN, MSN/MBA, MSN/MS)*

**District of Columbia**

The Catholic University of America, School of Nursing, *Washington (MSN, MA/MSM)*

Georgetown University, School of Nursing and Health Studies, *Washington (MS)*

The George Washington University, School of Nursing, *Washington (MSN)*

Howard University, Division of Nursing, *Washington (MSN)*

**Florida**

Barry University, Division of Nursing, *Miami Shores (MSN, MSN/MBA)*

Florida Agricultural and Mechanical University, School of Nursing, *Tallahassee (MSN)*

Florida Atlantic University, Christine E. Lynn College of Nursing, *Boca Raton (MSN)*

Florida Gulf Coast University, School of Nursing, *Fort Myers (MSN)*

Florida International University, Nursing Program, *Miami (MSN)*

Florida Southern College, School of Nursing & Health Sciences, *Lakeland (MSN, MSN/MBA)*

Florida State University, College of Nursing, *Tallahassee (MSN)*

Jacksonville University, School of Nursing, *Jacksonville (MSN, MSN/MBA)*

Kaplan University Online, The School of Nursing Online, *Fort Lauderdale (MSN)*

Keiser University, Nursing Programs, *Fort Lauderdale (MSN)*

Keiser University, Nursing Programs, *Fort Myers (MSN)*

Keiser University, Nursing Programs, *Jacksonville (MSN)*

Keiser University, Nursing Programs, *Lakeland (MSN)*

Keiser University, Nursing Programs, *Melbourne (MSN)*

Keiser University, Nursing Programs, *Miami (MSN)*

Keiser University, Nursing Programs, *Orlando (MSN)*

Keiser University, Nursing Programs, *Port St. Lucie (MSN)*

Keiser University, Nursing Programs, *Sarasota (MSN)*

Keiser University, Nursing Programs, *Tallahassee (MSN)*

Keiser University, Nursing Programs, *Tampa (MSN)*

Nova Southeastern University, College of Health Care Sciences, *Fort Lauderdale (MSN)*

University of Central Florida, College of Nursing, *Orlando (MSN)*

University of Florida, College of Nursing, *Gainesville (MSN, MSN/PhD)*

University of Miami, School of Nursing and Health Studies, *Coral Gables (MSN)*

University of North Florida, School of Nursing, *Jacksonville (MSN)*

University of Phoenix–North Florida Campus, College of Nursing, *Jacksonville (MSN, MSN/MHA, MSN/Ed D)*

University of Phoenix–South Florida Campus, College of Nursing, *Miramar (MSN, MSN/MBA, MSN/MHA)*

University of South Florida, College of Nursing, *Tampa (MS, MS/MPH)*

The University of Tampa, Department of Nursing, *Tampa (MSN)*

University of West Florida, Department of Nursing, *Pensacola (MSN)*

## Georgia

Albany State University, College of Sciences and Health Professions, *Albany (MSN)*

Armstrong Atlantic State University, Program in Nursing, *Savannah (MSN)*

Brenau University, College of Health and Science, *Gainesville (MSN)*

Clayton State University, Department of Nursing, *Morrow (MSN)*

Emory University, Nell Hodgson Woodruff School of Nursing, *Atlanta (MSN, MSN/MPH)*

Georgia College & State University, College of Health Sciences, *Milledgeville (MSN)*

Georgia Regents University, School of Nursing, *Augusta (MSN)*

Georgia Southern University, School of Nursing, *Statesboro (MSN)*

Georgia Southwestern State University, School of Nursing, *Americus (MSN)*

Georgia State University, Byrdine F. Lewis School of Nursing and Health Professions, *Atlanta (MSN)*

Kennesaw State University, School of Nursing, *Kennesaw (MSN)*

Georgia Baptist College of Nursing, *Atlanta (MSN)*

Thomas University, Division of Nursing, *Thomasville (MSN, MSN/MBA)*

University of North Georgia, Department of Nursing, *Dahlonega (MS)*

University of West Georgia, School of Nursing, *Carrollton (MSN)*

Valdosta State University, College of Nursing, *Valdosta (MSN)*

## Hawaii

Hawai`i Pacific University, College of Nursing and Health Sciences, *Honolulu (MSN, MSN/MBA)*

University of Hawaii at Manoa, School of Nursing and Dental Hygiene, *Honolulu (MS, MSN/MBA)*

University of Phoenix–Hawaii Campus, College of Nursing, *Honolulu (MSN, MSN/Ed D)*

## Idaho

Boise State University, Department of Nursing, *Boise (MSN, MSN/MS)*

Idaho State University, Department of Nursing, *Pocatello (MS)*

Northwest Nazarene University, School of Health and Science, *Nampa (MSN)*

## Illinois

Aurora University, School of Nursing, *Aurora (MSN)*

Benedictine University, Department of Nursing, *Lisle (MSN)*

Blessing–Rieman College of Nursing, *Quincy (MSN)*

Bradley University, Department of Nursing, *Peoria (MSN)*

DePaul University, School of Nursing, *Chicago (MS)*

Elmhurst College, Deicke Center for Nursing Education, *Elmhurst (MS, MSN/MBA)*

Governors State University, College of Health and Human Services, *University Park (MS)*

Illinois State University, Mennonite College of Nursing, *Normal (MSN)*

Lewis University, Program in Nursing, *Romeoville (MSN, MSN/MBA)*

Loyola University Chicago, Marcella Niehoff School of Nursing, *Maywood (MSN, MSN/MBA)*

McKendree University, Department of Nursing, *Lebanon (MSN, MSN/MBA)*

Millikin University, School of Nursing, *Decatur (MSN)*

Northern Illinois University, School of Nursing and Health Studies, *De Kalb (MS, MSN/MPH)*

North Park University, School of Nursing, *Chicago (MS, MSN/MA, MSN/MBA, MSN/MM)*

Olivet Nazarene University, Division of Nursing, *Bourbonnais (MSN)*

Resurrection University, *Chicago (MSN)*

Rush University, College of Nursing, *Chicago (MSN)*

Saint Anthony College of Nursing, *Rockford (MSN)*

Saint Francis Medical Center College of Nursing, Baccalaureate Nursing Program, *Peoria (MSN)*

Saint Xavier University, School of Nursing, *Chicago (MSN, MSN/MBA)*

Southern Illinois University Edwardsville, School of Nursing, *Edwardsville (MS)*

University of Illinois at Chicago, College of Nursing, *Chicago (MS, MS/MBA, MS/MPH)*

University of St. Francis, Leach College of Nursing, *Joliet (MSN)*

## Indiana

Anderson University, School of Nursing, *Anderson (MSN, MSN/MBA)*

Ball State University, School of Nursing, *Muncie (MS)*

Bethel College, School of Nursing, *Mishawaka (MSN)*

Goshen College, Department of Nursing, *Goshen (MSN)*

Indiana State University, Department of Nursing, *Terre Haute (MS)*

Indiana University–Purdue University Fort Wayne, Department of Nursing, *Fort Wayne (MS)*

Indiana University–Purdue University Indianapolis, School of Nursing, *Indianapolis (MSN)*

Indiana University South Bend, College of Health Sciences, *South Bend (MSN)*

Indiana Wesleyan University, School of Nursing, *Marion (MSN)*

Purdue University, School of Nursing, *West Lafayette (MS)*

Purdue University Calumet, School of Nursing, *Hammond (MS)*

University of Indianapolis, School of Nursing, *Indianapolis (MSN)*

University of Saint Francis, Department of Nursing, *Fort Wayne (MSN)*

University of Southern Indiana, College of Nursing and Health Professions, *Evansville (MSN)*

Valparaiso University, College of Nursing, *Valparaiso (MSN, MSN/MBA)*

## Iowa

Allen College, Program in Nursing, *Waterloo (MSN)*

Briar Cliff University, Department of Nursing, *Sioux City (MSN)*

Clarke University, Department of Nursing and Health, *Dubuque (MSN)*

Grand View University, Division of Nursing, *Des Moines (MS)*

Mount Mercy University, Department of Nursing, *Cedar Rapids (MSN)*

St. Ambrose University, Program in Nursing (BSN), *Davenport (MSN)*

The University of Iowa, College of Nursing, *Iowa City (MSN, MSN/MBA, MSN/MPH)*

## Kansas

Fort Hays State University, Department of Nursing, *Hays (MSN, MSN/Ed D)*

MidAmerica Nazarene University, Division of Nursing, *Olathe (MSN)*

Newman University, Division of Nursing, *Wichita (MS)*

Pittsburg State University, Department of Nursing, *Pittsburg (MSN)*

The University of Kansas, School of Nursing, *Kansas City (MS, MS/MHSA, MS/MPH)*

Washburn University, School of Nursing, *Topeka (MSN)*

## Kentucky

Bellarmine University, Donna and Allan Lansing School of Nursing and Health Sciences, *Louisville (Certificate of Completion, MSN, MSN/MBA)*

Eastern Kentucky University, Department of Baccalaureate and Graduate Nursing, *Richmond (MSN)*

Murray State University, Program in Nursing, *Murray (MSN)*

Northern Kentucky University, Department of Nursing, *Highland Heights (MSN)*

Spalding University, School of Nursing, *Louisville (MSN)*

University of Kentucky, College of Nursing, *Lexington (MSN)*

University of Louisville, School of Nursing, *Louisville (MSN)*

Western Kentucky University, School of Nursing, *Bowling Green (MSN)*

## Louisiana

Grambling State University, School of Nursing, *Grambling (MSN)*

Louisiana State University Health Sciences Center, School of Nursing, *New Orleans (MN)*

Loyola University New Orleans, School of Nursing, *New Orleans (MSN)*

McNeese State University, College of Nursing, *Lake Charles (MSN)*

Northwestern State University of Louisiana, College of Nursing and Allied Health, *Shreveport (MSN)*

Our Lady of the Lake College, Division of Nursing, *Baton Rouge (MSN)*
Southeastern Louisiana University, School of Nursing, *Hammond (MSN)*
Southern University and Agricultural and Mechanical College, School of Nursing, *Baton Rouge (MSN)*
University of Louisiana at Lafayette, College of Nursing, *Lafayette (MSN)*

**Maine**

Husson University, School of Nursing, *Bangor (MSN)*
Saint Joseph's College of Maine, Master of Science in Nursing Program, *Standish (MSN, MSN/MHA)*
University of Maine, School of Nursing, *Orono (MSN)*
University of Southern Maine, School of Nursing, *Portland (MS, MS/MBA)*

**Maryland**

Bowie State University, Department of Nursing, *Bowie (MSN)*
Coppin State University, Helene Fuld School of Nursing, *Baltimore (MSN)*
The Johns Hopkins University, School of Nursing, *Baltimore (MSN, MSN/MBA, MSN/MPH, MSN/PhD)*
Salisbury University, Nursing DNP Program, *Salisbury (MS)*
Towson University, Department of Nursing, *Towson (MS)*
University of Maryland, Baltimore, Master's Program in Nursing, *Baltimore (MS, MSN/MBA, MSN/MPH)*

**Massachusetts**

American International College, Division of Nursing, *Springfield (MSN)*
Boston College, William F. Connell School of Nursing, *Chestnut Hill (MS, MS/MA, MS/MBA, MSN/PhD)*
Curry College, Division of Nursing, *Milton (MSN)*
Elms College, Division of Nursing, *Chicopee (MSN)*
Emmanuel College, Department of Nursing, *Boston (MS)*
Endicott College, Major in Nursing, *Beverly (MSN)*
Fitchburg State University, Department of Nursing, *Fitchburg (MS)*
Framingham State University, Department of Nursing, *Framingham (MSN)*
MGH Institute of Health Professions, School of Nursing, *Boston (MS)*
Northeastern University, School of Nursing, *Boston (MS)*
Regis College, School of Nursing, Science and Health Professions, *Weston (MSN)*
Salem State University, Program in Nursing, *Salem (MSN, MSN/MBA)*
Simmons College, School of Nursing and Health Sciences, *Boston (MS)*
University of Massachusetts Amherst, School of Nursing, *Amherst (MS)*
University of Massachusetts Boston, College of Nursing and Health Sciences, *Boston (MS)*
University of Massachusetts Dartmouth, College of Nursing, *North Dartmouth (MS)*
University of Massachusetts Lowell, School of Nursing, *Lowell (MS)*
University of Massachusetts Worcester, Graduate School of Nursing, *Worcester (MS)*
Worcester State University, Department of Nursing, *Worcester (MS)*

**Michigan**

Andrews University, Department of Nursing, *Berrien Springs (MS)*
Eastern Michigan University, School of Nursing, *Ypsilanti (MSN)*
Ferris State University, School of Nursing, *Big Rapids (MSN, MSN/MBA)*
Grand Valley State University, Kirkhof College of Nursing, *Allendale (MSN)*
Madonna University, College of Nursing and Health, *Livonia (MSN, MSN/MBA)*
Michigan State University, College of Nursing, *East Lansing (MSN)*
Northern Michigan University, College of Nursing and Allied Health Science, *Marquette (MSN)*
Oakland University, School of Nursing, *Rochester (MSN)*
Saginaw Valley State University, College of Health and Human Services, *University Center (MSN)*
Spring Arbor University, Program in Nursing, *Spring Arbor (MSN, MSN/MBA)*
University of Detroit Mercy, McAuley School of Nursing, *Detroit (MSN)*
University of Michigan, School of Nursing, *Ann Arbor (MS, MSN/MBA, MSN/MPH)*
Wayne State University, College of Nursing, *Detroit (MSN)*
Western Michigan University, College of Health and Human Services, *Kalamazoo (MSN)*

**Minnesota**

Augsburg College, Program in Nursing, *Minneapolis (MA)*
Bethel University, Department of Nursing, *St. Paul (MA)*
Capella University, Nursing Programs, *Minneapolis (MSN)*
The College of St. Scholastica, Department of Nursing, *Duluth (MA)*
Concordia College, Department of Nursing, *Moorhead (MS)*
Minnesota State University Mankato, School of Nursing, *Mankato (MSN, MSN/MS)*
Minnesota State University Moorhead, School of Nursing and Healthcare Leadership, *Moorhead (MS)*
St. Catherine University, Department of Nursing, *St. Paul (MS)*
Walden University, Nursing Programs, *Minneapolis (MSN)*
Winona State University, College of Nursing and Health Sciences, *Winona (MS)*

**Mississippi**

Alcorn State University, School of Nursing, *Natchez (MSN)*
Delta State University, School of Nursing, *Cleveland (MSN)*
Mississippi University for Women, College of Nursing and Speech Language Pathology, *Columbus (MSN)*
University of Mississippi Medical Center, School of Nursing, *Jackson (MSN)*
University of Southern Mississippi, School of Nursing, *Hattiesburg (MSN)*
William Carey University, School of Nursing, *Hattiesburg (MSN)*

**Missouri**

Central Methodist University, College of Liberal Arts and Sciences, *Fayette (MSN)*
Cox College, Department of Nursing, *Springfield (MSN)*
Goldfarb School of Nursing at Barnes-Jewish College, *St. Louis (MSN)*
Graceland University, School of Nursing, *Independence (MSN)*
Maryville University of Saint Louis, Nursing Program, School of Health Professions, *St. Louis (MSN)*
Missouri Southern State University, Department of Nursing, *Joplin (MSN)*
Missouri State University, Department of Nursing, *Springfield (MSN)*
Missouri Western State University, Department of Nursing, *St. Joseph (MSN)*
Research College of Nursing, College of Nursing, *Kansas City (MSN)*
Saint Louis University, School of Nursing, *St. Louis (MSN)*
Southeast Missouri State University, Department of Nursing, *Cape Girardeau (MSN)*
Southwest Baptist University, College of Nursing, *Bolivar (MSN)*
University of Central Missouri, Department of Nursing, *Warrensburg (MS)*
University of Missouri, Sinclair School of Nursing, *Columbia (MSN, MSN/PhD)*
University of Missouri–Kansas City, School of Nursing and Health Studies, *Kansas City (MSN)*
University of Missouri–St. Louis, College of Nursing, *St. Louis (MSN)*
Webster University, Department of Nursing, *St. Louis (MSN)*

**Montana**

Montana State University, College of Nursing, *Bozeman (MN)*

**Nebraska**

Bryan College of Health Sciences, School of Nursing, *Lincoln (MS)*
Clarkson College, Master of Science in Nursing Program, *Omaha (MSN)*
College of Saint Mary, Division of Health Care Professions, *Omaha (MSN)*
Creighton University, School of Nursing, *Omaha (MSN)*
Nebraska Methodist College, Department of Nursing, *Omaha (MSN)*
Nebraska Wesleyan University, Department of Nursing, *Lincoln (MSN)*
University of Nebraska Medical Center, College of Nursing, *Omaha (MSN)*

**Nevada**

Touro University, School of Nursing, *Henderson (MSN)*
University of Nevada, Las Vegas, School of Nursing, *Las Vegas (MSN)*
University of Nevada, Reno, Orvis School of Nursing, *Reno (MSN, MSN/MPH)*

**New Hampshire**

Franklin Pierce University, Master of Science in Nursing, *Rindge (MSN)*

Rivier University, Division of Nursing, *Nashua (MS)*

University of New Hampshire, Department of Nursing, *Durham (MS)*

### New Jersey

The College of New Jersey, School of Nursing, Health and Exercise Science, *Ewing (MSN)*

Fairleigh Dickinson University, Metropolitan Campus, Henry P. Becton School of Nursing and Allied Health, *Teaneck (MSN)*

Felician College, Division of Nursing and Health Management, *Lodi (MSN, MA/MSM)*

Kean University, Department of Nursing, *Union (MSN, MSN/MPA)*

Monmouth University, Marjorie K. Unterberg School of Nursing, *West Long Branch (MSN)*

Ramapo College of New Jersey, Master of Science in Nursing Program, *Mahwah (MSN)*

Rutgers, The State University of New Jersey, Newark, Rutgers School of Nursing, *Newark (MSN, MSN/MPH)*

Saint Peter's University, Nursing Program, *Jersey City (MSN)*

Seton Hall University, College of Nursing, *South Orange (MSN, MSN/MA, MSN/MBA)*

Thomas Edison State College, School of Nursing, *Trenton (MSN)*

William Paterson University of New Jersey, Department of Nursing, *Wayne (MSN)*

### New Mexico

New Mexico State University, School of Nursing, *Las Cruces (MSN)*

University of New Mexico, College of Nursing, *Albuquerque (MSN)*

University of Phoenix–New Mexico Campus, College of Nursing, *Albuquerque (MSN, MSN/Ed D)*

### New York

Adelphi University, College of Nursing and Public Health, *Garden City (MS, MS/MBA)*

Binghamton University, State University of New York, Decker School of Nursing, *Vestal (MS)*

College of Mount Saint Vincent, Department of Nursing, *Riverdale (MSN)*

The College of New Rochelle, School of Nursing, *New Rochelle (MS)*

College of Staten Island of the City University of New York, Department of Nursing, *Staten Island (MS)*

Columbia University, School of Nursing, *New York (MS, MSN/MBA, MSN/MPH)*

Daemen College, Department of Nursing, *Amherst (MS)*

Dominican College, Department of Nursing, *Orangeburg (M Sc N)*

D'Youville College, School of Nursing, *Buffalo (MS)*

Excelsior College, School of Nursing, *Albany (MS)*

Hunter College of the City University of New York, Hunter-Bellevue School of Nursing, *New York (MS, MSN/MPA, MSN/MPH)*

Lehman College of the City University of New York, Department of Nursing, *Bronx (MS)*

Le Moyne College, Nursing Programs, *Syracuse (MS)*

Long Island University–LIU Brooklyn, School of Nursing, *Brooklyn (MS)*

Long Island University–LIU Post, Department of Nursing, *Brookville (MS)*

Mercy College, Programs in Nursing, *Dobbs Ferry (MS)*

Molloy College, Division of Nursing, *Rockville Centre (MS, MS/MBA)*

Mount Saint Mary College, Division of Nursing, *Newburgh (MS)*

New York University, College of Nursing, *New York (MS, MS/MPH, MSN/MPA)*

Pace University, Lienhard School of Nursing, *New York (MS)*

Roberts Wesleyan College, Division of Nursing, *Rochester (M Sc N)*

The Sage Colleges, Department of Nursing, *Troy (MS, MS/MBA)*

St. John Fisher College, Wegmans School of Nursing, *Rochester (MS)*

St. Joseph's College, New York, Department of Nursing, *Brooklyn (MS)*

State University of New York Downstate Medical Center, College of Nursing, *Brooklyn (MS, MS/MPH)*

State University of New York Institute of Technology, School of Nursing and Health Systems, *Utica (MS)*

State University of New York Upstate Medical University, College of Nursing, *Syracuse (MS)*

Stony Brook University, State University of New York, School of Nursing, *Stony Brook (MS)*

University at Buffalo, the State University of New York, School of Nursing, *Buffalo (MS)*

### North Carolina

Duke University, School of Nursing, *Durham (MSN, MSN/MBA)*

East Carolina University, College of Nursing, *Greenville (MSN)*

Gardner-Webb University, School of Nursing, *Boiling Springs (MSN, MSN/MBA)*

Lenoir-Rhyne University, Program in Nursing, *Hickory (MSN)*

Queens University of Charlotte, Presbyterian School of Nursing, *Charlotte (MSN, MSN/MBA)*

The University of North Carolina at Chapel Hill, School of Nursing, *Chapel Hill (MSN)*

The University of North Carolina at Charlotte, School of Nursing, *Charlotte (MSN)*

The University of North Carolina at Greensboro, School of Nursing, *Greensboro (MSN, MSN/MBA)*

The University of North Carolina Wilmington, School of Nursing, *Wilmington (MSN)*

Western Carolina University, School of Nursing, *Cullowhee (MS)*

Winston-Salem State University, Department of Nursing, *Winston-Salem (MSN)*

### North Dakota

North Dakota State University, Department of Nursing, *Fargo (MS)*

University of Mary, Division of Nursing, *Bismarck (MSN)*

University of North Dakota, College of Nursing, *Grand Forks (MS)*

### Ohio

Capital University, School of Nursing, *Columbus (MSN, MN/MBA, MSN/JD, MSN/MDIV)*

Case Western Reserve University, Frances Payne Bolton School of Nursing, *Cleveland (MSN, MSN/MA, MSN/MBA, MSN/PhD)*

Cedarville University, School of Nursing, *Cedarville (MSN)*

Chamberlain College of Nursing, *Columbus (MSN)*

Cleveland State University, School of Nursing, *Cleveland (MSN, MSN/MBA)*

Franciscan University of Steubenville, Department of Nursing, *Steubenville (MSN)*

Kent State University, College of Nursing, *Kent (MSN, MSN/MBA, MSN/MPA)*

Lourdes University, School of Nursing, *Sylvania (MSN)*

Malone University, School of Nursing, *Canton (MSN)*

Mount Carmel College of Nursing, Nursing Programs, *Columbus (MS)*

The Ohio State University, College of Nursing, *Columbus (MS, MS/MPH)*

Ohio University, School of Nursing, *Athens (MSN)*

Otterbein University, Department of Nursing, *Westerville (MSN)*

The University of Akron, School of Nursing, *Akron (MSN)*

University of Cincinnati, College of Nursing, *Cincinnati (MSN, MSN/MBA, MSN/PhD)*

University of Phoenix–Cleveland Campus, College of Nursing, *Independence (MSN)*

The University of Toledo, College of Nursing, *Toledo (MSN)*

Urbana University, College of Nursing and Allied Health, *Urbana (MSN)*

Ursuline College, The Breen School of Nursing, *Pepper Pike (MSN, MSN/MBA)*

Walsh University, Department of Nursing, *North Canton (MSN)*

Wright State University, College of Nursing and Health, *Dayton (MS, MS/MBA)*

Xavier University, School of Nursing, *Cincinnati (MSN, MSN/MBA, MSN/Ed D)*

### Oklahoma

Northeastern State University, Department of Nursing, *Tahlequah (MSN)*

Oklahoma Baptist University, School of Nursing, *Shawnee (MSN)*

Oklahoma City University, Kramer School of Nursing, *Oklahoma City (MSN, MSN/MBA)*

University of Central Oklahoma, Department of Nursing, *Edmond (MS)*

University of Oklahoma Health Sciences Center, College of Nursing, *Oklahoma City (MS)*

### Oregon

Oregon Health & Science University, School of Nursing, *Portland (MS, MN/MPH)*

University of Portland, School of Nursing, *Portland (MS)*

### Pennsylvania

Alvernia University, Nursing, *Reading (MSN)*

Bloomsburg University of Pennsylvania, Department of Nursing, *Bloomsburg (MSN, MSN/MBA)*

Carlow University, School of Nursing, *Pittsburgh (MSN)*

Cedar Crest College, Department of Nursing, *Allentown (MSN)*

Chatham University, Nursing Programs, *Pittsburgh (MSN)*
Clarion University of Pennsylvania, School of Nursing, *Oil City (MSN)*
DeSales University, Department of Nursing and Health, *Center Valley (MSN, MSN/MBA)*
Drexel University, College of Nursing and Health Professions, *Philadelphia (MSN)*
Duquesne University, School of Nursing, *Pittsburgh (MSN)*
Gannon University, Villa Maria School of Nursing, *Erie (MSN)*
Gwynedd Mercy University, School of Nursing, *Gwynedd Valley (MSN)*
Holy Family University, School of Nursing and Allied Health Professions, *Philadelphia (MSN)*
Immaculata University, Division of Nursing, *Immaculata (MSN)*
Indiana University of Pennsylvania, Department of Nursing and Allied Health, *Indiana (MS)*
La Roche College, Department of Nursing and Nursing Management, *Pittsburgh (MSN)*
La Salle University, School of Nursing and Health Sciences, *Philadelphia (MSN, MSN/MBA)*
Mansfield University of Pennsylvania, Department of Health Sciences–Nursing, *Mansfield (MSN)*
Marywood University, Department of Nursing, *Scranton (MSN, MSN/MPH)*
Millersville University of Pennsylvania, Department of Nursing, *Millersville (MSN)*
Misericordia University, Department of Nursing, *Dallas (MSN)*
Moravian College, Department of Nursing, *Bethlehem (MS)*
Neumann University, Program in Nursing and Health Sciences, *Aston (MS)*
Penn State University Park, School of Nursing, *University Park (MS, MSN/PhD)*
Robert Morris University, School of Nursing and Health Sciences, *Moon Township (MSN)*
Temple University, Department of Nursing, *Philadelphia (MSN)*
Thomas Jefferson University, Department of Nursing, *Philadelphia (MSN)*
University of Pennsylvania, School of Nursing, *Philadelphia (MSN, MSN/MBA, MSN/MPH, MSN/PhD)*
University of Pittsburgh, School of Nursing, *Pittsburgh (MSN)*
The University of Scranton, Department of Nursing, *Scranton (MSN)*
Villanova University, College of Nursing, *Villanova (MSN)*
West Chester University of Pennsylvania, Department of Nursing, *West Chester (MSN)*
Widener University, School of Nursing, *Chester (MSN, MSN/PhD)*
Wilkes University, Department of Nursing, *Wilkes-Barre (MS)*
York College of Pennsylvania, Department of Nursing, *York (MS)*

### Puerto Rico
University of Puerto Rico, Medical Sciences Campus, School of Nursing, *San Juan (MSN)*
University of the Sacred Heart, Program in Nursing, *San Juan (MSN)*

### Rhode Island
Rhode Island College, Department of Nursing, *Providence (MSN)*
University of Rhode Island, College of Nursing, *Kingston (MS)*

### South Carolina
Charleston Southern University, Wingo School of Nursing, *Charleston (MSN)*
Clemson University, School of Nursing, *Clemson (MS)*
Medical University of South Carolina, College of Nursing, *Charleston (MSN)*
University of South Carolina, College of Nursing, *Columbia (MSN)*

### South Dakota
South Dakota State University, College of Nursing, *Brookings (MS)*

### Tennessee
Aquinas College, School of Nursing, *Nashville (MSN)*
Austin Peay State University, School of Nursing, *Clarksville (MSN)*
Belmont University, School of Nursing, *Nashville (MSN)*
Carson-Newman University, Department of Nursing, *Jefferson City (MSN)*
East Tennessee State University, College of Nursing, *Johnson City (MSN)*
King College, School of Nursing, *Bristol (MSN, MSN/MBA)*
Lincoln Memorial University, Caylor School of Nursing, *Harrogate (MSN)*
Middle Tennessee State University, School of Nursing, *Murfreesboro (MSN)*
Southern Adventist University, School of Nursing, *Collegedale (MSN, MSN/MBA)*
Tennessee Technological University, Whitson-Hester School of Nursing, *Cookeville (MSN, M Sc N)*
Union University, School of Nursing, *Jackson (MSN)*
University of Memphis, Loewenberg School of Nursing, *Memphis (MSN)*
The University of Tennessee, College of Nursing, *Knoxville (MSN, MSN/PhD)*
The University of Tennessee at Chattanooga, School of Nursing, *Chattanooga (MSN)*
The University of Tennessee Health Science Center, College of Nursing, *Memphis (MSN)*
Vanderbilt University, Vanderbilt University School of Nursing, *Nashville (MSN, MSN/MDIV, MSN/MTS)*

### Texas
Angelo State University, Department of Nursing and Rehabilitation Sciences, *San Angelo (MSN)*
Baylor University, Louise Herrington School of Nursing, *Dallas (MSN)*
Lamar University, Department of Nursing, *Beaumont (MSN, MSN/MBA)*
Midwestern State University, Nursing Program, *Wichita Falls (MSN)*
Patty Hanks Shelton School of Nursing, *Abilene (MSN)*
Prairie View A&M University, College of Nursing, *Houston (MSN)*
Texas A&M International University, Canseco School of Nursing, *Laredo (MSN)*
Texas A&M University–Corpus Christi, College of Nursing and Health Sciences, *Corpus Christi (MSN)*
Texas A&M University–Texarkana, Nursing Department, *Texarkana (MSN)*
Texas Christian University, Harris College of Nursing, *Fort Worth (MSN)*
Texas State University–San Marcos, St. David's School of Nursing, *San Marcos (MSN)*
Texas Tech University Health Sciences Center, School of Nursing, *Lubbock (MSN)*
Texas Woman's University, College of Nursing, *Denton (MS, MS/MHA)*
University of Houston–Victoria, School of Nursing, *Victoria (MSN)*
University of Mary Hardin-Baylor, College of Nursing, *Belton (MSN)*
The University of Texas at Arlington, College of Nursing, *Arlington (MSN, MSN/MBA, MSN/MHA, MSN/MPH)*
The University of Texas at Austin, School of Nursing, *Austin (MSN, MSN/MBA)*
The University of Texas at Brownsville, Department of Nursing, *Brownsville (MSN)*
The University of Texas at El Paso, School of Nursing, *El Paso (MSN)*
The University of Texas at Tyler, Program in Nursing, *Tyler (MSN, MSN/MBA)*
The University of Texas Health Science Center at Houston, School of Nursing, *Houston (MSN, MSN/MPH)*
The University of Texas Health Science Center at San Antonio, School of Nursing, *San Antonio (MSN)*
The University of Texas Medical Branch, School of Nursing, *Galveston (MSN)*
The University of Texas–Pan American, Department of Nursing, *Edinburg (MSN)*
University of the Incarnate Word, Program in Nursing, *San Antonio (MSN)*
West Texas A&M University, Department of Nursing, *Canyon (MSN)*

### Utah
Brigham Young University, College of Nursing, *Provo (MS)*
University of Utah, College of Nursing, *Salt Lake City (MS)*
Weber State University, Program in Nursing, *Ogden (MSN)*
Western Governors University, Online College of Health Professions, *Salt Lake City (MS)*
Westminster College, School of Nursing and Health Sciences, *Salt Lake City (MSN)*

### Vermont
University of Vermont, Department of Nursing, *Burlington (MS)*

### Virginia
Eastern Mennonite University, Department of Nursing, *Harrisonburg (MSN)*
George Mason University, College of Health and Human Services, *Fairfax (MSN)*
Hampton University, School of Nursing, *Hampton (MS)*
James Madison University, Department of Nursing, *Harrisonburg (MSN)*
Jefferson College of Health Sciences, Nursing Education Program, *Roanoke (MSN)*
Liberty University, Department of Nursing, *Lynchburg (MSN)*

Lynchburg College, School of Health Sciences and Human Performance, *Lynchburg (MSN)*
Marymount University, School of Health Professions, *Arlington (MSN)*
Old Dominion University, Department of Nursing, *Norfolk (MSN)*
Radford University, School of Nursing, *Radford (MSN)*
Shenandoah University, Division of Nursing, *Winchester (MSN, MSN/MBA)*
University of Virginia, School of Nursing, *Charlottesville (MSN, MSN/MBA, MSN/PhD)*
Virginia Commonwealth University, School of Nursing, *Richmond (MS)*

### Washington

Gonzaga University, Department of Nursing, *Spokane (MSN)*
Pacific Lutheran University, School of Nursing, *Tacoma (MSN, MSN/MBA)*
Seattle Pacific University, School of Health Sciences, *Seattle (MSN)*
Seattle University, College of Nursing, *Seattle (MSN)*
University of Washington, School of Nursing, *Seattle (MN, MN/MPH)*
Washington State University College of Nursing, *Spokane (MN)*

### West Virginia

Marshall University, College of Health Professions, *Huntington (MSN)*
West Virginia University, School of Nursing, *Morgantown (MSN)*
West Virginia Wesleyan College, School of Nursing, *Buckhannon (MSN)*
Wheeling Jesuit University, Department of Nursing, *Wheeling (MSN)*

### Wisconsin

Alverno College, Division of Nursing, *Milwaukee (MSN)*
Bellin College, Nursing Program, *Green Bay (MSN)*
Concordia University Wisconsin, Program in Nursing, *Mequon (MSN)*
Edgewood College, Program in Nursing, *Madison (MS, MSN/MBA)*
Herzing University Online, Program in Nursing, *Milwaukee (MSN)*
Marian University, School of Nursing, *Fond du Lac (MSN)*
Marquette University, College of Nursing, *Milwaukee (MSN, MSN/MBA)*
University of Phoenix–Milwaukee Campus, College of Health and Human Services, *Milwaukee (MSN)*
University of Wisconsin–Eau Claire, College of Nursing and Health Sciences, *Eau Claire (MSN)*
University of Wisconsin–Green Bay, BSN–LINC Online RN–BSN Program, *Green Bay (MSN)*
University of Wisconsin–Milwaukee, College of Nursing, *Milwaukee (MN)*
University of Wisconsin–Oshkosh, College of Nursing, *Oshkosh (MSN)*
Viterbo University, School of Nursing, *La Crosse (MSN)*

### Wyoming

University of Wyoming, Fay W. Whitney School of Nursing, *Laramie (MS)*

## CANADA

### Alberta

Athabasca University, Centre for Nursing and Health Studies, *Athabasca (MN, MN/MHSA)*
University of Alberta, Faculty of Nursing, *Edmonton (MN)*
University of Calgary, Faculty of Nursing, *Calgary (MN)*
University of Lethbridge, Faculty of Health Sciences, *Lethbridge (M Sc)*

### British Columbia

Trinity Western University, Department of Nursing, *Langley (MSN)*
The University of British Columbia, Program in Nursing, *Vancouver (MSN, MSN/MPH)*
University of Northern British Columbia, Nursing Programme, *Prince George (M Sc N)*
University of Victoria, School of Nursing, *Victoria (MN)*

### Manitoba

University of Manitoba, Faculty of Nursing, *Winnipeg (MN)*

### New Brunswick

Université de Moncton, School of Nursing, *Moncton (M Sc N)*
University of New Brunswick Fredericton, Faculty of Nursing, *Fredericton (MN)*

### Newfoundland and Labrador

Memorial University of Newfoundland, School of Nursing, *St. John's (MN)*

### Ontario

Laurentian University, School of Nursing, *Sudbury (M Sc N)*
McMaster University, School of Nursing, *Hamilton (M Sc, MSN/PhD)*
Queen's University at Kingston, School of Nursing, *Kingston (M Sc)*
Ryerson University, Program in Nursing, *Toronto (MN)*
University of Ottawa, School of Nursing, *Ottawa (M Sc N)*
University of Toronto, Faculty of Nursing, *Toronto (MN)*
The University of Western Ontario, School of Nursing, *London (M Sc N)*
University of Windsor, Faculty of Nursing, *Windsor (M Sc N)*

### Quebec

McGill University, School of Nursing, *Montréal (M Sc)*
Université de Montréal, Faculty of Nursing, *Montréal (M Sc)*
Université de Sherbrooke, Department of Nursing, *Sherbrooke (M Sc)*
Université du Québec à Chicoutimi, Program in Nursing, *Chicoutimi (MSN, MS/MPH)*
Université du Québec à Rimouski, Program in Nursing, *Rimouski (M Sc N)*
Université du Québec à Trois-Rivières, Program in Nursing, *Trois-Rivières (MSN)*
Université du Québec en Outaouais, Département des Sciences Infirmières, *Gatineau (M Sc N)*
Université Laval, Faculty of Nursing, *Québec (MSN)*

### Saskatchewan

University of Saskatchewan, College of Nursing, *Saskatoon (MN)*

# MASTER'S FOR NON-NURSING COLLEGE GRADUATES

## U.S. AND U.S. TERRITORIES

### California

California State University, Dominguez Hills, Program in Nursing, *Carson (MSN)*
California State University, Fullerton, Department of Nursing, *Fullerton (MSN)*
California State University, Long Beach, School of Nursing, *Long Beach (MSN, MSN/MHA)*
California State University, Los Angeles, School of Nursing, *Los Angeles (MSN)*
Samuel Merritt University, School of Nursing, *Oakland (MSN)*
San Francisco State University, School of Nursing, *San Francisco (MSN)*
University of California, Los Angeles, School of Nursing, *Los Angeles (MSN, MSN/MBA)*
University of California, San Francisco, School of Nursing, *San Francisco (MS)*

### Connecticut

Yale University, School of Nursing, *New Haven (MSN, MSN/MPH, MSN/MDIV)*

### Hawaii

University of Hawaii at Manoa, School of Nursing and Dental Hygiene, *Honolulu (MS, MSN/MBA)*

### Illinois

DePaul University, School of Nursing, *Chicago (MS)*
University of Illinois at Chicago, College of Nursing, *Chicago (MS, MS/MBA, MS/MPH)*

### Maine

University of Southern Maine, School of Nursing, *Portland (MS, MS/MBA)*

### Massachusetts

MGH Institute of Health Professions, School of Nursing, *Boston (MS)*
Regis College, School of Nursing, Science and Health Professions, *Weston (MSN)*

### Nebraska

University of Nebraska Medical Center, College of Nursing, *Omaha (MSN)*

### New Jersey

Seton Hall University, College of Nursing, *South Orange (MSN, MSN/MA, MSN/MBA)*

### New York

Columbia University, School of Nursing, *New York (MS, MSN/MBA, MSN/MPH)*
Mercy College, Programs in Nursing, *Dobbs Ferry (MS)*

### North Carolina

Gardner-Webb University, School of Nursing, *Boiling Springs (MSN, MSN/MBA)*

### Ohio

Case Western Reserve University, Frances Payne Bolton School of Nursing, *Cleveland (MSN, MSN/MA, MSN/MBA, MSN/PhD)*

The Ohio State University, College of Nursing, *Columbus (MS, MS/MPH)*
The University of Toledo, College of Nursing, *Toledo (MSN)*

**Oklahoma**
University of Oklahoma Health Sciences Center, College of Nursing, *Oklahoma City (MS)*

**Pennsylvania**
Immaculata University, Division of Nursing, *Immaculata (MSN)*
Thomas Jefferson University, Department of Nursing, *Philadelphia (MSN)*
Wilkes University, Department of Nursing, *Wilkes-Barre (MS)*

**Tennessee**
University of Memphis, Loewenberg School of Nursing, *Memphis (MSN)*
Vanderbilt University, Vanderbilt University School of Nursing, *Nashville (MSN, MSN/MDIV, MSN/MTS)*

**Texas**
Angelo State University, Department of Nursing and Rehabilitation Sciences, *San Angelo (MSN)*
The University of Texas at Austin, School of Nursing, *Austin (MSN, MSN/MBA)*

**Vermont**
University of Vermont, Department of Nursing, *Burlington (MS)*

**Virginia**
University of Virginia, School of Nursing, *Charlottesville (MSN, MSN/MBA, MSN/PhD)*

**Wisconsin**
Marquette University, College of Nursing, *Milwaukee (MSN, MSN/MBA)*
University of Wisconsin–Milwaukee, College of Nursing, *Milwaukee (MN)*

**CANADA**

**Quebec**
McGill University, School of Nursing, *Montréal (M Sc)*

## MASTER'S FOR NURSES WITH NON-NURSING DEGREES

### U.S. AND U.S. TERRITORIES

**Alabama**
University of South Alabama, College of Nursing, *Mobile (MSN)*

**Arizona**
University of Phoenix–Online Campus, Online Campus, *Phoenix (MSN, MSN/MBA, MSN/MHA)*

**Arkansas**
Arkansas Tech University, Program in Nursing, *Russellville (MSN)*
University of Arkansas for Medical Sciences, College of Nursing, *Little Rock (MN Sc)*

**California**
California State University, Dominguez Hills, Program in Nursing, *Carson (MSN)*
Dominican University of California, Program in Nursing, *San Rafael (MSN)*
Holy Names University, Department of Nursing, *Oakland (MSN, MSN/MBA)*
Samuel Merritt University, School of Nursing, *Oakland (MSN)*
San Francisco State University, School of Nursing, *San Francisco (MSN)*
University of California, San Francisco, School of Nursing, *San Francisco (MS)*
University of San Francisco, School of Nursing, *San Francisco (MSN)*

**Connecticut**
Fairfield University, School of Nursing, *Fairfield (MSN)*
University of Hartford, College of Education, Nursing, and Health Professions, *West Hartford (MSN)*
University of Saint Joseph, Department of Nursing, *West Hartford (MS)*
Yale University, School of Nursing, *New Haven (MSN, MSN/MPH, MSN/MDIV)*

**Florida**
Florida International University, Nursing Program, *Miami (MSN)*
Florida Southern College, School of Nursing & Health Sciences, *Lakeland (MSN, MSN/MBA)*
University of South Florida, College of Nursing, *Tampa (MS, MS/MPH)*

**Illinois**
Resurrection University, *Chicago (MSN)*
Rush University, College of Nursing, *Chicago (MSN)*
University of Illinois at Chicago, College of Nursing, *Chicago (MS, MS/MBA, MS/MPH)*
University of St. Francis, Leach College of Nursing, *Joliet (MSN)*

**Indiana**
University of Saint Francis, Department of Nursing, *Fort Wayne (MSN)*

**Iowa**
Allen College, Program in Nursing, *Waterloo (MSN)*
The University of Iowa, College of Nursing, *Iowa City (MSN, MSN/MBA, MSN/MPH)*

**Kentucky**
Bellarmine University, Donna and Allan Lansing School of Nursing and Health Sciences, *Louisville (Certificate of Completion, MSN, MSN/MBA)*

**Louisiana**
Loyola University New Orleans, School of Nursing, *New Orleans (MSN)*

**Maine**
Husson University, School of Nursing, *Bangor (MSN)*
Saint Joseph's College of Maine, Master of Science in Nursing Program, *Standish (MSN, MSN/MHA)*
University of Southern Maine, School of Nursing, *Portland (MS, MS/MBA)*

**Massachusetts**
MGH Institute of Health Professions, School of Nursing, *Boston (MS)*
Regis College, School of Nursing, Science and Health Professions, *Weston (MSN)*
Salem State University, Program in Nursing, *Salem (MSN, MSN/MBA)*
Worcester State University, Department of Nursing, *Worcester (MS)*

**Michigan**
Eastern Michigan University, School of Nursing, *Ypsilanti (MSN)*
University of Detroit Mercy, McAuley School of Nursing, *Detroit (MSN)*

**Minnesota**
Metropolitan State University, College of Health, Community and Professional Studies, *St. Paul (MSN)*
Minnesota State University Mankato, School of Nursing, *Mankato (MSN, MSN/MS)*
St. Catherine University, Department of Nursing, *St. Paul (MS)*
Winona State University, College of Nursing and Health Sciences, *Winona (MS)*

**Mississippi**
Delta State University, School of Nursing, *Cleveland (MSN)*

**Missouri**
Saint Louis University, School of Nursing, *St. Louis (MSN)*

**Nebraska**
Nebraska Methodist College, Department of Nursing, *Omaha (MSN)*

**New Hampshire**
Franklin Pierce University, Master of Science in Nursing, *Rindge (MSN)*
Rivier University, Division of Nursing, *Nashua (MS)*
University of New Hampshire, Department of Nursing, *Durham (MS)*

**New Jersey**
The College of New Jersey, School of Nursing, Health and Exercise Science, *Ewing (MSN)*
Kean University, Department of Nursing, *Union (MSN, MSN/MPA)*
Monmouth University, Marjorie K. Unterberg School of Nursing, *West Long Branch (MSN)*
Rutgers, the State University of New Jersey, Newark, Rutgers School of Nursing, *Newark (MSN, MSN/MPH)*
Saint Peter's University, Nursing Program, *Jersey City (MSN)*
Seton Hall University, College of Nursing, *South Orange (MSN, MSN/MA, MSN/MBA)*
William Paterson University of New Jersey, Department of Nursing, *Wayne (MSN)*

**New Mexico**
New Mexico State University, School of Nursing, *Las Cruces (MSN)*

**New York**
Columbia University, School of Nursing, *New York (MS, MSN/MBA, MSN/MPH)*
Lehman College of the City University of New York, Department of Nursing, *Bronx (MS)*
Le Moyne College, Nursing Programs, *Syracuse (MS)*
Mercy College, Programs in Nursing, *Dobbs Ferry (MS)*
Pace University, Lienhard School of Nursing, *New York (MS)*

State University of New York Upstate Medical University, College of Nursing, *Syracuse (MS)*

### Ohio

The Ohio State University, College of Nursing, *Columbus (MS, MS/MPH)*

The University of Toledo, College of Nursing, *Toledo (MSN)*

Urbana University, College of Nursing and Allied Health, *Urbana (MSN)*

Wright State University, College of Nursing and Health, *Dayton (MS, MS/MBA)*

Xavier University, School of Nursing, *Cincinnati (MSN, MSN/MBA, MSN/Ed D)*

### Oklahoma

Oklahoma City University, Kramer School of Nursing, *Oklahoma City (MSN, MSN/MBA)*

### Pennsylvania

Bloomsburg University of Pennsylvania, Department of Nursing, *Bloomsburg (MSN, MSN/MBA)*

Holy Family University, School of Nursing and Allied Health Professions, *Philadelphia (MSN)*

Indiana University of Pennsylvania, Department of Nursing and Allied Health, *Indiana (MS)*

Moravian College, Department of Nursing, *Bethlehem (MS)*

Thomas Jefferson University, Department of Nursing, *Philadelphia (MSN)*

Widener University, School of Nursing, *Chester (MSN, MSN/PhD)*

### Tennessee

East Tennessee State University, College of Nursing, *Johnson City (MSN)*

Tennessee Technological University, Whitson-Hester School of Nursing, *Cookeville (MSN, M Sc N)*

University of Memphis, Loewenberg School of Nursing, *Memphis (MSN)*

### Texas

The University of Texas at Austin, School of Nursing, *Austin (MSN, MSN/MBA)*

The University of Texas at Brownsville, Department of Nursing, *Brownsville (MSN)*

### Vermont

University of Vermont, Department of Nursing, *Burlington (MS)*

### Virginia

Eastern Mennonite University, Department of Nursing, *Harrisonburg (MSN)*

Jefferson College of Health Sciences, Nursing Education Program, *Roanoke (MSN)*

University of Virginia, School of Nursing, *Charlottesville (MSN, MSN/MBA, MSN/PhD)*

### Washington

Gonzaga University, Department of Nursing, *Spokane (MSN)*

Pacific Lutheran University, School of Nursing, *Tacoma (MSN, MSN/MBA)*

Seattle Pacific University, School of Health Sciences, *Seattle (MSN)*

University of Washington, School of Nursing, *Seattle (MN, MN/MPH)*

### Wisconsin

Marquette University, College of Nursing, *Milwaukee (MSN, MSN/MBA)*

### Wyoming

University of Wyoming, Fay W. Whitney School of Nursing, *Laramie (MS)*

## CANADA

### Alberta

Athabasca University, Centre for Nursing and Health Studies, *Athabasca (MN, MN/MHSA)*

# RN TO MASTER'S

## U.S. AND U.S. TERRITORIES

### Alabama

Samford University, Ida V. Moffett School of Nursing, *Birmingham (MSN)*

Spring Hill College, Division of Nursing, *Mobile (MSN)*

The University of Alabama, Capstone College of Nursing, *Tuscaloosa (MSN, MSN/Ed D)*

The University of Alabama in Huntsville, College of Nursing, *Huntsville (MSN)*

### Arizona

The University of Arizona, College of Nursing, *Tucson (MSN)*

### Arkansas

Arkansas Tech University, Program in Nursing, *Russellville (MSN)*

University of Arkansas for Medical Sciences, College of Nursing, *Little Rock (MN Sc)*

University of Central Arkansas, Department of Nursing, *Conway (MSN)*

### California

Dominican University of California, Program in Nursing, *San Rafael (MSN)*

Loma Linda University, School of Nursing, *Loma Linda (MS)*

Mount St. Mary's College, Department of Nursing, *Los Angeles (MSN)*

National University, Department of Nursing, *La Jolla (MSN)*

Point Loma Nazarene University, School of Nursing, *San Diego (MSN)*

University of San Francisco, School of Nursing, *San Francisco (MSN)*

### Colorado

Aspen University, Graduate School of Health Professions and Studies, *Denver (MSN)*

Regis University, School of Nursing, *Denver (MS)*

### Connecticut

Sacred Heart University, Program in Nursing, *Fairfield (MSN)*

Southern Connecticut State University, Department of Nursing, *New Haven (MSN)*

University of Connecticut, School of Nursing, *Storrs (MS)*

### Delaware

University of Delaware, School of Nursing, *Newark (MSN)*

Wesley College, Nursing Program, *Dover (MSN)*

### Florida

Kaplan University Online, The School of Nursing Online, *Fort Lauderdale (MSN)*

Nova Southeastern University, College of Health Care Sciences, *Fort Lauderdale (MSN)*

University of Central Florida, College of Nursing, *Orlando (MSN)*

University of North Florida, School of Nursing, *Jacksonville (MSN)*

University of South Florida, College of Nursing, *Tampa (MS, MS/MPH)*

The University of Tampa, Department of Nursing, *Tampa (MSN)*

### Georgia

Albany State University, College of Sciences and Health Professions, *Albany (MSN)*

Brenau University, College of Health and Science, *Gainesville (MSN)*

Clayton State University, Department of Nursing, *Morrow (MSN)*

Georgia Southern University, School of Nursing, *Statesboro (MSN)*

Georgia State University, Byrdine F. Lewis School of Nursing and Health Professions, *Atlanta (MSN)*

Thomas University, Division of Nursing, *Thomasville (MSN, MSN/MBA)*

Valdosta State University, College of Nursing, *Valdosta (MSN)*

### Hawaii

Hawai`i Pacific University, College of Nursing and Health Sciences, *Honolulu (MSN, MSN/MBA)*

University of Hawaii at Manoa, School of Nursing and Dental Hygiene, *Honolulu (MS, MSN/MBA)*

### Idaho

Northwest Nazarene University, School of Health and Science, *Nampa (MSN)*

### Illinois

Blessing–Rieman College of Nursing, *Quincy (MSN)*

Bradley University, Department of Nursing, *Peoria (MSN)*

Lewis University, Program in Nursing, *Romeoville (MSN, MSN/MBA)*

Loyola University Chicago, Marcella Niehoff School of Nursing, *Maywood (MSN, MSN/MBA)*

McKendree University, Department of Nursing, *Lebanon (MSN, MSN/MBA)*

North Park University, School of Nursing, *Chicago (MS, MSN/MA, MSN/MBA, MSN/MM)*

Resurrection University, *Chicago (MSN)*

### Indiana

Anderson University, School of Nursing, *Anderson (MSN, MSN/MBA)*

Ball State University, School of Nursing, *Muncie (MS)*

Indiana University–Purdue University Indianapolis, School of Nursing, *Indianapolis (MSN)*

Valparaiso University, College of Nursing, *Valparaiso (MSN, MSN/MBA)*

**Iowa**

Allen College, Program in Nursing, *Waterloo (MSN)*

**Kansas**

The University of Kansas, School of Nursing, *Kansas City (MS, MS/MHSA, MS/MPH)*

**Kentucky**

Bellarmine University, Donna and Allan Lansing School of Nursing and Health Sciences, *Louisville (Certificate of Completion, MSN, MSN/MBA)*

University of Kentucky, College of Nursing, *Lexington (MSN)*

**Louisiana**

Loyola University New Orleans, School of Nursing, *New Orleans (MSN)*

University of Louisiana at Lafayette, College of Nursing, *Lafayette (MSN)*

**Maine**

Saint Joseph's College of Maine, Master of Science in Nursing Program, *Standish (MSN, MSN/MHA)*

University of Maine, School of Nursing, *Orono (MSN)*

University of Southern Maine, School of Nursing, *Portland (MS, MS/MBA)*

**Maryland**

Salisbury University, Nursing DNP Program, *Salisbury (MS)*

Stevenson University, Nursing Division, *Stevenson (MS)*

University of Maryland, Baltimore, Master's Program in Nursing, *Baltimore (MS, MSN/MBA, MSN/MPH)*

**Massachusetts**

Boston College, William F. Connell School of Nursing, *Chestnut Hill (MS, MS/MA, MS/MBA, MSN/PhD)*

Curry College, Division of Nursing, *Milton (MSN)*

Elms College, Division of Nursing, *Chicopee (MSN)*

MGH Institute of Health Professions, School of Nursing, *Boston (MS)*

Regis College, School of Nursing, Science and Health Professions, *Weston (MSN)*

Simmons College, School of Nursing and Health Sciences, *Boston (MS)*

Worcester State University, Department of Nursing, *Worcester (MS)*

**Michigan**

Ferris State University, School of Nursing, *Big Rapids (MSN, MSN/MBA)*

Saginaw Valley State University, College of Health and Human Services, *University Center (MSN)*

University of Michigan, School of Nursing, *Ann Arbor (MS, MSN/MBA, MSN/MPH)*

University of Michigan–Flint, Department of Nursing, *Flint (MSN)*

**Minnesota**

Metropolitan State University, College of Health, Community and Professional Studies, *St. Paul (MSN)*

Minnesota State University Mankato, School of Nursing, *Mankato (MSN, MSN/MS)*

Walden University, Nursing Programs, *Minneapolis (MSN)*

Winona State University, College of Nursing and Health Sciences, *Winona (MS)*

**Mississippi**

University of Mississippi Medical Center, School of Nursing, *Jackson (MSN)*

University of Southern Mississippi, School of Nursing, *Hattiesburg (MSN)*

**Missouri**

Cox College, Department of Nursing, *Springfield (MSN)*

Graceland University, School of Nursing, *Independence (MSN)*

Maryville University of Saint Louis, Nursing Program, School of Health Professions, *St. Louis (MSN)*

Missouri State University, Department of Nursing, *Springfield (MSN)*

Research College of Nursing, College of Nursing, *Kansas City (MSN)*

Webster University, Department of Nursing, *St. Louis (MSN)*

**Nebraska**

Clarkson College, Master of Science in Nursing Program, *Omaha (MSN)*

Nebraska Methodist College, Department of Nursing, *Omaha (MSN)*

Nebraska Wesleyan University, Department of Nursing, *Lincoln (MSN)*

University of Nebraska Medical Center, College of Nursing, *Omaha (MSN)*

**New Hampshire**

Franklin Pierce University, Master of Science in Nursing, *Rindge (MSN)*

Rivier University, Division of Nursing, *Nashua (MS)*

**New Jersey**

The College of New Jersey, School of Nursing, Health and Exercise Science, *Ewing (MSN)*

Fairleigh Dickinson University, Metropolitan Campus, Henry P. Becton School of Nursing and Allied Health, *Teaneck (MSN)*

Monmouth University, Marjorie K. Unterberg School of Nursing, *West Long Branch (MSN)*

Rutgers, The State University of New Jersey, Newark, Rutgers School of Nursing, *Newark (MSN, MSN/MPH)*

Seton Hall University, College of Nursing, *South Orange (MSN, MSN/MA, MSN/MBA)*

Thomas Edison State College, School of Nursing, *Trenton (MSN)*

**New York**

The College of New Rochelle, School of Nursing, *New Rochelle (MS)*

Daemen College, Department of Nursing, *Amherst (MS)*

D'Youville College, School of Nursing, *Buffalo (MS)*

Excelsior College, School of Nursing, *Albany (MS)*

Long Island University–LIU Brooklyn, School of Nursing, *Brooklyn (MS)*

New York University, College of Nursing, *New York (MS, MS/MPH, MSN/MPA)*

St. John Fisher College, Wegmans School of Nursing, *Rochester (MS)*

State University of New York Institute of Technology, School of Nursing and Health Systems, *Utica (MS)*

State University of New York Upstate Medical University, College of Nursing, *Syracuse (MS)*

Stony Brook University, State University of New York, School of Nursing, *Stony Brook (MS)*

**North Carolina**

Duke University, School of Nursing, *Durham (MSN, MSN/MBA)*

East Carolina University, College of Nursing, *Greenville (MSN)*

Gardner-Webb University, School of Nursing, *Boiling Springs (MSN, MSN/MBA)*

Lenoir-Rhyne University, Program in Nursing, *Hickory (MSN)*

Queens University of Charlotte, Presbyterian School of Nursing, *Charlotte (MSN, MSN/MBA)*

The University of North Carolina at Chapel Hill, School of Nursing, *Chapel Hill (MSN)*

The University of North Carolina at Charlotte, School of Nursing, *Charlotte (MSN)*

**North Dakota**

University of Mary, Division of Nursing, *Bismarck (MSN)*

**Ohio**

Capital University, School of Nursing, *Columbus (MSN, MN/MBA, MSN/JD, MSN/MDIV)*

Case Western Reserve University, Frances Payne Bolton School of Nursing, *Cleveland (MSN, MSN/MA, MSN/MBA, MSN/PhD)*

Franciscan University of Steubenville, Department of Nursing, *Steubenville (MSN)*

Lourdes University, School of Nursing, *Sylvania (MSN)*

The Ohio State University, College of Nursing, *Columbus (MS, MS/MPH)*

The University of Akron, School of Nursing, *Akron (MSN)*

Urbana University, College of Nursing and Allied Health, *Urbana (MSN)*

Xavier University, School of Nursing, *Cincinnati (MSN, MSN/MBA, MSN/Ed D)*

**Oklahoma**

Oklahoma City University, Kramer School of Nursing, *Oklahoma City (MSN, MSN/MBA)*

**Pennsylvania**

Alvernia University, Nursing, *Reading (MSN)*

Bloomsburg University of Pennsylvania, Department of Nursing, *Bloomsburg (MSN, MSN/MBA)*

Carlow University, School of Nursing, *Pittsburgh (MSN)*

Clarion University of Pennsylvania, School of Nursing, *Oil City (MSN)*

DeSales University, Department of Nursing and Health, *Center Valley (MSN, MSN/MBA)*

Drexel University, College of Nursing and Health Professions, *Philadelphia (MSN)*

Gannon University, Villa Maria School of Nursing, *Erie (MSN)*

Gwynedd Mercy University, School of Nursing, *Gwynedd Valley (MSN)*

La Roche College, Department of Nursing and Nursing Management, *Pittsburgh (MSN)*

La Salle University, School of Nursing and Health Sciences, *Philadelphia (MSN, MSN/MBA)*

Messiah College, Department of Nursing, *Mechanicsburg (MSN)*

Misericordia University, Department of Nursing, *Dallas (MSN)*

Thomas Jefferson University, Department of Nursing, *Philadelphia (MSN)*

University of Pittsburgh, School of Nursing, *Pittsburgh (MSN)*

The University of Scranton, Department of Nursing, *Scranton (MSN)*

Wilkes University, Department of Nursing, *Wilkes-Barre (MS)*

York College of Pennsylvania, Department of Nursing, *York (MS)*

### Rhode Island

University of Rhode Island, College of Nursing, *Kingston (MS)*

### South Carolina

Charleston Southern University, Wingo School of Nursing, *Charleston (MSN)*

### South Dakota

South Dakota State University, College of Nursing, *Brookings (MS)*

### Tennessee

Tennessee State University, Division of Nursing, *Nashville (MSN)*

Vanderbilt University, Vanderbilt University School of Nursing, *Nashville (MSN, MSN/MDIV, MSN/MTS)*

### Texas

Angelo State University, Department of Nursing and Rehabilitation Sciences, *San Angelo (MSN)*

Midwestern State University, Nursing Program, *Wichita Falls (MSN)*

Texas A&M University–Corpus Christi, College of Nursing and Health Sciences, *Corpus Christi (MSN)*

Texas Woman's University, College of Nursing, *Denton (MS, MS/MHA)*

University of Houston–Victoria, School of Nursing, *Victoria (MSN)*

The University of Texas at El Paso, School of Nursing, *El Paso (MSN)*

The University of Texas at Tyler, Program in Nursing, *Tyler (MSN, MSN/MBA)*

The University of Texas Health Science Center at San Antonio, School of Nursing, *San Antonio (MSN)*

West Texas A&M University, Department of Nursing, *Canyon (MSN)*

### Utah

University of Utah, College of Nursing, *Salt Lake City (MS)*

Western Governors University, Online College of Health Professions, *Salt Lake City (MS)*

### Vermont

University of Vermont, Department of Nursing, *Burlington (MS)*

### Virginia

Hampton University, School of Nursing, *Hampton (MS)*

Lynchburg College, School of Health Sciences and Human Performance, *Lynchburg (MSN)*

Old Dominion University, Department of Nursing, *Norfolk (MSN)*

Shenandoah University, Division of Nursing, *Winchester (MSN, MSN/MBA)*

University of Virginia, School of Nursing, *Charlottesville (MSN, MSN/MBA, MSN/PhD)*

Virginia Commonwealth University, School of Nursing, *Richmond (MS)*

### West Virginia

West Virginia University, School of Nursing, *Morgantown (MSN)*

Wheeling Jesuit University, Department of Nursing, *Wheeling (MSN)*

### Wisconsin

University of Wisconsin–Eau Claire, College of Nursing and Health Sciences, *Eau Claire (MSN)*

University of Wisconsin–Oshkosh, College of Nursing, *Oshkosh (MSN)*

## CANADA

### Alberta

University of Calgary, Faculty of Nursing, *Calgary (MN)*

### New Brunswick

Université de Moncton, School of Nursing, *Moncton (M Sc N)*

### Quebec

Université de Montréal, Faculty of Nursing, *Montréal (M Sc)*

Université du Québec à Chicoutimi, Program in Nursing, *Chicoutimi (MSN, MS/MPH)*

# CONCENTRATIONS WITHIN MASTER'S DEGREE PROGRAMS

## CASE MANAGEMENT

American Sentinel University, CO
Boise State University, ID
Carlow University, PA
Duke University, NC
The Johns Hopkins University, MD
Loyola University New Orleans, LA
Pacific Lutheran University, WA
Regis College, MA
Saint Peter's University, NJ
Samuel Merritt University, CA
San Francisco State University, CA
Seton Hall University, NJ
Shenandoah University, VA
Université de Moncton, NB
The University of Alabama, AL
University of Kentucky, KY
University of Nebraska Medical Center, NE
University of New Brunswick Fredericton, NB
Ursuline College, OH
Valdosta State University, GA
Washington State University College of Nursing, WA

## CLINICAL NURSE LEADER

Boise State University, ID
Brenau University, GA
California Baptist University, CA
California State University, Dominguez Hills, CA
Central Methodist University, MO
Cleveland State University, OH
The College of New Jersey, NJ
Cox College, MO
Creighton University, NE
Curry College, MA
Dominican University of California, CA
Drexel University, PA
East Tennessee State University, TN
Elmhurst College, IL
Fairfield University, CT
Florida Atlantic University, FL
The George Washington University, DC
Georgia Regents University, GA
Grand Valley State University, MI
Grand View University, IA
Hunter College of the City University of New York, NY
Illinois State University, IL
James Madison University, VA
Lynchburg College, VA
Marquette University, WI
MGH Institute of Health Professions, MA
Millikin University, IL
Montana State University, MT
Moravian College, PA
The Ohio State University, OH
Pacific Lutheran University, WA
Queens University of Charlotte, NC
Regis College, MA
Research College of Nursing, MO
Resurrection University, IL
Rush University, IL
Rutgers, The State University of New Jersey, Newark, NJ
Sacred Heart University, CT
Saginaw Valley State University, MI
Saint Anthony College of Nursing, IL
Saint Francis Medical Center College of Nursing, IL
Saint Xavier University, IL
Salem State University, MA
Seton Hall University, NJ
South Dakota State University, SD
Southern Connecticut State University, CT
Spring Hill College, AL
Texas Christian University, TX
Texas Woman's University, TX
Université de Montréal, QC
Université Laval, QC
The University of Alabama, AL
The University of Alabama at Birmingham, AL
The University of Alabama in Huntsville, AL
University of California, Los Angeles, CA
University of Connecticut, CT
University of Florida, FL
University of Mary Hardin-Baylor, TX
University of Maryland, Baltimore, MD
University of Massachusetts Amherst, MA
University of Nevada, Reno, NV
The University of North Carolina at Chapel Hill, NC
University of Oklahoma Health Sciences Center, OK
University of Pittsburgh, PA
University of Portland, OR
University of Rhode Island, RI
University of San Diego, CA
University of San Francisco, CA
University of Southern Maine, ME
The University of Tennessee Health Science Center, TN
The University of Texas Health Science Center at San Antonio, TX
The University of Texas Medical Branch, TX
University of the Incarnate Word, TX
The University of Toledo, OH
University of Toronto, ON
University of Virginia, VA
University of West Georgia, GA
University of Windsor, ON
University of Wisconsin–Milwaukee, WI
University of Wisconsin–Oshkosh, WI
Viterbo University, WI
Walsh University, OH
Western Governors University, UT
Western University of Health Sciences, CA
Wright State University, OH
Xavier University, OH

## CLINICAL NURSE SPECIALIST PROGRAMS

### Acute Care

Alvernia University, PA
Arizona State University at the Downtown Phoenix Campus, AZ
Colorado State University–Pueblo, CO
Indiana University–Purdue University Indianapolis, IN
The Johns Hopkins University, MD
King College, TN
Liberty University, VA
Loyola University Chicago, IL
McGill University, QC
Georgia Baptist College of Nursing, GA
Regis College, MA
Rhode Island College, RI
The Sage Colleges, NY
Seattle Pacific University, WA
Thomas Jefferson University, PA
Université de Montréal, QC
Université de Sherbrooke, QC
Université du Québec à Chicoutimi, QC
Université du Québec à Trois-Rivières, QC
Université Laval, QC
University of Arkansas, AR
University of Arkansas for Medical Sciences, AR
University of Calgary, AB
University of California, Los Angeles, CA
University of Central Florida, FL
University of Connecticut, CT
University of Illinois at Chicago, IL
University of Kentucky, KY
University of Manitoba, MB
University of Massachusetts Boston, MA
University of Missouri, MO
University of Nebraska Medical Center, NE
University of New Brunswick Fredericton, NB
University of Oklahoma Health Sciences Center, OK
University of Ottawa, ON
University of Pennsylvania, PA
University of San Diego, CA
University of South Alabama, AL
The University of Texas Health Science Center at Houston, TX
University of Toronto, ON
University of Virginia, VA
The University of Western Ontario, ON
Wayne State University, MI
Widener University, PA

### Adult Health

Alvernia University, PA
Alverno College, WI
Angelo State University, TX
Arizona State University at the Downtown Phoenix Campus, AZ
Arkansas State University, AR
Auburn University, AL
Auburn University at Montgomery, AL
Azusa Pacific University, CA
Boston College, MA
California Baptist University, CA
California State University, Fresno, CA
California State University, Long Beach, CA
Capital University, OH
The Catholic University of America, DC
The College of New Jersey, NJ
College of Staten Island of the City University of New York, NY
Creighton University, NE
DeSales University, PA
East Carolina University, NC
Eastern Michigan University, MI
Florida Southern College, FL
George Mason University, VA
Georgia State University, GA
Governors State University, IL
Grambling State University, LA
Grand Canyon University, AZ
Hunter College of the City University of New York, NY
Indiana University–Purdue University Indianapolis, IN

The Johns Hopkins University, MD
Kennesaw State University, GA
Kent State University, OH
King College, TN
La Salle University, PA
Lehman College of the City University of New York, NY
Lewis University, IL
Loma Linda University, CA
Long Island University–LIU Post, NY
Louisiana State University Health Sciences Center, LA
Loyola University Chicago, IL
Marquette University, WI
McGill University, QC
Georgia Baptist College of Nursing, GA
Michigan State University, MI
Minnesota State University Mankato, MN
Minnesota State University Moorhead, MN
Molloy College, NY
Mount Carmel College of Nursing, OH
Mount Saint Mary College, NY
Mount St. Mary's College, CA
Murray State University, KY
North Dakota State University, ND
Northern Illinois University, IL
Northwestern State University of Louisiana, LA
The Ohio State University, OH
Otterbein University, OH
Penn State University Park, PA
Purdue University Calumet, IN
Rhode Island College, RI
Rush University, IL
Ryerson University, ON
The Sage Colleges, NY
Saint Anthony College of Nursing, IL
St. John Fisher College, NY
St. Joseph's College, New York, NY
San Diego State University, CA
San Francisco State University, CA
Seattle Pacific University, WA
State University of New York Downstate Medical Center, NY
Stony Brook University, State University of New York, NY
Texas Christian University, TX
Thomas Jefferson University, PA
Troy University, AL
Union University, TN
Université de Montréal, QC
Université du Québec à Chicoutimi, QC
Université du Québec à Trois-Rivières, QC
Université Laval, QC
The University of Akron, OH
The University of Alabama in Huntsville, AL
University of Arkansas for Medical Sciences, AR
The University of British Columbia, BC
University of Calgary, AB
University of Cincinnati, OH
University of Colorado Colorado Springs, CO
University of Colorado Denver, CO
University of Delaware, DE
University of Illinois at Chicago, IL
The University of Iowa, IA
The University of Kansas, KS
University of Kentucky, KY
University of Louisiana at Lafayette, LA
University of Massachusetts Boston, MA
University of Massachusetts Dartmouth, MA
University of Missouri, MO
University of Nebraska Medical Center, NE
University of New Brunswick Fredericton, NB
University of New Hampshire, NH
University of North Florida, FL
University of Ottawa, ON
University of Pennsylvania, PA
University of Puerto Rico, Medical Sciences Campus, PR
University of San Diego, CA
The University of Scranton, PA
University of Southern Indiana, IN
The University of Texas at Austin, TX
The University of Texas Health Science Center at Houston, TX
The University of Texas–Pan American, TX
University of the Incarnate Word, TX
University of Toronto, ON
The University of Western Ontario, ON
University of Wisconsin–Eau Claire, WI
Ursuline College, OH
Valdosta State University, GA
Valparaiso University, IN
Western Connecticut State University, CT
Widener University, PA
Winona State University, MN
Wright State University, OH
York College of Pennsylvania, PA

### Cardiovascular

Alvernia University, PA
Creighton University, NE
McGill University, QC
Université de Montréal, QC
Université du Québec à Chicoutimi, QC
Université Laval, QC
The University of British Columbia, BC
University of Calgary, AB
University of California, San Francisco, CA
University of Illinois at Chicago, IL
University of Missouri, MO
University of Nebraska Medical Center, NE
University of New Brunswick Fredericton, NB
University of North Florida, FL
University of Ottawa, ON
University of Toronto, ON

### Community Health

Arizona State University at the Downtown Phoenix Campus, AZ
Augsburg College, MN
Binghamton University, State University of New York, NY
Bloomsburg University of Pennsylvania, PA
Boston College, MA
California State University, San Bernardino, CA
The Catholic University of America, DC
Cedarville University, OH
Cleveland State University, OH
D'Youville College, NY
Georgia Southern University, GA
Hawai`i Pacific University, HI
Hunter College of the City University of New York, NY
Jacksonville State University, AL
Kean University, NJ
Louisiana State University Health Sciences Center, LA
McGill University, QC
Mount Mercy University, IA
Mount St. Mary's College, CA
Northern Illinois University, IL
North Park University, IL
The Ohio State University, OH
Penn State University Park, PA
Rhode Island College, RI
Rush University, IL
Ryerson University, ON
The Sage Colleges, NY
Salem State University, MA
San Diego State University, CA
Seattle Pacific University, WA
Seattle University, WA
Stony Brook University, State University of New York, NY
Thomas Jefferson University, PA
Université de Moncton, NB
Université de Montréal, QC
Université de Sherbrooke, QC
Université du Québec à Chicoutimi, QC
Université du Québec à Rimouski, QC
Université du Québec à Trois-Rivières, QC
Université du Québec en Outaouais, QC
Université Laval, QC
University of Alaska Anchorage, AK
The University of British Columbia, BC
University of Calgary, AB
University of California, San Francisco, CA
University of Illinois at Chicago, IL
The University of Iowa, IA
University of Kentucky, KY
University of Maryland, Baltimore, MD
University of Massachusetts Dartmouth, MA
University of Michigan, MI
University of Missouri, MO
University of Nebraska Medical Center, NE
University of New Brunswick Fredericton, NB
The University of North Carolina at Charlotte, NC
University of North Florida, FL
University of Ottawa, ON
University of Puerto Rico, Medical Sciences Campus, PR
University of South Alabama, AL
University of Toronto, ON
University of Washington, WA
The University of Western Ontario, ON
Washington State University College of Nursing, WA
Wayne State University, MI
Wesley College, DE
William Paterson University of New Jersey, NJ
Worcester State University, MA
Wright State University, OH

### Critical Care

Alvernia University, PA
Indiana University–Purdue University Indianapolis, IN
Loyola University Chicago, IL
McGill University, QC
Murray State University, KY
Northwestern State University of Louisiana, LA
Purdue University Calumet, IN
Rush University, IL
The Sage Colleges, NY
San Diego State University, CA
Seattle Pacific University, WA
Stony Brook University, State University of New York, NY
Thomas Jefferson University, PA
Université du Québec à Chicoutimi, QC
Université du Québec à Rimouski, QC
Université du Québec à Trois-Rivières, QC

Université du Québec en Outaouais, QC
Université Laval, QC
University of Calgary, AB
University of California, San Francisco, CA
University of Cincinnati, OH
University of Kentucky, KY
University of Massachusetts Boston, MA
University of Missouri, MO
University of Nebraska Medical Center, NE
University of New Brunswick Fredericton, NB
University of North Florida, FL
University of Ottawa, ON
University of Puerto Rico, Medical Sciences Campus, PR
University of San Diego, CA
The University of Texas Health Science Center at Houston, TX
University of Toronto, ON
Wayne State University, MI
Widener University, PA

**Family Health**
Alvernia University, PA
Binghamton University, State University of New York, NY
Cedarville University, OH
Cox College, MO
Creighton University, NE
Loma Linda University, CA
McGill University, QC
Minnesota State University Mankato, MN
Misericordia University, PA
Missouri Southern State University, MO
Point Loma Nazarene University, CA
Ryerson University, ON
The Sage Colleges, NY
Saginaw Valley State University, MI
Saint Francis Medical Center College of Nursing, IL
Southern University and Agricultural and Mechanical College, LA
Université de Moncton, NB
Université de Montréal, QC
Université de Sherbrooke, QC
Université du Québec à Chicoutimi, QC
Université du Québec à Trois-Rivières, QC
Université Laval, QC
The University of British Columbia, BC
University of Calgary, AB
University of Illinois at Chicago, IL
University of Manitoba, MB
University of Massachusetts Lowell, MA
University of Nebraska Medical Center, NE
University of New Brunswick Fredericton, NB
University of Northern Colorado, CO
University of Ottawa, ON
University of South Alabama, AL
University of Toronto, ON
Valdosta State University, GA
Webster University, MO

**Forensic Nursing**
Alvernia University, PA
Cleveland State University, OH
Duquesne University, PA
Fitchburg State University, MA
Monmouth University, NJ
National University, CA
University of Ottawa, ON
Xavier University, OH

**Gerontology**
Alvernia University, PA
Alverno College, WI
Auburn University, AL
Auburn University at Montgomery, AL
Binghamton University, State University of New York, NY
Boston College, MA
California State University, Dominguez Hills, CA
California State University, Fresno, CA
Capella University, MN
Capital University, OH
College of Staten Island of the City University of New York, NY
Creighton University, NE
Florida Southern College, FL
Gwynedd Mercy University, PA
Indiana University–Purdue University Indianapolis, IN
The Johns Hopkins University, MD
Lehman College of the City University of New York, NY
Le Moyne College, NY
Lewis University, IL
McGill University, QC
Georgia Baptist College of Nursing, GA
Minnesota State University Moorhead, MN
Penn State University Park, PA
Point Loma Nazarene University, CA
Rush University, IL
The Sage Colleges, NY
Saint Francis Medical Center College of Nursing, IL
St. John Fisher College, NY
San Diego State University, CA
Seattle Pacific University, WA
Texas Christian University, TX
Université de Montréal, QC
Université de Sherbrooke, QC
Université du Québec à Chicoutimi, QC
Université du Québec à Rimouski, QC
Université Laval, QC
The University of Akron, OH
The University of British Columbia, BC
University of Calgary, AB
University of California, San Francisco, CA
University of Cincinnati, OH
University of Illinois at Chicago, IL
The University of Iowa, IA
The University of Kansas, KS
University of Kentucky, KY
University of Manitoba, MB
University of Massachusetts Boston, MA
University of Michigan, MI
University of Nebraska Medical Center, NE
University of New Brunswick Fredericton, NB
University of North Dakota, ND
University of North Florida, FL
University of Ottawa, ON
University of Puerto Rico, Medical Sciences Campus, PR
University of Rhode Island, RI
University of South Alabama, AL
The University of Texas Health Science Center at Houston, TX
University of Toronto, ON
Valparaiso University, IN
Widener University, PA
Wilkes University, PA

**Home Health Care**
Alvernia University, PA
Carlow University, PA
McGill University, QC
Thomas Jefferson University, PA
Université de Moncton, NB
Université du Québec à Chicoutimi, QC
Université du Québec à Trois-Rivières, QC
University of Michigan, MI
University of Missouri, MO
University of Ottawa, ON

**Maternity-newborn**
Creighton University, NE
Grambling State University, LA
Loma Linda University, CA
McGill University, QC
San Diego State University, CA
State University of New York Downstate Medical Center, NY
Troy University, AL
Université de Montréal, QC
Université du Québec à Chicoutimi, QC
Université du Québec à Trois-Rivières, QC
The University of British Columbia, BC
University of Calgary, AB
University of Connecticut, CT
University of Illinois at Chicago, IL
University of Missouri, MO
University of Nebraska Medical Center, NE
University of New Brunswick Fredericton, NB
University of North Florida, FL
University of Ottawa, ON
University of Puerto Rico, Medical Sciences Campus, PR
University of South Alabama, AL
University of Toronto, ON

**Medical-surgical**
Alvernia University, PA
Alverno College, WI
Angelo State University, TX
Azusa Pacific University, CA
Indiana University–Purdue University Indianapolis, IN
Loma Linda University, CA
McGill University, QC
Murray State University, KY
Point Loma Nazarene University, CA
Seattle Pacific University, WA
State University of New York Upstate Medical University, NY
Thomas Jefferson University, PA
Université de Montréal, QC
Université du Québec à Chicoutimi, QC
Université du Québec à Trois-Rivières, QC
University of Arkansas, AR
University of Calgary, AB
University of Central Arkansas, AR
University of Cincinnati, OH
University of Illinois at Chicago, IL
University of Kentucky, KY
University of Michigan, MI
University of Nebraska Medical Center, NE
University of New Brunswick Fredericton, NB
University of North Florida, FL
University of Ottawa, ON
University of San Diego, CA
University of Toronto, ON
University of Virginia, VA

**Occupational Health**
Université de Moncton, NB
Université de Montréal, QC
Université du Québec à Chicoutimi, QC
University of California, San Francisco, CA

University of Cincinnati, OH
University of Illinois at Chicago, IL
The University of Iowa, IA
University of Michigan, MI
University of Ottawa, ON
University of Toronto, ON

### Oncology

Alvernia University, PA
Case Western Reserve University, OH
Creighton University, NE
Gwynedd Mercy University, PA
Indiana University–Purdue University Indianapolis, IN
King College, TN
Loyola University Chicago, IL
McGill University, QC
Rutgers, The State University of New Jersey, College of Nursing, NJ
Seattle Pacific University, WA
Thomas Jefferson University, PA
Université de Montréal, QC
Université du Québec à Chicoutimi, QC
Université Laval, QC
The University of British Columbia, BC
University of California, San Francisco, CA
University of Kentucky, KY
University of Missouri, MO
University of Nebraska Medical Center, NE
University of New Brunswick Fredericton, NB
University of Ottawa, ON
University of Toronto, ON

### Palliative Care

Case Western Reserve University, OH
D'Youville College, NY
Le Moyne College, NY
Seattle Pacific University, WA
Université de Montréal, QC
Université Laval, QC
University of Missouri, MO
University of Ottawa, ON
University of San Diego, CA
University of Toronto, ON
Ursuline College, OH

### Parent-child

Azusa Pacific University, CA
California State University, Dominguez Hills, CA
Lehman College of the City University of New York, NY
Loma Linda University, CA
McGill University, QC
Seattle Pacific University, WA
Stony Brook University, State University of New York, NY
Université de Montréal, QC
Université du Québec à Chicoutimi, QC
Université Laval, QC
The University of British Columbia, BC
University of Calgary, AB
University of Kentucky, KY
University of Nebraska Medical Center, NE
University of New Brunswick Fredericton, NB
University of Ottawa, ON
University of Toronto, ON

### Pediatric

Arizona State University at the Downtown Phoenix Campus, AZ
Auburn University, AL
Auburn University at Montgomery, AL
Azusa Pacific University, CA
Boston College, MA
California State University, Fresno, CA
Creighton University, NE
Georgia State University, GA
Grambling State University, LA
Gwynedd Mercy University, PA
The Johns Hopkins University, MD
Kent State University, OH
Loma Linda University, CA
Marquette University, WI
McGill University, QC
Georgia Baptist College of Nursing, GA
Minnesota State University Mankato, MN
Rush University, IL
St. John Fisher College, NY
Seattle Pacific University, WA
Stony Brook University, State University of New York, NY
Texas Christian University, TX
Thomas Jefferson University, PA
Union University, TN
Université de Moncton, NB
Université du Québec à Chicoutimi, QC
Université du Québec à Trois-Rivières, QC
Université Laval, QC
The University of Akron, OH
University of Arkansas for Medical Sciences, AR
The University of British Columbia, BC
University of Calgary, AB
University of California, Los Angeles, CA
University of California, San Francisco, CA
University of Delaware, DE
University of Illinois at Chicago, IL
University of Kentucky, KY
University of Missouri, MO
University of Nebraska Medical Center, NE
University of New Brunswick Fredericton, NB
University of North Florida, FL
University of Ottawa, ON
University of Pennsylvania, PA
University of Puerto Rico, Medical Sciences Campus, PR
University of South Alabama, AL
The University of Tennessee, TN
University of Toronto, ON
Wright State University, OH

### Perinatal

Georgia State University, GA
Loma Linda University, CA
McGill University, QC
McMaster University, ON
San Francisco State University, CA
Stony Brook University, State University of New York, NY
Université du Québec à Chicoutimi, QC
Université du Québec à Trois-Rivières, QC
Université Laval, QC
The University of British Columbia, BC
University of Calgary, AB
University of California, San Francisco, CA
University of Illinois at Chicago, IL
University of Kentucky, KY
University of Manitoba, MB
University of Nebraska Medical Center, NE
University of Ottawa, ON
University of Toronto, ON

### Psychiatric/Mental Health

Arizona State University at the Downtown Phoenix Campus, AZ
Binghamton University, State University of New York, NY
California State University, Los Angeles, CA
Case Western Reserve University, OH
Colorado State University–Pueblo, CO
Georgia State University, GA
Gonzaga University, WA
Husson University, ME
McGill University, QC
Point Loma Nazarene University, CA
Rutgers, The State University of New Jersey, College of Nursing, NJ
The Sage Colleges, NY
Shenandoah University, VA
Stony Brook University, State University of New York, NY
Temple University, PA
Université de Moncton, NB
Université de Montréal, QC
Université du Québec à Chicoutimi, QC
Université du Québec à Rimouski, QC
Université du Québec à Trois-Rivières, QC
Université du Québec en Outaouais, QC
Université Laval, QC
The University of Akron, OH
University of Alaska Anchorage, AK
The University of British Columbia, BC
University of Calgary, AB
University of California, San Francisco, CA
University of Florida, FL
University of Hawaii at Manoa, HI
University of Illinois at Chicago, IL
The University of Iowa, IA
University of Kentucky, KY
University of Louisiana at Lafayette, LA
University of Massachusetts Lowell, MA
University of Michigan, MI
University of Nebraska Medical Center, NE
University of New Brunswick Fredericton, NB
University of North Dakota, ND
University of North Florida, FL
University of Ottawa, ON
University of Puerto Rico, Medical Sciences Campus, PR
University of Rhode Island, RI
University of South Alabama, AL
The University of Tennessee, TN
University of Toronto, ON
The University of Western Ontario, ON
Valdosta State University, GA
Wayne State University, MI
Wilkes University, PA

### Public Health

Delaware State University, DE
Eastern Kentucky University, KY
Hunter College of the City University of New York, NY
La Salle University, PA
Louisiana State University Health Sciences Center, LA
McGill University, QC
Mount Mercy University, IA
The Ohio State University, OH
Rush University, IL
Ryerson University, ON
Salem State University, MA
San Francisco State University, CA
Thomas Jefferson University, PA
Université de Moncton, NB
Université de Montréal, QC
Université du Québec à Chicoutimi, QC

Université du Québec à Trois-Rivières, QC
Université Laval, QC
The University of British Columbia, BC
University of Calgary, AB
University of Cincinnati, OH
University of Florida, FL
University of Hartford, CT
University of Illinois at Chicago, IL
University of Kentucky, KY
University of Maryland, Baltimore, MD
University of Missouri, MO
University of Nebraska Medical Center, NE
University of New Brunswick Fredericton, NB
University of North Dakota, ND
University of Ottawa, ON
The University of Texas at Brownsville, TX
University of Toronto, ON
The University of Western Ontario, ON
West Chester University of Pennsylvania, PA
Worcester State University, MA
Wright State University, OH

### Rehabilitation

McGill University, QC
Salem State University, MA
Université de Montréal, QC
Université du Québec à Chicoutimi, QC
Université du Québec en Outaouais, QC
Université Laval, QC
University of Calgary, AB
University of Missouri, MO
University of Ottawa, ON
University of Toronto, ON

### School Health

Azusa Pacific University, CA
Bloomsburg University of Pennsylvania, PA
California State University, Fullerton, CA
Kean University, NJ
Monmouth University, NJ
San Diego State University, CA
Université de Moncton, NB
Université du Québec à Chicoutimi, QC
University of Illinois at Chicago, IL
University of Missouri, MO
University of New Brunswick Fredericton, NB
University of Ottawa, ON
University of Toronto, ON
Wright State University, OH
Xavier University, OH

### Women's Health

Drexel University, PA
Georgia State University, GA
McGill University, QC
St. John Fisher College, NY
San Diego State University, CA
Seattle Pacific University, WA
Stony Brook University, State University of New York, NY
Université de Montréal, QC
Université du Québec à Chicoutimi, QC
The University of British Columbia, BC
University of Calgary, AB
University of Illinois at Chicago, IL
University of Kentucky, KY
University of Manitoba, MB
University of Missouri, MO
University of Nebraska Medical Center, NE
University of New Brunswick Fredericton, NB
University of North Florida, FL
University of Ottawa, ON
University of South Alabama, AL
University of Toronto, ON
The University of Western Ontario, ON
Valparaiso University, IN
Wesley College, DE

## HEALTH-CARE ADMINISTRATION

Adelphi University, NY
Baylor University, TX
Boise State University, ID
California State University, Long Beach, CA
Clarkson College, NE
The College of New Rochelle, NY
Daemen College, NY
Duke University, NC
Georgetown University, DC
The George Washington University, DC
Goldfarb School of Nursing at Barnes-Jewish College, MO
Gonzaga University, WA
Hampton University, VA
The Johns Hopkins University, MD
Kaplan University Online, FL
Kean University, NJ
Kent State University, OH
Lenoir-Rhyne University, NC
Loma Linda University, CA
Long Island University–LIU Brooklyn, NY
Loyola University New Orleans, LA
Mercy College, NY
MGH Institute of Health Professions, MA
MidAmerica Nazarene University, KS
Missouri Western State University, MO
Mount Mercy University, IA
The Ohio State University, OH
Pacific Lutheran University, WA
Regis College, MA
Regis University, CO
Resurrection University, IL
The Sage Colleges, NY
St. Ambrose University, IA
Salisbury University, MD
San Jose State University, CA
Seton Hall University, NJ
Southern Illinois University Edwardsville, IL
Southern University and Agricultural and Mechanical College, LA
Stevenson University, MD
Texas Woman's University, TX
Thomas University, GA
Towson University, MD
Université de Moncton, NB
Université du Québec en Outaouais, QC
Université Laval, QC
The University of Alabama at Birmingham, AL
The University of Alabama in Huntsville, AL
University of Alaska Anchorage, AK
University of Delaware, DE
University of Illinois at Chicago, IL
The University of Kansas, KS
University of Louisiana at Lafayette, LA
University of Maine, ME
University of Michigan, MI
University of Nebraska Medical Center, NE
University of Oklahoma Health Sciences Center, OK
University of Pennsylvania, PA
University of Phoenix–Bay Area Campus, CA
University of Phoenix–Hawaii Campus, HI
University of Phoenix–North Florida Campus, FL
University of Phoenix–Online Campus, AZ
University of Phoenix–Phoenix Campus, AZ
University of Phoenix–Sacramento Valley Campus, CA
University of Phoenix–San Diego Campus, CA
University of Phoenix–Southern Arizona Campus, AZ
University of Phoenix–Southern California Campus, CA
University of Phoenix–South Florida Campus, FL
The University of Texas at Arlington, TX
University of Toronto, ON
The University of Western Ontario, ON
University of Wisconsin–Green Bay, WI
Vanderbilt University, TN
Villanova University, PA
Western Governors University, UT
Wright State University, OH

## LEGAL NURSE CONSULTANT

Capital University, OH
Wilmington University, DE

## NURSE ANESTHESIA

Arkansas State University, AR
Bloomsburg University of Pennsylvania, PA
Boston College, MA
Bryan College of Health Sciences, NE
California State University, Fullerton, CA
Case Western Reserve University, OH
Clarkson College, NE
Columbia University, NY
DePaul University, IL
Drexel University, PA
Duke University, NC
East Carolina University, NC
Florida Gulf Coast University, FL
Florida International University, FL
Gannon University, PA
Georgetown University, DC
Georgia Regents University, GA
Goldfarb School of Nursing at Barnes-Jewish College, MO
La Roche College, PA
La Salle University, PA
Lincoln Memorial University, TN
Loma Linda University, CA
Louisiana State University Health Sciences Center, LA
Lourdes University, OH
Michigan State University, MI
Millikin University, IL
Murray State University, KY
National University, CA
Newman University, KS
Oakland University, MI
Old Dominion University, VA
Oregon Health & Science University, OR
Our Lady of the Lake College, LA
Rush University, IL
Rutgers, The State University of New Jersey, Newark, NJ
Samford University, AL
Samuel Merritt University, CA
Southern Illinois University Edwardsville, IL
State University of New York Downstate Medical Center, NY
Thomas Jefferson University, PA
Union University, TN
The University of Akron, OH
The University of Alabama at Birmingham, AL

University of Cincinnati, OH
The University of Iowa, IA
University of Miami, FL
University of Michigan–Flint, MI
The University of North Carolina at Charlotte, NC
The University of North Carolina at Greensboro, NC
University of North Dakota, ND
University of Pennsylvania, PA
University of Pittsburgh, PA
University of Puerto Rico, Medical Sciences Campus, PR
The University of Scranton, PA
University of South Florida, FL
The University of Tennessee, TN
The University of Tennessee at Chattanooga, TN
The University of Texas Health Science Center at Houston, TX
University of Toronto, ON
Villanova University, PA
Western Carolina University, NC
York College of Pennsylvania, PA
Youngstown State University, OH

## NURSE-MIDWIFERY

California State University, Fullerton, CA
Case Western Reserve University, OH
Columbia University, NY
East Carolina University, NC
Emory University, GA
Georgetown University, DC
James Madison University, VA
The Johns Hopkins University, MD
Marquette University, WI
New York University, NY
The Ohio State University, OH
Old Dominion University, VA
Oregon Health & Science University, OR
Radford University, VA
Rutgers, The State University of New Jersey, Newark, NJ
San Diego State University, CA
Shenandoah University, VA
State University of New York Downstate Medical Center, NY
Stony Brook University, State University of New York, NY
Texas Tech University Health Sciences Center, TX
University of California, San Francisco, CA
University of Cincinnati, OH
University of Colorado Denver, CO
University of Florida, FL
University of Illinois at Chicago, IL
University of Indianapolis, IN
The University of Kansas, KS
University of Michigan, MI
University of New Mexico, NM
University of Pennsylvania, PA
Vanderbilt University, TN
Wayne State University, MI
West Virginia Wesleyan College, WV
Yale University, CT

## NURSE PRACTITIONER PROGRAMS

### Acute Care

Allen College, IA
Arizona State University at the Downtown Phoenix Campus, AZ
Armstrong Atlantic State University, GA
Barry University, FL
California State University, Los Angeles, CA
Case Western Reserve University, OH
The Catholic University of America, DC
Colorado State University–Pueblo, CO
Columbia University, NY
Creighton University, NE
Drexel University, PA
Duke University, NC
Emory University, GA
Florida Gulf Coast University, FL
Georgetown University, DC
Goldfarb School of Nursing at Barnes-Jewish College, MO
Grand Canyon University, AZ
Indiana University–Purdue University Indianapolis, IN
The Johns Hopkins University, MD
Kent State University, OH
Loyola University Chicago, IL
Madonna University, MI
Marquette University, WI
Memorial University of Newfoundland, NL
MGH Institute of Health Professions, MA
New York University, NY
Northern Kentucky University, KY
Northwestern State University of Louisiana, LA
The Ohio State University, OH
Rhode Island College, RI
Rush University, IL
Rutgers, The State University of New Jersey, Newark, NJ
The Sage Colleges, NY
Saint Louis University, MO
San Diego State University, CA
Seton Hall University, NJ
Southern Adventist University, TN
Texas Tech University Health Sciences Center, TX
Texas Woman's University, TX
Thomas Jefferson University, PA
Université de Montréal, QC
The University of Akron, OH
The University of Alabama at Birmingham, AL
The University of Alabama in Huntsville, AL
University of Arkansas for Medical Sciences, AR
University of Calgary, AB
University of California, Los Angeles, CA
University of California, San Francisco, CA
University of Connecticut, CT
University of Florida, FL
University of Illinois at Chicago, IL
University of Kentucky, KY
University of Louisville, KY
University of Massachusetts Boston, MA
University of Massachusetts Worcester, MA
University of Miami, FL
University of Michigan, MI
University of Mississippi Medical Center, MS
University of Nebraska Medical Center, NE
University of Nevada, Reno, NV
University of New Brunswick Fredericton, NB
University of New Mexico, NM
University of Pennsylvania, PA
University of South Alabama, AL
University of South Carolina, SC
University of Southern Indiana, IN
University of South Florida, FL
The University of Texas at Arlington, TX
The University of Texas Health Science Center at Houston, TX
University of Toronto, ON
University of Virginia, VA
Vanderbilt University, TN
Virginia Commonwealth University, VA
Wayne State University, MI
Wright State University, OH
Yale University, CT

### Adult Health

Adelphi University, NY
Allen College, IA
Arizona State University at the Downtown Phoenix Campus, AZ
Armstrong Atlantic State University, GA
Azusa Pacific University, CA
Ball State University, IN
Bloomsburg University of Pennsylvania, PA
Boston College, MA
California State University, Long Beach, CA
California State University, Los Angeles, CA
Case Western Reserve University, OH
The Catholic University of America, DC
Clarkson College, NE
Clemson University, SC
The College of New Jersey, NJ
The College of St. Scholastica, MN
College of Staten Island of the City University of New York, NY
Columbia University, NY
Concordia University Wisconsin, WI
Creighton University, NE
Daemen College, NY
DePaul University, IL
Drexel University, PA
Duke University, NC
East Carolina University, NC
Eastern Michigan University, MI
Emory University, GA
Fairleigh Dickinson University, Metropolitan Campus, NJ
Felician College, NJ
Florida Agricultural and Mechanical University, FL
Florida Atlantic University, FL
Florida Gulf Coast University, FL
Florida International University, FL
Florida Southern College, FL
George Mason University, VA
The George Washington University, DC
Georgia State University, GA
Goldfarb School of Nursing at Barnes-Jewish College, MO
Gwynedd Mercy University, PA
Indiana University–Purdue University Fort Wayne, IN
Indiana University–Purdue University Indianapolis, IN
James Madison University, VA
The Johns Hopkins University, MD
Kaplan University Online, FL
Kennesaw State University, GA
Kent State University, OH
La Salle University, PA
Lewis University, IL
Loma Linda University, CA
Long Island University–LIU Brooklyn, NY
Loyola University Chicago, IL
Loyola University New Orleans, LA

Marian University, WI
Marquette University, WI
Maryville University of Saint Louis, MO
Medical University of South Carolina, SC
MGH Institute of Health Professions, MA
Michigan State University, MI
Molloy College, NY
Monmouth University, NJ
Mount Saint Mary College, NY
Neumann University, PA
Northern Illinois University, IL
Northern Kentucky University, KY
North Park University, IL
Oakland University, MI
The Ohio State University, OH
Otterbein University, OH
Penn State University Park, PA
Purdue University, IN
Quinnipiac University, CT
Regis College, MA
Research College of Nursing, MO
Rhode Island College, RI
The Richard Stockton College of New Jersey, NJ
Rush University, IL
Rutgers, The State University of New Jersey, Newark, NJ
The Sage Colleges, NY
St. Catherine University, MN
Saint Louis University, MO
Saint Peter's University, NJ
San Diego State University, CA
Seattle Pacific University, WA
Seton Hall University, NJ
Southern Adventist University, TN
Spalding University, KY
Spring Arbor University, MI
State University of New York Institute of Technology, NY
State University of New York Upstate Medical University, NY
Stony Brook University, State University of New York, NY
Temple University, PA
Texas Woman's University, TX
Thomas Jefferson University, PA
Université de Moncton, NB
Université Laval, QC
University at Buffalo, the State University of New York, NY
The University of Akron, OH
The University of Alabama at Birmingham, AL
University of Alberta, AB
University of Calgary, AB
University of California, Irvine, CA
University of California, Los Angeles, CA
University of California, San Francisco, CA
University of Central Arkansas, AR
University of Central Florida, FL
University of Cincinnati, OH
University of Colorado Colorado Springs, CO
University of Colorado Denver, CO
University of Delaware, DE
University of Florida, FL
University of Hawaii at Manoa, HI
University of Illinois at Chicago, IL
University of Indianapolis, IN
The University of Iowa, IA
The University of Kansas, KS
University of Kentucky, KY
University of Louisiana at Lafayette, LA
University of Louisville, KY
University of Massachusetts Boston, MA
University of Massachusetts Dartmouth, MA
University of Miami, FL
University of Michigan, MI
University of Michigan–Flint, MI
University of Missouri–St. Louis, MO
University of Nebraska Medical Center, NE
University of New Brunswick Fredericton, NB
University of New Hampshire, NH
The University of North Carolina at Charlotte, NC
The University of North Carolina at Greensboro, NC
University of Oklahoma Health Sciences Center, OK
University of Pennsylvania, PA
University of San Diego, CA
University of South Florida, FL
The University of Tampa, FL
The University of Texas at Arlington, TX
The University of Texas Health Science Center at Houston, TX
University of Toronto, ON
University of Vermont, VT
University of Wisconsin–Eau Claire, WI
Ursuline College, OH
Vanderbilt University, TN
Villanova University, PA
Viterbo University, WI
Washburn University, KS
Western Connecticut State University, CT
William Paterson University of New Jersey, NJ
Wilmington University, DE
Winona State University, MN
York College of Pennsylvania, PA

**Community Health**

Athabasca University, AB
Binghamton University, State University of New York, NY
Hunter College of the City University of New York, NY
The Ohio State University, OH
The Sage Colleges, NY
Université de Moncton, NB
The University of British Columbia, BC
University of Hawaii at Manoa, HI
University of Nebraska Medical Center, NE
University of New Brunswick Fredericton, NB
University of Virginia, VA
The University of Western Ontario, ON

**Family Health**

Albany State University, GA
Alcorn State University, MS
Allen College, IA
Angelo State University, TX
Arizona State University at the Downtown Phoenix Campus, AZ
Athabasca University, AB
Austin Peay State University, TN
Azusa Pacific University, CA
Ball State University, IN
Barry University, FL
Belmont University, TN
Binghamton University, State University of New York, NY
Bloomsburg University of Pennsylvania, PA
Boston College, MA
Bowie State University, MD
Brenau University, GA
Brigham Young University, UT
California State University, Dominguez Hills, CA
California State University, Fresno, CA
California State University, Long Beach, CA
California State University, Los Angeles, CA
California State University, Sacramento, CA
Carlow University, PA
Carson-Newman University, TN
Case Western Reserve University, OH
The Catholic University of America, DC
Cedarville University, OH
Clarion University of Pennsylvania, PA
Clarke University, IA
Clarkson College, NE
Clemson University, SC
The College of New Jersey, NJ
The College of New Rochelle, NY
The College of St. Scholastica, MN
Colorado State University–Pueblo, CO
Columbia University, NY
Concordia University Wisconsin, WI
Coppin State University, MD
Creighton University, NE
Delta State University, MS
DePaul University, IL
DeSales University, PA
Dominican College, NY
Drexel University, PA
Duke University, NC
Duquesne University, PA
D'Youville College, NY
East Carolina University, NC
Eastern Kentucky University, KY
East Tennessee State University, TN
Emory University, GA
Fairfield University, CT
Fairleigh Dickinson University, Metropolitan Campus, NJ
Felician College, NJ
Florida Atlantic University, FL
Florida Gulf Coast University, FL
Florida International University, FL
Fort Hays State University, KS
Franciscan University of Steubenville, OH
Gannon University, PA
Gardner-Webb University, NC
George Mason University, VA
Georgetown University, DC
The George Washington University, DC
Georgia College & State University, GA
Georgia Regents University, GA
Georgia Southern University, GA
Georgia State University, GA
Gonzaga University, WA
Goshen College, IN
Graceland University, IA
Grambling State University, LA
Grand Canyon University, AZ
Hampton University, VA
Hawai`i Pacific University, HI
Herzing University Online, WI
Holy Names University, CA
Howard University, DC
Hunter College of the City University of New York, NY
Husson University, ME
Illinois State University, IL
Indiana State University, IN
Indiana University–Purdue University Indianapolis, IN
Indiana University South Bend, IN
Indiana Wesleyan University, IN

Jacksonville University, FL
James Madison University, VA
The Johns Hopkins University, MD
Kaplan University Online, FL
Kennesaw State University, GA
Kent State University, OH
La Salle University, PA
Lehman College of the City University of New York, NY
Lewis University, IL
Lincoln Memorial University, TN
Loma Linda University, CA
Long Island University–LIU Brooklyn, NY
Long Island University–LIU Post, NY
Louisiana State University Health Sciences Center, LA
Loyola University Chicago, IL
Loyola University New Orleans, LA
Malone University, OH
Marshall University, WV
Marymount University, VA
Maryville University of Saint Louis, MO
McNeese State University, LA
Medical University of South Carolina, SC
Georgia Baptist College of Nursing, GA
MGH Institute of Health Professions, MA
Michigan State University, MI
Middle Tennessee State University, TN
Midwestern State University, TX
Millersville University of Pennsylvania, PA
Minnesota State University Mankato, MN
Misericordia University, PA
Mississippi University for Women, MS
Missouri State University, MO
Molloy College, NY
Monmouth University, NJ
Mount Carmel College of Nursing, OH
Murray State University, KY
New York University, NY
North Dakota State University, ND
Northern Arizona University, AZ
Northern Illinois University, IL
Northern Kentucky University, KY
Northern Michigan University, MI
North Park University, IL
Northwestern State University of Louisiana, LA
Oakland University, MI
The Ohio State University, OH
Ohio University, OH
Old Dominion University, VA
Olivet Nazarene University, IL
Oregon Health & Science University, OR
Otterbein University, OH
Pace University, NY
Pacific Lutheran University, WA
Patty Hanks Shelton School of Nursing, TX
Penn State University Park, PA
Pittsburg State University, KS
Prairie View A&M University, TX
Purdue University Calumet, IN
Quinnipiac University, CT
Radford University, VA
Regis College, MA
Regis University, CO
Research College of Nursing, MO
Rivier University, NH
Rush University, IL
Rutgers, The State University of New Jersey, Newark, NJ
Sacred Heart University, CT
The Sage Colleges, NY
Saginaw Valley State University, MI
Saint Anthony College of Nursing, IL
Saint Francis Medical Center College of Nursing, IL
St. John Fisher College, NY
Saint Louis University, MO
Saint Xavier University, IL
Salisbury University, MD
Samford University, AL
Samuel Merritt University, CA
San Francisco State University, CA
San Jose State University, CA
Seattle Pacific University, WA
Seattle University, WA
Shenandoah University, VA
Simmons College, MA
South Dakota State University, SD
Southeastern Louisiana University, LA
Southeast Missouri State University, MO
Southern Adventist University, TN
Southern Connecticut State University, CT
Southern Illinois University Edwardsville, IL
Southern University and Agricultural and Mechanical College, LA
Spalding University, KY
State University of New York Downstate Medical Center, NY
State University of New York Institute of Technology, NY
State University of New York Upstate Medical University, NY
Temple University, PA
Tennessee State University, TN
Tennessee Technological University, TN
Texas A&M International University, TX
Texas A&M University–Corpus Christi, TX
Texas State University–San Marcos, TX
Texas Tech University Health Sciences Center, TX
Texas Woman's University, TX
Thomas Jefferson University, PA
Troy University, AL
Union University, TN
Université de Moncton, NB
Université de Montréal, QC
University at Buffalo, the State University of New York, NY
The University of Alabama, AL
The University of Alabama at Birmingham, AL
The University of Alabama in Huntsville, AL
University of Alaska Anchorage, AK
University of Arkansas for Medical Sciences, AR
The University of British Columbia, BC
University of California, Davis, CA
University of California, Irvine, CA
University of California, Los Angeles, CA
University of California, San Francisco, CA
University of Central Arkansas, AR
University of Central Florida, FL
University of Central Missouri, MO
University of Cincinnati, OH
University of Colorado Colorado Springs, CO
University of Colorado Denver, CO
University of Connecticut, CT
University of Delaware, DE
University of Detroit Mercy, MI
University of Florida, FL
University of Hawaii at Manoa, HI
University of Illinois at Chicago, IL
University of Indianapolis, IN
The University of Iowa, IA
The University of Kansas, KS
University of Kentucky, KY
University of Louisville, KY
University of Maine, ME
University of Mary, ND
University of Mary Hardin-Baylor, TX
University of Massachusetts Boston, MA
University of Massachusetts Lowell, MA
University of Massachusetts Worcester, MA
University of Memphis, TN
University of Miami, FL
University of Michigan, MI
University of Mississippi Medical Center, MS
University of Missouri, MO
University of Missouri–St. Louis, MO
University of Nebraska Medical Center, NE
University of Nevada, Las Vegas, NV
University of Nevada, Reno, NV
University of New Brunswick Fredericton, NB
University of New Hampshire, NH
University of New Mexico, NM
The University of North Carolina at Charlotte, NC
The University of North Carolina Wilmington, NC
University of North Dakota, ND
University of Northern British Columbia, BC
University of Northern Colorado, CO
University of North Florida, FL
University of North Georgia, GA
University of Oklahoma Health Sciences Center, OK
University of Pennsylvania, PA
University of Phoenix–Hawaii Campus, HI
University of Phoenix–Online Campus, AZ
University of Phoenix–Phoenix Campus, AZ
University of Phoenix–Sacramento Valley Campus, CA
University of Phoenix–Southern Arizona Campus, AZ
University of Phoenix–Southern California Campus, CA
University of Rhode Island, RI
University of St. Francis, IL
University of Saint Francis, IN
University of Saint Joseph, CT
University of San Diego, CA
The University of Scranton, PA
University of South Alabama, AL
University of South Carolina, SC
University of Southern Indiana, IN
University of Southern Maine, ME
University of Southern Mississippi, MS
University of South Florida, FL
The University of Tampa, FL
The University of Tennessee, TN
The University of Tennessee at Chattanooga, TN
The University of Texas at Arlington, TX
The University of Texas at Austin, TX
The University of Texas at El Paso, TX
The University of Texas at Tyler, TX
The University of Texas Health Science Center at Houston, TX
The University of Texas Health Science Center at San Antonio, TX
The University of Texas Medical Branch, TX
The University of Texas–Pan American, TX
The University of Toledo, OH
University of Toronto, ON
University of Vermont, VT
University of Virginia, VA

University of Wisconsin–Eau Claire, WI
Ursuline College, OH
Vanderbilt University, TN
Villanova University, PA
Virginia Commonwealth University, VA
Viterbo University, WI
Wagner College, NY
Walden University, MN
Washburn University, KS
Washington State University College of Nursing, WA
Western Carolina University, NC
Western University of Health Sciences, CA
Westminster College, UT
West Texas A&M University, TX
West Virginia University, WV
Wheeling Jesuit University, WV
Widener University, PA
William Paterson University of New Jersey, NJ
Wilmington University, DE
Winona State University, MN
Winston-Salem State University, NC
Wright State University, OH
Yale University, CT

### Gerontology

Allen College, IA
Binghamton University, State University of New York, NY
Bloomsburg University of Pennsylvania, PA
Boston College, MA
California State University, Long Beach, CA
Case Western Reserve University, OH
Clemson University, SC
The College of St. Scholastica, MN
College of Staten Island of the City University of New York, NY
Concordia University Wisconsin, WI
Creighton University, NE
Daemen College, NY
Delta State University, MS
Duke University, NC
Fairleigh Dickinson University, Metropolitan Campus, NJ
Florida Agricultural and Mechanical University, FL
Florida Atlantic University, FL
George Mason University, VA
Hampton University, VA
Hunter College of the City University of New York, NY
James Madison University, VA
The Johns Hopkins University, MD
Lewis University, IL
Loma Linda University, CA
Medical University of South Carolina, SC
MGH Institute of Health Professions, MA
Michigan State University, MI
Mississippi University for Women, MS
Mount Carmel College of Nursing, OH
Oakland University, MI
The Ohio State University, OH
Rush University, IL
Rutgers, The State University of New Jersey, Newark, NJ
The Sage Colleges, NY
St. Catherine University, MN
Saint Louis University, MO
San Diego State University, CA
Seattle University, WA
Seton Hall University, NJ
Spring Arbor University, MI
State University of New York Institute of Technology, NY
Texas Tech University Health Sciences Center, TX
The University of Akron, OH
University of Alberta, AB
University of California, Irvine, CA
University of California, Los Angeles, CA
University of California, San Francisco, CA
University of Hawaii at Manoa, HI
University of Illinois at Chicago, IL
University of Indianapolis, IN
The University of Iowa, IA
The University of Kansas, KS
University of Kentucky, KY
University of Massachusetts Boston, MA
University of Massachusetts Lowell, MA
University of Massachusetts Worcester, MA
University of Miami, FL
University of Michigan, MI
University of Mississippi Medical Center, MS
University of Missouri, MO
University of Nebraska Medical Center, NE
University of New Brunswick Fredericton, NB
The University of North Carolina at Greensboro, NC
University of North Dakota, ND
University of Pennsylvania, PA
University of Rhode Island, RI
University of San Diego, CA
University of South Alabama, AL
University of Southern Mississippi, MS
University of South Florida, FL
The University of Tampa, FL
The University of Texas at Arlington, TX
The University of Texas Health Science Center at Houston, TX
The University of Texas Health Science Center at San Antonio, TX
The University of Texas Medical Branch, TX
University of Toronto, ON
University of Utah, UT
University of Wisconsin–Eau Claire, WI
Walden University, MN
Wayne State University, MI
Wilmington University, DE

### Neonatal Health

Arizona State University at the Downtown Phoenix Campus, AZ
Case Western Reserve University, OH
The College of New Jersey, NJ
Creighton University, NE
Duke University, NC
East Carolina University, NC
Loma Linda University, CA
Louisiana State University Health Sciences Center, LA
McGill University, QC
McMaster University, ON
The Ohio State University, OH
Regis University, CO
Rush University, IL
Saint Francis Medical Center College of Nursing, IL
South Dakota State University, SD
Stony Brook University, State University of New York, NY
Thomas Jefferson University, PA
The University of Alabama at Birmingham, AL
University of Calgary, AB
University of California, San Francisco, CA
University of Cincinnati, OH
University of Connecticut, CT
University of Florida, FL
University of Indianapolis, IN
The University of Iowa, IA
University of Louisville, KY
University of Missouri–Kansas City, MO
University of Missouri–St. Louis, MO
University of Nebraska Medical Center, NE
University of New Brunswick Fredericton, NB
University of Oklahoma Health Sciences Center, OK
University of Pennsylvania, PA
University of Pittsburgh, PA
University of South Alabama, AL
The University of Texas at Arlington, TX
The University of Texas Medical Branch, TX
University of Toronto, ON
Vanderbilt University, TN
Wayne State University, MI
West Virginia University, WV

### Occupational Health

The University of Alabama at Birmingham, AL
University of California, Los Angeles, CA
University of California, San Francisco, CA
University of Cincinnati, OH
University of Illinois at Chicago, IL
University of South Florida, FL
University of the Sacred Heart, PR

### Oncology

Case Western Reserve University, OH
Creighton University, NE
Duke University, NC
Thomas Jefferson University, PA
Université de Moncton, NB
University of Nebraska Medical Center, NE
University of South Florida, FL
University of Toronto, ON

### Pediatric

Arizona State University at the Downtown Phoenix Campus, AZ
Azusa Pacific University, CA
Boston College, MA
California State University, Fresno, CA
California State University, Long Beach, CA
California State University, Los Angeles, CA
Case Western Reserve University, OH
The Catholic University of America, DC
Colorado State University–Pueblo, CO
Columbia University, NY
Creighton University, NE
Drexel University, PA
Duke University, NC
Emory University, GA
Florida International University, FL
Georgia Regents University, GA
Georgia State University, GA
Grambling State University, LA
Gwynedd Mercy University, PA
Hampton University, VA
Indiana University–Purdue University Indianapolis, IN
The Johns Hopkins University, MD
Kent State University, OH
Lehman College of the City University of New York, NY
Loma Linda University, CA
Marquette University, WI
Medical University of South Carolina, SC
MGH Institute of Health Professions, MA

Mississippi University for Women, MS
Molloy College, NY
New York University, NY
Northern Kentucky University, KY
Northwestern State University of Louisiana, LA
The Ohio State University, OH
Purdue University, IN
Regis College, MA
Rush University, IL
St. Catherine University, MN
Saint Louis University, MO
Seton Hall University, NJ
Spalding University, KY
State University of New York Upstate Medical University, NY
Stony Brook University, State University of New York, NY
Temple University, PA
Texas Tech University Health Sciences Center, TX
Texas Woman's University, TX
Thomas Jefferson University, PA
The University of Akron, OH
The University of Alabama at Birmingham, AL
University of Arkansas for Medical Sciences, AR
University of California, Los Angeles, CA
University of California, San Francisco, CA
University of Cincinnati, OH
University of Colorado Denver, CO
University of Florida, FL
University of Hawaii at Manoa, HI
University of Illinois at Chicago, IL
The University of Iowa, IA
University of Kentucky, KY
University of Michigan, MI
University of Missouri, MO
University of Missouri–St. Louis, MO
University of Nebraska Medical Center, NE
University of New Brunswick Fredericton, NB
University of New Mexico, NM
University of Oklahoma Health Sciences Center, OK
University of Pennsylvania, PA
University of San Diego, CA
University of South Alabama, AL
University of South Florida, FL
The University of Tennessee, TN
The University of Texas at Arlington, TX
The University of Texas at Austin, TX
The University of Texas at Tyler, TX
The University of Texas Health Science Center at Houston, TX
The University of Texas Health Science Center at San Antonio, TX
The University of Texas–Pan American, TX
The University of Toledo, OH
University of Toronto, ON
University of Virginia, VA
Vanderbilt University, TN
Villanova University, PA
Wayne State University, MI
West Virginia University, WV
Wright State University, OH
Yale University, CT

### Primary Care

Arkansas State University, AR
Athabasca University, AB
Auburn University at Montgomery, AL
Azusa Pacific University, CA
California State University, Los Angeles, CA
California State University, Sacramento, CA
Duke University, NC
Eastern Michigan University, MI
Emory University, GA
Florida Atlantic University, FL
Florida Southern College, FL
Gonzaga University, WA
Hampton University, VA
Indiana University–Purdue University Fort Wayne, IN
The Johns Hopkins University, MD
Kennesaw State University, GA
Kent State University, OH
Loma Linda University, CA
Loyola University Chicago, IL
Madonna University, MI
McGill University, QC
Medical University of South Carolina, SC
MGH Institute of Health Professions, MA
New York University, NY
The Ohio State University, OH
Queen's University at Kingston, ON
Regis College, MA
Ryerson University, ON
Saint Louis University, MO
Seton Hall University, NJ
Simmons College, MA
Université de Moncton, NB
Université de Montréal, QC
Université du Québec à Chicoutimi, QC
Université du Québec à Trois-Rivières, QC
Université du Québec en Outaouais, QC
Université Laval, QC
The University of Akron, OH
The University of British Columbia, BC
University of Connecticut, CT
University of Indianapolis, IN
University of Manitoba, MB
University of Massachusetts Worcester, MA
University of Michigan, MI
University of Missouri, MO
University of Nebraska Medical Center, NE
University of New Brunswick Fredericton, NB
University of North Dakota, ND
University of North Florida, FL
University of Ottawa, ON
University of Pennsylvania, PA
University of San Diego, CA
University of Saskatchewan, SK
University of Toronto, ON
University of Virginia, VA
University of Windsor, ON
Wayne State University, MI

### Psychiatric/Mental Health

Allen College, IA
Arizona State University at the Downtown Phoenix Campus, AZ
Binghamton University, State University of New York, NY
Boston College, MA
California State University, Long Beach, CA
California State University, Los Angeles, CA
Case Western Reserve University, OH
The College of St. Scholastica, MN
Columbia University, NY
Creighton University, NE
Delta State University, MS
Drexel University, PA
Eastern Kentucky University, KY
Fairfield University, CT
Fairleigh Dickinson University, Metropolitan Campus, NJ
George Mason University, VA
Georgia State University, GA
Gonzaga University, WA
Hunter College of the City University of New York, NY
Indiana University–Purdue University Indianapolis, IN
Kent State University, OH
Lincoln Memorial University, TN
Loma Linda University, CA
McNeese State University, LA
MGH Institute of Health Professions, MA
Midwestern State University, TX
Mississippi University for Women, MS
Molloy College, NY
Monmouth University, NJ
New York University, NY
The Ohio State University, OH
Oregon Health & Science University, OR
Regis College, MA
Rivier University, NH
Rush University, IL
Rutgers, The State University of New Jersey, Newark, NJ
The Sage Colleges, NY
Saint Francis Medical Center College of Nursing, IL
Saint Louis University, MO
Seattle University, WA
Shenandoah University, VA
South Dakota State University, SD
Southeastern Louisiana University, LA
State University of New York Upstate Medical University, NY
Stony Brook University, State University of New York, NY
University at Buffalo, the State University of New York, NY
The University of Akron, OH
The University of Alabama, AL
The University of Alabama at Birmingham, AL
University of Alaska Anchorage, AK
University of Arkansas for Medical Sciences, AR
University of California, San Francisco, CA
University of Colorado Denver, CO
University of Florida, FL
University of Illinois at Chicago, IL
The University of Iowa, IA
The University of Kansas, KS
University of Kentucky, KY
University of Louisiana at Lafayette, LA
University of Louisville, KY
University of Massachusetts Lowell, MA
University of Michigan, MI
University of Mississippi Medical Center, MS
University of Missouri, MO
University of Missouri–Kansas City, MO
University of Nebraska Medical Center, NE
University of New Brunswick Fredericton, NB
University of North Dakota, ND
University of Pennsylvania, PA
University of St. Francis, IL
University of Saint Joseph, CT
University of San Diego, CA
University of South Alabama, AL
University of Southern Indiana, IN
University of Southern Maine, ME
University of Southern Mississippi, MS
The University of Tennessee, TN

The University of Texas at Arlington, TX
The University of Texas at Austin, TX
The University of Texas Health Science Center at Houston, TX
The University of Texas Health Science Center at San Antonio, TX
University of Vermont, VT
University of Virginia, VA
Vanderbilt University, TN
Virginia Commonwealth University, VA
Washington State University College of Nursing, WA
Wayne State University, MI
West Virginia Wesleyan College, WV
Winston-Salem State University, NC
Yale University, CT

### School Health

The College of New Jersey, NJ
Seton Hall University, NJ
University of Illinois at Chicago, IL

### Women's Health

Arizona State University at the Downtown Phoenix Campus, AZ
Boston College, MA
California State University, Fullerton, CA
California State University, Long Beach, CA
Case Western Reserve University, OH
Drexel University, PA
Emory University, GA
Florida Agricultural and Mechanical University, FL
Georgetown University, DC
Georgia State University, GA
Hampton University, VA
Indiana University–Purdue University Fort Wayne, IN
Kent State University, OH
Loyola University Chicago, IL
MGH Institute of Health Professions, MA
Northwestern State University of Louisiana, LA
The Ohio State University, OH
Old Dominion University, VA
Regis College, MA
Rutgers, The State University of New Jersey, Newark, NJ
Salem State University, MA
San Diego State University, CA
State University of New York Downstate Medical Center, NY
Stony Brook University, State University of New York, NY
Texas Woman's University, TX
The University of Alabama at Birmingham, AL
University of Cincinnati, OH
University of Colorado Denver, CO
University of Illinois at Chicago, IL
University of Indianapolis, IN
University of Louisville, KY
University of Missouri–St. Louis, MO
University of Nebraska Medical Center, NE
University of New Brunswick Fredericton, NB
University of Pennsylvania, PA
University of South Alabama, AL
The University of Texas Health Science Center at Houston, TX
Vanderbilt University, TN
Wayne State University, MI
Wesley College, DE
West Virginia University, WV

## NURSING ADMINISTRATION

Adelphi University, NY
Allen College, IA
American International College, MA
American Sentinel University, CO
Anderson University, IN
Arkansas State University, AR
Arkansas Tech University, AR
Aspen University, CO
Athabasca University, AB
Aurora University, IL
Austin Peay State University, TN
Azusa Pacific University, CA
Ball State University, IN
Barry University, FL
Bellarmine University, KY
Bellin College, WI
Bethel College, IN
Bethel University, MN
Binghamton University, State University of New York, NY
Blessing–Rieman College of Nursing, IL
Bloomsburg University of Pennsylvania, PA
Boise State University, ID
Bradley University, IL
Brandman University, CA
California State University, Chico, CA
California State University, Dominguez Hills, CA
California State University, Fullerton, CA
California State University, Long Beach, CA
California State University, Los Angeles, CA
California State University, Sacramento, CA
California State University, San Bernardino, CA
Capella University, MN
Capital University, OH
Carlow University, PA
Chatham University, PA
Clarkson College, NE
Clayton State University, GA
Clemson University, SC
The College of New Rochelle, NY
Creighton University, NE
Delta State University, MS
DeSales University, PA
Drexel University, PA
Duke University, NC
East Carolina University, NC
Eastern Mennonite University, VA
East Tennessee State University, TN
Edgewood College, WI
Elms College, MA
Emmanuel College, MA
Endicott College, MA
Excelsior College, NY
Fairleigh Dickinson University, Metropolitan Campus, NJ
Felician College, NJ
Ferris State University, MI
Florida Atlantic University, FL
Florida International University, FL
Florida Southern College, FL
Florida State University, FL
Fort Hays State University, KS
Framingham State University, MA
Franklin Pierce University, NH
Gannon University, PA
Gardner-Webb University, NC
George Mason University, VA
The George Washington University, DC
Georgia Southwestern State University, GA
Georgia State University, GA
Goldfarb School of Nursing at Barnes-Jewish College, MO
Gonzaga University, WA
Grand Canyon University, AZ
Hampton University, VA
Herzing University Online, WI
Holy Family University, PA
Holy Names University, CA
Hunter College of the City University of New York, NY
Idaho State University, ID
Illinois State University, IL
Immaculata University, PA
Indiana State University, IN
Indiana University of Pennsylvania, PA
Indiana University–Purdue University Fort Wayne, IN
Indiana University–Purdue University Indianapolis, IN
Indiana Wesleyan University, IN
Jacksonville University, FL
James Madison University, VA
Jefferson College of Health Sciences, VA
The Johns Hopkins University, MD
Kean University, NJ
Lamar University, TX
La Roche College, PA
La Salle University, PA
Lehman College of the City University of New York, NY
Le Moyne College, NY
Lewis University, IL
Loma Linda University, CA
Long Island University–LIU Brooklyn, NY
Louisiana State University Health Sciences Center, LA
Lourdes University, OH
Loyola University Chicago, IL
Madonna University, MI
Mansfield University of Pennsylvania, PA
Marquette University, WI
Marshall University, WV
Marywood University, PA
McGill University, QC
McKendree University, IL
McNeese State University, LA
Mercy College, NY
Metropolitan State University, MN
MGH Institute of Health Professions, MA
Middle Tennessee State University, TN
Molloy College, NY
Monmouth University, NJ
Moravian College, PA
Mount Carmel College of Nursing, OH
Mount Mercy University, IA
Mount St. Mary's College, CA
National University, CA
Nebraska Methodist College, NE
Nebraska Wesleyan University, NE
New Mexico State University, NM
New York University, NY
Northern Kentucky University, KY
North Park University, IL
Northwestern State University of Louisiana, LA
Nova Southeastern University, FL
The Ohio State University, OH
Ohio University, OH
Oklahoma City University, OK
Old Dominion University, VA
Otterbein University, OH

Our Lady of the Lake College, LA
Pacific Lutheran University, WA
Penn State University Park, PA
Pittsburg State University, KS
Prairie View A&M University, TX
Purdue University Calumet, IN
Queens University of Charlotte, NC
Regis College, MA
Regis University, CO
Research College of Nursing, MO
Resurrection University, IL
Roberts Wesleyan College, NY
Sacred Heart University, CT
The Sage Colleges, NY
Saginaw Valley State University, MI
St. Ambrose University, IA
Saint Francis Medical Center College of Nursing, IL
Saint Joseph's College of Maine, ME
Saint Peter's University, NJ
Saint Xavier University, IL
Salem State University, MA
Samford University, AL
San Diego State University, CA
San Francisco State University, CA
San Jose State University, CA
Seattle Pacific University, WA
Seton Hall University, NJ
Simmons College, MA
South Dakota State University, SD
Southeastern Louisiana University, LA
Southern Nazarene University, OK
Southwest Baptist University, MO
Spalding University, KY
State University of New York Institute of Technology, NY
Stevenson University, MD
Tennessee State University, TN
Tennessee Technological University, TN
Texas A&M International University, TX
Texas A&M University–Corpus Christi, TX
Texas A&M University–Texarkana, TX
Texas Tech University Health Sciences Center, TX
Texas Woman's University, TX
Thomas University, GA
Troy University, AL
Union University, TN
Université de Moncton, NB
Université de Montréal, QC
Université Laval, QC
University at Buffalo, the State University of New York, NY
The University of Akron, OH
The University of Alabama, AL
The University of Alabama at Birmingham, AL
University of Arkansas for Medical Sciences, AR
The University of British Columbia, BC
University of California, Los Angeles, CA
University of California, San Francisco, CA
University of Central Florida, FL
University of Cincinnati, OH
University of Colorado Denver, CO
University of Detroit Mercy, MI
University of Hartford, CT
University of Hawaii at Manoa, HI
University of Houston–Victoria, TX
University of Illinois at Chicago, IL
University of Indianapolis, IN
The University of Iowa, IA
The University of Kansas, KS
University of Kentucky, KY
University of Louisiana at Lafayette, LA
University of Manitoba, MB
University of Mary, ND
University of Memphis, TN
University of Michigan, MI
University of Mississippi Medical Center, MS
University of Missouri, MO
University of Mobile, AL
University of Nebraska Medical Center, NE
University of New Brunswick Fredericton, NB
University of New Mexico, NM
University of North Alabama, AL
The University of North Carolina at Charlotte, NC
The University of North Carolina at Greensboro, NC
University of Pennsylvania, PA
University of Phoenix–Bay Area Campus, CA
University of Phoenix–Cleveland Campus, OH
University of Phoenix–Hawaii Campus, HI
University of Phoenix–New Mexico Campus, NM
University of Phoenix–North Florida Campus, FL
University of Phoenix–Online Campus, AZ
University of Phoenix–Phoenix Campus, AZ
University of Phoenix–Sacramento Valley Campus, CA
University of Phoenix–San Diego Campus, CA
University of Phoenix–Southern Arizona Campus, AZ
University of Phoenix–Southern California Campus, CA
University of Phoenix–South Florida Campus, FL
University of Pittsburgh, PA
University of Puerto Rico, Medical Sciences Campus, PR
University of Rhode Island, RI
University of St. Francis, IL
University of San Diego, CA
University of South Alabama, AL
University of Southern Indiana, IN
University of Southern Maine, ME
University of Southern Mississippi, MS
The University of Tennessee, TN
The University of Texas at Arlington, TX
The University of Texas at Austin, TX
The University of Texas at Brownsville, TX
The University of Texas at El Paso, TX
The University of Texas at Tyler, TX
The University of Texas Health Science Center at Houston, TX
The University of Texas Health Science Center at San Antonio, TX
The University of Texas Medical Branch, TX
University of Toronto, ON
University of Vermont, VT
University of Virginia, VA
The University of Western Ontario, ON
University of West Florida, FL
University of West Georgia, GA
University of Windsor, ON
University of Wisconsin–Eau Claire, WI
University of Wisconsin–Green Bay, WI
Urbana University, OH
Valdosta State University, GA
Vanderbilt University, TN
Virginia Commonwealth University, VA
Walden University, MN
Washburn University, KS
Washington State University College of Nursing, WA
Waynesburg University, PA
Weber State University, UT
Webster University, MO
West Chester University of Pennsylvania, PA
Western Carolina University, NC
Western Governors University, UT
Western Kentucky University, KY
Western Michigan University, MI
Western University of Health Sciences, CA
West Texas A&M University, TX
West Virginia University, WV
West Virginia Wesleyan College, WV
Wheeling Jesuit University, WV
Wilkes University, PA
William Paterson University of New Jersey, NJ
Wilmington University, DE
Winona State University, MN
Wright State University, OH
Xavier University, OH

## NURSING EDUCATION

Adelphi University, NY
Albany State University, GA
Alcorn State University, MS
Allen College, IA
Alverno College, WI
American International College, MA
American Sentinel University, CO
Anderson University, IN
Andrews University, MI
Angelo State University, TX
Aquinas College, TN
Arkansas State University, AR
Aspen University, CO
Athabasca University, AB
Auburn University, AL
Auburn University at Montgomery, AL
Aurora University, IL
Austin Peay State University, TN
Azusa Pacific University, CA
Ball State University, IN
Barry University, FL
Bellarmine University, KY
Bellin College, WI
Belmont University, TN
Bethel College, IN
Bethel University, MN
Binghamton University, State University of New York, NY
Blessing–Rieman College of Nursing, IL
Boise State University, ID
Bowie State University, MD
Bradley University, IL
Brenau University, GA
Briar Cliff University, IA
Bryan College of Health Sciences, NE
California Baptist University, CA
California State University, Chico, CA
California State University, Dominguez Hills, CA
California State University, Fresno, CA
California State University, Fullerton, CA
California State University, Long Beach, CA
California State University, Los Angeles, CA
California State University, Sacramento, CA
California State University, San Bernardino, CA
Capella University, MN
Capital University, OH
Cardinal Stritch University, WI

Carlow University, PA
Carson-Newman University, TN
Case Western Reserve University, OH
Central Methodist University, MO
Charleston Southern University, SC
Chatham University, PA
Clarke University, IA
Clarkson College, NE
Clayton State University, GA
Clemson University, SC
Cleveland State University, OH
The College of New Rochelle, NY
College of Saint Mary, NE
Colorado State University–Pueblo, CO
Concordia College, MN
Concordia University Wisconsin, WI
Cox College, MO
Creighton University, NE
Daemen College, NY
Delaware State University, DE
Delta State University, MS
DeSales University, PA
Drexel University, PA
Duke University, NC
Duquesne University, PA
D'Youville College, NY
East Carolina University, NC
Eastern Kentucky University, KY
East Tennessee State University, TN
Edgewood College, WI
Elmhurst College, IL
Elms College, MA
Emmanuel College, MA
Endicott College, MA
Excelsior College, NY
Fairleigh Dickinson University, Metropolitan Campus, NJ
Felician College, NJ
Ferris State University, MI
Florida Atlantic University, FL
Florida International University, FL
Florida Southern College, FL
Florida State University, FL
Fort Hays State University, KS
Framingham State University, MA
Franciscan University of Steubenville, OH
Franklin Pierce University, NH
Gardner-Webb University, NC
George Mason University, VA
Georgia Southwestern State University, GA
Goldfarb School of Nursing at Barnes-Jewish College, MO
Gonzaga University, WA
Graceland University, IA
Grambling State University, LA
Grand Canyon University, AZ
Hampton University, VA
Hawai`i Pacific University, HI
Herzing University Online, WI
Holy Family University, PA
Holy Names University, CA
Howard University, DC
Husson University, ME
Idaho State University, ID
Immaculata University, PA
Indiana State University, IN
Indiana University of Pennsylvania, PA
Indiana University–Purdue University Fort Wayne, IN
Indiana University–Purdue University Indianapolis, IN
Indiana Wesleyan University, IN
Jacksonville University, FL
Jefferson College of Health Sciences, VA
Kaplan University Online, FL
Kent State University, OH
Lamar University, TX
La Roche College, PA
Lehman College of the City University of New York, NY
Le Moyne College, NY
Lenoir-Rhyne University, NC
Lewis University, IL
Liberty University, VA
Loma Linda University, CA
Long Island University–LIU Brooklyn, NY
Long Island University–LIU Post, NY
Louisiana State University Health Sciences Center, LA
Lourdes University, OH
Lynchburg College, VA
Mansfield University of Pennsylvania, PA
Marian University, WI
Marshall University, WV
Maryville University of Saint Louis, MO
McKendree University, IL
McNeese State University, LA
Memorial University of Newfoundland, NL
Georgia Baptist College of Nursing, GA
Mercy College, NY
Messiah College, PA
Metropolitan State University, MN
MGH Institute of Health Professions, MA
MidAmerica Nazarene University, KS
Middle Tennessee State University, TN
Midwestern State University, TX
Millersville University of Pennsylvania, PA
Millikin University, IL
Minnesota State University Mankato, MN
Minnesota State University Moorhead, MN
Misericordia University, PA
Missouri Southern State University, MO
Missouri State University, MO
Molloy College, NY
Monmouth University, NJ
Moravian College, PA
Mount Carmel College of Nursing, OH
Mount Mercy University, IA
Mount St. Mary's College, CA
Nebraska Methodist College, NE
Nebraska Wesleyan University, NE
Neumann University, PA
New York University, NY
North Dakota State University, ND
Northeastern State University, OK
Northern Illinois University, IL
Northern Kentucky University, KY
Northwestern State University of Louisiana, LA
Northwest Nazarene University, ID
Nova Southeastern University, FL
Oakland University, MI
Ohio University, OH
Oklahoma Baptist University, OK
Oklahoma City University, OK
Old Dominion University, VA
Oregon Health & Science University, OR
Otterbein University, OH
Our Lady of the Lake College, LA
Pace University, NY
Pacific Lutheran University, WA
Patty Hanks Shelton School of Nursing, TX
Pittsburg State University, KS
Point Loma Nazarene University, CA
Prairie View A&M University, TX
Queens University of Charlotte, NC
Ramapo College of New Jersey, NJ
Regis College, MA
Regis University, CO
Research College of Nursing, MO
Resurrection University, IL
Rivier University, NH
Robert Morris University, PA
Roberts Wesleyan College, NY
Rutgers, The State University of New Jersey, Newark, NJ
Sacred Heart University, CT
The Sage Colleges, NY
Saginaw Valley State University, MI
Saint Anthony College of Nursing, IL
St. Catherine University, MN
Saint Francis Medical Center College of Nursing, IL
St. John Fisher College, NY
St. Joseph's College, New York, NY
Saint Joseph's College of Maine, ME
Saint Louis University, MO
Salem State University, MA
Salisbury University, MD
Samford University, AL
San Diego State University, CA
San Jose State University, CA
Seattle Pacific University, WA
Seton Hall University, NJ
South Dakota State University, SD
Southeast Missouri State University, MO
Southern Adventist University, TN
Southern Connecticut State University, CT
Southern Illinois University Edwardsville, IL
Southern Nazarene University, OK
Southern University and Agricultural and Mechanical College, LA
Southwest Baptist University, MO
Spalding University, KY
Spring Arbor University, MI
State University of New York Institute of Technology, NY
Stevenson University, MD
Temple University, PA
Tennessee State University, TN
Tennessee Technological University, TN
Texas A&M University–Corpus Christi, TX
Texas A&M University–Texarkana, TX
Texas Christian University, TX
Texas Tech University Health Sciences Center, TX
Texas Woman's University, TX
Thomas Jefferson University, PA
Thomas University, GA
Touro University, NV
Towson University, MD
Troy University, AL
Union University, TN
Université de Moncton, NB
Université de Montréal, QC
The University of Alabama, AL
The University of Alabama at Birmingham, AL
University of Alaska Anchorage, AK
University of Arkansas, AR
University of Arkansas for Medical Sciences, AR
The University of British Columbia, BC
University of Central Arkansas, AR
University of Central Florida, FL
University of Central Missouri, MO
University of Central Oklahoma, OK

University of Detroit Mercy, MI
University of Hartford, CT
University of Hawaii at Manoa, HI
University of Houston–Victoria, TX
University of Indianapolis, IN
The University of Iowa, IA
University of Louisiana at Lafayette, LA
University of Louisville, KY
University of Maine, ME
University of Mary, ND
University of Mary Hardin-Baylor, TX
University of Massachusetts Worcester, MA
University of Memphis, TN
University of Mississippi Medical Center, MS
University of Missouri, MO
University of Missouri–Kansas City, MO
University of Missouri–St. Louis, MO
University of Mobile, AL
University of Nebraska Medical Center, NE
University of Nevada, Las Vegas, NV
University of Nevada, Reno, NV
University of New Brunswick Fredericton, NB
University of New Mexico, NM
University of North Alabama, AL
The University of North Carolina at Chapel Hill, NC
The University of North Carolina at Charlotte, NC
The University of North Carolina at Greensboro, NC
University of North Dakota, ND
University of Northern Colorado, CO
University of North Georgia, GA
University of Oklahoma Health Sciences Center, OK
University of Phoenix–Bay Area Campus, CA
University of Phoenix–Hawaii Campus, HI
University of Phoenix–New Mexico Campus, NM
University of Phoenix–North Florida Campus, FL
University of Phoenix–Online Campus, AZ
University of Phoenix–Phoenix Campus, AZ
University of Phoenix–Sacramento Valley Campus, CA
University of Phoenix–San Diego Campus, CA
University of Phoenix–Southern Arizona Campus, AZ
University of Phoenix–Southern California Campus, CA
University of Phoenix–South Florida Campus, FL
University of Portland, OR
University of Puerto Rico, Medical Sciences Campus, PR
University of Rhode Island, RI
University of St. Francis, IL
University of Saint Joseph, CT
University of San Diego, CA
University of Saskatchewan, SK
The University of Scranton, PA
University of South Alabama, AL
University of Southern Indiana, IN
University of Southern Maine, ME
University of South Florida, FL
The University of Texas at Arlington, TX
The University of Texas at Brownsville, TX
The University of Texas at El Paso, TX
The University of Texas at Tyler, TX
The University of Texas Health Science Center at Houston, TX
The University of Texas Health Science Center at San Antonio, TX
The University of Texas Medical Branch, TX
The University of Toledo, OH
University of Toronto, ON
University of Utah, UT
The University of Western Ontario, ON
University of West Florida, FL
University of West Georgia, GA
University of Wisconsin–Eau Claire, WI
University of Wisconsin–Oshkosh, WI
University of Wyoming, WY
Urbana University, OH
Ursuline College, OH
Valdosta State University, GA
Villanova University, PA
Viterbo University, WI
Wagner College, NY
Walden University, MN
Walsh University, OH
Washington State University College of Nursing, WA
Waynesburg University, PA
Weber State University, UT
Webster University, MO
West Chester University of Pennsylvania, PA
Western Carolina University, NC
Western Governors University, UT
Western Kentucky University, KY
Western Michigan University, MI
Westminster College, UT
West Texas A&M University, TX
West Virginia Wesleyan College, WV
Wheeling Jesuit University, WV
Widener University, PA
Wilkes University, PA
William Carey University, MS
William Paterson University of New Jersey, NJ
Wilmington University, DE
Winona State University, MN
Winston-Salem State University, NC
Worcester State University, MA
Xavier University, OH
York College of Pennsylvania, PA
Youngstown State University, OH

## NURSING INFORMATICS

Adelphi University, NY
American Sentinel University, CO
Anderson University, IN
Austin Peay State University, TN
Chatham University, PA
Duke University, NC
East Tennessee State University, TN
Excelsior College, NY
Fairleigh Dickinson University, Metropolitan Campus, NJ
Ferris State University, MI
Georgia Southwestern State University, GA
Georgia State University, GA
Kaplan University Online, FL
Le Moyne College, NY
Loyola University Chicago, IL
Middle Tennessee State University, TN
Molloy College, NY
National University, CA
New York University, NY
Northern Kentucky University, KY
Nova Southeastern University, FL
Regis College, MA
Rutgers, The State University of New Jersey, Newark, NJ
San Jose State University, CA
Tennessee State University, TN
Tennessee Technological University, TN
Thomas Jefferson University, PA
Troy University, AL
The University of Alabama at Birmingham, AL
University of Colorado Denver, CO
University of Illinois at Chicago, IL
The University of Iowa, IA
The University of Kansas, KS
University of Maryland, Baltimore, MD
University of Michigan, MI
University of Nebraska Medical Center, NE
University of New Brunswick Fredericton, NB
University of Pittsburgh, PA
University of San Diego, CA
University of Toronto, ON
University of Utah, UT
Ursuline College, OH
Vanderbilt University, TN
Walden University, MN
Waynesburg University, PA
Xavier University, OH

# DOCTORAL PROGRAMS

## U.S. AND U.S. TERRITORIES

### Alabama

Samford University, Ida V. Moffett School of Nursing, *Birmingham (DNP)*
Troy University, School of Nursing, *Troy (DNP)*
The University of Alabama, Capstone College of Nursing, *Tuscaloosa (DNP)*
The University of Alabama at Birmingham, School of Nursing, *Birmingham (DNP, PhD)*
The University of Alabama in Huntsville, College of Nursing, *Huntsville (DNP)*

### Arizona

Arizona State University at the Downtown Phoenix Campus, College of Nursing, *Phoenix (DNP)*
Northern Arizona University, School of Nursing, *Flagstaff (DNP)*
The University of Arizona, College of Nursing, *Tucson (PhD)*
University of Phoenix–Online Campus, Online Campus, *Phoenix (PhD)*

### Arkansas

Arkansas State University, Department of Nursing, *State University (DNP)*
University of Arkansas for Medical Sciences, College of Nursing, *Little Rock (DNP, PhD)*

### California

Azusa Pacific University, School of Nursing, *Azusa (PhD)*
Brandman University, School of Nursing and Health Professions, *Irvine (DNP)*
California State University, Fresno, Department of Nursing, *Fresno (DNP)*
California State University, Fullerton, Department of Nursing, *Fullerton (DNP)*
Loma Linda University, School of Nursing, *Loma Linda (DNP)*
Samuel Merritt University, School of Nursing, *Oakland (DNP)*
University of California, Davis, The Betty Irene Moore School of Nursing, *Davis (PhD)*
University of California, Irvine, Program in Nursing Science, *Irvine (PhD)*
University of California, Los Angeles, School of Nursing, *Los Angeles (PhD)*
University of California, San Francisco, School of Nursing, *San Francisco (PhD)*
University of San Diego, Hahn School of Nursing and Health Science, *San Diego (DNP, PhD)*
University of San Francisco, School of Nursing, *San Francisco (DNP)*
Western University of Health Sciences, College of Graduate Nursing, *Pomona (DNP)*

### Colorado

University of Colorado Colorado Springs, Beth-El College of Nursing and Health Sciences, *Colorado Springs (DNP)*
University of Colorado Denver, College of Nursing, *Aurora (DNP, PhD)*
University of Northern Colorado, School of Nursing, *Greeley (PhD)*

### Connecticut

Fairfield University, School of Nursing, *Fairfield (DNP)*
Quinnipiac University, School of Nursing, *Hamden (DNP)*
Sacred Heart University, Program in Nursing, *Fairfield (DNP)*
Southern Connecticut State University, Department of Nursing, *New Haven (EdD)*
University of Connecticut, School of Nursing, *Storrs (DNP, PhD)*
Yale University, School of Nursing, *New Haven (DNP, PhD)*

### Delaware

University of Delaware, School of Nursing, *Newark (PhD)*

### District of Columbia

The Catholic University of America, School of Nursing, *Washington (PhD)*
Georgetown University, School of Nursing and Health Studies, *Washington (DNP)*
The George Washington University, School of Nursing, *Washington (DNP)*

### Florida

Barry University, Division of Nursing, *Miami Shores (PhD)*
Florida Agricultural and Mechanical University, School of Nursing, *Tallahassee (PhD)*
Florida Atlantic University, Christine E. Lynn College of Nursing, *Boca Raton (DNP)*
Florida International University, Nursing Program, *Miami (DNP, PhD)*
Florida State University, College of Nursing, *Tallahassee (DNP)*
Jacksonville University, School of Nursing, *Jacksonville (DNP)*
University of Central Florida, College of Nursing, *Orlando (DNP, PhD)*
University of Florida, College of Nursing, *Gainesville (PhD)*
University of Miami, School of Nursing and Health Studies, *Coral Gables (PhD)*
University of South Florida, College of Nursing, *Tampa (DNP, PhD)*

### Georgia

Brenau University, College of Health and Science, *Gainesville (DNP)*
Emory University, Nell Hodgson Woodruff School of Nursing, *Atlanta (PhD)*
Georgia College & State University, College of Health Sciences, *Milledgeville (DNP)*
Georgia Regents University, School of Nursing, *Augusta (DNP, PhD)*
Georgia Southern University, School of Nursing, *Statesboro (DNP)*
Georgia State University, Byrdine F. Lewis School of Nursing and Health Professions, *Atlanta (PhD)*
Georgia Baptist College of Nursing, *Atlanta (DNP, PhD)*
University of West Georgia, School of Nursing, *Carrollton (EdD)*

### Hawaii

University of Hawaii at Manoa, School of Nursing and Dental Hygiene, *Honolulu (PhD)*

### Idaho

Idaho State University, Department of Nursing, *Pocatello (DNP, PhD)*

### Illinois

DePaul University, School of Nursing, *Chicago (DNP)*
Illinois State University, Mennonite College of Nursing, *Normal (DNP, PhD)*
Lewis University, Program in Nursing, *Romeoville (DNP)*
Loyola University Chicago, Marcella Niehoff School of Nursing, *Maywood (DNP, PhD)*
Millikin University, School of Nursing, *Decatur (DNP)*
Rush University, College of Nursing, *Chicago (PhD)*
Saint Francis Medical Center College of Nursing, Baccalaureate Nursing Program, *Peoria (DNP)*
Southern Illinois University Edwardsville, School of Nursing, *Edwardsville (DNP)*
University of Illinois at Chicago, College of Nursing, *Chicago (PhD)*
University of St. Francis, Leach College of Nursing, *Joliet (DNP)*

### Indiana

Ball State University, School of Nursing, *Muncie (DNP)*
Indiana State University, Department of Nursing, *Terre Haute (DNP)*
Indiana University–Purdue University Indianapolis, School of Nursing, *Indianapolis (PhD)*
Purdue University, School of Nursing, *West Lafayette (DNP)*
University of Indianapolis, School of Nursing, *Indianapolis (DNP)*
University of Southern Indiana, College of Nursing and Health Professions, *Evansville (DNP)*

### Iowa

Allen College, Program in Nursing, *Waterloo (DNP)*
Briar Cliff University, Department of Nursing, *Sioux City (DNP)*
The University of Iowa, College of Nursing, *Iowa City (PhD)*

### Kansas

The University of Kansas, School of Nursing, *Kansas City (PhD)*
Wichita State University, School of Nursing, *Wichita (DNP)*

### Kentucky

Bellarmine University, Donna and Allan Lansing School of Nursing and Health Sciences, *Louisville (DNP)*
Frontier Nursing University, Nursing Degree Programs, *Hyden (DNP)*
Northern Kentucky University, Department of Nursing, *Highland Heights (DNP)*
University of Kentucky, College of Nursing, *Lexington (PhD)*
University of Louisville, School of Nursing, *Louisville (PhD)*
Western Kentucky University, School of Nursing, *Bowling Green (DNP)*

### Louisiana

Louisiana State University Health Sciences Center, School of Nursing, *New Orleans (DNP)*

Loyola University New Orleans, School of Nursing, *New Orleans (DNP)*
Southeastern Louisiana University, School of Nursing, *Hammond (DNP)*
Southern University and Agricultural and Mechanical College, School of Nursing, *Baton Rouge (PhD)*

### Maine

University of Southern Maine, School of Nursing, *Portland (DNP)*

### Maryland

The Johns Hopkins University, School of Nursing, *Baltimore (DNP, PhD)*
Salisbury University, Nursing DNP Program, *Salisbury (DNP)*
University of Maryland, Baltimore, Master's Program in Nursing, *Baltimore (DNP, PhD)*

### Massachusetts

Boston College, William F. Connell School of Nursing, *Chestnut Hill (PhD)*
MGH Institute of Health Professions, School of Nursing, *Boston (DNP)*
Northeastern University, School of Nursing, *Boston (DNP)*
Regis College, School of Nursing, Science and Health Professions, *Weston (DNP)*
Simmons College, School of Nursing and Health Sciences, *Boston (DNP)*
University of Massachusetts Amherst, School of Nursing, *Amherst (PhD)*
University of Massachusetts Boston, College of Nursing and Health Sciences, *Boston (DNP, PhD)*
University of Massachusetts Dartmouth, College of Nursing, *North Dartmouth (PhD)*
University of Massachusetts Lowell, School of Nursing, *Lowell (DNP, PhD)*
University of Massachusetts Worcester, Graduate School of Nursing, *Worcester (PhD)*

### Michigan

Eastern Michigan University, School of Nursing, *Ypsilanti (PhD)*
Grand Valley State University, Kirkhof College of Nursing, *Allendale (DNP)*
Madonna University, College of Nursing and Health, *Livonia (DNP)*
Michigan State University, College of Nursing, *East Lansing (DNP, PhD)*
Saginaw Valley State University, College of Health and Human Services, *University Center (DNP)*
University of Michigan, School of Nursing, *Ann Arbor (PhD)*
University of Michigan–Flint, Department of Nursing, *Flint (DNP)*
Wayne State University, College of Nursing, *Detroit (DNP)*

### Minnesota

Capella University, Nursing Programs, *Minneapolis (DNP)*
The College of St. Scholastica, Department of Nursing, *Duluth (DNP)*
Metropolitan State University, College of Health, Community and Professional Studies, *St. Paul (DNP)*
Minnesota State University Mankato, School of Nursing, *Mankato (DNP)*
St. Catherine University, Department of Nursing, *St. Paul (DNP)*
University of Minnesota, Twin Cities Campus, School of Nursing, *Minneapolis (DNP, PhD)*
Walden University, Nursing Programs, *Minneapolis (DNP)*
Winona State University, College of Nursing and Health Sciences, *Winona (DNP)*

### Mississippi

Delta State University, School of Nursing, *Cleveland (DNP)*
Mississippi University for Women, College of Nursing and Speech Language Pathology, *Columbus (DNP)*
University of Mississippi Medical Center, School of Nursing, *Jackson (DNP)*
University of Southern Mississippi, School of Nursing, *Hattiesburg (PhD)*
William Carey University, School of Nursing, *Hattiesburg (PhD)*

### Missouri

Goldfarb School of Nursing at Barnes-Jewish College, *St. Louis (PhD)*
Graceland University, School of Nursing, *Independence (DNP)*
Maryville University of Saint Louis, Nursing Program, School of Health Professions, *St. Louis (DNP)*
Missouri State University, Department of Nursing, *Springfield (DNP)*
Saint Louis University, School of Nursing, *St. Louis (DNP, PhD)*
University of Missouri, Sinclair School of Nursing, *Columbia (PhD)*
University of Missouri–Kansas City, School of Nursing and Health Studies, *Kansas City (DNP, PhD)*
University of Missouri–St. Louis, College of Nursing, *St. Louis (DNP)*

### Montana

Montana State University, College of Nursing, *Bozeman (DNP)*

### Nebraska

Creighton University, School of Nursing, *Omaha (DNP)*
University of Nebraska Medical Center, College of Nursing, *Omaha (PhD)*

### Nevada

Touro University, School of Nursing, *Henderson (DNP)*
University of Nevada, Las Vegas, School of Nursing, *Las Vegas (DNP, PhD)*
University of Nevada, Reno, Orvis School of Nursing, *Reno (DNP)*

### New Jersey

Fairleigh Dickinson University, Metropolitan Campus, Henry P. Becton School of Nursing and Allied Health, *Teaneck (DNP)*
Rutgers, The State University of New Jersey, Newark, Rutgers School of Nursing, *Newark (DNP)*
Seton Hall University, College of Nursing, *South Orange (DNP)*
William Paterson University of New Jersey, Department of Nursing, *Wayne (DNP)*

### New Mexico

New Mexico State University, School of Nursing, *Las Cruces (PhD)*
University of New Mexico, College of Nursing, *Albuquerque (DNP, PhD)*

### New York

Adelphi University, College of Nursing and Public Health, *Garden City (PhD)*
Binghamton University, State University of New York, Decker School of Nursing, *Vestal (DNP, PhD)*
Columbia University, School of Nursing, *New York (PhD)*
Daemen College, Department of Nursing, *Amherst (DNP)*
Hunter College of the City University of New York, Hunter-Bellevue School of Nursing, *New York (DNP)*
Lehman College of the City University of New York, Department of Nursing, *Bronx (DNS)*
Molloy College, Division of Nursing, *Rockville Centre (PhD)*
New York University, College of Nursing, *New York (DNP, PhD)*
Pace University, Lienhard School of Nursing, *New York (DNP)*
The Sage Colleges, Department of Nursing, *Troy (DNS)*
St. John Fisher College, Wegmans School of Nursing, *Rochester (DNP)*
Stony Brook University, State University of New York, School of Nursing, *Stony Brook (DNP)*
University at Buffalo, the State University of New York, School of Nursing, *Buffalo (DNP, PhD)*

### North Carolina

Duke University, School of Nursing, *Durham (PhD)*
East Carolina University, College of Nursing, *Greenville (PhD)*
Gardner-Webb University, School of Nursing, *Boiling Springs (DNP)*
The University of North Carolina at Chapel Hill, School of Nursing, *Chapel Hill (DNP, PhD)*
The University of North Carolina at Greensboro, School of Nursing, *Greensboro (PhD)*

### North Dakota

North Dakota State University, Department of Nursing, *Fargo (DNP)*
University of North Dakota, College of Nursing, *Grand Forks (PhD)*

### Ohio

Case Western Reserve University, Frances Payne Bolton School of Nursing, *Cleveland (PhD)*
Cleveland State University, School of Nursing, *Cleveland (PhD)*
Kent State University, College of Nursing, *Kent (DNP, PhD)*
The Ohio State University, College of Nursing, *Columbus (DNP, PhD)*
The University of Akron, School of Nursing, *Akron (PhD)*
University of Cincinnati, College of Nursing, *Cincinnati (PhD)*
The University of Toledo, College of Nursing, *Toledo (DNP)*
Ursuline College, The Breen School of Nursing, *Pepper Pike (DNP)*

Walsh University, Department of Nursing, *North Canton (DNP)*

Wright State University, College of Nursing and Health, *Dayton (DNP)*

### Oklahoma

Oklahoma City University, Kramer School of Nursing, *Oklahoma City (DNP, PhD)*

University of Oklahoma Health Sciences Center, College of Nursing, *Oklahoma City (PhD)*

### Oregon

Oregon Health & Science University, School of Nursing, *Portland (PhD)*

University of Portland, School of Nursing, *Portland (DNP)*

### Pennsylvania

Chatham University, Nursing Programs, *Pittsburgh (DNP)*

Drexel University, College of Nursing and Health Professions, *Philadelphia (Dr NP)*

Duquesne University, School of Nursing, *Pittsburgh (PhD)*

Gannon University, Villa Maria School of Nursing, *Erie (DNP)*

Indiana University of Pennsylvania, Department of Nursing and Allied Health, *Indiana (PhD)*

Penn State University Park, School of Nursing, *University Park (PhD)*

Robert Morris University, School of Nursing and Health Sciences, *Moon Township (DNP)*

Temple University, Department of Nursing, *Philadelphia (DNP)*

Thomas Jefferson University, Department of Nursing, *Philadelphia (DNP)*

University of Pennsylvania, School of Nursing, *Philadelphia (PhD)*

University of Pittsburgh, School of Nursing, *Pittsburgh (PhD)*

Villanova University, College of Nursing, *Villanova (PhD)*

Waynesburg University, Department of Nursing, *Waynesburg (DNP)*

Widener University, School of Nursing, *Chester (PhD)*

York College of Pennsylvania, Department of Nursing, *York (DNP)*

### Rhode Island

University of Rhode Island, College of Nursing, *Kingston (PhD)*

### South Carolina

Medical University of South Carolina, College of Nursing, *Charleston (PhD)*

University of South Carolina, College of Nursing, *Columbia (DNP, PhD)*

### South Dakota

South Dakota State University, College of Nursing, *Brookings (PhD)*

### Tennessee

East Tennessee State University, College of Nursing, *Johnson City (DNP, PhD)*

Southern Adventist University, School of Nursing, *Collegedale (DNP)*

The University of Tennessee, College of Nursing, *Knoxville (PhD)*

The University of Tennessee at Chattanooga, School of Nursing, *Chattanooga (DNP)*

The University of Tennessee Health Science Center, College of Nursing, *Memphis (DNP)*

Vanderbilt University, Vanderbilt University School of Nursing, *Nashville (DNP, PhD)*

### Texas

Baylor University, Louise Herrington School of Nursing, *Dallas (DNP)*

Texas Christian University, Harris College of Nursing, *Fort Worth (DNP, DNP)*

Texas Tech University Health Sciences Center, School of Nursing, *Lubbock (DNP)*

Texas Woman's University, College of Nursing, *Denton (PhD)*

The University of Texas at Arlington, College of Nursing, *Arlington (PhD)*

The University of Texas at Austin, School of Nursing, *Austin (PhD)*

The University of Texas at Tyler, Program in Nursing, *Tyler (PhD)*

The University of Texas Health Science Center at Houston, School of Nursing, *Houston (PhD)*

The University of Texas Health Science Center at San Antonio, School of Nursing, *San Antonio (PhD)*

The University of Texas Medical Branch, School of Nursing, *Galveston (DNP)*

University of the Incarnate Word, Program in Nursing, *San Antonio (DNP)*

### Utah

University of Utah, College of Nursing, *Salt Lake City (PhD)*

### Virginia

George Mason University, College of Health and Human Services, *Fairfax (PhD)*

Hampton University, School of Nursing, *Hampton (PhD)*

James Madison University, Department of Nursing, *Harrisonburg (DNP)*

Marymount University, School of Health Professions, *Arlington (DNP)*

Old Dominion University, Department of Nursing, *Norfolk (DNP)*

Radford University, School of Nursing, *Radford (DNP)*

Shenandoah University, Division of Nursing, *Winchester (DNP)*

University of Virginia, School of Nursing, *Charlottesville (PhD)*

Virginia Commonwealth University, School of Nursing, *Richmond (PhD)*

### Washington

Seattle University, College of Nursing, *Seattle (DNP)*

University of Washington, School of Nursing, *Seattle (DNP, PhD)*

Washington State University College of Nursing, *Spokane (PhD)*

### West Virginia

West Virginia University, School of Nursing, *Morgantown (DNP, PhD)*

### Wisconsin

Concordia University Wisconsin, Program in Nursing, *Mequon (DNP)*

Marquette University, College of Nursing, *Milwaukee (DNP, PhD)*

University of Phoenix–Milwaukee Campus, College of Health and Human Services, *Milwaukee (PhD)*

University of Wisconsin–Eau Claire, College of Nursing and Health Sciences, *Eau Claire (DNP)*

University of Wisconsin–Madison, School of Nursing, *Madison (PhD)*

University of Wisconsin–Milwaukee, College of Nursing, *Milwaukee (PhD, DNP, DNP)*

University of Wisconsin–Oshkosh, College of Nursing, *Oshkosh (DNP)*

Viterbo University, School of Nursing, *La Crosse (DNP)*

### Wyoming

University of Wyoming, Fay W. Whitney School of Nursing, *Laramie (DNP)*

## CANADA

### Alberta

University of Alberta, Faculty of Nursing, *Edmonton (PhD)*

University of Calgary, Faculty of Nursing, *Calgary (PhD)*

### British Columbia

The University of British Columbia, Program in Nursing, *Vancouver (PhD)*

University of Victoria, School of Nursing, *Victoria (PhD)*

### Manitoba

University of Manitoba, Faculty of Nursing, *Winnipeg (PhD)*

### Ontario

McMaster University, School of Nursing, *Hamilton (PhD)*

Queen's University at Kingston, School of Nursing, *Kingston (PhD)*

University of Ottawa, School of Nursing, *Ottawa (PhD)*

University of Toronto, Faculty of Nursing, *Toronto (PhD)*

The University of Western Ontario, School of Nursing, *London (PhD)*

### Quebec

McGill University, School of Nursing, *Montréal (PhD)*

Université de Montréal, Faculty of Nursing, *Montréal (PhD)*

Université de Sherbrooke, Department of Nursing, *Sherbrooke (PhD)*

Université Laval, Faculty of Nursing, *Québec (PhD)*

### Saskatchewan

University of Saskatchewan, College of Nursing, *Saskatoon (PhD)*

# POSTDOCTORAL PROGRAMS

## U.S. AND U.S. TERRITORIES

### Alabama

The University of Alabama at Birmingham, School of Nursing, *Birmingham*

### Arkansas

University of Arkansas for Medical Sciences, College of Nursing, *Little Rock*

### California

University of California, Davis, The Betty Irene Moore School of Nursing, *Davis*

University of California, Los Angeles, School of Nursing, *Los Angeles*

University of California, San Francisco, School of Nursing, *San Francisco*

### Colorado

University of Colorado Denver, College of Nursing, *Aurora*

### Connecticut

University of Connecticut, School of Nursing, *Storrs*

Yale University, School of Nursing, *New Haven*

### Illinois

University of Illinois at Chicago, College of Nursing, *Chicago*

### Indiana

Indiana University–Purdue University Indianapolis, School of Nursing, *Indianapolis*

### Iowa

The University of Iowa, College of Nursing, *Iowa City*

### Kansas

The University of Kansas, School of Nursing, *Kansas City*

### Maryland

The Johns Hopkins University, School of Nursing, *Baltimore*

### Massachusetts

University of Massachusetts Boston, College of Nursing and Health Sciences, *Boston*

### Michigan

University of Michigan, School of Nursing, *Ann Arbor*

### Nebraska

University of Nebraska Medical Center, College of Nursing, *Omaha*

### New York

Columbia University, School of Nursing, *New York*

### North Carolina

The University of North Carolina at Chapel Hill, School of Nursing, *Chapel Hill*

### Ohio

Case Western Reserve University, Frances Payne Bolton School of Nursing, *Cleveland*

### Oregon

Oregon Health & Science University, School of Nursing, *Portland*

### Pennsylvania

Penn State University Park, School of Nursing, *University Park*

University of Pennsylvania, School of Nursing, *Philadelphia*

University of Pittsburgh, School of Nursing, *Pittsburgh*

### South Carolina

Medical University of South Carolina, College of Nursing, *Charleston*

University of South Carolina, College of Nursing, *Columbia*

### Tennessee

Vanderbilt University, Vanderbilt University School of Nursing, *Nashville*

### Utah

University of Utah, College of Nursing, *Salt Lake City*

### Virginia

University of Virginia, School of Nursing, *Charlottesville*

### Washington

University of Washington, School of Nursing, *Seattle*

### Wisconsin

University of Wisconsin–Madison, School of Nursing, *Madison*

## CANADA

### British Columbia

The University of British Columbia, Program in Nursing, *Vancouver*

University of Northern British Columbia, Nursing Programme, *Prince George*

### Ontario

University of Ottawa, School of Nursing, *Ottawa*

University of Toronto, Faculty of Nursing, *Toronto*

The University of Western Ontario, School of Nursing, *London*

### Quebec

McGill University, School of Nursing, *Montréal*

Université de Montréal, Faculty of Nursing, *Montréal*

Université de Sherbrooke, Department of Nursing, *Sherbrooke*

Université Laval, Faculty of Nursing, *Québec*

# Online Programs

## ONLINE BACCALAUREATE PROGRAMS

Adventist University of Health Sciences, FL
Albany State University, GA
Alcorn State University, MS
Allen College, IA
American Public University System, WV
Angelo State University, TX
Appalachian State University, NC
Arizona State University at the Downtown Phoenix Campus, AZ
Arkansas State University, AR
Arkansas Tech University, AR
Ashland University, OH
Aurora University, IL
Bethel College, KS
Blessing–Rieman College of Nursing, IL
Bluefield State College, WV
Boise State University, ID
Bon Secours Memorial College of Nursing, VA
Brenau University, GA
Caldwell College, NJ
California State University, Dominguez Hills, CA
Carson-Newman University, TN
Central Methodist University, MO
Chamberlain College of Nursing, MO
Charleston Southern University, SC
Clarion University of Pennsylvania, PA
Clarkson College, NE
Clayton State University, GA
Cleveland State University, OH
College of Coastal Georgia, GA
The College of St. Scholastica, MN
Colorado Christian University, CO
Colorado Mesa University, CO
Columbus State University, GA
Cox College, MO
Creighton University, NE
Cumberland University, TN
Davenport University, MI
East Carolina University, NC
Eastern Illinois University, IL
Eastern Michigan University, MI
Eastern New Mexico University, NM
East Tennessee State University, TN
ECPI University, VA
Ferris State University, MI
Finlandia University, MI
Fitchburg State University, MA
Florida Atlantic University, FL
Florida International University, FL
Fort Hays State University, KS
Francis Marion University, SC
Frostburg State University, MD
Gannon University, PA
Gardner-Webb University, NC
George Mason University, VA
Georgia College & State University, GA
Georgia Southern University, GA
Georgia Southwestern State University, GA
Grand Canyon University, AZ
Great Basin College, NV
Herzing University Online, WI
Hondros College, OH
Howard University, DC
Illinois State University, IL
Indiana State University, IN
Indiana University Northwest, IN
Indiana University–Purdue University Indianapolis, IN
Jacksonville State University, AL
Jacksonville University, FL
Kettering College, OH
Lakehead University, ON
Lamar University, TX
Lander University, SC
La Roche College, PA
Lees-McRae College, NC
Lehman College of the City University of New York, NY
Loyola University New Orleans, LA
Marian University, IN
McKendree University, IL
Mercy College, NY
Mercy College of Ohio, OH
Methodist College, IL
Michigan State University, MI
MidAmerica Nazarene University, KS
Middle Tennessee State University, TN
Minnesota State University Moorhead, MN
Minot State University, ND
Mississippi University for Women, MS
Missouri State University, MO
Montana State University–Northern, MT
Morehead State University, KY
Morningside College, IA
Mount Aloysius College, PA
Mount Carmel College of Nursing, OH
Nevada State College at Henderson, NV
Newman University, KS
New Mexico Highlands University, NM
New Mexico State University, NM
Nipissing University, ON
Northeastern State University, OK
Northern Arizona University, AZ
Northwestern State University of Louisiana, LA
Nova Southeastern University, FL
The Ohio State University, OH
Ohio University, OH
Oklahoma Panhandle State University, OK
Our Lady of the Lake College, LA
Penn State University Park, PA
Pittsburg State University, KS
Presentation College, SD
Purdue University Calumet, IN
Queens University of Charlotte, NC
Radford University, VA
Ramapo College of New Jersey, NJ
Rivier University, NH
Robert Morris University, PA
Roberts Wesleyan College, NY
Ryerson University, ON
Saint Louis University, MO
St. Petersburg College, FL
St. Vincent's College, CT
Sentara College of Health Sciences, VA
Silver Lake College of the Holy Family, WI
Slippery Rock University of Pennsylvania, PA
South Dakota State University, SD
Southeastern Louisiana University, LA
Southeast Missouri State University, MO
Southern Adventist University, TN
Southern Arkansas University–Magnolia, AR
Southwestern Oklahoma State University, OK
State University of New York at Plattsburgh, NY
State University of New York College of Technology at Alfred, NY
State University of New York College of Technology at Delhi, NY
State University of New York Empire State College, NY
State University of New York Institute of Technology, NY
Stevenson University, MD
Tabor College, KS
Texas A&M Health Science Center, TX
Texas A&M University–Corpus Christi, TX
Texas Tech University Health Sciences Center, TX
Texas Tech University Health Sciences Center-El Paso, TX
Texas Woman's University, TX
Touro University, NV
Trocaire College, NY
University at Buffalo, the State University of New York, NY
The University of Akron, OH
University of Arkansas for Medical Sciences, AR
University of Arkansas–Fort Smith, AR
University of Central Florida, FL
University of Central Missouri, MO
University of Colorado Colorado Springs, CO
University of Colorado Denver, CO
University of Delaware, DE
University of Illinois at Chicago, IL
University of Indianapolis, IN
University of Louisiana at Lafayette, LA
University of Louisiana at Monroe, LA
University of Louisville, KY
University of Maine at Fort Kent, ME
University of Mary, ND
University of Maryland, Baltimore, MD
University of Massachusetts Amherst, MA
University of Massachusetts Boston, MA
University of Michigan–Flint, MI
University of Missouri, MO
University of Missouri–Kansas City, MO
University of Missouri–St. Louis, MO
University of North Alabama, AL
The University of North Carolina Wilmington, NC
University of North Georgia, GA
University of Phoenix–Online Campus, AZ
University of Phoenix–Phoenix Campus, AZ
University of Phoenix–Sacramento Valley Campus, CA
University of Phoenix–Southern Arizona Campus, AZ
University of Phoenix–South Florida Campus, FL
University of Phoenix–West Florida Campus, FL
University of St. Francis, IL
University of Saint Francis, IN
University of Saint Mary, KS
University of San Francisco, CA
University of Sioux Falls, SD
University of South Carolina Aiken, SC
University of South Carolina Upstate, SC
University of Southern Indiana, IN
University of Southern Mississippi, MS
University of South Florida, FL
The University of Tennessee at Chattanooga, TN

The University of Tennessee Health Science Center, TN
The University of Texas at Brownsville, TX
The University of Texas at Tyler, TX
University of the Incarnate Word, TX
The University of Toledo, OH
University of Utah, UT
University of Wisconsin–Green Bay, WI
University of Wisconsin–Oshkosh, WI
University of Wyoming, WY
Urbana University, OH
Utica College, NY
Villanova University, PA
Walden University, MN
Western Carolina University, NC
Western Governors University, UT
Western Illinois University, IL
Western New Mexico University, NM
Wheeling Jesuit University, WV
Wichita State University, KS
Wilmington University, DE

## ONLINE ONLY BACCALAUREATE PROGRAMS

Adventist University of Health Sciences, FL
American Public University System, WV
Bluefield State College, WV
Chamberlain College of Nursing, MO
Clarion University of Pennsylvania, PA
Cox College, MO
Eastern Illinois University, IL
Eastern New Mexico University, NM
Florida Atlantic University, FL
Frostburg State University, MD
Herzing University Online, WI
Hondros College, OH
Kettering College, OH
La Roche College, PA
Loyola University New Orleans, LA
Methodist College, IL
Minnesota State University Moorhead, MN
Montana State University–Northern, MT
New Mexico Highlands University, NM
Northeastern State University, OK
Oklahoma Panhandle State University, OK
St. Vincent's College, CT
Slippery Rock University of Pennsylvania, PA
State University of New York College of Technology at Delhi, NY
State University of New York Empire State College, NY
Stevenson University, MD
Tabor College, KS
Texas Tech University Health Sciences Center, TX
Trocaire College, NY
University of Arkansas–Fort Smith, AR
University of Louisiana at Monroe, LA
University of Missouri–Kansas City, MO
University of North Alabama, AL
University of North Georgia, GA
University of Saint Mary, KS
The University of Tennessee at Chattanooga, TN
The University of Texas at Brownsville, TX
The University of Texas at Tyler, TX
Walden University, MN
Western Governors University, UT
Western New Mexico University, NM

## ONLINE MASTER'S DEGREE PROGRAMS

Albany State University, GA
Alcorn State University, MS
Allen College, IA
American International College, MA
Angelo State University, TX
Aspen University, CO
Athabasca University, AB
Austin Peay State University, TN
Ball State University, IN
Baylor University, TX
Bellin College, WI
Benedictine University, IL
Brandman University, CA
Briar Cliff University, IA
California State University, Chico, CA
California State University, Dominguez Hills, CA
California State University, Fullerton, CA
Cedarville University, OH
Central Methodist University, MO
Charleston Southern University, SC
Chatham University, PA
Clarkson College, NE
Clayton State University, GA
Cleveland State University, OH
Cox College, MO
Delta State University, MS
Drexel University, PA
Duke University, NC
Duquesne University, PA
East Carolina University, NC
Eastern Mennonite University, VA
East Tennessee State University, TN
Excelsior College, NY
Fairleigh Dickinson University, Metropolitan Campus, NJ
Felician College, NJ
Ferris State University, MI
Fitchburg State University, MA
Florida Atlantic University, FL
Florida State University, FL
Gardner-Webb University, NC
George Mason University, VA
Georgetown University, DC
Georgia College & State University, GA
Georgia Regents University, GA
Georgia Southwestern State University, GA
Gonzaga University, WA
Graceland University, IA
Grand Canyon University, AZ
Hampton University, VA
Herzing University Online, WI
Idaho State University, ID
Illinois State University, IL
Indiana State University, IN
Indiana University–Purdue University Fort Wayne, IN
Indiana University–Purdue University Indianapolis, IN
Indiana Wesleyan University, IN
Jacksonville State University, AL
Jacksonville University, FL
The Johns Hopkins University, MD
Kent State University, OH
Lamar University, TX
La Roche College, PA
Lewis University, IL
Liberty University, VA
Loyola University Chicago, IL
Loyola University New Orleans, LA
Lynchburg College, VA
Mansfield University of Pennsylvania, PA
McKendree University, IL
McNeese State University, LA
Medical University of South Carolina, SC
Memorial University of Newfoundland, NL
Mercy College, NY
Messiah College, PA
Metropolitan State University, MN
Michigan State University, MI
MidAmerica Nazarene University, KS
Middle Tennessee State University, TN
Midwestern State University, TX
Minnesota State University Moorhead, MN
Missouri State University, MO
Nebraska Methodist College, NE
New Mexico State University, NM
Northeastern State University, OK
Northern Arizona University, AZ
Northern Kentucky University, KY
Northwest Nazarene University, ID
Nova Southeastern University, FL
The Ohio State University, OH
Old Dominion University, VA
Olivet Nazarene University, IL
Pace University, NY
Penn State University Park, PA
Purdue University Calumet, IN
Queens University of Charlotte, NC
Ramapo College of New Jersey, NJ
Regis University, CO
Research College of Nursing, MO
Roberts Wesleyan College, NY
Rush University, IL
Rutgers, The State University of New Jersey, Newark, NJ
Sacred Heart University, CT
Saint Francis Medical Center College of Nursing, IL
Saint Joseph's College of Maine, ME
Saint Louis University, MO
Saint Xavier University, IL
Samford University, AL
Seton Hall University, NJ
Simmons College, MA
South Dakota State University, SD
Southeastern Louisiana University, LA
Southern Adventist University, TN
Southwest Baptist University, MO
Spring Arbor University, MI
Spring Hill College, AL
State University of New York Institute of Technology, NY
Stevenson University, MD
Tennessee State University, TN
Tennessee Technological University, TN
Texas A&M University–Corpus Christi, TX
Texas Christian University, TX
Texas State University–San Marcos, TX
Texas Tech University Health Sciences Center, TX
Texas Woman's University, TX
Touro University, NV
Troy University, AL
The University of Alabama, AL
The University of Alabama in Huntsville, AL
The University of Arizona, AZ
University of Arkansas, AR
University of Central Arkansas, AR
University of Central Missouri, MO
University of Cincinnati, OH

University of Colorado Colorado Springs, CO
University of Colorado Denver, CO
University of Delaware, DE
University of Florida, FL
University of Hawaii at Manoa, HI
University of Indianapolis, IN
The University of Kansas, KS
University of Louisiana at Lafayette, LA
University of Mary, ND
University of Maryland, Baltimore, MD
University of Massachusetts Amherst, MA
University of Memphis, TN
University of Michigan–Flint, MI
University of Missouri, MO
University of Missouri–St. Louis, MO
University of Nevada, Las Vegas, NV
University of New Mexico, NM
University of North Alabama, AL
The University of North Carolina at Charlotte, NC
The University of North Carolina at Greensboro, NC
University of North Dakota, ND
University of Northern Colorado, CO
University of Oklahoma Health Sciences Center, OK
University of Phoenix–New Mexico Campus, NM
University of Phoenix–Online Campus, AZ
University of Phoenix–Phoenix Campus, AZ
University of Phoenix–Southern Arizona Campus, AZ
University of Phoenix–South Florida Campus, FL
University of Pittsburgh, PA
University of St. Francis, IL
University of San Francisco, CA
University of Southern Indiana, IN
The University of Texas at Arlington, TX
The University of Texas at Brownsville, TX
The University of Texas at El Paso, TX
The University of Texas at Tyler, TX
The University of Texas Medical Branch, TX
University of Toronto, ON
University of Utah, UT
University of West Florida, FL
University of West Georgia, GA
University of Wisconsin–Green Bay, WI
University of Wisconsin–Oshkosh, WI
University of Wyoming, WY
Vanderbilt University, TN
Walden University, MN
Walsh University, OH
Western Carolina University, NC
Western Governors University, UT
Western University of Health Sciences, CA
West Virginia University, WV
Wheeling Jesuit University, WV
Wilmington University, DE
Wright State University, OH

## ONLINE ONLY MASTER'S DEGREE PROGRAMS

Albany State University, GA
American International College, MA
Angelo State University, TX
Aspen University, CO
Austin Peay State University, TN
Ball State University, IN
Baylor University, TX
Benedictine University, IL
Briar Cliff University, IA
California State University, Chico, CA
California State University, Dominguez Hills, CA
Central Methodist University, MO
Charleston Southern University, SC
Chatham University, PA
Clarkson College, NE
Clayton State University, GA
Cleveland State University, OH
Cox College, MO
Delta State University, MS
Duquesne University, PA
Eastern Mennonite University, VA
Excelsior College, NY
Ferris State University, MI
Fitchburg State University, MA
Florida State University, FL
Gardner-Webb University, NC
Georgetown University, DC
Georgia College & State University, GA
Georgia Southwestern State University, GA
Gonzaga University, WA
Graceland University, IA
Herzing University Online, WI
Idaho State University, ID
Illinois State University, IL
Indiana State University, IN
Jacksonville State University, AL
Lamar University, TX
La Roche College, PA
Liberty University, VA
Loyola University Chicago, IL
Lynchburg College, VA
Mansfield University of Pennsylvania, PA
McNeese State University, LA
Medical University of South Carolina, SC
Memorial University of Newfoundland, NL
Messiah College, PA
Minnesota State University Moorhead, MN
Missouri State University, MO
Nebraska Methodist College, NE
New Mexico State University, NM
Northeastern State University, OK
Northern Arizona University, AZ
Northwest Nazarene University, ID
Nova Southeastern University, FL
Old Dominion University, VA
Queens University of Charlotte, NC
Ramapo College of New Jersey, NJ
Saint Francis Medical Center College of Nursing, IL
Saint Joseph's College of Maine, ME
Saint Louis University, MO
Seton Hall University, NJ
Southern Adventist University, TN
Spring Arbor University, MI
Spring Hill College, AL
Stevenson University, MD
Tennessee Technological University, TN
Texas A&M University–Corpus Christi, TX
Texas Christian University, TX
Texas State University–San Marcos, TX
Texas Tech University Health Sciences Center, TX
Touro University, NV
The University of Alabama, AL
University of Central Arkansas, AR
University of Central Missouri, MO
University of Colorado Colorado Springs, CO
University of Louisiana at Lafayette, LA
University of Massachusetts Amherst, MA
University of Missouri, MO
University of Nevada, Las Vegas, NV
University of New Mexico, NM
University of North Alabama, AL
University of Northern Colorado, CO
University of Southern Indiana, IN
The University of Texas at Brownsville, TX
The University of Texas at El Paso, TX
The University of Texas at Tyler, TX
The University of Texas Medical Branch, TX
University of West Florida, FL
University of West Georgia, GA
University of Wisconsin–Green Bay, WI
University of Wisconsin–Oshkosh, WI
University of Wyoming, WY
Vanderbilt University, TN
Walden University, MN
Walsh University, OH
Western Governors University, UT
Western University of Health Sciences, CA
West Virginia University, WV
Wheeling Jesuit University, WV

## ONLINE DOCTORAL DEGREE PROGRAMS

Allen College, IA
Arkansas State University, AR
Ball State University, IN
Binghamton University, State University of New York, NY
Briar Cliff University, IA
California State University, Fresno, CA
The Catholic University of America, DC
Chatham University, PA
Concordia University Wisconsin, WI
Delta State University, MS
Drexel University, PA
Duquesne University, PA
Georgia College & State University, GA
Georgia Southern University, GA
Graceland University, IA
Hampton University, VA
Idaho State University, ID
Indiana State University, IN
James Madison University, VA
Kent State University, OH
Lewis University, IL
Loyola University New Orleans, LA
Medical University of South Carolina, SC
Georgia Baptist College of Nursing, GA
Missouri State University, MO
New Mexico State University, NM
North Dakota State University, ND
Northern Arizona University, AZ
Northern Kentucky University, KY
Old Dominion University, VA
Radford University, VA
Rush University, IL
Saint Francis Medical Center College of Nursing, IL
Samford University, AL
Seton Hall University, NJ
Southern Adventist University, TN
Southern Connecticut State University, CT
Texas Christian University, TX
Touro University, NV
Troy University, AL
University at Buffalo, the State University of New York, NY
The University of Alabama, AL
The University of Alabama in Huntsville, AL

The University of Arizona, AZ
University of Colorado Colorado Springs, CO
University of Florida, FL
University of Hawaii at Manoa, HI
University of Indianapolis, IN
The University of Kansas, KS
University of Michigan–Flint, MI
University of Nevada, Las Vegas, NV
University of Nevada, Reno, NV
University of New Mexico, NM
University of North Dakota, ND
University of Northern Colorado, CO
University of Phoenix–Online Campus, AZ
University of St. Francis, IL
The University of Tennessee, TN
The University of Tennessee at Chattanooga, TN
The University of Tennessee Health Science Center, TN
The University of Texas Medical Branch, TX
University of the Incarnate Word, TX
The University of Toledo, OH
University of West Georgia, GA
University of Wisconsin–Milwaukee, WI
Virginia Commonwealth University, VA
Walden University, MN
Walsh University, OH
Western University of Health Sciences, CA
Winona State University, MN
Wright State University, OH
Yale University, CT

## ONLINE ONLY DOCTORAL DEGREE PROGRAMS

Allen College, IA
Arkansas State University, AR
Ball State University, IN
Briar Cliff University, IA
California State University, Fresno, CA
Chatham University, PA
Concordia University Wisconsin, WI
Delta State University, MS
Drexel University, PA
Duquesne University, PA
Georgia College & State University, GA
Georgia Southern University, GA
Graceland University, IA
Hampton University, VA
Idaho State University, ID
Indiana State University, IN
James Madison University, VA
Lewis University, IL
Loyola University New Orleans, LA
Medical University of South Carolina, SC
Georgia Baptist College of Nursing, GA
New Mexico State University, NM
Northern Arizona University, AZ
Old Dominion University, VA
Radford University, VA
Rush University, IL
Saint Francis Medical Center College of Nursing, IL
Samford University, AL
Southern Adventist University, TN
Southern Connecticut State University, CT
Texas Christian University, TX
Touro University, NV
Troy University, AL
The University of Alabama, AL
The University of Alabama in Huntsville, AL
The University of Arizona, AZ
University of Colorado Colorado Springs, CO
University of Hawaii at Manoa, HI
University of Indianapolis, IN
University of Michigan–Flint, MI
University of Nevada, Las Vegas, NV
University of Nevada, Reno, NV
University of North Dakota, ND
University of Northern Colorado, CO
University of Phoenix–Online Campus, AZ
University of St. Francis, IL
The University of Tennessee, TN
The University of Tennessee at Chattanooga, TN
The University of Tennessee Health Science Center, TN
The University of Texas Medical Branch, TX
University of the Incarnate Word, TX
University of West Georgia, GA
University of Wisconsin–Milwaukee, WI
Virginia Commonwealth University, VA
Walden University, MN
Walsh University, OH
Western University of Health Sciences, CA
Winona State University, MN
Wright State University, OH
Yale University, CT

# Continuing Education Programs

## U.S. and U.S. Territories

### Alabama

Auburn University, School of Nursing, *Auburn University*

Jacksonville State University, College of Nursing and Health Sciences, *Jacksonville*

Samford University, Ida V. Moffett School of Nursing, *Birmingham*

The University of Alabama at Birmingham, School of Nursing, *Birmingham*

The University of Alabama in Huntsville, College of Nursing, *Huntsville*

University of Mobile, School of Nursing, *Mobile*

University of North Alabama, College of Nursing and Allied Health, *Florence*

### Arizona

Arizona State University at the Downtown Phoenix Campus, College of Nursing, *Phoenix*

Grand Canyon University, College of Nursing and Health Sciences, *Phoenix*

University of Phoenix–Online Campus, Online Campus, *Phoenix*

University of Phoenix–Phoenix Campus, College of Nursing, *Tempe*

University of Phoenix–Southern Arizona Campus, College of Social Sciences, *Tucson*

### Arkansas

Harding University, College of Nursing, *Searcy*

University of Arkansas, Eleanor Mann School of Nursing, *Fayetteville*

University of Arkansas for Medical Sciences, College of Nursing, *Little Rock*

### California

Azusa Pacific University, School of Nursing, *Azusa*

Brandman University, School of Nursing and Health Professions, *Irvine*

California State University, Bakersfield, Program in Nursing, *Bakersfield*

California State University, Chico, School of Nursing, *Chico*

California State University, Fresno, Department of Nursing, *Fresno*

Dominican University of California, Program in Nursing, *San Rafael*

Pacific Union College, Department of Nursing, *Angwin*

Point Loma Nazarene University, School of Nursing, *San Diego*

San Diego State University, School of Nursing, *San Diego*

San Francisco State University, School of Nursing, *San Francisco*

University of California, Davis, The Betty Irene Moore School of Nursing, *Davis*

University of California, Irvine, Program in Nursing Science, *Irvine*

University of California, Los Angeles, School of Nursing, *Los Angeles*

University of Phoenix–Sacramento Valley Campus, College of Nursing, *Sacramento*

University of Phoenix–Southern California Campus, College of Nursing, *Costa Mesa*

### Colorado

University of Colorado Colorado Springs, Beth-El College of Nursing and Health Sciences, *Colorado Springs*

University of Colorado Denver, College of Nursing, *Aurora*

### Connecticut

Fairfield University, School of Nursing, *Fairfield*

University of Connecticut, School of Nursing, *Storrs*

University of Hartford, College of Education, Nursing, and Health Professions, *West Hartford*

### Delaware

University of Delaware, School of Nursing, *Newark*

Wesley College, Nursing Program, *Dover*

### Florida

Florida Agricultural and Mechanical University, School of Nursing, *Tallahassee*

Florida Gulf Coast University, School of Nursing, *Fort Myers*

St. Petersburg College, Department of Nursing, *St. Petersburg*

University of Miami, School of Nursing and Health Studies, *Coral Gables*

University of South Florida, College of Nursing, *Tampa*

The University of Tampa, Department of Nursing, *Tampa*

### Georgia

Kennesaw State University, School of Nursing, *Kennesaw*

Valdosta State University, College of Nursing, *Valdosta*

### Illinois

Lewis University, Program in Nursing, *Romeoville*

Olivet Nazarene University, Division of Nursing, *Bourbonnais*

Rush University, College of Nursing, *Chicago*

Saint Xavier University, School of Nursing, *Chicago*

Southern Illinois University Edwardsville, School of Nursing, *Edwardsville*

University of Illinois at Chicago, College of Nursing, *Chicago*

### Indiana

Indiana State University, Department of Nursing, *Terre Haute*

Indiana University Kokomo, Indiana University School of Nursing, *Kokomo*

Indiana University–Purdue University Indianapolis, School of Nursing, *Indianapolis*

Marian University, School of Nursing, *Indianapolis*

Purdue University, School of Nursing, *West Lafayette*

University of Southern Indiana, College of Nursing and Health Professions, *Evansville*

Valparaiso University, College of Nursing, *Valparaiso*

### Iowa

Allen College, Program in Nursing, *Waterloo*

Briar Cliff University, Department of Nursing, *Sioux City*

Clarke University, Department of Nursing and Health, *Dubuque*

Grand View University, Division of Nursing, *Des Moines*

Luther College, Department of Nursing, *Decorah*

Mount Mercy University, Department of Nursing, *Cedar Rapids*

St. Ambrose University, Program in Nursing (BSN), *Davenport*

The University of Iowa, College of Nursing, *Iowa City*

### Kansas

Pittsburg State University, Department of Nursing, *Pittsburg*

The University of Kansas, School of Nursing, *Kansas City*

Washburn University, School of Nursing, *Topeka*

### Kentucky

Bellarmine University, Donna and Allan Lansing School of Nursing and Health Sciences, *Louisville*

Kentucky Christian University, School of Nursing, *Grayson*

Midway College, Program in Nursing (Baccalaureate), *Midway*

Murray State University, Program in Nursing, *Murray*

Northern Kentucky University, Department of Nursing, *Highland Heights*

Spalding University, School of Nursing, *Louisville*

University of Kentucky, College of Nursing, *Lexington*

University of Louisville, School of Nursing, *Louisville*

Western Kentucky University, School of Nursing, *Bowling Green*

### Louisiana

Dillard University, Division of Nursing, *New Orleans*

Louisiana State University Health Sciences Center, School of Nursing, *New Orleans*

McNeese State University, College of Nursing, *Lake Charles*

Nicholls State University, Department of Nursing, *Thibodaux*

Northwestern State University of Louisiana, College of Nursing and Allied Health, *Shreveport*

Our Lady of the Lake College, Division of Nursing, *Baton Rouge*

University of Louisiana at Lafayette, College of Nursing, *Lafayette*

University of Louisiana at Monroe, Nursing, *Monroe*

### Maine

Saint Joseph's College of Maine, Master of Science in Nursing Program, *Standish*

University of New England, Department of Nursing, *Biddeford*

University of Southern Maine, School of Nursing, *Portland*

**Maryland**

The Johns Hopkins University, School of Nursing, *Baltimore*

University of Maryland, Baltimore, Master's Program in Nursing, *Baltimore*

**Massachusetts**

Anna Maria College, Department of Nursing, *Paxton*

Boston College, William F. Connell School of Nursing, *Chestnut Hill*

Endicott College, Major in Nursing, *Beverly*

Framingham State University, Department of Nursing, *Framingham*

MCPHS University, School of Nursing, *Boston*

Northeastern University, School of Nursing, *Boston*

Regis College, School of Nursing, Science and Health Professions, *Weston*

Salem State University, Program in Nursing, *Salem*

University of Massachusetts Amherst, School of Nursing, *Amherst*

University of Massachusetts Boston, College of Nursing and Health Sciences, *Boston*

University of Massachusetts Dartmouth, College of Nursing, *North Dartmouth*

University of Massachusetts Worcester, Graduate School of Nursing, *Worcester*

Worcester State University, Department of Nursing, *Worcester*

**Michigan**

Grand Valley State University, Kirkhof College of Nursing, *Allendale*

Madonna University, College of Nursing and Health, *Livonia*

Michigan State University, College of Nursing, *East Lansing*

Northern Michigan University, College of Nursing and Allied Health Science, *Marquette*

Oakland University, School of Nursing, *Rochester*

Saginaw Valley State University, College of Health and Human Services, *University Center*

Western Michigan University, College of Health and Human Services, *Kalamazoo*

**Minnesota**

Bemidji State University, Department of Nursing, *Bemidji*

Minnesota State University Mankato, School of Nursing, *Mankato*

University of Minnesota, Twin Cities Campus, School of Nursing, *Minneapolis*

**Mississippi**

University of Mississippi Medical Center, School of Nursing, *Jackson*

**Missouri**

Cox College, Department of Nursing, *Springfield*

Missouri State University, Department of Nursing, *Springfield*

Missouri Western State University, Department of Nursing, *St. Joseph*

Saint Louis University, School of Nursing, *St. Louis*

University of Missouri, Sinclair School of Nursing, *Columbia*

University of Missouri–Kansas City, School of Nursing and Health Studies, *Kansas City*

University of Missouri–St. Louis, College of Nursing, *St. Louis*

**Nebraska**

Clarkson College, Master of Science in Nursing Program, *Omaha*

Nebraska Methodist College, Department of Nursing, *Omaha*

University of Nebraska Medical Center, College of Nursing, *Omaha*

**Nevada**

University of Nevada, Las Vegas, School of Nursing, *Las Vegas*

**New Hampshire**

Saint Anselm College, Department of Nursing, *Manchester*

**New Jersey**

College of Saint Elizabeth, Department of Nursing, *Morristown*

Fairleigh Dickinson University, Metropolitan Campus, Henry P. Becton School of Nursing and Allied Health, *Teaneck*

Monmouth University, Marjorie K. Unterberg School of Nursing, *West Long Branch*

Ramapo College of New Jersey, Master of Science in Nursing Program, *Mahwah*

Rutgers, The State University of New Jersey, *Newark*

**New Mexico**

New Mexico State University, School of Nursing, *Las Cruces*

**New York**

Adelphi University, College of Nursing and Public Health, *Garden City*

Binghamton University, State University of New York, Decker School of Nursing, *Vestal*

Columbia University, School of Nursing, *New York*

Elmira College, Program in Nursing Education, *Elmira*

Hunter College of the City University of New York, Hunter-Bellevue School of Nursing, *New York*

Lehman College of the City University of New York, Department of Nursing, *Bronx*

Molloy College, Division of Nursing, *Rockville Centre*

New York University, College of Nursing, *New York*

The Sage Colleges, Department of Nursing, *Troy*

State University of New York Downstate Medical Center, College of Nursing, *Brooklyn*

State University of New York Institute of Technology, School of Nursing and Health Systems, *Utica*

State University of New York Upstate Medical University, College of Nursing, *Syracuse*

Stony Brook University, State University of New York, School of Nursing, *Stony Brook*

**North Carolina**

Queens University of Charlotte, Presbyterian School of Nursing, *Charlotte*

The University of North Carolina at Chapel Hill, School of Nursing, *Chapel Hill*

Winston-Salem State University, Department of Nursing, *Winston-Salem*

**Ohio**

Case Western Reserve University, Frances Payne Bolton School of Nursing, *Cleveland*

Cleveland State University, School of Nursing, *Cleveland*

Kent State University, College of Nursing, *Kent*

The Ohio State University, College of Nursing, *Columbus*

Otterbein University, Department of Nursing, *Westerville*

Shawnee State University, Department of Nursing, *Portsmouth*

The University of Akron, School of Nursing, *Akron*

University of Cincinnati, College of Nursing, *Cincinnati*

The University of Toledo, College of Nursing, *Toledo*

Urbana University, College of Nursing and Allied Health, *Urbana*

Wright State University, College of Nursing and Health, *Dayton*

**Oklahoma**

Oklahoma City University, Kramer School of Nursing, *Oklahoma City*

University of Oklahoma Health Sciences Center, College of Nursing, *Oklahoma City*

**Oregon**

Linfield College, School of Nursing, *McMinnville*

Oregon Health & Science University, School of Nursing, *Portland*

**Pennsylvania**

Alvernia University, Nursing, *Reading*

Carlow University, School of Nursing, *Pittsburgh*

DeSales University, Department of Nursing and Health, *Center Valley*

Drexel University, College of Nursing and Health Professions, *Philadelphia*

Duquesne University, School of Nursing, *Pittsburgh*

Holy Family University, School of Nursing and Allied Health Professions, *Philadelphia*

La Roche College, Department of Nursing and Nursing Management, *Pittsburgh*

La Salle University, School of Nursing and Health Sciences, *Philadelphia*

Marywood University, Department of Nursing, *Scranton*

Moravian College, Department of Nursing, *Bethlehem*

Mount Aloysius College, Division of Nursing, *Cresson*

Penn State University Park, School of Nursing, *University Park*

Temple University, Department of Nursing, *Philadelphia*

Thomas Jefferson University, Department of Nursing, *Philadelphia*

University of Pennsylvania, School of Nursing, *Philadelphia*

University of Pittsburgh, School of Nursing, *Pittsburgh*

Villanova University, College of Nursing, *Villanova*

Widener University, School of Nursing, *Chester*

Wilkes University, Department of Nursing, *Wilkes-Barre*

**Puerto Rico**

Universidad Adventista de las Antillas, Department of Nursing, *Mayagüez*

University of Puerto Rico, Mayagüez Campus, Department of Nursing, *Mayagüez*

University of Puerto Rico, Medical Sciences Campus, School of Nursing, *San Juan*

**Rhode Island**

Salve Regina University, Department of Nursing, *Newport*

**South Carolina**

University of South Carolina, College of Nursing, *Columbia*

**South Dakota**

South Dakota State University, College of Nursing, *Brookings*

**Tennessee**

East Tennessee State University, College of Nursing, *Johnson City*

Southern Adventist University, School of Nursing, *Collegedale*

Tennessee State University, Division of Nursing, *Nashville*

Union University, School of Nursing, *Jackson*

The University of Tennessee, College of Nursing, *Knoxville*

**Texas**

Lamar University, Department of Nursing, *Beaumont*

Midwestern State University, Nursing Program, *Wichita Falls*

Patty Hanks Shelton School of Nursing, *Abilene*

Tarleton State University, Department of Nursing, *Stephenville*

Texas A&M University–Corpus Christi, College of Nursing and Health Sciences, *Corpus Christi*

Texas Christian University, Harris College of Nursing, *Fort Worth*

The University of Texas at Arlington, College of Nursing, *Arlington*

The University of Texas at Brownsville, Department of Nursing, *Brownsville*

The University of Texas Health Science Center at Houston, School of Nursing, *Houston*

The University of Texas Health Science Center at San Antonio, School of Nursing, *San Antonio*

**Virginia**

George Mason University, College of Health and Human Services, *Fairfax*

Jefferson College of Health Sciences, Nursing Education Program, *Roanoke*

Old Dominion University, Department of Nursing, *Norfolk*

Shenandoah University, Division of Nursing, *Winchester*

**Washington**

Pacific Lutheran University, School of Nursing, *Tacoma*

University of Washington, School of Nursing, *Seattle*

Washington State University College of Nursing, *Spokane*

**West Virginia**

Fairmont State University, School of Nursing and Allied Health Administration, *Fairmont*

Shepherd University, Department of Nursing Education, *Shepherdstown*

West Virginia University, School of Nursing, *Morgantown*

**Wisconsin**

Alverno College, Division of Nursing, *Milwaukee*

Milwaukee School of Engineering, School of Nursing, *Milwaukee*

University of Wisconsin–Eau Claire, College of Nursing and Health Sciences, *Eau Claire*

University of Wisconsin–Madison, School of Nursing, *Madison*

University of Wisconsin–Oshkosh, College of Nursing, *Oshkosh*

Viterbo University, School of Nursing, *La Crosse*

Wisconsin Lutheran College, Nursing Program, *Milwaukee*

## CANADA

**British Columbia**

British Columbia Institute of Technology, School of Health Sciences, *Burnaby*

Thompson Rivers University, School of Nursing, *Kamloops*

Vancouver Island University, Department of Nursing, *Nanaimo*

**Manitoba**

University of Manitoba, Faculty of Nursing, *Winnipeg*

**New Brunswick**

Université de Moncton, School of Nursing, *Moncton*

University of New Brunswick Fredericton, Faculty of Nursing, *Fredericton*

**Nova Scotia**

St. Francis Xavier University, Department of Nursing, *Antigonish*

**Ontario**

Laurentian University, School of Nursing, *Sudbury*

Ryerson University, Program in Nursing, *Toronto*

University of Toronto, Faculty of Nursing, *Toronto*

University of Windsor, Faculty of Nursing, *Windsor*

York University, School of Nursing, *Toronto*

**Quebec**

Université de Montréal, Faculty of Nursing, *Montréal*

Université du Québec à Rimouski, Program in Nursing, *Rimouski*

Université du Québec en Outaouais, Département des Sciences Infirmières, *Gatineau*

Université Laval, Faculty of Nursing, *Québec*

**Saskatchewan**

University of Saskatchewan, College of Nursing, *Saskatoon*

# ALPHABETICAL LISTING OF INSTITUTIONS

In this index, the page locations of the profiles are printed in regular type, the displays are in *italics,* and the two-page descriptions are in **bold** type.

# NOTES

# NOTES

# NOTES

# NOTES